HYPERTENSION:
MECHANISMS AND MANAGEMENT

HYPERTENSION:
MECHANISMS AND MANAGEMENT
THE TWENTY-SIXTH HAHNEMANN SYMPOSIUM

Edited by

GADDO ONESTI, M.D.

Professor of Medicine
Hahnemann Medical College and Hospital
Philadelphia, Pennsylvania

KWAN EUN KIM, M.D.

Associate Professor of Medicine
Hahnemann Medical College and Hospital
Philadelphia, Pennsylvania

JOHN H. MOYER, M.D.

Professor of Medicine
Hahnemann Medical College and Hospital
Philadelphia, Pennsylvania

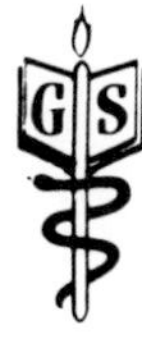

GRUNE & STRATTON, ***New York and London***

Library of Congress Cataloging in Publication Data
Main entry under title:

Hypertension: mechanisms and management.

Includes bibliographical references.
1. Hypertension. I. Onesti, Gaddo, ed. II. Kim,
Kwan Eun, 1933—ed. III. Moyer, John Henry, ed.
IV. Hahnemann Medical College and Hospital of Phila-
delphia. [DNLM: 1. Hypertension—Congresses.
WG 340 H9956 1971]
RC685.H8H8 616.1'32 73–1934
ISBN 0–8089–0790–5

Grune & Stratton, Inc.
111 Fifth Avenue
New York, New York 10003

Library of Congress Catalog Card Number 73–1934
International Standard Book Number 0–8089–0790–5
Printed in the United States of America

This book is dedicated to

CHARLES S. CAMERON, M.D.

Provost, Hahnemann Medical College and Hospital

As Dean of the Medical College from 1957 to 1962, and as President until 1971, he has worked devotedly to advance medical education at all levels. Through the honesty, integrity and modest approach to life that have characterized his dedication to that cause, he has inspired the faculty throughout these years and provided the leadership under which Hahnemann has achieved preeminence in the field of continuing education.

Acknowledgment

We wish to express appreciation to Hoechst Pharmaceutical Company; Merck Sharp & Dohme, Division of Merck & Co., Inc.; and Geigy Pharmaceuticals, Division of CIBA-GEIGY Corporation, who have made major grants in support of this scientific endeavor. In addition, we are grateful to Boehringer Ingelheim Limited, U.S.; Searle & Company; Strasenburgh Laboratories, Pharmaceutical Division of Pennwalt Corporation; the Upjohn Company; and Merck Sharp & Dohme International, all of whom have also made substantial contributions. Their aid has been invaluable to the success of this symposium.

Our thanks also go to Mrs. Sage Cordell and her staff for their assistance in the administrative conduct of this symposium, and to Mrs. Edith Schwager for her editorial assistance.

Gaddo Onesti, M.D.
Kwan Eun Kim, M.D.
John H. Moyer, M.D.

Contents

VI. Recent Advances in Drug Thrapy

VII. Adrenal Hypertension

VIII. Renal Hypertension

IX. Miscellaneous Hypertension

X. Complications and Special Considerations in the Treatment of Hypertension

Contributors

WILLIAM B. ABRAMS, M.D.
Vice-president,—Clinical Research, Ayerst Laboratories, New York, N. Y.; Clinical Associate Professor of Medicine, College of Medicine and Dentistry of New Jersey, Newark, New Jersey

BARBRO ANDERSSON
Electron microscopy Technician, Department of Pathology, Lenox Hill Hospital, New York, N. Y.

AARON H. ANTON, PH.D.
Professor of Anesthesiology and Pharmacology, Department of Anesthesiology and Department of Pharmacology, Case-Western Reserve University, Cleveland, Ohio

D. A. ARCHER, M.B., CH.B.
Research Fellow, Department of Clinical Pharmacology, Royal Postgraduate Medical School, University of London, London, England

LELAND L. ATKINS, M.D.
The Medical Associates Clinic, Memphis, Tennessee

GIORGIO BACCELLI, M.D.
Assistant Professor of Medicine, and Investigator, Cardiovascular Research Institute, University of Milan School of Medicine, Milan, Italy

BENJAMIN BACHARACH, M.D.
Jefferson Medical College and Hospital, Philadelphia, Pennsylvania

LESLIE BAER, M.D.
Assistant Professor of Medicine, Columbia University, College of Physicians and Surgeons, New York, N. Y.

STANLEY BANACH, M.D.
Nephrologist, Department of Medicine, Allentown Hospital Association, Allentown, Pennsylvania

HERBERT BENSON, M.D.
Associate Professor of Medicine, Harvard Medical School; Program Director, Harvard General Clinical Research Center, Thorndike Memorial and Channing Laboratories, Boston, Massachusetts

EDWARD G. BIGLIERI, M.D.
Medical Service, San Francisco General Hospital; Professor, Department of Medicine, University of California at San Francisco, San Francisco, California

KLAUS D. BOCK, M.D.
Professor of Medicine, and Head, Division of Renal and Hypertensive Disease, Medizinische Klinik, Klinikum der Ruhruniversitaet, Essen, West Germany

JOSEPH J. BOOKSTEIN, M.D.
Professor of Radiology, University of Michigan Medical Center, Ann Arbor, Michigan

ROGER BOUCHER, PH.D.
Professor of Medicine, University of Montreal Medical School, Montreal, Canada

ALBERT N. BREST, M.D.
Professor of Medicine, and Head, Division of Cardiology, Jefferson Medical College and Hospital, Philadelphia, Pennsylvania

JAN BROD, M.D., D.SC.
Professor of Medicine, Medical School of Hanover, Hanover, West Germany

BENNIE BROOKS
Laboratory Supervisor, University of Tennessee Medical Units, Memphis, Tennessee

HANS R. BRUNNER, M.D.
Assistant Professor of Medicine, Columbia University, College of Physicians and Surgeons, New York, N. Y.

FRITZ R. BÜHLER, M.D.
Research Associate of Medicine, Columbia University, College of Physicians and Surgeons, New York, N. Y.

C. J. BULPITT, M.B., CH.B.
Lecturer in Clinical Pharmacology, Royal Postgraduate Medical School, University of London, London, England

LAWRENCE W. BYERS, PH.D.
Associate Professor of Biochemistry, University of Tennessee Medical Units; Associate Clinical Chemist, Department of Pathology, Baptist Memorial Hospital, Memphis, Tennessee

PAUL J. CANNON, M.D.
Associate Professor of Medicine, Columbia University, College of Physicians and Surgeons; Associate Attending Physician, Columbia-Presbyterian Medical Center, New York, N. Y.

CHARLES A. CHIDSEY, M.D.
Associate Professor of Medicine and Pharmacology, Departments of Medicine and Pharmacology, and Head, Division of Clinical Pharmacology, University of Colorado Medical Center, Denver, Colorado

JAY N. COHN, M.D.
Chief, Hypertension and Clinical Hemodynamics, Veterans Administration Hospital; Professor of Medicine, Georgetown University School of Medicine, Washington, D.C.

THOMAS G. COLEMAN, PH.D.
Associate Professor, Department of Physiology and Biophysics, University of Mississippi School of Medicine, Jackson Mississippi

JEROME W. CONN, M.D.
Louis Harry Newburgh Distinguished University Professor of Internal Medicine and Director of the Department of Endocrinology and Metabolism and the Metabolism Research Unit, University of Michigan Medical School, Ann Arbor, Michigan

JAY W. CONSTANTINE, PH.D.
Department of Pharmacology, Medical Research Laboratories, Pfizer, Inc., Groton, Connecticut

ALLEN W. COWLEY, JR., PH.D.
Assistant Professor, Department of Physiology and Biophysics, University of Mississippi School of Medicine, Jackson, Mississippi

LEWIS K. DAHL, M.D.
Senior Scientist, Medical Department, Brookhaven National Laboratory, Upton, New York

SIDNEY L. DALE, M.S.
Section of Endocrinology and Metabolism, Robert Dawson Evans Department of Clinical Research, Boston University School of Medicine, Boston, Massachusetts

MARIE M. DALY, PH.D.
Associate Professor of Biochemistry, Albert Einstein College of Medicine, Bronx, New York

R. C. DAVIDSON, M.D.
Assistant Professor of Medicine, University of Washington School of Medicine, Seattle, Washington

JAMES O. DAVIS, PH.D., M.D.
Professor and Chairman, Department of Physiology, University of Missouri School of Medicine, Columbia, Missouri

THOMAS R. DAWBER, M.D.
Associate Professor of Medicine, Boston University School of Medicine, Boston, Massachusetts

JACQUES DE CHAMPLAIN, M.D., PH.D.
Associate Professor, Department of Physiology, Research Center in Neurosciences, University of Montreal, Quebec, Canada

QUENTIN B. DEMING, M.D.
Professor of Medicine, Albert Einstein College of Medicine, Bronx, New York

COLIN T. DOLLERY, M.B., CH.B.
Professor of Clinical Pharmacology, Royal Postgraduate Medical School, University of London, London, England

HARRIET P. DUSTAN, M.D.
Vice Chairman, Research Division, The Cleveland Clinic Foundation and The Cleveland Clinic Educational Foundation, Cleveland, Ohio

KARL ENGELMAN, M.D.
Associate Professor of Medicine and Pharmacology, and Chief, Section on Hypertension and Clinical Pharmacology, University of Pennsylvania School of Medicine, Philadelphia, Pennsylvania

K. F. FAIRLEY, M.D.
Inpatient Physician, University Department of Medicine, Royal Melbourne Hospital, Victoria, Australia

CARLOS M. FERRARIO, M.D.
Staff member, Research Division, The Cleveland Clinic Foundation, Cleveland, Ohio; Established Investigator, American Heart Association

FRANK A. FINNERTY, JR., M.D.
Professor, Departments of Medicine and Obstetrics/Gynecology, Georgetown University School of Medicine; Chief, Cardiovascular Research, Georgetown University Medical Division, D.C. General Hospital, Washington, D.C.

Annette Fitz, M.D.
Assistant Professor of Medicine, Department of Medicine, College of Medicine, University of Iowa, Iowa City, Iowa

Ralph P. Forsyth, Ph.D.
Associate Professor of Medical Psychology in Residence, Department of Psychiatry, and Associate Member, Cardiovascular Research Institute, University of California, San Francisco, California

Edward D. Freis, M.D.
Professor of Medicine, Georgetown University School of Medicine; Senior Medical Investigator, Veterans Administration Hospital, Washington, D.C.

Edward D. Frohlich, M.D.
Professor of Medicine, Physiology, and Biophysics, Division of Hypertension, College of Medicine, The University of Oklahoma Health Sciences Center, Oklahoma City, Oklahoma

Thomas E. Gaffney, M.D.
Professor and Chairman, Department of Pharmacology; Professor of Medicine, College of Medicine, Medical University of South Carolina, Charleston, South Carolina

Arunabha Ganguly, M.D.
Division of Endocrinology, Department of Medicine, Stanford University School of Medicine, Stanford, California

Robert Gaunt, Ph.D.
CIBA, Geigy Corporation, Summit, New Jersey

Jacques Genest, C.C., M.D.
Scientific Director, Clinical Research Institute of Montreal; Professor of Medicine, University of Montreal and McGill University Medical Schools; Chief, Neurology-Hypertension Service, University of Montreal, Hotel-Dieu Hospital, Montreal, Quebec, Canada

Ray W. Gifford, Jr., M.D.
Head, Department of Hypertension and Nephrology, The Cleveland Clinic Foundation, Cleveland, Ohio

Leon I. Goldberg, M.D., Ph.D.
Professor of Medicine (Clinical Pharmacology) and Professor of Pharmacology; Director of the Clinical Pharmacology Program, Emory University School of Medicine, Atlanta, Georgia

Thomas B. Gottlieb, M.D.
Department of Medicine, University of Colorado Medical Center, Denver, Colorado

Mary Jane Gray, M.D., D.M.S.
Professor of Obstetrics and Gynecology, University of Vermont College of Medicine; Attending Staff, Medical Center Hospital of Vermont, Burlington, Vermont

Ashton Graybiel, M.D., Captain USN (ret.)
U.S. Naval School of Aerospace Medicine, Naval Air Station, Pensacola, Florida

James A. Greco, M.D.
Clinical Senior Instructor in Medicine, Hahnemann Medical College and Hospital, Philadelphia, Pennsylvania; Codirector, Division of Nephrology and Hypertension, Department of Medicine, Monmouth Medical Center, Long Branch, New Jersey

Roger J. Grekin, M.D.
Section of Endocrinology and Metabolism, Robert Dawson Evans Department of Clinical Research, Boston University School of Medicine, Boston, Massachusetts

Arthur Grollman, Ph.D., M.D.
Professor of Experimental Medicine, Department of Pathology, The University of Texas Southwestern Medical School; National Civilian Consultant, The Surgeon General, U.S. Air Force; Senior Attending Physician, Parkland Memorial Hospital; Attending Physician, St. Paul Hospital, Dallas; Consultant in Internal Medicine, Baylor University, Veterans Administration, Wilford Hall, USAF, Gaston Episcopal and Shannon West Texas Hospitals

Maurizio Guazzi, M.D.
Associate Professor of Medicine, and Investigator, Cardiovascular Research Institute, University of Milan School of Medicine, Milan, Italy

NABIL H. GUIHA, M.D.
Trainee in Cardiovascular Physiology and Pharmacology, Veterans Administration Hospital and Georgetown University School of Medicine, Washington, D.C.

NIROO GUPTA, M.D.
Fellow, Department of Medicine (Clinical Pharmacology), Emory University School of Medicine, Atlanta, Georgia

ARTHUR C. GUYTON, M.D.
Chairman and Professor, Department of Physiology and Biophysics, University of Mississippi School of Medicine, Jackson, Mississippi

CHARLES E. HALL, PH.D.
Professor, Department of Physiology, University of Texas Medical Branch, Galveston, Texas

O. HALL, M.SC.
Research Associate Professor, Department of Physiology, University of Texas Medical Branch, Galveston, Texas

WILLIAM R. HARLAN, M.D.
Professor of Medicine and Community Health Sciences, Duke University Medical Center, Durham, North Carolina

ROBERT E. HARRIS, PH.D.
Professor of Medical Psychology, Department of Psychiatry, and Member, Cardiovascular Research Institute, University of California, San Francisco

W. F. HEALE, M.B.
Renal Research Fellow, University Department of Medicine, Royal Melbourne Hospital, Victoria, Australia

VOLKER H. HEIMSOTH, M.D.
Chief Resident, Division of Renal and Hypertensive Disease, Medizinische Klinik, Klinikum der Ruhruniversitaet, Essen, West Germany

ROBERT H. HEPTINSTALL, M.D.
Baxley Professor of Pathology and Director of the Department of Pathology, The Johns Hopkins University School of Medicine and Hospital, Baltimore, Maryland

HANS-JÜRGEN HESS, PH.D.
Department of Medicinal Chemistry, Medical Research Laboratories, Pfizer, Inc., Groton, Connecticut

ROGER B. HICKLER, M.D.
Professor and Chairman, Department of Medicine, University of Massachusetts Medical School; Chief, Medical Division, The Memorial Hospital, Worcester, Massachusetts

JUNICHI IWAI, M.D.
Associate Scientist, Medical Department, Brookhaven National Laboratory, Upton, New York

WILLIAM B. KANNEL, M.D.
Director, Framingham Heart Study; Consultant, Cushing Hospital; Research Associate, Boston University; Lecturer in Preventative Medicine, Harvard University, Cambridge, Massachusetts

PAUL KEZDI, M.D.
Director, Cox Heart Institute, Kettering Medical Center, Kettering, Ohio

KWAN EUN KIM, M.D.
Associate Professor of Medicine, Hahnemann Medical College and Hospital, Philadelphia, Pennsylvania

PRISCILLA KINCAID-SMITH, M.D.
Reader in Medicine and Physician in Charge, Renal Unit, University Department of Medicine, Royal Melbourne Hospital, Victoria, Australia

WALTER M. KIRKENDALL, M.D.
Professor and Director, Program in Internal Medicine, University of Texas Medical School, Houston, Texas

J. DIANNE KIRSHMAN
Department of Medicine, Columbia University College of Physicians and Surgeons, New York, N. Y.

ABBIE I. KNOWLTON, M.D.
Assistant Professor of Medicine, Columbia University, College of Physicians and Surgeons, New York, N. Y.

KNUD D. KNUDSEN, M.D.
Scientist, Medical Department, Brookhaven National Laboratory, Upton, New York

WALTER KOBINGER, M.D.
Pharmacological Department, Arzneimittelforschung Ges. m.b.H., Vienna, Austria

R. KARL KORDENAT, M.S.
Staff Physiologist, Cox Heart Institute, Kettering Medical Center, Kettering, Ohio

OTTO KÜCHEL, M.D., SC.D.
Senior Investigator, Clinical Research Institute of Montreal; Professor of Medicine, University of Montreal and McGill University Medical Schools; Member of the Service of Nephrology and Hypertension, Hotel-Dieu Hospital, Montreal, Quebec, Canada

JOHN H. LARAGH, M.D.
Professor of Clinical Medicine, Department of Medicine, Columbia University, College of Physicians and Surgeons, New York, N. Y.

BYRON E. LEACH, PH.D.
Professor of Biochemistry, University of Tennessee Medical Units; Clinical Chemist, Department of Pathology, Baptist Memorial Hospital, Memphis, Tennessee

J. F. LIARD, M.D.
Fellow of the Fonds National de la Recherche Scientifique, Switzerland

PER LUND-JOHANSEN, M.D.
Associate Professor of Medicine, Medical Department A, University of Bergen School of Medicine, Bergen, Norway

GIUSEPPE MANCIA, M.D.
Assistant Professor of Medicine, and Investigator, Cardiovascular Research Institute, University of Milan School of Medicine, Milan, Italy

R. DAVIS MANNING, JR., M.S.
Research Associate, Department of Physiology and Biophysics, University of Mississippi School of Medicine, Jackson, Mississippi

MORTON H. MAXWELL, M.D.
Clinical Professor of Medicine, University of California Medical Center, Los Angeles; Director, Nephrology and Hypertension Service, Cedars-Sinai Medical Center, Los Angeles; Chairman, Cooperative Study of Renovascular Hypertension, Los Angeles, California

LAWRENCE J. MCCORMACK, M.D., M.S. PATH.
Chairman, Division of Laboratory Medicine, The Cleveland Clinic Foundation, Cleveland, Ohio

JAMES W. MCCUBBIN, M.D.
Staff member, Research Division, The Cleveland Clinic Foundation, Cleveland, Ohio

WILFRED K. MCSHANE, B.S.
Department of Pharmacology, Medical Research Laboratories, Pfizer Inc., Groton, Connecticut

JAMES C. MELBY, M.D.
Section of Endocrinology and Metabolism, Robert Dawson Evans Department of Clinical Research, Boston University School of Medicine, Boston, Massachusetts

MILTON MENDLOWITZ, M.D.
The Joe Lowe and Louise Price Professor of Medicine, Mount Sinai School of Medicine of the City University of New York; Attending Physician, The Mount Sinai Hospital, New York, N. Y.

PETER MERGUET, M.D.
Chief Resident, Division of Renal and Hypertensive Disease, Medizinische Klinik, Klinikum der Ruhruniversitaet, Essen, West Germany

J. MILUTINOVIC, M.D.
Instructor in Medicine, University of Washington School of Medicine, Seattle, Washington

ROBERT E. MITCHELL, CAPTAIN USN (MC)
U. S. Naval School of Aerospace Medicine, Naval Air Station, Pensacola, Florida

SHAKIL MOHAMMED, M.D., PH.D.
Associate Professor of Pharmacology, University of Cincinnati College of Medicine, Cincinnati, Ohio

JOHN H. MOYER, M.D.
Professor of Medicine, Hahnemann Medical College and Hospital, Philadelphia, Pennsylvania

E. ERIC MUIRHEAD, M.D.
Professor of Pathology and Clinical Professor of Medicine, University of Tennessee Medical Units; Director, Department of

Pathology, Baptist Memorial Hospital, Memphis, Tennessee

MARTIN S. NEFF, M.D.
Assistant Clinical Professor of Medicine, Mount Sinai College of Medicine of the City University of New York; Assistant Attending Physician, City Hospital at Elmhurst, New York, N. Y.

ROGER A. NORMAN, JR., M.S.
Research Associate, Department of Physiology and Biophysics, University of Mississippi School of Medicine, Jackson, Mississippi

WOJCIECH NOWACZYNSKI, D.SC.
Professor of Medicine, University of Montreal Medical School, Montreal, Quebec, Canada

ALBERT OBERMAN, M.D.
Professor of Public Health and Associate Professor of Medicine, University of Alabama in Birmingham Medical Center, Birmingham, Alabama

GADDO ONESTI, M.D.
Professor of Medicine, Hahnemann Medical College and Hospital, Philadelphia, Pennsylvania

JAMES C. ORCUTT
Department of Pharmacology, University of Colorado Medical Center, Denver, Colorado

VIRGILIO PAZ-MARTINEZ, M.D.
Associate Professor of Medicine, University Los Andes, Merida, Venezuela

W. STANLEY PEART, M.D., F.R.S., F.R.C.P.
Professor of Medicine, Medical Unit, St. Mary's Hospital, London, England

JAMES A. PITCOCK, M.D.
Clinical Assistant Professor of Pathology, University of Tennessee Medical Units; Associate Pathologist, Department of Pathology, Baptist Memorial Hospital, Memphis, Tennessee

RICHARD G. PLUSS, M.D.
Department of Medicine, University of Colorado Medical Center, Denver, Colorado

PHILIP J. PRIVITERA, PH.D.
Associate Professor of Pharmacology, College of Medicine, Medical University of South Carolina, Charleston, South Carolina

JOHN P. RAPP, D.V.M., PH.D.
Assistant Director, Penrose Research Laboratory, Philadelphia Zoological Society; Department of Pathology, University of Pennsylvania Medical School, Philadelphia, Pennsylvania

DAVID W. RICHARDSON, M.D.
Professor of Medicine and Chairman, Division of Cardiology, Medical College of Virginia, Virginia Commonwealth University, Richmond, Virginia

CHARLES W. ROBERTSON, M.D.
Associate Clinical Professor of Surgery, Boston University School of Medicine; Visiting Surgeon, University Hospital, Boston, Massachusetts

J. C. ROCHA, M.D.
Division of Nephrology, Universidade Estadual de Campinas, Campinas, Sao Paulo, Brazil

ERNESTO RODRIGUERA, M.D.
Trainee in Cardiovascular Physiology and Pharmacology, Veterans Administration Hospital and Georgetown University School of Medicine, Washington, D.C.

MORRIS SCHAMBELAN, M.D.
Assistant Professor of Medicine in Residence, Medical Service, San Francisco General Hospital, University of California, San Francisco, California

ALLAN B. SCHWARTZ, M.D.
Division of Nephrology and Hypertension, Department of Medicine, Hahnemann Medical College and Hospital; Chief, Nephrology Section, Hahnemann Division, Philadelphia General Hospital, Philadelphia, Pennsylvania

ALEXANDER SCRIABINE, M.D.
Department of Pharmacology, Merck Institute for Therapeutic Research, West Point, Pennsylvania

BELDING H. SCRIBNER, M.D.
Professor of Medicine, University of Washington School of Medicine, Seattle, Washington

ALFRED M. SELLERS, M.D.
Associate Professor of Medicine, University of Pennsylvania School of Medicine and Hospital, Philadelphia, Pennsylvania

NORMAN M. SIMON, M.D.
Associate Professor of Medicine, Northwestern University-McGraw Medical Center; Attending Physician, Passavant Memorial Hospital and Veterans Administration Research Hospitals, Chicago, Illinois; Member, Executive Committee, Cooperative Study of Renovascular Hypertension

ROBERT F. SLIFKIN, M.D.
Clinical Associate in Medicine, Mount Sinai College of Medicine of the City University of New York; Assistant Attending Physician, City Hospital at Elmhurst, New York, N. Y.

JOSEPH W. SMILEY, M.D.
Clinical Senior Instructor, Division of Nephrology and Hypertension, Department of Medicine, Hahnemann Medical College and Hospital; Associate Attending Physician, Department of Medicine, Mercy Catholic Medical Center, Philadelphia, Pennsylvania

SIR F. HORACE SMIRK, K.B.E., M.D., D.SC.
Emeritus Professor of Medicine, Wellcome Medical Research Institute; Department of Medicine, University of Otago Medical School, Dunedin, New Zealand

I. SANFORD SMITH, M.D.
Fellow, Division of Nephrology and Hypertension, Department of Medicine, Hahnemann Medical College and Hospital, Philadelphia, Pennsylvania

REGINALD H. SMITHWICK, M.D.
Professor of Surgery (Emeritus), Boston University School of Medicine; Consultant, University Hospital; Board of Consultation, Massachusetts General Hospital, Boston, Massachusetts

SHELDON C. SOMMERS, M.D.
Director of Laboratories, Lenox Hill Hospital; Clinical Professor of Pathology, Columbia University, College of Physicians and Surgeons, New York, N. Y.; Clinical Professor of Pathology, University of Southern California School of Medicine, Los Angeles, California

J. WILLIAM SPICKLER, PH.D.
Head, Physiology and Biology Section, Cox Heart Institute, Kettering Medical Center, Kettering, Ohio

J. R. STOCKIGT, M.D.
Bay Area Heart Association Research Fellow, Departments of Medicine and Physiology, University of California, San Francisco, California; Wellcome Trust Fellow in Medicine, St. Mary's Hospital, London, England; Downie Metabolic Unit, Alfred Hospital, Melbourne, Victoria, Australia

CHARLES SWARTZ, M.D.
Professor of Medicine, and Director, Division of Nephrology and Hypertension, Department of Medicine, Hahnemann Medical College and Hospital, Philadelphia, Pennsylvania

ROBERT C. TARAZI, M.D.
Staff Member, Research Division, The Cleveland Clinic Foundation and The Cleveland Clinic Educational Foundation, Cleveland, Ohio

CAROLINE BEDELL THOMAS, M.D.
Professor Emeritus of Medicine, The Johns Hopkins University School of Medicine, Baltimore, Maryland

T. BUDYA TJANDRAMAGA, M.D., M.SC.
Instructor in Medicine (Clinical Pharmacology), Department of Medicine, Emory University School of Medicine, Atlanta, Georgia

LOUIS TOBIAN, M.D.
Professor of Internal Medicine, Chief of Hypertension-Nephrology Unit, University of Minnesota Hospital, Minneapolis, Minnesota

GEORGE W. VETROVEC, M.D.
Health Sciences Division, Medical College of Virginia, Virginia Commonwealth University, Richmond, Virginia

JOHN V. WEIL, M.D.
Associate Professor of Medicine, University of Colorado Medical Center, Denver, Colorado

JACK P. WHISNANT, M.D.
Chairman, Department of Neurology, Mayo Clinic; Professor of Neurology, Mayo Graduate School of Medicine, University of Minnesota, Rochester, Minnesota

LESLIE WIENER, M.D.
Associate Professor of Medicine, Jefferson Medical College and Hospital, Philadelphia, Pennsylvania

WILLIAM C. WILLIAMSON, M.D.
Health Sciences Division, Medical College of Virginia, Virginia Commonwealth University, Richmond, Virginia

THOMAS E. WILSON, M.S.
Section of Endocrinology and Metabolism, Robert Dawson Evans Department of Clinical Research, Boston University School of Medicine, Boston, Massachusetts

ROBERT L. WOLF, M.D.
Assistant Clinical Professor of Medicine, Mount Sinai School of Medicine of the City University of New York; Assistant Attending Physician, Mount Sinai Hospital, New York, N. Y.

HARVEY WOLINSKY, M.D., PH.D.
Assistant Professor of Medicine and Pathology, Albert Einstein College of Medicine, Bronx, New York

ALBERTO ZANCHETTI, M.D.
Professor of Medicine, and Associate Director, Cardiovascular Research Institute, University of Milan School of Medicine, Milan, Italy

VINCENT J. ZARRO, M.D., PH.D.
Associate Professor of Pharmacology, and Assistant Professor of Medicine, Hahnemann Medical College and Hospital, Philadelphia, Pennsylvania

Preface

In December of 1959, the first Hahnemann Symposium on Hypertensive Vascular Disease was held in Philadelphia. It was followed in 1961 by the second Hahnemann Symposium on Hypertensive Disease. Ten years later, this third symposium was organized—initially stimulated through the interest of Sir F. Horace Smirk of New Zealand. He made a number of suggestions which became the cornerstone of the program. On the basis of these suggestions the format was developed by the current editors in association with Dr. Albert N. Brest, who left Hahnemann during the structuring of the program to become Director of the Division of Cardiology at Thomas Jefferson University. A group of 146 internationally known authorities participated in the program.

The accomplishments of the twelve years that had passed since the first of these symposia are evidenced by the different emphasis that was placed on the biochemistry and mechanisms of hypertensive vascular disease. Since that first symposium, many studies have been completed and new data added to our understanding of the epidemiology and role of environmental factors in hypertension Probably the greatest fund of new information has been produced by the observations made on the role of the renin-aldosterone system and electrolyte metabolism in blood pressure regulation.

It is now quite evident that blood pressure reduction prolongs life and reduces morbidity in patients with essential hypertension. These same conclusions were drawn at the first symposium, but were not based on the solid facts and conclusive data that are now available through long-term follow-up treatment programs. Although different and more effective drugs are now available, the basic understanding and application of general pharmacodynamics have changed very little. Nonetheless, the drugs now available are easier to use, have fewer side effects, and therefore are more therapeutically efficacious, although survey studies indicate that less than half of the people with high blood pressure are under treatment and probably only half of these receive adequate treatment. This emphasizes the continuing need for education of physicians responsible for the treatment of hypertension. In addition, probably the most remarkable therapeutic improvement in any of the cardiovascular diseases over the past ten years has been in the medical treatment of essential hypertension. This symposium presents a comprehensive review of the hypertensive mechanisms, methods available for therapy, and complications associated with the disease.

Gaddo Onesti, M.D.
Kwan Eun Kim, M.D.
John H. Moyer, M.D.

Part I. BLOOD PRESSURE MEASUREMENT AND DEFINITION OF HYPERTENSION

METHODS OF BLOOD PRESSURE RECORDING: 1733–1971

By HERBERT BENSON, M.D.

HISTORICAL ASPECTS OF BLOOD PRESSURE MEASUREMENT

EVERY VESSEL through which blood flows has a blood pressure equal to the product of the blood flow in and the resistance of that vessel. Thus, different systemic and pulmonary venous and arterial blood pressures are present. These differences between the pressures in various blood vessels were appreciated more than 500 years ago by the medieval artist Giovanni di Paolo (1403–1483).[1] In his painting of the beheading of St. John the Baptist, he portrayed three streams of blood from the severed neck: one dripping and two spurting. This chapter will deal only with the measurement of one of these types of blood pressure: systemic arterial blood pressure.

Systemic arterial pressure was not quantifiably measured until approximately 300 years after di Paolo's painting when the Reverend Stephen Hales, in 1733, performed his classic investigations on the horse.[2]

> In December I caused a *mare* to be tied down alive on her back; she was 14 hands high, and about 14 years of age, had a fistula on her withers, was neither very lean nor yet lusty: having laid open the left crural artery about 3 inches from her belly, I inserted into it a brass pipe whose bore was 1/16 of an inch in diameter; and to that, by means of another brass pipe which was fitly adapted to it, I fixed a glass tube, of nearly the same diameter, which was 9 feet in length: then untying the ligature on the artery, the blood rose in the tube 8 feet 3 inches perpendicular above the level of the left ventricle of the heart: but it did not attain to its full height at once; it rushed up about half way in an instant, and afterwards gradually at each pulse 12, 8, 6, 4, 2 and sometimes 1 inch: when it was at its full height, it would rise and fall at and after each pulse, 2, 3, or 4 inches . . . .

After approximately another 100 years, Poiseuille in 1828 connected a mercury-filled U tube to a cannulated artery.[3] Because mercury is 13.6 times more dense than blood or water, the column in the tube was raised to a considerably smaller height and the indoor measurement of blood pressure became feasible. Since that time, millimeters of mercury, or mm Hg, have been the standard units of blood pressure measurement.

Little was known concerning the presence or significance of elevated systemic arterial blood pressure, systemic hypertension, until Richard Bright noted cardiac hypertrophy and observed that an ". . . altered quality of the blood affords irregular and unwanted stimulus to the organ (heart) immediately. . . ."[4] Subsequently, in 1968, George Johnson stated:[5]

> . . . It cannot be supposed that the great hypertrophy of the left ventricle, which is often found in cases of chronic Bright's disease, is a direct result solely of the resistance offered by the renal arteries. We must look for the cause of this hypertrophy rather in the fact that the blood, in consequence of degeneration of the kidney, being contaminated by urinary excreta and otherwise deteriorated, is impeded in its transit through the minute arteries throughout the body. We have evidence of such an impediment in the full, hard, throbbing pulse, which is a very common phenomenon in the advanced stage of chronic Bright's disease.

From the Thorndike and Channing Laboratories, Harvard Medical Unit, Boston City Hospital, and the Department of Medicine, Harvard Medical School, Boston, Massachusetts.

Supported in part by Grants HE 10539–04 and SF 57–135 from the National Institutes of Health and Grant RR–76 from the General Clinical Research Centers Program of the Division of Research Resources.

Frederick Henry Horatio Akhbar Mahomed noted that hypertension may precede the albuminuria of Bright's disease [6] and later, he was probably the first to describe what is now termed essential hypertension: [7]

> . . . If in nephritis it be said that the high arterial pressure produces hypertrophy of the heart and thickening of the arteries, then let it be admitted that under all circumstances in which high arterial pressure can be proved to exist as a permanent condition it produces, or tends to produce, the same general cardio-vascular changes.
>
> . . . Therefore, we may justly assume that if the persistence of high arterial pressure produces these cardio-vascular changes, then also the accompanying kidney changes may be anticipated in individuals subject to this condition; in other words, these individuals are the subjects of chronic Bright's disease. *But these symptoms of high pressure are not infrequently met with at all ages; they are even seen in young adults enjoying apparently good health. Are we to say that these are suffering from chronic Bright's disease? No, certainly not.* [Italics added.]

Huchard, a professor of medicine in Paris, described arterial hypertension as the cause of atherosclerosis.[8] Much later, in the late 1940s, prospective epidemiologic investigations were started which ultimately established that elevated systemic arterial blood pressure increased the risk of coronary artery disease and cerebrovascular accidents.[9,10] The more recent studies of E. D. Freis and his collaborators clearly demonstrated that this increased risk is lessened by lowering blood pressure.[11,12] Therefore, the measurement of blood pressure is of great importance in order to discover the presence of asymptomatic hypertension before more overt disease becomes manifest and also to monitor subsequent preventative, controlled antihypertensive therapy.

Measurement of Systemic Arterial Blood Pressure

Systemic arterial blood pressure may be measured either directly or indirectly. Direct blood pressure measurement requires the cannulation of an artery and is the ultimate standard of blood pressure. Indirect blood pressure measurements are made bloodlessly without cannulation and are valid insofar as they approximate the data from direct measurements. This chapter describes historic and current methods of both the direct and indirect measurement of systemic arterial blood pressure. For a more extensive review, the excellent recent monograph by L. A. Geddes is highly recommended.[13]

The Direct Measurement of Blood Pressure

Direct *mean* arterial pressure was measured by both Hales and Poiseuille because the inertia and resistance of the fluid column in the tubes prevented accurate representation of systolic and diastolic blood pressures. The accurate direct recording of systolic and diastolic blood pressure was first made possible by the rapidly responding system of Marey and Chauveau in 1861, in which pressure was transmitted to a rubber membrane and thence through a tube to a tambour writing lever.[13] Subsequently, rapidly responding manometers or pressure-sensitive transducers were developed which employ either optical, electrolytic, electro-optical, capacitance, inductive, mechano-electronic tube, or strain-gauge devices.[13] These devices are connected on one side to an intra-arterial catheter or needle and on the other usually to an electronic amplifier and recorder.

Currently, strain-gauge transducers are used most commonly in direct measurements of arterial blood pressure. The strain-gauge transducer is based on the principle that when a wire is stretched by a force or pressure (force per unit area) a change occurs in the resistance of that wire. Since the change in resistance is proportional to the pressure, accurate measurements of blood pressure are possible after calibration. Most strain-gauge transducers are removed from the actual site of pressure measurement, but recently small catheter-tip, strain-gauge transducers have become available.[13] These catheter-tip transducers are desirable since they eliminate many of the kinetic energy and pressure wave artifacts secondary to the presence of a catheter and fluid column between the transducer and site of measurement.[14,15] Electro-optical catheter-tip transducers are also now being used.[13,16]

Routine direct measurement of arterial blood pressure, although the most accurate method available, is not feasible. It carries a small but potentially serious morbidity. However, 24-

hour ambulatory human direct blood pressure has been safely monitored.[17] At the present time, direct blood pressure recordings serve as the standard against which indirect blood pressure monitoring systems should be tested and as a means of monitoring in-hospital blood pressures when required. Direct blood pressure recordings are also usually necessary in hemodynamic investigations.

The Indirect Measurement of Blood Pressure

Toward the end of the nineteenth century, early indirect blood pressure-measuring devices were designed by von Basch, Potain, and Marey.[13] Three principles employed in these instruments were important in the subsequent development of other indirect devices: (*1*) application of counterpressure occludes an artery and the occlusion is made manifest by the disappearance of the distal pulse; (*2*) oscillations appear from the artery to which counterpressure is being applied, and the amplitude of the oscillations varies with the amount of counterpressure; (*3*) a limb pales when adequate pressures are applied to it, and its normal hues return when the counterpressure is removed.[13]

Most currently used indirect blood pressure devices employ a bladder and cuff to produce arterial occlusion. The cuff consists of material which can be wrapped around and stabilized on an extremity. The bladder is encased within the cuff. The cuff and bladder are placed over a compressible artery and, routinely, the occluding bladder pressure is raised, usually by an air-inflation system, to pressures greater than arterial systolic. Bladder pressure is then gradually decreased while one or more of the pressure-induced changes in the underlying artery is measured. These induced arterial changes are related to systolic, diastolic, and perhaps mean arterial blood pressure. The proper size of the occluding bladder depends upon the size of the extremity. A bladder width equal to 40 percent of the circumference of the extremity has been recommended.[13] A proper length of the bladder is more difficult to specify,[13] but some feel that the standard 22- to 26-cm bladder is too short and that a 30- to 40-cm bladder obviates any risk of placing the bladder too distant from the compressible artery.[13,18] In extremely obese patients, the validity of even very wide bladders has been questioned and only direct measurement deemed accurate.[19]

The palpatory and flush methods were two of the earliest and simplest methods of measuring blood pressure indirectly by use of the occluding cuff.[13] After brachial arterial occlusion, systolic pressure is indicated by the cuff-bladder pressure at the palpated appearance of radial pulsations. Some experienced clinicians have been able also to palpate diastolic blood pressure by noting the disappearance of arterial vibrations as bladder pressure is progressively decreased.[20] Seventy-nine percent of the systolic and 89 percent of the diastolic blood pressures obtained by the palpatory method were within ±4 mm Hg of those obtained by the standard auscultatory techniques.[20] The flush method is used now primarily to measure systolic blood pressure in infants and small children. Blood is expelled from an extremity by wrapping it tightly in an elastic bandage. The pressure in the bladder and cuff, which were previously applied proximal to the elastic bandage, is raised above systolic blood pressure. Then, the bandage is removed and bladder pressure slowly decreased. The bladder pressure at which rubor (flush) first appears in the blanched extremity is indicatory of systolic blood pressure. Flush-method systolic blood pressures averaged about 10 mm Hg below those obtained by auscultation.[21]

The auscultatory technique of indirectly measuring blood pressure is the most widely used because of its relative accuracy and ease of interpretation for both systolic and diastolic pressures without extensive equipment. The occluding cuff and bladder are usually placed around the arm. The pressure within the occluding bladder is easily visualized from a connected aneroid or mercury manometer. When bladder pressure decreases to systolic blood pressure, a sound is heard through a stethoscope placed over the brachial artery distal to the cuff. As bladder pressures reach and pass below diastolic pressure, the sounds first become muffled and finally disappear. Korotkoff was the first to describe this method and the sounds now carry his name.[22] The origin of the Korotkoff sounds has been extensively investigated. They are thought by most investigators to be secondary to rapid changes beneath and distal to the cuff sufficient to impart sonic vibrations to the arterial wall and surrounding tissues and also to flow phenomena or both.[13,23,24] In subjects in whom proper attention is given to the ratio of bladder size to arm size, the auscultatory method yields systolic blood pressures which are on the average 5 mm Hg below direct systolic pressure.[13] Using the muffling criterion for diastolic blood pressure, diastolic blood pressures obtained by the auscultatory technique are about 8 mm Hg higher than those measured directly.[13] In many instances, the Korotkoff sounds do not disappear until pressures well below diastolic are reached.[13] In low blood flow states when blood pressure is low and the intensity of the Korotkoff sounds decreased, auscultatory blood pressure may be obtained by inserting the diaphragm piece of the stethoscope under the lower edge of the blood pressure cuff instead of its customary placement distal to the cuff.[25] Korotkoff sounds may be detected automatically and efficiently by using electronic microphones and recording both pressures and sounds. If the microphones are placed wholly within the cuff, sounds can be detected from practically any location on the upper arm and are essentially the same as those obtained from the antecubital fossa.[26] Further, extraneous sounds may be largely eliminated by using the R wave of the electrocardiogram (ECG) as a reference point and by selectively receiving auditory signals over the artery only when the pulse transmitted from the left ventricle is expected to be present.[13,27,28]

The oscillometric technique of indirectly measuring systemic arterial blood pressure enjoyed wide acceptance around the turn of the twentieth century.[13] As the cuff-bladder pressure decreases from above systolic to below diastolic blood pressure, oscillations appear in the bladder and are transmitted to a manometer and recording device. The first oscillations appear at a bladder pressure greater than direct systolic pressures. The oscillations progressively increase in amplitude as bladder pressure further decreases. Then, with additional decreases in bladder pressure, the oscillations sharply decrease in amplitude and finally disappear.[13] The oscillometric method accurately measures systolic blood pressure when two adjacent cuffs are used. The bladder of the distal cuff is inflated to approximately 40 mm Hg and maintained at that pressure. The bladder of the proximal cuff is inflated to a pressure greater than systolic and then progressively decreased. Systolic pressure is indicated by appearance of the first oscillations in the distal cuff. The oscillometric equivalent to direct diastolic blood pressure has been debated for many years. Erlanger in 1904 was the first to suggest that bladder pressure at which the maximum oscillations *decrease abruptly* corresponds to diastolic blood pressure.[29] Recently, this has been confirmed using the contralateral arm as a reference: decreased amplitude of 20 percent or more than the largest oscillation corresponds

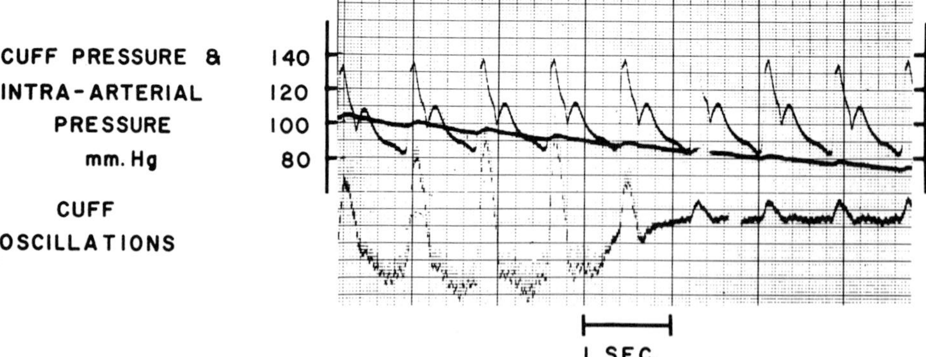

FIG. 1.—Comparison of human intra-arterial blood pressure (mm Hg) with the pressure (mm Hg) of a bladder within a cuff on the contralateral arm and also with the oscillations from that arm cuff. Cuff oscillations markedly decreased in amplitude when the decreasing pressure within the cuff-bladder reached intra-arterial diastolic blood pressure.

to auscultatory muffling.[30] Abrupt decreased amplitude of the maximum oscillation at diastolic blood pressure has also been supported by recent intraarterial comparisons [31] (Fig. 1). Although the maximum oscillations had been considered to be present at a pressure equal to direct diastolic pressure for many years, this relation could not be substantiated.[13] However, some experimental evidence exists showing that maximal oscillations are present at *mean* arterial pressure.[32] If maximal oscillations do indeed represent mean pressure, the oscillometric method is the only indirect measure of mean arterial pressure in existence.

An ultrasonic method as a more recent technique for indirect measurement of blood pressure, was first proposed by Ware in 1965.[33] A standard bladder and cuff are applied to an extremity. Small transmitting and receiving crystals are mounted on the skin over an artery and under the cuff. An ultrasonic beam from an ultrasound oscillator is directed to the transmitting crystal and thence to the artery. The reflected ultrasound is recorded or listened to from the receiving crystal. When the bladder of the occluding cuff is inflated above systolic blood pressure, and so long as the underlying artery is collapsed, the reflected ultrasound is of constant frequency. As bladder pressure decreases below systolic blood pressure, the arterial wall rapidly opens and closes, and the reflected ultrasound rapidly changes its frequency depending on whether the wall is moving toward or away from the wave source (the so-called Doppler effect). When these movements of the arterial wall are no longer present at pressures equal to and below diastolic, the reflected ultrasound is again relatively constant and can be readily distinguished from that produced by the opening and closing artery.[13,34–37] The ultrasonic method has distinct advantages: Blood pressure can be measured during low flow states when Korotkoff sounds are frequently heard with great difficulty; [38] it is applicable to humans of all sizes; [13,39] it is not influenced by environmental noise.[13] However, the ultrasonic method depends upon the accurate, stable placement of the transmitting and receiving crystals over an artery. If the crystals shift position, the measurements will no longer be accurate. The automated systems employing Korotkoff sounds and oscillations are much less dependent upon accurate placement.

The so-called phase shift method is another indirect blood pressure measurement which employs cuffs.[40] Three side-by-side occluding cuffs are placed on the upper arm and inflated. A change in volume of the cuffs is measured by a pressure transducer and recorded. As pressure within the cuffs decreases, the time necessary for blood to travel between the proximal and distal cuffs varies from 30 to 100 msec with a progressively smaller time delay between the proximal and distal cuffs. At diastolic blood pressure, a time delay between cuffs of less than 1 msec is experienced. This marked phase shift at diastolic blood pressure appears to correlate to a diastolic pressure lower than that of auscultatory muffling, but higher than disappearance. Direct arterial comparisons are needed for verification.

Tonometry is an indirect blood pressure-measuring technique which does not employ cuffs. Based on the principle that displacement of a force-sensitive transducer over a superficial artery can be made linearly proportional to the arterial blood pressure, the technique has the advantage of continuous, instantaneous recording of blood pressure.[41] However, absolute immobility of the force-sensitive device and extremity is required for accurate measurements and presents a major problem.

Many limitations exist for indirect blood pressure-monitoring systems. Several indirect systems are sufficiently accurate for clinical use, but no such system yields absolute measurements. In practically all indirect systems the subject must not move the area where the monitor is placed lest artifactual signals be produced. Further, the direct monitoring measurements are continuous, and few heartbeat-to-heartbeat pressure variation problems are encountered. With the exception of tonometric measurements, the indirect methods yield intermittent data which may not be representative of direct pressures over a given period unless the indirect measurements are repeated several times and the pressure in the occluding bladder is slowly and regularly decreased. The use of a constant cuff-pressure system obviates many of these problems of indirect systems.[27,42] The bladder of the constant cuff-pressure system is inflated to and *maintained* at systolic or diastolic pressure for 50 consecutive heart beats and then deflated. Korotkoff sounds are recorded from a crystal microphone. The ECG is also recorded and an electronic coincidence circuit detects the number of R waves followed by a Korotkoff sound. For example, during the measurement of systolic blood pressure, when cuff-bladder pressure exceeds brachial artery systolic pressure, no Korotkoff sound is produced; when cuff-bladder pressure is less than brachial artery systolic pressure, a Korotkoff sound is present. Median systolic blood pressure during the inflation is equal to cuff-bladder pressure when approximately 50 percent of the Korotkoff sounds are noted, e.g., when between 14 and 36 Korotkoff sounds per cycle of 50 heartbeats are present. If less than 14 Korotkoff sounds are present, indicating cuff pressure exceeds systolic arterial pressure for most of the trial, the cuff pressure is decreased 4 mm Hg for the next cuff inflation. If more than 36 Korotkoff sounds are present, indicating that cuff pressure is lower than arterial pressure for most of the trial, the cuff pressure is increased by 4 mm Hg. Thus, median systolic pressure can be tracked and recorded. Diastolic pressure can be measured also by the same system. Further, not only can this constant cuff pressure use Korotkoff sounds as a signal, but varying amplitude of heartbeat-to-heartbeat oscillations may be used.[43] Thus, the constant cuff-pressure system allows averaging of either systolic or diastolic blood pressure over a specified number of heartbeats.

Recent advances have also been made in the indirect recording of ambulatory human blood pressure.[44-46] These data are perhaps most important at the present time since a casual blood pressure measurement represents only 1/1400 of the total day's blood pressures and often samples only several heartbeats. In this context, the routine measurement of blood pressure in the physician's office is an inadequate sample, especially when therapy is to be initiated or changed depending upon its results. Further, such ambulatory human blood pressure data are required to establish normal 24-hour values and to relate these to the presence or absence of disease parameters.

Conclusions

If we are to understand better the pathogenesis and manage the therapy of hypertension, continued advances in the methods of recording of blood pressure will be required. However, with the fact in mind that humans did not evolve and were not designed to have their blood pressure readily measured, the technologic progress made from Hales's original measurements in 1733 to the present is truly encouraging.

Acknowledgment

The helpful suggestions of Walter H. Abelmann and the editorial assistance of Barbara R. Marzetta are gratefully acknowledged.

References

1. Pickering, G.: Systemic arterial blood pressure. *In* Fishman, A. P., and Richards, D. W. (Eds.): Circulation of the Blood. New York: Oxford, 1964, pp. 487–541.
2. Hales, S.: Statical essays: containing haemastatics; or, an account of some hydraulic and hydrostatical experiments made on the blood and blood-vessels of animals. *As reprinted in* Willius, F. A. and Keys, T. E. (Eds.): Cardiac Classics. New York: Dover, 1941, pp. 129–133.
3. Poiseuille, J. L. M.: Recherches sur la force du coeur aortique. Extraits des Theses soutennues dans les Trois Facultes de Medecine de France. Arch. Gen. Med. 18:550, 1828.
4. Bright, R.: Tabular view of the morbid appearances in 100 cases connected with albuminous urine. With observations. Guys Hosp. Rep. 1:380, 1836.
5. Johnson, G. I.: On certain points in the anatomy and pathology of Bright's disease of the kidney. II. On the influence of the minute blood-vessels upon the circulation. Med.-Chir. Trans. 51:57, 1868, as quoted in reference 1.
6. Mahomed, F. A.: The etiology of Bright's disease and the pre-albuminuric stage. Med.-Chir. Trans. 57:197, 1874.
7. Mahomed, F. A.: Some clinical aspects of chronic Bright's disease. Guys Hosp. Rep. (3rd. Ser.) 24:363, 1879.
8. Huchard, H.: Maladies du Coeur et des Vaisseaux. Paris: Doin, 1889, as quoted in Reference 1.
9. Kannel, W. B., Dawber, T. R., Kagen, A., Revotskie, N., and Stokes, J.: Factors of risk in the development of coronary heart disease —six-year follow-up experience. Ann. Intern. Med. 55:33, 1961.
10. Kannel, W. B., Schwartz, M. J., and McNamara, P. M.: Blood pressure and risk of cor-

onary heart disease: The Framingham study. Chest 56:43, 1969.

11. Freis, E. D., and the Veterans Administration Cooperative Study Group on Antihypertensive Agents: Effects of treatment on morbidity in hypertension: Results in patients with diastolic blood pressures averaging 115 through 129 mm Hg. JAMA 202:1028, 1967.
12. Freis, E. D., and the Veterans Administration Cooperative Study Group on Antihypertensive Agents: Effects of treatment on morbidity in hypertension: Results in patients with diastolic blood pressure averaging 90 through 114 mm Hg. JAMA 213:1143, 1970.
13. Geddes, L. A.: The Direct and Indirect Measurement of Blood Pressure. Chicago: Year Book, 1970.
14. Kanai, H., Iizuka, M., and Sakamoto, K.: One of the problems in the measurement of blood pressure by catheter-insertion: Wave reflection at the tip of the catheter. Med. Biol. Eng. 8:483, 1970.
15. Manktelow, R. T., and Baird, R. J.: A practical approach to accurate pressure measurements. J. Thorac. Cardiovasc. Surg. 58:122, 1969.
16. Lindstrom, L. H.: Miniaturized pressure transducer intended for intravascular use. I.E.E.E. Trans. Biomed. Eng. BME-17:207, 1970.
17. Bevan, A. T., Honour, A. J., and Stott, F. H.: Direct arterial pressure recording in unrestricted man. Clin. Sci. 36:329, 1969.
18. King, G. E.: Taking the blood pressure. JAMA 209:1902, 1969.
19. Kvols, L. K., Rohlfing, B. M., and Alexander, J. K.: A comparison of intra-arterial and cuff blood pressure measurements in very obese subjects. Cardiovasc. Res. Cent. Bull. 7:118, 1969.
20. Segall, H. N.: A note on the measurement of diastolic and systolic blood pressure by the palpation of arterial vibrations (sounds) over the brachial artery. Can. Med. Assoc. J. 42: 311, 1940.
21. Goldring, D., and Wohltmann, H.: Flush method for blood pressure determinations in newborn infants. J. Pediat. 40:285, 1952.
22. Korotkoff, N. S.: On the subject of methods of determining blood pressure. Voen. Med. Zh. 11:365, 1905.
23. Tavel, M. E., Faris, J., Nasser, W. K., Feigenbaum, H., and Fisch, C.: Korotkoff sounds. Observations on pressure-pulse changes underlying their formation. Circulation 39:465, 1969.
24. Ur, A., and Gordon, M.: Origin of Korotkoff sounds. Am. J. Physiol. 218:524, 1970.
25. Zahir, M., and Gould, L.: A new method for measurement of blood pressure in clinical shock. Am. Heart J. 79:572, 1970.
26. Geddes, L. A., and Moore, A. G.: The efficient detection of Korotkoff sounds. Med. Biol. Eng. 6:603, 1968.
27. Shapiro, D., Tursky, B., Gershon, E., and Stern, M.: Effects of feedback and reinforcement on the control of human systolic blood pressure. Science 163:588, 1969.
28. Lagerwerff, J. M., and Luce, R. S.: Artifact suppression in indirect blood pressure measurements. Aerosp. Med. 41:1157, 1970.
29. Erlanger, J.: A new instrument for determining the minimum and maximum blood-pressures in man. Johns Hopkins Hosp. Res. 12: 53, 1904.
30. Benson, H., and Herd, J. A.: Oscillometric measurement of arterial blood pressure. Circulation 40 (Suppl. III): 43, 1969.
31. Benson, H.: Unpublished data.
32. Posey, J. A., Geddes, L. A., Williams, H. and Moore, A. G.: The meaning of the point of maximum oscillations in cuff pressure in the indirect measurement of blood pressure. Part I. Cardiovasc. Res. Cent. Bull. 8:15, 1969.
33. Ware, R. W.: New approaches to the indirect measurement of human blood pressure. Presented at the Third National Biomed. Sci. Instr. Symp. Instr. Soc. of Amer., paper BM-65, Dallas, Texas, April 19–21, 1965.
34. Morgan, J. L., Kemmerer, W. T., and Halber, M. D.: Doppler shifted ultrasound. History and applications in clinical medicine. Minn. Med. 52:503, 1969.
35. Kirby, R. R., Kemmerer, W. T., and Morgan, J. L.: Transcutaneous Doppler measurement of blood pressure. Anesthesiology 31:86, 1969.
36. Kemmerer, W. T., Ware, R. W., Stegall, H. F., Morgan, J. L., and Kirby, R.: Blood pressure measurement by Doppler ultrasonic detection of arterial wall motion. Surg. Gynec. Obstet. 131:1141, 1970.
37. Hochberg, H. M., and Salomon, H.: Accuracy of an automated ultrasound blood pressure monitor. Curr. Ther. Res. 13:129, 1971.
38. Waltemath, C. L., and Preuss, D. D.: Determination of blood pressure in low-flow states by the Doppler technique. Anesthesiology 34: 77, 1971.
39. Hochberg, H. M., and Saltzman, M. B.: Accuracy of an ultrasound blood pressure instrument in neonates, infants, and children. Curr. Ther. Res. 13:482, 1971.
40. Gruen, W.: An assessment of present automated methods of indirect blood pressure

measurement. Ann. N.Y. Acad. Sci. 147:107, 1968.

41. Stein, P. D., and Blick, E. F.: Arterial tonometry for the atraumatic measurement of arterial blood pressure. J. Appl. Physiol. 30: 593, 1971.
42. Tursky, D., Shapiro, D., and Schwartz, G. E.: Automated constant cuff-pressure system to measure average systolic and diastolic blood-pressure in man. I.E.E.E. Trans. Biomed. Eng. 19:271, 1972.
43. Benson, H.: Unpublished data.
44. Kain, H. K., Hinman, A. T., and Sokolow, M.: Arterial blood pressure measurements with a portable recorder in hypertensive patients. I. Variability and correlation with "casual" pressures. Circulation 30:882, 1964.
45. Werdegar, D., Sokolow, M., and Perloff, D. B.: Portable recordings of blood pressure: A new approach to assessments of the severity and prognosis of hypertension. Trans. Assoc. Life Ins. Med. Dir. Am. 51:93, 1967.
46. Riess, W. F., Werdegar, D. and Sokolow, M.: Blood pressure responses to daily life events. Trans. Assoc. Life Ins. Med. Dir. Am. 51:116, 1967.

Normal and Raised Arterial Pressure: What is Hypertension?

By Colin T. Dollery, M.B.

THE SYSTEMIC arterial pressure is the driving pressure of the capillary circulation throughout the body. The level at which this pressure is set varies greatly in different individuals and at different times. It is low during sleep and high during emotional stress or heavy muscular exercise. The range of pressure recorded in healthy, normal young adults during a 24-hour period ranges from 65 mm Hg systolic during sleep to over 170 mm Hg systolic during maximal exercise. This variability makes it hard to characterize an individual by a single reading of blood pressure.

There are physiologic reasons why the blood pressure had to be held within certain limits. Glomerular filtration ceases if the mean arterial pressure falls much below 60 mm Hg because it is a pressure filtration system. Very low pressures in the upright position also impair blood flow to the eyes, the brain, and the arms extended above the head. These factors set a lower limit to blood pressure during activity. Levels of pressure which are much higher than the minimum do not necessarily convey any biological disadvantage, but the higher the level of pressure, the greater the long-term risk of vascular disease. If the pressure rises to very high levels there is short-term risk of left ventricular failure, cerebral hemorrhage, and arteriolar necrosis which may lead to early death. Thus physiologic considerations set some limits to "normal" blood pressure but these are so wide as to be of little practical value.

Because of its variability, efforts have been made to standardize the circumstances of blood pressure recording to secure more uniform results. Examples include measurements made during pentobarbital-induced sleep for the "basal" blood pressure recording of Smirk [1] and averaging a number of daytime readings obtained with Sokolow's portometer.[2] Both these authors claim advantages for their method, but neither has been widely adopted because of their complexity. Data obtained by life insurance companies and by epidemiologists suggest that a single casual reading of blood pressure obtained at an interview is as satisfactory in predicting prognosis as the more complex methods.[3] It is important that precautions be taken to avoid bias and digit preference if this reading is required for exact purposes.[4]

Against this background, trying to define a normal level of blood pressure is exceedingly difficult. At one extreme, no doctor would have any doubt that a patient with a blood pressure of 260/160 mm Hg and bilateral papilledema and cotton-wool spots in the fundus had a potentially lethal disease called malignant hypertension. At the other extreme lies a symptomless young man or woman who is found at a routine examination to have a blood pressure of 150/90 mm Hg, a value which many physicians would consider to be of no significance.

Changes of Pressure with Time

On average the blood pressure is higher in older people than it is in the young. The rate of rise with age is neither constant for different individuals nor for the two sexes. Those with higher levels of blood pressure at the start of a period of observation will rise faster over the succeeding years. Miall predicted from his studies in Wales that if a man had a diastolic pressure 20 mm Hg higher than average at the age of 40, he would have a diastolic pressure 35 mm Hg higher than the average for that age by the time he reached 60 years.[5] For some individuals and in some communities there is little rise in pressure with age so it is difficult to speak of that rise as being "normal." Lovell in Oceania [6] and Shaper [7] in East Africa, among many others, have identified communities and tribes in which there is little if any rise in blood pressure with age. There is some evidence that

From the Department of Clinical Pharmacology, Royal Postgraduate Medical School, University of London, London, England.

when these individuals become "westernized" their pressure levels are higher than before.

The increment of blood pressure with age observed in most Caucasian and Negro communities may only reflect the duration of exposure to environmental factors that raise blood pressure.

Attempts to define normal or raised levels of blood pressure based upon such data have an uncertain basis. The answer to such a basic question of whether the normal level of pressure changes with age depends upon the community and the sample chosen to define it. It has been suggested that a useful operational decision as to whether hypertension is present would be to select those whose blood pressure fell above the 95th percentile for their age in the community under study. When this proposal is interpreted in the light of relative risk of developing vascular disease, it loses most of its attractions, for risk is related to level of pressure, not just above the 95th percentile but throughout the range.

As it is traditional to separate normality from disease much effort has been spent in trying to find an acceptable definition which will allow everyone to be defined either as "normal" or "hypertensive." Different authors have sought to separate normal from abnormal by a consideration of inheritance, etiology, clinical features, and risk. It is necessary to give brief consideration to each of these before dismissing all save the last.

Classification by Inheritance

There is a multiplicity of evidence that inheritance affects the level of blood pressure in both man and experimental animals. Pickering and his colleagues showed that there was a resemblance between pressure levels of propositi and their first-degree relatives with a coefficient of resemblance of about 0.2.[8] Miall and Oldham concluded that a regression of 0.287 for systolic pressure and 0.224 for diastolic pressure fits the relationship between propositi and their first-degree relatives.[9] Pickering concluded that inheritance of blood pressure was polygenic and that essential hypertension represents a type of disease, not generally recognized, in which the deviation from the norm is quantitative and qualitative. This view was disputed by Platt who pointed out the high degree of resemblance of blood pressure in identical twins.[10] Platt attempted to demonstrate a break in the distribution curve of blood pressures that would divide the hypertensives from the normals, but further work suggests that much of this break was an artifact induced by digit preference and avoidance in the original recordings.[11]

The weight of evidence is strongly in favor of the polygenic theory, and in any case the inheritance of blood pressure is not strong enough to be of any value in deciding whether a particular individual is constitutionally "hypertensive." If Pickering is right this is a wrongly formulated question.

Classification by Clinical Features

Many patients with high blood pressure are free of symptoms and physical signs apart from the pressure level itself. A small proportion of patients are suffering immediate consequences of a high pressure level such as retinal cotton-wool spots or left ventricular failure. A somewhat larger proportion have suffered late complications of atheromatous vascular disease such as a myocardial infarction or stroke when they present to a doctor. It is tempting to classify patients according to the organ damage they have suffered at the time of first presentation. There are many features that can be used: clinical signs of heart failure, or cardiac hypertrophy; changes in the peripheral pulses; retinal vascular disease. These clinical findings can be supplemented by the results of investigations which throw additional light upon the state of the heart and kidneys.

Classification systems have been constructed that rely both upon pressure level and complications to provide an index of severity.[13] The most widely used is the classification of Keith, Wagener, and Barker.[14] I have argued that grades I and II of this classification have outlived their usefulness, but grades III and IV undoubtedly identify a group in urgent need of treatment and having a poor prognosis without it.[15] However, atheromatous complications do not have the same prognostic significance and are not solely related to blood pressure. A patient without symptoms who has a high pressure level may be felled by a cerebral hemorrhage although his present state does not assign him to a severe category. A classification based upon such criteria is too heterogeneous and has too little prognostic value to serve a useful purpose. If we reserve the diagnosis of hypertensive disease to those who have suffered complications, we resign any chance of preventing them in those who have most to gain, the patients who have no symptoms or signs.

Classification by Cause

Many causes of a raised blood pressure have been discovered. They include many different types of renal disease, mineralocorticoid excess, disorders of the central nervous system, and abnormalities of the circulation. Can hypertension be regarded in the same light as fever and be classified by its causes?

There are two main reasons why such a classification breaks down. The first is that no cause can be ascertained in the majority of individuals whose blood pressure lies in the higher part of the range. In a study of 229 patients with "hypertension" who were under 40 years old, no cause could be found in two thirds of them.[12] The second reason is that the adverse effects of a high blood pressure are usually a consequence of the pressure level itself, and the causative factor is not of special importance except in the small proportion of patients with a surgically correctable etiology.

Classification by Risk

If no cause of a high blood pressure can be identified and the patient has survived any complications thus far, only one question remains and it is the most important. What is the future outlook?

This question was asked and to some extent answered by life insurance companies surprisingly soon after the introduction of the sphygmomanometer. The accumulated experience of the American life insurance companies was published in 1959 and should be compulsory reading for anyone who is interested in the treatment of hypertension.[3] The essential message of this massive study was that elevations of blood pressure that many would consider trivial greatly increased the risk of premature death from disease of the heart, brain, or kidneys. Furthermore, it established that risk was graded with level of pressure throughout the range examined. In terms of risk the normal range of blood pressure has no meaning.

Prospective epidemiologic studies have established that high blood pressure is one of several factors that significantly affect the risk of developing vascular disease.[16,17] These include blood lipids, smoking habit, age, sex, body weight, and physical activity as well as blood pressure. Such measurements have been used to calculate the relative risk of coronary heart disease in different groups of people.[18,19] The risk of vascular disease is much greater if an individual lies in the upper part of the distribution for several of these risk factors than for only one or two.

If the level of blood pressure is very high, it is the dominant consideration but in milder cases all of the relevant factors should be taken into account before a decision is made about treatment. For example, it would not be particularly logical to initiate treatment of a mildly raised blood pressure and ignore the fact that the patient was a heavy cigarette smoker.

It is much more important to think about patients in this way than it is to lose time pondering whether or not hypertension is an appropriate label to apply to them.

References

1. Smirk, F. H.: High Arterial Pressure. Oxford: Blackwell, 1957.
2. Sokolow, M., Werdegar, D., Kain, H. K., and Hinman, A. T.: Relationship between level of blood pressure measured casually and by portable recorders and severity of complications in essential hypertension. Circulation 34:279, 1966.
3. Society of Actuaries: Build and Blood Pressure Study. Chicago: Society of Actuaries, 1959.
4. Rose, G. A., Holland, W. W., and Crowley, E. A.: A sphygmomanometer for epidemiologists. Lancet 1:296, 1964.
5. Miall, W. E., and Lovell, H. G.: Relation between change of blood pressure and age. Br. Med. J. 2:660, 1967.
6. Lovell, R. R. H.: Race and blood pressure with special reference to Oceania. *In* Stamler, J., Stamler, R., and Pullman, T. N. (Eds.): The Epidemiology of Hypertension. New York: Grune & Stratton, 1967, p. 122.
7. Shaper, A. G.: Blood pressure studies in East Africa. *In* Stamler, J., Stamler, R., and Pull-

man, T. N. (Eds.): The Epidemiology of Hypertension. New York: Grune & Stratton, 1967, p. 139.

8. Pickering, G. W.: High Blood Pressure. Oxford: Blackwell, 1968, p. 264.
9. Miall, W. E., and Oldham, P. D.: The heredity factor in arterial blood pressure. Br. Med. J. 1:75, 1963.
10. Platt, R.: Heredity in hypertension. Lancet 1:899, 1963.
11. Humerfelt, S. B.: Methodology of blood pressure recording. *In* Gross, F. (Ed.): Antihypertensive Therapy, Principles and Practice. An International Symposium. Berlin: Springer, 1966, p. 212.
12. Breckenridge, A., Preger, L., Dollery, C. T., and Laws, J. W.: Hypertension in the young. Q. J. Med. 36:549, 1967.
13. World Health Organization: Arterial hypertension and ischaemic heart disease: preventive aspects. Report of an expert committee. WHO Tech. Rep. Ser. 231, 1962.
14. Keith, N. M., Wagener, H. P., and Barker, N. W.: Some different types of essential hypertension: Their course and prognosis. Am. J. Med. Sci. 197:332, 1939.
15. Wise, G. N., Dollery, C. T., and Henkind, P.: The Retinal Circulation. New York: Harper & Row, 1971.
16. Kannel, W. B., Dawber, T. K. R., Kagan, A., Revotskie, N., and Stokes, J.: Factors of risk in the development of coronary heart disease—Six year follow-up experience. The Framingham Study. Ann. Intern. Med. 55:33, 1961.
17. Doyle, J. T., Heslins, S., Hilleboe, H. E., Formel, P. F., and Korns, R. F.: Prospective study of degenerative cardiovascular disease in Albany. Report of three years experience. I. Ischemic heart disease. Am. J. Public Health 47:25, 1957.
18. Truett, J., Cornfield, J., and Kannel, W.: Multivariate analysis of the risk of coronary heart disease. J. Chronic Dis. 20:511, 1967.
19. Buzina, R., Keys, A., Mohacek, I., Marinkovic, M., Hahn, A., et al.: Coronary heart disease in seven countries. Part V. Five-year follow-up in Dalmatia and Slavonia. Circulation 41–42 (Suppl. 1):40, 1970.

Casual, Basal, and Supplemental Blood Pressures

By Sir F. Horace Smirk, K.B.E., M.D., Sc.D.

Over 30 years ago my colleague Alam and I [1,2] found that with emotional desensitization to the procedure of blood pressure measurement, by repeating the measurements regularly and monotonously under very quiet conditions, the blood pressure fell, often to below 100 mm Hg systolic in healthy young males.

Although the level of the blood pressure, as ordinarily measured, would vary in the same person from one day to another, yet, under unstimulating conditions, as described, the blood pressure usually fell to a level which was almost constant for the individual. In the state of comfortable monotony, subjects often drifted into sleep. Sleep had very little immediate effect on the blood pressure, but we found in other experiments that deep sleep does reduce the blood pressure further.

We began talking about "basal blood pressures," but soon found that Addis [3] had already introduced the term in 1922. In 1939 a committee of the American Heart Association and the Cardiac Society of Great Britain and Ireland [4] followed the recommendation of Addis [3] that for a basal pressure the patient should be prepared as for a basal metabolic rate.

Our method of rest and emotional desensitization alone produced somewhat lower results than the Addis method. By combining the Addis method and our ritual of emotional desensitization, still lower blood pressure levels were obtained.

Our present technique for basal blood pressure,[5] slightly modified, is as follows:

1. The patient is assured that measurements of the blood pressure will not be the prelude to painful or frightening procedures.
2. The patient is given 100 to 200 mg of pentobarbitone to ensure a night's rest.
3. In the morning, bladder and bowels are emptied but only if desired.
4. A technician or doctor then enters the single room in which the patient has been sleeping and, without conversation, measures the blood pressure regularly, monotonously, at half-minute to 1-minute intervals for 15 minutes.

It is important that no other persons should enter the room while the test is in progress, the observer should sit quietly by the patient throughout the test, and the patient should have been asked not to speak but to relax as completely as possible, physically and mentally. Even quiet conversation can raise the blood pressure.[6] The mean of the two lowest blood pressures obtained by this technique is the basal blood pressure. For the blood pressure as ordinarily measured, and without special precautions, we devised the term "casual blood pressure." We used the term "supplemental pressure" for the casual blood pressure minus the basal blood pressure.

When we speak of supplemental pressures in this way, it is important to remember that the supplemental pressures referred to are those derived from casual pressures taken in a clinical setting. They do not refer to the supplemental pressures which may exist under conditions of physical exertion or under long-continued emotional stress.

To get the most reliable estimates of the basal blood pressure the physician in charge must use some imaginative insight. Basal levels of the blood pressures will not be obtained if noises of patient distress are coming from an adjacent cubicle, nor if the subject is worried about getting late to work, nor, in a male, if an attractive, scented female appears with the sphygmomanometer.

The basal blood pressure taken under good conditions is almost a physiologic constant. In hypertensives the basal blood pressure is more

---

From Wellcome Medical Research Institute, Department of Medicine, Medical School, Dunedin, New Zealand.

Supported by a grant from the Medical Research Council of New Zealand, Wellington, New Zealand.

variable than in normotensives, but is much less variable than the casual blood pressure.[7]

The supplemental blood pressure is the variable or labile part of the blood pressure and is dependent upon the state of metabolic, physical, and emotional activity at the time of measuring the blood pressure.

Relationship Between Basal and Supplemental Blood Pressures and Prognosis

In a series of 315 untreated hypertensives, mostly assembled before active hypotensive drugs became available, we studied the casual, basal, and supplemental pressures and other factors which concern prognosis.[8]

A follow-up study of the patients was made 5 years and again 8 years after the initial investigation. There was a strong positive correlation between the original height of the basal blood pressure and subsequent mortality. Patients with a high basal blood pressure (systolic or diastolic) had a much greater mortality than those whose basal blood pressures were low, whereas possession of a high supplemental pressure (systolic or diastolic) did not increase the 5- or 8-year mortality.

The casual blood pressure is, therefore, the sum of the important basal blood pressure and the supplemental or labile part of the blood pressure which, within an 8-year period, shows no tendency to influence the prognosis adversely.

For individual prognosis basal pressures give better results than casual pressures, as shown in Figure 1. Eighteen groups of female hypertensive patients were selected so that each group contained a patient who died in the 5-year follow-up period (dots) together with all the available patients within the same age range who had similar levels of the casual systolic blood pressure and survived (triangles). The position of the symbols (dots and triangles) in relation to the scale indicates the corresponding basal systolic blood pressure levels of the individual patients within the 18 groups, these being displayed along the 18 vertical lines.

In 26 out of 36 instances the survivors had lower basal systolic blood pressures than those (with similar casual systolic pressures) who

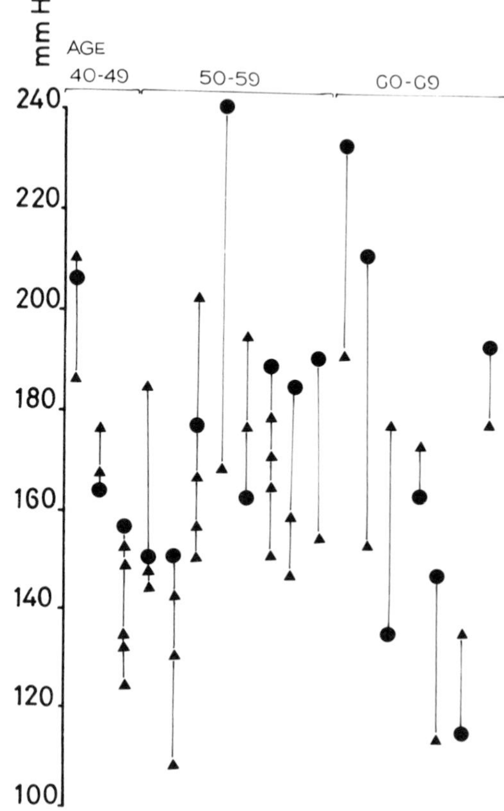

Fig. 1.—Out of a series of 107 untreated female hypertensives aged 40 to 69, all of retinal grading 1 or 2, all followed for a period of 5 years, it was possible to select 18 groups. Within each group the hypertensive patients were alike in that, at the outset of the follow-up period, they were in the same age range, had closely similar systolic blood pressures, and were alike in the number, if any, of the hypertensive complications experienced.

Within such matched groups, having similar casual systolic blood pressures, a comparison is made between the basal systolic pressures (ordinates) of those who died (**large dots**) and those who survived in the 5-year period (**triangles**). The symbols relating to each of the 18 matched groups are arranged for comparison along 18 **vertical lines.** At similar levels of age and casual systolic pressures, low basal pressures were associated with a better chance of survival.

died and in 10 out of 36 they had higher basal systolic pressures. In Figure 2, which shows results in 18 groups of female hypertensives selected for similar ages and casual diastolic

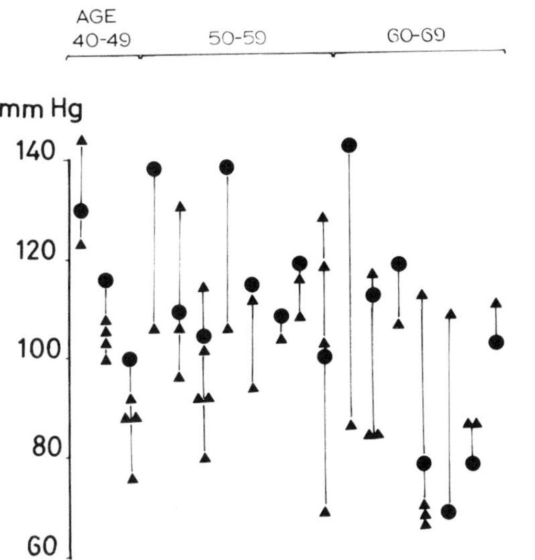

FIG. 2.—Arrangements are the same as those established for Figure 1 except that the comparison made here is of the relationship of basal diastolic pressures in 18 groups of hypertensive females matched groups, those with lower basal diastolic level of the casual diastolic pressure and number, if any, of hypertensive complications. Within the matched groups those with lower basal diastolic pressures were associated with a better chance of a 5-year survival.

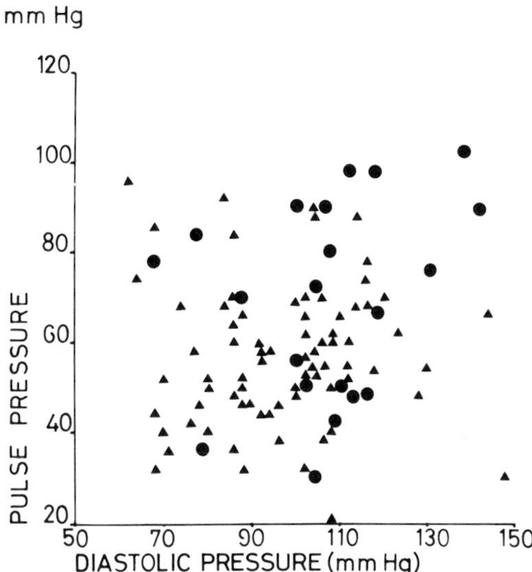

FIG. 3.—The relationship of the 5-year mortality to basal pulse pressures (*ordinates*) and basal diastolic pressures (*abscissae*) is shown for untreated female hypertensives, aged 40 to 69, retinal grades 1 or 2. The pulse pressures of those who died (**large dots**) are in general higher than the pulse pressures of those who survived (**triangles**).

pressures, the survivors had a lower basal diastolic blood pressure than those who died in 30 out of 42 patients and a higher basal diastolic pressure in 12 out of 42. A similar relationship is found in males.

The Build and Blood Pressure Study of the American Society of Actuaries [9] has demonstrated clearly that the eventual mortality is related to the systolic as well as to the diastolic blood pressure.

RELATIONSHIP BETWEEN PULSE PRESSURE AND SURVIVAL

If we wish to examine that part of the systolic blood pressure which does not contain the diastolic pressure then we should turn to the pulse pressure which, of course, is systolic minus diastolic pressure. The basal pulse pressure is more closely related to mortality than the casual pulse pressure.

If we subdivide our female hypertensives (Fig. 3) by levels of the basal pulse pressure,

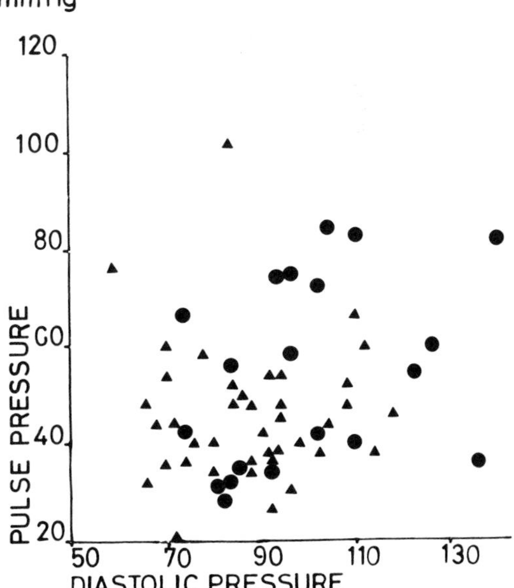

FIG. 4.—The relationship of the 5-year mortality to the basal pulse pressures (*ordinates*) and basal diastolic pressures (*abscissae*) is shown for untreated males, aged 40 to 49, retinal grades 1 or 2. In general the pulse pressures of those who died (**large dots**) are higher than the pulse pressures of those who survived (**triangles**).

those with pulse pressures above 80 mm Hg had a mortality of 53 percent, those with pressures between 60 and 79 mm Hg, 17 percent; and those with pressures under 60 mm Hg, 15.4 percent. In males (Fig. 4) pulse pressures above 80 mm Hg were associated with a mortality of 80 percent; pressures between 60 and 79 mm Hg, 63 percent; and pressures under 60 mm Hg, 22 percent. Taking males and females together, the rate of mortality of those with a pulse pressure of 60 mm Hg or more was 37 percent and of those with pressures of under 60 mm Hg was 21 percent.

Basal pulse pressures above 60 mm Hg are associated with an unusually high 5-year mortality even when a comparison is made with patients who have similar levels of the basal diastolic pressure.

Relationship of Basal and Supplemental Pressures to the Pathogenesis of Hypertension

Basal and supplemental pressures are almost independent variables in the sense that possession by an individual of a high or a low basal blood pressure hardly influences the expectation of that individual having a high or low supplemental pressure.[8]

These variables being almost independent, it is likely that basal and supplemental pressures have a different pathogenesis. Some support for this statement comes from the results of a study of casual, basal, and supplemental pressures in 519 first-degree relatives of substantial hypertensives and 290 controls considered to be representative of the general population.[10]

Figure 5 shows that in males the basal systolic and diastolic pressures both rise with age. In females (not shown) they also rise with age.

In both males and females the rise in the basal blood pressure with age is greater in the first-degree relatives of substantial hypertensives than in controls considered to be representative of the general population.

In males the supplemental pressure does not rise appreciably with age whereas a rise occurs in females. But neither in males nor in females is there any appreciable difference between levels of the supplemental pressures of the first-degree relatives and controls.

There is good evidence that the level of the supplemental blood pressure is under a variety of influences. It seems probable that any condition—physical, metabolic or emotional—increasing the cardiac output will tend to raise the supplemental blood pressure. There are numerous studies which show that physical and emotional activity increase the blood pressure above basal or resting casual blood pressure levels.

Regarding the pathogenesis of the basal blood pressure, there is evidence that a part at least of the basal blood pressure is neurogenically maintained. In hypertensives and in normotensives Doyle and Smirk [11] found that, even in the horizontal posture, large doses of a ganglion-blocking drug such as hexamethonium reduce the blood pressure to well below the basal level, and do so by blocking nervous impulses. They had a series of 55 persons whose basal blood pressures and hexamethonium-floor pressures were both available. The mean of the basal systolic pressures was

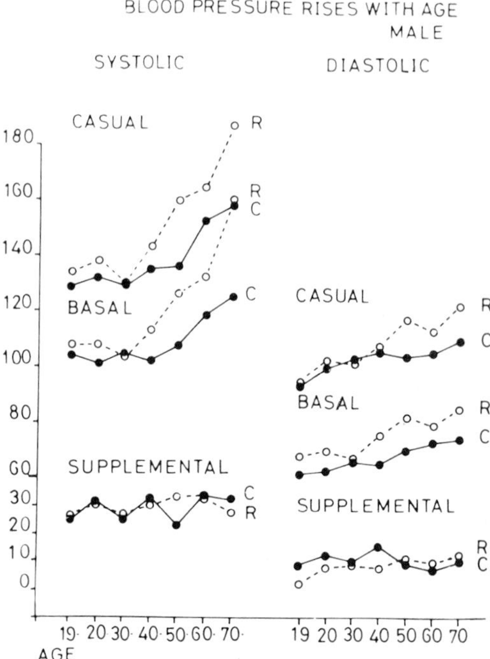

Fig. 5.—Comparison of the casual, basal, and supplemental blood pressures of the first-degree male relatives (**R**) of substantial hypertensives with controls (**C**) representative of the general population. Age groups (*abscissae*); blood pressures measured in millimeters of mercury (*ordinates*). (From Smirk, F. H.,[10] with permission.)

180.6 mm Hg and of the hexamethonium-floor systolic pressures 146.0 mm Hg systolic. The mean of the basal diastolic pressures was 115 mm Hg and of the hexamethonium-floor diastolic pressures 97.0 mm Hg. It would appear that the basal blood pressure is maintained to some degree by the discharge of nerve impulses which have to pass through sympathetic ganglia.

In most hypertensives even large doses of ganglion-blocking drugs do not reduce the blood pressure in the horizontal posture to the level attained in normals after ganglionic blockade.[11] It will be noted in Figures 6 and 7 that in the absence of pressor drugs the hexamethonium falls in pressure and the hexamethonium-floor pressures (systolic in Fig. 6, diastolic in Fig. 7) are ordinarily appreciably larger in the hypertensives (large dots) than in the normotensives (small dots). It seems reasonable to suppose that at least a part of the blood pressure increase above the normal in hypertension is maintained by factors which are not dependent upon neurogenic impulses.

There are interactions between the neurogenically and nonneurogenically maintained parts of the blood pressure as may be seen in the following experiments. The nonneurogenically maintained part of the blood pressure may be raised experimentally either in animals or in man. We have shown [11,12] that if the blood pressure is raised by the administration of norepinephrine, S-methyl-*iso*-thiourea or angiotensin, then the fall of blood pressure in response to the administration of large doses of hexamethonium is smaller after than it was before administration of the pressor agent (Figs. 6 and 7). It seems that the administration of a humoral pressor agent leads to a decrease in the neurogenically maintained fraction of the blood pressure as the result of homeostasis. The injected pressor agent raises the nonneurogenically maintained part of the blood pressure, and homeostatic mechanisms

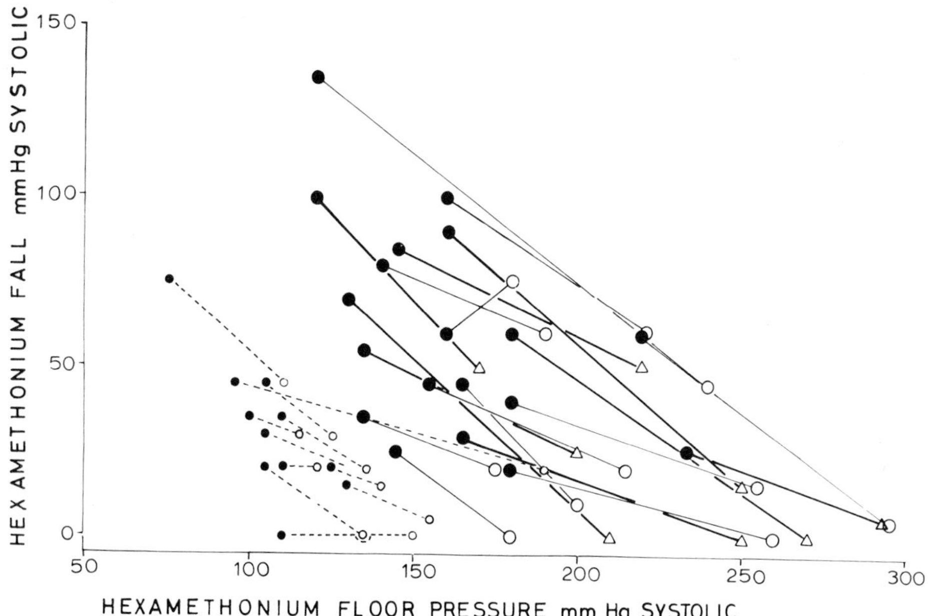

FIG. 6.—Effect of pressor drugs on systolic pressure responses to hexamethonium in hypertensive patients (**large dots**) and in normotensive patients (**small dots**). The **lines** joining two dots indicate that the two results were obtained on the same person, one in the absence of pressor-drug infusion (**black circles**) and one during infusion of angiotensin (**white circles**) or norepinephrine (**triangles**). (From Smirk, F. H.: The neurogenically maintained component in hypertension. Circ. Res. 27 (Suppl. 2):55, 1970, by permission of the American Heart Association, Inc.)

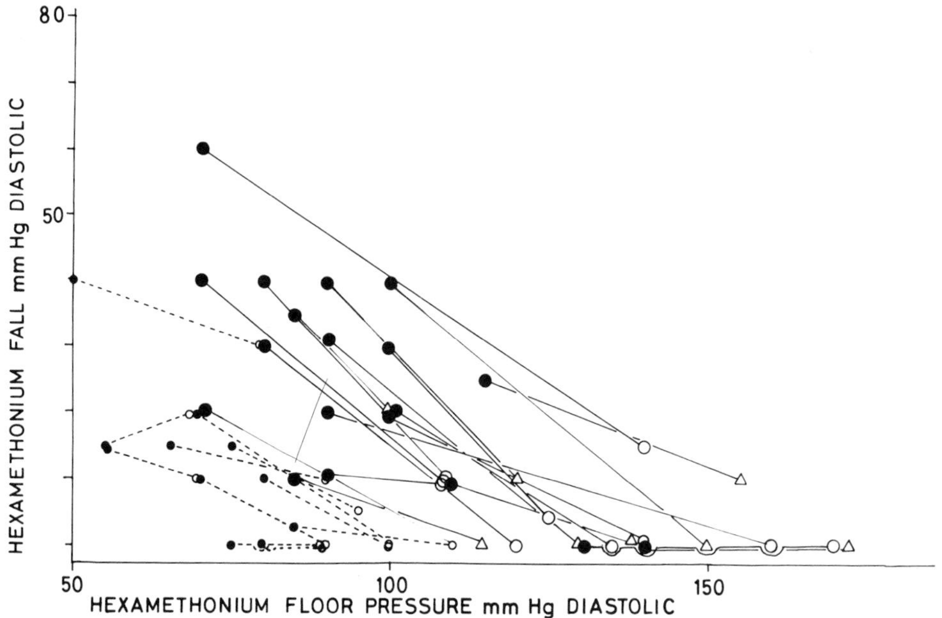

FIG. 7.—Effect of pressor drugs on diastolic pressures responses to hexamethonium in hypertensive patient (**large dots**) and in normotensive patients (**small dots**). The lines joining two dots indicate that the two results were obtained on the same person, one in the absence of pressor-drug infusion (**black circles**) and one during infusion of angiotensin (**white circles**) or norepinephrine (**triangles**). (From Smirk, F. H. The neurogenically maintained component in hypertension. Circ. Res. 27 (Suppl. 2):55, 1970, by permission of the American Heart Associaciation, Inc.)

respond by reducing the neurogenically maintained part of the blood pressure. There is less neurogenic tone to be removed and ganglionic blockade leads to a smaller fall in blood pressure.

One may conclude that, not only the supplemental, but also the basal blood pressure is determined by the operation of more than one factor.

The hexamethonium-floor pressure is not only raised above the normal in essential hypertension but also in experimental renal hypertension of rats and in rats from our spontaneously hypertensive rat colony.[13]

SUMMARY

1. The casual blood pressure may be subdivided into the basal blood pressure taken under standard basal conditions, and the supplemental pressure which is the casual minus the basal blood pressure.

2. The basal and supplemental pressures are almost independent variables, any slight interrelationship being inverse.

3. In the first-degree relatives of substantial hypertensives, males and females, there is a rise of the basal blood pressure with age which is greater than in controls thought to be representative of the general population.

4. In females the mean supplemental pressure shows a distinct rise with age whereas in males age has comparatively little influence on the level of the supplemental blood pressure.

5. Neither in males nor in females does there appear to be any important difference between the supplemental pressures of controls and the first-degree relatives of hypertensives.

6. The 5- and 8-year mortalities are closely related to the systolic and diastolic basal blood pressures but, if anything, somewhat negatively related to the supplemental blood pressure.

7. The supplemental blood pressure arises as the result of physical, emotional, and metabolic stimuli which raise the blood pressure above the

basal level. Many of these are environmental. Emotional stimuli may also be endogenous.

8. The basal blood pressure may be subdivided into neurogenically maintained parts and nonneurogenically maintained parts.

9. When pressor drugs such as norepinephrine, angiotensin, or S-methyl-*iso*-thiourea are administered the nonneurogenically maintained part of the blood pressure is increased and this leads to a homeostatic decrease in the neurogenically maintained part.

Acknowledgments

The author is much indebted to Mrs. Joy Tomlin who has been responsible for the secretarial work. Professor F. O. Simpson, of the Dunedin Hospital hypertensive clinic, has always been most helpful to me in the discussion of problems in the field of hypertension. I am grateful to Dr. John Hunter, Professor of Medicine in the Medical School, Dunedin, for generous facilities within the Wellcome Medical Research Institute.

References

1. Alam, G. M., and Smirk, F. H.: Casual and basal blood pressures. I. In British and Egyptian men. Br. Heart J. 5:152, 1943.
2. Alam, G. M., and Smirk, F. H.: Casual and basal blood pressures. II. In essential hypertension. Br. Heart J. 5:156, 1943.
3. Addis, T.: Blood pressure and pulse rate levels. Arch. Intern. Med. 29:539, 1922.
4. Committee for the Standardization of Blood Pressure Readings of the American Heart Association and of the Cardiac Society of Great Britain and Ireland. Standard method for taking and recording blood pressure readings. JAMA 113:294, 1939.
5. Smirk, F. H.: High Arterial Pressure. Oxford: Blackwell, 1957, pp. 11–20, 63–77, and 212.
6. Ulrych, M.: Changes of general haemodynamics during stressful mental arithmetic and non-stressing quiet conversation and modification of the latter by beta-adrenergic blockade. Clin. Sci. 36:453, 1969.
7. Kilpatrick, J. A.: The variation of casual, basal and supplemental blood pressure in health and in essential hypertension. Br. Heart J. 10:48, 1948.
8. Smirk, F. H., Veale, A. M. O., and Alstad, K.: Basal and supplemental blood pressures in relationship to life expectancy and hypertension symptomatology. N. Z. Med. J. 58:711, 1959.
9. Build and Blood Pressure Study 1959. Chicago: Society of Actuaries, 1959, pp. 133, 142.
10. Smirk, F. H.: Blood pressure in families: Preliminary communication. N. Z. Med. J. 71:355, 1970.
11. Doyle, A. E., and Smirk, F. H.: The neurogenic component in hypertension. Circulation 12:974, 1955.
12. Smirk, F. H.: The neurogenically maintained component in hypertension. Circ. Res. 27 (Suppl. 2): 55, 1970.
13. Phelan, E. L.: Cardiovascular reactivity in rats with spontaneous inherited hypertension and constricted renal artery hypertension. Am. Heart J. 71:50, 1966.

Etiologic Classification of Hypertension

By Kwan Eun Kim, M.D.

An ETIOLOGIC CLASSIFICATION of hypertension is valuable because it defines specific clinical syndromes, their diagnosis, pathogenesis, and rational treatment. A tentative etiologic classification is shown in Table 1 to give the reader a framework within which to work. The possible pathogenesis of secondary hypertension not covered in detail elsewhere in this book will be discussed briefly in this chapter.

Systolic blood pressure is determined by two main factors. The first is stroke volume. Any condition increasing stroke volume may raise systolic blood pressure. The second determinant of systolic blood pressure is the compliance of the aorta and its large branches. A decrease in compliance, i.e., a reduction in elasticity, of the aorta and its branches will increase systolic blood pressure. This is usually due to atherosclerotic changes in the aorta and its main branches. It is, therefore, common to find high systolic blood pressure (e.g., 180 mm Hg) with normal diastolic blood pressure (e.g., 80 mm Hg) in elderly subjects.

Diastolic blood pressure is primarily determined by total peripheral vascular resistance, predominantly regulated by the resistance of small arteries and arterioles.

Patients with combined systolic and diastolic hypertension can be divided into two main groups: those with primary (essential) or with secondary hypertension. When a specific cause of high blood pressure cannot be identified, the term "essential hypertension" is used; patients with this type of hypertension still constitute the majority of hypertensives. As medical knowledge progresses, we expect that other underlying causes of hypertension will be uncovered, and many patients now thought to have essential hypertension will turn out to have secondary hypertension. The bulk of patients with hypertension form a fairly uniform group for which no well-defined etiologic process has been delineated. The genetic patterns, epidemiology, environmental factors, hemodynamic alterations, and clinical and pathologic manifestations of essential hypertension are discussed extensively in subsequent chapters.

Secondary hypertension can be arbitrarily divided into groups according to the organ system which causes high blood pressure.

Renal Hypertension

Renal hypertension (i.e., renal parenchymal and renal vascular) is the most common cause of secondary hypertension. The majority of patients with acute glomerulonephritis have hypertension. In chronic renal parenchymal diseases including chronic glomerulonephritis, hypertension usually occurs in the late stage of the diseases. Any renal parenchymal disease or renal involvement associated with systemic disease may cause hypertension. The precise pathophysiology of renal parenchymal hypertension has not been uncovered. The hemodynamics, renin-angiotensin system, vasopressor and vasodepressor substances, neurogenic factors, and management of renal hypertension are extensively discussed in subsequent chapters.

Dynamic renal artery stenosis is not only the most common cause of renovascular hypertension but is also the most common cause of surgically curable hypertension. The different anatomic and pathologic types of renal artery stenosis have been recently reviewed.[1,2]

Renal infarction may be caused by emboli to the main renal artery or one of its branches. Emboli of the renal artery usually originate from the heart in patients with valvular heart disease, particularly in those with chronic atrial fibrillation. Atheromatous materials from the aorta may cause renal artery embolism and renal infarction. Dissecting aneurysm of the aorta or dissecting aneurysm of the renal artery in patients with renal artery occlusive disease may also cause renal infarction.

From the Division of Nephrology and Hypertension, Department of Medicine, Hahnemann Medical College and Hospital, Philadelphia, Pennsylvania.

TABLE 1.—*Etiologic Classification of Hypertension*

- I. Systolic Hypertension
  - A. Increased stroke volume
    1. Bradycardia with complete heart block
    2. Aortic insufficiency
    3. Arteriovenous fistula
    4. Patent ductus arteriosus
    5. Thyrotoxicosis
    6. Anemia
    7. Others
  - B. Decreased compliance (decreased distensibility) of the aorta and its large branches (atherosclerosis)
- II. Combined Systolic and Diastolic Hypertension
  - A. Primary hypertension (essential hypertension)
  - B. Secondary hypertension
    1. Renal hypertension
       - a. Renal parenchymal hypertension
         - (1) Acute and chronic glomerulonephritis
         - (2) Chronic pyelonephritis
         - (3) Polycystic kidney disease
         - (4) Radiation nephritis
         - (5) Other primary renal parenchymal diseases
         - (6) Renal involvement associated with systemic diseases (e.g., diabetic nephropathy, gouty nephropathy and collagen vascular diseases)
       - b. Renovascular hypertension
         - (1) Renal artery stenosis
         - (2) Renal infarction
         - (3) Renal arterial aneurysm
         - (4) Renal arteriovenous fistula
    2. Adrenal hypertension
       - a. Primary aldosteronism
       - b. Cushing's syndrome
       - c. Congenital adrenogenital syndrome (11-β-hydroxylase and 17-α-hydroxylase defects)
       - d. Pheochromocytoma
    3. Neurogenic hypertension
       - a. Rapidly rising intracranial pressure (cerebral hemorrhage, head trauma, lead encephalopathy)
       - b. Bulbar poliomyelitis
       - c. Acute intermittent porphyria
       - d. Guillain-Barré syndrome
    4. Miscellaneous hypertension
       - a. Coarctation of aorta
       - b. Toxemia of pregnancy
       - c. Hypercalcemia
       - d. Myxedema

Renal artery aneurysms may occur in association with renal artery occlusive disease or may occur independently. It would seem that the majority of aneurysms of the renal artery are asymptomatic and an association with hypertension is more frequently seen in those patients with renal artery aneurysms who also have occlusive disease of one or both renal arteries than in those patients who do not have concomitant occlusive disease.[3]

Renal arteriovenous fistulas may be congenital or acquired. The acquired type occurs after trauma, particularly from penetrating wounds, but also from iatrogenic trauma such as nephrolithotomy, partial nephrectomy, or renal biopsy. Renal arteriovenous fistula may also occur in association with renal carcinoma. It has been suggested that the hypertension may be based on renal ischemia distal to the fistula.[4]

ADRENAL HYPERTENSION

Adrenal hypertension both cortical and medullary will be discussed at great length in subsequent chapters. The recent advances in evaluating the biochemical metabolism of the adrenal cortex and medulla combined with our ability to measure the components of the renin-angiotensin-aldosterone system have greatly improved our diagnostic skill and management of adrenal hypertension.

NEUROGENIC HYPERTENSION

Cushing[5] originally showed that an increase in intracranial pressure caused hypertension. Many subsequent reports have documented the occurrence of hypertension when intracranial pressure rises very rapidly as with head trauma and lead encephalopathy. Fremont-Smith and Merritt[6] found no correlation between blood pressure and cerebrospinal fluid pressure. Therefore, it seems important that the rise of intracranial pressure should be fairly rapid to raise blood pressure.

The association of hypertension and tachycardia in patients with poliomyelitis has been ascribed to a variety of causes such as anoxia and hypercapnea,[7] emotional factors,[8] disease of the reticular formation,[9,10] and the invasion of brainstem autonomic structures.[11]

There are different theories about the pathogenesis of hypertension in porphyric neuropathy.[12–14] Kezdi[14] failed to raise blood pressure in a patient with porphyria by injecting procaine into the carotid sinus. Therefore, he concluded that the patient's hypertension was due to a paralysis of the carotid sinus nerves together with the glossopharyngeal nerves and that their inhibitory mechanism was suspended.

Hypertension has been noted[15,16] in association with the Guillain-Barré syndrome. Like other neurogenic hypertension, the pathogenesis of hypertension in the Guillain-Barré syndrome has not been clearly defined. Mitchell and Meilman[17] suggested that a pathologic alteration of sympathetic nervous system, whereby high levels of pressor amines were produced, was the mechanism of hypertension in a case with Guillain-Barré syndrome. In contrast, Lichtenfeld[16] found normal values of urinary catecholamine and vanillylmandelic acid (VMA) on five occasions in two patients with Guillain-Barré syndrome during the hypertensive state. However, he noted that autonomic dysfunction occurred frequently in the form of either excessive or inadequate activity of the sympathetic and/or parasympathetic systems.

Miscellaneous Hypertension

When a specific organ responsible for hypertension cannot be identified, the hypertensive state is termed "miscellaneous hypertension." Toxemia of pregnancy and oral contraceptive agents and hypertension are discussed in subsequent chapters.

The frequency of the association of hypercalcemia with hypertension is not known. Lemann and Donatelli[18] reported 35 percent of patients in their review of hyperparathyroidism were hypertensive. They suggested that hypertension could be related to renal damage resulting from hypercalcemia superimposed on minimal benign nephrosclerosis or to chronic pyelonephritis associated with nephrolithiasis. Moore and Smith[19] found that the infusion of 15 mg of calcium per kilogram of body weight over a 4-hour period resulted in a systolic blood pressure rise of at least 30 mm Hg in nine of 19 patients and two patients had severe hypertensive responses that forced discontinuation of the test. The rapid onset of the hypertension suggests that it was correlated with a direct effect of the calcium ion rather than renal damage. Earll, Kurtzman, and Moser[20] also noted three consecutive cases of hypercalcemic hypertension in which the patients' blood pressures returned to normal when the hypercalcemia remitted. There is also experimental evidence that the calcium ion directly increases peripheral vascular resistance.[21,22]

Myxedema has been described as a cause of hypertension. Fuller and associates[23] noted that 22 of 77 patients with myxedema associated with hypertension became normotensive with only restoration of euthyroidism and without antihypertensive therapy. Ronan and Weintraub[24] reported a patient with myxedema associated with hypertension who became normotensive with replacement therapy and then reverted back to a hypertensive state when thyroid therapy was withheld. Hemodynamic studies demonstrated that an elevated peripheral resistance was the dominant feature in producing the hypertension. In contrast, Attarian[25] reported that of the 24 hypertensive myxedematous patients he studied, 18 remained hypertensive despite adequate thyroid replacement therapy, two became normotensive, and four were lost to follow-up.

It would seem that a certain number of patients with myxedema associated with hypertension become normotensive when they become euthyroid after thyroid therapy.

References

1. McCormack, L. J., Poutasse, E. F., Meaney, T.F., Noto, T. J., Jr., and Dustan, H. P.: A pathologic-arteriographic correlation of renal artery disease. Am. Heart J. 72:188, 1966.
2. Harrison, E. G., Jr., and McCormack, L. J.: Pathologic classification of renal artery disease in renovascular hypertension. Mayo Clin. Proc. 46:161, 1971.
3. Popowniak, K. L., Gifford, R. W., Jr., Straffon, R. A., Meaney, T. F., and McCormack, L. J.: Aneurysms of the renal artery. Postgrad. Med. 40:255, 1966.
4. Maldonado, J. E., and Sheps, S. G.: Renal arteriovenous fistula. Postgrad. Med. 40:263, 1966.
5. Cushing, H.: The blood pressure reaction of acute cerebral compression illustrated by cases of intracranial hemorrhage. Am. J. Heart Sci. 125:1017, 1903.

6. Fremont-Smith, F., and Merritt, H. H.: Relationship of arterial blood to cerebrospinal pressure in man. Arch. Neurol. Psychiat. 30: 1309, 1933.
7. Minnesota poliomyelitis research commission. Bulbar forms of poliomyelitis. JAMA 134: 757, 1947.
8. Ruskin, A., Beard, O. W., and Schaffer, R. L.: "Blast hypertension." Am. J. Med. 4:228, 1948.
9. Tyler, H. R., and Dawson, D.: Hypertension and its relation to the nervous system. Ann. Intern. Med. 55:681, 1961.
10. Kemp, E.: Arterial hypertension in poliomyelitis. Acta Med. Scand. 157:109, 1957.
11. McDowell, F. H., and Plum, F.: Arterial hypertension associated with acute anterior poliomyelitis. N. Engl. J. Med. 245:241, 1951.
12. Waldenström, J.: Studien über porphyrie. Acta Med. Scand. Suppl. 82:1, 1937.
13. Barker, A. B., and Watson, C. J.: The central nervous system in porphyria. J. Neuropathol. Exp. Neurol. 4:68, 1945.
14. Kezdi, P.: Neurogenic hypertension in man in porphyria. Transient hypertension and tachycardia caused by disruption of the carotid sinus; review of buffer nerve mechanism. Arch. Intern. Med. 94:122, 1954.
15. Haymaker, W., and Kernohan, J. W.: The Landry-Guillain-Barré syndrome. Medicine 28:59, 1949.
16. Lichtenfeld, P.: Autonomic dysfunction in the Guillain-Barré syndrome. Am. J. Med. 50:772, 1971.
17. Mitchell, P. L., and Meilman, E.: The mechanism of hypertension in the Guillain-Barré syndrome. Am. J. Med. 42:986, 1967.
18. Lemann, J., Jr., and Donatelli, A. A.: Calcium intoxication due to primary hyperparathyroidism. A medical and surgical emergency. Ann. Intern. Med. 60:447, 1964.
19. Moore, W. T., and Smith, L. H., Jr.: Experience with a calcium infusion test in parathyroid disease. Metabolism 12:447, 1963.
20. Earll, J. M., Kurtzman, N. A., and Moser, R. H.: Hypercalcemia and hypertension. Ann. Intern. Med. 64:378, 1966.
21. Overbeck, H. W., Molnar, J. I., and Haddy, F. J.: Resistance to blood flow through the vascular bed of the dog forelimb. Local effects of sodium, potassium, calcium, magnesium, acetate, hypertonicity and hypotonicity. Am. J. Cardiol. 8:533, 1961.
22. Haddy, F. J., Scott, J. B., Florio, M., Daugherty, R. M., Jr., and Huizenga, J. N.: Local vascular effects of hypokalemia, alkalosis, hypercalcemia and hypomagnesemia. Am. J. Physiol. 204:202, 1963.
23. Fuller, H., Jr., Spittell, J. A., Jr., McConahey, W. M., and Schirger, A.: Myxedema and hypertension. Postgrad. Med. 40:425, 1966.
24. Ronan, J. A., Jr., and Weintraub, A. M.: Hypertension and myxedema. Case report and a review of the literature. Med. Ann. D. C. 39:78, 1970.
25. Attarian, E.: Myxedema and hypertension. N.Y. State J. Med. 63:2801, 1963.

Part II. HEMODYNAMICS OF ESSENTIAL HYPERTENSION

RELATIONSHIP OF FLUID AND ELECTROLYTES TO ARTERIAL PRESSURE CONTROL AND HYPERTENSION: QUANTITATIVE ANALYSIS OF AN INFINITE-GAIN FEEDBACK SYSTEM

By ARTHUR C. GUYTON, M.D., THOMAS G. COLEMAN, PH.D., ALLEN W. COWLEY, JR., PH.D., ROGER A. NORMAN, JR., M.S., R. DAVIS MANNING, JR., M.S., AND J. F. LIARD, M.D.

TO STABILIZE arterial pressure for very short periods of time (seconds) or equally well for long periods of time (months), the body utilizes several different arterial pressure control systems. For instance, if the arterial pressure is decreased instantaneously from a normal value to a very low value, the nervous system reflexes come into play within seconds to increase the pressure nearly back to normal. Furthermore, several different nervous reflex systems exist for this purpose, most importantly the baroreceptor reflex, the chemoreceptor reflex, and the ischemic response of the central nervous system (CNS). These operate most effectively in different pressure ranges, the baroreceptors between 80 and 180 mm Hg,[1] the chemoreceptors between 40 and 80 mm Hg,[2] and the CNS ischemic response from 50 mm Hg downward.[3]

On the other hand, if the pressure abnormality lasts for days or weeks the nervous system reflexes, in general, fail to provide the necessary long-term pressure compensation because of adaptation of either the receptors or the effectors in the nervous system feedback loops. For instance, within 3 to 4 days after an acute but continued increase in arterial pressure, the baroreceptors adapt all the way back to their original activity level and are thereafter useless in correcting the original abnormality in arterial pressure. Therefore, still a different set of control systems is required.

At least three nonnervous system pressure control mechanisms begin to act within minutes and can probably provide continuing service as pressure controllers for many hours or days. These are (*1*) the renin-angiotensin-vasoconstrictor system which responds by release of renin, formation of angiotensin, and vasoconstriction when the arterial pressure falls below normal,[4] (*2*) the stress relaxation mechanism in which the blood vessels either slowly dilate in response to excess pressure or slowly contract in response to low pressure, thereby changing the pressure back toward normal,[5] and (*3*) the capillary fluid-shift mechanism in which excess capillary pressure causes loss of fluid volume from the circulation, or decreased capillary pressure causes fluid to be absorbed from the interstitial spaces into the circulation [6]—this effect usually helps to return arterial pressure back toward normal.

Finally come the very long-term adjustments in arterial pressure that do not make much headway for the first few hours but which continue to act for days, weeks, months, or indefinitely. One of these is the effect of the adrenal glands to secrete aldosterone when the arterial pressure falls below normal [7] or to decrease the secretion of aldosterone when the arterial pressure rises too high. These effects begin within minutes but do not have a significant effect on arterial pressure regulation until many hours of salt and water retention or excretion have occurred.

In addition to the indirect stimulation of water and salt retention by the aldosterone

From the Department of Physiology and Biophysics, University of Mississippi School of Medicine, Jackson, Mississippi.

Supported by research grants-in-aid from the United States Public Health Service and the American Heart Association.

mechanism, arterial pressure also plays a direct role in determining water and salt balance. Indeed, this mechanism is so important that it will serve as the theme of most of the remainder of this chapter. Basically, experiments in laboratories throughout the world [8–10] have demonstrated that the urinary output of water and salt decreases markedly when the arterial pressure is reduced below normal. Conversely, an increase in arterial pressure drastically increases urinary output of water and salt—e.g., an increase in pressure from 100 to 200 mm Hg increases urinary output of both water and salt six- to eightfold. Therefore, whenever arterial pressure falls too low, an automatic system for building up the body fluids occurs, and the arterial pressure returns toward normal; or whenever the arterial pressure rises too high, automatic loss of water and salt from the body returns the pressure downward again toward normal. Though this system is slow to act, being almost completely subjugated to the rapidly acting nervous system controls and the intermediately acting systems during the first few hours to days, nevertheless, there is compelling evidence that the renal body-fluid feedback system for control of arterial pressure becomes progressively more powerful with time, until its so-called "feedback gain" reaches infinity.[11] Therefore, over a period of many days to weeks or months one would expect this system to take over completely from all the other pressure control systems in the final determination of long-term level of arterial pressure. To explain this concept in more detail, and also to show the interrelationships between different ones of the pressure control systems, we will present, first, a quantitative analysis of arterial pressure control and then discuss specifically the importance of the infinite gain feedback concept that is applicable to the renal body-fluid feedback system for control of arterial pressure.

Systems Analysis of Arterial Pressure Control and Hypertension

Basic Feedback Control Loop of the Renal Body-Fluid–Arterial Pressure Control System

Figure 1 illustrates a control system diagram of the basic renal body-fluid–arterial pressure

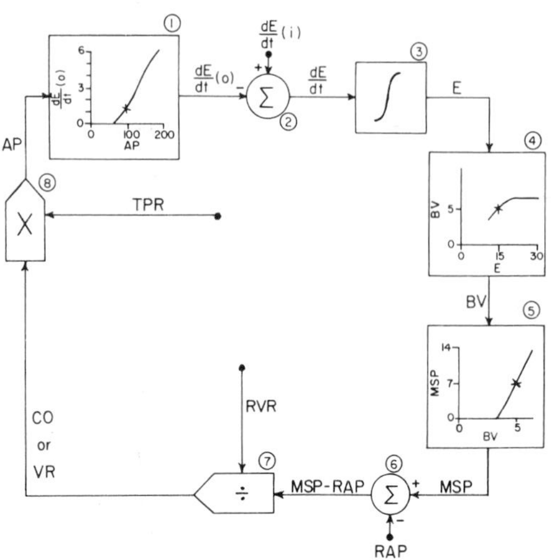

FIG. 1.—Basic system diagram for the renal body-fluid mechanism of arterial pressure control. (From Guyton, A. C., and Coleman, T. G.,[14] with permission.)

control system. The elements of this system are represented by the blocks numbered 1 through 8, and the respective blocks have the following meanings.

Block 1 shows the effect of arterial pressure (AP) on output of extracellular fluid (dE/dt(0)). Careful study of this block shows that at an arterial pressure of 100 mm Hg approximately 1 ml of urine is excreted by the kidneys each minute, and since urine has a water and electrolyte composition very similar to that of extracellular fluid, this represents approximately the rate of extracellular fluid loss from the body. Note, however, that increasing the arterial pressure from 100 to 200 mm Hg increases output of extracellular fluid about sixfold, while on the other hand, decreasing the arterial pressure to 60 mm Hg causes the output essentially to cease.

Block 2 summates the output of extracellular fluid plus the intake (dE/dt(i)). The output from this block (dE/dt) represents the rate of change of the extracellular fluid volume.

Block 3 represents integration of the rate of change of extracellular fluid volume, or, in other words, block 3 is an accumulator. The output from block 3 is the actual extracellular fluid volume (E) at any given time.

Block 4 shows the relationship between extracellular fluid volume and blood volume

(BV). This illustrates that at a normal extracellular fluid volume of 15 liters, the blood volume is approximately 5 liters. Increasing the extracellular fluid volume up to a value of about 22 liters increases the blood volume to about 7 liters. However, a further increase in extracellular fluid volume does not further increase blood volume because, at levels above 22 liters, essentially all of the excess fluid leaks rapidly into the interstitial spaces for reasons that have been explained in detail elsewhere;[12] basically, above 22 liters of extracellular fluid the interstitial fluid pressure rises above atmospheric pressure, and in the positive pressure range the compliance of the tissue spaces suddenly increases 25-fold or more.

Block 5 shows the effect of blood volume on mean systemic pressure (MSP) which is the filling pressure of the systemic circulation with blood. At a normal blood volume of 5 liters, the mean systemic pressure is approximately 7 mm Hg, and this falls to zero at a blood volume of about 3.5 liters or rises to double normal values at a blood volume of about 6.5 liters.

Block 6 calculates the pressure gradient for venous return (MSP − RAP). That is, the mean systemic pressure, which is the filling pressure of the peripheral circulation, tends to force blood toward the heart, while the right atrial pressure (RAP) tends to oppose blood return to the heart. It has been shown both mathematically and experimentally[13] that venous return is approximately proportional to the difference between these two values, which is called the pressure gradient for venous return.

Block 7 calculates venous return by dividing the pressure gradient for venous return by the resistance to venous return (RVR). The resistance to venous return is mainly the resistance in the veins, but resistances in all other segments of the circulation play lesser roles. The total resistance to venous return is an algebraic summation of all these, in accordance with definite mathematical laws that have been developed elsewhere.[13]

Block 8 calculates arterial pressure by multiplying venous return (VR) or cardiac output (CO) (which are equal to each other) times total peripheral resistance (TPR).

Significance of the Renal Body-Fluid Control Loop. Now let us see how the control loop in Figure 1 operates to control arterial pressure. First, assume that arterial pressure increases above the normal value. Block 1 shows that the output of extracellular fluid from the body would be increased to more than the person's intake of extracellular fluid. This excess output causes the rate of change of extracellular fluid volume (dE/dt) to become negative, and the output of block 3, extracellular fluid volume, continues to fall so long as dE/dt is less than zero. As a result, blood volume, mean systemic pressure, pressure gradient for venous return, venous return, cardiac output, and arterial pressure all also continue to fall. That is, all factors in the cycle continue to change until there is absolute balance between intake and output of extracellular fluid. When this state has been achieved, arterial pressure will be exactly back where it started. Note that the factor which determines when a new state of equilibrium will be achieved is the rate of change of extracellular fluid volume (dE/dt). So long as this is either negative or positive, all the factors in the circuit will be changing and will be causing dE/dt to reapproach the zero value. Once it has reached the zero value, a new steady state will have been achieved and will continue until some new abnormality appears somewhere in the circuit to throw the system out of balance.

However, the circuit of Figure 1 describes only one of the arterial pressure control mechanisms. Therefore, if one should attempt to use this circuit by itself to predict the effects of different factors on arterial pressure control, he would be likely to find predictions that are not true. For instance, this control loop, taken by itself, indicates that arterial pressure can never rise above normal without there also being simultaneous increases in cardiac output, mean systemic pressure, blood volume, and extracellular fluid volume. Since we know that none of these is *necessarily* increased when the arterial pressure increases, it is almost useless to use this control loop by itself to analyze the basic control of arterial pressure. Therefore, let us expand the basic system by adding still other control factors.

Effect of Reflexes, Heart Function, and Autoregulation on Circulatory Control

Figure 2 illustrates an expansion of Figure 1 showing addition of several other control fac-

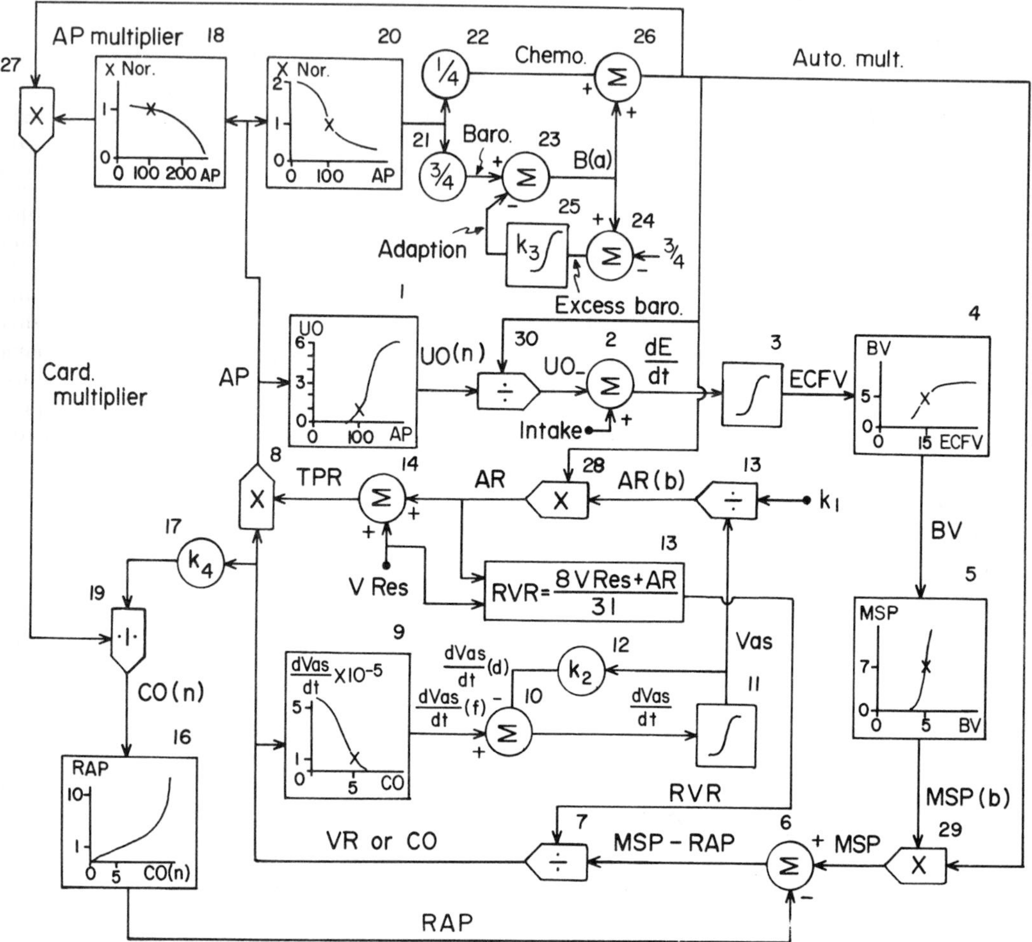

FIG. 2.—An expanded system diagram for control of arterial pressure, utilizing the basic renal body-fluid system of Figure 1 plus the roles of the heart, of the baroreceptor and chemoreceptor reflexes, and of autoregulation. (Modified from Guyton, A. C., and Coleman, T. G.,[14] with permission.)

tors to the circulatory model. A detailed discussion of these additions to the analysis has been presented previously[14] and will not be repeated here. However, the significance of these additions to the control circuit is essentially that mentioned below.

Since right atrial pressure is one of the determinants of venous return, it is important in any analysis of circulatory function to show how it is controlled. Basically, when excess load is applied to the heart, either in the form of excess blood flow entering the heart (blocks 16, 17, and 19) or in the form of too high a pressure load on the output side of the heart (blocks 16, 18, 19, and 27), blood begins to dam up in the right atrium, and the right atrial pressure begins to rise. The output of block 16 gives the resultant right atrial pressure.

Blocks 20 through 26 show that whenever the arterial pressure rises above normal, output from the baroreceptors increases, and output from the chemoreceptors decreases. Both of these effects, in turn, summate in the brain to decrease sympathetic activity and increase parasympathetic activity. Thus, the output of block 26, called the *autonomic multiplier,* represents these autonomic effects, and they in turn act at several points in the circuit to modify circulatory control, acting on heart function (blocks 16, 19, and 27), acting on arterial resistance, total peripheral resistance, and resistance to venous return (blocks 13, 14, and 28), acting on mean systemic pressure (block 29), and acting on renal output (block 30).

Finally, the phenomenon of autoregulation also plays a role in control of the circulation. When cardiac output increases above that required for tissue nutrition, the excess blood flow to the tissues causes progressive constriction of the peripheral blood vessels.[15] This, in turn, increases the arterial resistance and, as a result, increases both total peripheral resistance and resistance to venous return. These effects are illustrated in blocks 9 through 15.

Use of the Control System to Predict Arterial Pressure Control. Now that the additional controls have been added to the basic renal body-fluid mechanism for arterial pressure control, one can use the overall systems analysis of Figure 2 for at least some reasonably accurate predictions of arterial pressure control. Let us compare some actual experimental results with predictions from the systems analysis.

The left side of Figure 3 illustrates average effects on circulatory parameters occurring in six dogs during the onset of salt-loading hypertension as measured in previous studies.[16] In the initial portion of the experiment, 70 percent of the renal mass had already been removed 2 weeks previously by resecting both poles of one kidney plus the entire second kidney. Then salt and water were infused intravenously at a rate four times the animals' normal rates of intake. The effect of the extra water and salt was to increase the extracellular fluid volume and blood volume. Note in Figure 3 that the right atrial pressure, stroke volume, cardiac output, and arterial pressure all began to increase immediately while heart rate decreased. The total peripheral resistance also decreased for the first few days but then began to rise. As the total peripheral resistance rose, right atrial pressure, stroke volume, and cardiac output all decreased back toward normal, and heart rate rose back toward normal. However, arterial pressure remained elevated. Thus, as the steady state approached, essentially every factor returned near to normal except total peripheral resistance and arterial pressure, both of which were elevated.

Now, let us perform the same experiment on the computer using the systems analysis of Figure 2. The right side of Figure 3 illustrates the results from this computer simulation experiment showing exactly the same directional changes and nearly the same temporal and quantitative changes in all the different parameters. However, values are not exactly equivalent, illustrating that the analysis in Figure 2 is nearly complete enough, but not quite, to explain all events that take place in arterial pressure regulation under the conditions of this experiment.

Both the experimental results and the computer analysis demonstrate that retention of water and salt causes hypertension by first increasing cardiac output. The total peripheral resistance actually falls during the first few days but rises later. Consequently, one can come to the conclusion that the increase in total peripheral resistance in this type of hypertension is secondary to the increase in arterial pressure and is not the primary event that causes the rise in arterial pressure.[11,14,16,17] Another way of looking at these results is to state that the arterial pressure rises first and the total peripheral resistance then increases to cause a decrease in cardiac output. In other words, it is cardiac output that is affected by the total peripheral resistance and not arterial pressure. This concept will be borne out in more detail as we go more deeply into this quantitative analysis of arterial pressure regulation.

A Complex Systems Analysis for Arterial Pressure Regulation

Figure 4 illustrates still a much more complex analysis of circulatory function that can be used for analyzing arterial pressure regulation. It is impossible to explain this complex analysis here, but the reader can refer to a previous explanation of this diagram[18] if he cares to go more deeply into it. Figure 4 merely shows the different elements that have been considered in this overall analysis of circulatory function, including such fundamental circulatory factors as basic circulatory dynamics, autonomic control of the circulation, aldosterone control, angiotensin control, tissue fluids, electrolytes, kidney function, oxygen transport to the tissues, and others.

Significance of the Complex Analysis. Using the more complex analysis of Figure 4 to study arterial pressure control, one can begin to for-

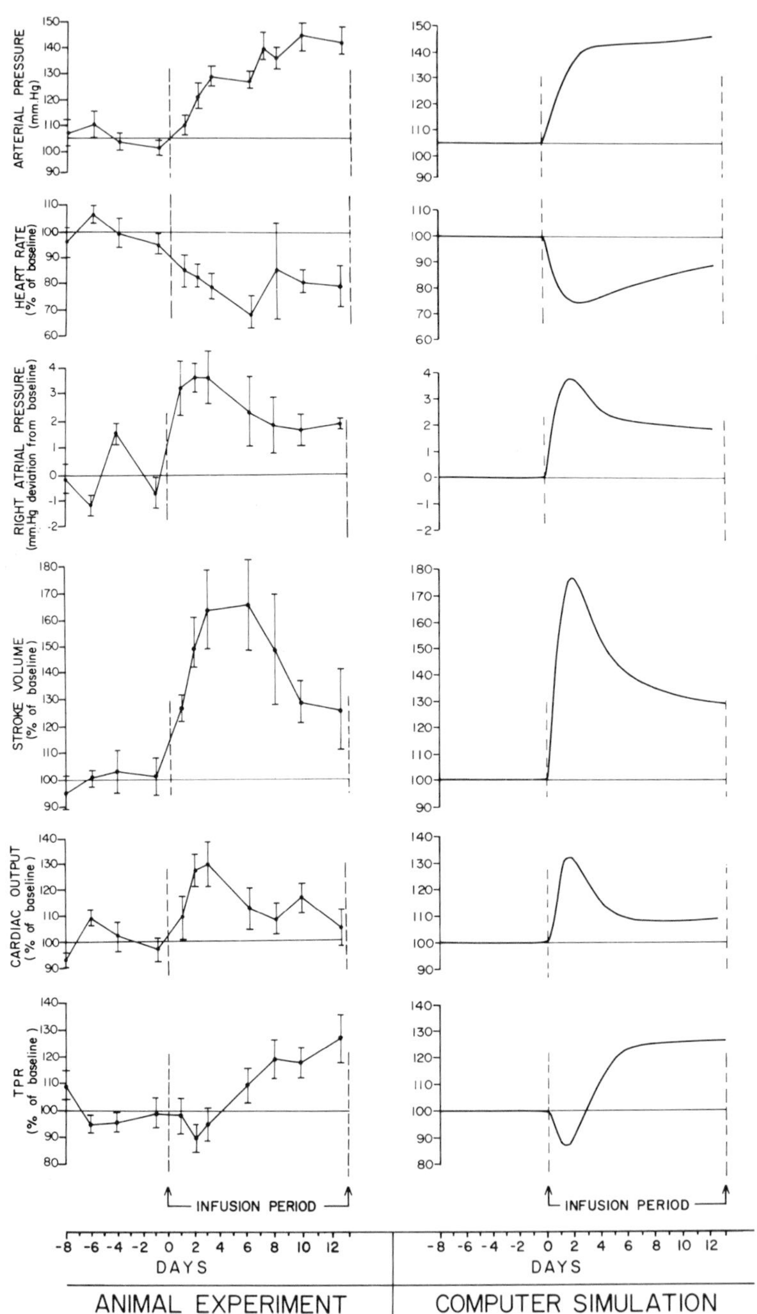

FIG. 3.—*Left,* Sequential changes in different parameters of circulatory function in a series of six dogs in which 70 percent of the renal mass had been removed and intravenous infusion of saline at a rate of 2 to 3 liters per day was given for 13 days.

Right, Computer simulation, using the systems analysis of Figure 2, of the same experiment as that seen on the *left* in dogs. Note that the changes in all of the parameters of circulatory function are essentially the same as those found in the animals. (Heart rate is calculated in the simulation to change in proportion to changes in the autonomic multiplier.)

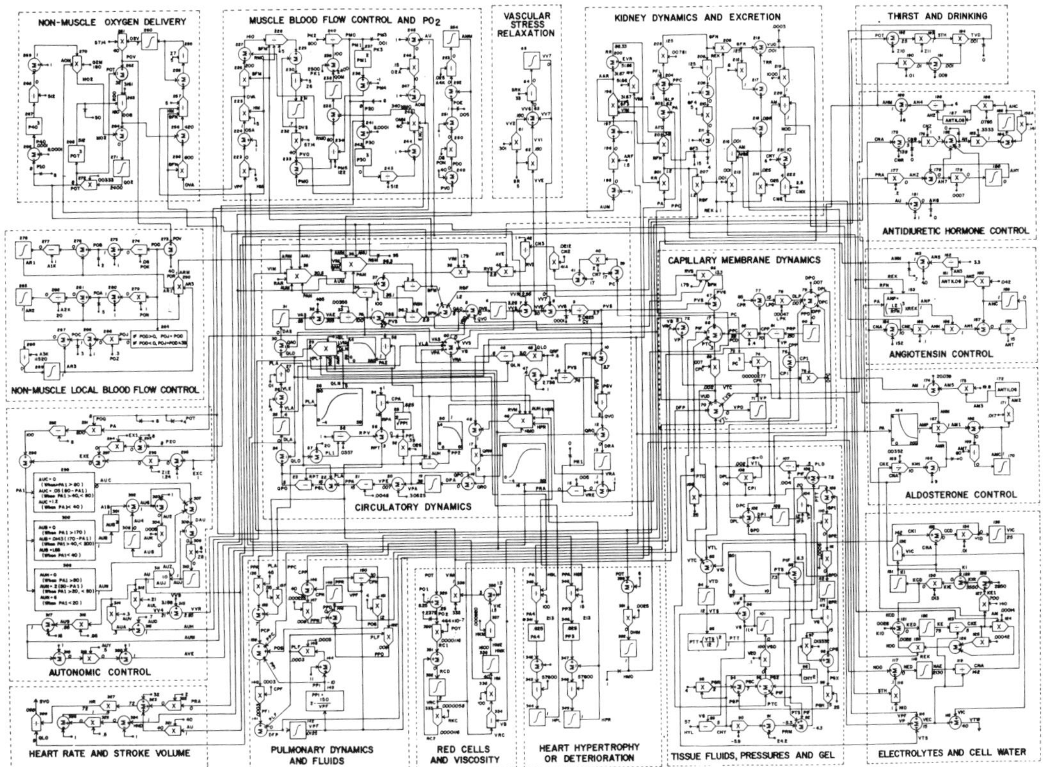

FIG. 4.—A complex analysis of circulatory function and of the roles of different circulatory control elements in the regulation of arterial pressure. (From Guyton, A. C., Coleman, T. G., and Granger, H. J.,[18] with permission.)

mulate the roles of still other factors besides those already considered in arterial pressure regulation, such as the roles of angiotensin, aldosterone, antidiuretic hormone, oxygen delivery to the tissues, effect of oxygen on local vascular resistance, hypertrophy of the heart, specific abnormalities of renal function, several separate types of nervous system reflex feedback responses, etc.

Figure 5 illustrates the effects that the computer predicts from the complex systems analysis in Goldblatt hypertension—i.e., in a human being with sudden renal artery constriction in both kidneys. Note the sequence of changes in extracellular fluid volume, blood volume, heart rate, total peripheral resistance, arterial pressure, angiotensin secretion, and urine output. These changes are almost exactly the same as those reported by Bianchi, Tenconi, and Lucca [19] for changes in circulatory dynamics following closure of Goldblatt clamps in dogs in which the clamps had been implanted previously so that it was not necessary to perform an operation to close the clamp. Indeed, the results in Figure 5 were computed in the exact form shown prior to referring to Bianchi's studies. Both the computer studies and those of Bianchi show the biphasic responses illustrated in some of the curves, such as in cardiac output and in total peripheral resistance. And both also show that, in the initial phases of Goldblatt hypertension, total peripheral resistance is increased markedly as a result of angiotensin secretion, while in the latter phases of Goldblatt hypertension, the arterial pressure is elevated primarily secondarily to body fluid changes. However, the continued secretion of angiotensin decreases the total capacitance of the circulatory system and increases the total peripheral resistance, these two effects causing less blood volume and less cardiac output in this type of hypertension in comparison with the salt-loading type of hypertension.

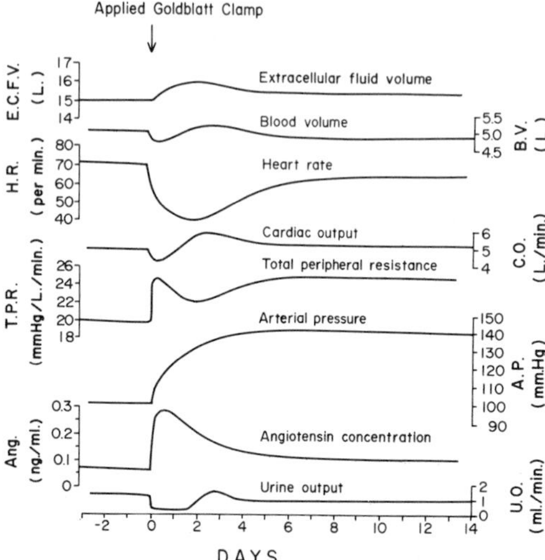

FIG. 5.—Computer simulation of Goldblatt hypertension, utilizing the complex analysis of Figure 4. *Left,* normal values and, following the **arrow,** the sequential effects caused by applying a Goldblatt clamp to each of the two kidneys in a hypothetical human being. (For this simulation, the section on angiotensin in Fig. 4 was expanded to provide additional detail.)

THE INFINITE GAIN OF THE RENAL BODY-FLUID FEEDBACK CONTROL SYSTEM

Though it has been necessary to develop the very complex systems analysis of Figure 4 so that we could determine with increasing precision how different arterial pressure control systems interact with each other, such an analysis is not necessary for a general understanding of the quantitative factors important in regulation of arterial pressure. Indeed, one small portion of the total analysis overrides all the remainder in determining the final level of arterial pressure regulation. This small portion, the balance between intake and output of fluid and electrolytes plus the effect of arterial pressure on renal output, is the basis of a so-called "infinite-gain" arterial pressure feedback system. For long-term control of arterial pressure, this infinite-gain system inundates the other pressure feedback controls. Therefore, this portion of the overall systems analysis deserves detailed comment in the following paragraphs.

The principle of infinite gain is discussed in more mathematical terms in the section entitled "Appendix." However, the significance of infinite gain is the following: The only arterial pressure control system that has been found to have infinite gain—defined as a control system capable of adjusting the pressure *all the way back to its control level*—is the renal body-fluid mechanism. Indeed, the maximum gain found for any of the other pressure control systems has been approximately 10 to 15,[3] which is the gain of the nervous system-induced pressure response caused by ischemia of the brain when the arterial pressure falls to 20 to 30 mm Hg. The usual baroreceptor system has a gain of approximately 7,[20] and the gain of the renin-angiotensin-vasoconstrictor system has been measured to be only 1.6.[4] Since all these mechanisms compete to control the arterial pressure, their relative values in overall control of pressure are determined by the ratios of their gains; and because the gain of the renal body-fluid system is infinite for long-term regulation of arterial pressure while all the others are finite, the relative ratios of the gain of the renal body-fluid system to the gains of all of the others is also infinity. This means simply that the renal body-fluid system does not merely dominate long-term arterial pressure regulation by a factor of 75, 80, or 90 percent but, instead, dominates it by a factor of 100 percent. Obviously, there are chances of error in being so completely positive about this 100-percent dominance, but thus far, in attempting for several years, both mathematically and in animal experiments, to find these chances of error, we still have not done so.[11,14,16,18]

Determinants of Long-term Arterial Pressure Control. Figure 6 illustrates the essential determinants of long-term arterial pressure control in all three of the analyses presented thus far (Figs. 1, 2, and 4). It shows in block 1 the effect of arterial pressure on renal output of water and electrolytes, which is actually output of extracellular fluid (dE/dt(0)). And block 2 illustrates the balance between *net* intake of water and electrolytes (dE/dt(i)), i.e., intake minus nonrenal output, and the renal output of water and electrolytes. The output of this block is the rate of change of extracellular fluid volume (dE/dt). In discussion of the simple systems analysis of Figure 1, it was pointed out that the renal body-fluid feedback system for control of arterial pressure always readjusts it-

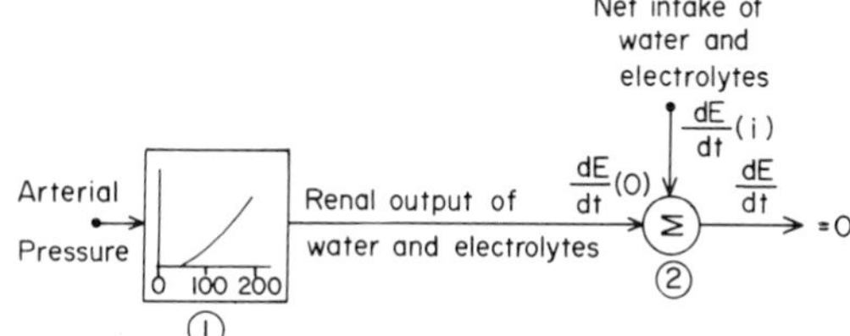

FIG. 6.—The basic determinants of long-term arterial pressure regulation. See the text for further information.

self to a steady state in which the rate of change of extracellular fluid volume (dE/dt) becomes zero. Therefore, if we simply set dE/dt to equal zero, as illustrated in Figure 6, we can then work backward from this point to denote those factors that determine arterial pressure.

One can see immediately that there are only two factors operative between the zero point in Figure 6 ($dE/dt = 0$) and arterial pressure. These are (*1*) the net intake of water and electrolytes (intake minus nonrenal output) and (*2*) the effect of arterial pressure on renal output of water and electrolytes. Obviously, these two elements can be broken down into subelements. However, on close analysis, one can also readily understand that the only factors that can affect the long-term level of arterial pressure are those factors that affect one of the above two elements.

Let us first discuss the net intake of water and electrolytes. This is determined by the intake of water and electrolytes in fluids or food minus the nonrenal loss of water and electrolytes such as in sweat, in insensible loss of water, in the feces, and in fluids lost in abnormal ways, i.e., from burns, expectoration, vomiting, dialysis, etc. Thus, these factors are limited and are easily understood; in any given human being they usually remain relatively constant. However, from one human being to another, one frequently finds markedly differing intakes of water and salt, which, therefore, are an important factor in arterial pressure determination.

The second set of factors affecting arterial pressure are those that alter the relationship between arterial pressure and renal output of water and electrolytes. In other words, essentially anything that can alter renal excretory function has the possibility of affecting the final control level of arterial pressure. Most of these factors are well known; some of these are:

1. Pathologic decrease in renal mass
2. Constriction of the renal arteries or afferent arterioles
3. Stimulation of the kidneys by aldosterone to increase salt and water reabsorption
4. Effect of angiotensin on renal function
5. Effect of sympathetic stimulation to cause decreased urinary output at any given arterial pressure
6. Effect of antidiuretic hormone to reduce urinary output
7. Effect of any other vasoconstrictor or vasodilator agent to decrease or increase urinary output of water and salt
8. Effect of increased venous pressure or increased intrarenal pressure to alter urinary output.

Thus, one finds it possible to delineate within a very narrow range those factors that can possibly increase or decrease the long-range level of arterial pressure. On the other hand, every single one of the factors illustrated in the complex systems analysis of Figure 4 can alter arterial pressure temporarily—for seconds, minutes, days, or even weeks at a time; but, in the long run, unless these factors have an effect on the kidneys to alter output of water and salt, or unless they in some other way alter the salt and water balance, they theoretically would play no role in the final determined level of arterial pressure.

Lack of Correlation of Arterial Pressure with Parameters of Circulatory Function. One of the most important results of the overall analysis of arterial pressure regulation is an understanding of the roles played by such important circulatory parameters as total peripheral resistance, cardiac output, and blood volume in the regulation of arterial pressure. None of these factors are represented between the arterial pressure point and the zero point in Figure 6. Therefore, none of them, from a mathematical point of view, are independent determinants of the final level at which the arterial pressure will stabilize in the steady state. However, they are all dependent variables in the system, which can be explained as follows: If ever the arterial pressure falls too low and the output of the kidneys becomes less than the net intake of fluid and electrolytes, then water and electrolytes are retained, thus increasing extracellular fluid volume. This also increases blood volume, cardiac output, and total peripheral resistance (the total peripheral resistance being increased because of excess flow through the tissues, which causes resultant local vascular constriction). All of these factors continue to increase until the arterial pressure rises to that value which causes equilibrium between output and net intake of water and salt. In other words, each of these factors is automatically adjusted to a new value in accordance with the dictates of the renal body-fluid feedback system.

Thus, one can see easily that it is only those effects illustrated in Figure 6 that are the determinants of the final level of arterial pressure, while other factors—total peripheral resistance, cardiac output, blood volume, and many others—are merely dependent variables in the system. Since they are variables they may or may not be correlated with arterial pressure.

An outstanding example of the lack of correlation between arterial pressure and the operators is the effects that occur when an arteriovenous fistula is opened or closed. Initial opening of an arteriovenous fistula decreases total peripheral resistance markedly and, therefore, decreases arterial pressure instantaneously. However, within seconds the arterial pressure returns most of the way back toward normal, and it returns entirely to normal within a day or two.[21] These effects are illustrated in the computer study shown in Figure 7, utilizing the complex systems analysis of Figure 4. Note that when the arteriovenous fistula was opened, the total peripheral resistance was reduced essentially to N/2. The cardiac output rose approximately 75 percent within seconds. After the almost instantaneous circulatory reflex readjustments, the arterial pressure was about 12 mm Hg below normal—not 50 mm Hg below normal as would be expected if arterial pressure correlated proportionately with total peripheral resistance. Urine output fell to a very low value, and during the ensuing day extracellular fluid volume increased, blood volume increased, and cardiac output rose to exactly 2N. This increase in cardiac output also returned the arterial pressure to its normal level. Yet, note that the dependent variables

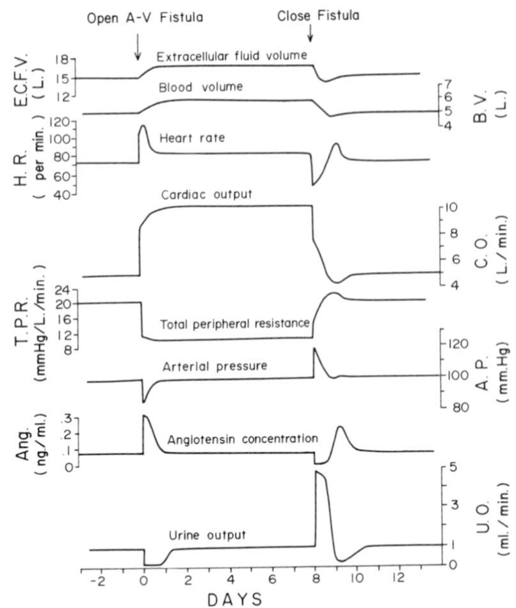

FIG. 7.—Computed effects, utilizing the complex systems analysis of Figure 4, that occur in the circulation when a large arteriovenous fistula is opened. *Left,* normal values recorded before the fistula was opened at zero days and closed at 8 days. Note that despite marked changes in total peripheral resistance, cardiac output, and other factors, the arterial pressure returned exactly to normal.

in the system—total peripheral resistance, cardiac output, heart rate, blood volume, and extracellular fluid volume—are all still very abnormal. Therefore, none of these factors correlates with arterial pressure.

Conversely, when the fistula was closed so that total peripheral resistance returned back toward normal, there was rapid loss of fluid from the body during the first day, and all of the same variables that had been abnormal the day previously returned within 2 days to exactly their normal levels. The initial effect on arterial pressure of closing the arteriovenous fistula, even though the total peripheral resistance was essentially doubled, was to raise the pressure only 15 percent (after the instantaneous reflex readjustments had occurred), but the pressure, too, returned precisely to normal within 2 days.

The events illustrated in Figure 7 have also been demonstrated in studies of arteriovenous fistulas in human beings [21] and animals.[22] The importance of these results is that arterial pressure is always regulated back to that level dictated by (*1*) the kidneys and (*2*) the net intake of water and salt. Since neither of these two effects is altered when an arteriovenous fistula is opened or closed, the arterial pressure, after an initial period of readjustment, returns precisely to its normal value. On the other hand, the dependent variables are altered drastically either upon opening or upon closing the fistula.

Summary

Though we have discussed both simple and complex quantitative analyses of arterial pressure regulation, the principal point of this chapter is that only a small portion of all the elements in the analyses is responsible for final determination of the long-term arterial pressure level. This portion is the relationship between arterial pressure and the body's balance of water and salt. Factors that can affect this balance are changes in intake of water and salt, changes in nonrenal output of water and salt, and changes in kidney function. The mathematical analyses show that only these factors are determinants of the long-term level of arterial pressure. On the other hand, such other factors as total peripheral resistance, cardiac output, blood volume, and extracellular fluid volume are dependent variables in the overall system. Therefore, they may or may not correlate with changes in arterial pressure, depending on the causes of the changes. Furthermore, they are adjusted upward or downward by the renal body-fluid feedback mechanism until the arterial pressure stabilizes at that level dictated by the determinant factors noted above.

The importance of this study is that it separates those factors that are truly determinants of long-term regulation of arterial pressure from those other factors—such as total peripheral resistance, cardiac output, blood volume, etc.—which play manipulative roles in making the arterial pressure go up or down but are not part of the determinative complex.

Appendix

The Infinite-Gain Principle Applied to Arterial Pressure Regulation. Earlier we pointed out that the renal body-fluid mechanism for control of arterial pressure will automatically adjust the outputs of water and salt to exactly equal their intakes, i.e., until the rate of change of extracellular fluid volume (dE/dt) becomes exactly equal to zero. In calculating the gain of a feedback system, one calculates the ratio of the original abnormality to the final abnormality. In the case of the renal body-fluid feedback mechanism for control of arterial pressure, the final abnormality is always exactly zero for the balance between intake and output of water and salts. Therefore, the rate of change of extracellular fluid volume, dE/dt, is controlled with infinite gain because it always returns in the steady state exactly back to its original value of zero. That is, any original abnormality, which is a finite value, divided by zero gives infinity.

Now, we can apply this same principle to the control of arterial pressure. If the intake of water and salt is constant, if the nonrenal output of water and salt is constant, and if the nonarterial, pressure-dependent, functional capabilities of the kidneys remain constant, the only factor that can then affect dE/dt is the arterial pressure. When dE/dt becomes adjusted to its steady-state value of zero, the arterial pressure will also have adjusted to a steady-state value. Now assume that the arterial pressure is decreased; dE/dt immediately becomes positive, and a cycle of events is initiated, as described in the explanation of Figure 1, which will eventually return arterial pressure exactly back to its original level, i.e., back to that level at which dE/dt becomes zero once again. Therefore, the original abnormality of arterial pressure is a finite value and the final abnormality is zero because the arterial pressure is returned exactly to the point from which it started. Here again, one finds a state of infinite gain. It should be realized, however, that arterial pressure is controlled with infinite gain only with the above three qualifications, namely, (*1*) constant intake of water and salt, (*2*) constant nonrenal output of water and salt, and (*3*) constant nonarterial, pressure-dependent, functional capabilities of the kidneys.

Note especially that dE/dt is controlled with infinite gain always. On the other hand, it is only after the above three conditions have been defined that arterial pressure is also controlled with infinite gain. Consequently, it is the definitions of the three qualifications above that are the determinants of the long-term level of arterial pressure.

References

1. Korner, P. I.: Integrative neural cardiovascular control. Physiol. Rev. 51:312, 1971.
2. Heymans, C., and Neil, E.: Reflexogenic Areas of the Cardiovascular System. Boston: Little, Brown, 1959.
3. Sagawa, K., Taylor, A. E., and Guyton, A. C.: Dynamic performance and stability of cerebral ischemic pressor response. Am. J. Physiol. 201:1164, 1961.
4. Cowley, A. W., Jr., Miller, J. P., and Guyton, A. C.: Open-loop analysis of the renin-angiotensin system in the dog. Circ. Res. 28: 568, 1971.
5. Guyton, A. C., and Crowell, J. W.: Cardiac deterioration in shock: I. Its progressive nature. Int. Anesthesiol. Clin. 2:159, 1964.
6. Guyton, A. C., Lindley, J. E., Touchstone, R. N., Smith, C. M., Jr., and Batson, H. M., Jr.: Effects of massive transfusion and hemorrhage on blood pressure and fluid shifts. Am. J. Physiol. 163:525, 1950.
7. Davis, J. O., Carpenter, C. C. J., Ayers, C. L., Holman, J. E., and Bahn, R. C.: Evidence for secretion of an aldosterone-stimulating hormone by the kidney. J. Clin. Invest. 40:684, 1961.
8. Selkurt, E. E.: Effects of pulse pressure and mean arterial pressure modification on renal hemodynamics and electrolyte and water excretion. Circulation 4:541, 1951.
9. Thurau, K., and Deetzen, P.: Die Diurese bei arteriellen Drucksteigerungen. Pfluegers Arch. 274:567, 1962.
10. Fourcade, J. C., Navar, L. G., and Guyton, A. C.: Possibility that angiotensin resulting from unilateral kidney disease affects contralateral renal function. Nephron 8:1, 1971.
11. Guyton, A. C., and Coleman, T. G.: A quantitative analysis of the pathophysiology of hypertension. Circ. Res. 24:1, 1969.
12. Guyton, A. C., Granger, H. J., and Taylor, A. E.: Interstitial fluid pressure. Physiol. Rev. 51:527, 1971.
13. Guyton, A. C.: Circulatory Physiology: Cardiac Output and Its Regulation. Philadelphia: Saunders, 1963.
14. Guyton, A. C., and Coleman, T. G.: Long-term regulation of the circulation: Interrelationships with body fluid volumes. *In* Reeve, B. and Guyton, A. C. (Eds.): Physical Bases of Circulatory Transport: Regulation and Exchange. Philadelphia: Saunders, 1967.
15. Granger, H. J., and Guyton, A. C. Autoregulation of the total systemic circulation following destruction of the central nervous system in the dog. Circ. Res. 25:379, 1969.
16. Coleman, T. G., and Guyton, A. C.: Hypertension caused by salt loading in the dog. III. Onset transients of cardiac output and other circulatory variables. Circ. Res. 25:153, 1969.
17. Ledingham, J. M., and Cohen, R. D.: Changes in the extracellular fluid volume and cardiac output during the development of experimental renal hypertension. Can. Med. Assoc. J. 90:292, 1964.
18. Guyton, A. C., Coleman, T. G., and Granger, H. J.: Circulation: Overall regulation. Ann. Rev. Physiol. 34:13, 1972.
19. Bianchi, G., Tenconi, L. T., and Lucca, R.: Effect in the conscious dog of constriction of the renal artery of the sole remaining kidney on the hemodynamics, sodium balance, body fluid volumes, plasma renin concentration and pressor responsiveness to angiotensin. Clin. Sci. 38:741, 1970.
20. Dobbs, W. A., Prather, J. W., and Guyton, A. C.: Relative importance of nervous control of cardiac output and arterial pressure. Am. J. Cardiol. 27:507, 1971.
21. Holman, E.: Arteriovenous aneurysm: Abnormal communication between arterial and venous circulations. New York: Macmillan, 1937.
22. Warren, J. V., Nickerson, J. L., and Elkin, D. C.: The cardiac output in patients with arteriovenous fistulas. J. Clin. Invest. 30:210. 1951.

Regional Blood Flow in Essential Hypertension

By Jan Brod, M.D., Sc.D.

FOR MANY YEARS it had been well accepted that, in essential hypertension, heart rate, stroke volume, and cardiac output were not different from normal. This led to the conclusion that the basic hemodynamic disturbance was in the raised total peripheral vascular resistance.

In 1936, Prinzmetal and Wilson [1] studied the blood flow through the upper extremities by occlusion plethysmography in essential hypertension. They found that the blood flow did not differ from normal and concluded that the increased vascular resistance was distributed regularly all over the circulation. In that study, however, the hand, with its different vascular reactivity, had been included in the plethysmograph; the possibility, therefore, could not be excluded that blood flows in different areas were different and compensated for each other when total vascular resistance was estimated.

For this reason, in 1942 Abramson and Fierst [2] excluded the hand from their study of the circulation of the upper extremities and reported a marked increase in blood flow through the forearm of hypertensive patients. The same findings were reported for the leg. In addition, the studies of Goldring et al.,[3] Smith et al.,[4,5] and of Brod [6] established that in the early stages of essential hypertension, renal plasma flow may be decreased. These contrasting findings supported the conclusion that changes in vascular resistances and in distribution of cardiac output in essential hypertension were different in different parts of the circulation.

The studies of Hejl in 1957 [7] and those of Brod and his co-workers in 1962 [8] introduced a different concept of the basic hemodynamics of essential hypertension. The calculated total peripheral resistance was found to cover a wide range of values, from low normal to markedly elevated. The hemodynamic pattern of high cardiac output (with a statistically demonstrable rise in heart rate) and a normal peripheral vascular resistance was first recognized in juvenile hypertensive patients. These subjects probably represented the early stages of essential hypertension. This characteristic hemodynamic pattern was subsequently confirmed by several laboratories.[9-14] (See chapter entitled "Hemodynamic Alterations in Essential Hypertension.")

It should not be concluded, however, that a total peripheral vascular resistance within the normal range represents a normal state of the peripheral vascular bed. The increase in mean arterial pressure in these juvenile hypertensive patients is the result of a vascular bed that fails to adjust when the high cardiac output is ejected into it.

Figure 1 correlates the total peripheral vascular resistance with renal vascular resistance in normotensive subjects and in patients with essential hypertension. At any level of total peripheral vascular resistance, the values of renal vascular resistance in essential hypertension are above those of the normotensive subjects. This demonstrates a state of vasoconstriction of the renal circulation in essential hypertension.

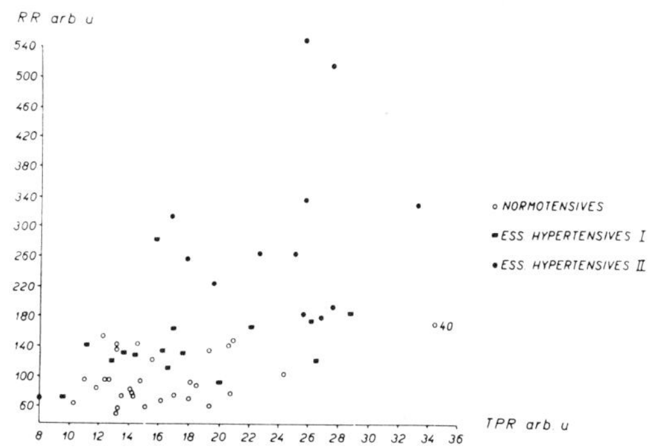

Fig. 1.—Correlation of total peripheral vascular resistance and renal vascular resistance, in normotensive subjects and in subjects with essential hypertension. **TPR**, total peripheral resistance; **RR**, renal vascular resistance; **arb.u.**, arbitrary resistance units.

From the Abteilung für Nephrologie, Krankenhaus Oststadt, Hannover, Germany.

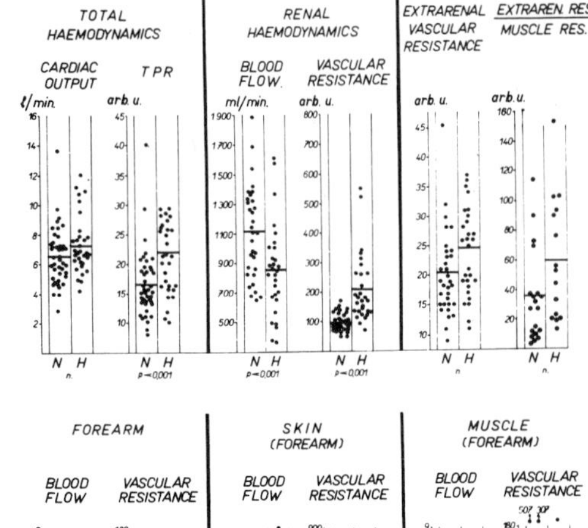

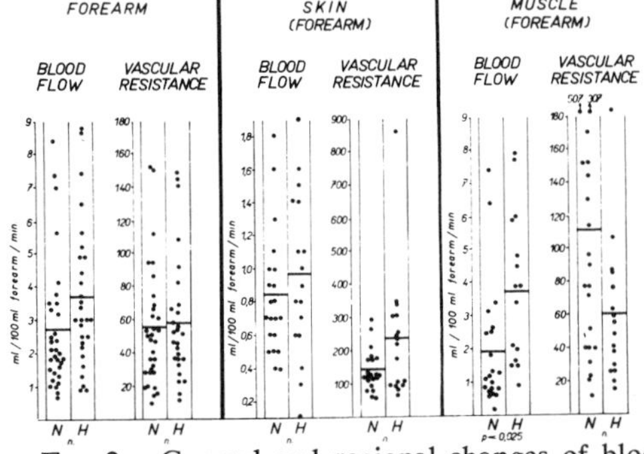

FIG. 2.—General and regional changes of blood flow and vascular resistance in normotensive subjects (**N**) and patients with essential hypertension (**H**). **TPR,** total peripheral vascular resistance; **arb. u.,** arbitrary units.

The normalization of the decreased renal blood flow by the administration of pyrogens [5] or hypnotics [15] and a decrease of the elevated renal vascular resistance during sleep [16] suggests that the high renal vascular resistance of essential hypertension is, at least in part, of a functional nature.

Cerebral blood flow,[17] splanchnic blood flow,[18] and skin blood flow [19,20] have been found to be normal in patients with essential hypertension. In the presence of an increased pressure, vascular resistance, therefore, is elevated in these areas of the circulation.

In contrast, the studies of Abramson and Fierst [2] had demonstrated a higher than normal blood flow through forearm and leg in a mixed group of hypertensive patients. Brod and his co-workers in 1962 demonstrated that this was not a passive consequence of the high perfusion pressure but a true decrease of vascular tone in the muscle.[8]

Coronary blood flow is reported to be increased in essential hypertension. When expressed per 100 gm of heart, however, the coronary blood flow is within the limits of normal. For this reason, Bing interpreted the high values of coronary flow in essential hypertension to be the result of left ventricular hypertrophy.[21] The early occurrence of atherosclerotic changes in the coronary arteries of hypertensive patients may result in severe increase in coronary vascular resistance.[22]

These studies suggest that from the early stages of essential hypertension, the vascular resistances in different regions of the body are different from both a qualitative and a quantitative standpoint. Figure 2 summarizes the results of our studies in 1960 and 1962.[8,23] The following parameters were measured simultaneously: cardiac output (dye-dilution method), intra-arterial pressure (brachial artery), renal blood flow (clearance of para-aminohippurate), muscle blood flow (occlusion plethysmography). In addition, splanchnic vascular resistance was estimated from the ratio, extrarenal vascular resistance:muscle vascular resistance. It is evident from Figure 2 that the scatter of values of cardiac output and total peripheral vascular resistance is greater in hypertensive than in normotensive subjects. Although the mean cardiac output in hypertensives is not significantly different from controls, it is noteworthy that some of the highest resting cardiac outputs were recorded in the hypertensive patients. Their corresponding total peripheral resistance values were in the lowest range. The hemodynamic changes in the individual regional vascular beds are more uniform. In essential hypertension, renal, skin, and splanchnic vascular beds are in a state of constriction while the vascular bed of the skeletal muscles is in a state of relaxation.

Total peripheral vascular resistance is, of course, the result of a balance of the vascular resistances in the individual regions. When total peripheral resistance is normal or even low in early essential hypertension, it is suggested that the vasoconstriction of the kidneys, skin, and splanchnic region is well compensated for by a vasodilation in the muscles. With the duration of the disease, the total peripheral vascular resistance of essential hypertensives starts to rise because of further increase in resistance in the renal vascular bed and in other constricted areas. This is due, in part, to the development of vascular sclerotic changes, but also, in part, to the adaptation phenomenon of the arteriolar wall described by Folkow, Grimby, and Thulesius.[24] According to this interpretation, the vascular wall responds to functional overload with an increase in the wall/lumen ratio. At this point, the elevated cardiac output starts to return to normal.

Caliva, Napodano, and Lyons [25] and Walsh, Hyman, and Maronde [26] found the capacitance vessels in early essential hypertension in a state of constriction. The diminished venous distensibility may be one factor in the mechanism of increased cardiac output in young hypertensive patients.

From a pathophysiologic standpoint, only factors producing these described hemodynamic changes may be considered possible causes of essential hypertension. The hemodynamic effect of angiotensin, suspected for many years as a possible cause of essential hypertension, is a redistribution of cardiac output in favor of the muscles.[27] Angiotensin also reduces the venous distensibility.[28,29] However, it regularly decreases cardiac output and heart rate and elevates total peripheral resistance. Angiotensin, therefore, has not been demonstrated to produce the hemodynamic changes of early essential hypertension: increase in cardiac output, increase in heart rate, and normal total peripheral vascular resistance.

The hemodynamic effects of norepinephrine are qualitatively similar to the ones produced by angiotensin.[27] A pathophysiologic role of norepinephrine in essential hypertension is, therefore, difficult to accept.

In contrast, the hemodynamic pattern of essential hypertension is entirely similar to the acute hemodynamic changes induced by emotional stress in man. These human hemodynamic responses are mediated by the same mechanism as the defense reaction in dogs and cats.[30]

Figure 3 summarizes the acute hemodynamic changes induced in man by emotional (mental arithmetic) and cold stimuli. Similarly to what is observed in essential hypertension, with emotional or cold stimuli, the cardiac output may increase, remain unchanged, or even decrease, while total peripheral resistance falls, remains unchanged, or increases. However, the increase in blood pressure speaks in favor of a vascular bed that is unyielding to a given cardiac output. The cardiac output is distributed exactly the same way as in essential hypertension, with a shift of blood from the kidneys, viscera, and

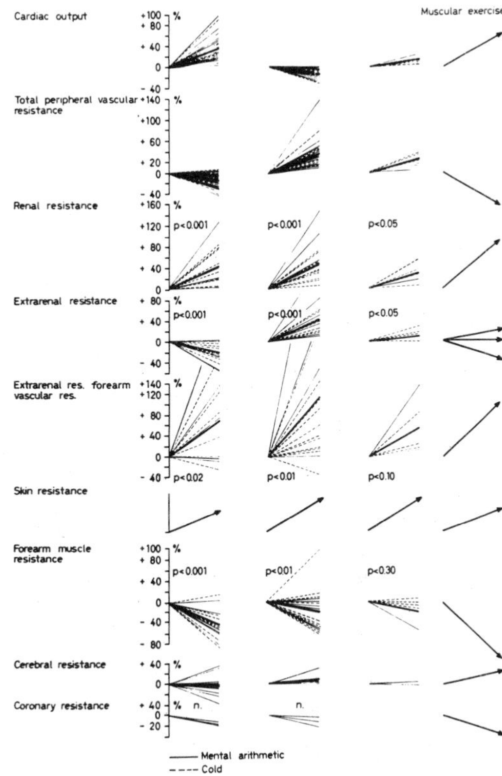

FIG. 3.—Summary of the changes of the cardiac output, total peripheral vascular resistance, and regional hemodynamics following emotional (mental arithmetic) and cold-pressor stimuli. Every **dashed line** is the result in one subject. **Thick full lines** indicate the average change. The data are divided arbitrarily into three columns according to the mutual behavior of the cardiac output and total peripheral vascular resistance. The regional changes are, however, analogous in all three columns. The vascular resistances are calculated as ratios: mean blood pressure:flow. The ratio, extrarenal vascular resistance:muscular resistance, is an indicator of the behavior of the splanchnic vascular bed, which, apart from muscles, represents the largest extrarenal vascular region. The **arrows** in the line of skin resistance indicate the result of an investigation on a separate group of subjects. On the *right,* the **arrows** indicate hemodynamic changes during muscular exercise, which are analogous to those during the pressor reactions. (From Brod et al.,[31] with permission.)

skin to the skeletal muscles.[31] Similarly, the venous bed becomes less distensible.[32] Unlike angiotensin or other pressor agents, stimulation of the hypothalamic defense area appears to suppress the vagal cardioinhibitory mechanism.

Stimulation of the hypothalamic defense area in the cat results in a rise in blood pressure and vasodilatation of the muscle. This vasodilatation is mediated in part by the sympathetic cholinergic fibers,[33,34] and in part by circulating epinephrine.[35] For a final demonstration that an unregulated defense reaction is involved in the pathophysiology of the early stage of essential hypertension, it will be necessary to demonstrate that the decreased vascular tone in the skeletal muscle is mediated by cholinergic sympathetic fibers and by circulating epinephrine. This is our next step in the investigation of this problem.

REFERENCES

1. Prinzmetal, M., and Wilson, C.: The nature of the peripheral resistance in arterial hypertension with special reference to the vasomotor system. J. Clin. Invest. 15:63, 1936.
2. Abramson, D. I., and Fierst, S. M.: Resting blood flow and peripheral vascular responses in hypertensive subjects. Am. Heart J. 23:84, 1942.
3. Goldring, W., Chasis, H., Ranges, H. A., and Smith, H. W.: Effective renal blood flow in subjects with essential hypertension. J. Clin. Invest. 20:637, 1941.
4. Smith, H. W., Goldring, W., Chasis, H., and Ranges, H. A.: Observations on the effective renal blood flow and functional excretory mass in man, with special reference to essential hypertension. Am. J. Physiol. 123:189, 1938.
5. Smith, H. W., Goldring, W., and Chasis, H.: Role of the kidney in the genesis of hypertension. Bull. N. Y. Acad. Med. 19:449, 1943.
6. Brod, J.: Klinická Fysiologie a Pathologie Ledvin. (Clinical Physiology and Pathology of the Kidneys.) Prague: Spol. čes. lek., 1949.
7. Hejl, Z.: Changes in cardiac output and peripheral resistance during simple stimuli influencing blood pressure. Cardiologia 31:375, 1957.
8. Brod, J., Fencl, V., Hejl, Z., Jirka, J., and Ulrych, M.: General and regional hemodynamic pattern underlying essential hypertension. Clin. Sci. 23:339, 1962.
9. Finkielman, S., Worcel, M., and Agrest, A.: Hemodynamic patterns in essential hypertension. Circulation 31:356, 1965.
10. Widimský, J., Fejfarová, M., Exnerová, M., Dejdar, R., and Pirk, F.: Juvenilní hypertense (Juvenile hypertension). Thomayerova sbírka, 358. Prague: State Medical Publishing House.
11. Sannerstedt, R.: Hemodynamic response to exercise in patients with arterial hypertension. Acta Med. Scand. 180 (Suppl. 458):1, 1966.
12. Eich, R. R., Cuddy, R. R., Smulyan, H., and Lyons, R. H.: Hemodynamics in labile hypertension. A follow-up study. Circulation 34: 299, 1966.
13. Bello, C. T., Sewy, R. W., Harakal, C., and Hillyer, P. N.: Relationship between clinical severity of disease and hemodynamic patterns in essential hypertension. Am. J. Med. Sci. 253:194, 1967.
14. Julius, S., and Conway, S.: Hemodynamic studies in patients with borderline blood pressure elevation. Circulation 38:282, 1968.
15. Ratner, N. A.: O roli počečnogo faktora v patogeneze gipertoni: Vestn. Akad. Nauk SSSR 10:39, 1958.
16. Brod, J., and Fencl, V.: Diurnal variation of systemic and renal hemodynamics in normal subjects and in hypertensive disease. Cardiologia 31:494, 1957.
17. Kety, S. S., Hafkenschiel, J. H., Jeffers, W. A., Leopold, I. H., and Shenkin, H. A.: The blood flow, vascular resistance, and oxygen consumption of the brain in essential hypertension. J. Clin. Invest. 27:511, 1948.
18. Culbertson, J. W., Wilkins, R. W., Ingelfinger, F. J., and Bradley, S. E.: The effect of the upright posture upon hepatic blood flow in normotensive and hypertensive subjects. J. Clin. Invest. 30:305, 1951.
19. Pickering, G. W.: The peripheral resistance in persistent arterial hypertension. Clin. Sci. 2:209, 1936.
20. Stewart, H. J., Evans, W. F., Haskell, H. S., and Brown, H.: The peripheral blood flow and skin temperatures in hypertension. Am. Heart J. 31:617, 1946.
21. Bing, R. J.: The coronary circulation in health and disease as studied by coronary sinus catheterization. Bull. N.Y. Acad. Med. 27: 407, 1951.
22. Ganz, V.: Unpublished results, 1966.
23. Brod, J.: Essential hypertension. Hemodynamic observations with a bearing on its pathogenesis. Lancet 1:733, 1960.
24. Folkow, B., Grimby, G., and Thulesius, O.: Adaptive structural changes of the vascular

walls in hypertension and their relation to the control of the peripheral resistance. Acta Physiol. Scand. 44:255, 1958.

25. Caliva, F. S., Napodano, R. M., and Lyons, R. H.: Digital hemodynamics in the normotensive and hypertensive states. Circulation 28:261, 1963.

26. Walsh, S. A., Hyman, C., and Maronde, R. F.: Venous distensibility in essential hypertension. Cardiovasc. Res. 3:338, 1969.

27. Brod, J., Hejl, Z., Hornych, A., Jirka, J., Šlechta, V., and Buríanová, B.: Comparison of the haemodynamic effects of equipressor doses of intravenous angiotensin and noradrenaline in man. Clin. Sci. 36:161, 1969.

28. dePasquale, N. P., and Burch, G. E.: Effect of angiotensin II on the intact forearm veins of man. Circ. Res. 13:239, 1963.

29. Finnerty, F. A.: Hemodynamics of angiotensin in man. Circulation 25:255, 1962.

30. Brod, J.: Haemodynamic basis of acute pressor reactions and hypertension. Br. Med. J. 25:227, 1963.

31. Brod, J., Fencl, V., Hejl, Z., and Jirka, J.: Circulatory changes underlying blood pressure elevation during acute emotional stress (mental arithmetic) in normotensive and hypertensive subjects. Clin. Sci. 23:339, 1959.

32. Brod, J., Pirerovsky, I., Ulrych, M., and Linhart, J.: Effect of emotional stress (mental arithmetic) on venous circulation. Meeting of Int. Soc. of Hypertension, Oxford, 1970.

33. Eliasson, S., Lindgren, P., and Uvnas, B.: Representation in hypothalamus and the motor cortex in the dog of the sympathetic vasodilator outflow to the skeletal muscles. Acta Physiol. Scand. 27:18, 1952.

34. Barcroft, H., Brod, J., Hejl, Z., Hirsjarvi, E. A., and Kitchin, A. H.: The mechanism of the vasodilatation in the forearm muscle during stress (mental arithmetic). Clin. Sci. 19:4, 1960.

35. Konzett, H., Strieder, N., and Ziegler, E.: Die Wirkung eines Beta-Rezeptorenblockers auf emotionell bedingte Kreislaufreaktionen, insbesondere auf die Durchblutung des Unterarmes. Wien. Klin. Wochenschr. 80:953, 1968.

Hemodynamic Alterations in Essential Hypertension

By Per Lund-Johansen, M.D.

When the hemodynamic alterations in essential hypertension were discussed by Peterson [1] at the second Hahnemann Symposium on Hypertension 10 years ago, he stated that if the behavior of the various parts of the circulatory system were well understood, it would probably be possible to describe hemodynamics with one page of equations. If anybody had hoped that this would be done by Peterson's successor on that chapter at the next symposium a decade later, they will be very disappointed.

Instead, I will briefly review the most important findings in the hemodynamic studies performed in subjects with essential hypertension during the last decade.

The Heart in Early Essential Hypertension

Until 1960 most studies on the hemodynamics in essential hypertension were done by heart catheterization and included usually small groups of subjects, mainly with established hypertension of long duration. The common finding was that the elevated systemic blood pressure was caused by an increased total peripheral resistance, while the cardiac output was normal so long as heart failure was not present.[2–5] From a pathogenetic point of view, the heart was not of much interest.

However, not all subjects with essential hypertension had an increased total peripheral resistance at rest. In some, mainly younger subjects, the increased pressure was maintained by an increased cardiac output while the calculated total peripheral resistance was normal.[4,6] Furthermore, observations in experimental renal hypertension in rats suggested that, in the starting phase of the hypertensive process, the cardiac output might be elevated and the total peripheral resistance normal, but this increased later as a secondary phenomenon.[7,8]

From Medical Department A, University of Bergen School of Medicine, Bergen, Norway.

These ideas contributed to renewed interest in hemodynamics in essential hypertension. New percutaneous techniques made studies of central hemodynamics more simple, and during the last decade several studies from many parts of the world have appeared (Argentine,[9] the United States,[10–17] the USSR,[18] Norway,[19] Sweden,[20] France,[21] Czechoslovakia,[22] Holland,[23] and Japan [24]). These studies have shown that the hemodynamic alterations in essential hypertension show a varied picture with regard to the mechanism responsible for the pressure elevation. The alterations are clearly dependent upon the stage of the disease and the age of the subject.

I will first discuss the findings in what is supposed to be early essential hypertension. It is of course difficult to find subjects with well-documented essential hypertension of very short duration. Most investigators have studied young subjects with mild pressure elevation without complications (WHO stage I)[25] and compared them with age-matched controls and with older hypertensive subjects in whom the hypertension was known or supposed to have lasted longer.

At rest, in the supine position, most investigators have found that in subjects below the age of 40, with a mean arterial pressure around 100 to 110 at the time of study, the cardiac index is significantly higher than in controls.[10,13,15,19,20,21,24,26] Table 1 summarizes recent data from various parts of the world.[10,15,21,26] The similarity between the control values should be noted. In all these studies the hypertensive groups have a high cardiac output and a calculated total peripheral resistance not significantly different from controls. Individual variations are, however, great. Studies at rest performed in the sitting position in young subjects with mild hypertension have also revealed a high cardiac index,[19,20] but in a similar study in subjects with borderline hypertension, who had high cardiac index in the supine position,

TABLE 1.—*Mean Values for Cardiac Index (CI), Mean Arterial Blood Pressure (MAP), Total Peripheral Resistance Index (TPRI), Heart Rate (HR) and Stroke Index (SI) in Subjects with Labile or Mild Essential Hypertension in the Supine Position at Rest* *

Author(s), Year, Country	*n*	*MAP (mm Hg)*	*CI (liters per minute per* m^2*)*	*TPRI (dyn per second per* cm^{-5} m^2*)*	*HR (beats per minute)*	*SI (milliliters per stroke per* m^2*)*
Bello, Sevy, and Harakal [10] 1965, United States	11	108 (91)	4.10 (3.29)	2107 (2212)	81 (74)	51 (44)
Frohlich, Tarazi, and Dustan 1969, United States	9	106 (93)	3.53 (3.05)	2402 (2439)	77 (68)	46 (45)
Safar et al.[21] 1970, France	23	105 (86)	4.09 (3.15)	2099 (2221)	80 (72)	51 (44)
Julius et al.[26] 1971, United States	77	100 (83)	3.79 (3.31)	2216 (2088)	76 (67)	50 (50)
Lund-Johansen 1971, Norway	25	102 (84)	4.14 (3.45)	1971 (1948)	75 (63)	56 (55)

* Mean values for control groups are in parentheses.

the cardiac index became normal in the sitting position.[16]

Most investigators have found that the high resting cardiac output is due to an increase in heart rate.[13,19,20,26] Only one large study reports a normal heart rate and a very marked increase in stroke index.[9] These subjects were older and had considerably higher pressure than the subjects in the other series. In two studies both stroke volume and heart rate were increased.[10,21]

The high resting cardiac index in subjects with suggested early essential hypertension needs some comment. The cardiac index is high when compared with age-matched controls or older subjects with more advanced hypertension. However, the cardiac output in relation to oxygen consumption is normal. This is demonstrated in the study by Julius and Conway [16] and was also found by Sannerstedt [20] and Lund-Johansen.[19] This clearly separates the circulatory system in mild essential hypertension from the circulation in the hyperkinetic heart syndrome described by Gorlin [27] where a low arteriovenous oxygen difference is common. In this syndrome a true luxury perfusion takes place but this is not present in early essential hypertension where the arteriovenous oxygen difference is normal.[19,20]

The mechanisms behind the high cardiac output, high heart rate, and increased oxygen consumption in subjects with mild or labile essential hypertension are unknown. No clinical or biochemical findings suggesting a thyrotoxic state have been demonstrated.[19,20]

An increased activity in the sympathetic nervous system has been discussed but to my knowledge definite proof for this is still lacking.

An increased responsiveness of the beta-receptors in the heart has been suggested.[28] The effect of beta-blockade with propranolol in subjects with borderline hypertension has been studied.[28] The heart rate remained elevated after blockade and the authors conclude that the elevation of heart rate is not mediated through the beta-adrenergic system and may result from decreased parasympathetic inhibition or from different intrinsic myocardial pacing.

The role of parasympathetic inhibition in the hyperkinetic type of borderline hypertension has been studied recently.[29] After atropine administration, the difference in cardiac output and heart rate disappeared. However, the subjects responded to propranolol with a decrease in heart rate, and the authors conclude that patients with borderline hypertension and hyperkinetic circulation simultaneously exhibit an increase of sympathetic and decrease of parasympathetic tone.

Studies of the circulatory system in such subjects during sleep could perhaps unveil a possible effect of nervousness alone. While studies during sleep in established hypertension have been published,[30,31] it has not been possible to find such data in early hypertension.

Thus, it might be concluded that the heart pump in what is supposed to be early essential hypertension is hyperkinetic compared to normal controls but not in relation to metabolic demands. The heart rate is increased. The mechanisms behind these disturbances are still unknown but an imbalance between the sympathetic and parasympathetic tone probably plays a role.

Total Peripheral Resistance in Early Essential Hypertension

One may ask if the total peripheral resistance really is normal in early essential hypertension even though it does appear so from most studies at rest. It of course may be argued that if the total peripheral resistance were normal, the resistance vessels should have adapted to the high cardiac output with dilatation, thus keeping the blood pressure normal.

These considerations will become more clear if the circulatory system is studied under conditions which greatly increase blood flow, such as during muscular exercise. To avoid excessive rise in blood pressure, the resistance vessels must then dilate at least in some parts of the body.[12,16,17,19,20]

Because of differences in methods, it is difficult to compare data from the various studies during muscular exercise directly. I will therefore elucidate the changes in the hemodynamics by personal data. Table 2 shows the age distribution of hypertensives and controls, studied in our laboratory since 1964. All but four of the subjects below 50 years belong to WHO stage I (no complications). In the age group 50 to 59 years, 14 were in stage I and 11 in stage II (signs of cardiovascular hypertrophy). The subjects were studied during steady-state exercise on an ergometer bicycle at 300-, 600-, and 900-kpm per minute loads.[19] The habitual physical activity in hypertensives and controls did not differ. All were previously untreated and actively working at the time of the study. The results from the two youngest age groups

Table 2.—*Age Distribution in Subjects Studied Hemodynamically at Rest and During Exercise*

Age group (in years)	*Normotensive controls*	*Hypertensives*		*Total of Groups A and B*
		Group A	*Group B*	
17–29	11	19	16	35
30–39	11	17	12	29
40–49	11	25	23	48
50–59	0	7	18	25
Total				

Hypertensive group A data published in 1967,[19] group B subjects studied later.

showed that in transition from rest to exercise, the cardiac index, heart rate, stroke volume, and mean arterial pressure increased both in hypertensives and controls, as seen in Figure 1. During muscular exercise the cardiac index was no longer higher than in controls in any age group but tended to be lower. The heart rate remained increased but the stroke volume was significantly reduced in all ages. It is possible that this difference in stroke volume represents the first sign of incipient cardiac insufficiency in hypertension.[32] The total peripheral resistance was now clearly increased also in the youngest group (Fig. 1). This was present already at the lowest work level, 300 kpm per minute. In other words, as soon as the mild hypertensive subject performs even moderate muscular exercise, the circulatory system is changed from a high output and a normal resistance pattern to a normal or subnormal output and high resistance pattern. The rise in blood pressure in these patients during exercise was similar to the rise in the controls when related to oxygen consumption. When compared to the blood flow (Fig. 1), the rise was steeper than in the controls; the steepest rise was seen in the oldest group. This was reflected in the calculated total peripheral resistance (Fig. 1).

Most of these findings have been made in exercise studies on ergometer bicycle by other groups.[12,20] In a study on treadmill in young subjects with labile essential hypertension,[17] an impaired cardiac pump function was found only at maximal work level in a few of the

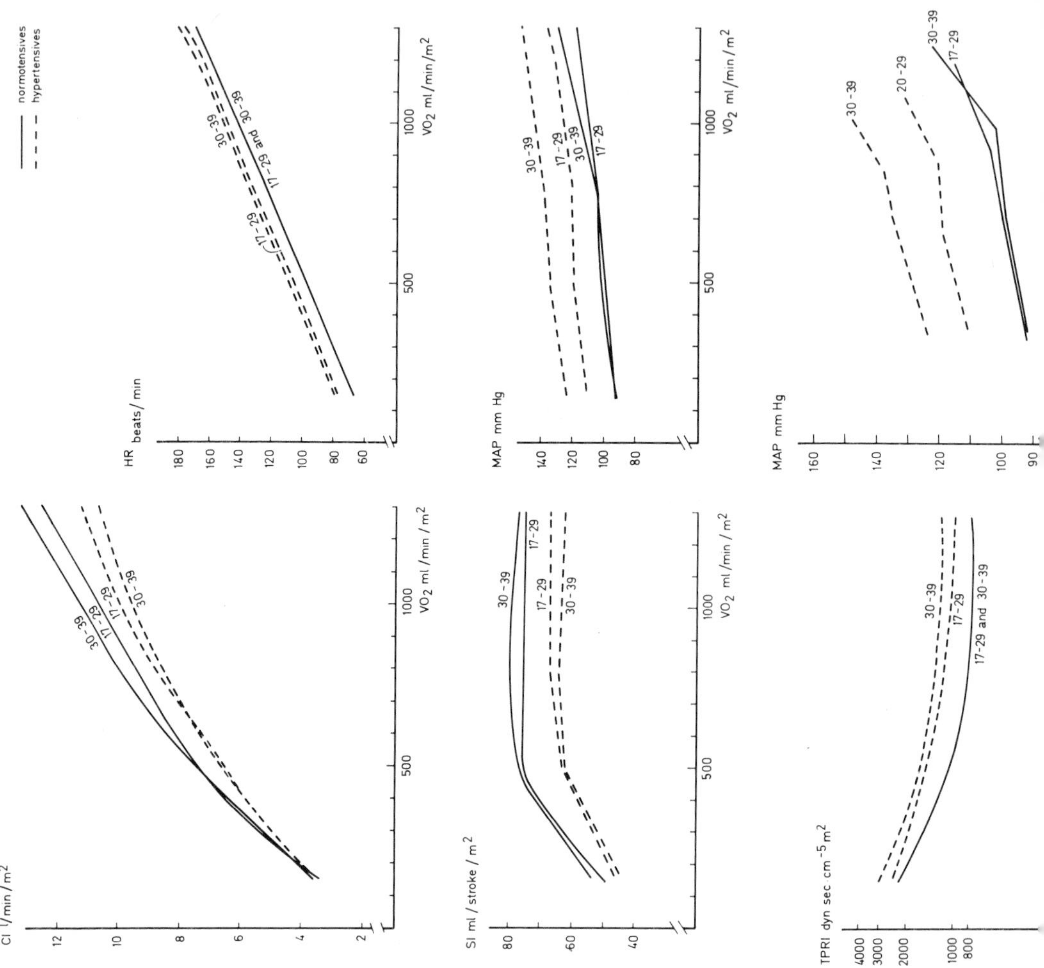

FIG. 1.—Hemodynamic changes at rest and during exercise in subjects with essential hypertension in WHO stage I, aged 17 to 29 and 30 to 39 years, compared to normotensive controls. **CI,** cardiac index; **HR,** heart rate; **SI,** stroke index; **MAP,** mean arterial pressure; **TPRI,** total peripheral resistance index; **VO_2,** oxygen consumption. Mean values.

subjects. The total peripheral resistance was increased at all work levels.

A disturbed total peripheral resistance in borderline hypertension has also been demonstrated by beta-blockers in subjects with that condition.[26] After blockade, the cardiac output drops and the total peripheral resistance increases more than in controls.

Thus even if the calculated total peripheral resistance was not different from controls at rest, it is evident from these studies that it is nevertheless already abnormal in subjects supposed to have early essential hypertension.

Hemodynamic Alterations in Established Hypertension of Longer Duration

In subjects with established essential hypertension of long duration, but without clinical heart failure, the results from recent years are in agreement with earlier findings. At rest, the high arterial pressure is maintained by an increased total peripheral resistance in the presence of a normal or low cardiac index.[12,18–20] With increasing clinical severity of the disease, the cardiac index tends to be very low and total peripheral resistance very high.[19,20] Essentially the same is found during muscular exercise.[12,19,20] Exercise studies also demonstrate that in established essential hypertension the circulatory system might be hypokinetic even if no clinical signs of heart failure are present (Fig. 2). Since subjects with this hemodynamic pattern represent the majority of those who are treated with antihypertensive drugs, I would like to emphasize that the rational therapy would be to use drugs which lower total peripheral resistance and do not depress car-

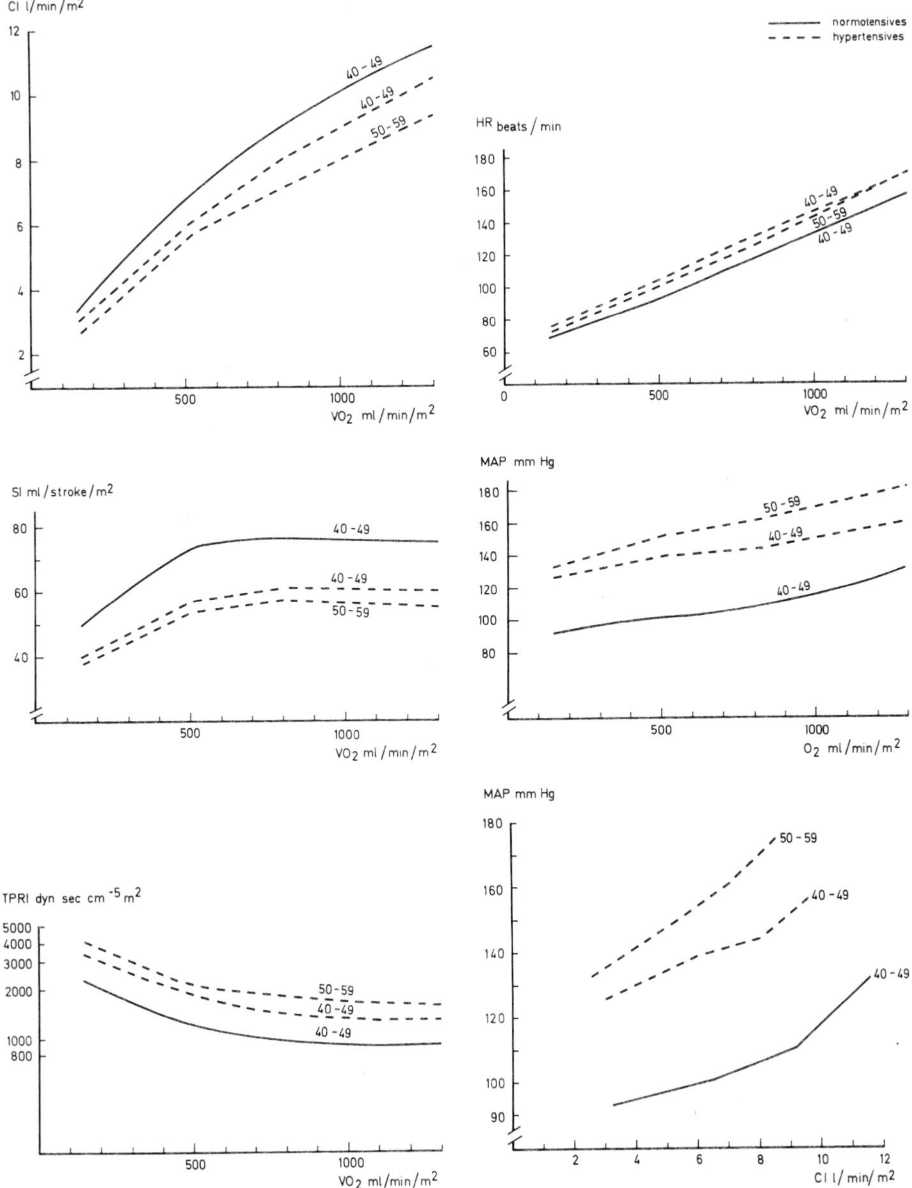

FIG. 2.—Hemodynamic changes at rest and during exercise in subjects with essential hypertension aged 40 to 49 years (WHO stage I) and aged 50 to 59 years (WHO stage I or II) compared to normotensive controls aged 40 to 49 years. **CI,** cardiac index; **HR,** heart rate; **SI,** stroke index; **MAP,** mean arterial pressure; **TPRI,** total peripheral resistance index; **VO_2,** oxygen consumption.

diac output further, either at rest or during exercise.[33,34] This seems even more important in subjects with long-standing hypertension and with complications in various organs. In such subjects the cardiac index at rest is very low and total peripheral resistance is usually very high.[19,20] During exercise a marked reduction in heart-pump function is usually found together with an increase in pulmonary artery pressure.[3] The arteriovenous oxygen difference is increased, demonstrating the disproportion between the cardiac pump function and the metabolic demands.[3]

Changes in Regional Circulation

The regional circulation in essential hypertension is less well studied than the central hemodynamics, probably because of the technical difficulties of such an investigation. Systematic studies of the circulatory pattern in various parts of the body, at different ages, and with hypertension in different stages are lacking.

A review of studies at rest and during exercise has been given recently by Amery,[35] who has also performed an extensive study of muscle blood flow in hypertensive and normotensive subjects of different ages.[36] He found that the muscle blood flow (measured by ^{133}Xe) after maximum ischemic exercise was increased in hypertensives in all ages, and so was the vascular resistance but to a lesser extent than in the rest of the body. Essentially the same conclusions were made by Conway [37] in an earlier plethysmographic study of the circulation in the forearm. The greatest increase in resistance was seen in patients with the most severe hypertension.

The renal blood flow is sometimes increased in early essential hypertension.[38] In established and more severe hypertension the renal blood flow is reduced and the resistance increased, probably more than in the rest of the body.[22,35] Studies of the splanchnic circulation and the cerebral circulation have revealed an increase in the resistance assumed to be of the same order as in the rest of the body.[35] (See chapter entitled "Regional Blood Flow in Essential Hypertension.")

The Capacitance Vessels in Essential Hypertension

A diminished distensibility of the capacitance vessels has been suggested in essential hypertension.[39] This could result in sharp rises in cardiac output when the plasma volume was suddenly increased, and be of importance in the pathogenesis of hypertension. Several studies of the effect of dextran infusion in subjects with essential hypertension in various stages have been published but the results have been conflicting.[19,26,39] A marked increase in central venous pressure and cardiac output in mild hypertension was reported by Ulrych, Hofman, and Hejl.[39] In my own study [19] the rise in central venous pressure in such subjects was normal but the increase in cardiac output was somewhat greater than in normotensive controls and hypertensives of older age. Recently Julius et al.[26] found no greater cardiac output rise in subjects with borderline essential hypertension after similar dextran infusion. Welner and Groen [40] have drawn attention to a strong influence of the psychic condition of the subject during such studies and it is possible that this can explain some of the differences. The majority of the subjects studied by Julius et al.[26] had participated in earlier hemodynamic studies. Thus it seems reasonable to conclude that the evidence in favor of a diminished distensibility of the capacitance vessels in essential hypertension is rather scanty.

Changes in Plasma Volume

Abnormalities in the plasma volume could of course be of importance for the hemodynamic alterations in hypertension.

In subjects with mild or borderline hypertension, a decreased plasma volume has been found in some studies [10,41] but not in another.[42] In subjects with established hypertension with diastolic levels above 100 to 105 mm Hg, a decreased plasma volume was found in some studies [42,43] but not in others.[44,45] One study reports a greater diurnal variation in plasma volume in hypertensives than in normal controls.[44]

It must be concluded that the data on the changes in plasma volume at present are conflicting. A strict selection of untreated subjects grouped according to sex, age, pressure level, hypertensive stage, and, if possible, duration of the hypertension should be made in future studies.

Conclusions

It is concluded that the hemodynamic picture in what we call essential hypertension is different in groups of subjects of different ages with different degrees of pressure elevation and with different degrees of complications. In subjects supposed to be in the early stage of the disease, the cardiac output is usually high and the calculated total peripheral resistance is normal. However, studies changing the relationship between blood flow and resistance, such as muscular exercise, demonstrate that the peripheral resistance is abnormal early—i.e., in subjects in their twenties. In subjects with established hypertension in older age with or without complications and with long duration of hypertension, the blood flow is normal or low at rest and also low during exercise. The peripheral resistance is high. In subjects with clinical heart failure the flow is very low and resistance very high, both at rest and during work. The crucial question is whether all subjects really represent individuals with the same disease in various stages. A few observations have offered support to the theory that such a change in the hemodynamics really takes place [11,14] but more extensive studies will be necessary before this problem is finally solved. A better understanding of the hemodynamic background in essential hypertension will hopefully contribute to a more physiologic approach in the reduction of the blood pressure with antihypertensive drugs.[33,34]

References

1. Peterson, L. H.: Hemodynamic alterations in essential hypertension. *In* Brest, A. N., and Moyer, J. H. (Eds.): Hypertension: Recent Advances. Philadelphia: Lea & Febiger, 1961, pp. 45–52.
2. Freis, E. D.: Hemodynamics of hypertension. Physiol. Rev. 40:27, 1960.
3. Taylor, S. H., Donald, K. W., and Bishop, J. M.: Circulatory studies in hypertensive patients at rest and during exercise. Clin. Sci. 16:351, 1957.
4. Varnauskas, E.: Studies in hypertensive cardiovascular disease with special reference to cardiac function. Scand. J. Clin. Lab. Invest. 7(Suppl. 17):1, 1955.
5. Werkø, L., and Lagerløf, H.: Studies on the circulation in man. IV. Cardiac output and blood pressure in the right auricle, right ventricle and pulmonary artery in patients with hypertensive cardiovascular disease. Acta Med. Scand. 133:427, 1949.
6. Fejfar, Z., and Widimsky, J.: Juvenile hypertension. *In* Cort, J. H., Fencl, V., Hejl, Z., and Jirka, J. (Eds.): The Pathogenesis of Essential Hypertension. Prague: State Medical Publishing House, 1961, pp. 33–42.
7. Ledingham, J. M., and Cohen, R. D.: The role of the heart in the pathogenesis of renal hypertension. Lancet 2:979, 1963.
8. Wilson, C.: Etiological considerations in essential hypertension. *In* Brest, A. N., and Moyer, J. H. (Eds.): Hypertension: Recent Advances. Philadelphia: Lea & Febiger, 1961, pp. 64–71.
9. Finkielman, S., Worcel, M., and Agrest, A.: Hemodynamic patterns in essential hypertension. Circulation 31:356, 1965.
10. Bello, C. T., Sevy, R. W., and Harakal, C.: Varying hemodynamic patterns in essential hypertension. Am. J. Med. Sci. 250:24, 1965.
11. Bello, C. T., Sevy, R. W., Harakal, C., and Hillyer, P. N.: Relationship between clinical severity of disease and hemodynamic patterns in essential hypertension. Am. J. Med. Sci. 253:194, 1967.
12. Amery, A., Julius, S., Whitlock, L. S., and Conway, J.: Influence of hypertension on the hemodynamic response to exercise. Circulation 36:231, 1967.
13. Eich, R. H., Peters, R. J., Cuddy, R. P., Smulyan, H., and Lyons, R. H.: The hemodynamics in labile hypertension. Am. Heart J. 63:188, 1962.
14. Eich, R. H., Cuddy, R. P., Smulyan, H., and Lyons, R. H.: Hemodynamics in labile hypertension. Circulation 34:299, 1966.
15. Frohlich, E. D., Tarazi, R. C., and Dustan, H. P.: Re-examination of the hemodynamics of hypertension. Am. J. Med. Sci. 257:9, 1969.
16. Julius, S., and Conway, J.: Hemodynamic studies in patients with borderline blood pressure elevation. Circulation 38:282, 1968.
17. Levy, A. M., Tabakin, B. S., and Hanson, J. S.: Hemodynamic responses to graded treadmill exercise in young untreated labile hypertensive patients. Circulation 35:1063, 1967.

18. Glazer, G. A.: A study of some haemodynamic parameters in essential hypertension. Cor Vasa 5:165, 1963.
19. Lund-Johansen, P.: Hemodynamics in early essential hypertension. Acta Med. Scand. 181(Suppl. 482):1, 1967.
20. Sannerstedt, R.: Hemodynamic response to exercise in patients with arterial hypertension. Acta Med. Scand. 180(Suppl. 458):1, 1966.
21. Safar, M., Fendler, J.–P., Weil, B., Idatte, J.–M., Beuve-Mery, P., and Milliez, P.: Étude hémodynamique de l'hypertension artérielle labile. Presse Med. 78:111, 1970.
22. Brod, J., Fencl, V., Hejl, Z., Jirka, J., and Ulrych, M.: General and regional haemodynamic pattern underlying essential hypertension. Clin. Sci. 23:339, 1962.
23. Birkenhäger, W. H., van Es, L. A., Houwing, A., Lamers, H. J., and Mulder, A. H.: Studies on the lability of hypertension in man. Clin. Sci. 35:445, 1968.
24. Kuramoto, K., Murata, K., Yazaki, Y., Ikeda, M., and Nakao, K.: Hemodynamics in the juvenile hypertension with special reference to the response to propranolol. Jap. Circ. J. 32:981, 1968.
25. Expert Committee: Arterial hypertension and ischaemic heart disease. Preventive aspects. WHO Tech. Rep. Ser. 231:1962.
26. Julius, S., Pascual, A. V., Sannerstedt, R., and Mitchell, C.: Relationship between cardiac output and peripheral resistance in borderline hypertension. Circulation 43:382, 1971.
27. Gorlin, R.: The hyperkinetic heart syndrome. JAMA 182:823, 1962.
28. Sannerstedt, R., Julius, S., and Conway, J.: Hemodynamic responses to tilt and beta-adrenergic blockade in young patients with borderline hypertension. Circulation 42:1057, 1970.
29. Julius, S., Pascual, A. V., and London, R.: Role of parasympathetic inhibition in the hyperkinetic type of borderline hypertension. Circulation 46:413, 1971.
30. Bristow, J. D., Honour, A. J., Pickering, T. G., and Sleight, P.: Cardiovascular and respiratory changes during sleep in normal and hypertensive subjects. Cardiovasc. Res. 3:476, 1969.
31. Khatri, I. M., and Freis, E. D.: Hemodynamic changes during sleep in hypertensive patients. Circulation 39:785, 1969.
32. Lund-Johansen, P.: Physiological symptoms and signs of ICIN in arterial hypertension; changes in the physiological data announcing failure. *In* European Society of Cardiology. Symposium on incipient cardiac insufficiency. Basle: Sandoz Ltd., 1970, pp. 119–125.
33. Lund-Johansen, P.: Hemodynamic changes in long-term diuretic therapy of essential hypertension. Acta Med. Scand. 187:509, 1970.
34. Gilmore, E., Weil, J., and Chidsey, C.: Treatment of essential hypertension with a new vasodilator in combination with beta-adrenergic blockade. N. Engl. J. Med. 282:521, 1970.
35. Amery, A.: Hemodynamic changes during exercise in hypertensive patients. *In* Rosselli, M. (Ed.): Malattie Cardiovascolari. Florence: 1969, pp. 227–245.
36. Amery, A., Bossaert, H., and Verstracle, M.: Muscle blood flow in normal and hypertensive subjects. Am. Heart J. 78:211, 1969.
37. Conway, J.: A vascular abnormality in hypertension. A study of blood flow in the forearm. Circulation 27:520, 1963.
38. Hollenberg, N. K., and Adams, D. F.: Hypertension and intrarenal perfusion patterns in man. Am. J. Med. Sci. 261:232, 1971.
39. Ulrych, M., Hofman, J., and Hejl, Z.: Cardiac and renal hyperresponsiveness to acute plasma volume expansion in hypertension. Am. Heart J. 68:193, 1964.
40. Welner, A., and Groen, J. J.: Effect of a simple deconditioning procedure on the diuretic and natriuretic response of hypertensive patients to a hypertonic salt load. Circulation 35:260, 1967.
41. Julius, S., Pascual, A. V., Reilly, K., and London, R.: Abnormalities of plasma volume in borderline hypertension. Arch. Intern. Med. 127:116, 1971.
42. Tarazi, G., Frohlich, E. D., and Dustan, H. P.: Plasma volume in men with essential hypertension. N. Engl. J. Med. 278:762, 1968.
43. Tibblin, G., Bergentz, S.–E., Bjure, J., and Wilhelmsen, L.: Hematocrit, plasma protein, plasma volume, and viscosity in early hypertensive disease. Am. Heart J. 72:165, 1966.
44. Cranston, W. I., and Brown, W.: Diurnal variation in plasma volume in normal and hypertensive subjects. Clin. Sci. 25:107, 1963.
45. Hansen, J.: Blood volume and exchangeable sodium in essential hypertension. Acta Med. Scand. 184:517, 1968.

VASCULAR REACTIVITY IN SYSTEMIC ARTERIAL HYPERTENSION

By MILTON MENDLOWITZ, M.D.

THE RELATION of increased vascular reactivity to the genesis of hypertension is a subject which has been debated for many years but is still unsettled. I shall try to point out some of the reasons for the disagreements and then describe the historic development of the subject including observations and views from my own laboratory.

One of the major reasons for investigative differences in this area can be attributed to deficiencies in physiologic theory with reference to vascular function. For example, the physiologists had long sought to define changes in vascular caliber from changes in pressure-flow ratio.[1] This, however, became flawed by the discovery that viscosity increased at low rates of flow [2] and vasoconstriction shifted the relationship to the right on the horizontal pressure axis because of critical closing pressure, a portion of the intravascular pressure keeping the vessel open at low rates of flow and balancing the force of vasoconstriction at higher rates of flow.[3] Therefore, this portion of intravascular pressure was not expended in the propulsion of blood. Since interpretation of vascular caliber changes from changes in pressure-flow ratios depended to some extent on rate of flow, Poiseuille's law apparently became inapplicable under several conditions: (*1*) at low rates of flow caused by changing apparent viscosity; (*2*) with vasoconstriction because of critical closing pressure changes in proportion to the vasoconstriction; (*3*) at very high rates of flow in large vessels because of turbulence;[4] and (*4*) in capillaries because of variable deformation of red cells.[5]

Because of these apparently insuperable imponderables, the physiologists fell back on measurements of pressure as such or of peripheral resistance [6] which is merely a ratio of pressure to flow or, what is worse, percentage changes in these values from which the actual events in any given vascular bed were inferred. Using such methods, Wilkins and Eichna [7] came to the conclusion that there was no increase in responsiveness to infused norepinephrine in essential hypertension whereas Doyle and Black [8] concluded that there was an increase. Both groups measured pressure changes only at that time.

Where flow and pressure are measured together, however, there has been fairly general agreement that responsiveness to vasoactive substances is increased in essential hypertension. This has been found in various vascular beds [9–14] and in the systemic circulation as a whole.[10,15] It is not true of the kidney [16] or the retina and the brain [17–20] where response to norepinephrine is relatively feeble, and response to 100 percent oxygen inhalation is less than normal in patients with essential hypertension.

What is still disputed is whether the increase in reactivity is a cause or an effect of the hypertension. Those who favor the latter hypothesis point out that structural narrowing of vascular lumina and increase in wall thickness is an effect or at least a feature of hypertension and that increase in the pressure-flow ratio with a given rate of infusion of a vasoactive substance may merely be a function of this structural change and may not represent a true increase in sensitivity to the hormone.[21] More recently another group of workers came to the same conclusion from studies of norepinephrine dose-response peripheral-resistance curves.[22] My own studies [23–25] and those of others [10,13,26] favor the hypothesis that increased reactivity is a causative factor in essential hypertension.

As to the physiologic theory of vascular function, it must be realized that the pressure-flow ratio or resistance is an index of vascular caliber only. Also, the relationship between re-

---

From the Department of Medicine, Mount Sinai School of Medicine, City University of New York, New York, New York.

Supported by Grant HE-05802 from the National Heart and Lung Institute, National Institutes of Health.

sistance and vascular caliber is curvilinear, rising more steeply as vascular caliber decreases. If the starting levels are different, therefore, absolute resistance changes do not accurately reflect absolute caliber changes. What is more, several factors are frequently disregarded in measurement of resistance changes. These include viscosity,[27] critical closing pressure factors,[28] turbulence,[29] and erythrocyte deformation factors.[30] Measurement of percentage changes in resistance attempts to correct for different starting resistances but does not correct for the curvilinearity of the relationship or for these other factors and often obscures real absolute differences between groups. In comparing hypertensive and normotensive groups another factor must be taken into account. Even if caliber changes could be estimated accurately, the intravascular pressure against which such changes take place must also be reckoned with. It is clear that more vasoconsfrictive force and physical work will be required to produce a given caliber change if the intravascular pressure is high than if it is low.

To overcome most of these difficulties, a frame of reference for the digit [9,31] was established as follows: The movement, with increasing grades of vasoconstriction, of the pressure axis intercept of the pressure-flow plot at different levels of perfusing pressure was measured and recorded. Also, the venous pressure in the digit at heart level was determined and its change with decreasing rates of flow could be calculated. The pressure-flow plot at intermediate rates of flow under these conditions was rectilinear and Poiseuille's law could be applied to the slope, provided the flow rate was above the level where the ratio began to curve because of viscosity, red cell deformation, and closing pressure factors and was below the level where the ratio was modified by turbulence. What is more, in the digit most of the flow is through arteriovenous anastomoses which are almost exclusively under adrenergic sympathetic control and the caliber of the vessels is such that turbulence is almost nonexistent under normal conditions and red cell deformation is a minor factor. The calorimeter was ideal for measuring flow in the digit since nearly all of it is surface flow, and flow per square centimeter of skin and nail is easily determined and accurate if room temperature is kept within 26 to 29 C.[32]

Caliber changes in terms of Poiseuille's law can only be accurately determined in a single tube of a uniform radius throughout its length. This difficulty was overcome by determining the caliber of an average anterior digital artery and extending it to a length such that its resistance changes were the same as those which usually obtain in half of a vasodilated terminal digit. Whatever took place in the digital circulation was then translated into changes in this model. Since internal vascular surface area, caliber and pressure changes could thus be determined in the model, the force and work of vasoconstriction could be calculated as well. These measurements could also take into account the intravascular pressure against which the caliber changes took place and the vasomotor changes in hypertensive and normotensive groups could be compared. The absolute values are undoubtedly incorrect but the relative difference between the two groups cannot be properly estimated in any other known way. Resistance changes, as such, also show differences between the two groups [9] but these are less than work changes probably because the inaccuracies already referred to in the measurement of resistance changes obscure real existing differences.

In 1957 we established that there is increased reactivity to norepinephrine in inherited essential hypertension in these terms.[9,31] This has recently been confirmed in the same terms by Moldovan et al.[33] The test is called digital vascular reactivity (DVR). Meanwhile, Duff published a paper demonstrating increased reactivity in the hand in essential hypertension to intra-arterially administered epinephrine.[11] The work on the digit was confirmed much later by Miyahara using the plethysmograph to measure blood flow.[10] Doyle and Fraser [13] demonstrated increased responsiveness in forearm muscle, Moulton, Spencer, and Willoughby [14] in calf muscle, and Barany [12] in proximal skin in essential hypertension. Increased responsiveness in the systemic circulation as a whole was demonstrated by Tuckman, Mendlowitz, and Naftchi [15] and also by Miyahara.[10] In the renal circulation, however, no increased reactivity could be demonstrated by Gombos et al.[16] and they inferred that systemic reactivity as a whole was not increased. There is also no clear evidence of increased responsiveness in the brain or in the retina in essential hypertension.[17–20]

In the digit [34] and in forearm muscle [13] increased responsiveness in essential hypertension was also found to angiotensin II and in the digit to tyramine.[35] It is now known that angiotensin II does affect the sympathetic nervous system, in addition to its other effects [36] and that tyramine releases endogenous norepinephrine from its sympathetic neural stores.[37] Miyahara also demonstrated increased reactivity in the systemic circulation to angiotensin II.[10] It is clear, then, that the preponderance of the evidence established the fact that vascular responsiveness to various vasoactive substances, especially those affecting vascular receptors and the sympathetic nervous system and also those that release endogenous norepinephrine, is increased in essential hypertension.

Other evidence accumulated to favor the theory that the increase in responsiveness in essential hypertension was etiologic rather than an effect of the hypertension or a structural concomitant. We studied a large number of patients with renal hypertension and renovascular hypertension whose reactivity was normal.[38] Yet it is well known that such hypertension produces vascular smooth-muscle hypertrophy and narrowing of the vascular bed. In the digit, such changes are also produced by Raynaud's disease both of the vasospastic and obstructive types and here, too, the reactivity was either normal or only slightly increased.[29] Also, the most extensive vascular changes in essential hypertension take place in the kidney, where hypertrophy and intimal changes are more marked than anywhere else in the body. Yet in this organ, reactivity to norepinephrine was not found to be increased in essential hypertension [16] in contrast to the increase found in many other vascular beds of the systemic circulation.

Several other findings suggested that the increased reactivity might be a causal factor which was biochemical in nature. For one thing, reactivity could be changed by various hormones and drugs. Prednisone increased it in normotensive subjects and left it unchanged in hypertensive patients.[40] This occurred within 3 weeks. Aldosterone and salt increased responsiveness in hypertensive patients in 3 days but had only a slight effect on normotensive subjects.[41] Guanethidine and methyldopa decreased blood pressure but increased responsiveness in 2 weeks of administration to hypertensive patients.[42] Thiazides [43] or spironolactone,[44] on the other hand, decreased both blood pressure and responsiveness in such patients. Increased reactivity could also be demonstrated in inherited essential prehypertension. Doyle and Fraser demonstrated it in the children of hypertensive parents [45] and we found increased digital vascular reactivity in some women who were normotensive but had a history of toxemia of pregnancy, suggesting that they were prehypertensive.[46]

The first direct evidence of a biochemical defect peculiar to essential hypertension came from our laboratory. Gitlow et al. infused tritiated norepinephrine (^{3}H-norepinephrine) intravenously into normotensive and hypertensive subjects and found that the labeled hormone and its metabolites disappeared from the plasma more rapidly in patients with essential hypertension.[47] Later, Wolf, Mendlowitz, and Roboz [48] gave a single bolus of ^{3}H-norepinephrine intravenously and measured the specific activity of normetanephrine in a 24-hour urine specimen collected after the injection. More ^{3}H-normetanephrine was excreted by the essential hypertensive patients than by normal subjects and if the amount given was divided by the specific activity of normetanephrine, this value was lower in the hypertensive group. They called this test the apparent norepinephrine secretion rate (ANESR). If one fifth of that dose was given, Gitlow et al.[49] showed that one could separate the normotensive from the hypertensive group by counting tritium only in the 24-hour urine specimen collected after the injection. The hypertensive patient excreted more than 62 percent of the administered dose and the normotensive less than 62 percent. This test was designated tritiated norepinephrine uptake (TNEU).

What is more, both the Gitlow and the Wolf groups began to study a number of renal and renovascular patients in whom the tests fell into the normal range. The correlation of these tests with the reactivity tests thus far appears to be quite good and investigators continue to establish the specificity of the tests for the diagnosis of inherited essential hypertension.

The importance of dosage in this type of testing cannot be overemphasized. Both Gitlow et al.[50] and DeQuattro and Sjoerdsma [51] could not find any difference between normotensive and hypertensive subjects in the specific activity of norepinephrine and vanillylmandelic acid, as measured in the urine after infusion with either ^{3}H-norepinephrine or tritiated levo-dihydroxyphenylalanine (^{3}H-dopa). This might have been caused from the labeling of large nonspecific muscle and liver stores which obscured the more specific metabolism of the tracer. Both groups did report profound effects on urinary-specific activity of catecholamines and their metabolites when such drugs as reserpine, guanethidine, pargyline, etc., were administered.[51,52] Substances which inhibit vascular smooth-muscle contraction directly, such as guancydine [53] and prostaglandin A_1[54] decreased digital vascular reactivity but had no effect on TNEU. Engelman, Portnoy, and Sjoerdsma [55] found increased plasma levels of the catecholamines in both essential hypertension and psychotic states although norepinephrine was not separated from epinephrine in most of these studies. They used a sensitive double-isotope method for measuring the minute amounts of these hormones in the plasma. Nestel [56] found increased blood pressure response in essential hypertension to standardized psychic stress and also increased output of norepinephrine in the urine with such stress. Lorimer et al.[57] confirmed the increased rise in blood pressure but could not confirm the increase in urinary norepinephrine in essential hypertension, using a different standardized stress.

One of the major difficulties in the area of specific testing for inherited essential hypertension began to appear soon after the reactivity test was described and has since also surfaced in relation to the biochemical testing. Although most patients with specific types of hypertension had tests for inherited essential hypertension which were normal, some had elevated DVR, TNEU, and decreased ANESR tests, characteristics of essential hypertension. This happened most frequently in patients with renovascular hypertension, patients with pyelonephritis and hypertension, and more recently in some patients with primary aldosteronism.

The probable explanation for this came from an unexpected source, namely, epidemiologic studies. It became apparent that hypertension was probably the most common chronic disease in the world. It is estimated that from 10 to 15 percent of the population either has or will have hypertension; [58] 80 percent or more of these patients are afflicted with inherited essential hypertension, so that on the basis of chance alone, mixed cases of specific secondary and inherited primary essential hypertension would not be uncommon. However, essential hypertension predisposes to several of the more specific varieties of high blood pressure. It predisposes to atherosclerosis [59] and hence to the most common form of renovascular hypertension which is caused by an atherosclerotic plaque in the renal artery. It predisposes to pyelonephritis [60] and it is now believed that it may predispose to primary as well as to secondary hyperaldosteronism, since after the tumor or hyperplasia is removed and the hyperaldosteronism cured, hypertension recurs in about 50 percent of patients,[62] particularly in those with hyperplasia and less so in those with adenomas. There is also a form of hypertension which is caused by anxiety only.[63] It is sporadic and apt to appear under stressful conditions and particularly during examination by a physician. Tests for inherited essential hypertension are negative and blood pressures self-determined at home are normal in this condition. Hypertension may be identified in some patients by the exaggerated reaction to administration of a beta-adrenergic stimulator [64] although this test is not widely used. This condition too, may be superimposed on true inherited essential hypertension and there may also be a predisposition factor here, in addition to chance association. In these special diseases, namely pyelonephritis, renovascular obstruction, primary aldosteronism, and anxiety hypertension, the incidence of mixed cases may approach 30 or 40 percent; and this should not be surprising.

One other condition may produce increased reactivity in the absence of essential hypertension, namely, Cushing's syndrome.[65] This disease, however, is recognizable from its clinical manifestations as well as by various testing procedures. It must also be emphasized that testing for pheochromocytoma should always precede that for essential hypertension and that the DVR is contraindicated whereas the other tests (TNEU, ANESR) are difficult to interpret in the presence of this disease.[66]

To return to the subject of vascular reactivity, the question may now be asked as to how increased reactivity and its biochemical concomitants are related etiologically to essential hypertension which is fundamentally hereditary, even though it can be modified by environmental factors. The hereditary nature of the disease is generally accepted. It is known that if two parents have essential hypertension, two out of three of the children will probably develop it. If only one parent has the disease, about one out of three of the children will inherit it. Also, the concordance in identical twins is nearly 100 percent.[62] What is disputed is whether the inheritance of hypertension is uni-[69] or multigenic[70] but it must be remembered that many epidemiologic studies do not sift out the more specific types of hypertension in the population and do not compare groups at the ages where its incidence is greatest, namely from 45 to 60. Even crude estimates during this age period reveal a double peak in the distribution curve of blood pressure.[69]

Whatever the genetic abnormality, however, it must cause an alteration in a protein or proteins. These proteins may be involved in the sympathetic neural storage mechanism or in the arteriolar smooth-muscle receptor–contractile system or both. On the other hand, the altered protein may influence this area indirectly by influencing electrolyte balance, for example. Since prostaglandin A_1 inhibits contraction of vascular smooth muscle directly and has no effect on TNEU,[54] it is probably not involved in the etiology of inherited essential hypertension, provided this aspect of catecholamine metabolism is considered to be causal. This does not preclude the possibility of a deficiency in prostaglandins A_1 or E_1 being a factor in renal or renovascular hypertension. All this, of course, is speculative but it seems clear that an abnormality does exist at the sympathetic neural storage or smooth-muscle receptor–contractile sites or both which is an initiating factor in the disease we know as essential hypertension.

Summary

In most systemic vascular beds and in the systemic circulation as a whole, vascular reactivity to vasoactive substances acting directly or indirectly on the sympathetic neural and vascular receptor complex is increased in inherited essential hypertension.

Since such increased reactivity is present early in the course of the disease and even in essential prehypertension and is associated with certain abnormalities of catecholamine metabolism, it is probably etiologic.

Since 10 to 15 percent of the population has or will have inherited essential hypertension and since this disease predisposes to renovascular hypertension and pyelonephritis and probably anxiety hypertension and primary as well as secondary hyperaldosteronism, mixed cases of essential hypertension together with these special types of hypertension comprise from 30 to 50 percent of these special cases. In the pure cases, however, digital vascular reactivity and catecholamine metabolism are normal.

Inherited essential hypertension is probably caused by an abnormal gene, or genes, producing an abnormal protein, or proteins, which either directly or indirectly affect the systemic sympathetic neural or vascular receptor–contractile sites or both.

References

1. Poiseuille, J. L. M.: Recherches experimentales sur le mouvement des liquides dans les tubes de très petits diamètres. C. R. Acad. Sci. [D] (Paris) 11:961, 1041, 1840; 12:113, 1841.
2. Whittaker, S. R. F., and Winton, F. R.: The apparent viscosity of blood flow in the isolated hindlimb of the dog, and its variation with corpuscular concentration. J. Physiol. 78:339, 1933.
3. Girling, F.: Vasomotor effects of electrical stimulation. Am. J. Physiol. 170:131, 1952.
4. Reynolds, O.: An investigation of the circumstances which determine whether the motion of water shall be direct or sinuous, and the law of resistance in parallel channels. Philos. Trans. 174:935, 1883.
5. Chien, S., Usami, S., Dellenback, R. J., and Gregerson, M. I.: Shear dependent deformation of erythrocytes in rheology of human blood. Am. J. Physiol. 219:166, 1970.

6. Green, H. D., Lewis, R. N., Nickerson, N. D., and Heller, A. L.: Blood flow, peripheral resistance and vascular tonus, with observations on the relationship between blood flow and cutaneous temperature. Am. J. Physiol. 141: 518, 1944.
7. Wilkins, R. W., and Eichna, L. W.: Blood flow to forearm and calf; effect of changes in arterial pressure on blood flow to limbs under controlled vasodilation in normal and hypertensive subjects. Johns Hopkins Med. J. 68: 477, 1941.
8. Doyle, A. E., and Black, H.: Reactivity to pressor agents in hypertension. Circulation 12:974, 1955.
9. Mendlowitz, M., and Naftchi, N.: Work of digital vasoconstriction produced by infused norepinephrine in primary hypertension. J. Appl. Physiol. 13:247, 1958.
10. Miyahara, M.: Catecholamines and hemodynamic changes in hypertension. Jap. Circ. J. 30:157, 1966.
11. Duff, R. S.: Some characteristics of peripheral arterioles in human hypertension. *In* Harington, M. (Ed.): Hypotensive Drugs. New York: Pergamon Press, 1956, pp. 196–203.
12. Barany, F. L.: Reactivity of the skin vessels to noradrenaline and angiotensin in arterial hypertension. Scand. J. Clin. Lab. Invest. 15: 317, 1963.
13. Doyle, A. E., and Fraser, J. R. E.: Vascular reactivity in hypertension. Circ. Res. 9:755, 1961.
14. Moulton, R., Spencer, A. G., and Willoughby, D. A.: Noradrenaline sensitivity in hypertension measured with radioactive sodium techniques. Br. Heart J. 20:224, 1958.
15. Tuckman, J., Mendlowitz, M., and Naftchi, N. E.: Systemic vascular reactivity to *l*-norepinephrine. In manuscript.
16. Gombos, E. A., Hulet, W. H., Bopp, P., Goldring, W., Baldwin, D. S., and Chasis, H.: Reactivity of renal and systemic circulation to vasoconstrictor agents in normotensive and hypertensive subjects. J. Clin. Invest. 41:203, 1962.
17. Hickam, J. B., and Frayser, R.: Studies of the retinal circulation in man. Observations on vessel diameter, arteriovenous oxygen difference and mean circulation tone. Circulation 33:302, 1966.
18. Dollery, C. T., Hill, D. W., and Hodge, J. V.: The response of normal retinal blood vessels to angiotensin and noradrenaline. J. Physiol. 165:500, 1963.
19. Lowe, R. D.: *In* Altman, P. L. and Dittmer, D. S. (Eds.): Biological Handbooks. Respiration and Circulation. Bethesda, Md.: Fed. Am. Soc. Exp. Biol., 1971, p. 450.
20. Greenfield, J. C., Jr., and Trindull, G. T.: Effect of norepinephrine, epinephrine and angiotensin on blood flow in the internal carotid artery of man. J. Clin. Invest. 47:1672, 1968.
21. Redleaf, P. D., and Tobian, L.: The question of hyper-responsiveness in hypertension. Circ. Res. 6:185, 1958.
22. Sivertsson, R., and Olander, R.: Aspects of the nature of increased vascular resistance and increased "reactivity" to noradrenaline in hypertensive subjects. Life Sci. [I] 7:1291, 1968.
23. Mendlowitz, M., Wolf, R. L., and Gitlow, S. E.: Catecholamine metabolism in essential hypertension. Am. Heart J. 79:401, 1970.
24. Mendlowitz, M.: The biology of hypertension. *In* Bittar, E. (Ed.): The Biological Basis of Medicine. New York: Academic Press, 1970, Vol. 6, p. 143.
25. Mendlowitz, M.: Etiology of hypertension. *In* Brest, A. N., and Moyer, J. H. (Eds.): Cardiovascular Disorders. Philadelphia: Davis, 1968, p. 929.
26. Crout, J. R.: Sympathetic and adrenal medullary factors in hypertension. *In* Moyer, J. H. (Ed.): Hypertension. Philadelphia: Saunders, 1959, p. 159.
27. Whittaker, S. R. F., and Winton, F. R.: The apparent viscosity of blood flowing in isolated hindlimb of the dog, and its variation with corpuscular concentration. J. Physiol. 78:339, 1933.
28. Pappenheimer, J. R., and Maes, J. P.: A quantitative measure of the vasomotor tone in the hindlimb muscles of the dog. Am. J. Physiol. 137:187, 1942.
29. McDonald, D. A.: Blood flow in arteries. London: Arnold, 1960.
30. Gregerson, M. I., Bryant, C. A., Mannerle, W. E., Usami, S., and Chien, S.: Flow characteristics of human erythrocytes through polycarbonate sieves. Science 157:25, 1967.
31. Mendlowitz, M., Torosdag, A., and Sharney, L.: The force and work of digital arteriolar vasoconstriction in hypertension. J. Appl. Physiol. 10:436, 1957.
32. Eurman, G. H., and Mendlowitz, M.: The relationship between skin temperature and the difference between mouth and radial or digital arterial blood temperature. J. Appl. Physiol. 5:579, 1953.
33. Moldovan, T., Idu, S. M., Anastasiu, R., and Mihei, N.: Muscle and red cell electrolytes in essential hypertension; correlations with digital vascular reactivity; the effects of hy-

drochlorothiazide. Z. Kreislaufforsch. (In press).

34. Mendlowitz, M., Naftchi, N. E., Wolf, R. L., and Gitlow, S. E.: Reactivity of the digital blood vessels to angiotensin II in normotensive and hypertensive subjects. Am. Heart J. 62:221, 1961.
35. Mendlowitz, M., Naftchi, N. E., Tuckman, J., Gitlow, S. E., and Wolf, R. L.: The effects of tyramine on the digital circulation in normotensive and hypertensive subjects. Chest 52: 709, 1967.
36. McCubbin, J. W., and Page, I. H.: Neurogenic component of chronic renal hypertension. Science 139:210, 1963.
37. Burn, J. H., and Rand, M. J.: The action of sympathomimetic amines treated with reserpine. J. Physiol. 144:314, 1958.
38. Mendlowitz, M., Naftchi, N., Wolf, R. L., and Gitlow, S. E.: Vascular responsiveness in hypertensive and hypotensive states. Geriatrics 20:797, 1965.
39. Mendlowitz, M., and Naftchi, N.: The digital circulation in Raynaud's disease. Am. J. Cardiol. 4:580, 1959.
40. Mendlowitz, M., Naftchi, N., Weinreb, H. L., and Gitlow, S. E.: Effect of prednisone on digital vascular reactivity in normotensive and hypertensive subjects. J. Appl. Physiol. 16:89, 1961.
41. Mendlowitz, M., Naftchi, N. E., Bobrow, E. B., Wolf, R. L., and Gitlow, S. E.: The effect of aldosterone on electrolytes and on digital vascular reactivity to *l*-norepinephrine in normotensive, hypertensive and hypotensive subjects. Am. Heart J. 65:93, 1963.
42. Mendlowitz, M., Naftchi, N. E., Wolf, R. L., and Gitlow, S. E.: The effects of guanethidine and of alpha-methyldopa on the digital circulation in hypertension. Am. Heart J. 69:731, 1965.
43. Mendlowitz, M., Naftchi, N., Gitlow, S. E., and Wolf, R. L.: The effect of chlorothiazide and its congeners on the digital circulation in normotensive subjects and in patients with essential hypertension. Ann. N.Y. Acad. Sci. 88:964, 1960.
44. Mendlowitz, M., Naftchi, N. E., Gitlow, S. E., and Wolf, R. L.: The effect of spironolactone on digital vascular reactivity in essential hypertension. Am. Heart J. 76:795, 1968.
45. Doyle, A. E., and Fraser, J. R. E.: Essential hypertension and inheritance of vascular reactivity. Lancet 2:509, 1961.
46. Mendlowitz, M., Altchek, A., and Naftchi, N.: The work and force of digital vasoconstriction in normotensive and hypertensive pregnant women. Am. J. Obstet. Gynec. 76:673, 1958.
47. Gitlow, S. E., Mendlowitz, M., Kruk, E., Wilk, S., Wolf, R. L., and Naftchi, N.: Norepinephrine metabolism in essential hypertension. J. Clin. Invest. 42:934, 1963.
48. Wolf, R. L., Mendlowitz, M., and Roboz, J.: A new test for primary hypertension: The apparent norepinephrine secretion rate in normotensive and hypertensive man. (Abstract.) J. Clin. Invest. 46:1134, 1967.
49. Gitlow, S. E., Mendlowitz, M., Bertani, L. M., Wilk, E. K., and Glabman, S.: Tritium excretion of normotensive and hypertensive subjects following administration of tritiated norepinephrine. J. Lab. Clin. Med. 73:129, 1969.
50. Gitlow, S. E., Mendlowitz, M., Wilk, E., Wilk, S., and Bertani, L. M.: Unpublished observations.
51. DeQuattro, V., and Sjoerdsma, A.: Catecholamine turnover in normotensive and hypertensive man: Effects of adrenergic drugs. J. Clin. Invest. 47:2359, 1968.
52. Gitlow, S. E., Mendlowitz, M., Wilk, E. K., and Wilk, S.: Effects of guanethidine and reserpine on norepinephrine metabolism of normal human subjects. Circulation 36(Suppl. II):121, 1967.
53. Russo, C., and Mendlowitz, M.: The effect of guancydine on blood pressure, vascular reactivity and norepinephrine uptake in essential hypertension. (Abstract.) Fed. Proc. 29:447, 1971.
54. Stricker, J., Mendlowitz, M., Russo, C., Gitlow, S. E., and Bertani, L. M.: The effect of continuous intravenous prostaglandin A_1 infusion in patients with essential hypertension. (Abstract.) Clin. Res. 19:713, 1971.
55. Engelman, K., Portnoy, B., and Sjoerdsma, A.: Plasma catecholamine concentration in patients with hypertension. Circ. Res. 26–27 (Suppl. I):141, 1970.
56. Nestel, P. J.: Blood pressure and catecholamine excretion after mental stress in labile hypertension. Lancet 1:692, 1969.
57. Lorimer, A. R., MacFarlane, P. W., Provan, G., Duffy, T., and Larrie, T. D. V.: Blood pressure and catecholamine response to "stress" in normotensive and hypertensive subjects. Cardiovasc. Res. 5:169, 1971.
58. Stamler, J., Stamler, R., and Pullman, T. N.: The Epidemiology of Hypertension. New York: Grune & Stratton, 1967.
59. Deming, Q. B., and Daly, M. M.: The relationship of atherosclerosis to hypertension. *In*

Moyer, J. H. (Ed.): Hypertension. Philadelphia: Saunders, 1959, p. 95.

60. Shapiro, A. P., Sapira, J. D., and Scheib, E. T.: Development of bacteruria in a hypertensive population. A 7-year follow-up study. Ann. Intern. Med. 74:861, 1971.
61. Mendlowitz, M.: The problem of mass screening for hypertension. Mt. Sinai J. Med. N. Y. 38:474, 1971.
62. Biglieri, E. G., Schambelan, M., Slaton, P. E., and Stockigt, J. R.: The intercurrent hypertension of primary aldosteronism. Circ. Res. 27(Suppl. I):195, 1970.
63. Suck, A. F., Mendlowitz, M., Wolf, R. L., Gitlow, S. E., and Naftchi, N. E.: Identification of essential hypertension in patients with labile blood pressures. Chest 59:402, 1971.
64. Frohlich, E., Terrazi, R., Dustan, H.: Hyperdynamic β-adrenergic circulatory state. Arch. Intern. Med. 123:1, 1969.
65. Mendlowitz, M., Gitlow, S. E., and Naftchi, N.: Work of digital vasoconstriction produced by infused norepinephrine in Cushing's syndrome. J. Appl. Physiol. 13:252, 1958.
66. Mendlowitz, M.: A practical approach to diagnosis and treatment of hypertension. Geriatrics 27:105, 1972.
67. Wollheim, E.: Die essentielle Hypertonie als nosologische Einheit und ihre Differentialdiagnose. Verh. Dtsch. es. Kreislaufforsch. 28: 59, 1962.
68. Vander Molen, R., Brewer, J., Honeyman, M. S., Morrison, J., and Hoobler, S. W.: A study of hypertension in twins. Am. Heart J. 79:454, 1970.
69. Platt, R.: The nature of essential hypertension. Lancet 2:55, 1959.
70. Pickering, G. W.: High Blood Pressure, 2nd edition. New York: Grune & Stratton, 1968.

Part III. GENETICS, EPIDEMIOLOGY, AND ENVIRONMENTAL FACTORS IN ESSENTIAL HYPERTENSION

Experimental Genetic Hypertension

By Sir F. Horace Smirk, K.B.E., M.D., D.Sc.

ABOUT 20 YEARS AGO we began selective breeding from our ordinary stock Wistar rats with the aim of obtaining a colony of rats with spontaneous hypertension. Early on we had failures and had to make a fresh start, but by the eighth year Smirk and Hall [1] were able to report a rise of systolic tail blood pressures to about 18 mm above controls. Now, 15 years after starting the successful breeding program, we have an inbred strain of frank hypertensives.

Phelan [2] has traced the effect of selection for high blood pressures in our sublines a, c, and d since 1955. The rate of increase of the blood pressure has been approximately 2 mm Hg per generation. Since 1969 the mean systolic blood pressures have been in the region of 170 mm Hg when taken under light ether anesthesia; this is 50 mm Hg above the controls.

Now there is no difficulty in obtaining by selection a group of rats with blood pressures, developed spontaneously, of 190 mm Hg or more. It has been shown by successful reciprocal skin grafts that our subline a is a pure strain.

Okamoto and Aoki [3] from Japan have since found a spontaneously hypertensive male rat in their stock colony. This was mated with a female rat with an overaverage blood pressure. From these they bred, selecting for high blood pressure. By the F_3 generation they had achieved blood pressures (unanesthetized) of 177 mm Hg. This contrasts remarkably with our breeding experience, for after our initial failure the New Zealand colony took about 15 years and as many as 27 generations of inbreeding to obtain similar blood pressure levels under light ether anesthesia. Furthermore, in the Japanese male rats (F_{13}) blood pressures were about 14 mm Hg higher than their controls at 5 weeks. By contrast, rats from our New Zealand colony had blood pressures about 24 mm Hg higher than the controls at this time and were near to their top level, reaching a mean systolic blood pressure about 170 mm Hg by 8 weeks.

Such differences, and others to be mentioned later, make it likely that there are at least two distinctive genotypes, both leading to frank spontaneous hypertension and pathologic changes such as cardiac enlargement (Fig. 1), polyarteritis nodosa, advanced renal damage, and occasionally medial necrosis of arterioles. To these two genotypes must be added the salt-sensitive and salt-insensitive rat strains developed by Dahl, Heine, and Tassinari,[4] the former developing severe hypertension when 8 percent of salt is present in the food.

In baby rats from our hypertensive colony the mean blood pressure at the second day of postnatal life is somewhat above that of controls but the difference is significant.[5] By the sixth week the average blood pressure is up to 160 mm Hg or more, controls being about 118 mm Hg and the mean systolic blood pressure does not usually rise much higher than 175 mm Hg as age advances.

Frank hypertension is present in our genetic hypertensive rat colony by the seventh week of postnatal life, corresponding to about one fourteenth of the life span. This would be equivalent to about age 5 years in man. Clearly the hypertension is not geriatric. At 6 weeks the

From Wellcome Medical Research Institute, Department of Medicine, Medical School, Dunedin, New Zealand.

Supported by grants from the Life Insurance Medical Research Fund of Australia and New Zealand and by Grant HE-10942 from the National Heart and Lung Institute (U.S.A.) and by the Medical Research Council of New Zealand, Wellington, New Zealand.

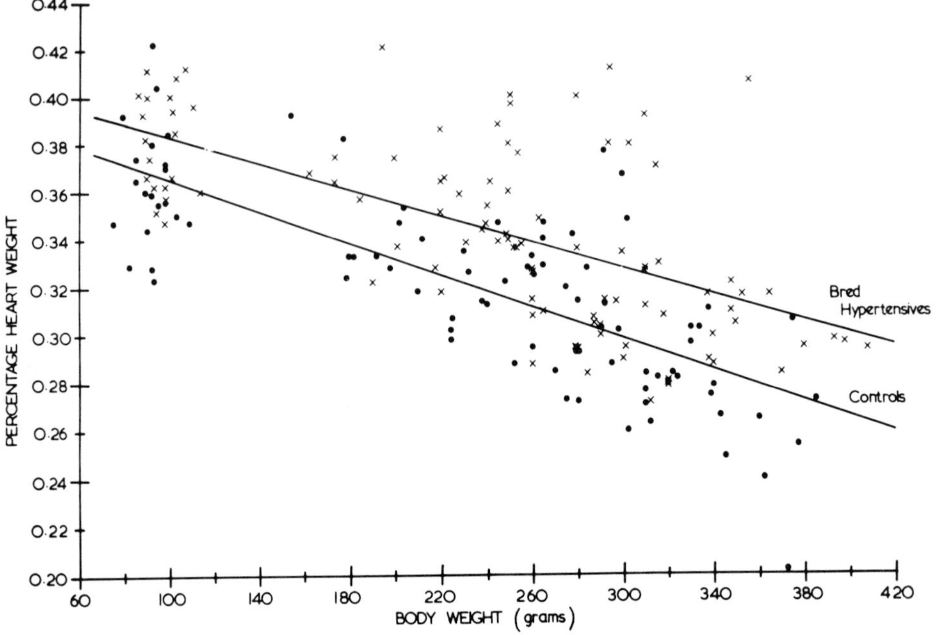

FIG. 1.—Relation between body weight and heart weight per 100 gm of body weight in rats with spontaneous genetic hypertension (**crosses**) and controls (**dots**). The difference is highly significant ($P < 0.001$). Even at a body weight of 100 gm, roughly corresponding to an age of 7 weeks, the difference is still significant ($0.02 < P < 0.05$). (From Phelan, E. L., and Smirk, F. H.,[6] with permission.)

average heart rate is increased: 400 per minute in hypertensives and 368 in normotensive controls.[6] The rats seem healthy and superficially resemble normotensive controls; but careful testing reveals some psychologic differences between the hypertensives and the normotensives.

There is evidence that the pathogenesis of the hypertension of our genetic hypertensive rats, when young, is not the same as that of experimental Goldblatt hypertension for the following reasons: up to the age of 2 or 3 months no difference from normal controls has been observed in the renal parenchyma by light microscopy. The caliber of the main renal blood vessels was studied using mercury as the radiopaque medium.[7] Main branches of the renal artery are shown in some detail by x-rays. Independent assessment by two observers revealed no consistent difference between the renal blood vessels of genetic hypertensive and control rats. No difference was observed in the juxtaglomerular granulations by Simpson.[8] In short, up to the age of 3 months there is no evidence of frank renal pathology.

Phelan and Wong [9] showed that Goldblatt-hypertensive rats with a renal artery clip differ from genetic hypertensive rats matched by age, weight, and approximately equal blood pressures, in that only the Goldblatt hypertensives show the well-known elevation above normal concentrations of sodium, potassium, and water in the thoracic aorta. The electrolyte and water concentrations in the thoracic aortas of our genetic hypertensive rats are much below the concentrations found in experimental renal hypertensives and, indeed, do not differ much from the normal (Table 1). Hence, we may conclude that if some esoteric change in the kidneys is responsible for the genetic hypertension, it cannot be the same esoteric renal change which, in the case of Goldblatt hypertension, has so long eluded discovery.

McKenzie and Phelan [10] showed that in our genetic hypertensive rats aged 120 days the plasma and the renal renin were less than in

TABLE 1.—*Water and Electrolytes in Aortas of Hypertensive Rats*

Group (no.)	*Percentage of Water in Fresh Aorta*	*Sodium (mEq per kg)*	*Potassium (mEq per kg)*
Renal hypertensive (31)	70.2 ± 0.8	305 ± 14	131 ± 6
Genetic hypertensive (15)	66.1 ± 0.3	245 ± 2.7	92 ± 1.7
Control (40)	65.9 ± 0.2	236 ± 1.4	93.7 ± 1.2

control rats. Correspondingly in patients with uncomplicated essential hypertension, Hollenberg et al.[11] and many others found that the rate of renin secretion was extremely low, being unmeasurable in three out of seven patients. Hollenberg et al. found that with increasing grades of renal vascular injury there was a corresponding increase in the renin activity of arterial plasma from 1.1 ± 0.5 in the absence of vascular damage to 1.9 ± 1.4, through 5.3 ± 1.1 up to 13.5 ± 1.7 ng of angiotensin per milliliter of plasma per 3 hours incubation with the increasing grades of vascular injury.

Before the blood pressures in our genetic hypertensive rats had risen to their present high level we compared the effects of maximal doses of hexamethonium in genetic hypertensives and controls. The blood pressures fell to the same level.[12,13] Also, the peripheral resistance of perfused, innervated, limb blood vessels of controls and genetic hypertensives fell to the same level with similar treatment.[12] We concluded that the blood pressure increase in the genetic hypertensive rats at this early date was neurogenically maintained, either because there were more nerve impulses, or because the reactivity of the blood vessels to nerve impulses was increased above the normal. This experiment has been repeated recently by Phelan [14] and Smirk [15] because the blood pressure of our genetic hypertensive rats has risen to a higher level. We find that now, after hexamethonium administration, the blood pressure in the genetic hypertensives does not fall to as low a level as in the controls. It seems that a nonneurogenically maintained element has been added on to the neurogenically maintained part of the blood pressure increase (Table 2). The hexamethonium floor blood pressure was 80.1 mm Hg in the genetic hypertensives, 91.8 mm Hg in renal hypertensives, and 67.5 mm Hg in the controls.[14] The blood pressures of the genetic hypertensives and renal hypertensives were similar before hexamethonium administration, and this experiment shows that in Goldblatt hypertension the neurogenically maintained part of the blood pressure is relatively smaller and the nonneurogenically maintained part relatively higher in renal than in the genetic hypertensives.

A difference between the renal and genetic hypertensives is that when matched for age, weight, and blood pressure the pressor responses to pitressin are larger in the renal hypertensives than in the genetic hypertensive rats.[14]

Still another difference is that brain catecholamines are raised in our genetically hypertensive rats but not in renal hypertensive rats.[16]

When the isolated mesenteric blood vessels of our genetic hypertensive rats and control rats are perfused either with saline or with blood, the perfusion-pressure baseline is distinctly greater in the genetic hypertensives than in the controls (Table 3). This difference in the perfusion-pressure baseline persists when sodium nitroprusside (50 μg per milliliter) is

TABLE 2.—*Blood Pressures (mm Hg) of Genetic Hypertensive (GH), Renal Hypertensive (RH), and Control Normotensive (C) Rats before and after Full Doses of Hexamethonium Bromide (HMB)*

	GH	*RH*	*C*	*GH−C*	*RH−C*
Before HMB	156.5	158.5	122.0	34.5	36.5
HMB floor	80.1	91.8	67.5	12.6	24.3
HMB fall	76.4	66.7	54.5	21.9	12.2

From Phelan, E. H., and Smirk, F. H.[6]

TABLE 3.—*Pressure Baselines of Isolated Perfused Mesenteric Arteries from Genetic Hypertensive (GH) and Control Normotensive (C) Rats*

	Baseline Perfusion Pressures (mm Hg)	
	GH	*C*
1. Blood perfusion no drugs	40.1 ± 2.2	32.4 ± 1.2
2. Saline perfusion no drugs	27.4 ± 0.9	23.2 ± 0.9
3. Saline perfusion plus 50 μg per milliliter of sodium nitroprusside	26.3 ± 0.9	21.4 ± 0.9
4. Saline perfusion plus 50 μg per milliliter of sodium nitroprusside—intestine removed	18.1 ± 1.1	13.7 ± 0.6

The perfusion rate was 1 ml per minute for blood and 2 ml per minute for physiologic saline. Differences between GH and C rats are significant, $p < 0.005$ or 0.001.

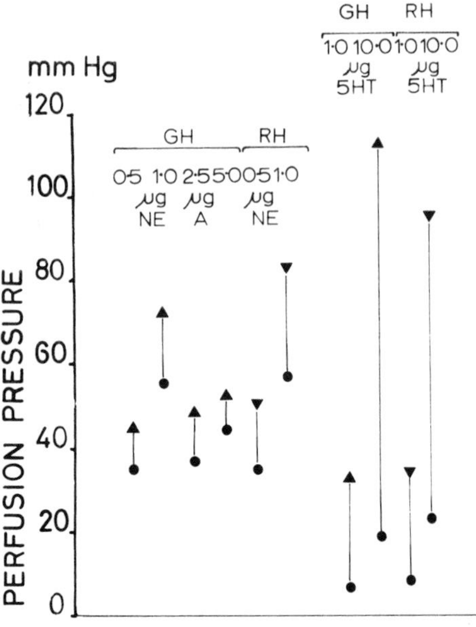

FIG. 2.—In mesenteric blood vessels perfused at 2 ml per minute with physiologic saline a comparison is made of the rises in perfusion pressure resulting from close injections of norepinephrine (**NE**), angiotensin (**A**) and 5-hydroxytryptamine (**5HT**) in genetic hypertensive (**GH**), renal hypertensive (**RH**) rats, and controls. Responses of controls are indicated in all instances by a **dot**, of genetic hypertensives by a **triangle with apex up**, and of renal hypertensives by a **triangle with apex down.**

It will be noted that the difference between the responses of controls and hypertensives is very much larger when the vasoconstrictor is 5-hydroxytryptamine than when it is norepinephrine or angiotensin.

added to the perfusion fluid; indicating that an increase in the peripheral resistance of the mesenteric blood vessels has taken place which does not depend on the contractile activity of the vascular smooth muscle.[20]

The response of perfused blood vessels to pressor drugs is of interest. Limb blood vessels and mesenteric blood vessels from our genetic hypertensive rats and from renal hypertensive rats, perfused with artificial media or with blood at a constant rate, responded to such pressor agents as epinephrine, norepinephrine, angiotensin, and 5-hydroxytryptamine, by larger rises in the peripheral resistance in the blood vessels from hypertensives than in the blood vessels from controls.[17–22]

Clearly, in the hypertensives there is an increase in the responsiveness of these perfused vascular beds and this may be part of the pathogenesis. We have some evidence [21] which is interesting, but not conclusive, suggesting that there may be an increase in the responses of vascular smooth muscle (Fig. 2). The mean responses of the hypertensives to norepinephrine and angiotensin were no more than 50 percent above the mean responses of controls. When, however, 5-hydroxytryptamine was used as the vasoconstrictor agent the responses of the hypertensives were now as large as 420 to 730 percent of the responses of controls. It is difficult to explain this in terms of a structural difference between the mesenteric arteries of hypertensives and normotensives. A possibility is an increase of the reactivity of smooth muscle to 5-hydroxytryptamine in the hypertensives.

It was noted that bilateral adrenalectomy in genetic hypertensives and controls with subsequent administration of 1% salt solution in the drinking fluid causes a fall in the blood pressure in both, but a difference in blood pressure between the two groups of rats is maintained, and within a period of 5 to 8 weeks the blood pressures have risen gradually to the original levels.[23] Aoki[24] found that adrenalectomy abolished the hypertension in rats from their colony.

Hypophysectomy[25] led to a fall of blood pressure in hypertensives and controls which persisted in our experiments for at least 4 months, but throughout the 4 months the blood pressure remained higher in the genetic hypertensives.

In our genetic hypertensive rats, cardiac hypertrophy, periarteritis nodosa, and advanced renal damage[6,7] may occur spontaneously, whereas such occurrences are most exceptional early in life in our stock colony. The pathologic changes, however, are of the same kind as those encountered in other types of rat hypertension, for example, by placing a clip on the renal artery.

Recently, in man, I studied about 519 first-degree relatives of substantial hypertensives and about 290 controls thought to be representative of the general population.[26] The rise with age of the blood pressure was greater in the first-degree relatives than in controls, indicating that in man the rise with age is influenced to an important degree by genetic factors as it is in our rats with spontaneous hypertension.

It was found[27] that blood pressure-raising procedures, when applied to the rats with genetic hypertension, gave rise to a higher eventual blood pressure level than the same procedure did when applied to normotensive controls. Furthermore, the occurrence of hypertensive disease such as periarteritis nodosa and gross structural changes in the kidneys was much more frequent in the genetic hypertensives subjected to such treatment than in the controls.[27]

The procedures which have been tried are: unilateral nephrectomy; subtotal nephrectomy,[27] in which half of one kidney and the whole of the opposite kidney are removed; the administration of 1.4% salt solution as drinking fluid;[28] the administration of 1% salt solution as drinking fluid after unilateral nephrectomy or the application of a clip to one renal artery.[27]

Unilateral nephrectomy was performed on 24 rats with genetic hypertension and mean preoperative systolic pressure of 160 mm Hg, and on 22 normotensive controls with mean preoperative pressure of 118 mm Hg. Tap water was the drinking fluid. After 5 months the blood pressure in the genetic hypertensives had risen to 170 mm Hg and after 7 months the mean systolic pressure ranged from 180 to 190 mm Hg. The corresponding mean systolic blood pressures for controls were 122 mm Hg at 5 months and 122 mm Hg (on two occasions 130 mm Hg) after 7 months. At 8 months, seven genetic hypertensives and two controls had died. Although the rise of blood pressure after unilateral nephrectomy was slow in the genetic hypertensive rats it amounted to an average of 25 mm Hg, whereas there was no significant rise of blood pressure in the controls.

A three-quarter nephrectomy causes similar blood pressure increases in genetic hypertensives and also in controls, being of the order of 40 mm Hg. This increase developed within 3 months.

The mortalities were increased when, after unilateral nephrectomy, 1% salt solution was used as drinking fluid. There was a 90.5-percent

TABLE 4.—*Mean Systolic Blood Pressure in Rats (in mm Hg ± S.D.) after 1.4% Sodium Chloride as Drinking Fluid*

Group	*Before Giving Added Salt*	*Highest after Giving Added Salt*	*Final*
Genetic Hypertensives			
Expt. 1	153.8 ± 10.4	171.3 ± 8.9	155.9 ± 11.7
Expt. 2	148.3 ± 4.2	187.5 ± 15.9	165.7 ± 20.8
Control			
Expt. 1	114.4 ± 9.5	137.6 ± 5.8	117.7 ± 13.6
Expt. 2	113.9 ± 10.1	141.5 ± 15.6	113.8 ± 13.5

TABLE 5.—*Number of Rats Exhibiting Periarteritis Nodosa after 1.4% Sodium Chloride as Drinking Fluid*

Group	*Definite Periar-teritis Nodosa*	*Possible Early Periar-teritis Nodosa*	*No Periar-teritis Nodosa*
Genetic hypertensive	14	1	12
Controls	0	3	15

mortality in 9 weeks among 21 genetic hypertensives receiving this treatment as against 29.5 percent of 17 controls.

Application of a clip to one renal artery increased the blood pressures in both genetic hypertensive and control rats but the mean blood pressure increase was no greater in genetic hypertensives than in the controls.

In rats aged less than 12 months, 1.4% salt solution administered as drinking fluid usually causes the blood pressure of both hypertensive and control rats to increase (Table 4). The rises are variable in magnitude but the hypertensives, starting from a higher level, not infrequently attain blood pressures in excess of 200 mm Hg. There were many more examples of periarteritis nodosa among the hypertensives than among the controls (Table 5).

These experiments were performed before blood pressures in our genetic hypertensive colony had risen to their present high levels.

The extent to which genetic and environmental factors are responsible for the high blood pressure of essential hypertension has been much debated. The above observations show that blood pressure-raising stimuli superimposed on high blood pressures of genetic origin may lead to important further increases in the blood pressure level and the development of advanced hypertensive disease.

ACKNOWLEDGMENT

The author is much indebted to Mrs. Joy Tomlin who has been responsible for the secretarial work. Professor F. O. Simpson, of the Dunedin Hospital Hypertensive Clinic, has been most helpful to me in the discussion of problems in the field of hypertension. I am grateful to Dr. John Hunter, Professor of Medicine in the Medical School, Dunedin, for his permission to use the facilities of the Wellcome Medical Research Institute.

REFERENCES

1. Smirk, F. H., and Hall, W. H.: Inherited hypertension in rats. Nature (London) 182:727, 1958.
2. Phelan, E. L.: Genetic and autonomic factors in inherited hypertension. Circ. Res. 27 (Suppl. 2):65, 1970.
3. Okamoto, K., and Aoki, K.: Development of a strain of spontaneously hypertensive rats. Jap. Circ. J. 27:282, 1963.
4. Dahl, L. K., Heine, M., and Tassinari, L.: Role of genetic factors in susceptibility to experimental hypertension due to chronic excess salt ingestion. Nature (London) 194:480, 1962.
5. Jones, D. R., and Dowd, D. A.: Development of elevated blood pressure in young genetically hypertensive rats. Life Sci. 9:247, 1970.
6. Phelan, E. L., and Smirk, F. H.: Cardiac hypertrophy in genetically hypertensive rats. J. Path. Bact. 80:445, 1960.
7. Smirk, F. H., and Phelan, E. L.: Kidneys of rats with genetic hypertension. J. Path. Bact. 89:57, 1965.
8. Simpson, F. O. (Personal communication), cited by Smirk, F. H. and Phelan, E. L.: The kidneys of rats with genetic hypertension. J. Path. Bact. 89:57, 1965.
9. Phelan, E. L., and Wong, L. C. K.: Sodium, potassium and water in the tissues of rats with genetic hypertension and constricted renal artery hypertension. Clin. Sci. 35:487, 1968.
10. McKenzie, J. K., and Phelan, E. L.: Plasma and renal renin in the N.Z. strain of genetic hypertensive and random-bred control rats. Proc. Univ. Otago Med. Sch. 47:23, 1969.
11. Hollenberg, N. K., Epstein, M., Basch, R. I., Couch, N. P., Hickler, R. B., and Merrill, J. P.: "No man's land" of the renal vasculature. An arteriographic and hemodynamic assessment of the interlobar and arcuate arteries in essential and accelerated hypertension. Am. J. Med. 47:855, 1969.
12. Laverty, R., and Smirk, F. H.: Observations on the pathogenesis of spontaneous inherited hypertension and constricted renal-artery hypertension in rats. Circ. Res. 9:455, 1961.
13. Phelan, E. L., Eryetisher, I., and Smirk, F. H.: Observations on the responses of rats with spontaneous hypertension and control rats to pressor drugs and to hexamethonium. Circ. Res. 10:817, 1962.

14. Phelan, E. L.: Cardiovascular reactivity in rats with spontaneous inherited hypertension and constricted renal artery hypertension. Am. Heart J. 71:50, 1966.
15. Smirk, F. H.: The neurogenically maintained component in hypertension. Circ. Res. 27 (Suppl. 2):55, 1970.
16. Robertson, A. A., Hodge, J. V., Laverty, R., and Smirk, F. H.: Tissue catecholamine levels in normotensive, genetically hypertensive and renal hypertensive rats. Aust. J. Exp. Biol. Med. Sci. 46:689, 1968.
17. Restall, P. A., and Smirk, F. H., cited in Smirk, F. H.: The pathogenesis of essential hypertension. Br. Med. J. 2:23, 1949.
18. McQueen, E. G.: Vascular reactivity in experimental renal and renoprival hypertension. Clin. Sci. 15:523, 1956.
19. Laverty, R.: Increased vascular reactivity in rats with genetic hypertension. Proc. Univ. Otago Med. Sch. 39:23, 1961.
20. McGregor, D. D., and Smirk, F. H.: Vascular responses in mesenteric arteries from genetic and renal hypertensive rats. Am. J. Physiol. 214:1429, 1968.
21. McGregor, D. D., and Smirk, F. H.: Vascular responses to 5-hydroxytryptamine in genetic and renal hypertensive rats. Am. J. Physiol. 219:687, 1970.
22. Laverty, R., McGregor, D. D., and McQueen, E. G.: Vascular reactivity in experimental hypertension. N.Z. Med. J. 67:303, 1968.
23. Nolla-Panades, J., and Smirk, F. H.: Effect of bilateral adrenalectomy on the blood pressure of rats with spontaneous inherited hypertension. Australas. Ann. Med. 13:320, 1964.
24. Aoki, K.: Experimental studies on the relationship between endocrine organs and hypertension in spontaneously hypertensive rats. III. Role of the endocrine organs and hormones. Jap. Heart J. 5:57, 1964.
25. Sirette, N. E., and Smirk, F. H.: Unpublished observations.
26. Smirk, F. H.: Blood pressure in families: Preliminary communication. N.Z. Med. J. 71:355, 1970.
27. Smirk, F. H.: Unpublished observations.
28. Smirk, F. H.: Effect of added sodium chloride on genetic hypertensive and control rats. Proc. Univ. Otago Med. Sch. 41:29, 1963.

Genetic Pattern of Hypertension in Man

By Caroline Bedell Thomas, M.D.

In the previous chapter, Sir Horace Smirk described a form of hypertension in rats in which the hereditary factor is clear cut, and Dr. Dahl will present, in this part of the symposium, experimental evidence that the interaction of an environmental factor with a particular genetic endowment can result in severe and even lethal hypertension. In man, the genetic contribution to hypertension is much more difficult to evaluate.

One difficulty arises from the fact that the pathogenesis of hypertensive arterial disease itself is still obscure. We know that elevation of blood pressure may result from neurogenic, endocrine, renal, or psychogenic factors acting singly or in combination, but it is not yet determined whether "essential hypertension" is a unitary disorder in which the pathway from a specific cause to the end result, although complex, may ultimately be traced, or whether it embraces a number of pathogenetic configurations, some beginning in one area and some in another, so that there is no common genetic factor but rather multiple mechanisms. Another problem is that essential hypertension rarely exists in pure form, but is intertwined with atherosclerosis, particularly with coronary atherosclerosis, so that in real life one is usually observing a mixture of the two.

There is general agreement about the basic facts of blood pressure distribution in the populations of Western countries:

1. There are more values above the mean than below it, so that the frequency distribution of both systolic and diastolic pressure is skewed.
2. This skewing increases with age.
3. The blood pressure rise with age is greater in some individuals than others.
4. In a small proportion of the population, blood pressure does not rise at all with age.
5. There is a sex difference in blood pressure distribution. In youth, blood pressure is higher in males, whereas the rise with age is greater in females, so that after middle age, blood pressure is higher in females.[1]

First I shall discuss the main positions taken by leaders in the controversy concerning inheritance. One school of thought, of which the protagonist is Platt, believes that heredity is the main cause of essential hypertension. In his view, hypertension is a specific disorder of middle age reflecting the operation of a single autosomal gene. At first Platt postulated that this gene is dominant, so that there are two populations, one normotensive and one hypertensive.[2] In youth, the blood pressure distribution of the hypertensive population almost overlaps that of the normotensive population, accounting for the slight skewing or bulge to the right of the distribution curve. As blood pressure in the hypertensives rises with age, this skewing becomes more and more marked.

Morrison and Morris's study of London busmen supports this hypothesis.[3] Considering early death as a crude indication of the presence or absence of hypertension, they classified the busmen by their parents' length of life. The systolic blood pressure of bus drivers whose parents lived to old age (65 or over) showed a roughly normal distribution with a single peak, whereas that of bus drivers with a parent dead in middle age (40 to 64) showed a bimodal distribution. They considered that these findings fitted the single dominant gene hypothesis, since sons of a hypertensive parent would be expected to segregate into normotensive and hypertensive groups, while sons of normotensive parents would be mostly normotensive. More recently, Platt has modified his hypothesis.[4] According to his current theory, the gene for hypertension exhibits incomplete dominance, so that there are not two but three populations:

1. Those who do not inherit the hypertensive gene from either parent are homozygous for normotension; in them, blood pressure rises little if at all with increasing years.

From the Department of Medicine, The Johns Hopkins University School of Medicine, Baltimore, Maryland.

2. Those who inherit the hypertensive gene from one parent have the heterozygous form of hypertension; this results in a moderate elevation of blood pressure.

3. Those who inherit the hypertensive gene from both parents have the homozygous form of hypertension; this results in severe hypertension.

He supports his hypothesis with studies of the blood pressures in siblings of patients with severe hypertension and with twin studies.

The other viewpoint, championed by Pickering, considers that blood pressure is determined by a multiplicity of genetic and environmental factors, all more or less equal in importance and operating in a more or less independent fashion.[1,5] Thus, what is called essential hypertension represents, not a disease entity, but rather that section of the population with arterial pressures higher than an arbitrarily selected value and having no disease to which this pressure can be attributed. In Pickering's view, essential hypertension represents a quantitative rather than a qualitative deviation from the norm. Blood pressure is inherited as a graded characteristic like height, and the manner and degree of inheritance are the same whether the pressure is below the norm or far enough above it to constitute essential hypertension. Pickering emphasizes that there is no natural division between normal and abnormal pressures; any attempt to divide pressures sharply into normal and abnormal is artificial. Also, he considers that studies of family histories yield results of doubtful value, since these histories are usually indicative of structural arterial disease rather than pure hypertension.

To compare the arterial pressure of first-degree relatives of various ages and both sexes, Roberts devised an age- and sex-adjusted score, a numerical value for the extent to which an individual's arterial pressure exceeds or is less than the expected norm. Using this method, Hamilton et al., and later Miall and Oldham, found a positive correlation between the arterial pressure of index cases and their first-degree relatives.[6,7] From their data, they concluded that the inheritance of arterial pressure is quantitative, or polygenic. When they examined the relationship between index cases with severe hypertension and their first-degree relatives, however, they found a much smaller correlation, so that in the patients with the severest cases of hypertension they considered the contribution of inheritance to be smaller, not larger, than in the mildly affected patients and in the population at large. Thus Pickering infers that the role of environment is of exceptional importance in severe hypertension.

This conclusion seems open to criticism on several grounds:

1. The age- and sex-adjusted scores are based on the assumption that there is, in fact, only one population, for which the variances were plotted against age. If there were actually two or three populations, their divergence with age would lead to an increase in total variance. But the Roberts method "adjusts" for any change in variance, thus robbing us of a powerful test of the single-locus hypothesis.

2. Age and sex adjustment was made to age 60, one of two ages where the variance curves for systolic and diastolic pressures of the two sexes crossed. Since an appreciable proportion of the population dies of cardiovascular disease and other causes before age 60, the use of blood pressure means and variances from the residual population as a point for standardizing the age- and sex-adjusted scores is open to question. It would seem more reasonable to have adjusted the scores to age 25, the other age at which the variance curves for the two sexes crossed.

3. The smaller correlation between patients with severe hypertension and their first-degree relatives may result from the fact that the index cases were *selected* for severe hypertension. It is not surprising, therefore, that the blood pressures of relatives show a regression toward the mean. Also, all of the index cases with severe hypertension were necessarily living, whereas many first-degree relatives with the severest cardiovascular disease had undoubtedly died. When the blood pressure data for relatives of the propositi are examined, many of the parents were not represented.[4,5,7]

The controversy over the meaning of the shape of the distribution curves, which might be called the "Battle of the Bulge," has diminished somewhat. Platt[8] has conceded that the inheritance of hypertension might be multifactorial, although he is still convinced that heredity is paramount, while Pickering [1] is at a loss to explain the pathogenesis of the severest cases of hypertension on the basis of allelomorphic genes.

Murphy, Thomas, and Bolling explored the two hypotheses in some detail insofar as this is possible in young white males, but did not resolve the problem.[9] In a population of 1091 white male medical students, they found that both systolic and diastolic pressure showed positive skewness and excessive kurtosis, which were considerably reduced by logarithmic transformation. Theoretical statistical considerations led to the conclusion that blood pressure might well be determined by the combined effects of a considerable number of factors, no one of them dominating, the effects compounding multiplicatively. However, the competing hypothesis, that there is one main factor operating in the midst of a number of minor sources of "noise," is also a possibility, since there might be two normal distributions with different means, the smaller of them being concealed in the upper part of the larger curve. Judged by the systolic pressure, about 74 percent of the population was in one curve, 25 percent in the other. The means calculated for the resting blood pressure of the left-hand population were 112.8 mm Hg systolic and 69.4 mm Hg diastolic and for the right-hand population were 118.5 and 73.8 mm Hg. These relatively small differences in mean pressure for the two groups in youth may well increase markedly toward middle life when clinical hypertension becomes recognizable.

Now let us consider other approaches to the question of inherited hypertension in man. Twin studies have shown a high degree of correlation between the blood pressure levels of monozygotic twins. Smirk's plot of the systolic and diastolic pressures of identical twins, based on reports by different investigators, gives striking visual proof of their resemblance.[10] Blood pressures of dizygotic twins show much lower correlations. More recently, Platt has reported strong concordance of blood pressure in three sets of identical twins with severe essential hypertension.[4]

Our own findings are based on carefully obtained family histories. As part of the Study of the Precursors of Hypertension and Coronary Heart Disease, we have studied the occurrence of hypertension in three generations: a population of former medical students, now physicians; their parents, aunts, and uncles; and their grandparents.[11]

Detailed studies were reported in 1955, when the index population consisted of 262 Johns Hopkins medical students at a mean age of 25.5 years. The 532 parents were at a mean age of 55; over 90 percent were living. There were 1,595 parental siblings; the mean age of those living was also 55 years, but 7 percent of parental siblings had died between the ages of 18 and 40 whereas only 1 percent of parents had died so young. Those dying under age 40 were classified as "unknown." Seventeen percent of the 1,064 grandparents were living; the mean age for grandparents, living and dead, was 70 years. Comparison of the ages of affected and unaffected parents and grandparents did not show conspicuous differences. Diagnoses were primarily based on physicians' statements and death certificates.

Hypertensive parents had more than twice as much hypertension among their siblings as normotensive parents (Fig. 1). Where hypertension and coronary disease or both were treated as a single disorder, the pattern was

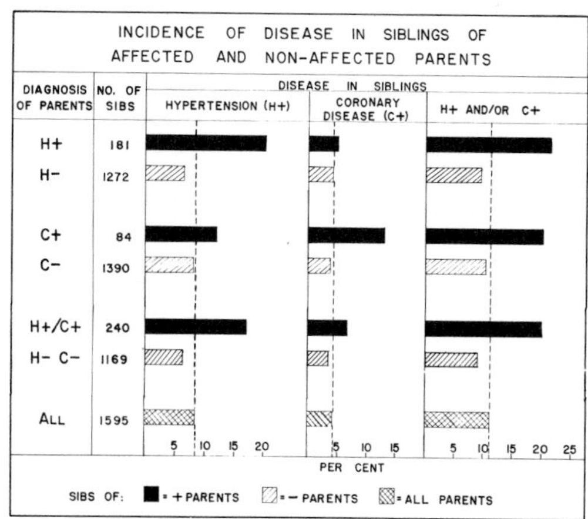

FIG. 1.—Incidence of hypertension, coronary artery disease, and the two disorders combined among the siblings of affected and unaffected parents of medical students. The **broken lines** indicate the percentage incidence for each disorder in the total population of siblings. (From Thomas, C. B., and Cohen, B. H.,[11] with permission.)

similar. This method of classification most accurately divides the population into those affected by and those free from arterial cardiovascular disease. In this figure, the many highly significant comparisons point to the fact that siblings of individuals *with* hypertension or coronary artery disease or both are affected more often by some form of these disorders than are siblings of unaffected individuals.

We then compared the occurrence of hypertension in two generations according to three types of mating in the grandparents' generation (Fig. 2). According to whether both, one or neither grandparent had hypertension, there was a significant descending gradation in the prevalence of hypertension in their offspring (the parents, aunts, and uncles of the medical students). When hypertension and coronary disease were considered together as one disorder, this gradation was even more striking. No gradation in the opposite direction was found in any of the comparisons. This gradation in disorder rates among the offspring of three types of mating is consistent with the Mendelian law of segregation, in that the greatest proportion of affected persons was always found among the offspring of two affected persons and the smallest proportion among the offspring of two unaffected individuals. However, a like effect would occur with a polygenic pattern of inheritance.

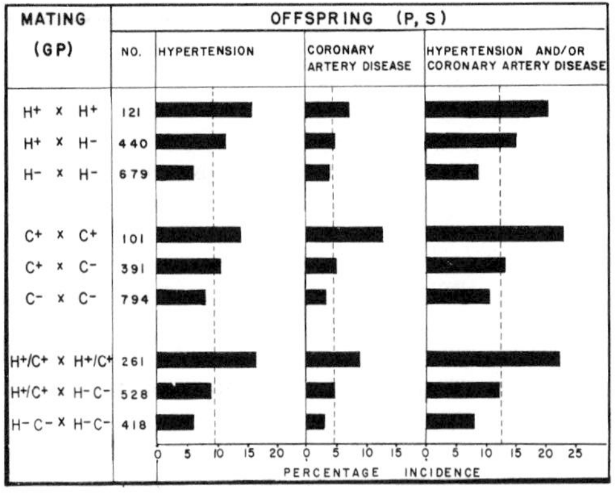

FIG. 2.—The comparative incidence of hypertension and coronary artery disease, and the two disorders combined among the offspring of three types of mating: both marital partners affected, one partner affected, and neither partner affected. In this two-generation comparison, data for the three types of mating came from the grandparents' generation (**GP**); their offspring were the parents of the medical students and the parental siblings (**P, S**). The **broken lines** indicate the percentage incidence for each disorder in the total population of offspring. (From Thomas, C. B., and Cohen, B. H.,[11] with permission.)

At the end of these early analyses, in which my colleague Bernice H. Cohen played an important role, we examined the findings to see if they were consistent with any simple genetic pattern. Comparisons were made of the observed disorder rates among the offspring of the three types of mating and the rates to be expected in the presence of a single dominant gene or a single recessive gene. Theoretical values were derived by Snyder's formula which applied population methods to genetic analysis. The estimated corrected incidences in the grandparents' generation were used as the best basis for the gene frequency values. A correction factor which took into account the disparity in age between the generations was applied so that theoretical values might be comparable to observed values in the offspring at an age when expression was not yet complete. None of the sets of observed values showed a very good fit with the corresponding expected values, however, whether calculated on the basis of a dominant or a recessive gene. The application of Snyder's formula was therefore inconclusive, neither verifying nor disproving the presence of a single autosomal gene for hypertension. In view of its apparent relationship to coronary disease, also a familial disorder, a more complex etiology, possibly involving multiple genetic factors with modifying environmental agents, was suggested.

In a two-generation comparison of the subjects themselves and their parents, medical students at a mean age of 23 were grouped on the basis of parental hypertension.[12] When the blood pressures of offspring of two affected parents, one affected parent, and two unaffected parents were compared, a significant descending gradation was found in regard to both systolic and diastolic pressure levels. Fourteen subjects with two hypertensive parents had mean resting pressures of 121.9 systolic and 70.6 mm Hg diastolic, whereas 377 students with two normotensive parents had mean pressures of 112.9 and 68.6 mm Hg respectively (Table 1). Those with one hypertensive par-

TABLE 1.—*Mean Resting Blood Pressure of Medical Students with Different Parental Histories*

History of Parental Hypertension	*Number of Subjects*	*Systolic Pressure*	*Diastolic Pressure*
Both parents affected	14	121.9	70.6
One parent affected	194	114.6	70.2
Neither parent affected	377	112.9	68.6
p		<.005	<.05

ent had the intermediate values of 114.6 and 70.2 mm Hg. The difference in systolic pressure was highly significant at the 0.005 level, whereas the difference in diastolic pressure was significant at the 0.05 level.

In 1969, we reported preliminary findings on 16 subjects who developed doctor-diagnosed hypertension at a mean age of 36.5 years.[13] Forty-four percent of their parents had been hypertensive, in contrast to 14 percent of the parents of their age-matched controls. Thus these two-generation comparisons of parents and subjects support the grandparent-parental generation findings. When the resting blood pressure of the future hypertensives (then in medical school) was plotted against norms for the entire student population, 13 of the 16 fell in the high range, that is, above the 80th percentile, or fourth quintile (Fig. 3). Nevertheless, their resting pressures at that time did not seem impressive, since the 80th percentile fell at 120 mm Hg for systolic and at 75 mm Hg for diastolic pressure. Only one of the 16 future hypertensives had had both systolic and diastolic pressures above the 90th percentile; his blood pressure was 132/82.

As an example of the impossibility of separating hypertension from coronary artery disease in some instances, let me cite a pair of identical twins whose hypertensive cardiovascular disease was well documented (Table 2). Twin A was my patient for most of the last 6 years of his life. The history of Twin B, who lived at a distance, was obtained from his physicians, family members, and the autopsy report.

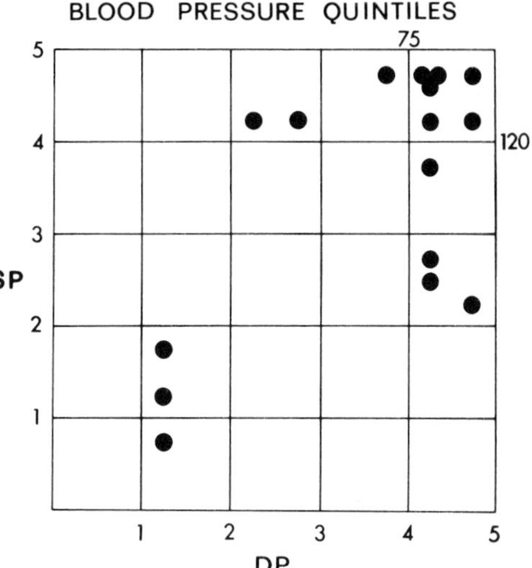

FIG. 3.—The resting blood pressures in medical school of 16 subjects who later developed clinical hypertension plotted against the norms for 1082 white male medical students. The fourth quintiles (80th percentiles) fall at 120 mm Hg systolic pressure (**SP**) and 75 mm Hg diastolic pressure (**DP**). (From Thomas, C. B.,[13] with permission.)

The twins' family history was remarkable. Their father had had severe hypertension in his late 30s, suffered a stroke at 40, and died of a second stroke 2 months later. Their mother, now 71, has had benign hypertension for over 30 years. The twins' only sibling, a brother 5 years younger, has also had benign hypertension since around the age of 30; now 42, he is doing well on antihypertensive treatment, but developed mild diabetes at 38. Hypertension and diabetes are said to "run in the family" on both the paternal and maternal sides; the twins' maternal aunt is said to be dying of diabetes mellitus.

The twins were always unusually healthy and vigorous, excelling in football and other sports in high school and college. At age 18, on his college entrance physical examination, Twin A was told he had elevated blood pressure; he was hospitalized for study, but no cause for his hypertension was found. Nonetheless, at 19, both twins were inducted into the United States Air Force, attended Officers Candidate School, and became lieutenants. In 1946, at age 22, their discharge physical examinations on the same day showed that their heights were identi-

TABLE 2.—*Life Histories of Identical Twins*

Age	*Circumstances*	*Twin A*	*Twin B*
18	College entry	Hypertension	Normal
19	Entered U.S.A.F.	B.P. suspect	Normal
22	Discharge P.E. from U.S.A.F.	B.P. 124/86; Ht. 65 inches Wt. 156	B.P. 136/80; Ht. 65 inches Wt. 169
36	Intensive chemotherapy started	B.P. 234/170; malignant hypertension	B.P. 260/140; asymptomatic hypertension
41–39		Hemiparesis	Myocardial infarction
42–43	Actively working Postmortem	Sudden death Coronary occlusion	Sudden death Coronary occlusion

Abbreviations used: B.P., blood pressure; Ht., height; P.E., physical examination; Wt., weight.

cal and their blood pressures, which were very similar, were in the high normal range.

On returning to college and afterward, Twin A had repeated difficulties on physical examinations because of transitory blood pressure elevation, but got by each hurdle until age 32, when he was finally turned down for life insurance. Twin B was also turned down for insurance because of hypertension at about the same time. During the next 4 years, both were started on antihypertensive therapy but lapsed because they felt so well. Then, at age 36,

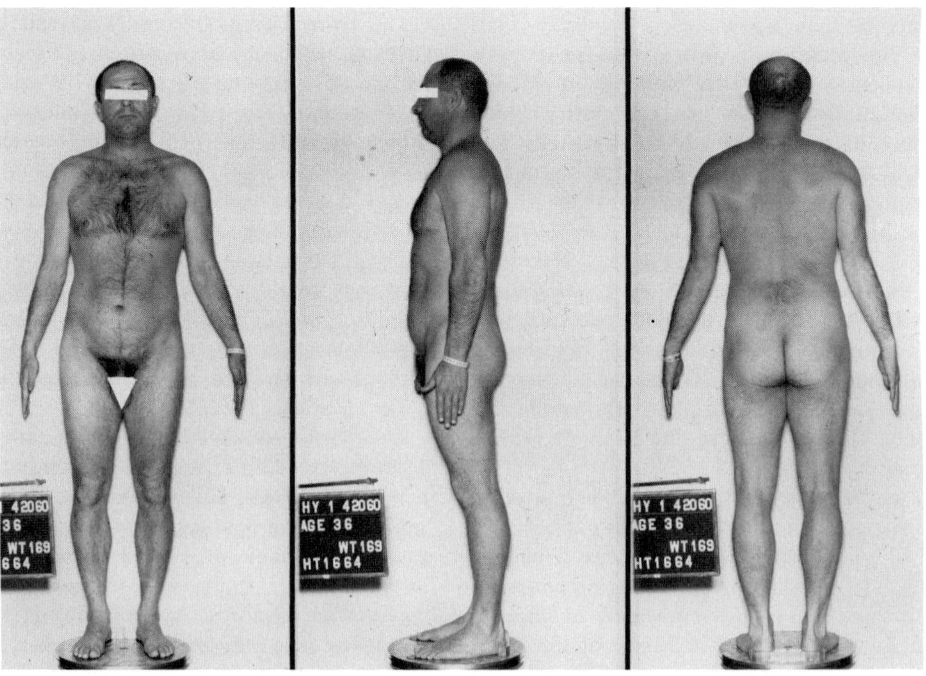

FIG. 4.—Constitutional photograph of Twin A at age 36. Somatotype dominant mesomorphy, 4–6–1.

Twin A developed blurred vision and retinal hemorrhages and was found to have malignant hypertension. Learning this, Twin B, still asymptomatic, returned to his physician, who found that Twin B, too, had severe hypertension. From then on, the excessively high blood pressure levels of both twins were reduced by vigorous antihypertensive therapy. Both twins had hypercholesteremia, with cholesterol levels over 300 mg per 100 ml on repeated occasions. Both were overweight; both were mesomorphic (Fig. 4). Both were fathers of large families, hard workers, and heavy cigarette smokers.

At 41, Twin A had transitory hemiparesis, but soon was working as hard as ever. Eight months later, at age 42, he died instantly at home, having disregarded pain down his left arm 4 days before. Twin B had recovered from a myocardial infarction at 39 but had died suddenly at age 43 while on an automobile trip. Coronary occlusion was confirmed at postmortem examination in both twins.

It is hard to avoid the conclusion that there is a large hereditary component in this constellation of disorders. Nevertheless, the problem remains: in these twins, and in others like them, is one dealing with a single disorder or several? Does one gene and its alleles control blood pressure while others independently control hypercholesteremia, body build, coronary artery disease, obesity, and diabetes, or is there a more fundamental genetic defect which, in some individuals, controls this whole spectrum of appearances? In our family studies, hypertension was found to occur in various combinations with coronary disease, obesity, and diabetes in the same individual from 2 to 10 times as often as would be expected by chance.[11] In a different disorder, Cushing's syndrome, combinations of hypertension, obesity, diabetes, coronary disease, and hypercholesteremia are frequently found without being thought of as separate disease entities.

In the end, I must conclude that our knowledge of genetic patterns in hypertension is far from complete. From the evidence, the case for inheritance is strong, but the mode of inheritance remains uncertain. In severe hypertension, genes governing blood pressure may interact with genes governing lipid levels, so that a vicious circle is created—as blood pressure rises, atherosclerosis increases, and as arteries become narrower, higher blood pressure levels ensue. Quite possibly, there are several major causes of essential hypertension rather than one. Not until these problems are solved will patterns of inheritance be clearly understood.

References

1. Pickering, G.: High Blood Pressure. New York: Grune & Stratton, 1968.
2. Platt, R.: Heredity in hypertension. Q. J. Med. 16:111, 1947.
3. Morrison, S. L., and Morris, J. N.: Epidemiological observations on high blood-pressure without evident cause. Lancet 2:864, 1959.
4. Platt, R.: Heredity in hypertension. Lancet 1:899, 1963.
5. Hamilton, M., Pickering, G. W., Roberts, J. A. F., and Sowry, G. S. C.: The aetiology of essential hypertension. 4. The role of inheritance. Clin. Sci. 13:273, 1954.
6. Hamilton, M., Pickering, G. W., Roberts, J. A. F., and Sowry, G. S. C.: The aetiology of essential hypertension. 2. Scores for arterial blood pressures adjusted for differences in age and sex. Clin. Sci. 13:37, 1954.
7. Miall, W. E., and Oldham, P. D.: A study of arterial blood pressure and its inheritance in a sample of the general population. Clin. Sci. 14:459, 1955.
8. Platt, R.: The natural history and epidemiology of essential hypertension. Practitioner 193:5, 1964.
9. Murphy, E. A., Thomas, C. B., and Bolling, D. R.: The precursors of hypertension and coronary disease: Statistical consideration of distributions in a population of medical students. II. Blood pressure. Johns Hopkins Med. J. 120:1, 1967.
10. Smirk, F. H.: High Arterial Pressure. Springfield, Illinois: Thomas, 1957.
11. Thomas, C. B., and Cohen, B. H.: The familial occurrence of hypertension and coronary artery disease with observations concerning obesity and diabetes. Ann. Intern. Med. 42: 90, 1955.
12. Thomas, C. B., Ross, D. C., and Higinbothom, C. Q.: Precursors of hypertension and coronary disease among healthy medical students: Discriminant function analysis. II. Using parental history as the criterion. Bull. Johns Hopkins Hosp. 115:246, 1964.
13. Thomas, C. B.: Developmental patterns in hypertensive cardiovascular disease: Fact or fiction? Bull. N. Y. Acad. Med. (Second Series) 45:831, 1969.

Epidemiology of Essential Hypertension: A Survey of Significance

By Arthur Grollman, Ph.D., M.D.

LIKE MANY OTHER WORDS, "epidemiology" has changed in meaning over the years. Originally the term was defined as "that branch of medical science which treats of epidemics," [1] but it is now considered to be "a science that deals with the incidence, distribution, and control of disease in a population" [2] regardless of the nature of the disease. It has also been defined as "the field of science dealing with the relationships of the various factors which determine the frequencies and distributions of an infectious process, a disease, or a physiological state in a human community." [3] This definition also may require further modification to include "a critical evaluation of measures directed at the treatment of disease as well as its prevention and, therefore, by implication the study of its prognosis." [4] The common feature underlying all epidemiologic techniques remains their dependence on the group rather than upon the individual or the cell as the working unit.[5]

Most epidemiologic surveys of hypertension have included any condition characterized by an elevation in blood pressure as within the domain of their interest rather than limiting themselves to a consideration of the disease entity—hypertensive cardiovascular disease. Such surveys, accordingly, suffer from the fact that they deal with a hemodynamic variable rather than with a disease entity and hence are of limited significance insofar as essential hypertension is concerned. To attain more meaningful results one must limit oneself to a consideration of a specific disease.[6]

The present chapter deals primarily with the incidence, distribution, and clinical course of essential hypertension as they bear on the pathogenesis of this disorder and its relation to other disorders associated with an elevation in blood pressure.

A small percentage of the patients considered formerly to be suffering from essential hypertension have been shown to owe their elevated blood pressure to such surgically remediable disorders as chromaphil cell tumors, hyperaldosteronism, renovascular abnormalities, etc. It has been suggested, therefore, that essential hypertension represents a pathogenetically heterogeneous group of disorders rather than a single entity. There is a mass of clinical and experimental evidence to indicate, however, that this is not the case and that essential hypertension does represent a disease entity amenable to definition.[6,7] Although the diagnosis of essential hypertension in its incipient stages may be difficult, the disorder has certain unique clinical and pathologic features which make it recognizable, at least in its more advanced stages.

Clinically, essential hypertension is characterized by an elevated systolic and diastolic pressure which is insidious in its development but is apparent in many patients during childhood.[8–10] In its more advanced stage it is accompanied by a normal cardiac output; the elevated blood pressure is accordingly due to an increased peripheral resistance.[11] (See the chapter entitled "Hemodynamic Alterations in Essential Hypertension.") During most of its course, essential hypertension is accompanied by no apparent symptoms of complaint; only in the later stages with the onset of cardiac, cerebral, and renal failure do physical manifestations of the disorder appear.

The diagnosis of essential hypertension has been applied only to patients with no evidence of renal disease, but it is our opinion that it, like the so-called "secondary hypertension" of chronic glomerulonephritis and other renal diseases, is also renal in origin. Both are ascribable to the loss of that function of the kidney which is concerned in the maintenance of the normotensive state.[12] Hypertension of renal

From the Laboratory for Experimental Medicine, Department of Pathology, University of Texas Southwestern Medical School, Dallas, Texas.

Aided by Grant 71–1113 from the American Heart Association and the Lilien K. Christy Bequest.

origin may also arise, however, from conditions which cause the kidney to secrete a pressor agent.[13] This form of hypertension differs in its clinical features from the other types and is remediable by removal of the affected kidney or correction of the vascular or other defect responsible for its appearance.

The characteristics of essential hypertension which permit its recognition are cardiac enlargement and arteriolar sclerosis, the pathologic hallmarks of the disease. There is accordingly no difficulty in identifying the patient with essential hypertension at autopsy without any knowledge as to his blood pressure during life.

Experimental studies have contributed greatly to establishing essential hypertension as a disease entity secondary to kidney dysfunction. Not only has it been possible to reproduce the disease in various species of laboratory animals by manipulation of the kidney, but colonies of hypertensive rats and rabbits have been developed by selective inbreeding which follow the same clinical course and manifest the hemodynamic and pathologic features of essential hypertension as it occurs spontaneously in the human being.[14–16] (See the chapter entitled "Salt, Heredity and Hypertension.")

Diagnosis

To obtain useful epidemiologic data, exact diagnosis of the disease is obviously necessary. In the case of essential hypertension this involves several difficulties. Not only is the taking of the blood pressure subject to considerable error [17] but the lability of this hemodynamic variable, the fact that it is elevated in a variety of physiologic and pathologic conditions, and other factors render the blood pressure alone an inadequate indicator of the presence or severity of essential hypertension.[6] It is not surprising, therefore, that an elevation in blood pressure in the absence of renal excretory insufficiency as the criterion for diagnosing the disorder has furnished conflicting epidemiologic data.

In our present state of knowledge it is impossible to diagnose essential hypertension with certainty prior to the appearance of structural complications of the disease. Arbitrarily, certain levels of blood pressure have been adopted as criteria for establishing the diagnosis. Incipient and mild hypertension are excluded, while subjects with an elevated blood pressure from other causes are included in the survey. Anxiety and emotional disturbances may be associated with appreciable increases in the blood pressure and give rise to so-called labile hypertension which may remain unaltered over many years. Arteriosclerosis involving the smaller arteries and arterioles may increase the peripheral resistance sufficiently to induce an elevated diastolic pressure and thus mimic essential hypertension insofar as the level of the blood pressure is concerned.[18] When essential hypertension has developed to a degree in which its diagnosis may be established with relative certainty, complications—particularly myocardial insufficiency and arteriosclerosis—appear which complicate the clinical picture. Arteriosclerosis, in particular, whether primary or secondary to hypertension may initiate, if it involves the kidney, a vicious cycle so that one is dealing with a combination of two diseases—i.e., hypertension and atherosclerosis—rather than with a single entity.[19]

Despite the above-mentioned vitiating factors, epidemiologic studies have yielded data which confirm the concepts regarding the pathogenesis of hypertension as derived from many experimental and clinical studies, contributed to a better understanding of essential hypertension, and suggested approaches to its therapeutic management.

Genetic Factors

There is a strong hereditary predisposition to the development of hypertension. Platt,[20] for example, showed that 40 percent of siblings of patients with severe essential hypertension had a diastolic pressure above 110 mm Hg. Experimental studies suggest that environmental influences during fetal life may also induce the disorder.[21] Dietary, toxic, and other environmental factors during postnatal life may induce renal changes and the development of essential hypertension.[22,23] Pyelonephritis and other disturbances of the kidney may also give rise to hypertension and be mistakenly diagnosed as essential hypertension. Reliance on the blood pressure alone in the absence of urinary changes for the diagnosis may thus lead to the inclusion of other forms of renal hypertension in epidemiologic surveys of essential hypertension.

A genetic tendency to essential hypertension is not only present in the human being but also in other animals.[14–16] The total variation of hypertension from inherited genetic causes is estimated to be 33 percent in the human, 15 percent in rats, and 20 percent in mice. There is some controversy regarding the number of loci concerned in hypertension in the human. Platt [20] suggested that a single dominant gene determines the presence of the disease and the variation in blood pressure. Pickering [24] views the disorder as a quantitative deviation rather than as a unique entity. He considers the hypertensive population as being at the upper range of a Gaussian distribution curve, the inheritance of which is polygenic and the expression of which depends on environmental factors. Epidemiologic studies in human populations have been conducted primarily on the assumption of a polygenic inheritance but the available evidence indicates that this assumption may be erroneous.

Schlager [25] found that after four generations of selection in mice, the mean blood pressure changes which he observed could not be due to different alleles at the same locus since the selected genotype was the same. He concluded that different alleles contributed to the original gene pool and that on the basis of the genetic selection theory the difference between mean systolic blood pressure of the two inbred strains of mice was due to the action of at least three loci.

In man, the hereditary mechanism for essential hypertension is not explicable by multifactorial inheritance or by the action of a single dominant gene but is best explained as a result of the action of a single gene with incomplete dominance and a frequency of about 0.24. In its homozygous form, severe hypertension results; in the heterozygous form, a more moderate degree of the disease occurs.[20] Offspring of parents both of whom suffer from essential hypertension develop the most intense form of the disease.

In support of the hereditary nature of essential hypertension are observations on its incidence in twins. Prevalence of the disease in identical-twin samples resembles that in the population at large and its ultimate development is heavily dependent on genetic influences with an increased concordance of hypertension in monozygotic twins.[26–28] The occasional occurrence of hypertension in only one of identical twins may be attributed to its nongenetic environmental acquisition.[29]

Incidence and Racial Distribution

If essential hypertension is an inherited genetic disorder with environmental factors also playing a role in its pathogenesis, one would anticipate that the incidence of the disease would vary in different population groups. Despite the difficulties attending such studies,[5,17,30,31] epidemiologic surveys indicate that this is indeed the case. The Cuni Indians of the San Blas Islands, the Melanesian Gaus of Fiji, the Micronesian Abiangs of the Gilbert Islands, certain natives of New Guinea, and other small aboriginal groups appear to be free of essential hypertension.[32–35]

Much attention has been directed to the incidence of hypertension in the Negro in Africa and his descendants in the Western hemisphere. Since the Africans are not racially homogeneous it is not surprising that the incidence of hypertension among them should vary. Thus the incidence of hypertension in Kenya is low [36,37] but high among the Bantu and West Africans.[38] It is reported as being only moderately increased among rural Nigerians [39] but high in the natives of Uganda and central and south Africa.[40] The fact that the incidence of hypertension is essentially the same in the Congo,[41] where the American Negro originated, as in his descendants in the Caribbean islands, Central America, and the United States,[42–44] is strong evidence of the importance of genetic rather than environmental influences on the incidence of essential hypertension. There is also a positive correlation between the blood pressure and pigmentation of the American Negro as measured by skin reflectance.[45]

The increased incidence of hypertension in the American Negro, a minority in an economically advanced society, must be considered as genetically determined rather than as a result of environmental influences. The Maoris, who also comprise a minority of a population that is otherwise of European ancestry, manifest blood pressures which are similar to those of other New Zealanders.[17]

The incidence of essential hypertension in Caucasians is about 5 to 7 percent as opposed to about 20 to 30 percent in the American Negro. The suggestion that part of this difference between Negroes and white races is attributable to anxiety of Negroes when faced with a medical examination is scarcely tenable in view of the autopsy data and the fact that hypertensive heart disease diagnosed on electrocardiographic and radiographic criteria is more common among Negroes than among Caucasians.[42,45] The relative incidence of hypertension in three racial groups residing in Panama—Caucasian, Negro, and San Blas Indian—is about 5, 30, and zero percent, respectively, but is increased by acquired renal infection absent in the San Blas Indian living on his native islands.[46]

Role of Salt Intake in Pathogenesis of Hypertension

The fact that drastic restriction of sodium intake reduces the blood pressure in both man and the experimental animal [47] and that the administration of large doses of salt accelerates development of hypertension in animals [48] has suggested that differences in dietary sodium may contribute to differences in the incidence of hypertension.[49] Epidemiologic observations have led to divergent results: some indicating that a habitually high-salt intake is accompanied by a high incidence of hypertension in certain populations, while others show no correlation between the salt intake and the level of the blood pressure.[50,51]

In two South Pacific Polynesian populations, Prior et al.[52] found that although their observations were compatible with the hypothesis that a high-salt intake and high blood pressure are related, other differences between the two groups could explain the observed variation in the incidence of essential hypertension in the two populations.

Behavioral Factors in Pathogenesis of Hypertension

The fact that psychologic stimuli provoke a marked rise in mean arterial blood pressure suggested that behavioral factors might play a role in the pathogenesis of hypertension. The physical and intellectual activity and the stresses of normal daily life cause an elevation of the arterial blood pressure but this subsides quickly and represents simply a hemodynamic homeostatic alteration. It would not necessarily follow that stimuli which activate somatomotor, visceral, and endocrine adaptive responses should induce a permanent elevation in blood pressure. There is, in fact, pertinent evidence to indicate that anxiety and other repeated stimuli in neither the experimental animal nor in man lead to chronic hypertension.[53,54]

In the early stages of essential hypertension, before one is able to diagnose the presence of the disease with certainty, a greater rise in blood pressure may follow a given stimulus than in the normal, but neurotic individuals may also respond in a similar way and nevertheless do not develop hypertension over the course of many years.[53] The discrepancy in the available data is attributable to the inability to differentiate so-called "labile" hypertension in the individual with incipient stages of the disease from the rise caused by psychogenic factors. The same objection may be raised to the finding of some increased cardiac outputs in early labile hypertension. That such elevations in blood pressure and cardiac output occur in response to psychogenic stimuli has long been known [55] but unless such patients are followed over many years and demonstrated to develop essential hypertension, the conclusion that these elevations represent an early stage of this disease is unjustified.

Clinical Considerations

Epidemiologic studies of certain clinical features of essential hypertension have yielded data which contribute to a better understanding of the nature of the disease and approaches to its management.[6,56,57]

Age and Sex

Essential hypertension usually does not manifest itself at birth but first appears at age 20 to 60 depending on its severity. In patients with a severe degree of the disease the elevation in blood pressure and complications of the disease become evident at a young age and even during childhood or adolescence.[8–10] In most populations, the systolic and diastolic pressures rise with age with a more rapid rate of increase in the systolic level after the age of 50 and a positive skewness of the frequency-distribution curve.[58] This phenomenon is attributable to the increase in severity of atherosclerosis with age.

In populations in which both essential hypertension and atherosclerosis are infrequent, the blood pressure declines with age [35,58] as a result of decreased cardiovascular activity.[55] The changes in blood pressure with age, observed when normotensive, atherosclerotic, and hypertensive individuals are included (as is usually the case in epidemiologic studies), will result in overlapping skewed curves which have no significance insofar as the natural history of essential hypertension is concerned.[59–61]

The available data on the effect of sex on the level of the blood pressure and on the prognosis in hypertension is complicated by the different incidence of atherosclerosis in the two sexes. In early adult life, the blood pressure tends to be lower in women than in men. After the age of 45 when atherosclerosis becomes more pronounced in the female, there is a steep rise in blood pressure and the mean pressure becomes higher in women than in men. In general, the trend for diastolic pressure is the same in men and women till early middle age.

Prognosis

Actuarial tables indicate that an elevation in blood pressure of moderate or severe degree with or without symptoms carries a large risk of complications, particularly of stroke and heart failure, regardless of whether the elevation be diastolic, due to hypertensive disease, or systolic, secondary to atherosclerosis.[62] The highest mortality rate is found in the group with the highest systolic and lowest diastolic pressures. In this group the mortality exceeds that in the group with an elevation in both systolic and diastolic pressure of only a moderate degree. The explanation for this apparent anomaly, which is confirmed in the Framingham study,[63,64] is to be found in the fact that the high systolic and low diastolic pressure reflects a high degree of atherosclerosis. Bechgaard [57] found that a diastolic pressure over 100 mm Hg in men and 110 mm Hg in women under the age of 40, or over 105 mm Hg in men and 115 mm Hg in women over 40, was associated with a mortality 2.5 times that of normotensives of the corresponding age.

Despite the poor prognosis presented in the above-cited data, untreated patients with essential hypertension may have a mean life span of about 20 years after the onset of the disease.[56] In fact, the casually obtained blood pressure has little prognostic value; patients with marked elevation in blood pressure often survive for more than 35 years with a period of uncomplicated disease lasting about 15 years before organic complications appear.[65] About 74 percent of these complications are cardiac, 42 percent renal, and 32 percent retinal; with more than half of the subjects dying of heart disease—usually congestive heart failure— 10 to 15 percent of cerebrovascular accidents, and 10 percent of renal failure.[56,66,67] Malignant hypertension occurs in less than 5 percent.[68]

Effects of Treatment

It is obviously difficult to determine the significance of therapy in essential hypertension which has a variable and at times good prognosis. Since atherosclerosis contributes to the high mortality of patients with an elevated blood pressure, it is impossible in most patients to decide whether death was due to essential hypertension or the associated atherosclerosis.

No treatment is available which counteracts the basic defect responsible for essential hypertension. It is now widely believed, however, that use of the drugs which lower the blood pressure results in a prolonged survival and mitigation of the complications of essential hypertension.[69,70] Treatment is of unquestioned value in prolonging survival in malignant hypertension and is probably of value in hypertensive encephalopathy and congestive heart failure associated with hypertension. In malignant hypertension 1-year survival has increased from less than 20 percent to 50 to 80 percent and 5-year survival from less than 1 percent to 20 to 50 percent.[68,71] Necropsy reveals healing of the necrotizing arteriolitis characteristic of the malignant phase of hypertension.[72]

The most encouraging data in support of the

beneficial effect of lowering the blood pressure have been obtained in a cooperative study by the United States Veterans Administration.[73] In this study, the risk of developing a morbid event over a 5-year period was reduced from 55 to 18 percent by treatment of patients with diastolic blood pressures averaging 90 to 114 mm Hg. The degree of benefit was related to the level of the prerandomization blood pressure. Terminating morbid events occurred in 35 patients of the control as compared to nine in the treated group. Treatment was more effective in preventing congestive heart failure and stroke than in preventing the complications of coronary artery disease.

Aurell and Hood,[74] in a smaller series of uncontrolled patients, and Hamilton,[75] in a controlled trial, have also claimed to have reduced mortality and morbidity from stroke but not from ischemic heart disease in hypertensive men and women under 65. On the other hand, a review of the literature by Dickinson [76] led him to conclude that the medical treatment of hypertension has not affected the death rate from strokes; in many series, stroke as a specific cause of death in hypertension was actually increased considerably, despite the prevention of death from cardiac and renal failure.

Active treatment has caused a virtual disappearance of the previous dominant cause of death, congestive failure, and sharply diminished uremia as a cause of death, whereas myocardial infarction remains frequent. Cerebrovascular accident has apparently increased sharply, accounting for 46 percent of deaths,[74–77] except in the Veterans Administration study.[73] It is difficult to know whether drug treatment actually provokes cerebral infarction [76] or whether it increases the proportion of deaths due to stroke simply by preventing other complications.

Conclusions

Despite the difficulties attending epidemiologic studies of essential hypertension, certain conclusions may be drawn from the available data. Such studies indicate that essential hypertension represents a clinical entity which in most cases is an inherited congenital disorder with a variable racial incidence. Environmental influences may play an etiologic role through teratogenic influences during fetal life and by postnatal influences which affect the kidney, particularly in those predisposed to the disease.

Epidemiologic studies give no support for the theory that essential hypertension is a consequence of acculturation or of such environmental influences as economic status, climate, or psychogenic stress. There is no evidence to indicate that essential hypertension represents a Pavlovian-conditioned, persistent alarm reaction, or that it is caused by alterations in baroreceptor or other neurogenic cardiovascular regulators or to the presence of renin or circulating pressor agents. There is also no valid evidence to indicate that the sex hormones are concerned in its development. Although a given level of blood pressure has a graver prognostic significance in the male than in the female, the average age of death in both sexes is essentially the same. The development of hypertension secondarily to eclampsia has been attributed to an autoimmune reaction affecting the kidney.[78]

There is good evidence to indicate that lowering of the blood pressure by the available drugs greatly prolongs life in malignant hypertension and mitigates the complications of the disease. The available methods of treatment, however, leave much to be desired and must await the availability of therapeutic measures which counter the basic defect responsible for the disease rather than merely mitigate one of its manifestations, viz., the elevated blood pressure.

References

1. Murray, J. A. H.: A New English Dictionary on Historical Principles. Oxford: Clarendon Press, 1897.
2. Webster's Third New International Dictionary. Springfield, Mass.: Merriam, 1967.
3. Maxcy, K. F.: *In* Dorland's Medical Dictionary, 23rd ed. Philadelphia: Saunders, 1963, p. 459.
4. Acheson, E. D.: Epidemiology. Br. Med. Bull. 27:1, 1971.
5. Clark, E. G.: An epidemiologic approach to the study of essential hypertension. *In* A Symposium on Essential Hypertension: An Epidemiologic Approach to the Elucidation of Its Natural History in Man. Boston: Wright & Proctor, 1951, pp. 17–20.

6. Grollman, A.: The natural history of essential hypertension. Cardiovasc. Clin. 1:1, 1969.
7. Grollman, A.: A unitary concept of experimental and clinical hypertensive cardiovascular disease. Perspect. Biol. Med. 2:208, 1959.
8. Takeuchi, J.: Etiology of juvenile hypertension. Jap. Circ. J. 30:178, 1966.
9. Londe, S., Bourgoignie, J. J., Robson, A. M., and Goldring, D.: Hypertension in apparently normal children. J. Pediat. 78:569, 1971.
10. Zinner, S. H., Levy, P. S., and Kass, E. H.: Familial aggregation of blood pressure in childhood. N. Engl. J. Med. 284:401, 1971.
11. Finkielman, S., Worcel, M., and Agrest, A.: Hemodynamic patterns in essential hypertension. Circulation 31:356, 1965.
12. Grollman, A.: The pathogenesis of hypertensive cardiovascular disease. Acta Clin. Belg. 18:183, 1963.
13. Grollman, A.: Pathogenesis of hypertension and implications for its therapeutic management. Clin. Pharmacol. Ther. 10:755, 1969.
14. Smirk, F. H., and Hall, W. H.: Inherited hypertension in rats. Nature 182:727, 1958.
15. Okamoto, K. and Kyuzo, A.: Development of a strain of spontaneously hypertensive rats. Jap. Circ. J. 27:282, 1963.
16. Alexander, N., Tibbs, W. J., and Drury, D. R.: Cold pressor responses in family responses of rabbits with spontaneous hypertension. Proc. Soc. Exp. Biol. Med. 95:356, 1957.
17. Evans, J. G., and Rose, G.: Epidemiology of hypertension. Br. Med. Bull. 27:37, 1971.
18. Conway, J.: Could hardening of arteries lead to diastolic hypertension? Hypertension 7: 113, 1959.
19. Grollman, A.: The pathogenesis and treatment of hypertension. J. Am. Geriatr. Soc. 1:223, 1953.
20. Platt, R.: Heredity in hypertension. Lancet 1:899, 1963.
21. Grollman, E. F., and Grollman, A.: The teratogenic induction of hypertension. J. Clin. Invest. 41:710, 1962.
22. Schroeder, H. A.: Mechanisms of Hypertension. Springfield, Ill.: Thomas, 1957, pp. 141–202.
23. Grollman, A., and White, F. N.: Induction of renal hypertension in rats and dogs by potassium or choline deficiency. Am. J. Physiol. 193:144, 1958.
24. Pickering, G. W.: Inheritance of high blood pressure. *In* Bock, K. D. and Cottier, P. T. (Eds.): Essential Hypertension. Berlin: Springer, 1960, pp. 30–38.
25. Schlager, G.: Genetic control of blood pressure by more than one pair of alleles. Proc. Soc. Exp. Biol. Med. 136:863, 1971.
26. Frohlich, K.: Jugenliche Zwillinge mit arteriellen Hochdruck. Med. Klin. 33:1196, 1937.
27. Hames, C. G., McDonough, J. R., and Elliott, J. L.: Hypertension in identical twins. Lancet 2:585, 1964.
28. Vander Molen, R., Brewer, G., Honeyman, M. S., Morrison, J., and Hoobler, S. W.: A study of hypertension in twins. Am. Heart J. 79:454, 1970.
29. Friedman, M., and Kasanin, J. S.: Hypertension in only one of identical twins. Arch. Intern. Med. 72:767, 1943.
30. Bays, R. P., and Scrimshaw, N. S.: Facts and fallacies regarding blood pressure of different regional and racial groups. Circulation 8:655, 1953.
31. Hart, J. T.: Semicontinuous screening of a whole community for hypertension. Lancet 2:223, 1970.
32. Kean, B. H.: The blood pressure of the Cuni Indians. Am. J. Trop. Med. Hgy. 24: 341, 1944.
33. Maddocks, I.: Possible absence of essential hypertension in two complete Pacific Island populations. Lancet 2:396, 1961.
34. Whyte, H. M.: Body fat and blood pressure of natives in New Guinea: Reflections on essential hypertension. Aust. Ann. Med. 7:36, 1958.
35. Lowenstein, F. W.: Blood pressure in relation to age and sex in the tropics and sub-tropics: A review of the literature and an investigation into two tribes of Brazil Indians. Lancet 1: 389, 1961.
36. Donnison, C. P.: Blood pressure in the African native. Lancet 1:6, 1929.
37. Vint, F. W.: Post-mortem findings in natives of Kenya. East Afr. Med. J. 13:332, 1937.
38. Schrire, V.: The racial incidence of heart disease at Groote Schuur Hospital, Cape Town. II. Hypertension and valvular disease of the heart. Am. Heart J. 56:742, 1958.
39. Akinkugbe, O. O., and Ojo, A. O.: The systemic blood pressure in a rural Nigerian population. Trop. Geogr. Med. 20:347, 1968.
40. Williams, A. W.: Heart disease in native population of Uganda: Hypertensive heart disease. East Afr. Med. J. 21:328, 1944.
41. Du Bois, A.: Note sur la tension artérielle chez les indigènes congolais. Ann. Soc. Belg. Med. Trop. 12:133, 1932.

42. Phillips, J. H. and Burch, G. E.: A review of cardiovascular diseases in the white and Negro races. Medicine 39:241, 1960.
43. Schneckloth, R. E., Corcoran, A. C., Stuart, K. L., and Moore, F. E.: Arterial pressure and hypertensive disease in a West Indian Negro population: Report of survey in St. Kitts, West Indies. Am. Heart J. 63:607, 1962.
44. Kean, B. H., and Hammill, J. F.: Anthropathology of arterial tension. Arch. Intern. Med. 83:355, 1949.
45. Boyle, E., Jr.: Biological patterns in hypertension by race, sex, bodyweight, and skin color. JAMA 213:1637, 1970.
46. Taylor, C. E.: The racial distribution of nephritis and hypertension in Panama. Am. J. Pathol. 21:1031, 1945.
47. Grollman, A., Harrison, T. R., Mason, M. F., Baxter, J., Crampton, J., and Reichsman, F.: Sodium restriction in the diet for hypertension. JAMA 129:533, 1945.
48. Meneely, G. R.: Salt. Am. J. Med. 16:1, 1954.
49. Dahl, L. K.: Possible role of chronic excess salt consumption in pathogenesis of essential hypertension. Am. J. Cardiol. 8:571, 1961.
50. Maddocks, I.: Dietary factors in the genesis of hypertension. *In* Nutrition, Proceedings of the Sixth International Congress. Edinburgh: Livingstone, 1964.
51. Isaacson, L. D., Modlin, M., and Jackson, W. P. U.: Sodium intake and hypertension. Lancet 1:946, 1963.
52. Prior, I. A. M., Evans, J. G., Harvey, H. P. B., Davidson, B. H., and Lindsey, M.: Sodium intake and blood pressure in two Polynesian populations. N. Engl. J. Med. 279:515, 1968.
53. Wheeler, E. O., White, P. D., Reed, E. W., and Cohen, M. E.: Neurocirculatory asthenia (anxiety neurosis, effort syndrome, neurasthenia): A twenty year follow-up study of 173 patients. JAMA 142:878, 1950.
54. Lee, R. E., and Schneider, R. F.: Hypertension and arteriosclerosis in executive and nonexecutive personnel. JAMA 167:1447, 1958.
55. Grollman, A.: The Cardiac Output of Man in Health and Disease. Springfield, Ill.: Thomas, 1932, pp. 117–121.
56. Perera, G. A.: Hypertensive vascular disease: description and natural history. J. Chronic Dis. 1:33, 1955.
57. Bechgaard, P.: The natural history of benign hypertension. *In* Bock, K. D. and Cottier, P. T. (Eds.): Essential Hypertension. Berlin: Springer, 1960, p. 198.
58. Maddocks, I.: Blood pressure in Melanesians. Med. J. Aust. 1:1123, 1967.
59. Stamler, J., Lindberg, H. A., Berkson, D. M., Shaffer, A., Miller, W., and Poindexter, A.: Epidemiologic analysis of hypertension and hypertensive disease in the labor force of a Chicago utility company. Hypertension 7:23, 1959.
60. Masters, A., Marks, H. H., and Dack, S.: Hypertension in people over forty. JAMA 121:1251, 1943.
61. Platt, R.: The nature of essential hypertension. *In* Bock, K. D. and Cottier, P. T. (Eds.): Essential Hypertension. Berlin: Springer, 1960, pp. 39–44.
62. Mathieson, H. S.: The prognosis in arterial hypertension. Acta Med. Scand. 147(Suppl. 287):89, 1954.
63. Kannel, W. B., Wolf, P. A., Verter, J., and McNamara, P. M.: Epidemiologic assessment of the role of blood pressure in stroke. The Framingham study. JAMA 214:301, 1970.
64. Gordon, T. and Schwartz, M. J.: Systolic versus diastolic blood pressure and risk of coronary heart disease. Am. J. Cardiol. 27: 335, 1971.
65. O'Hare, J. P. and Holden, R. B.: Longevity in benign essential hypertension. JAMA 149: 1453, 1952.
66. Evelyn, K. A.: The natural course of essential hypertension in man. *In* Clark, E. G. (Ed.): A Symposium on Essential Hypertension Sponsored by the Commonwealth of Massachusetts. Boston: Wright & Potter, 1951, pp. 66–89.
67. Edwards, J. C.: Management of Hypertensive Disease. St. Louis, Mo.: Mosby, 1960.
68. Hood, B., Örndahl, G., and Björk, S.: Survival and mortality in malignant (Grade IV) and Grade III hypertension. Acta Med. Scand. 187:291, 1970.
69. Leishman, A. W. D.: Merits of reducing high blood pressure. Lancet 1:1284, 1963.
70. Moyer, J. H., and Brest, A. N.: The changing outlook for the patient with hypertension. Am. J. Cardiol. 17:673, 1966.
71. Harington, M., Kincaid-Smith, P., and McMichael, J.: Results of treatment of malignant hypertension: a seven year experience in 94 cases. Br. Med. J. 2:969, 1959.
72. Dorph, S., Leth, A., Degnbol, B., and From, A.: Visceral changes in severe hypertension and their response to drug treatment. Acta Med. Scand. 187:411, 1970.
73. Veterans Administration Cooperative Study Group: Effects of treatment on morbidity in hypertension. JAMA 213:1143, 1970.

74. Aurell, M., and Hood, B.: Cerebral hemorrhage in a population after a decade of active acute hypertensive treatment. Acta Med. Scand. 176:377, 1964.
75. Hamilton, M.: Selection of patients for antihypertensive therapy. *In* Gross, F. (Ed.): Antihypertensive Therapy. Berlin: Springer, 1966, pp. 196–211.
76. Dickinson, C. J.: Neurogenic Hypertension. Oxford: Blackwell, 1965, pp. 135–140.
77. Ueda, H., Nakajima, K., Takeda, T., and Ikeda, T.: Effectiveness of prolonged antihypertensive treatment on survival of patients with essential hypertension. Jap. Heart J. 5: 399, 1964.
78. Irino, T., Okuda, T., and Grollman, A.: Changes induced in the glomeruli of the kidney of rats by placental extracts as observed with the electron microscope. Am. J. Pathol. 50:421, 1967.

A 30-Year Study of Blood Pressure in a White Male Cohort

By William R. Harlan, M.D., Albert Oberman, M.D., Robert E. Mitchell (MC), and Ashton Graybiel, M.D.

TIME IS A CRITICAL dimension missing from most epidemiologic studies of blood pressure. Most of our knowledge about arterial pressure is derived from observations of acute physiologic alterations or from cross-sectional studies of populations at single points in time. Despite obvious needs for such information in clinical management, little data are available about changes in pressure with age and the effects of hereditary and environmental factors. In the absence of longitudinal data many questions are posed about what constitutes "physiologic" rises in arterial pressure with age, the causes of these increases, optimal times for surveillance, and the risk of modest blood pressure increments. We have had the unusual opportunity of following a cohort of white male naval flight trainees from early adulthood throughout middle age, a total of 30 years, and of seeking answers to some of these questions. Despite the rather select nature of the group, we believe that the information gleaned from this study provides some insights into longitudinal aspects of arterial pressure.

Materials and Methods

The study group consists of survivors of a cohort of 1,056 white males who were physically qualified for naval flight training in 1940. The mean age in 1940 was 24 years and all except 13 were between 20 and 30 years of age. The initial evaluation was performed to validate a number of physiologic and psychologic tests for preselecting successful flight trainees. Dr. Ashton Graybiel, one of the original investigators recruited from the Harvard Fatigue Laboratory, appreciated the potential of making serial observations on the group and initiated follow-up evaluations in 1951, 1957, 1964, and 1970 under the auspices of the U.S. Naval Aerospace Medical Research Institute, with participation by the U.S. Public Health Service, Federal Aviation Agency, and National Aeronautics and Space Administration. The methodology utilized in each evaluation is detailed in two monographs,[1,2] and only aspects of testing pertinent to blood pressure are described here.

Follow-up examinations were obtained on 85, 98, and 88 percent of the survivors in 1951, 1958, and 1964, respectively and only four men have been lost entirely to follow-up. The current examination cycle began in 1970 and is nearly complete now with more than 80 percent examined.

Blood pressures were recorded with a standard adult cuff and mercury sphygmomanometer midway through the physical examination with the patient in the supine, seated, and standing positions. Diastolic pressure was taken as the fifth phase although both fourth- and fifth-phase changes were recorded. In addition to these casual blood pressures, basal pressures were recorded in 1940 and 1970 after the patient had been fasted overnight and permitted to rest supine 20 to 40 minutes in a dark soundproof room. After three successive pressures were recorded in this manner, a cold pressor test was performed by immersing the hand opposite the cuffed arm in ice water for 1 minute and recording blood pressure every 30 seconds thereafter for 5 minutes.[3] To minimize number bias, blood pressures were recorded by machine in 1970 and by a number-hiding technique in 1964.

Standard statistical methods were used for analysis of data. Both systolic and diastolic pressures were analyzed. The correlates of each were similar and the majority of data presented here relate to systolic pressure, but the results are equally valid for diastolic pressure.

From the Departments of Medicine and Community Health Sciences, Duke University, Durham, North Carolina, and the U.S. Naval Aerospace Medical Research Institute, Pensacola, Florida.

Standard procedures were used for other measurements, and these methods are described in several monographs.[1,2]

Results and Discussion

Despite the rigorous selection criteria and rather homogeneous nature of the group, the distribution of blood pressures recorded during the 30 years of study is remarkably similar to several cross-sectional studies of larger and more representative population samples (Fig. 1). The distributions at the two age extremes, 24 years and 54 years, are similar to distributions reported in cross-sectional studies of other American groups [4] and those reported from England.[5] The mean systolic and diastolic pressures of the group increased over the 30-year interval and the distribution became skewed toward higher values. On inspection or by statistical analysis one can find no natural segmentation into two groups—one with "normal" blood pressures and one with "high" blood pressures. Thus, there is no support for the arguments of Platt [6] that a population, if followed long enough, will develop a biomodal distribution of blood pressure and the high group could be defined as having high blood pressure on a statistical basis rather than on the present arbitrary basis. This does not imply that the skewing to higher pressures is innocuous because it is common. As well documented elsewhere and in this study, these higher pressures are associated with measurable alterations in target organs and the increased risk of cardiovascular and cerebrovascular disease. Rather, the pattern of blood pressure distribution suggests strongly that multiple factors are involved in the pathogenesis and that at least some of these factors require time—or some aspect of the aging process—for their expression.

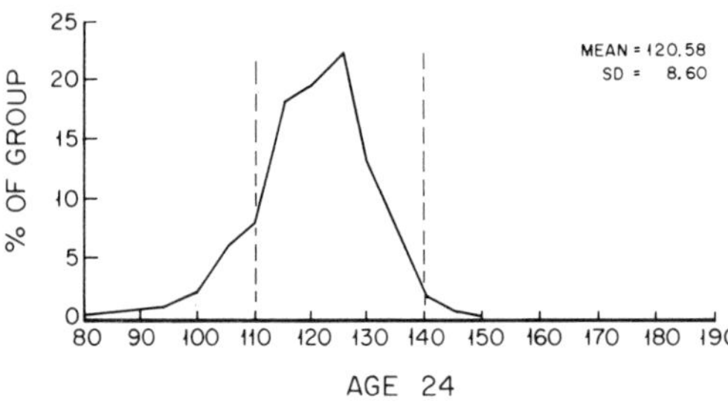

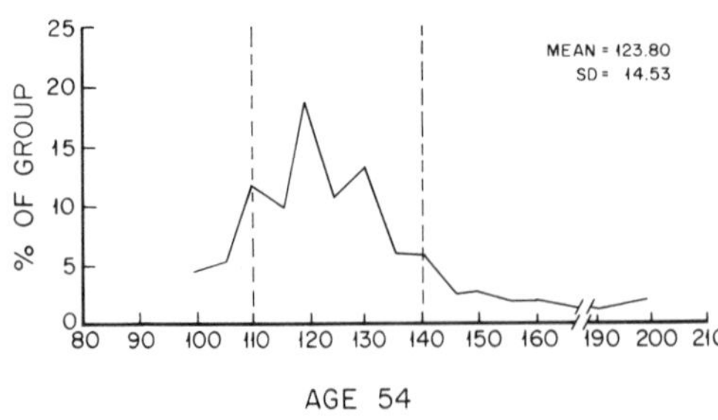

Fig. 1.—Frequency distribution curves for systolic blood pressures in the same cohort at 24 and 54 years of age. The **dashed lines** are used to emphasize the skewing of blood pressures to higher values with increasing age.

More pertinent to the longitudinal observations in this study are questions related to individual blood pressure changes with time. Does the blood pressure increase in all individuals with age or only in particular individuals? What factors can be identified as being related to these interval changes? What intervals are critical in surveillance of individuals? Can individuals at greatest risk of developing high blood pressure be identified before the development of elevated pressure?

An increase in blood pressure is not an inevitable consequence of increasing age. Approximately half of this cohort experienced a rise of 3 mm Hg or less in systolic or diastolic blood pressure during the 30-year follow-up (Fig. 2). The changes in systolic and diastolic pressures from age 24 to 54 years are plotted on the abscissa and the number of individuals experiencing this change are plotted on the ordinate. There is no clear segmentation of interval blood pressure change; rather the change assumes a fairly normal distribution for both systolic and diastolic pressures. Some striking increases in pressure occurred, with 12 percent having systolic increases of more than 24 mm Hg or diastolic increases of more than 18 mm Hg.

When does the pattern of change become apparent and does this help us to devise national intervals for surveillance of the population? In Figure 3, we have arbitrarily divided the cohort into three groups based on the systolic blood pressure at age 54. The division into high, middle, and low ranges of blood pressure is arbitrary and there is no particular reason for making this particular division since

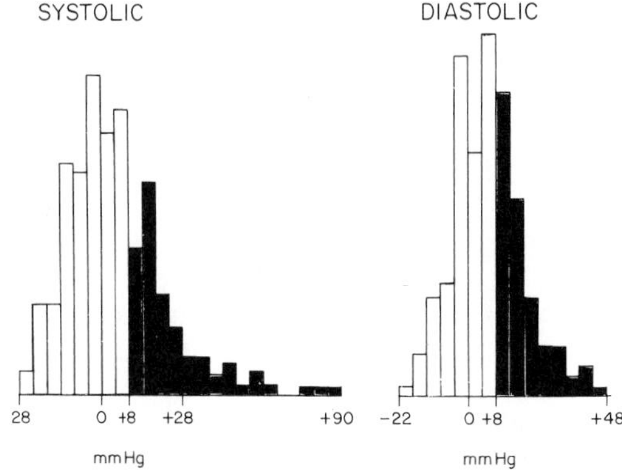

FIG. 2.—Distribution of change in blood pressure from age 24 to 54. See text for explanation.

separation into four or five groups would yield similar results. It is apparent from Figure 3 that the group with the lower blood pressures at age 54 actually experienced an interval drop in blood pressure. On the other hand, the upper group had higher blood pressures on each examination and the differences became more marked as the group grew older. No particular trend is apparent for the middle group. The vertical lines at each age indicate the standard error. From these observations it is clear that the differences in blood pressure between the groups are statistically significant at each examination except age 24 when the study began. At that age there were no statistically significant differences although there was an apparent trend for the high group at age 54 to have higher pressures at age 24.

An important collateral question is the relationship between the interval change in pressure and the final pressure attained. Our results (Fig. 4) agree with those of Miall and Lovell [7] and indicate that the greatest increment of blood pressure occurred in individuals with the higher pressures at age 36 and the higher final pressures at age 54. In Figure 4 the interval change in systolic pressure (on ordinate) is shown for each decile of mean systolic pressure, i.e., the mean pressure for all examinations for a particular individual.[8] It is apparent that the higher the blood pressure, the greater the increment; further, that there is a significant group with lower pressures who experience no increment with time. This finding is compatible with a self-perpetuating mechanism for blood pressure elevation wherein an elevated pressure activates or resets a process within the body to cause further increases in pressure. The available data from this study and from Miall and Lovell are compatible with this thesis but provide no direct evidence for a causal relationship.

Two salient features emerge from these data. First, age per se is not related to increase in arterial pressure. The data of Miall and Lovell [7] collected in South Wales confirm that there is no age-related increase for some men and women during an 8-year longitudinal study, and the data collected by Stamler [8] are similar. Data from more primitive societies provide a further dimension since only a minority have a rise in blood pressure with age. Some features of particular groups—either hereditary

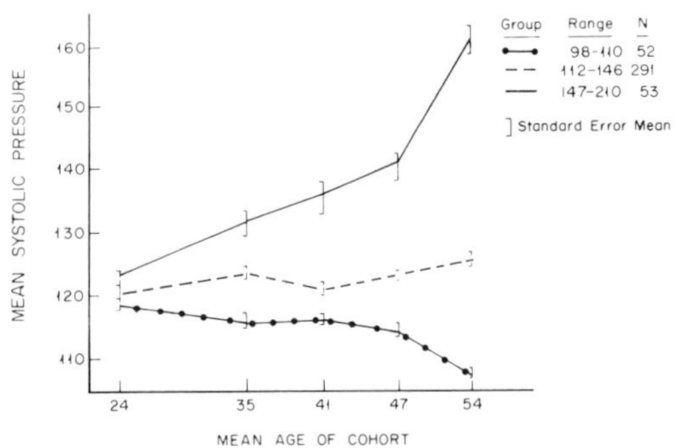

FIG. 3.—Trend of systolic pressure in cohort separated by systolic pressure at age 54. See text for explanation.

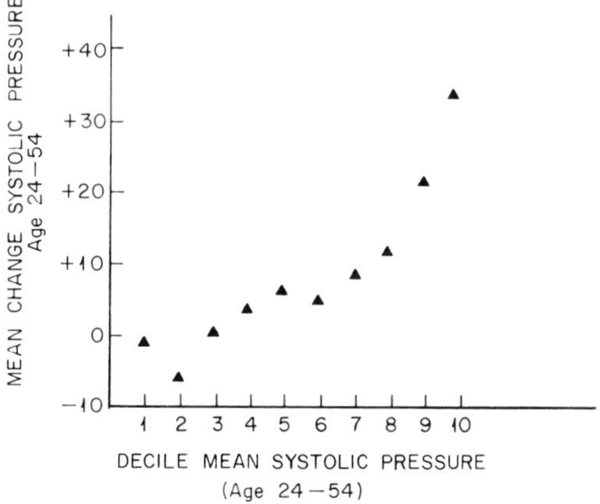

FIG. 4.—Mean change of systolic pressure by level of mean systolic pressure from mean age 24 to 54. See text for explanation.

or environmental influences—must explain the differential effect seen with aging. Second, the subsequent rate of rise in blood pressure relates directly to the pressure attained. Stated somewhat differently, those with higher pressures experience greater interval rises in arterial pressure and those with lower pressures either experience a decline or a lesser increment during the observation interval. Parenthetically, it should be noted that this is not a statistical artifact. Actually, the tendency would be for regression toward the mean and not a progressive increment or decrement. Further, the use of a standardized pressure for each individual [7,9] makes the relationship even stronger, although statistically one would expect some decrease in the strength of this relationship using this technique if the relationship were spurious.

Because this initial increase in pressure may have importance in activating a self-perpetuating mechanism it deserves particular attention. An interesting aspect of our study is the observation that this relationship was striking from age 36 onward but was not obvious on the first examination at age 24 (Fig. 3). Several explanations may be offered. The individuals in this group were rigorously selected and those with high blood pressure and excess weight were eliminated. This selection would emphasize subsequent changes in blood pressure and weight as the group assumed the characteristics of the general population. This implies that the influences operative from age 24 to 36 in this cohort are similar to those operative in the general population, although less obvious in a general population because the changes occur more gradually. Miall and Lovell [7] also found a steep initial increment in blood pressure in males between 10 and 30 years of age but no particular comment was directed to this finding. Since most studies of blood pressure focus on older groups, this early and perhaps critical change may be missed. Whatever the explanation for this early increment, once the initial rise occurs it appears that a self-perpetuating process is set in motion.

What characterizes the individuals who develop high blood pressure? As indicated above, blood pressure itself is important. There was a relationship between casual blood pressure at age 24 and subsequent blood pressures ($r = 0.19$, $p < .01$) but a significantly higher correlation was found between basal blood pressure at age 24 and subsequent casual blood pressures ($r = 0.32$, $p < .01$).[10] Thus, minimizing extraneous influences probably increases the validity and predictive capacity of blood pressures recorded early in life.

The relationship between blood pressure variability and response to stressful stimuli was examined to explore the possibility that altered neurogenic control may be related to initially transient and then later permanent elevations of blood pressure. The cold pressor test has been suggested as an appropriate measure of vascular reactivity and was performed on 385 men in this group during the initial examination.[11] The response of systolic and diastolic pressure at age 24 was then compared with blood pressures measured during subsequent examinations. The results at age 54 are shown in Table 1. The systolic response at age 24 was divided into deciles and compared with systolic and diastolic blood pressure 30 years later. No relationship between cold pressure response and subsequent blood pressure is apparent and this is confirmed by statistical analysis. Similar results were obtained when blood pressures at other ages were examined and when diastolic response to cold stress was examined.[11] Additionally, we could find no relationships between the cold pressor responses in 1940 and in 1970. Our negative results could be the result of the selection process which eliminated most hyper-

TABLE 1.—*Cohort Blood Pressure at Age 54 Related to Systolic Cold Pressor Response by Decile at Age 24*

Systolic Cold Pressor Responses Mean Age 24			*Mean Blood Pressures Age 54*	
Decile	*Range*	*N*	*Systolic*	*Diastolic*
1	38–50	15	128.7 ± 18	80.6 ± 11
2	25–28	18	123.7 ± 15	78.8 ± 10
3	22–24	17	127.3 ± 17	81.1 ± 7
4	20–21	12	126.5 ± 19	80.7 ± 12
5	16–18	16	127.4 ± 23	80.6 ± 12
6	14–15	17	133.5 ± 22	80.1 ± 8
7	11–13	13	129.7 ± 19	79.9 ± 10
8	10	12	133.1 ± 20	80.8 ± 9
9	66–9	15	126.3 ± 16	79.4 ± 8
10	(–8)–5	16	134.3 ± 21	84.2 ± 11

tensive subjects and perhaps some hyperresponsive subjects. However, the responses of our group were similar to the responses found in normal subjects by Hines [4] and there was no apparent elimination of hyperresponders. We conclude that cold stress may test the functional adequacy of the sympathetic nervous control of blood pressure, but it does not predict those who will subsequently develop elevated arterial pressure.

What other features characterize the individuals with serial increments in pressure and eventual development of elevated pressures? Weight stands out as the factor of greatest importance aside from blood pressure measurements (Table 2). The data in Table 2 are representative of several analyses. We have made an arbitrary division of the group into thirds depending on the blood pressure at age 54 and determined what characteristics have a significant and independent relationship to blood pressure. The influence of weight on blood pressure was statistically significant on every examination except the initial evaluation at age 24 when the men were at ideal weight following selection into the program. As might be expected there was also a significant relationship between interval blood pressure change and interval weight change. The greatest increase in weight occurred between 24 and 36 years of age and concomitantly the blood pressure increment was greatest during this interval. Although several measurements of adiposity, including skinfold-thickness, somatotype, and anthropometric measurements were made, none was found to be superior to interval weight gain. Furthermore, as discussed previously, once an elevation of arterial pressure becomes apparent there is a tendency for successive increments to increase and for the blood pressure to rise still higher. Whether weight gain is the primary feature or even a definite causal factor in the initial rise certainly cannot be determined from these data, but a controlled therapeutic trial of weight reduction in a young group would provide a test of this possibility.

TABLE 2.—*Characteristics of Individuals Grouped by Blood Pressure at Age 54*

Variable	*Systolic Blood Pressure* Lower Third	Middle Third	Upper Third
Weight change in pounds (age 24–54)	14	21	25
Glucose 2h p 75 gm meal (mg per 100 ml)	113	114	136
Weekly alcohol intake (oz.)	8.4	11.9	13.4
Parental longevity	+	±	—

No significant differences: uric acid, somatotype, postglucose meal serum insulin, cholesterol

No independent differences: fasting serum insulin, very low-density lipoproteins, triglyceride

Other factors were apparently related to blood pressure increase. Parental longevity bears a clear relationship to blood pressure. If one or both parents died before age 65 the blood pressure was significantly higher than if both parents survived to later ages.[9] This influence was present even at age 24 when a weight relationship to blood pressure was not apparent. It should be noted, however, that the significance of family history was not demonstrable until the group achieved a mean age of 42 years and sufficient parental mortality experience had occurred. The further interesting point is the interaction between weight change and parental longevity and their relationship to blood pressure. This interaction is most striking in the group with greater than 20 pounds gain in weight and short-lived parents, and there seems to be a potential effect.[9]

Other features associated with increasing blood pressure include abnormal carbohydrate tolerance as measured either by plasma glucose or insulin following challenge with a 75-gm glucose meal, alcohol intake, and the very low-density (SF 20–400 or pre-beta) lipoproteins. All of these characteristics are related to adiposity but postchallenge glucose and alcohol intake appear to make contributions independent of this relationship to weight. A number of other factors did not make independent contributions toward explaining either blood pressure increments or the blood pressure at age 54. These factors are listed in part in Table 2.

The important end points are morbidity and mortality from arterial pressure and not the levels of pressure attained. Several measurements have permitted us to examine the relationship between blood pressure trends and damage to the organs affected by increased blood pressure. Some general statements can be made from data presented in detail elsewhere.[12] Measurement of target organ change revealed subtle but statistically significant changes in transverse diameter of the heart, electrocardiograms (ECGs), and evaluation of the ocular fundus. These changes were continuous throughout the entire range of blood pressures and no threshold for damage was apparent. Furthermore, these changes were related to both systolic and diastolic pressures although the relationships were generally stronger with diastolic pressures. As expected, factors other than blood pressure also contribute to target organ changes and this reflects the well-recognized multifactorial pathogenesis of arteriosclerotic complications. Body weight, lipoproteins, and carbohydrate tolerance were the other important factors interacting with blood pressure to produce these changes. The pattern of blood pressure rise was also important. The greatest morbidity changes were present in individuals with progressive increases in arterial pressure during the 30 years of follow-up. Transient elevations during a single examination (blood pressure variability) had no significant relationships to organ changes. Thus, our experience suggests that the absolute arterial pressure and serial incremental changes are more important than transient elevations in determining organ damage. Further, there is no threshold pressure for expression of organ damage and, therefore, even mild increases in blood pressure are important. These studies reveal a further value in making serial measurements of target organ function. Such changes, though subtle and apparent only on serial measurements, can provide a quantifiable basis for initiating treatment or become end points in therapeutic trials in treatment of mild blood pressure increase where mortality and overt morbidity are uncommon.

Finally, one may ask whether these studies provide useful information that will predict those who have a greater risk of developing high blood pressure and what constitutes optimal monitoring of the population. The preceding discussion focused on a retrospective analysis of data from the vantage point of the "final" blood pressure at age 54. If, on the other hand, one views the data prospectively from age 24, a somewhat different perspective develops. Of identified features at age 24 only one, the relative ranking in blood pressure distribution, emerges as a significant predictor of future high blood pressure. The family history at this age had not sufficient time to develop in parents or siblings and was of no value. Tests of blood pressure variability such as the cold pressor test apparently have little validity. Of the blood pressures recorded at this early age, the basal blood pressure had the greatest predictive value. Thus, serial surveillance for blood pressure trends and for weight changes and the response of blood pressure to weight increments emerge as the primary factors to be followed in young populations.

In this group, important pressure changes occurred between 24 years and 36 years. Although we have no data on the rapidity of change during this 12-year interval, there is obvious value in frequent blood pressure and weight determinations during this period when weight gain is maximal and the first and perhaps critical increment of blood pressure occurs. Based on these observations, greatest attention should be directed toward monitoring young adults in their early 20s with blood pressures above the mean and those who experience weight gain. One can only venture an estimate about the best intervals for observations but perhaps every third year would be sufficient. Of course, discovery of elevated blood pressures and associated weight increases on any examination would call for more frequent observations as would detection of a clear upward trend of pressure. The observation interval could perhaps be longer (perhaps 5 years) after age 35 in those whose pressures remain below the mean although it is also clear from this study that the incidence of high blood pressure continues to be significant throughout the fourth and fifth decades and there is no age below 60 years when hypertension is not a clear potential. Furthermore, the relationship of weight gain to blood pressure remains important throughout adult life and, coupled with the frequently associated carbohydrate intolerance, these facets represent risk factors for high blood pressure and demand more frequent surveillance when present. More frequent attention is necessary for those with pressures above the mean and in whom incremental changes have been found in early adult life.

As a final statement, the caveat expressed in the introduction bears repetition. This study provided a longitudinal perspective of blood pressure based on a group of rigorously selected white males who were relatively homogeneous in psychologic and physiologic traits. Although this limits the direct application of these observations to less highly selected groups, it nevertheless represents a strength of the study in that confounding variable and extraneous influences were minimized, and the trends that emerge from a homogeneous group could be expected to be even stronger where greater variations are present.

References

1. McFarland, R. A., and Franzen, R.: The Pensacola study of naval aviators: Final summary report. Report No. 38. Washington, D.C.: Civil Aeronautics Administration Division of Research, 1944.
2. Oberman, A., Mitchell, R. E., and Graybiel, A.: Thousand Aviator Study Methodology. Monograph II, U.S. Naval School of Aviation Medicine. Pensacola, Florida, 1965.
3. Hines, E. A., Jr. and Brown, G. E.: The cold pressor test for measuring reactibility of blood pressure: Data concerning 571 normal and hypertensive subjects. Am. Heart J. 11:1, 1936.
4. National Center for Health Statistics: Blood Pressures of Adults by Age and Sex. Vital and Health Statistics, publication no. 1,000, ser. 11, no. 5, Washington, D.C.: Public Health Service, 1964.
5. Robinson, S. C., and Brucer, M.: Range of normal blood pressure: Statistical and clinical study of 11,383 persons. Ann. Intern. Med. 64:409, 1939.
6. Platt, R.: Nature of essential hypertension. Lancet 2:55, 1959.
7. Miall, W. E., and Lovell, H. G.: Relation between change of blood pressure and age. Br. Med. J. 2:660, 1967.
8. Stamler, J.: Discussion (on the Natural History of Hypertension and Hypertensive Disease). *In* Cort, J. H., French, V., Heil, Z., and Jirka, J.: Pathogenesis of Essential Hypertension, Prague Symposium, 1960. New York: Macmillan, 1962, p. 67.
9. Oberman, A., Lane, N. E., Harlan, W. R., Graybiel, A., and Mitchell, R. E.: Trends in systolic blood pressure in the thousand aviator cohort over a twenty-four year period. Circulation 36:812, 1967.
10. Harlan, W. R., Osborne, R. K., and Graybiel, A.: A longitudinal study of blood pressure. Circulation 26:530, 1962.
11. Harlan, W. R., Osborne, R. K. and Graybiel, A.: Prognostic value of the cold pressor test and the basal blood pressure. Am. J. Cardiol. 13:683, 1964.
12. Oberman, A., Harlan, W. R., Smith, M., and Graybiel, A.: The cardiovascular risk associated with different levels and types of elevated blood pressure. Minn. Med. 52:1283, 1969.

Hypertensive Cardiovascular Disease: The Framingham Study

By William B. Kannel, M.D., and Thomas R. Dawber, M.D.

Cardiovascular diseases constitute the main underlying cause of mortality and morbidity in the United States. These diseases are not necessarily the inevitable concomitants of aging but rather the culmination of a chain of events evolving over several decades. Elevated blood pressure is one of the most common and most potent precursors of coronary heart disease, stroke, and congestive failure.

Importance of Hypertension

Cardiac hypertrophy and eventual failure may be the direct result of elevated blood pressure. In addition, every major manifestation of atherosclerosis has been found to occur in marked excess among hypertensive persons. Risk of developing these diseases has been shown to be proportional to the blood pressure status of persons followed prospectively over decades at Framingham and elsewhere. At Framingham, subjects with hypertension were found subsequently to develop coronary disease, brain infarctions, intermittent claudication, and congestive heart failure at a rate about three times that of normotensive persons (Fig. 1). This warrants a detailed examination of the role of hypertension in the development of cardiovascular disease. Such an examination requires the study of the evolution of hypertension from the presymptomatic state into various cardiovascular sequelae. Examination of data from the Framingham study in which a cohort of 5,209 men and women has been followed biennially for the development of cardiovascular disease permits such an investigation.[1]

Prevalence

Not only is hypertension a potent contributor to cardiovascular morbidity and mortality, but it is an extremely common finding in otherwise healthy individuals. Estimates made by the National Health Survey in 1962 indicate that about 26 million persons in the United States have hypertension or hypertensive heart disease. When hypertension is defined in terms of blood pressure readings of 150/100 mm Hg or greater, 20 percent of men and women aged 45 to 54 years are found to be afflicted.[2] Evidence from surveys in Georgia and Chicago indicates that approximately half of this is undetected and about half of recognized hypertension is not under treatment.[3,4] In only a small percentage can a specific cause be identified; the vast majority have essential hypertension of unknown cause. Prevalence estimates from Framingham are presented in Figure 2.

Accurate, acceptable incidence, e.g., the appearance of hypertension in persons known to be previously normotensive, is scarce. Examination of trends in blood pressure in persons under observation for long periods in Framingham suggests that hypertension is a high-prevalence but low-incidence disease in persons over age 30. Very few entirely normo-

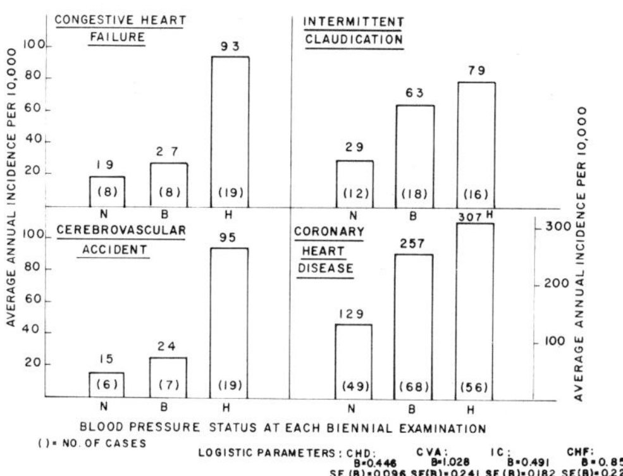

Fig. 1.—Average annual incidence of cardiovascular disease according to blood pressure status at each biennial examination of men 35 to 64 years of age in the Framingham study. (From Shurtleff, D.,[37] with permission.)

From the Framingham Heart Disease Epidemiology Study, Framingham, Massachusetts, and the Department of Medicine, Boston University School of Medicine, Boston, Massachusetts.

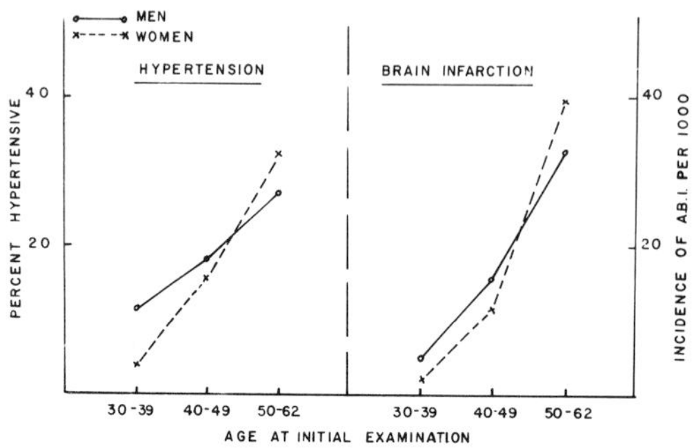

FIG. 2.—Prevalence of hypertension and incidence of atherothrombotic brain infarction by age and sex in men and women 30 to 62 years of age at entry in the Framingham study.

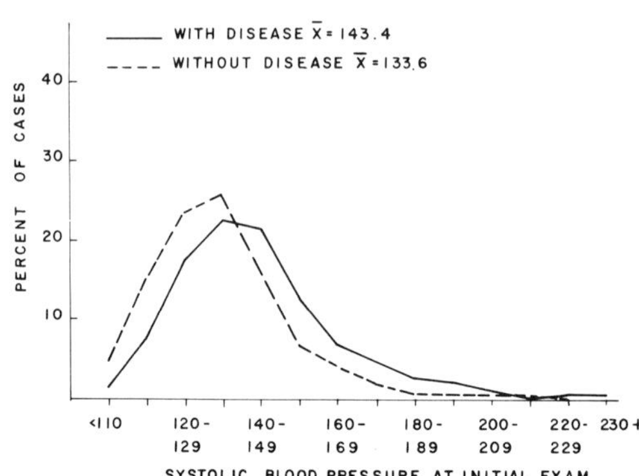

FIG. 3.—Distribution of systolic blood pressure in men 30 to 49 years of age at initial examination according to whether coronary heart disease, cerebrovascular accident, congestive heart failure, or intermittent claudication developed in 18-year follow-up of the Framingham study.

tensive persons have developed sustained "hypertension" under observation in this population, aged 30 to 62 years at the time of initial examination. Although one might conclude from reports in medical literature that specific causes of hypertension are extremely common, it is clear that over 90 percent is unexplained "essential" or "primary" hypertension.

Definitions

Before diagnosable organ involvement appears, hypertension is manifested only by the physical findings of elevated blood pressure. The determination of the point at which normotension changes to hypertension is to a large extent arbitrary. This problem can be handled in a statistical manner, e.g., values 2 S.D. above the mean are regarded as abnormal. Another approach is to examine the blood pressure distribution of those who eventually develop organ involvement compared to those who have remained free of pathologic findings. In the Framingham study average values of systolic and diastolic blood pressure were only slightly higher in those who later developed cardiovascular sequelae than in those who remained free of them. The mean systolic value in men 30 to 49 years old who subsequently developed coronary heart disease was 144 mm Hg systolic (93 mm Hg diastolic) compared to 137 mm Hg (87 mm Hg diastolic) for those who remained free (Fig. 3). The distribution curves of the two groups overlap to such an extent that it is not possible to discriminate persons in one group from those in the other. Although the differences attain a high level of statistical significance for population groups, such differences applied to individuals have little meaning.

Thus, we must reject the concept that hypertension is a categorical entity to be distinguished from normotension and treat blood pressure as the continuous variable it is. Elevated pressure readings now considered clinically unimportant may have serious implications when accompanied by elevated blood lipids (Fig. 4) or ECG abnormalities. Blood pressure is best treated as one ingredient of an atherogenic profile based on the measurement of a number of risk factors.

Role of Hypertension in Atherosclerosis

Hypertension appears to promote accelerated atherogenesis as well as to precipitate myocardial failure and stroke. Age-sex trends in blood pressure may to a large extent explain the converging incidence of atherosclerotic disease in the sexes with advancing age (Fig. 5). The pathogenesis of atherosclerosis is a complex process resulting from the interplay of many factors. Focal anatomic factors, dynamics of flow, arterial caliber, and the integrity of the vascular intima appear to determine the site of the lesions.[5–7] Thus, angulation or tortuosity producing turbulence of flow and impingement of the blood stream on the arterial wall favors early localization of lesions. However, the architecture of the arterial circulation is only

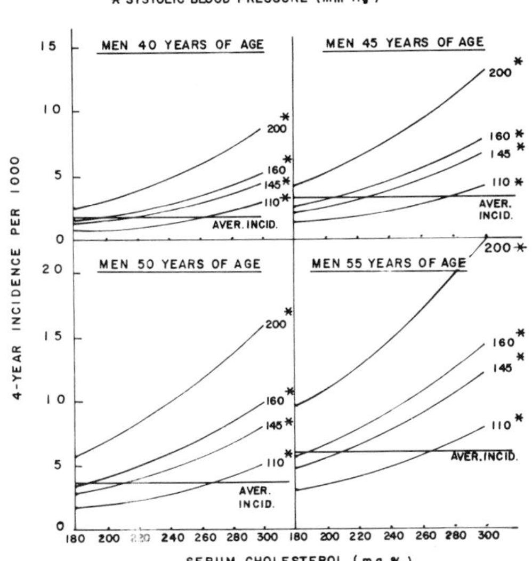

FIG. 4.—Four-year incidence of coronary heart disease according to serum cholesterol concentration at specified levels of systolic blood pressure in men 40 to 55 years of age in the Framingham study. (From Gordon, T., and Verter, J.,[38] with permission.)

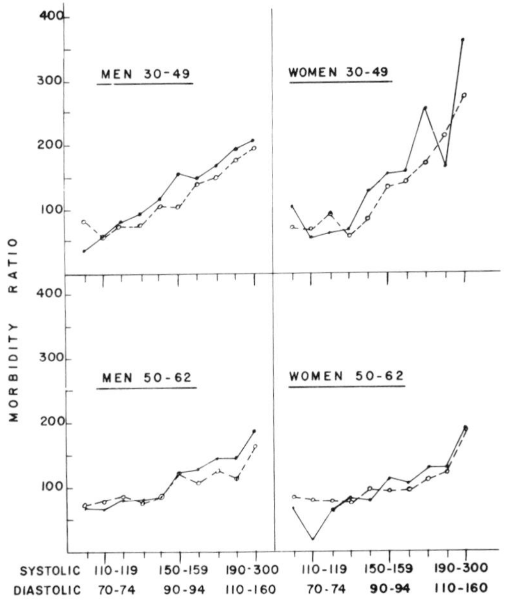

FIG. 5.—Relative risk of cardiovascular disease according to systolic and diastolic blood pressures in men and women 30 to 62 years of age, in 18-year follow-up of the Framingham study.

one determinant of atheroma formation. Risk is proportional to blood lipid and pressure level. Veins and pulmonary arteries can be quite tortuous and except in rare instances escape atheromatosis. The level of blood pressure is a crucial factor in producing atherosclerosis. Below some critical level of pressure, atherosclerosis does not develop. When the pressure is raised, regardless of the reason, atheromas appear even in parts of the circulation normally "immune." In general, the closer the origin of an artery to the aorta, the more likely will atherosclerosis develop.

Direct evidence in support of this hypothesis is provided by animal experiments which have conclusively demonstrated that lipid-induced atherosclerosis can be accelerated by also raising the blood pressure of the animal.[8–10] The human counterpart of this experiment is provided by prospective epidemiologic evidence that at any blood lipid value, risk of coronary heart disease and atherothrombotic brain infarction is directly proportional to the blood pressure level. Even elevated blood lipid values impose little risk at low blood pressure values. A combination of elevated values of both is, however, ominous.

There may well be pressures below which atherosclerosis does not develop, e.g., in the pulmonary arteries or the venous circulation. It would therefore seem wise to keep systemic arterial pressures as low as practicable. All available evidence suggests that the cardiovascular diseases attributable to hypertension depend on the degree of elevation, its duration, and the rate of increase in its severity. There is no suggestion of a critical level of blood pressure at which cardiovascular disease incidence suddenly accelerates.

Blood pressure makes an independent contribution to the development of cardiovascular disease. Hypertension is second to none of the factors contributing to coronary morbidity and mortality.[11] A comparison of univariate and multivariate regression coefficients shows that all the other factors which are related to cardiovascular incidence and also to hypertension account for no more than a small percentage of its effect.

A distinct gradient of risk of coronary heart disease can be shown in relation to blood pressure status even after exclusion of persons with obesity, gout, abnormal lipids, diabetes, or electrocardiographic abnormalities. However, persons with elevated blood pressure are at greater relative risk when these conditions are present.

Systolic versus Diastolic Blood Pressure

Systemic hypertension is said to exist when the mean arterial pressure is elevated due to a rise in both systolic and diastolic pressure secondary to increased peripheral resistance. It is usually associated with a normal cardiac output. In a small percentage of patients there may be hypervolemia or increased viscosity due to erythrocythemia. Elevated *diastolic* pressure has been considered the sine qua non of hypertension. Elevated systolic blood pressure is usually attributed to decreased compliance of the aortic wall often associated with aging. Such an elevation may be observed in severe bradycardia, thyrotoxicosis, fever, anemia, aortic regurgitation, arteriovenous shunts, and the hyperkinetic syndrome. Physiologically it is a consequence of an elevated stroke volume, accompanied by a rapid diastolic runoff, rather than increased peripheral resistance as found in "true" hypertension.

An examination of the gradients of risk of mortality and of the development of the major cardiovascular sequelae in relation to systolic and diastolic pressure does not reveal that diastolic pressure plays a more important role.[12] On the contrary, elevated systolic blood pressure appears to make a greater contribution than diastolic pressure (Table 1).

To some extent the argument is academic, since in the general population the two components of the blood pressure are highly correlated.[12] Further data are required to assess the importance of *isolated* systolic blood pressure elevation. However, failure to show a diminishing impact of systolic pressure with advancing age brings into question the concept that isolated systolic pressure elevation in the aged is innocuous. A comparison of subjects having coronary heart disease with those remaining free of this disease shows no decrease in the influence of systolic pressure with advancing age (Fig. 4). A recent study assessing the cardiovascular consequences of systolic hypertension in the elderly supports this contention.[13]

Systolic blood pressure as measured casually has proved to be a powerful determinant of cardiovascular morbidity or mortality at any age, in either sex. In fact, this measurement is as useful as any other parameter of blood pressure. Limited data from the Framingham study show that women with diastolic pressures below 90 mm Hg have a distinct gradient of risk proportional to systolic pressure. Disorders characterized by a wide pulse pressure and a disproportionate rise in systolic blood pressure (e.g., complete heart block, aortic regurgitation, thyrotoxicosis and anemia) are also characterized by eventual myocardial hy-

TABLE 1.—*A 16-Year Follow-up Study of Subjects 45 to 74 Years of Age Showing Average Standardized Regression Coefficient for Cardiovascular Morbidity and Mortality–Systolic versus Diastolic Blood Pressure*

	CHD	*CVA*	*I.C.*	*CHF*	*CHD death*	*Other C-V Dis. Death*	*Overall Mortality*
Men							
Systolic blood pressure	0.340	0.581	0.238	0.648	0.370	0.465	0.309
Diastolic blood pressure	0.271	0.552	−0.115 *	0.466	0.283	0.196 *	0.214
Women							
Systolic blood pressure	0.447	0.535	0.550	0.688	0.368	0.583	0.250
Diastolic blood pressure	0.386	0.478	0.491	0.611	0.265	0.403	0.154

From Gordon, T., Sorlie, P., and Kannel, W. B.,[39] with permission.
* Not statistically significant.
CHD, coronary heart disease; CVA, cerebrovascular accident; I.C., intermittent claudication; C-V Dis., cardiovascular disease.

pertrophy and decompensation. However, since they may also be accompanied by myocardial disease it is difficult to determine if the systolic pressure load on the ventricle is entirely responsible. Isolated systolic blood pressure in the aged may only be a sign of arteriosclerosis rather than the cause of it.

Not only clinical cardiovascular disease, but myocardial hypertrophy itself is distinctly related to casual systolic blood pressure level. Regardless of the method used to measure cardiac hypertrophy, the degree of hypertrophy as assessed at Framingham was no more closely related to diastolic than systolic pressure.

Labile Blood Pressure

Blood pressure is normally a labile measurement since it represents a response to numerous physiologic demands. However, in some individuals the vascular bed overreacts to many stimuli. In general the higher the level of blood pressure the greater the degree of lability observed. Physicians have long suspected that fixed diastolic hypertension is preceded by a period of labile hypertension. It is generally considered unnecessary to treat hypertension manifested only as labile hypertension. Basal pressures which minimize lability rather than casual pressures are frequently used to determine the need for therapy. However, experience in the Framingham study demonstrates clearly that casual blood pressure values are distinctly related to the rate of development of every major sequela of hypertension (Fig. 1). Casual blood pressure elevations should not be too readily dismissed.

Determinants of Elevated Blood Pressure

A variety of host and environmental factors has been suggested as causally related to essential hypertension, but such relationships have yet to be firmly established. Factors incriminated include: an inability to cope with psychic stimuli, altered sensitivity of baroreceptors so that they perceive elevated pressures as "normal," excessive salt intake beginning early in life in susceptible persons, autonomic imbalance, trace metals, prostaglandin deficiency, and hereditary and racial influences, among others.

It appears unlikely that a single major "cause" will be uncovered which alone can account for the bulk of essential hypertension. There is much to suggest that an overreactive vascular response to nervous stress mediated through the autonomic nervous system may be responsible. Many biochemical and physiologic phenomena have been noted in hypertension, but it is still not clear what initiates the renal ischemia, adrenal secretory abnormalities, abnormal salt and water metabolism, increased vascular sensitivity, decreased barostat sensitivity, and abnormal secretion of a variety of hormonal substances such as renin, angiotensin, and aldosterone. It is not even clear to what extent these are compensatory mechanisms or primary disturbances.

Heredity—Familial and Host Factors

Predisposition to essential hypertension is regarded by many as an inherited characteristic, and there is evidence to support this contention. Certain racial groups seem unusually susceptible, particularly to the accelerated type of hypertension. Age-sex trends, familial aggregation, and variable resistance to sequelae all bear on the possibility of genetic influences in essential hypertension. A relationship to obesity and blood hemoglobin values could reflect either genetic or environmental influences in hypertension.

Familial Aggregation

There is evidence to suggest that propensity to essential hypertension is familial. Assessment of the familial aggregation of the disease can serve to test familial host and environmental influences. Population studies have demonstrated a modest but highly significant correlation of the blood pressure of siblings.[14] Twin studies have suggested a genetic explanation by revealing a closer correspondence of pressures among identical than fraternal twins. Blood pressure correlation between types of twins was higher than among siblings. This repeatedly demonstrated familial aggregation of blood pressure has been variously interpreted as supporting an inherited mechanism of blood pressure regulation.[15]

Nevertheless, environmental as well as genetic factors could explain the clustering of

TABLE 2.—*Mean Systolic Blood Pressure in Wives and Sisters of Men Classified According to Systolic Blood Pressure in the Framingham Heart Study*

Systolic Blood Pressure of Men	*Average Systolic Blood Pressure of Wives*	*Average Systolic Blood Pressure of Sisters*
82–111	121	128
112–119	120	129
120–131	129	132
132–147	134	131
148–167	133	138
168+	139	158

hypertension in families. After all, families share more than genes; the blood pressures of spouses tend toward similarity in proportion to the duration of the marriage.[14] The correlation of the blood pressure of a parent to that of the child tends to be greatest in families where spouse aggregation is also present.[14] Data from Framingham also reveal a modest correlation of the blood pressures of spouses and siblings (Table 2). The wives and sisters of men with higher blood pressures also tend to have elevated pressures. The correlation with the sister's pressure is somewhat greater than that with the spouse, although both correlations are of a low order (Table 3). This suggests (*1*) a greater genetic than environmental influence; (*2*) early environment has a greater impact than environmental influence; or (*3*) early environment has a greater impact than later environment. Recently, Zinner et al. have extended the findings of familial aggregation of blood pressure to include children in the 2- to 14-year range.[16] This tends to favor a genetic basis for hypertension. However, the

TABLE 3.—*Correlation of Systolic Pressures Between Spouses and Siblings*

	No.	*Correlation Coefficient*
Husbands versus wives	339	0.0926
Husbands versus sisters	339	0.1976 *
Wives versus husbands	258	0.1296 *
Wives versus brothers	258	0.1708 *

* Significant at 5-percent level.

possibility that early environmental influences may lead to hypertension later in life is not ruled out. In any event, the findings of Zinner et al. suggest that the process of essential hypertension, and ultimately its influence on cardiovascular disease, has its roots very early in life.

A rise in blood pressure with age is accepted as a normal phenomenon in most populations. Longitudinal data from Framingham show a progressive rise in pressures as persons grow older. However, a claim is made that the pressures of truly normotensive persons do not rise appreciably with age.[17] Whether the blood pressure rise with age observed in most populations is the result of an increasing incidence of "hypertensive disease," a biologic concomitant of aging that affects some more than others, a time-dose product of precursors, or progression of disease incurred in youth is not clear.

Further insight into the causes of essential hypertension will more surely arise from investigations conducted early in life. Factors initiating hypertension may differ from those sustaining it once established. Intensive study of the children of hypertensives may reveal the causes of hypertension in the adult.

Investigation of whether the changes in persons' pressures over time are correlated with their initial values has been carried out in the Framingham study among 5,209 men and women followed 12 years. This study has revealed that the tendency of systolic pressure to increase with age is largely independent of the initial pressure after age 30. Opinions to the contrary appear to stem from a misinterpretation of the regression properties of longitudinal data.

Almost all data tend to show lower pressures in women than in men at younger ages. Patterns of obesity, changes in blood hematocrit, and loss of ovarian function with advancing age may explain to some extent why pressures in women overtake and exceed those of men. However, no satisfactory explanation for this phenomenon is readily available. Overall death rates for hypertensive cardiovascular disease do not differ markedly by sex.[18]

Race

The reported differences in death rates attributed to hypertension according to skin color are reasonably consistent. Nonwhites have an appreciably higher rate of hypertension than whites. This difference becomes less pronounced with advanced age.[19] Between age 20 and 70 the prevalence of hypertensive heart disease is higher in each decade in nonwhites than in whites, with rates for nonwhites running almost four times as high as those of whites. The National Health Examination Survey found that Negro adults had blood pressures higher than whites (5.6 mm Hg systolic; 4.0 mm Hg diastolic). Since there were only six Negro families in the Framingham cohort this subject could not be studied.

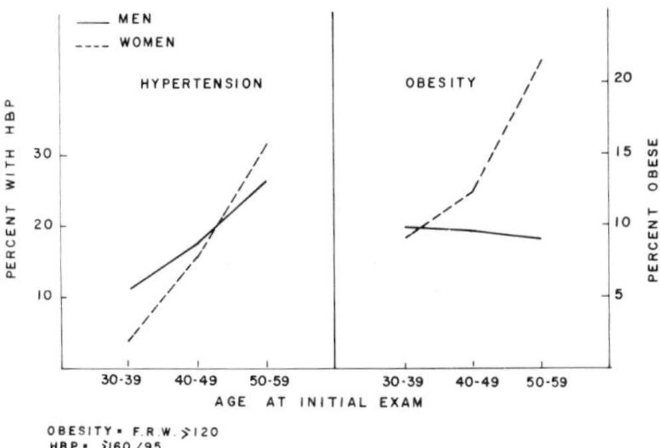

FIG. 6.—Prevalence of obesity and hypertension according to age and sex in men and women 30 to 59 years of age in the Framingham study. (From Kannel, W. B., et al.,[21] with permission.)

Obesity

A relationship between hypertension and excess body weight has long been recognized.[20] However, very little prospective data exist, particularly from general population samples, concerning the relation of changes in body weight to corresponding blood pressure values or to subsequent development of hypertension. Whether it is adiposity per se or some other associated factor that is primarily responsible for the higher pressures in the obese has not been established. The obesity-blood pressure correlation has been further clouded by the possible existence of an artifact in indirect blood pressure measurement related to the cushioning effect of adipose tissue in the upper arm.

The relationship of relative weight, adiposity, and arm girth to indirect blood pressure levels and to the subsequent rate of development of "hypertension" has been explored in Framingham. The independent contribution of arm girth, relative weight, and adiposity to current blood pressure and also to development of hypertension has been evaluated.[21]

Age trends in blood pressure and in obesity suggest a relationship between the two (Fig. 6). Both obesity and hypertension are less prevalent in women than men under age 50; beyond that age the converse is true. Not only is there a higher prevalence of hypertension in the obese, but its prevalence tends to increase quantitatively in proportion to the degree of overweight in each sex (Table 4). The average blood pressure increases in proportion to relative weight from the lowest to the highest weights recorded. However, the correlation between relative weight and blood pressure is modest ($r = 0.30$), indicating that while in-

TABLE 4.—*Prevalence of Hypertension at Initial Examination According to Relative Weight*

	Men			*Women*		
	Percentage Hypertensive			*Percentage Hypertensive*		
Relative Weight	*30–39*	*40–49*	*50–59*	*30–39*	*40–49*	*50–59*
<85	3	2	13	1	9	18
85–99	5	14	22	1	10	27
100–114	14	19	26	5	17	26
≥ 115	27	35	47	17	28	46

Reproduced from Kannel, W. B. et al.,[21] with permission.

Hypertension: ≥ 160 mm Hg systolic or ≥ 95 mm Hg diastolic on two blood pressure readings.

Framingham relative weight equals the percentage of median weight of population in each sex.

TABLE 5.—*Relation of Systolic Blood Pressure to Relative Weight in Men 30 to 50 Years of Age*

	Free of Coronary Heart Disease			Developed Coronary Heart Disease		
Age	*No.*	*Corre-lation*	*Regres-sion*	*No.*	*Corre-lation*	*Regres-sion*
30–39	786	0.313	0.364	31	0.383	0.421
40–49	693	0.251	0.353	74	0.452	0.764
50–59	514	0.212	0.368	99	0.267	0.554
Total	1993	0.259	0.370	204	0.291	0.534

Regressions and correlations are significantly different from zero in each coronary heart disease category
* Ten-year follow-up.

creased body weight may be a significant contributor to elevated blood pressure it is far from its chief determinant (Table 5). Relative weight, however, does appear to account for about 10 percent of the variance in blood pressure in the population. It is of interest that the correlation is higher in those who go on to develop coronary heart disease.

Changes in weight beyond the age of musculoskeletal growth in a sedentary population such as that in Framingham reflect principally changes in the size of the adipose tissue depot. Observation of the corresponding change in blood pressure in relation to the greatest gain and loss in weight for each subject during a 12-year period of observation revealed a substantial increase in pressure when the subjects gained weight, and a corresponding decrease with weight loss. The relationship was more striking in men than women.

Skinfold thickness provides a more direct measure of adiposity than does relative weight. Systolic pressure shows a distinct tendency to rise in proportion to skinfold thickness (Table

TABLE 6.—*Relation of Systolic Blood Pressure to Skinfold Thickness*

Age at Fourth Biennial Examination	*Subscapular Skinfold Thickness*			
	Men		*Women*	
	Regression	*Correlation*	*Regression*	*Correlation*
29–39	0.703	0.175	1.036	0.246
40–49	1.026	0.196	1.318	0.228
50–59	0.212	0.032	1.216	0.179
Total	0.634	0.120	1.520	0.251
Age at Fourth Biennial Examination	*Triceps Skinfold Thickness*			
	Men		*Women*	
	Regression	*Correlation*	*Regression*	*Correlation*
29–39	0.366	0.092	0.612	0.181
40–49	0.433	0.096	0.368	0.078
50–59	0.405	0.065	0.829	0.147
Total	0.352	0.071	0.720	0.145

Regressions and correlation coefficients are significantly different from zero except for men 55 to 64.

TABLE 7.—*Relation of Forearm Blood Pressure to Relative Weight in Men and Women 44 to 75 Years Old*

Relative Weight	*No.*	*Mean Systolic Blood Pressure*	*Percentage Hypertensive*
66–91	537	134	11.8
92–100	535	139	17.7
101–109	547	139	24.0
110–164	578	153	35.7

From Kannel, W. B. et al.,[21] with permission.
Trends are significant at 5-percent level.

6). The correlations and regression coefficients were modest but significant ($p = 0.05$). This was true whether the thickness was measured at the triceps or subscapular area. Correlations were higher for women than men. Pressures also rose in proportion to arm girth.

However, the relation of hypertension to adiposity cannot be attributed to a fat arm artifact since the blood pressure increased with relative weight even when the blood pressure was obtained with the cuff placed about the forearm (Table 7). In addition, blood pressures in the forearm and upper arm were similar regardless of the degree of adiposity.

Not only is *existing* hypertension related to relative weight, but initially normotensive obese subjects were found to *subsequently* develop hypertensive cardiovascular disease at an increased rate (Table 8). Relative weight at initial examination and weight gain after age 25 were shown to be related to subsequent

TABLE 8.—*An 8-Year Follow-up Study of Men and Women * 30 to 59 Years of Age Showing Risk of Developing Hypertensive Cardiovascular Disease According to Relative Weight*

Relative Weight	*8-Year Incidence of Hypertension †*		
	Observed	*Expected*	*Morbidity*
<90	22	45.5	48
90–109	83	81.4	102
110–119	22	17.7	125
≥ 120	26	8.1	320
	8-Year Incidence of Hypertensive Cardiovascular Disease ‡		
	Observed	*Expected*	*Morbidity*
<119	11	16.8	65
≥ 120	7	1.0	684

From Kannel, W. B. et al.,[21] with permission.
Morbidity ratio: observed cases per expected cases × 100.
* Normotensive at initial examination (< 140/90 mm Hg).
† Hypertension: ≧ 150/95 mm Hg.
‡ Hypertensive cardiovascular disease equals high blood pressure plus cardiac enlargement on x-ray or ECG.

development of hypertensive cardiovascular disease.[21] Evidently more than an immediate effect of adiposity is involved since normotensive obese persons had a tendency to later excess development of hypertension. The possibility of some unknown factor which promotes both adiposity and hypertension is suggested by the finding that lean hypertensives were also subject to subsequent excess development of

TABLE 9.—*Risk of Developing Obesity According to Blood Pressure Status of Men and Women 30 to 59 Years of Age*

Blood Pressure Status at Entry	*Men*			*Women*		
	Incidence of Obesity		*Morbidity Ratio (Observed/ Expected ×100)*	*Incidence of Obesity*		*Morbidity Ratio (Observed/ Expected ×100)*
	Observed	*Expected*		*Observed*	*Expected*	
Normotensive	54	68.6	79	81	108.6	75
Borderline	54	53.2	102	74	57.8	128
Hypertensive	36	22.3	162	37	25.6	145

From Kannel, W. B. et al.,[21] with permission.

TABLE 10.—*Correlation of Systolic and Diastolic Blood Pressure with Hemoglobin*

Correlation of Hemoglobin and:		*30–34*	*35–39*	*40–44*	*45–49*	*50–54*	*55–59*	*60–64*
Men	*No.*	*180*	*465*	*386*	*400*	*336*	*319*	*171*
Systolic blood pressure		0.13	0.18	0.04	0.12	0.09	0.08	0.07
Diastolic blood pressure		0.21	0.21	0.11	0.19	0.18	0.19	0.14
Women	*No.*	*208*	*548*	*526*	*436*	*435*	*385*	*201*
Systolic blood pressure		0.08	0.05	0.17	0.11	0.17	0.15	0.14
Diastolic blood pressure		0.14	0.14	0.18	0.14	0.18	0.20	0.20

Characteristics observed at second biennial examination (or at examination 1 if value at examination 2 was missing). Framingham study.

obesity (Table 9). Hypertensives had twice the risk of obesity of normotensives.

The evidence from previous investigations and the data from Framingham lead to the conclusion that development of adiposity is associated with a rise in blood pressure. Whether this is due solely to the accumulation of adiposity, some other attribute of body build, or some unknown factors related to both hypertension and obesity is not clear. While adiposity is certainly not the principal determinant of essential hypertension, it must be considered a significant contributor to elevated blood pressure. The widely accepted practice of prescribing weight reduction in overweight hypertensives seems amply justified. At least some hypertension may be prevented by avoidance of obesity.

Blood Hemoglobin

Within the normal range of blood hemoglobin values, excluding persons with polycythemia, there is a modest but statistically significant correlation between hemoglobin values and blood pressure (Table 10). At all ages, in both sexes, the correlation is higher for diastolic than systolic pressure, suggesting a relationship to peripheral resistance. These modest correlations translate into sizable differences in the prevalence of hypertension. There is a twofold gradient in prevalence within the normal range of blood hemoglobin (Table 11). The pathogenetic mechanisms remain obscure, although erythropoietin elaboration by an ischemic kidney may be postulated. The blood hematocrit influences its viscosity,

TABLE 11.—*Prevalence of Hypertension in Men and Women from 30 to 62 Years of Age According to Hemoglobin Level at Initial Examination*

Men		*Women*	
Hemoglobin (Grams per 100 ml)	*Percentage Hypertensive*	*Hemoglobin (Grams per 100 ml)*	*Percentage Hypertensive*
<12	16	<11	12
12–13.9	16	11–12.9	13
14–15.9	18	13–14.9	20
≥ 16	27	≥ 15	37

oxygen-carrying capacity, dynamics of flow, and possibly its clotting characteristics. A high hematocrit could also reflect a contraction of the blood plasma compartment. This association between hematocrit and blood pressure was also noted in the Evans County, Georgia study.[22]

Genetically determined conditions such as gout and diabetes are known to be associated with an increased incidence of hypertension, but hardly account for more than a fraction of the essential hypertension encountered in the general population.

Environmental Influences

A number of factors have been identified which appear to contribute to the occurrence of the cardiovascular diseases common to hypertensives. These include a rich diet, lack of physical activity, and cigarette smoking.[23] Obesity is primarily a product of overeating and lack of exercise. Except for obesity the search for potent environmental contributors to hypertension has been rewarded by little success.

Geographic variation in prevalence, secular trends, stratification by social class, income, education, urban-rural differences, and occupational variations are generally taken as evidence that environmental influences are at work. Such evidence for hypertension is inconclusive and inconsistent, and interpretation of such data is at best speculative.

Geographic Variation

The geographic variations in hypertension reported both within the United States and around the world, while interesting, are difficult to accept at face value.[19] Overall mortality from cardiovascular disease, to which hypertension contributes in large measure, is higher in the eastern and far western states, with lower mortality in the central and mountain regions. Death rates appear to be higher in large cities than in rural districts, but these do not entirely account for reported regional variations. Migration from high mortality areas does not appear to confer immunity. The National Health Examination Survey did not note differences between places of different population size or urban-rural differences although it did confirm regional differences. However, very impressive urban-rural differences have been noted in prevalence of hypertension in a carefully studied population sample in Puerto Rico.[24] The relative immunity of this rural population is still unaccounted for although the explanation may lie in the fact that the rural dwellers were leaner, more physically active, agrarian in occupation, and led a more quiet life than city dwellers. There is much to suggest that hypertension is a disease of industrialization and urbanization.

Secular Trends

Downward trends in death rates attributed to hypertension and hypertensive cardiovascular diseases over the past two decades suggest: (*1*) that these conditions are occurring less frequently; (*2*) that antihypertensive therapy is significantly effective; or (3) that diseases formerly attributed to hypertension are now being classified under another rubric. Between 1950 and 1967 age-adjusted death rates from hypertensive cardiovascular disease fell from 55.6 to 23.3 per 100,000 population.[25] However, since this decline has probably been going on since 1940, before effective antihypertensive agents were available, it seems likely that some other influence has been operative. Paffenbarger et al. found a downward trend in hypertensive death rates in Memphis between 1920 and 1960 and concluded that whatever the etiology of hypertensive disease, these diseases are being reported less frequently.[26] The roles of death certification and changing nosological rules in determining these downward trends are not clear. The present practice of listing sudden death as due to coronary heart disease as opposed to the previous custom of listing it as a cerebral hemorrhage is a good example. There is a strong clinical impression held by practicing physicians that hypertension, particularly severe hypertension, is less frequent than it was 20 years ago.

Physical Activity

There has been some suggestion that physical activity protects against the occurrence of hypertension. Since physically active people tend to be leaner, lower pressures would be expected on that account. On the other hand,

TABLE 12.—*Correlation of Living Habits with Systolic Blood Pressure*

	Men Simple Correlation			Women Simple Correlation		
Variable	*30–39*	*40–49*	*50–59*	*30–39*	*40–49*	*50–59*
Physical activity	—0.095	0.037	—0.100*	—0.050	—0.064	—0.023
Coffee	—0.065	—0.050	—0.078	—0.133*	—0.058	—0.042
Alcohol	0.067	—0.090*	0.071	0.091	0.085	0.104
Cigarettes	—0.065	—0.029	—0.117*	—0.101	—0.016	—0.045*

From Dawber, T. R. et al.,[27] with permission.
* Significant at 5 percent level.

systolic pressure levels equivalent to those of severe hypertension have been recorded during strenuous physical exertion. Some degree of hypertrophy may also be found in athletes. However, there is no evidence that transient pressure elevations induced by exercise persist after the exercise ceases. In fact, observations in the Framingham study suggest the blood pressure in physically active people may be slightly lower (Table 12). In the relatively sedentary population in Framingham the correlation between blood pressure and physical activity was virtually zero.[27] This would suggest that if there is an effect of increased physical activity it is slight and nevertheless beneficial. Possibly a leaner body habitus may explain this benefit. Peripheral adaptive changes of physical training in the skeletal muscles may play a role.

Job Stress

A variety of claims has been made concerning the influence of occupation on blood pressure. These have generally been inconsistent and difficult to interpret. The National Health Examination Survey found hypertension and hypertensive heart disease varied by occupation.[28] Professional occupations have also been incriminated.

In Framingham, no consistent pattern of blood pressure differences was observed in occupational subgroups presumed to reflect differences in job stress. Blood pressures were no different in relation to job responsibility (i.e., supervisor versus laborer), whether individuals were self-employed or working for others, or whether they were holding down one or multiple jobs (Table 13).

TABLE 13.—*Hypertensive Status of Men and Women According to Job Situation*

	Percentage of Hypertensives at Examination 4					
	Type of Employment				No. of Jobs *	
Age	*Self-*	*Other*	*Profes-sional*	*Laborer*	*One*	*More*
Men						
40–49	6.0	5.8	6.1	5.3	5.7	6.3
50–59	17.1	15.1	11.8	15.7	15.3	17.2
60–69	19.0	22.4	23.3	23.9	21.4	21.6 †
Women						
40–49	7.2	6.8	6.7	6.1	7.3	6.9
50–59	18.5	15.0	8.3	19.7	18.1	15.2
60–69	36.3	34.2	25.8	35.8	35.8	34.0

* Number of jobs held at one time. Housewife considered one job.
† Retired but working.

Education

The level of education achieved materially affects many aspects of life style. There is a suggestion in Framingham that those who achieved a higher level of schooling tended to have lower pressures.[27] This was particularly evident in the older age groups. Whether this reflects different weight patterns, adherence to antihypertensive therapy or psychosocial influences is difficult to state. This negative association of hypertension has also been reported in the National Health Survey.

Emotional Stress

Emotional stimuli are capable of producing profound transient elevations of blood pressure. Although it may be reasonable to hypothesize that these elevations may result in sustained hypertension, positive proof is lacking. Persons with hypertension are alleged to have different personality make-ups from normotensive individuals. That many of these personality assessments have been made after the fact makes interpretation difficult. The problems of defining and quantitating emotional stress have made the investigation of the role of this variable extremely complex.

Tobacco Smoking

Inhalation of tobacco smoke produces transient but distinct effects on the cardiovascular system. These effects are similar to those observed after the administration of nicotine. They include an increase in pulse rate, cardiac output, blood pressure, and peripheral resistance.[29] Contrary to expectation, however, neither at Framingham nor elsewhere is there evidence of any lasting effect. The distribution of pressures at Framingham was unrelated to cigarette-smoking status. There was, if anything, a slight but consistent negative correlation in every age-sex group (Table 12). These findings do not rule out the possibility that the immediate transient effects of tobacco smoking including increased myocardial irritability, effects on clotting, and on hemoglobin, may trigger lethal coronary attacks or precipitate a stroke. The cigarette habit has been shown to be associated with a distinct increase in risk of sudden death, myocardial infarction, brain infarction, and intermittent claudication.[23]

Coffee and Tea

Caffein is one of the few drugs consumed as part of the normal diet. The effects of caffein on the cardiovascular system are variable, but the usual net effect is a slight rise in blood pressure associated with an increase in cardiac output. As with cigarettes, the correlation with blood pressure is practically zero (Table 12). A conclusion that these transient effects are not translated into any lasting hypertensive effect is warranted.

Alcohol

No consistent effect of alcohol on blood pressure has been noted. In nondrinkers small amounts may produce transient elevations of cardiac output, pulse rate, and blood pressure.[30] This effect is less pronounced in habitual consumers of alcohol.[31] The distribution of blood pressures of persons using alcohol in the Framingham cohort was not significantly different from those who abstained.[27] Although male "heavy" alcohol consumers (one third of a bottle per day) appeared to have somewhat higher pressures, the correlation of blood pressure and alcohol intake throughout the range of intakes, however, was close to zero (Table 12).

Salt Intake

Salt has been implicated in the development of hypertension for a great many years. Since the turn of the century it has been customary to limit salt intake in the care of hypertensive patients. Restriction of salt intake to less than 200 mg daily was the first effective means of lowering blood pressure.[32] Geographic variation in the prevalence of hypertension has been noted to be related to the per-capita salt intake of the area. Eskimos, consuming 4 gm, had the lowest pressures; Americans averaging 10 gm, intermediate; and Japanese with 26 gm, the highest.[33] Rat experiments show that feeding large amounts of salt to susceptible strains for long periods beginning early in life can induce hypertension.[34] Simultaneous increase in potassium intake has been alleged to have a protective effect. Americans consume at least ten times the salt they require, often excreting 10 to 15 gm in the urine, while obligatory losses amount to only 5 to 35 mg.

TABLE 14.—*Proportion of Persons Reporting High Salt Intake According to Blood Pressure Quartiles*

Systolic Blood Pressure Quartile	*Percentage on High Salt Intake* *			
	Men		*Women*	
	37–49	*50–69*	*37–49*	*50–69*
1	32.4	40.8	12.9	0
2	30.0	25.0	11.8	23.5
3	34.0	37.5	14.3	7.4
4	25.6	44.8	10.0	9.5

From Dawber, T. R. et al.,[27] with permission.

* High intake is used to describe those who routinely add salt before tasting food and those who prefer salty food.

A crude assessment of dietary salt intake in Framingham revealed no relation between salt intake and blood pressure (Table 14). A failure to demonstrate any relationship between 24-hour sodium excretion and blood pressure confirmed this observation (Table 15). It is interesting that there is some relationship between relative weight and sodium excretion. The Framingham population was on a relatively high sodium intake. Even those with the lowest intake were well above the 200-mg intake per day below which therapeutic lowering of blood pressure can be achieved. Thus, the failure to establish a relationship between sodium intake and blood pressure in this population does not negate the possibility that in populations with much lower intakes of sodium such a relationship might be found. In the Framingham study the ratio of sodium to potassium excreted was unrelated to blood pressure.

That salt intake early in life may be important in persons susceptible to hypertension is still a strong possibility. This relationship warrants further investigation. Of all the environmental factors affecting the level of blood pressure a salt intake below 200 mg per 100 cc has the greatest impact.

Diet

Overeating in general, and of meat proteins in particular, has been incriminated as a cause of hypertension. No indication of any relation between blood pressure level and total daily calorie consumption or the nutrient composition of the diet with regard to protein, fat, or cholesterol was noted in the Framingham cohort (Table 16).

Clinical Implications

In 1970 approximately two million deaths occurred in the United States; half were due to diseases of the heart and blood vessels, including strokes. While only 7 percent of these deaths were *directly* attributed to hypertensive cardiovascular disease, it is clear that hypertension is a major contributor to stroke and coronary mortality as well. In addition, it is estimated that "hypertension" is reported in death certification in fewer than one fifth of the deaths in which it was known to be present. Together, cardiovascular and cerebrovascular diseases account for half the annual toll of mortality in the United States. The National Health Survey found that hypertensive heart disease is the most prevalent cardiac condition, afflicting 10.5 million people.

Because of ignorance of the etiologic factors responsible for hypertension in the general population, no effective measures for the primary prevention of hypertension can be recommended with any degree of assurance. Certain

TABLE 15.—*24-Hour Urine Sodium Excretion Compared to Blood Pressure and Relative Weight in Men*

Sodium Excretion (grams of sodium chloride)	*No.*	*Age*	*Mean Blood Pressure*	*Relative Weight*
<8 gm	41	44	131/85	101
8–10.4 gm	55	44	139/89	107
10.5–12.9 gm	45	44	137/87	107
>13 gm	44	45	139/88	112

TABLE 16.—*Mean Daily Intake of Nutrients According to Systolic Pressure*

	Daily Nutrient Intakes							
	Men				Women			
Systolic Pressure Quartiles	*Calories*	*Protein (grams)*	*Fat (grams)*	*Choles-terol (milli-grams)*	*Calories*	*Protein (grams)*	*Fat (grams)*	*Choles-terol (milli-grams)*
Q_1	3300	124	143	705	2225	91	102	532
Q_2	3285	128	144	686	2145	83	97	438
Q_3	3295	127	142	668	2250	92	100	489
Q_4	3160	122	130	645	2279	92	102	500

From Dawber et al.,[27] with permission.

persons appear to be more highly vulnerable. Included are Negroes, persons with gout and diabetes, close relatives of hypertensives, women who have had toxemia of pregnancy, the obese, persons with labile blood pressure elevation, and those with high hemoglobin values and rapid pulse rates. Whether weight reduction, tranquilizers, or salt restriction in such persons or in the general population will decrease the incidence of hypertension is unknown. However, periodic surveillance of the well population or of vulnerable persons can allow early detection and management of hypertension so that its deadly cardiovascular sequelae can be delayed. No other major contributor to cardiovascular disease is as easily detected and as readily controllable. Other major risk factors contributing to cardiovascular disease such as obesity, cigarette smoking, lack of exercise, and improper diet can be recognized and dealt with by the intelligent and motivated potential victim, but there is no possibility for this in persons with hypertension unless this disorder is detected.

Hypertension, more than any other factor demonstrated to contribute to cardiovascular morbidity and mortality, deserves serious attention from those concerned with the major cardiovascular killers. There is no longer reason to doubt that persons with either moderate or severe hypertension benefit from measures which lower their blood pressure.[35] The optimal time to begin such management is still in doubt, but evidence would suggest that the earlier in life this is undertaken the better. To date there is no concrete evidence that the same benefits will accrue for those with mild hypertension without organ damage. Further research to determine if such is the case is urgently needed, for it is here that the greatest potential for achieving a substantial lowering of hypertensive cardiovascular morbidity and mortality lies. Awaiting the onset of fixed diastolic hypertension of severe degree or involvement of the heart, brain or kidneys before instituting treatment does not appear logical.

Excluding curable forms of hypertension, the nature of the blood pressure elevation, its height, whether sustained or labile, its rate of progression, the condition of the arterioles in the optic fundi, and the extent of damage in other target organs is of fundamental concern in deciding the urgency of treatment. However, the patient with essential hypertension may remain asymptomatic for many years.

Few guidelines are available for assessing the importance of hypertensive disease, and the factors which influence its impact on the cardiovascular apparatus are not well understood. Identification of factors which influence the rate of evolution of presymptomatic hypertension into symptomatic overt cardiovascular disease has considerable relevance for prevention and for providing an understanding of pathogenesis. The course and prognosis of essential hypertension as it occurs in the general population have been only partially appreciated from numerous studies of "hypertensive" patients in clinical series. Such appraisals lack information on most of the presymptomatic segments of the hypertensive population and on those dying too suddenly to reach medical attention. They also suffer from incomplete follow-up. Prospective epidemiologic study of a reasonably representative sample of the general population in Framingham under continuous, routine periodic medical surveillance provides a less distorted appraisal of the serious impact of hypertension as a force of morbidity and mortality. Factors which influence the rate of development of cardiovascular morbidity and mortality have been identified. Factors which make a given blood pressure elevation particularly dangerous have been delineated. Although the seriousness of an elevated pressure is largely a function of its level, the other identified factors that markedly influence risk of cardiovascular morbidity and mortality must be taken into account. Elevated pressure, whether predominantly systolic or diastolic, labile or fixed, in either sex, at any age, assumes increasingly grave significance when attended by abnormal blood lipids, impaired glucose tolerance, cardiac enlargement on x-ray, left ventricular hypertrophy (LVH) on ECG, a high normal hemoglobin value, obesity, and the cigarette habit. Risk mounts precipitously when these appear and becomes grave when an elevated blood urea nitrogen (BUN), albuminuria, or eye-ground changes occur. Multiple factors are involved in the genesis of hypertensive cardiovascular and cerebrovascular disease; and blood pressure elevation is best conceptualized as one ingredient of a cardiovascular disease profile. Management of "mild hypertension" becomes urgent when the aforementioned harbingers of coronary attacks, strokes, and congestive failure appear.

Effective prophylaxis is hampered by a number of misconceptions concerning the natural history of "essential hypertension." It is not a disease which begins late in life; women do not tolerate it well; moderate, labile, and systolic elevations are not innocuous at any age; it does not generally cause symptoms until target-organ involvement occurs. Many physicians consider it meddlesome to intervene before hypertension becomes fixed and target-organ involvement appears. They are justifiably concerned about the possible hazards of long-term antihypertensive therapy with drugs known to have potentially serious side effects. However, labile, moderate hypertension often does not require potent, potentially harmful, antihypertensive agents. Before severe, fixed diastolic hypertension with involvement of the heart, brain, or kidneys appears, weight reduction, salt restriction, sedation or the mildest antihypertensive agents or both may be all that is required.

The advisability of lowering blood pressures in patients with cardiovascular disease or in those suspected of having it—particularly cerebrovascular disease, coronary disease, and renal artery disease—has long been debated. Despite the availability of effective and relatively safe antihypertensive agents their use in such individuals has been restricted for fear of producing further impairment of blood flow and reduced perfusion of already ischemic organs. Evidently the benefits of such therapy outweigh the hazards, as indicated by the Veterans Administrative Cooperative Study, which has clearly demonstrated the efficacy of controlling severe and moderate hypertension in preventing strokes, congestive failure, and renal insufficiency.

While the relation of hypertension to the development of cardiovascular disease is well established, there is much that remains to be learned about the pathogenetic mechanisms involved. Even after target-organ involvement has occurred, control of hypertension has been shown to decrease subsequent mortality and morbidity. Heightened cerebrovascular resistance and decreased cerebral blood flow can actually be returned toward normal by antihypertensive treatment.[36] Thus, in persons presumed to have a compromised circulation and at high risk of cardiovascular catastrophes and strokes, prudent control of hypertension may actually improve hemodynamics and remove the precipitating factor of hypertension.

Meanwhile, approximately half of the 21 million hypertensives in the United States go undetected and half of those detected go untreated. Furthermore, only about half of those receiving treatment have their pressures held down to reasonably normotensive values. Now that hypertension is a more manageable condition, evaluation and sustained management of the hypertensive have assumed greater importance. To implement effective prophylactic management of presymptomatic essential hypertension, guidelines for therapy based on knowledge of the factors which enhance the cardiovascular morbidity and mortality in the hypertensive are required. This evaluation must be possible at an office level if it is to be widely applied. These criteria can be met. The foregoing data can provide a basis for formulating such guidelines, and evaluation and follow-up require nothing more than ordinary office procedures and simple laboratory tests. It would seem reasonable to monitor blood pressure periodically throughout life, particularly in persons with a family history of hypertension, and to institute multifactoral corrective measures promptly.

Blood pressure should be controlled initially by hygienic measures such as weight reduction, exercise, and avoidance of rich, high-caloric, and salty foods. If it is refractory to these measures and of severe and fixed degree or rapidly progressive or accompanied by factors shown to adversely affect its course, effective antihypertensive agents are available. These, if effectively and prudently used, can control hypertension with minimal hazard and will delay the onset of congestive failure, strokes, and possibly coronary heart disease. Research is urgently needed to determine the efficacy and possible hazards of the currently available agents to control milder and labile degrees of hypertension. However, even these milder degrees of hypertension are associated with a substantial cardiovascular mortality and at the very least are a forerunner of more severe hypertension. Not all moderate hypertension is necessarily innocuous. Risk of cardiovascular consequences varies over a wide range depending on associated findings. Those that require intervention can be readily distinguished from those that merely require watching. Because such hypertension is more easily and safely controlled, prophylactic management of early as well as late hypertensive disease would seem both rational and justified.

References

1. Dawber, T. R., Meadors, G. F., and Moore, F. E., Jr.: Epidemiological approaches to heart disease: The Framingham Study. Am. J. Public Health 41:279, 1951.
2. Gordon, T., and Devine, B.: Hypertension and hypertensive heart disease in adults. U.S. 1960–1962. Vital and Health Statistics, Series 11, No. 13, 966.
3. Wilbur, J. A., Barrow, J. G.: Reducing elevated blood pressure experience found in a community. Minn. Med. 52:97, 1969.
4. Wood, J. E., Barrow, J. G., Gifford, R. W., Kirkendall, W., Lee, R. E., Williamson, H., Wilbur, J. A., and Stamler, J. J.: Intersociety Report III. Cardiovascular disease—long-term care. Guidelines for detection, diagnosis and management of hypertensive populations. Circulation 44:A26; A237, 1971.
5. Texon, M.: The hemodynamic concept. Concepts of atherosclerosis. Am. J. Cardiol. 5: 291, 1960.
6. Young, W., Gofman, J. W., Tandy, R., Malamud, N., and Waters, E. S.: The quantitation of atherosclerosis. I. Relationship to artery size. Am. J. Cardiol. 6:288, 1960.
7. Sako, Y.: Effects of turbulent blood flow and hypertension on experimental atherosclerosis. JAMA 179:36, 1962.
8. Deming, Q. B., Mosbach, E. H., Bevans, M. D., Daly, M. M., Akell, L. L., Martin, E., Brun, L. M., Halpern, E., and Kaplan, R.: Blood pressure, cholesterol content of serum and tissues and atherosclerosis in the rat. J. Exp. Med. 107:581, 1958.
9. Moses, C.: Development of atherosclerosis in dogs with hypercholesterolemia and chronic hypertension. Circ. Res. 2:243, 1954.
10. Bronte-Stewart, B., and Heptinstal, R. H.: The relationship between experimental hypertension and cholesterol-induced atheroma in rabbits. J. Pathol. 68:407, 1954.
11. Truett, J., Cornfield, J., Kannel, W. B.: A multivariate analysis of the risk of coronary heart disease in Framingham. J. Chronic Dis. 20:511, 1967.
12. Kannel, W. B., Gordon, T., and Schwartz, M. J.: Systolic versus diastolic blood pressure and risk of coronary heart disease. The Framingham Study. Am. J. Cardiol. 273:335, 1971.
13. Friedman, G. D., Loveland, D. B., and Ehrlich, S. P.: Relationship of stroke to other cardiovascular disease. Circulation 38:533, 1968.
14. Winkelstein, W., Jr., Kanter, S., Ibraham, M., and Sackett, D. L.: Familial aggregation of blood pressure. Preliminary Report. JAMA 195:848, 1966.
15. Pickering, G. W.: Inheritance of high blood pressure. *In* Pickering, G. W. (Ed.): Essential Hypertension. An International Symposium. Berlin: Springer, 1960.
16. Zinner, S. H., Levy, P. S., and Kass, E. H.: Familial aggregation of blood pressure in children. N. Engl. J. Med. 284:402, 1971.

17. Miall, W. E.: Implications of the relation between blood pressure and age. Milbank Mem. Fund. 47:107, part 2, 1969.
18. Cardiovascular Diseases in the U.S.: Facts and Figures. New York: American Heart Association and National Heart Institute, 1965.
19. Gordon, T.: Blood pressure of adults by race and area. U. S. 1960–1962. Vital and Health Statistics, series 11, No. 5, 1964.
20. Pickering, G. W.: High Blood Pressure. Churchill: London, 1955.
21. Kannel, W. B., Brand, N., Skinner, J. J., Dawber, T. R., and McNamara, P. M.: The relation of adiposity to blood pressure and development of hypertension. Ann. Intern. Med. 67:48, 1967.
22. McDonough, J. R., Hames, E. G., and Garrison, G. E.: The relationship of hematocrit to cardiovascular states of health in the Negro and white population of Evans County, Georgia. J. Chronic Dis. 18:243, 1965.
23. Kannel, W. B., Dawber, T. R., and McNamara, P. M.: Detection of the coronary-prone adult. The Framingham Study. J. Iowa Med. Soc. 56:25, 1966.
24. Garcia-Palmieri, M.: Personal communication.
25. Cardiovascular Diseases in the U.S.: Facts and Figures. New York: American Heart Association and National Heart Institute, 1965, p. 18.
26. Paffenbarger, R. S., Jr., Milling, R. N., and Poe, N. D.: Trends in death rates from hypertensive disease in Memphis, Tennessee, 1920–1960. J. Chronic Dis. 19:847, 1966.
27. Dawber, T. R., Kannel, W. B., Kagan, A., Donabedian, R. K., McNamara, P. M., and Pearson, G.: Environmental factors in hypertension. *In* Stamler, J., Stamler, R., and Pullman, T. N. (Eds.): Epidemiology of Hypertension. New York: Grune & Stratton, 1967, pp. 255–288.
28. Gordon, T., and Devine, B.: Hypertension and hypertensive heart disease in adults. U.S. 1960–1962. Vital and Health Statistics. Series 11, No. 13, 1966.
29. Larson, P. S., Hoag, H. B., Silvette, H.: Tobacco—Experimental and Clinical Studies. Baltimore: Williams & Wilkins, 1961.
30. Grollman, A.: The action of alcohol, caffein, and tobacco on the cardiac output (and its related functions) of normal man. J. Pharmacol. Exp. Ther. 39:313, 1930.
31. Abelman, W. H., Kowalski, H. J., and McNeely, W. F.: The circulation of the blood in alcohol addicts. Q. J. Stud. Alcohol 15:1, 1954.
32. Grollman, A.: The relationship of salt and diet to diastolic hypertension. Am. J. Cardiol. 9:700, 1962.
33. Dahl, L. K., and Love, R. A.: Etiological role of sodium chloride in essential hypertension in humans. JAMA 164:397, 1957.
34. Dahl, L., Heine, M., and Tassinari, L.: Effects of chronic excess salt ingestion. Evidence that genetic factors play an important role in susceptibility to experimental hypertension. J. Exp. Med. 115:1173, 1962.
35. Freis, E. D.: Veterans Administration Cooperative Study Group on Antihypertensive Agents. Effects of treatment on morbidity in hypertension. JAMA 202:1028, 1967; 213: 1143, 1970.
36. Meyer, J. S., Sawada, T., Kitamura, A., and Tayada, M.: Cerebral blood flow after control of hypertension in stroke. Neurology 18: 772, 1968.
37. Shurtleff, D.: Some characteristics related to the incidence of cardiovascular disease and death: Framingham Study, 16-year follow-up. *In* Kannel, W. B., and Gordon, T. (Eds.): The Framingham Study: An Epidemiological Investigation of Cardiovascular Disease. Washington, D.C.: U.S. Govt. Printing Office, 1970, Sect. 26.
38. Gordon, T., and Verter, J.: Serum cholesterol, systolic blood pressure and Framingham relative weight as discriminators of cardiovascular disease. *In* Kannel, W. B., and Gordon, T. (Eds.): The Framingham Study: An Epidemiological Investigation of Cardiovascular Disease. Washington, D.C.: U.S. Government Printing Office, 1969, Sect. 23.
39. Gordon, T., Sorlie, P., and Kannel, W. B.: Coronary heart disease, atherothrombotic brain infarction, intermittent claudication—A multivariate analysis of some factors related to their incidence: The Framingham Study, 16-year follow-up. *In* Kannel, W. B., and Gordon, T. (Eds.): The Framingham Study: An Epidemiological Investigation of Cardiovascular Disease. Washington, D.C.: U.S. Govt. Printing Office, 1971, Sect. 27.

Salt, Heredity, and Hypertension

By Knud D. Knudsen, M.D., Junichi Iwai, M.D., and Lewis K. Dahl, M.D.

THE THREE WORDS in the title are all common and may have different meanings in different contexts.

Here, "salt" is table salt, sodium chloride, and although the sodium ions of its crystals cause the problems that concern us, it is right and proper, when dealing with the public health aspect, to talk of salt in the food rather than of "sodium." The sodium originally present is of minor importance; it is the large amounts of salt added during processing which are of concern.

The first Hahnemann Symposium on Hypertensive Disease devoted whole sections to the role of salt in causation and treatment, and although the concepts have been modified they have not fundamentally changed in the last 13 years. Some of the positions taken in 1958 are still tenable.[1] No evidence has been forthcoming that man needs or benefits from any sodium over and above what he gets in unadulterated food. In the delightful introduction to his paper, Meneely stated the case succinctly: ". . . salt is a condiment, not an aliment."[2] Most of the epidemiologic and clinical evidence linking a high-salt intake to hypertension was also available at that time.[3–7] Epidemiologic evidence is summarized in Figure 1.[8] Clinical evidence continues to accumulate. Among patients with uncomplicated essential hypertension admitted to our metabolic ward, 20 to 30 percent demonstrate a significant improvement on salt restriction, only. We keep these patients in caloric balance on a constant low-salt diet and constant fluid intake, and when we observe them on high-salt intake, salt is given in water, not in the food. If all people reacted alike, there would be no argument. Fortunately, a majority seem to be able to eat salt to their heart's desire with no obvious penalty to pay and, unfortunately, there are many patients whose blood pressure remains high despite severe salt restriction. Salt is, therefore, a factor in hypertensive disease, but is neither sufficient to explain the pathogenesis, nor necessary to maintain established disease. Other factors exist and we must postulate an interaction of factors to explain the observation.

We are on record as favoring a ban on the addition of salt to processed baby foods.[9–12] This position is not contradictory to anything said here. It is based on a firm conviction that this addition is unnecessary and that it is a contamination which will prove harmful to a large number of the recipients. The fact that we cannot answer "whom" or "how many" is irrelevant. Recommendations must often be made on less than complete information and our bias must be the Hippocratic aphorism, "First, do no harm!"

"Heredity" is an overworked word, but it did not figure conspicuously in the first Hahnemann Symposium on Hypertension. The only title suggesting emphasis on genetics was "Epidemiology of primary hypertension with par-

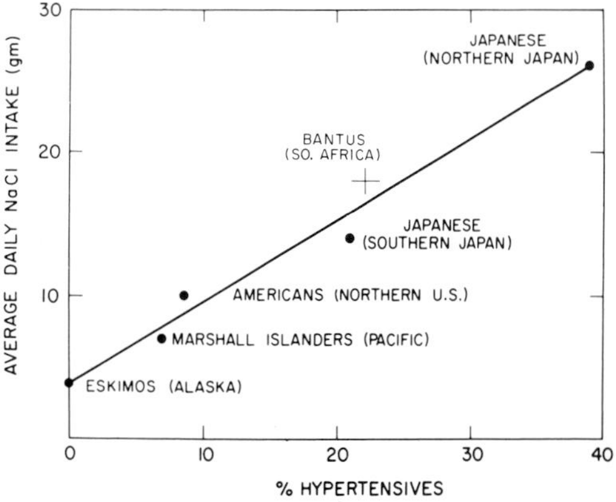

Fig. 1.—Correlation of average daily salt (NaCl) intakes with prevalence of hypertension in different geographic areas and among different races. (From Knudsen, K. D., and Dahl, L. K.,[8] with permission.)

This work was supported primarily by the U.S. Atomic Energy Commission; partial support was received from U.S.P.H.S. (HE 13408–01) and a grant-in-aid of the American Heart Association (AHA 70–772) supported by the Dutchess County (N.Y.) Heart Association.

From the Medical Department of Brookhaven National Laboratory, Upton, New York.

ticular reference to racial susceptibility," a paper presented by Dr. Marvin Moser.[13] In a panel discussion on basic concepts Grollman said, "An important aspect of the subject that I think ought to be discussed is the fact that many believe that hypertension is an inheritable disease." In the exchange which followed, everyone seemed to take the hereditary aspect for granted.[14]

In the second Hahnemann Symposium on Hypertension, hereditary factors are indexed seven times, mostly from passing remarks during discussion of other matters. In this year's Symposium, there are at least six contributions in which genetic concepts probably are a significant topic. Hence, our concern about, if not our knowledge of, the hereditary aspect must have increased during the last decade.

"Hypertension" will refer to blood pressure levels. When etiology, pathogenesis, or clinical correlates of hypertensive disease are considered they will be named explicitly.

The thesis in this paper is that genetic factors determine who will, and who will not, tolerate a high-salt intake. This is only a specific case of the general observation that phenotype is the end-product of genetic factors interacting with a given environment.

Figure 2 illustrates our way of thinking. The

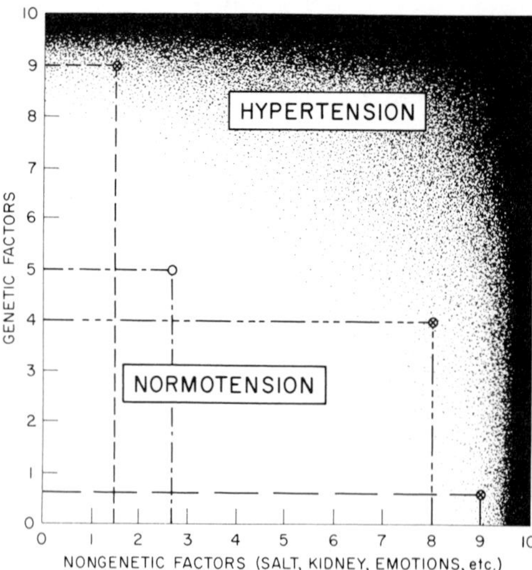

FIG. 2.—Diagram to suggest possible relative roles of genetic and nongenetic factors in hypertension. (From Dahl, L. K., Heine, M., and Tassinari, L.,[15] with permission.)

person with a high genetic susceptibility needs little prodding from the environment to develop his disease. On the other hand, if the external forces are overwhelming, even the genetically resistant person succumbs.[15]

Figure 2 is, of course, an illustration only but the concept has been developed into a tool for the study of heredity, particularly by British investigators.

Two words, "liability" and "heritability," must be introduced to develop this thesis. In quantitative genetics they are precise concepts, and involve subtleties which can be appreciated only by working with the definitions. They cannot be used in the general sense suggested by a dictionary. Liability as a genetic concept was introduced by Falconer [16] to express the whole combination of external and genetic circumstances that makes an individual more or less likely to develop a disease. Heritability is the additive genetic variance alone as a proportion of phenotypic variance. It expresses the extent to which the phenotypes exhibited by parents are transmitted to their offspring. It therefore determines the correlation between relatives.[16] Emphasis here is on variance, which is used in the sense defined in statistics, and also on additive. When genes interact, the degree of genetic determination may be larger than the heritability.

Heritability is of particular importance for our purpose for two reasons. First, it will predict the correlation between relatives. If we measure blood pressure in a population the regression coefficient of relatives on propositi, b, is related to heritability, h^2, by the equation

$$h^2 = b/r$$

where r is the coefficient of relationship. For monozygotic twins $r = 1.0$ and for the first-degree relatives $r = 0.5$. In the latter case we have

$$h^2 = 2b.$$

Secondly, Falconer [16] has developed a method based on the liability concept whereby heritability can be estimated from incidence data alone and which permits a comparison of epidemiologic surveys, even when criteria for diagnosis differ. His method has been applied to diseases as different as clubfoot and schizophrenia and is also applicable to hypertension.

Blood pressures are measured on a scale which is convenient for instrumentation; it is not a scale appropriate for statistical analysis of variance. (Distributions are skewed. Variances are not constant. There is a selection against high pressures.) Many transforms have been proposed; none as yet is entirely satisfactory.[17] Miall and Oldham [18] used a conversion to scores which intended to correct for age and sex.[19] Acheson and Fowler have discussed the value and the limitations of this particular transform.[20] They concluded that the regressions calculated from these scores were artificially low. The regression coefficients calculated by Miall and Oldham for all first-degree relatives on all propositi was about 0.3, which could correspond to a heritability factor of 0.6 for blood pressure in these populations. This, according to Acheson and Fowler, is then a lower limit for this estimate. If we apply Falconer's analysis to the data of Søbye [21] we get values for h^2 from 0.5 to 1.3 as we work out the heritability for each table he presented. Vander Molen's data on dizygotic twins [22] gives $h^2 = 1.0$ for systolic pressure, $h^2 = 1.3$ for diastolic pressure. From measurements on 23 monozygotic twins from three studies [22–24] we calculate $h^2 = 0.76$ for systolic pressure.

The estimates of heritability are admittedly lacking in precision, but they suggest that in these populations most of the variance in blood pressure is caused by genetic factors. If there is a large element of dominance and genetic interaction, the so-called degree of genetic determination is even stronger than the value suggested by heritability calculations.

What does this mean? In some excellent articles by Carter, he emphasized that "the heritability may vary from one population to another. . . . Even when the real heritability of a condition is high . . . it is still well worth searching for the environmental component. Protection from the environmental component may prevent the onset of disease even if there is a strong genetic liability. Further, the search for the environmental component in aetiology may often be most economically made in those known to be genetically predisposed." [25,26]

We shall leave considerations of the human experience and devote the rest of our time to hypertension in rats. Returning to the first Hahnemann Symposium, Dr. Grollman continued the remark on heredity quoted above [14] by saying, "Hypertension seems to be a purely human disease; it rarely occurs in other animals, except in the presence of obvious renal lesions." This situation is dramatically changed today. There are at least three strains of rats where elevated blood pressure depends on hereditary factors. They may have microscopic changes in the kidney when hypertension is manifest, but there is no obvious renal lesion. The first of these strains was reported by Smirk and Hall in 1958,[27] the next from our laboratory in 1962,[28] and then by Okamoto and Aoki in 1963.[29] We shall restrict our comments to our own experience.

Meneely and his associates demonstrated that rats developed hypertension when salt was added to their chow; [30] a standard dose-response was apparent in that as the average salt intake of groups increased, the average blood pressure of the respective groups increased correspondingly (Fig. 3). These results were strikingly similar to those seen in our epidemiologic studies of the human disease.[31]

When we fed salt to the rats we were struck by the wide varieties of response within a given level of salt intake.[32] This suggested a genetic rather than a technical variance, and we therefore started mating members at either extreme

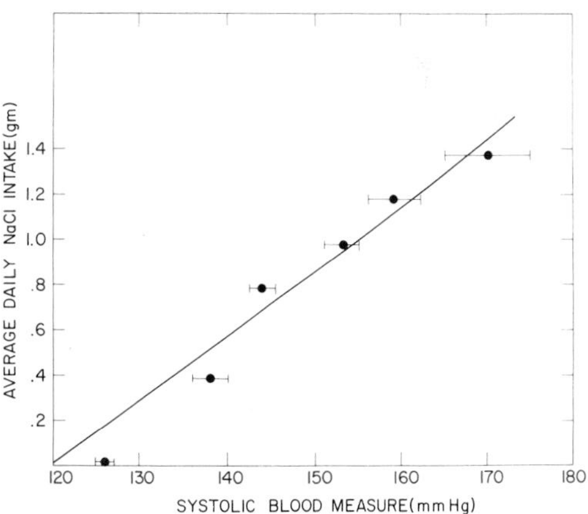

FIG. 3.—Correlation between average daily salt (NaCl) intake and mean (± S.E.) systolic blood pressure of rats after 12 months on various levels of salt intake. Recalculated from the findings of Meneely et al.[30] Each of six colonies of rats was fed chow containing different (but constant) levels of salt. The blood pressures after 1 year show that as average salt intake increased, average blood pressure also increased.

of the response range. Within a few generations we had two colonies which we have since kept breeding and studying. Within one colony—we called it the resistant or R strain—the members generally evinced a lack of response to high salt intake, and the average blood pressure of a group was not significantly increased by this diet.[32] In the other colony—the sensitive or S strain—moderate amounts of salt in the diet would produce a significant rise in blood pressure, and high-salt intake would lead to malignant hypertension and death within a few months.[33,34]

The results were so startling that they immediately raised a number of questions:

1. Was this disease the same as essential hypertension in man?
2. Was the resistance or sensitivity or both carried over to other means of producing hypertension, or was it a specifically salt-related trait?
3. What were the mechanisms by which salt produced this effect?
4. How many genes were involved?

The first question is still too vaguely phrased to be answered. Indeed, if we focus on the endpoint, i.e., blood pressure only, we cannot even tell whether essential hypertension in man is one or many diseases. To this end we must study etiology and pathogenesis, which lead to questions 2, 3, and 4. Half an answer to the first question is that no known particular feature of the disease in rats sets it apart from human hypertension.

The answer to the second question is yes; in addition to the high-salt diet, the S-strain rats are more sensitive than R-strain rats to unilateral renal artery constriction, adrenal enucleation, Doca-salt, cortisone, and uninephrectomy.[35,36] Hence, in these rats, increased susceptibility to one kind of hypertension implied an increased susceptibility to several other kinds. We must assume some common denominator for all these forms of experimental hypertension regardless of cause.

The third question, of course, is crucial. Among other mechanisms, we have postulated, and tried to identify, a humoral factor which we believe to be produced by the S-strain rat kidney. We have found that in the development of salt-induced and of Goldblatt hypertension in S-strain rats this factor can be transferred across a parabiosis junction and induce hypertension in co-twins from the R strain.[37–39] At this time we are exploring the possibility that the S factor is identical to a renin inhibitor which occurs under the same set of circumstances.[40] Interestingly enough, Goldblatt-hypertensive, R-strain rats do not appear to produce this factor. Goldblatt operation is the one exception to the rule that S-strain rats are more sensitive than R-strain rats. Rats from both strains develop equivalent blood pressure levels after this procedure, but R-strain rats do not induce hypertension in parabiotic co-twins. Hence, although Goldblatt hypertension has the same cause and reaches the same level in the two strains, the pathogenesis may have differences which depend on the genetic endowment.

We can answer question 4 with an estimate: The number of major genes involved is at least two, possibly no more than four. We will review briefly the observations on which this estimate is based.[41]

1. Rats from neither S nor R strains reproduce the traits faithfully. If the breeding is left to chance, the average blood pressure of both colonies tends to drift toward the middle. Hence, neither strain seems to be homozygous for the desired traits, and a continuous selection is needed to keep the strains at optimum response.
2. Variance within litters is smaller than variance within colonies.

Both these observations suggest that more than one gene is involved. We undertook a crossbreeding experiment to arrive at an estimate of the number of genes.[41] We mated R- with S-strain rats. The offspring—the F_1 generation—were mated among themselves to produce the F_2 rats, and with members of the parent strains to obtain backcrosses (BR) and (BS).

Figure 4 shows the average blood pressures over an observation period of 1 year on a high-salt intake.

The experiment pictured in Figure 4 shows in a microcosm all the complexities which face us in the study of human populations which have to be resolved before major progress can be expected.

Our blood pressure scale is not appropriate for analysis of variance. The distributions are

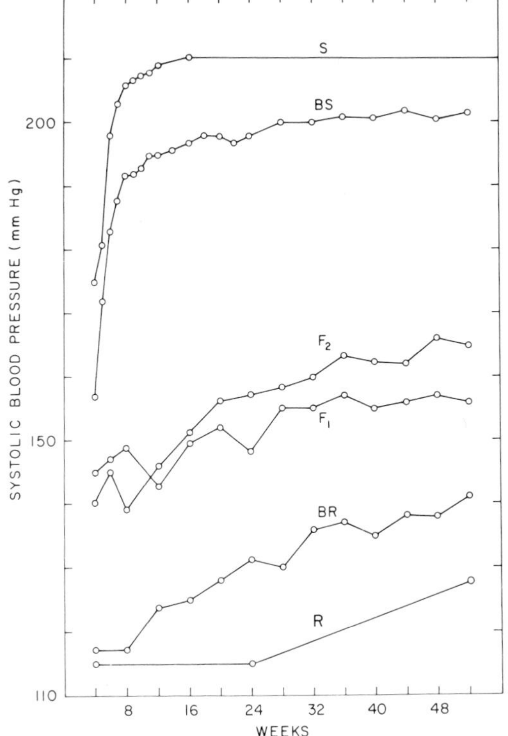

FIG. 4.—Average blood pressures of different rat populations on a uniform high-salt (8 percent NaCl in chow) diet during a year of observation. The **curves** represent average cumulative systolic blood pressure for each cross. Cumulative blood pressures include the last blood pressure taken when animal was in good health, and this value is carried forward whether an animal survived 6 weeks or 12 months on the regimen. Note that no S-strain rat survived beyond the 16th week. **S,** Sensitive strain; **R,** resistant strain; $\mathbf{F_1}$, R×S; $\mathbf{F_2}$, $F_1 \times F_1$; **BS,** $F_1 \times$S; **BR,** $F_1 \times$R. Although **R, BR,** $\mathbf{F_1}$, and $\mathbf{F_2}$ showed significant differences in blood pressure based on sex (males higher than females), the values have been pooled for the purpose of this graph which illustrates the definite genetic influence on the reaction to salt intake. (From Knudsen, K. D. et al.,[41] with permission.)

skewed and variance increases with increasing average blood pressure.

A logarithmic transform of the values will normalize the distributions sufficiently to resolve this problem. A physiologist may be hesitant to accept such arbitrary manipulations of data but the statisticians reply that there is nothing physiologic about the numbers we use —they merely represent another arbitrary scale imposed on us by our instruments.

There is a sex influence on the expressions of the genes: while the effects seem to be additive in the male, the female repressed the expression of the high blood pressure genes, which requires that we analyze the sexes separately.

There is a negative selection. Hypertensive rats die young. If among three rats at 6 weeks two have a blood pressure of 130 mm Hg, the third has a pressure of 200 mm Hg and dies shortly thereafter; if after 36 weeks one of the two surviving rats has a blood pressure of 200 mm Hg, while the other is still normotensive—how do we quantify this information? In the given example, we can at least give a ranking and use nonparametric statistics, but it is easy to conjure situations where even a ranking list is difficult to establish. Where does this leave us? Our reliance on blood pressure data to classify intensity of disease is inadequate since it excludes all information about mortality and morbidity. We believe that if progress is to be made in this line of research, we must abandon arguments as to whether blood pressure distributions are unimodal or bimodal and adopt Falconer's concept of a hypothetical liability scale which covers all aspects of the disease. Since no such scale has yet been devised, we must base our calculations on incidence data rather than on distribution curves.

We have no great expectations that large-scale population studies will lead to new levels of insight; we expect that intensive studies, rather than extensive, will be the order of the day. Progress will depend on identification of specific metabolic aberrations and the study of their inheritance and relation to hypertensive disease. An example of this is Dr. Rapp's report on 18-hydroxy-deoxycorticosterone. (See chapter entitled "Inheritance of 18-Hydroxy-deoxycorticosterone Formation in Genetic Hypertension in Rats.") When a sufficient number of such studies is available, we may start on the task of interrelating and correlating their causes and effects into an integrated picture.

REFERENCES

1. Dahl, L. K.: Sodium as an etiologic factor in hypertension. *In* Moyer, J. H. (Ed.): Hypertension. The First Hahnemann Sympo-

sium in Hypertensive Disease. Philadelphia: Saunders, 1959, pp. 262–268.

2. Meneely, George R.: The effect of salt and other electrolytes in hypertension. *In* Moyer, J. H. (Ed.): Hypertension. The First Hahnemann Symposium in Hypertensive Disease. Philadelphia: Saunders, 1959, pp. 250–261.
3. Dahl, L. K., and Love, R. A.: Evidence for relationship between sodium (chloride) intake and human essential hypertension. Arch. Intern. Med. 94:525, 1954.
4. Dahl, L. K., and Love, R. A.: Etiological role of sodium chloride intake in essential hypertension in humans. JAMA 164:397, 1957.
5. Dahl, L. K.: Salt intake and salt need. N. Engl. J. Med. 258:1152; 1205, 1958.
6. Dahl, L. K., Silver, L., and Christie, R. W.: The role of salt in the fall of blood pressure accompanying reduction in obesity. N. Engl. J. Med. 258:1186, 1958.
7. Dahl, L. K.: Possible role of salt intake in the development of essential hypertension. *In* Cottier, P. and Bock, K. D. (Eds.): Essential Hypertension, An International Symposium. Bern: Springer, 1960, pp. 53–65.
8. Knudsen, K. D., and Dahl, L. K.: Essential hypertension: Inborn error of sodium metabolism? Postgrad. Med. J. 42:148, 1966.
9. Dahl, L. K., Heine, M., and Tassinari, L.: High salt content of the western infant's diet: Possible relationship to hypertension in the adult. Nature 198:1204, 1963.
10. Dahl, L. K.: Salt in commercial baby foods. (Letter to the editor). Nutr. Rev. 26:124, 1968.
11. Dahl, L. K.: Salt in processed baby foods. (Guest editorial). Am. J. Clin. Nutr. 21:787, 1968.
12. Dahl, L. K., Heine, M., Leitl, G., and Tassinari, L.: Hypertension and death from consumption of processed baby foods by rats. Proc. Soc. Exp. Biol. Med. 133:1405, 1970.
13. Moser, M.: Epidemiology of primary hypertension with particular reference to racial susceptibility. *In* Moyer, J. H. (Ed.): Hypertension. The First Hahnemann Symposium in Hypertensive Disease. Philadelphia: Saunders, 1959, pp. 72–74.
14. Grollman, A.: Discussion. *In* Moyer, J. H. (Ed.): Hypertension. The First Hahnemann Symposium in Hypertensive Disease. Philadelphia: Saunders, 1959, pp. 175–176.
15. Dahl, L. K., Heine, M., and Tassinari, L.: Effects of chronic excess salt ingestion. Further demonstration that genetic factors influence the development of hypertension: Evidence from experimental hypertension due to cortisone and to adrenal regeneration. J. Exp. Med. 122:533, 1965.
16. Falconer, D. S.: The inheritance of liability to certain diseases, estimated from the incidence among relatives. Ann. Hum. Genet. 29:51, 1965.
17. Murphy, E. A., Thomas, C. B., and Bolling, D. R.: The precursors of hypertension and coronary disease: Statistical consideration of distributions in a population of medical students. Johns Hopkins Med. J. 120:1, 1967.
18. Miall, W. E., and Oldham, P. D.: A study of arterial blood pressure and its inheritance in a sample of the general population. Clin. Sci. 17:409, 1958.
19. Hamilton, M., Pickering, G. W., Roberts, J. A. F., and Sowry, G. S. C.: The aetiology of essential hypertension. II. Scores for arterial blood pressures adjusted for differences in age and sex. Clin. Sci. 13:37, 1954.
20. Acheson, R. M., and Fowler, G. B.: On the inheritance of stature and blood pressure. J. Chronic Dis. 20:731, 1967.
21. Søbye, P.: Heredity in essential hypertension and nephrosclerosis. A genetic clinical study of 200 propositi suffering from nephrosclerosis. *In* Opera ex Domo Biological Hereditarial Humanae Universitatis Hafniensis, vol. 16. Copenhagen: Munksgaard, 1948, pp. 89–97.
22. Vander Molen, R., Brewer, G., Honeyman, M. S., Morrison, J., and Hoobler, S. W.: A study of hypertension in twins. Am. Heart J. 79:454, 1970.
23. Šimon, J., Topinka, I., Sova, J., Barcal, R., Levy, L., and Kulich, Vl.: Twin studies from the view of the heredity of hypertensive disease. *In* Opatrný, K. and Sobotka, P. (Eds.): Genetics in Clinical Medicine. Symposium held in Plzeň, Czechoslovakia. Plzeň, Czechoslovakia: Medical Faculty, Charles University, 1968, pp. 13–18.
24. Hines, E. A., Jr., McIlhaney, M. L., and Gage, R. P.: A study of twins with normal blood pressures and with hypertension. Trans. Assoc. Am. Physicians 70:282, 1957.
25. Carter, C. O.: Genetics of common disorders. Br. Med. Bull. 25:52, 1969.
26. Carter, C. O.: An ABC of medical genetics. VI. Polygenic inheritance and common disease. Lancet I:1252, 1969.
27. Smirk, F. H., and Hall, W. H.: Inherited hypertension in rats. Nature 182:727, 1958.
28. Dahl, L. K., Heine, M., and Tassinari, L.: Role of genetic factors in susceptibility to experimental hypertension due to chronic excess salt ingestion. Nature 194:480, 1962.

29. Okamoto, K., and Aoki, K.: Development of a strain of spontaneously hypertensive rats. Jap. Circ. J. 27:282, 1963.
30. Meneely, G. R., Tucker, R. G., Darby, W. J., and Auerbach, S. H.: Chronic sodium chloride toxicity in the albino rat. II. Occurrence of hypertension and of a syndrome of edema and renal failure. J. Exp. Med. 98:71, 1955.
31. Meneely, G. R., and Dahl, L. K.: Hypertension and its treatment. Electrolytes in hypertension: the effects of sodium chloride—The evidence from animal and human studies. Med. Clin. North Am. 45:271, 1961.
32. Dahl, L. K., Heine, M., and Tassinari, L.: Effects of chronic excess salt ingestion. Evidence that genetic factors play an important role in susceptibility to experimental hypertension. J. Exp. Med. 115:1173, 1962.
33. Dahl, L. K., Knudsen, K. D., Heine, M. A., and Leitl, G. J.: Effects of chronic excess salt ingestion. Modification of experimental hypertension in the rat by variations in the diet. Circ. Res. 22:11, 1968.
34. Dahl, L. K., and Schackow, E.: Effects of chronic excess salt ingestion: Experimental hypertension in the rat. Proceedings of the International Symposium on Angiotensin, Sodium and Hypertension, Oct. 1963, Quebec. Can. Med. Assoc. J. 90:155, 1964.
35. Dahl, L. K., Heine, M., and Tassinari, L.: Effects of chronic excess salt ingestion. Role of genetic factors in both DOCA-salt and renal hypertension. J. Exp. Med. 118:605, 1963.
36. Dahl, L. K., Heine, M., and Tassinari, L.: Effects of chronic excess salt ingestion. Further demonstration that genetic factors influence the development of hypertension. Evidence from experimental hypertension due to cortisone and to adrenal regeneration. J. Exp. Med. 122:533, 1965.
37. Dahl, L. K., Knudsen, K. D., Heine, M., and Leitl, G.: Effects of chronic excess salt ingestion. Genetic influence on the development of salt hypertension in parabiotic rats: Evidence for a humoral factor. J. Exp. Med. 126:687, 1967.
38. Iwai, J., Knudsen, K. D., Dhal, L. K., Heine, M., and Leitl, G.: Genetic influence on the development of renal hypertension in parabiotic rats. Evidence for a humoral factor. J. Exp. Med. 129:507, 1969.
39. Knudsen, K. D., Iwai, J., Heine, M., Leitl, G., and Dahl, L. K.: Genetic influence on the development of renoprival hypertension in parabiotic rats. Evidence that a humoral hypertensinogenic factor is produced in kidney tissue of hypertension-prone rats. J. Exp. Med. 130:1353, 1969.
40. Iwai, J., Knudsen, K. D., and Dahl, L. K.: Genetic influence on the renin-angiotensin system. Evidence for a renin inhibitor in hypertension-prone rats. J. Exp. Med. 131:543, 1970.
41. Knudsen, K. D., Dahl, L. K., Thompson, K., Iwai, J., Heine, M., and Leitl, G.: Effects of chronic excess salt ingestion: Inheritance of hypertension in the rat. J. Exp. Med. 132: 976, 1970.

Conditioned Modifications of Blood Pressure

By Herbert Benson, M.D.

ELEVATED SYSTEMIC arterial blood pressure is related to environmental conditions which require continuous behavioral and physiologic adjustments.[1] The physiologic, autonomic nervous system adjustments to our environment evolved and stabilized many thousands of years ago. These autonomic evolutionary responses, such as the hypothalamic defense-alarm or fight-or-flight reaction of Cannon,[2] lead to a hypertensive response. This previously suitable response is now often inappropriate and may lead to permanent hypertension, especially since our environment has changed and is becoming more complex and unpredictable at an accelerating pace.[3] Since the apparently ever-continuing environmental changes are not readily altered, better prevention and perhaps therapy of related diseases such as hypertension might be achieved by altering the pathophysiologic autonomic responses of an individual to his environment.[1] This chapter discusses the production and alteration of hypertension through classical and operant conditioning techniques.

Classical Conditioning

The autonomic nervous system's hypertensive response may be elicited by classical conditioning techniques. Classical Pavlovian conditioning techniques related to the role of the central nervous system in hypertension have been extensively studied in the USSR.[4] Repeated blood pressure elevations (the unconditioned response), are elicited by painful sensory stimulation (the unconditioned stimulus) associated with a light or tone signal (the conditioned stimulus). Later presentation of the conditioned stimulus alone, the light or tone, produces acute elevations of blood pressure (conditioned response). The sequence may be restated: (*1*) Conditioned stimulus (light) associated with unconditioned stimulus (painful sensory stimulation) → unconditioned response (blood pressure elevation); (*2*) conditioned stimulus (light) → conditioned response (blood pressure elevation).[1]

Conditioned pressor responses in dogs are of large magnitude and resistant to extinction procedures in which the conditioned stimulus is presented without reinforcement by unconditioned stimuli.[4] Similar results have been obtained in the United States. Pressor and hypertensive responses in dogs have been conditioned to tone signals followed by electric shock. Once developed, the conditioned hypertensive response to the tone signals is retained for over 1 year without intervening training.[5]

"Experimental neurosis," produced by the simultaneous presentation of conflicting excitatory and inhibitory conditioned stimuli, leads to elevations in systemic arterial blood pressure in monkeys.[4] These results are consistent with the Russian neurogenic theory of essential hypertension which emphasizes the role of "psychic stress" and "emotional trauma." However, "experimental neurosis" does not consistently lead to behavioral disturbances or elevated blood pressures. Combination of a positive conditioned stimulus (a light) for food with an aversive stimulus (an airblast or shock) do not produce hypertension in the cat.[6] Complete inhibition of the conditioned feeding response occurred in all but one animal. Excessive neurotic behavior did not develop. However, acute anxiety limited to the experimental cage was observed as well as the adaptive behavor such as avoidance of the food box.[1,6]

Operant Conditioning

In operant conditioning, the occurrence of specific environmental events is made contin-

---

From Thorndike Memorial and Channing Laboratories, Harvard Medical Unit, Boston City Hospital, and the Department of Medicine, Harvard Medical School, Boston, Massachusetts.

Supported in part by Grants HE 10539–04 and SF 57–135 from the National Institutes of Health and Grant RR–76 from the General Clinical Research Centers Program of the Division of Research Resources.

gent upon specific behavioral responses. Environmental events that increase the probability of a specific behavioral response are known as reinforcers.[7] Through appropriate scheduling of reinforcers, a large number of behavioral responses can be brought under reliable stimulus control. For example, in the presence of a light (the stimulus), an animal can be trained to tap or press a key or bar (the behavioral response) which leads to the presentation of food (the reinforcer).[1]

Elevated systemic arterial blood pressure accompanies the performance of several operant conditioning schedules. Training unanesthetized adolescent rhesus monkeys to press a lever to avoid shock on various programed schedules for 15 days produced a concomitant increase in intra-arterial blood pressure.[8] Systolic and diastolic pressures were sustained at higher levels and for longer periods in those animals working on longer or more complex schedules. After 7 and 12 months, training on shock-avoidance schedules for 12 to 15 hours per day produced marked elevations in intra-arterial systolic and diastolic pressures.[9] No consistent relationship existed between patterns of bar-pressing or number of shocks received and the level of arterial pressure. In yet another series of experiments, unanesthetized squirrel monkeys were trained to press a key a fixed number of times to turn off a light associated with a noxious stimulus.[10] Eventually, four of six monkeys had sustained elevations in mean arterial blood pressure before, during, and after experimental sessions in the experimental chamber. The authors concluded that operant conditioning schedules that continuously exerted strong control over an animal's behavior also induced marked persistent elevations in systemic mean arterial blood pressure. Further investigations established that these sustained elevations in mean arterial pressure were present not only in the experimental chamber when the animals' behavior was under scheduled control, but also 24 hours a day when the animals were within their own cages before and after the experimental sessions.[11] In one monkey with behaviorally induced hypertension, renal pathologic changes consistent with severe hypertension were present.[12] More recently, elevated systemic arterial blood pressure in male rhesus monkeys has been reported after 3 to 5 days of training on shock-avoidance schedules.[13] In these experiments, the elevations of blood pressure after several hours were secondary to increased cardiac output, while those after 72 hours were secondary to increased total peripheral resistance. Changes in the resistance of skeletal muscle blood vessels were closely related to the increased total peripheral resistance.

Another type of operant conditioning experiments makes the reinforcement of feedback *directly dependent upon blood pressure changes*, rather than upon another behavioral response such as key-pressing. The reinforcement of increases and decreases in systolic blood pressure with escape or avoidance of electric shock or both in curarized rats produced reliable blood pressure changes in the rewarded direction.[14] Much smaller, but statistically significant, changes in systolic blood pressure also occurred in the reinforced direction in non-curarized rats.[15] Unanesthetized rhesus monkeys were trained to raise diastolic blood pressure by operant conditioning techniques employing avoidance of electric shock.[16] In unanesthetized squirrel monkeys, sustained elevations of mean arterial blood pressure ensued when increases in blood pressure per se prevented the delivery of noxious stimuli.[17] Further, sustained *depressions* of the elevated mean arterial blood pressure could be achieved in these same monkeys by training under a schedule in which decreases in blood pressure prevented the delivery of noxious stimuli.

In man, healthy normotensive subjects could be trained to decrease their systolic blood pressure with the use of operant conditioning-feedback techniques.[18,19] The decreases in systolic blood pressure averaged 4 mm Hg, but were statistically significant. No consistent increases in systolic pressure were achieved. Operant conditioning techniques have also been employed in normal subjects to both increase and decrease diastolic pressure.[20] Diastolic blood pressure decreases ranged from 2 to 10 mm Hg while increases ranged from 2 to 18 mm Hg. Increased and decreased diastolic pressures were associated with increased and decreased heart rates respectively.

Recently, decreased systolic blood pressure through operant conditioning techniques has been achieved in patients with essential hypertension.[21] The diagnosis of essential hypertension was established by exclusion of the known causes of hypertension by complete medical evaluations including renal arteriography in two patients. All patients were ambulatory and attending the Hypertension Clinic of the Boston City Hospital. The patients' average age was 47.9 years and there were five males and two females. Six of the seven were taking antihypertensive medications which were not altered during the experimental sessions. The patients were told they would be paid five dollars per session to come to the behavioral laboratory and have their blood pressure measured automatically for approximately 1 hour while they sat quietly. They were also informed that the procedures might be of value in lowering their blood pressure.

The methods were similar to those employed in normotensive subjects.[18,19] A 13-cm-wide cuff was wrapped around the left arm and inflated to a given pressure by a regulated, low-pressure, compressed-air source. The cuff was connected by tubing to a Statham strain-gauge pressure transducer. The electric output of the strain gauge was recorded on one channel of a Beckman polygraph. The output of a crystal microphone, placed under the cuff and over the brachial artery, recorded Korotkoff sounds on a second channel of the polygraph. The electrocardiogram (ECG) was also recorded on another channel. Increases or decreases in systolic pressure with each heartbeat relative to the cuff pressure could be ascertained by setting the cuff at a constant pressure, close to systolic blood pressure. When cuff pressure exceeded brachial artery systolic pressure, no Korotkoff sound was present; when cuff pressure was less than brachial artery systolic pressure, a Korotkoff sound was produced. During each trial, the cuff was inflated for 50 consecutive heartbeats (which were recorded automatically from the ECG) and then deflated. The absence or presence of a Korotkoff sound was recorded within 300 msec after the R wave of the ECG. Median systolic blood pressure during the trial was equal to cuff pressure when between 14 and 36 Korotkoff sounds per cycle of 50 heartbeats were produced. The cuff pressure was decreased 4 mm Hg for the next cycle if fewer than 14 Korotkoff sounds were present, indicating that the cuff pressure exceeded systolic arterial pressure for most of the trial. The cuff pressure was increased by 4 mm Hg if more than 36 Korotkoff sounds were present, indicating that cuff pressure was lower than arterial pressure for most of the trial. Median systolic pressure could thus be tracked throughout each session.

The patients were studied on consecutive weekdays, and during each session, the median systolic blood pressure was measured for 30 trials. Between the trials, the cuff was deflated for 30 to 45 seconds. There were 5 to 16 control sessions for each patient during which median systolic blood pressure was recorded with no feedback or reinforcement of lowered pressure. The control pressures therefore represented median systolic blood pressure of between 7,500 and 22,500 heartbeats.

During the 25 conditioning trials, relatively lowered systolic pressure, indicated by the absence of a Korotkoff sound, was fed back to the patient by presentation of a 100-msec flash of light and a simultaneous 100-msec tone of moderate intensity. The patients were told they should try to make the tone and light appear since they were desirable. As a reward, a photographic slide, equivalent to five cents, was

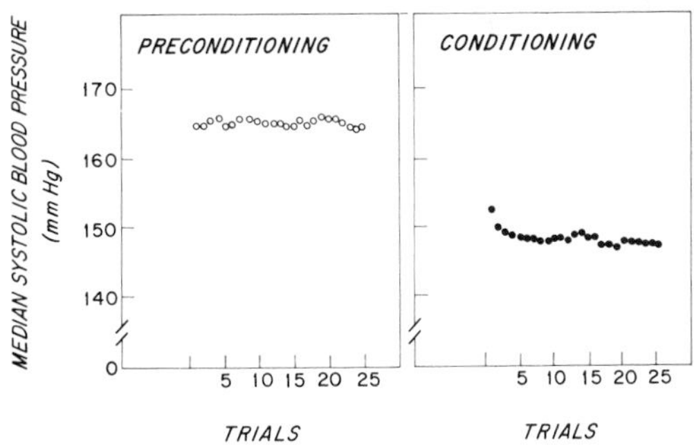

FIG. 1.—Median systolic blood pressure in preconditioning and conditioning trials. Each circle represents the average pressure of the seven patients in each of the last 25 trials in a session. The last five preconditioning and conditioning sessions are represented. The preconditioning sessions are represented by **open circles;** the conditioning sessions, by **closed circles.** Median systolic blood pressure was lower in the conditioning sessions than in the preconditioning sessions. Further, blood pressure decreased within the conditioning sessions, but did not do so within the preconditioning sessions.

shown for 5 seconds after each 20 presentations of tones and lights. The slides consisted of reminders of the amount of money earned and scenic pictures. The conditioning sessions continued until no further reductions in blood pressure occurred in five consecutive sessions.

Average median systolic blood pressure in the seven patients was 164.9 mm Hg during the last five control sessions. As an index of the effectiveness of training, pressures in the last five conditioning sessions were used. The average median systolic blood pressure decreased to 148.4 mm Hg ($p < 0.02$) during these conditioning sessions (Fig. 1). Systolic blood pressure decreased 3.5, 33.8, 29.2, 16.5, 16.1, 0, and 17.3 mm Hg in the individual patients. No consistent changes in heart rate were present in the patients during the blood pressure changes. Since these changes were measured only in the behavioral laboratory, therapeutic value cannot be evaluated. The lowering of diastolic and mean arterial blood pressure in patients with essential hypertension remains to be investigated.

Conclusion

In man and animals, predictable, reproducible systolic and diastolic arterial blood pressure changes occur during classical or operant conditioning experiments or both. It is hoped that conditioning techniques will be of value in altering the pathophysiologic autonomic nervous system responses which might result in and also which might perpetuate hypertension.

Acknowledgment

The helpful suggestions of Walter H. Abelmann and the editorial assistance of Barbara R. Marzetta are gratefully acknowledged.

References

1. Gutmann, M. C., and Benson, H.: Interaction of environmental factors and systemic arterial blood pressure: A review. Medicine 50:543, 1971.
2. Cannon, W. B.: The emergency function of the adrenal medulla in pain and the major emotions. Am. J. Physiol. 33:356, 1914.
3. Toffler, A.: Future Shock. New York: Random House, 1970.
4. Simonson, E., and Brožek, J.: Russian research on arterial hypertension. Ann. Intern. Med. 50:129, 1959.
5. Dykman, R. A., and Gantt, W. H.: Experimental psychogenic hypertension: Blood pressure changes conditioned to painful stimuli (schizokinesis). Johns Hopkins Med. J. 107: 72, 1960.
6. Shapiro, A. P., and Horn, P. W.: Blood pressure, plasma pepsinogen, and behavior in cats subjected to experimental production of anxiety. J. Nerv. Ment. Dis. 122:222, 1955.
7. Skinner, B. F.: Science and Human Behavior. New York: Macmillan, 1953.
8. Forsyth, R. P.: Blood pressure and avoidance conditioning. A study of 15-day trials in the rhesus monkey. Psychosom. Med. 30:125, 1968.
9. Forsyth, R. P.: Blood pressure responses to long-term avoidance schedules in the restrained rhesus monkey. Psychosom. Med. 31:300, 1969.
10. Herd, J. A., Morse, W. H., Kelleher, R. T., and Jones, J. G.: Arterial hypertension in the squirrel monkey during behavioral experiments. Am. J. Physiol. 217:24, 1969.
11. Grose, S. A., Herd, J. A., Morse, W. H., and Kelleher, R. T.: Behavioral hypertension in the squirrel monkey. Fed. Proc. 30:549, 1971.
12. Benson, H., Herd, J. A., Morse, W. H., and Kelleher, R. T.: Behaviorally induced hypertension in the squirrel monkey. Circ. Res. 26–27 (Suppl. I):I-21, 1970.
13. Forsyth, R. P.: Regional blood-flow changes during 72-hour avoidance schedules in the monkey. Science 173:546, 1971.
14. DiCara, L. V., and Miller, N. E.: Instrumental learning of systolic blood pressure responses by curarized rats: Dissociation of cardiac and vascular changes. Psychosom. Med. 30:489, 1968.
15. Pappas, B. A., DiCara, L. V., and Miller, N. E.: Learning of blood pressure responses in the noncurarized rat: Transfer to the curarized state. Physiol. Behav. 5:1029, 1970.
16. Plumlee, L. A.: Operant conditioning of increases in blood pressure. Psychophysiology 6:283, 1969.
17. Benson, H., Herd, J. A., Morse, W. H., and Kelleher, R. T.: Behavioral induction of arterial hypertension and its reversal. Am. J. Physiol. 217:30, 1969.
18. Shapiro, D., Tursky, B., Gershon, E., and Stern, M.: Effects of feedback and reinforcement on the control of human systolic blood pressure. Science 163:588, 1969.
19. Shapiro, D., Tursky, B., and Schwartz, G. E.: Control of blood pressure in man by operant conditioning. Circ. Res. 26–27 (Suppl. I.): I-27, 1970.

20. Shapiro, D., Schwartz, G. E., and Tursky, B.: Control of diastolic blood pressure in man by feedback and reinforcement. Psychophysiology 9:296, 1972.

21. Benson, H., Shapiro, D., Tursky, B., and Schwartz, G. E.: Decreased systolic blood pressure through operant conditioning techniques in patients with essential hypertension. Science 173:740, 1971.

Personality and Emotional Stress in Essential Hypertension in Man

By Robert E. Harris, Ph.D., and Ralph P. Forsyth, Ph.D.

The Pressor Effect of Emotion-provoking Situations

THE PRESSOR effects of brief, laboratory-arranged episodes of emotional stress can be amply documented. For example, Hardyck, Singer, and Harris [1] reported that interviews concerning personal history and current life situation in a group of hypertensive women produced mean increments in blood pressure of 40 mm Hg systolic and 20 mm Hg diastolic averaged over about 30 determinations in a 1-hour period. There were large variations between subjects and from moment to moment for each subject. These latter variations were found to be systematically related to the degree to which the subject became emotionally involved with the interviewer and with the topics being discussed, i.e., the individual differences in blood pressure responsivity correlated with behavioral differences in emotional responsivity.

To extend such findings to longer periods of observation and to naturally occurring life situations, a semiautomatic, portable, blood pressure recorder was developed. Blood pressures are recorded on a preset schedule, usually every half hour as the subjects go about their ordinary activities outside the laboratory. Even though wearing the recorder places some constraints on the subject's usual behavior and interactions with other people, it seems likely that the obtained values, averaged over a 2- or 3-day period, may be more representative of his usual blood pressure than those obtained in a physician's office. Furthermore, the record permits analysis of the events occurring at times when the pressures are unusually high or low. For this purpose the subject keeps a log of his activities and after each measurement checks a list of adjectives describing several moods or attitudes: anxiety, hostility, depression, and the feeling of time pressure (negative affects), and alertness and contentment (positive affects). Sokolow et al.[2] have reported that in 50 hypertensive patients the pressure was significantly higher when negative affects were reported in the logs. Intraindividual correlations between pressure and negative affects over the 20 or more recordings during the day were positive for most of the patients, and reached high levels of statistical significance in some. It may be noted that these patients tended to be drawn from lower socioeconomic and educational levels; it is possible that the relationships might be higher in subjects who are verbally more skillful and more observant of their own behavior.

The ranges of these intradaily variations are large. A group of male office workers and executives were followed for 2 days through their largely sedentary workdays and into the evenings. The mean of their daily averages was 130/76 mm Hg, and the range was about 50/30 for the average subject and for some subjects was higher than 80/50. Subjects with higher than average pressures and greater than average variabilities reached very high absolute levels of pressure, certainly within the range which, if obtained in a physician's office, would be called clinically significant.

The relevance of such stress-induced pressor episodes for the pathogenesis of essential hypertension has often been discounted because the primary mediator of the pressure change has been thought to be an increase in cardiac output without peripheral vasoconstriction. Only long-term studies will settle the point definitively, but in the meantime, some indirect evidence may be cited.

Brod et al.[3] have shown that at least in some subjects the pressure increase accompanying a mental arithmetic task is mediated by increases in renal and total peripheral resistance, not by cardiac output alone.

Folkow,[4] working with the Okamoto strain of spontaneously hypertensive rats, has shown

From the Department of Psychiatry and the Cardiovascular Research Institute, University of California, San Francisco, California.

Supported in part by National Institutes of Health Program-Project Grant HE-06285.

that cardiac output is high in the early development of elevated pressures, and that drug-induced suppression of cardiac output delays the onset of hypertension.

It is also possible that short-acting stressors have different hemodynamic effects from more prolonged ones. Recently, Forsyth [5] has shown that rhesus monkeys show significant increases in mean pressure on a continuous 72-hour schedule requiring shock-avoidance behavior. Utilizing a radioactively labeled microsphere method, he measured regional blood flows and resistance at four points after baseline measurements. At 20 minutes into the stressful period the cardiac output rose and total peripheral resistance decreased. Progressively, at 4, 24, and 72 hours the cardiac output decreased and resistance increased. The predominant regional change was a progressive decrease in flow to skeletal muscle which accounted for most of the change in total peripheral resistance. Renal flow was significantly lowered throughout the 72-hour period. These results are summarized in Figure 1.

Thus it seems reasonable to hypothesize that some persons by virtue of their personality characteristics are especially prone to over-respond in emotion-provoking situations, and hence to be subject to greater frequencies, magnitudes, and durations of pressor episodes which, integrated over time, may lead to blood pressures which are sustained at high levels by mechanisms as yet unknown.

The Psychosomatic Hypothesis

The modern era of inquiry into psychosomatic relations may be dated to the late 1930s, when Alexander and his colleagues were utilizing the clinical psychiatric interview to investigate the psychodynamics of conditions such as duodenal ulcer, asthma, and essential hypertension among others. Constellations of psycho-

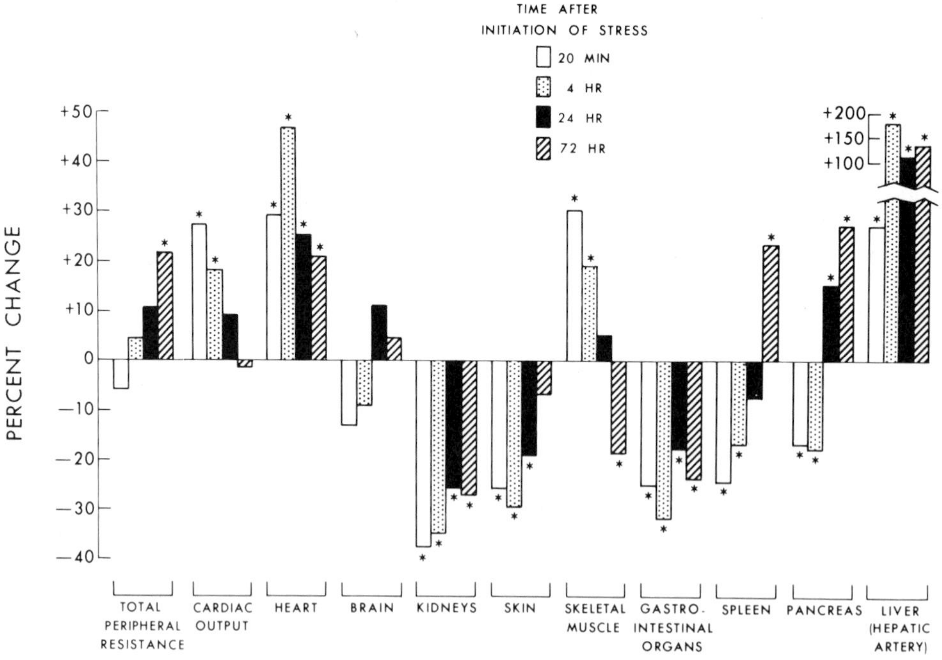

Fig. 1.—Mean percentage changes, compared to the baseline measurement in the total peripheral resistance, cardiac output, and regional fractions of cardiac output in five monkeys in nine major organs during the 72-hour stress period. The gastrointestinal tract includes the stomach, small and large intestines, and cecum. An asterisk (*) indicates significance levels of $P < 0.05$ compared to control-group changes, by use of the Mann-Whitney U test. (Reprinted with permission from Forsyth, R. P.: Science 173:546–548, August 6, 1971. Copyright 1971 by The American Association for the Advancement of Science.)

logic factors were found for each syndrome. In hypertensive patients the core problem seemed to be impulses toward aggression and the management and control of hostility, a theme which has remained a consistent one in the literature. Recognizing the limitations inherent in the interview, Alexander, French, and Pollock [6] undertook their "psychosomatic specificity study." Typescripts of interviews with patients representing seven different conditions, one of which was essential hypertension, were carefully edited by internists to eliminate any material concerning physical symptoms, onset or course or other medical cues which might reveal the diagnoses. A panel of psychoanalysts then judged each of the protocols, and made inferences concerning which syndrome was represented. All of the conditions were correctly identified beyond a chance level. Hypertension, along with peptic ulcer, was judged correctly somewhat less frequently than the other conditions, but still significantly better than chance. A group of internists, not psychoanalytically trained, studied the same typescripts, and were successful in identifying only about 25 percent of the patients (where chance would be 14), considerably less than the psychoanalysts, indicating that the editing of the typescripts for medical cues had been largely successful, and that the psychologic materials as interpreted by the analysts permitted valid inferences about the diagnoses. The formulation of the personality pattern of the hypertensive which provided the basis for the correct identifications by the psychoanalytic panel had as its core a continuous struggle against expressing hostile aggressive feelings and difficulty in asserting oneself. After an often stormy childhood with attacks of rage and aggression, more submissive, compliant attitudes develop. Overly conscientious, responsible attitudes result in increased feelings of resentment, demanding in turn greater and greater control of hostile feelings. A vicious circle develops, leading to a chronic state of psychologic tension.

Other investigators using different methods have reported consistent findings. Two studies in which hypertensives were sharply differentiated from other kinds of patients, and in which no obvious extraneous cues account for the results may be cited as illustrative.

Singer [7] interviewed female hypertensives and other patients presented in random order. They were being seen in a psychophysiologic experiment and were almost completely immobilized by pickups for skin resistance, finger and face temperatures, arm volume, heart rate, blood pressure, and breathing rate. Thus the observer was limited mainly to verbal, vocal, and facial cues. After a very brief introduction, she administered a mental arithmetic task for 4 minutes, then left the experimental room and registered her opinion as to the identity of the subject, e.g., hypertensive or control. After another baseline period she conducted an interview concerning life history and current life situation, following which she made a second guess. She was correct in 70 percent of her identifications after mental arithmetic and in 85 percent after the interview, both values well beyond a chance level. The bases for her judgments were the extent to which the subjects experienced the task as challenging and threatening and how involved emotionally they became.

Recently Sapira et al. [8] have reported highly significant differences in the responses of hypertensives and controls to brief films of physician-patient interactions. In a postfilm interview and questionnaire, objective analyses indicated that the hypertensives had misperceived or misinterpreted the films in an effort to screen out potentially emotion-provoking stimuli and thereby to protect themselves from their cardiovascular reactivity. Singer [7] has also reported such self-protective, buffering efforts in some hypertensive patients whom she described as "defended" as opposed to "pressured," those patients who respond overtly and strongly to external stimuli. In a follow-up study initiated before the advent of effective antihypertensive medication, the defended patients were found to have longer survival times, suggesting a kind of "wisdom of the body" in their efforts to reduce their inputs from disruptive and potentially damaging stimuli.

Such findings demonstrate that hypertensives differ from normotensives in personality functioning; however, their relevance to the pathogenesis of hypertension may be questioned on at least two grounds.

First, those hypertensives who present themselves at medical facilities or those who are recruited as research subjects from wards and clinics may differ in personality from those not so referred. For instance, hypochondriacal concern or noncompliance with therapeutic regimens may be selective factors which are not related to the level of the pressure. Many cases of high blood pressure are discovered in symptom-free persons in population surveys and in routine physical examinations; Robinson [9] has shown that such persons score lower on inventories of neuroticism than identified patients.

Second, the personality characteristics found to be associated with hypertension may be secondary or incidental to a number of factors, e.g., to central nervous system impairment due to elevated pressure; to the patient's knowledge that he has a condition which may shorten his life or impose on him a treatment regimen with undesirable side effects, etc.

To meet these objections we have studied nonpatient groups selected to represent the extremes of the normal range of blood pressure. We have also examined the natural history of blood pressure, looking at rates of rise with age and ages of onset of high pressures for what implications they might have for the nature of the factors that tend to raise the pressure.

Blood Pressure Changes with Age

At the second Hahnemann symposium on hypertension a decade ago, Sokolow and Harris [10] summarized the information on the changes in blood pressure with age which could be inferred from cross-sectional samples. Since then Harris [11] has reported longitudinal data on individuals. The subjects were life insurance company employees whose pressures were measured during annual physical examinations. Scatter plots relating blood pressure to age were constructed from pressures recorded annually beginning in early adult life and extending for periods ranging up to 40 years. Examination of several hundred employees indicated that both systolic and diastolic pressures could be well fitted by straight lines, and that no other simple function would better fit more of the persons. Accordingly, linear regression coefficients, representing the slopes or rates of rise in mm Hg per year were computed for 242 persons who were observed from ages 25 to 30 or earlier until ages 50 to 54 or later. The means were 0.59 mm Hg per year systolic and 0.42 diastolic. The distributions are shown in Figure 2. Both distributions are continuous, slightly skewed positively, with no distinct breaks at any point. There is no evidence for bimodality in the distributions, i.e., there is no small subset of persons whose pressures rise rapidly in contrast to a larger proportion who show little or no rise with age. The inference seems warranted that in most persons both systolic and diastolic pressures rise with age, more so in some persons than others.

To examine the significance of relatively high pressures in early adult life (prehypertension), the tenth of the employees with the highest pressures at age 30 to 34 were selected, and their pressures for the preceding and later 5-year periods were computed. A similar procedure was followed for the tenth with the lowest pressures and for a group from the middle of the distribution. The results are shown in Figure 3. It can be seen that the

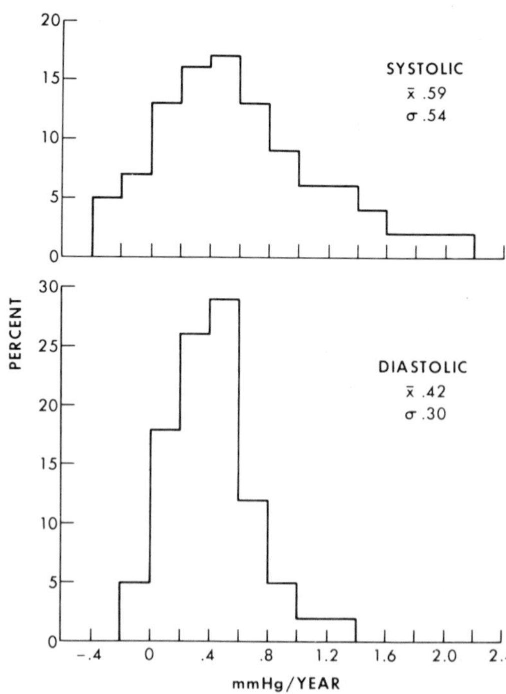

Fig. 2.—Distributions of slopes (regression coefficients) representing rates of increase in pressure from ages 25 to 30 to 50 to 54. (Reprinted from Singer, M. T.,[7] with permission.)

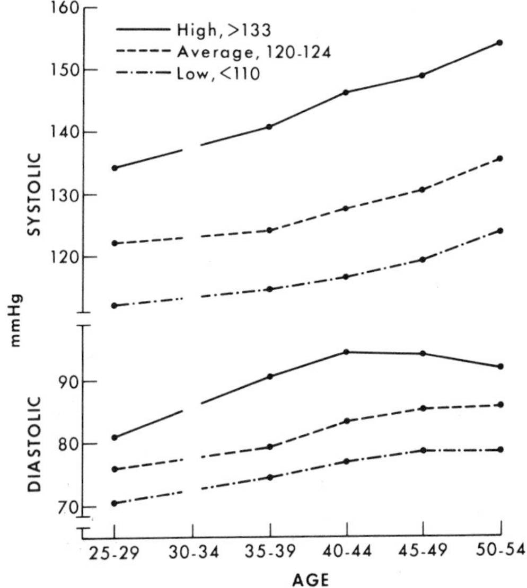

FIG. 3.—Blood pressure changes with age in persons selected for high, average, and low systolic pressures at ages 30 to 34. (Reprinted from Singer, M. T.,[7] with permission.)

groups maintain their separation throughout the period of observation. In fact, the curves tend to diverge, the slopes (regression coefficients) of the persons with high blood pressures being significantly steeper than those of the other groups. It may be inferred that whatever factors tend to produce relatively high pressures at ages 30 to 34 have already operated to produce high pressures at earlier ages and continue to operate to produce even higher pressures in later life.

In summary of these findings, it may be said concerning the factors which tend to raise the pressure with age that:

1. They have been present and showed their influence in early adult life but with no clear date of onset.

2. They operate over the whole range of pressures observed in early adult life, although somewhat more on persons with higher than lower pressures.

3. They operate to produce a linear rate of increase in the pressure, cumulatively, over time, by small increments.

Based on these considerations and those concerning the previously discussed selective factors which may make diagnosed hypertensives atypical of persons with high blood pressure, we have synopsized the way in which psychologic factors may influence the pathogenesis of hypertension in Figure 4. The vertical axis is an age scale, and starts at birth to suggest the possibility of genetic factors in the development of both personality and blood pressure and their possible linkage, and continues through the years of adult life to accommodate the longitudinal data just presented. The horizontal axis represents possible causal sequences, with interacting environmental and personality factors on the left, mediated by neural, humoral, and vascular factors in the middle, to result over time in increasing blood pressure on the right. To trace causal chains according to such a synopsis would require very extended longitudinal observations on large samples of the normal

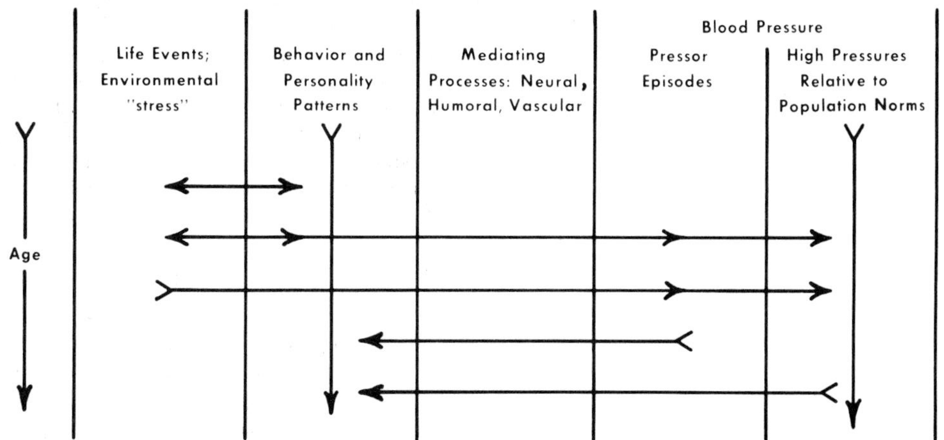

FIG. 4.—Mediational and temporal chains in the psychophysiology of blood pressure.

population. Short of such studies, it is possible to examine personality factors associated with the upper end of the range of blood pressure, looking for similarities in various groups which otherwise differ, most importantly, in age, but also in sex, educational level, occupation, etc.

Personality Functioning Associated with High Blood Pressure

In studying "normal" persons selected to represent the extremes of the range of blood pressure we have used a variety of psychologic methods, but have found the interview to be the most productive. The interview may be used to gather information on the life history and to assess the overall stressfulness of a person's environment and his typical ways of meeting problems. Also, the interview itself may be treated as a stressor, and the subject's manner of coping noted. Studies have usually been double-blind: the subjects have not known the reasons for their inclusion in the study, and the identification of the subjects as high or low on the blood pressure continuum was withheld from the interviewers until their personality assessment was completed.

A group of college women, selected because of their high pressures recorded during a physical examination at the time of their first registration, were studied while undergraduates, followed up 4 years later and again at 11 years.[12,13] At average age 30 they continued to be higher than matched controls on the blood pressure criterion, but their pressures were below what are usually considered significant levels.

Interview data as recorded by four different observers on the two follow-up occasions were recorded on rating scales and Q-sort items, the results being simplified by factor-analyzing the items which significantly differentiated between the groups. Four factors emerged:

1. Failure to achieve sex- and age-appropriate roles as defined by conventional cultural norms; an adjustment-normality factor
2. Forced responsiveness; an overreadiness to respond overtly to many kinds of stimuli; irritability, anxiety, restlessness
3. Hostility; a low threshold for perceiving hostility in others, to retaliate, and to behave in ways which provoke anger in other people
4. Aroused vigilance; a covert but unremitting kind of anxious, tense, defensive, attitude toward other people; perseverated emotional response

The subjects with the higher pressures scored higher on each of these factors, and to extrapolate to their probable social environments, it seems likely that they find many real life situations stressful.

Similar findings emerged from studies of United States Air Force officers who were exposed to 3 days of psychologic assessment procedures. Subjects within the total sample with the highest casual pressures ($x = 155/90$ mm Hg) were found to be dominant, assertive, decisive, task-oriented and generally effective in leadership roles. However, when they were matched with other officers who had similar leadership qualities but lower pressures ($x = 130/77$) they tended to have narrow ranges of interests, low thresholds for perceiving threat, challenge, and hostility in other people and were described as overcontrolling, rigid, stereotyped, and obtuse in social relations. Apparently their high needs for achievement and leadership roles had been at the expense of broader personality development. Again, as with the college women, it may be inferred that many of their everyday interactions are associated with high levels of emotional arousal.

A group of men, average age 58, whose blood pressures had been recorded annually since early adult life were selected to be representative of the distributions of pressures and rates of rise with age from a sample of several hundred insurance company employees. They completed biographical information forms and participated in 1- to 2-hour life history interviews. Health history was avoided by design. A subsample was interviewed by a second observer after they had worn an automatic blood pressure recorder for 2 days. They were a remarkably stable group: their average duration of employment with the same company was 36 years, and they had been married an average of 30 years. Their occupational levels ranged from relatively unskilled clerical work to high executive positions. Personality and behavior during the interviews clearly differentiated the higher and lower pressures. Subjects with higher pressures were rated as being emotionally more responsive, but also as being guarded, apprehensive, and unwilling to talk about themselves. Although seemingly poised, they were rated as fixedly hostile in their personal interactions, with a readiness, not often expressed, for verbal and physical aggression. They seemed to be warding off stimuli which might be the occasion for a strong emotional response. It should be noted that this is a sample of survivors of a cohort composed more than three decades earlier; other persons entering employment at the same time may have had more centrifugal tendencies, vocationally, maritally, and otherwise, and perhaps would show different correlates of elevated pressures, including a shorter life span.

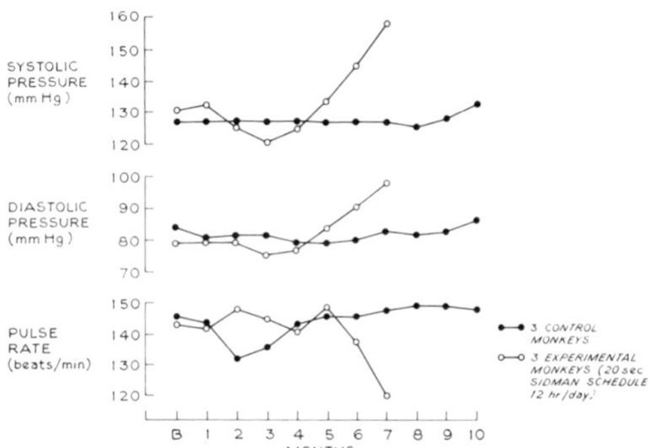

FIG. 5.—Baseline and monthly means (N=700 each month for each monkey) of arterial pressures and pulse rate for combined groups of three control and three experimental monkeys.

STRESS-INDUCED EXPERIMENTAL HYPERTENSION IN ANIMALS

To infer causal relations through long chains such as those hypothesized in Figure 4 is hazardous, but the plausibility of the psychosomatic hypothesis is enhanced by recent demonstrations that high blood pressure can be produced in animals through stressful environmental stimulation. Forsyth and Harris [14,15] exposed rhesus monkeys to conditioning schedules which required the animal to press a lever to avoid shock within 5-, 7-, or 20-second intervals for 12 or 16 hours per day. Pressure was measured through chronically implanted arterial catheters. All monkeys showed pressure increases when first introduced to the schedules. In three animals the pressure decreased for 3 months and then rose over a 4-month period to an average of about 160/100 mm Hg. Baseline levels had been about 130/80 mm Hg. Pressures were higher throughout the day, not just during the shock-avoidance hours. In two other animals on the more demanding 5- and 7-second schedules the initial rise was sustained, and after 5 months in one animal and 8 months in the other the pressure rose to new higher levels. Heart rate remained unchanged or decreased as the pressure rose. The data are shown in Figures 5 and 6. Behavioral changes in the form of irritability and hyperactivity preceded the blood pressure rises by several months. In this connection it may be pointed out that Folkow [4] reports that the Okamotu strain of hypertensive rats tend to be "choleric" in temperament, excitable from early ages onward, and resistant and combative in the blood pressure-measuring procedure. Other reports of experimental animal hypertension include these of Herd et al.[16] in the squirrel monkey following various conditioning procedures, and Henry, Meehan, and Stephens [17] in mice by a variety of environmental manipulations.

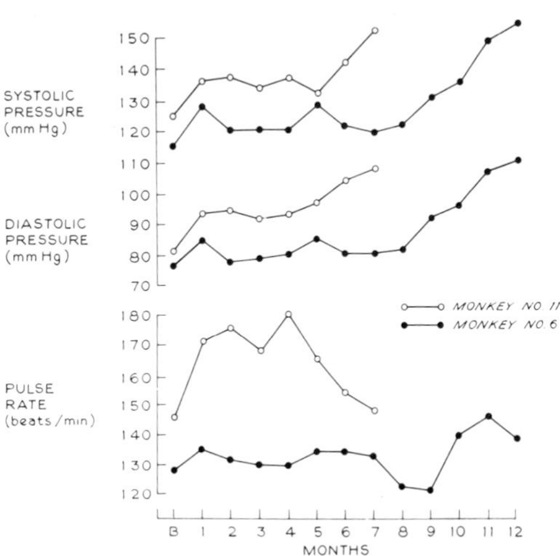

FIG. 6.—Baseline and monthly means (N=700 each month) of arterial pressures and pulse rates for two monkeys on 5- and 7-second Sidman avoidance schedules. (Reprinted from Forsyth, R. P.,[14] with permission.)

Summary and Interpretation

In summary it may be said: hypertensives and persons with high blood pressure relative to population norms but not so diagnosed differ from persons with lower pressures in personality functioning. At several ages and in both sexes persons with the higher pressures seem to experience many kinds of personal interactions as stressful and as the occasion for emotional arousal. Thus it seems likely that they experience emotional upsets more often, more intensely and for longer times than other persons, and that these upsets are accompanied by vasopressor episodes and possibly other neurogenic-humoral influences on peripheral vascular processes.

Such a formulation accords well with the neurogenic hypothesis of essential hypertension suggested by Folkow and Neil.[18] They propose a corticothalamic mechanism which, if engaged often enough over long periods of time, may act as an efficient trigger factor in the development of adaptive structural changes in the peripheral vasculature, for example, a hypertrophic increase in the ratio of wall to lumen.

It is suggested here that such a neurogenic hypothesis can readily be extended to a psychogenic hypothesis by adding afferent inputs and central integrative functions, or in psychologic language, the experience of stressful life situations.

References

1. Hardyck, C., Singer, M. T., and Harris, R. E.: Transient changes in affect and blood pressure. Arch. Gen. Psychiat. 7:15, 1962.
2. Sokolow, M., Werdegar, D., Perloff, D. B., Cowan, R. M., and Brenenstuhl, H.: Preliminary studies relating portably recorded blood pressures to daily life events in patients with essential hypertension. *In* Koster, W., Musaph, H., and Visser, P. (Eds.): Psychosomatics in Essential Hypertension. New York: Karger, 1970. As cited in Bibl. Psychiatr. 144:164, 1970.
3. Brod, J., Fencl, V., Hejl, Z., and Jirka, J.: Circulatory changes underlying blood pressure elevation during acute emotional stress (mental arithmetic) in normotensive and hypertensive subjects. Clin. Sci. 18:269, 1959.
4. Folkow, B.: Unpublished lecture given at the Cardiovascular Research Institute, University of California, San Francisco, California, Nov. 1971.
5. Forsyth, R. P.: Regional blood-flow changes during 72-hour avoidance schedules in the monkey. Science 173:546, 1971.
6. Alexander, F., French, T. M., and Pollock, G. H. Psychosomatic Specificity, Vol. 1. Chicago: University of Chicago Press, 1968.
7. Singer, M. T.: Enduring personality styles and responses to stress. Trans. Assoc. Life Ins. Med. Dir. of Am. LI:150, 1968.
8. Sapira, J. D., Scheib, E. T., Moriarty, R. and Shapiro, A. P.: Differences in perception between hypertensive and normotensive populations. Psychosom. Med. 33:239, 1971.
9. Robinson, J. O.: A possible effect of selection on the test scores of a group of hypertensives. J. Psychosom. Res. 8:239, 1964.
10. Sokolow, M., and Harris, R. E.: The natural history of hypertensive disease. *In* Brest, A. N., and Moyer, J. H. (Eds.): Hypertension, Recent Advances: The Second Hahnemann Symposium on Hypertensive Disease. Philadelphia: Lea & Febiger, 1961, pp. 3–17.
11. Harris, R. E.: Long-term studies of blood pressure recorded annually, with implications for the factors underlying essential hypertension. Trans. Assoc. Life Ins. Med. Dir. LI: 130, 1968.
12. Harris, R. E., Sokolow, M., Carpenter, L. G., Freedman, M. and Hunt, S. P.: Response to psychologic stress in persons who are potentially hypertensive. Circulation 7:874, 1953.
13. Kalis, B. L., Harris, R. E., Bennett, L. F., and Sokolow, M.: Personality and life history factors in persons who are potentially hypertensive. J. Nerv. Ment. Dis. 132:457, 1961.
14. Forsyth, R. P.: Blood pressure responses to long-term avoidance schedules in the restrained rhesus monkey. Psychosom. Med. 31:300, 1969.
15. Forsyth, R. P., and Harris, R. E.: Circulatory changes during stressful stimuli in rhesus monkeys. Circ. Res. 26–27 (Suppl. 1):13, 1970.
16. Herd, J. A., Morse, W. H., Kelleher, R. T., and Jones, L. G.: Arterial hypertension in the squirrel monkey during behavioral experiments. Am. J. Physiol. 217:24, 1969.
17. Henry, J. P., Meehan, J. P., and Stephens, P. M.: The use of psychosocial stimuli to induce systolic hypertension in mice. Psychosom. Med. 29:408, 1967.
18. Folkow, B., and Neil, E.: Circulation. New York: Oxford, 1971.

The Effect of Sleep on Experimental Hypertension

By Alberto Zanchetti, M.D., Giorgio Baccelli, M.D., Maurizio Guazzi, M.D., and Giuseppe Mancia, M.D.

When we began our studies of the effects of sleep on the circulation, we were looking for an experimental design by which to test the real importance of the neural control of circulation in baseline conditions and in absence of biasing factors such as anesthesia, acute surgical procedures, etc. The cardiovascular changes occurring during sleep were described, first in reference to simple measurements (blood pressure and heart rate),[1,2] and later on attention was paid to cardiac output [3] and regional blood flows.[4] Demonstration that these changes, or at least some of these changes, were mediated by neural mechanisms was given.[5] Finally the cardiovascular effects of sleep were studied in two types of hypertension, one caused by manipulating the neural control of circulation (sino-aortic deafferentation),[1,6,7] and the other by primarily acting upon the kidney (experimental renovascular hypertension).[7,8]

So far as sleep is concerned, suffice it to say at this point that we have studied only natural sleep,[9,10] in cats placed in a sound-attenuating cage with a large unidirectional window for visual observation. The wakefulness-sleep cycle was scored by continuous polygraphic recording, simultaneously with hemodynamic measurements. As quiet wakefulness (QW) we defined a state during which the animal quietly lay in a curled position, with the eyes half closed and the head slightly elevated from the floor, as signaled by a moderate activity in the neck electromyogram; the electro-oculogram periodically showed some slow movement of the eyes, and the electroencephalogram (EEG) alternated runs of desynchronized activity with a few bursts of spindles and rare slow waves. Synchronized sleep (SS) was scored whenever the cat, always in a curled position, was more fully relaxed on the cage floor, with the head

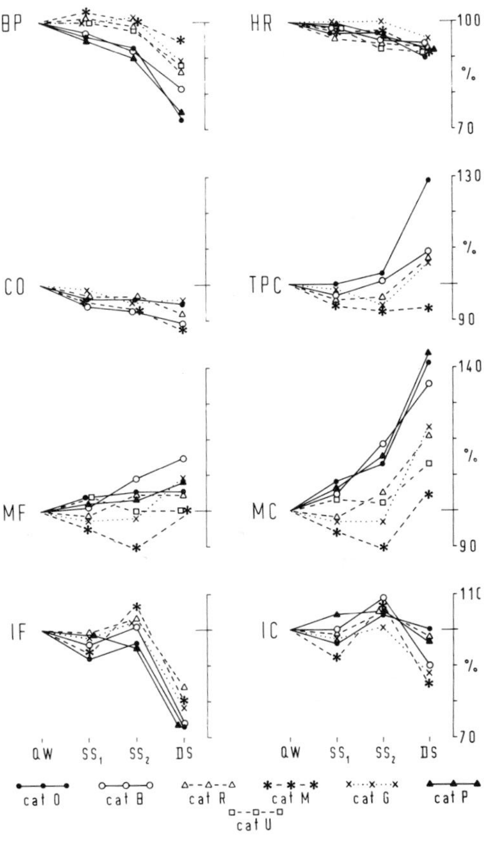

Fig. 1.—Percentage changes of cardiovascular variables throughout wakefulness-sleep cycle, referred to baselines in quiet wakefulness. **QW,** quiet wakefulness; **SS$_1$,** early period of synchronized sleep; **SS$_2$,** later period of synchronized sleep; **DS,** desynchronized sleep; **BP,** mean blood pressure; **HR,** heart rate; **CO,** cardiac output, **TPC,** total peripheral conductance; **MF** and **MC,** superior mesenteric flow and conductance; **IF** and **IC,** left external iliac flow and conductance. Different symbols refer to seven cats studied, identified at bottom of figure. Each symbol is mean of 60 measurements performed in six wakefulness-sleep cycles. (From Mancia, G. et al.,[4] with permission.)

From the Cardiovascular Research Institute, University of Milan School of Medicine, and the Center for Cardiovascular Research, National Research Council, Milan, Italy.

lying on the floor (lesser activity in the neck electromyogram) and the eyes completely closed (no electro-oculographic activity). The EEG showed continuous high-amplitude, slow waves. Intermediate periods, which were difficult to classify either as QW or SS, were considered as transition stages and were not selected for study. Desynchronized sleep (which corresponds to human REM sleep and dreaming) was quite easy to identify: the cat looked completely relaxed, generally lying on one side, the neck electromyogram showed no or little tonic activity; there were bursts of rapid eye movements (prominently recorded in the electro-oculogram) and of body twitches (also recorded in the neck and hindlimb electromyograms); the EEG showed low-voltage, fast activity.

Normotensive Cats

Figure 1 shows a detailed picture of cardiovascular manifestations of sleep in seven cats carrying an indwelling arterial cannula and electromagnetic flow probes on the ascending aorta, superior mesenteric artery, and external iliac artery, so that arterial pressure, heart rate, cardiac output, total peripheral conductance, as well as changes in a visceral vascular bed and in a musculocutaneous one could be simultaneously assessed.[4] Data are expressed as percentage changes of base lines in QW. Circulation was only modestly influenced by SS, both in periods closer in time to waking (SS_1) and in periods immediately preceding the desynchronized phase (SS_2), while clear-cut significant changes always occurred during de-

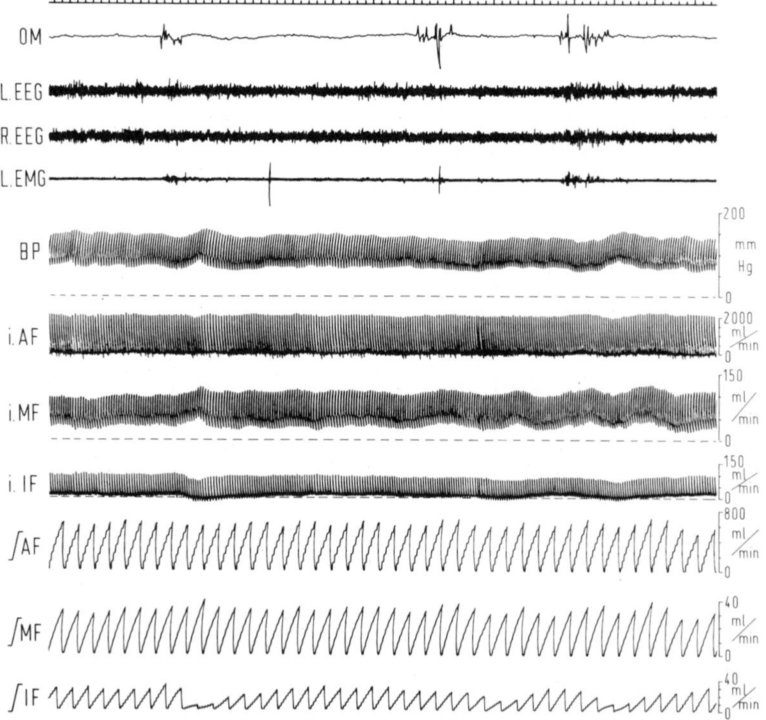

Fig. 2.—Original tracings from a DS episode in cat G, showing several phasic manifestations. From above downward: time (1 and 5 seconds); **OM,** ocular movements; **L.EEG** and **R.EEG,** electroencephalograms from left and right hemispheres; **L.EMG,** electromyogram from left hindlimb; **BP,** arterial blood pressure; **i.AF,** instantaneous flow through ascending aorta; **i.MF,** instantaneous flow through superior mesenteric artery; **i.IF,** instantaneous flow through left external iliac artery; **∫AF, ∫MF, ∫IF:** 2-second integrations of above flows. Calibrations on right. (From Mancia, G. et al.,[4] with permission.)

synchronized sleep (DS). Mean arterial pressure slightly and inconstantly decreased during SS but invariably fell in DS. Heart rate and cardiac output modestly decreased during SS, and were no further affected, or very mildly affected by DS. Total peripheral conductance either could slightly decrease or slightly increase in SS, but it almost invariably increased in the desynchronized stage signaling a definite overall vasodilatation. Mesenteric flow and conductance were variably influenced by SS in different cats, but DS always brought about a highly significant mesenteric vasodilatation. Finally, the external iliac bed was also slightly and variously affected during SS, but showed an unexpected constriction during the desynchronized stage. In summary, vasomotor regulation seems to be modestly disturbed during SS, while it is strongly modified by DS. During this stage, however, there is not a simple unidirectional readjustment, but muscle vasoconstriction coexists with the predominant visceral vasodilatation. Moreover, during DS cardiovascular changes of sudden development and short duration (called phasic phenomena [11]) can often be observed superimposed upon the slower ones we have just described. Figure 2 shows how they involve blood pressure, heart rate, mesenteric vessels, and particularly the iliac bed, where these phasic waves of vasoconstriction can be quite evident.[4] Phasic phenomena are generally time-locked with bursts of rapid eye movements and muscle twitches.

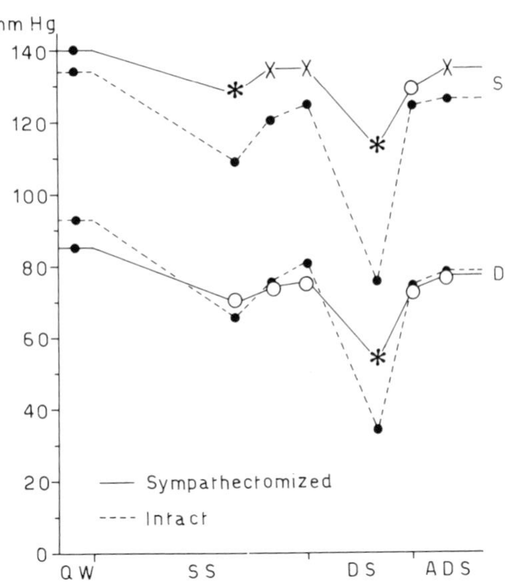

FIG. 3.—Changes in systolic **(S)** and diastolic **(D)** blood pressure during the wakefulness-sleep cycle in cats subjected to total sympathectomy **(continuous lines)** as compared to cats with intact sympathetic system **(interrupted lines)**. Each mark represents the mean of 40 measurements (10 in each of four cats). The first mark represents average blood pressures during quiet wakefulness **(QW)**, the second the lowest values recorded during synchronized sleep **(SS)**, the third the pressure levels at the time of onset of desynchronized sleep **(DS)**, the fourth the lowest values reached during DS, the fifth the levels immediately following DS, the last mark the blood pressures 10 minutes after termination of DS **(ADS)**. The time scale of the abscissa represents the average duration of a typical wakefulness-sleep cycle. Statistically significant differences between sympathectomized and nonsympathectomized animals are indicated by **X** ($P < 0.01$) or * ($P < 0.001$). **Hollow circles** indicate nonsignificant differences ($P > 0.05$). (From Baccelli, G., et al.,[5] with permission.)

NEURAL REGULATION OF CIRCULATION DURING SLEEP

It is important to prove, at this time, that the cardiovascular changes observed during SS and DS are really caused by neural mechanisms. Indeed, the blood pressure falls that occur during both stages of sleep are very greatly reduced by bilateral thoracolumbar sympathectomy [5] (Fig. 3). Figure 4 shows that the small decrease in blood pressure still occurring after sympathectomy is almost exclusively caused by a persistent decrease in cardiac output (apparently a nonneural change), while the conspicuous reduction in total peripheral resistance is almost completely nullified by sympathectomy.[5] Finally, Figure 5 also indicates that regional blood flow changes occurring during DS are no longer observed after adrenergic blockade by bretylium (Baccelli, Mancia and Zanchetti, unpublished experiments). The conclusion that cardiovascular changes during sleep are caused by a fall in sympathetic vasoconstrictor tone is in keeping with electrophysiological evidence showing a marked reduction in the electrical activity of sympathetic nerves during DS.[12,13]

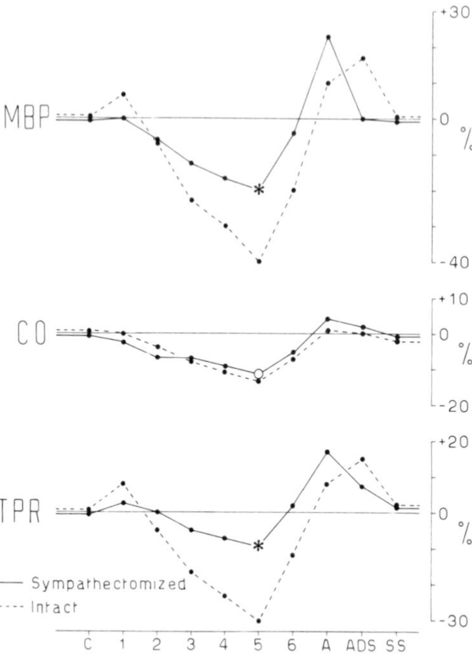

FIG. 4.—Changes in mean blood pressure **(MBP)**, cardiac output **(CO)**, and total peripheral resistance **(TPR)** during DS in cats subjected to total sympathectomy **(continuous lines)** as compared to cats with intact sympathetic system **(interrupted lines)**. Mean values of 20 episodes (sympathectomized animals) and 40 episodes (intact animals) at the following periods indicated on the abscissas: **C**, control during SS; **1**, onset of DS; **2**, beginning of hypotension; **3**, increase of hypotension; **4**, further increase of hypotension; **5**, lowest pressure values during DS; **6**, toward the end of DS; **A**, arousal from DS; **ADS**, 1 minute after A; **SS**, reappearance of synchronized sleep. On the ordinates all cardiovascular measurements expressed as percentage changes referred to **C**. Statistical symbols are the same as in Figure 3. (From Baccelli, G. et al.,[5] with permission.)

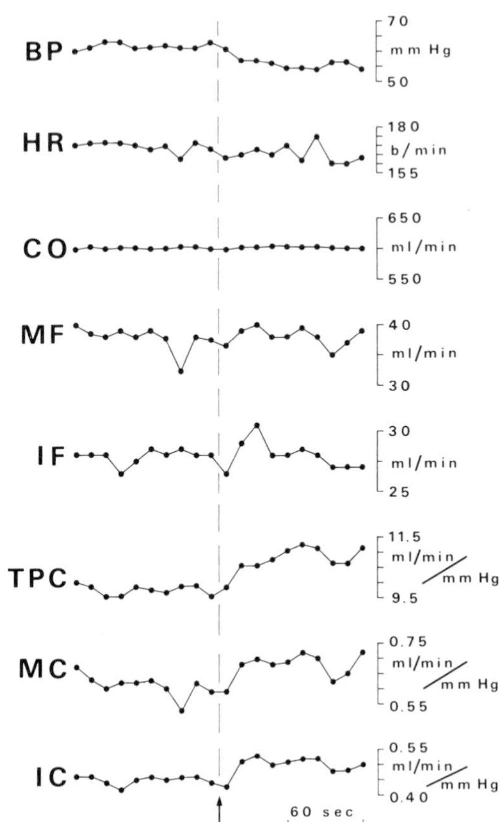

FIG. 5.—Abolition of cardiovascular manifestations of DS by previous intravenous administration of bretylium. Means of measurements taken during five sleep episodes. Each **dot** represents the value for 4 consecutive seconds out of every 12. The **arrow** and **vertical interrupted line** mark the beginning of DS. **BP,** mean blood pressure; **HR,** heart rate; **CO,** cardiac output; **MF,** superior mesenteric flow; **IF,** external iliac flow; **TPC,** total peripheral conductance; **MC,** superior mesenteric conductance; **IC,** external iliac conductance. (Based on unpublished observations by Baccelli, Mancia, and Zanchetti.)

Neurogenic Hypertension Induced by Sino-aortic Deafferentation

When cats are studied during quiet wakefulness in unrestrained conditions, it is apparent that bilateral sino-aortic denervation causes a definite but moderate increase in arterial pressure, which is about 20 mm Hg higher after interruption of sino-aortic reflexes than before.[1,6] Considerably higher pressures can sometimes be observed during excitement. (See Ferrario, McCubbin, and Page [14] for similar observations in the dog.) The cardiovascular changes induced by sleep, and particularly by DS, are markedly affected by sino-aortic deafferentation, however. We were soon struck by the profound fall in blood pressure during DS in these animals, so that the blood pressure commonly attained lower levels than before deafferentation.[1,6] Figure 6, based on the unpublished experiments of Baccelli, Mancia, and Zanchetti, summarizes recent experiments which provide detailed evidence concerning

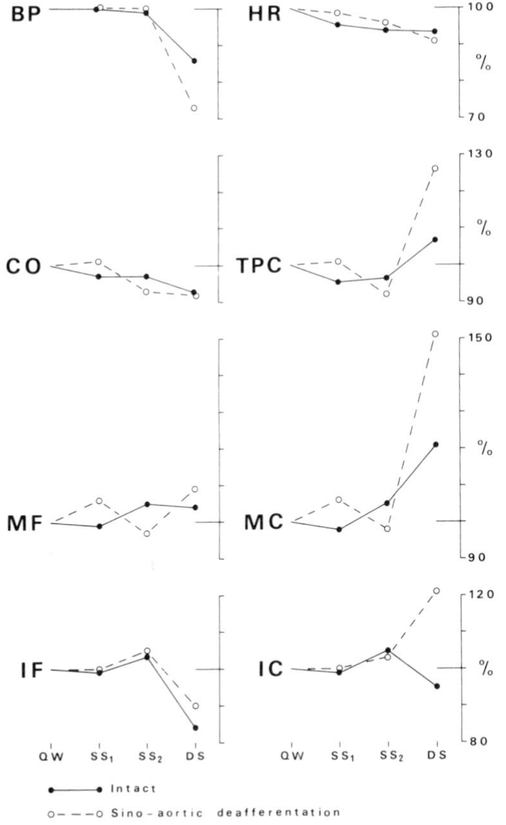

FIG. 6.—Cardiovascular manifestations of desynchronized sleep in cat **R** before **(filled circles, continuous lines)** and after sino-aortic deafferentation **(hollow circles, interrupted lines).** Each symbol is mean of 60 measurements performed in six wakefulness-sleep cycles. Percentage changes referred to baselines in QW. Abbreviations are the same as those in Figure 5. (Based on unpublished observations of Baccelli, Mancia, and Zanchetti.)

both synchronized and desynchronized sleep. Even after sino-aortic deafferentation the circulation was quite modestly influenced by synchronized sleep. Mean blood pressure levels remained practically unaffected, despite the usual slight decrease in cardiac output, resulting in a small and nonsignificant decrease in total vascular conductance. Variable nonsignificant changes were observed in mesenteric and iliac conductances as well. On the whole, SS was associated with small cardiovascular changes both before and after interruption of sino-aortic reflexes. Only during DS were the effects of sino-aortic deafferentation fully displayed. Though the reduction in heart rate and cardiac output during the desynchronized stage was not greater after than before deafferentation, blood pressure fell much more markedly, accompanied by a conspicuous overall vasodilatation (see also [3]). Sino-aortic deafferentation not only made overall vasodilatation and visceral vasodilatation more striking, but rendered the vasodilatation a more diffuse phenomenon. Indeed, even the iliac bed, which had shown a trend toward vasoconstriction before interruption of sino-aortic reflexes, became vasodilated, as if the vasoconstrictive influences normally active on muscle blood vessels during desynchronized sleep were overcome by the more general and marked suppression of vasoconstrictor tone occurring after sino-aortic deafferentation.

What is the mechanism by which animals with sino-aortic deafferentation, despite their higher blood pressure level during wakefulness, have a definitely exaggerated fall in pressure and a much greater vasodilatation during desynchronized sleep? Section of sino-aortic nerves interrupts both baroceptive and chemoceptive afferents. Experiments carried out with selective baroceptive or chemoceptive denervation [15,16] showed (Fig. 7) that the background of higher blood pressure and vasomotor tone caused by interruption of baroceptive reflexes was only partially responsible for the exaggerated blood pressure fall. Arterial pressure and vasomotor tone could attain levels actually lower than those occurring in the intact normotensive animal only when chemoceptive reflexes were inactivated, and their buffer action on the depressor vasodilator influence of sleep was abolished.

EXPERIMENTAL RENOVASCULAR HYPERTENSION

If we now turn to another and much more severe type of hypertension, that induced by bilateral clamping of the renal arteries, we can see [7,8] (Fig. 8) that also in these animals mean blood pressure decreases during SS and more markedly during the desynchronized stage, but always remains at much higher hypertensive levels than in intact animals during similar stages of sleep. These observations suggest that part of the blood pressure control in the renal hypertensive animal is neurogenic, but are also

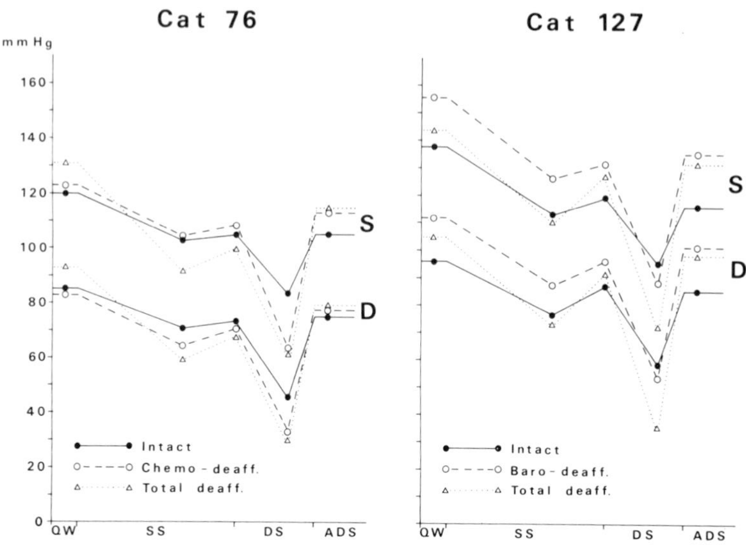

FIG. 7.—Effect of selective chemoceptive deafferentation (*left*) and of selective baroceptive deafferentation (*right*) on changes in systolic **(S)** and diastolic **(D)** blood pressure during the wakefulness-sleep cycle. *Left:* Cat 76, studied with intact reflexes **(filled circles, continuous lines),** then after selective chemoceptive deafferentation **(hollow circles, interrupted lines),** and finally after completion of sino-aortic deafferentation **(hollow triangles, dotted lines).** *Right:* Cat 127, studied with intact reflexes **(filled circles, continuous lines),** then after selective baroceptive deafferentation **(hollow circles, interrupted lines),** and finally after completion of sino-aortic deafferentation **(hollow triangles, dotted lines).** On both sides, each mark indicates the mean of 10 measurements under each condition of the wakefulness-sleep cycle. Other abbreviations as in Figure 3. (Based on an unpublished figure from Guazzi, M., Baccelli, G., and Zanchetti, A.[15])

compatible with the opinion that the largest component of renovascular hypertension is maintained by humoral factors. However, if renal artery clamping is followed by sino-aortic deafferentation, the neurogenic component of renal hypertension, as judged from the fall in pressure during sleep, appeared to be much greater than the one which could be assessed when the sino-aortic reflexes were intact. Indeed, the blood pressure fall became dramatically exaggerated not only because baseline pressure during QW had further and conspicuously increased, but also because blood pressure attained very low levels during DS. Figure 8 shows that, at least during this stage of sleep, the cat with renal artery stenosis and sino-aortic deafferentation can no longer be defined as a hypertensive animal.[7,8]

These findings are a very strong indication that maintenance of the high blood pressure of renovascular animals largely depends on neural vasomotor activity. This conclusion, however, may seem to contrast with the demonstration, in 1937, that total sympathectomy does not prevent development of hypertension in animals with renal artery stenosis.[17] Quite recently, Guazzi, Ellsworth, and Freis,[18] by studying the blood pressure effect of sleep in sympathectomized renovascular cats, have shown that these animals are hypertensive after sympathectomy as much as when the sympathetic system is intact, but that sympathectomy abolishes all blood pressure fall during sleep, even the deep fall normally occurring after sino-aortic deafferentation (Fig. 9). Thus, these experiments indicate that, though renal hypertension can depend on sympathetic mechanisms, it does not necessarily depend on them in all conditions. If neural mechanisms are apparently involved when the

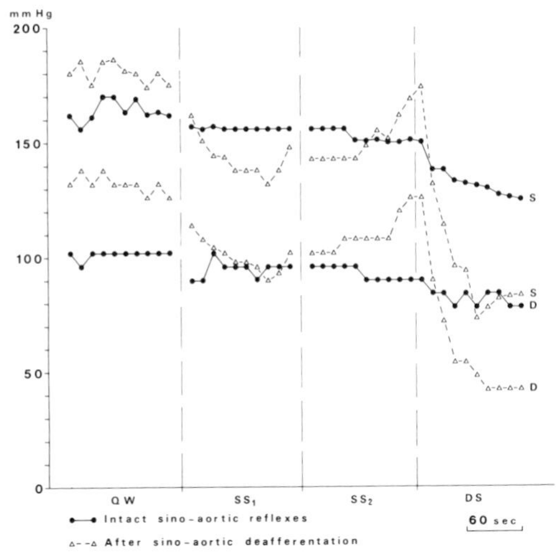

FIG. 8.—Changes in systolic **(S)** and diastolic **(D)** blood pressure during the wakefulness-sleep cycle in a cat with renovascular hypertension before **(filled circles, continuous lines)** and after sino-aortic deafferentation **(hollow triangles, interrupted lines).** Each symbol is the mean of five measurements taken at regular intervals (every 12 seconds) during five wakefulness-sleep cycles. Other abbreviations as in Fig. 1. (Based on an unpublished figure from Zanchetti, A., Guazzi, M., and Baccelli, G.[8])

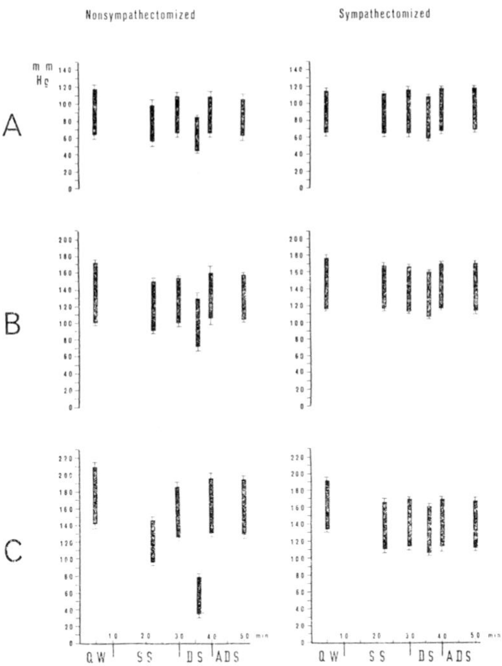

FIG. 9.—Averages and standard errors of the mean of systolic and diastolic arterial pressure during the wakefulness-sleep cycle in a group of five nonsympathectomized (*left*) versus a group of seven sympathectomized (*right*) cats. *A,* before renal arterial clipping; *B,* 2 to 4 weeks after clipping; *C,* 1 week after subsequent sino-aortic deafferentation. **QW,** quiet wakefulness; **SS,** synchronized sleep; **DS,** desynchronized sleep; **ADS,** after termination of **DS.** (Based on an unpublished figure from Guazzi, M., Ellsworth, O. T., and Freis.[18])

sympathetic system is intact, other mechanisms are likely to take over and maintain the hypertension when the sympathetic influences are chronically excluded. It seems reasonable, at the moment, to assume that suppression of the neural control of circulation by an enduring irreversible procedure such as sympathectomy is not an ideal method for assessing the neurogenic component of renovascular or other types of hypertension, as circulatory homeostasis is apparently capable of substituting neural for other types of mechanisms of circulatory control, and can therefore maintain the hypertension. This shift from one mechanism to others cannot occur when the suppression of sympathetic activity is short-lasting and reversible, as during sleep. It appears therefore that the study of cardiovascular changes during natural sleep is, for the moment, the most convenient physiologic method for studying the contribution of neural influences in circulatory control in the normotensive and hypertensive animal.[19]

REFERENCES

1. Guazzi, M., and Zanchetti, A.: Blood pressure and heart rate during natural sleep of the cat, and their regulation by carotid sinus and aortic reflexes. Arch. Ital. Biol. 103:789, 1965.
2. Guazzi, M., Mancia, G., Kumazawa, T., Baccelli, G., and Zanchetti, A.: Effects of cardiac denervation on blood pressure and heart rate during natural sleep in the cat. Cardiovasc. Res. 2:265, 1968.
3. Kumazawa, T., Baccelli, G., Guazzi, M., Mancia, G., and Zanchetti, A.: Hemodynamic patterns during desynchronized sleep in intact cats and in cats with sino-aortic deafferentation. Circ. Res. 24:923, 1969.

4. Mancia, G., Baccelli, G., Adams, D. B., and Zanchetti, A.: Vasomotor regulation during sleep in the cat. Am. J. Physiol. 220:1086, 1971.
5. Baccelli, G., Guazzi, M., Mancia, G., and Zanchetti, A.: Neural and non-neural mechanisms influencing circulation during sleep. Nature 223:184, 1969.
6. Guazzi, M., and Zanchetti, A.: Carotid sinus and aortic reflexes in the regulation of circulation during sleep. Science 148:397, 1965.
7. Zanchetti, A., Guazzi, M., and Baccelli, G.: Influence of sleep on circulation in normal and hypertensive animals. *In* Gross, F. (Ed.): Antihypertensive Therapy. Heidelberg: Springer, 1966, pp. 74–95.
8. Zanchetti, A., Guazzi, M., and Baccelli, G.: Role of sino-aortic reflexes in the regulation of experimental renal hypertension during natural sleep. *In* Kezdi, P. (Ed.): Baroreceptors and Hypertension. Oxford: Pergamon, 1967, pp. 387–400.
9. Zanchetti, A.: Brain stem mechanisms of sleep. Anesthesiology 28:81, 1967.
10. Jouvet, M.: Neurophysiology of the states of sleep. Physiol. Rev. 47:117, 1967.
11. Gassel, M. M., Ghelarducci, B., Marchiafava, P. L., and Pompeiano, O.: Phasic changes in blood pressure and heart rate during the rapid eye movement episodes of desynchronized sleep in unrestrained cats. Arch. Ital. Biol. 102:530, 1964.
12. Iwamura, Y., Uchino, Y., Ozawa, S., and Torii, S.: Spontaneous and reflex discharge of a sympathetic nerve during "para-sleep" in decerebrate cat. Brain Res. 16:359, 1969.
13. Baust, W., Weidinger, H., and Kirchner, F.: Sympathetic activity during natural sleep and arousal. Arch. Ital. Biol. 106:379, 1968.
14. Ferrario, C. M., McCubbin, J. W., and Page, I. H.: Hemodynamic characteristics of chronic experimental neurogenic hypertension in unanesthetized dogs. Circ. Res. 24:911, 1969.
15. Guazzi, M., Baccelli, G., and Zanchetti, A.: Carotid body chemoceptors: Physiological role in buffering fall in blood pressure during sleep. Science 153:206, 1966.
16. Guazzi, M., Baccelli, G., and Zanchetti, A.: Reflex chemoceptive regulation of arterial pressure during natural sleep in the cat. Am. J. Physiol. 214:969, 1968.
17. Freeman, N. E., and Page, I. H.: Hypertension produced by constriction of the renal artery in sympathectomized dogs. Am. Heart J. 14:405, 1937.
18. Guazzi, M., Ellsworth, O. T., and Freis, E. D.: Influence of the adrenergic system in renovascular hypertension. Cardiovasc. Res. 5:71, 1971.
19. Zanchetti, A.: Neural factors and catecholamines in experimental hypertension. *In* Zanchetti, A. (Ed.): Neural and Psychological Mechanisms in Cardiovascular Disease. Milan: Il Ponte, 1972, pp. 15–31.

Effect of Sleep on Blood Pressure in Patients with Hypertension

By David W. Richardson, M.D., George W. Vetrovec, M.D., and William C. Williamson, M.D.

Sleep is a natural event of universal occurrence during which long periods of unconsciousness and minimal interaction with the external environment are punctuated by shorter episodes of peculiar consciousness, dreaming. By comparison with periods of wakefulness in which the subject confronts his surroundings, sleep provides a baseline of minimal consciousness from which the short-term effects of patient-environment interaction can be judged. This chapter reports the changes in arterial blood pressure during wakefulness and sleep in hypertensive men and women, first during a day or more of life with minimal restriction, and second during sleep monitored electroencephalographically to estimate the depth of sleep and to signal the occurrence of specific events such as arousal and dreams. In addition, the effect of sleep on the sensitivity of the arterial baroreceptor reflex is briefly reviewed.

Changes in Blood Pressure During Sleep in Unrestricted Subjects

In 11 hypertensive patients, arterial blood pressure was monitored for at least 24 hours using a plastic cannula in a brachial artery, a commercially available transducer and radiotelemeter whose fidelity has been described previously,[1] and a small portable pump which perfused the cannula to prevent its clotting. Figure 1 shows a typical record. Nine of the patients had no demonstrable cause of hypertension. Two (W.R. and E.C.) had stenosis of a renal artery demonstrated arteriographically, but in neither was the ratio of renin concentrations between the two renal veins greater than 1.5. No patient had hemorrhagic or exudative retinopathy at the time of the study. Most studies were carried out with the patients housed in a private room of the Clinical Research Center or hotel unit of the hospital. In three subjects, we recorded blood pressure for two 24-hour periods, and in two of these the patient was at home during the second day. All stated that they sleep reasonably well; no other evidence of the depth of sleep is available. Each patient went to bed at his usual hour, none used sedative drugs on the night of the study, and each had omitted antihypertensive drugs for a sufficiently long period (1 to 2 weeks) for their effects to dissipate.

Table 1 compares for each subject the blood pressure averaged over the hours of sleep with the average for the remainder of the 24 hours, during which he was awake. The group's average systolic pressure fell from 177.6 awake to 161.9 mm Hg during sleep, a change of 15.7 mm Hg (S.E. 4.6 mm Hg) or 9 percent. Their average diastolic pressure fell from 98.3 mm Hg awake to 87.2 asleep, a change of 12.1 mm Hg (S.E. 2.3 mm Hg) or 11 percent. In three patients, pressures averaged over the entire period of sleep were not lower than the average for the rest of the 24 hours. These changes were significantly smaller than those observed in a group of eight healthy medical students and physicians observed under similar circumstances whose pressures fell from 130.2/75.5 awake to 102.5/57.9 mm Hg asleep, changes of 27.7/17.6 mm Hg or 21/23 percent.

To estimate the maximal effect of the stresses of an "ordinary" day in a patient's life, including arterial puncture and frequent visits by physicians but no other investigative or therapeutic measures, the average pressure for the hour in which blood pressure was highest was compared with the pressure averaged over the hour during sleep when blood pressure was lowest (see Table 2). For the group of 11 hy-

From the Medical College of Virginia, Health Sciences Division, Virginia Commonwealth University, Richmond, Virginia.

This study was supported by grants from the Richmond and Virginia Heart Associations and by Grants 5 T07 RR00016 and M 01 RR6509 from the National Institutes of Health.

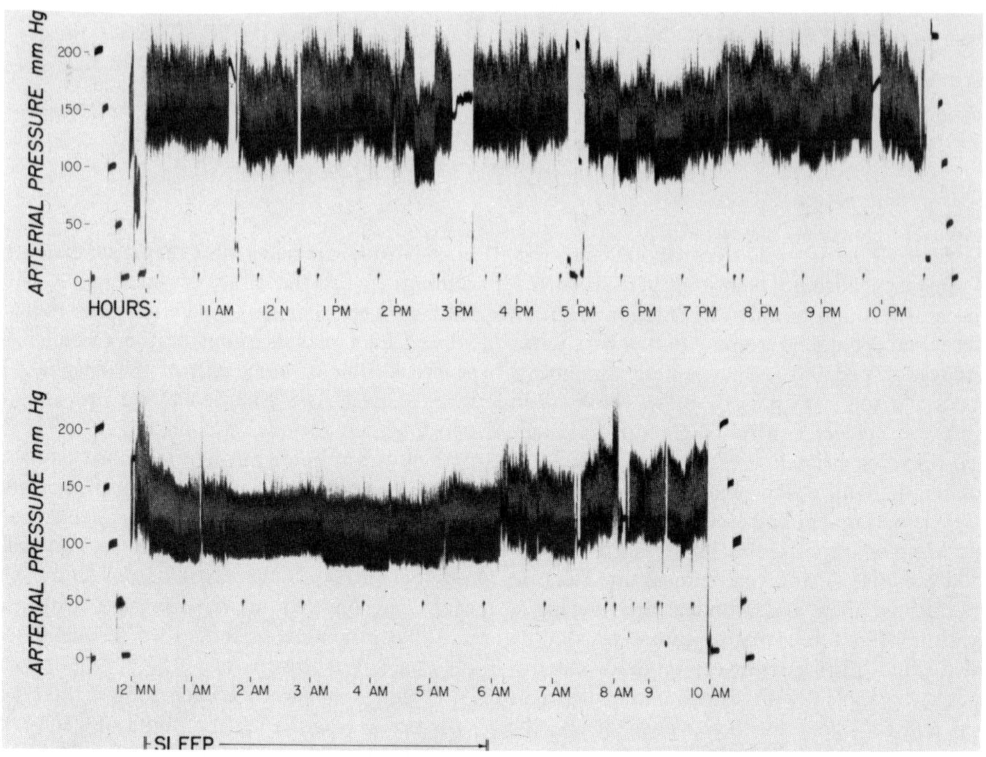

FIG. 1.—Intra-arterial pressure recorded by telemetry for 24 hours in a 37-year-old hypertensive woman. The *top* of each black band indicates systolic pressure, the *bottom* diastolic.

TABLE 1.—*Effect of Sleep on Blood Pressure in Unrestricted Hypertensive Humans*

					Pressure—mm Hg (Average ± SD)			
					Systolic		*Diastolic*	
Patient	*Sex*	*Age*	*Location*	*Hours of Sleep*	*Awake*	*Asleep*	*Awake*	*Asleep*
1. CA	M	57	Hospital	3	222 ± 15	222 ± 23	116 ± 7	100 ± 19
2. DJ	F	37	Hospital	8½	253 ± 10	231 ± 18	149 ± 5	136 ± 6
3. WR	M	57	Hospital	4	212 ± 14	215 ± 10	108 ± 9	97 ± 5
4. WS	M	55	Hospital	6	232 ± 17	202 ± 8	125 ± 12	103 ± 6
5. PT	F	48	Hospital	6	186 ± 19	158 ± 8	99 ± 7	85 ± 6
6. JD	F	26	Hospital	6	160 ± 9	121 ± 13	92 ± 9	69 ± 10
7. NH	M	29	Hospital	6	146 ± 6	135 ± 6	86 ± 5	78 ± 5
8. CB	M	31	Hospital	5	131 ± 13	106 ± 9	75 ± 9	60 ± 9
9. BD	F	34	Hospital	7	175 ± 10	147 ± 7	92 ± 4	81 ± 3
9. BD	F	34	Hospital	6	167 ± 16	156 ± 6	87 ± 9	84 ± 5
10. LS	M	45	Hospital	4	123 ± 5	134 ± 1	75 ± 4	81 ± 1
10. LS	M	45	Home	6	148 ± 14	163 ± 4	87 ± 7	93 ± 2
11. EC	F	37	Hospital	5	177 ± 8	148 ± 12	101 ± 6	87 ± 6
11. EC	F	37	Home	6	153 ± 7	127 ± 7	84 ± 5	68 ± 3
Mean					177.6	161.9	98.3	87.2
S.E.					10.5	10.7	5.5	5.0

TABLE 2.—*Average Blood Pressure during the Hours of Wakefulness When Pressure Was Highest and the Hour of Sleep When Pressure Was Lowest*

		Systolic Pressure (mm Hg)			*Diastolic Pressure (mm Hg)*		
Patient	*Location*	*Awake*	*Asleep*	*Decrease*	*Awake*	*Asleep*	*Decrease*
1	Hospital	244	199	45	125	80	45
2	Hospital	265	210	55	148	128	20
3	Hospital	237	204	33	120	90	30
4	Hospital	253	198	55	146	105	41
5	Hospital	236	145	91	114	78	36
6	Hospital	173	104	69	96	56	40
7	Hospital	162	128	34	92	72	20
8	Hospital	158	93	65	88	49	39
9	Hospital	197	138	59	103	78	25
9	Hospital	192	148	44	102	78	24
10	Hospital	136	117	19	83	71	12
10	Home	173	156	17	100	88	12
11	Hospital	187	137	50	110	81	29
11	Home	168	121	47	92	65	27
Mean		198.6	149.9	48.7	108.5	79.9	28.6
S.E.		10.9	10.3	5.3	5.4	5.2	2.8

pertensive patients, blood pressure during the hour of sleep with lowest pressure averaged 49/29 mm Hg (24/26%) below that present during the hour of highest waking pressure.

Bevan, Honour, and Stott,[2] using a portable photographic recorder in unrestricted patients, found smaller changes in intra-arterial pressure attributable to sleep. Pressure averaged over the hours of sleep was lower than the average during the waking hours by 9/2 mm Hg (5/2%) in eight patients with essential hypertension without retinopathy, and by 20/9 mm Hg (8/6%) in four patients in the malignant phase. All their subjects were in the hospital, presumably in large wards; it is possible that they slept less well than did ours.

Changes in Blood Pressure During Sleep Monitored Electroencephalographically

Ten untreated hypertensive patients, three of whom had retinal hemorrhages or exudates, slept without sedatives for one night in a dark, quiet room while blood pressure, EEG, and eye movements were recorded in an adjacent room, as described previously.[1] The group's average blood pressure behaved as follows: awake, in the second minute of recording, 208 ± 10 (S.E.)/111 ± 6; awake, in the minute just before sleep began, 194 ± 10/103 ± 6; asleep, in the minute during which blood pressure was lowest, 172 ± 9/90 ± 6; awake, in the first minute after waking in the morning, 205 ± 10/109 ± 6 mm Hg. Thus the maximal change in blood pressure between sleep and apprehension (arterial puncture) was 37/20 mm Hg. Though each of these ten subjects presented both electroencephalographic and behavioral evidence of sleep lasting 4 to 7 hours, the fall in blood pressure was less than that observed (Table 2) in subjects without EEG monitoring, which restricts movement and may have interfered with sleep to some extent.

Changes in cardiac output during sleep in hypertensive patients have been observed by two groups of investigators, with conflicting results. Khatri and Freis [3] noted decrease in mean intra-arterial blood pressure and in cardiac output of 9 percent in 14 patients with established hypertension. Bristow and his colleagues [4] studied nine hypertensives and, finding an insignificant decrease in cardiac output but 12 percent decrease in mean arterial pressure during sleep, attributed the fall in blood pressure to reduced peripheral resistance. Both groups made these observations during nondreaming sleep. The changes in blood pressure and cardiac output were rather small in both studies, and the differing conclusions about change in peripheral resistance may have resulted from different samples of the hypertensive population. At present I am unable to draw a firm conclusion about the mechanism responsible for the large fall in blood pressure observed in some patients during sleep, whether decrease in cardiac output or in peripheral vasoconstriction.

Events During Sleep

Dreams

External observers recognize dreaming in man by the concurrence of (*1*) disappearance of synchronized cortical electrical activity, (*2*) marked decrease in skeletal muscular electrical activity, (*3*) behavioral evidence of sleep, i.e., unawareness of the external environment; and (*4*) bursts of rapid eye movements (REM). Subjects awakened during or just after a period in which these four criteria occur together describe dreams vividly, whereas subjects awakened from other stages of sleep deny dreaming. During such episodes of REM sleep, we [1] usually found little change in blood pressure in normal or hypertensive subjects, though occasional episodes (bad dreams?) were associated with marked elevation in pressure and heart rate. Khatri and Freis,[3] on the other hand, observed rise in mean arterial pressure of 13 percent, from 109 to 122 mm Hg in 13 episodes of REM sleep in 11 hypertensive subjects, and similar changes in pressure in normotensive people. In the hypertensive subjects, cardiac output did not change during dreams despite the rise in blood pressure, which presumably resulted from peripheral vasoconstriction.

Brief Waking

Periods of wakefulness as brief as 15 seconds, recognized by appearance of alpha rhythm, the nine-cycle-per-second synchronized waves characteristic of relaxed wakefulness, were always accompanied by rise in blood pressure, which averaged 15/11 mm Hg in hypertensive subjects, and a like amount in normal people. Within 1 minute after awaking in the morning, blood pressure averaged only 4/2 mm Hg below its value during the first minutes of recording before sleep in our hypertensive patients.[1] Thus sleep-induced reduction in blood pressure is rapidly reversible.

Baroreceptor Activity During Sleep

Bristow, Sleight, and their colleagues [4,5] have shown that the arterial baroreceptor reflex is reset during sleep, that is, blood pressure is lower but heart rate is also lower, whereas the sensitivity of the reflex, that is, the decrease in heart rate for a given increase in arterial pressure, tends to be increased during sleep and especially during REM (dream) sleep. These changes were observed in hypertensive and normotensive subjects. They were not the result of the decrease in mean arterial pressure which accompanies sleep, since despite gradual elevation of pressure to the presleep level by infusion of angiotensin, the decrease in heart rate accompanying abrupt further increase in arterial pressure was still greater than during wakefulness.[5] The changes in baroreceptor reflex activity presumably reflect sleep-induced alteration in central neural activity.

Summary

Arterial blood pressure falls during sleep in hypertensive and in normal subjects. The change in blood pressure between the hour of wakefulness when blood pressure was highest and the hour of sleep when blood pressure was lowest averaged 49/29 mm Hg in 11 hypertensive patients monitored by telemetry for at least 24 hours of ordinary (for patients) life. This change is an estimate of the short-term pressor effect of the interaction between the mind and the environment in hypertensive man.

Changes in cardiac output and peripheral resistance in man during sleep are at present uncertain because of conflicting results by different investigators.

Dreaming is usually not associated with major changes in blood pressure. Even brief arousal is accompanied by prompt rise in pressure.

The baroreceptor reflex is promptly reset during sleep, operating around the lower steady pressure characteristic of the sleep state with increased sensitivity, especially during dreams.

References

1. Richardson, D. W., Honour, A. J., and Goodman, A. C.: Changes in arterial pressure during sleep in man. *In* Wood, J. E., III (Ed.): Hypertension. Vol. 16, Neural Control of the Circulation. New York: American Heart Association, 1968, p. 62.
2. Bevan, A. T., Honour, A. J., and Stott, F. H.: Direct arterial pressure recording in unrestricted man. Clin. Sci. 36:329, 1969.
3. Khatri, I. M., and Freis, E. D.: Hemodynamic changes during sleep in hypertensive patients. Circulation 39:785, 1969.
4. Bristow, J. D., Honour, A. J., Pickering, T. G., and Sleight, P.: Cardiovascular and respiratory changes during sleep in normal and hypertensive subjects. Cardiovasc. Res. 3:476, 1969.
5. Smyth, H. S., Sleight, P., and Pickering, G. W.: Reflex regulation of arterial pressure during sleep in man. Circ. Res. 24:109, 1969.

The Influence of Sodium on the Sympathetic System in Relation to Experimental Hypertension

By Jacques de Champlain, M.D., Ph.D.

The regulation of blood pressure involves the interaction of various systems and factors.[1] Hypertensive diseases could result from a variety of dysfunctions occurring at any point in this pressure-regulatory mechanism.[2] Among systems and factors which have been most often studied and proposed as triggering mechanisms in various forms of hypertensive diseases are: the pressor renal system; the endocrine system, especially in regard to the adrenal cortex and medulla; the sympathetic nervous system; the ionic balance mainly involving sodium and potassium or both; genetic predispositions; and emotional stress. However, it has been possible to recognize a specific etiologic cause for an elevated blood pressure in relatively few cases of clinical hypertension such as hypertensions associated with tumors of the adrenal cortex or medulla, with renal artery stenosis, or with a coarctation of the aorta. In the majority of patients the etiology has remained unknown or at most controversial.

There have been several indications in the literature that sodium or other ions might be implicated in the physiopathology of various forms of hypertension. Although ionic disturbances in vascular tissues involving sodium, potassium, and probably calcium appear to be an almost constant phenomenon associated with the rise in blood pressure it is still unsettled whether these changes play a determinant role in the initiation of hypertension or are secondary to elevated blood pressure.[3] Nevertheless, these changes could play a significant role in the chronic stage of hypertension since they are likely to influence the contraction of arteriolar smooth muscle [4,5] or else the vascular reactivity to pressor substances or to nerve stimulation.[6] Moreover, since many of the metabolic events responsible for impulse conduction and synaptic transmission as well as for the uptake, storage, release, and action of amines are ion-dependent,[7–12] it is probable that an ionic disturbance could alter the function of the sympathetic nervous system.

The increased sensitivity to catecholamine in most cases of hypertension [13] and the observation that most hypotensive drugs also alter the disposition of catecholamine or the activity of the sympathetic nervous system [14–16] constitute strong indirect evidence that the sympathetic nervous sysem may play an important role in the pathogenesis and maintenance of elevated blood pressure.

Since 1965, our interest in collaboration with Axelrod, Krakoff, and Mueller has been mainly focused on the study of relationship between the sympathetic nervous system and the variations of blood pressure induced by various sodium intakes ranging from sodium depletion to sodium loading in combination with the administration of deoxycorticosterone (DCA). These studies have permitted us to clearly establish that sodium balance directly or indirectly influences the activity of sympathetic fibers and adrenal medulla, and that these functional changes may be responsible for the variations in blood pressure under these experimental conditions.

The Role of Sympathetic Nervous System in Experimental Hypertension

Uninephrectomized male Sprague-Dawley rats were used for our studies. Animals were made hypertensive by weekly subcutaneous injection of deoxycorticosterone (DCA) pivalate (10 mg per week) and by giving a solution of 1% sodium chloride to drink at will. Animals so treated showed a significant increase in blood pressure during the second week of treatment and reached levels between 180 and 200 mm

From the Department of Physiology, Research Center in Neurosciences, University of Montreal, Montreal, Quebec, Canada.

Hg after 6 weeks of treatment.[17] Animals were studied at various times up to 10 weeks after the beginning of treatment. The recording of systolic blood pressure and the various methods used in these studies have been previously published in detail.[17] A systematic study of various functions of the sympathetic nerve endings was undertaken especially in regard to the uptake, storage, turnover, subcellular distribution, and metabolism of norepinephrine in various peripheral organs of these hypertensive rats.

Five minutes after administration of tritiated norepinephrine, the neuronal uptake as well as the uptake into the storage vesicles was found to be normal in various sympathetically innervated, peripheral organs of Doca-hypertensive animals in vivo and in vitro.[17–19] The retention and storage of norepinephrine was markedly reduced in these hypertensive animals however. One hour after injection, the amount of tritiated norepinephrine retained in the heart, intestine, skeletal muscle, spleen, and kidney was markedly reduced in hypertensive animals. Endogenous norepinephrine levels were also significantly lower in the same tissues of hypertensive animals (Fig. 1). The retention of norepinephrine as well as endogenous norepinephrine contents was normal in organs having a parenchymatous sympathetic innervation such as the salivary gland and the vas deferens.

A highly significant inverse relationship could be established between the level of systolic blood pressure and the capacity of the heart to retain tritiated norepinephrine (Fig. 2). A similar inverse relationship was also made between the systolic blood pressure and the endogenous norepinephrine content of the hearts of normotensive and hypertensive rats.[16] Since this relationship is significant even in the hearts of normotensive animals within the normal range of blood pressure, it appears that the greater decrease in norepinephrine retention or in endogenous norepinephrine levels observed in hypertensive animals might be caused by the same mechanism regulating the blood

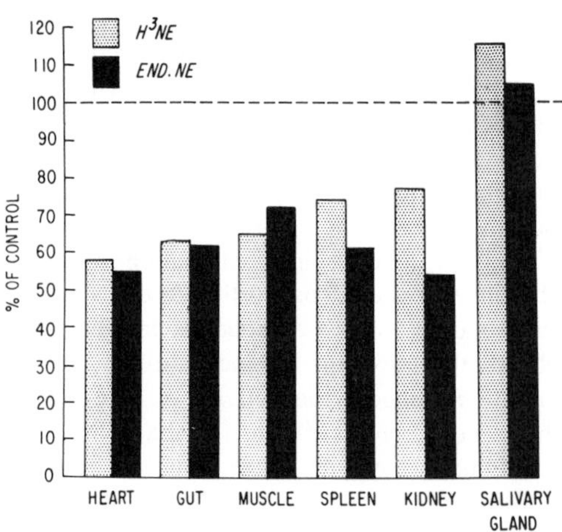

FIG. 1.—Retention of ³H-norepinephrine **(H³NE)** 1 hour after intravenous injection of 25 μCi of the tritiated amine and the endogenous norepinephrine levels **(END. NE)** in various tissues of Doca-hypertensive rats (7 weeks). Each bar represents the mean of 10 to 16 values. The results are expressed in percentages of the values found in normotensive control rats. With the exception of the heart and kidney, in which the values were expressed per total organ, in all the other tissues the results were calculated per gram of wet tissue. (From de Champlain, J., Krakoff, L. R., and Axelrod, J.: Catecholamine metabolism in experimental hypertension in the rat. Circ. Res. 20:136, 1967, by permission of The American Heart Association, Inc.)

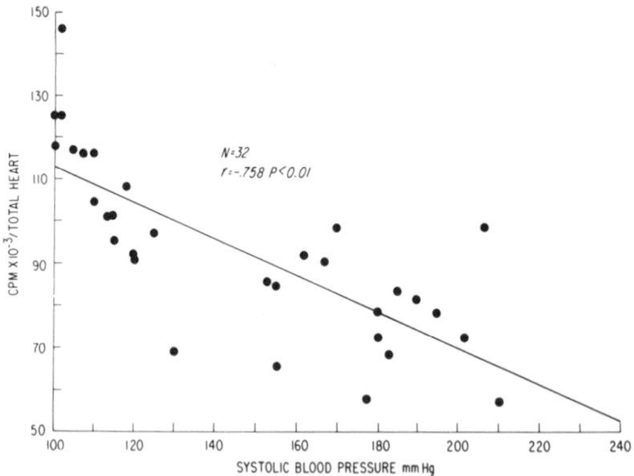

FIG. 2.—Correlation between the systolic blood pressure and the amount of tritiated norepinephrine retained in the hearts of normotensive and hypertensive rats 1 hour after the injection of 25 μCi of ³H-norepinephrine. The inverse relationship between the systolic blood pressure and the retention of ³H-norepinephrine was not only significant for the normotensive and hypertensive animals combined but was also significant within each group of animals. (From de Champlain, J., Krakoff, L. R., and Axelrod, J.: Catecholamine metabolism in experimental hypertension in the rat. Circ. Res. 20:136, 1967, by permission of The American Heart Association, Inc.)

pressure in normotensive animals. This defect in retention and storage of norepinephrine in Doca- and sodium-hypertensive animals has been confirmed recently by others.[20–23] The inverse relationship between the capacity of the heart to retain tritiated norepinephrine and the level of systolic blood pressure has also been confirmed.[21]

The reduced retention and storage of norepinephrine can be explained by an increased turnover of norepinephrine in the sympathetic peripheral fibers. This conclusion was reached after we utilized various techniques to estimate the turnover in these fibers. After injection of tracer doses of tritiated norepinephrine, the specific activity of norepinephrine fell more rapidly in the hearts of hypertensive rats so that the half-life of norepinephrine was found to be 32 percent shorter in these animals.[19] After inhibition of tyrosine hydroxylase by α-methyltyrosine, the rate of decline of norepinephrine content was markedly accelerated in the heart, slightly accelerated in the spleen and intestine, and normal in salivary glands of hypertensive rats. Moreover, the tritiated norepinephrine formed from tritiated dopamine decreased significantly faster from the heart of hypertensive rats thus indicating that the newly formed norepinephrine is utilized more rapidly in hypertensive rats.[24]

It appears that this increase in norepinephrine turnover might play an important role in the pathogenesis of this form of hypertension since it was found, in experiments made early in the course of treatment with Doca and sodium, that the increase in turnover rate preceded the development of hypertension.[25] In animals treated for 1 week with Doca and sodium, the capacity to retain norepinephrine was reduced by 26 percent over a 24-hour period although the blood pressure was not significantly increased and endogenous norepinephrine levels were still normal in treated animals (Table 1). Using the same methodology, Louis and his co-workers [22] found a slight, but not significant, reduction of about 20 percent in the capacity of the heart to retain norepinephrine in similarly treated animals before the development of hypertension.

In view of these important changes in the turnover rate, the activity of tyrosine hydroxylase, which is the limiting step in the biosynthesis of norepinephrine,[26] was indirectly estimated by measuring the capacity of the nerve fibers to convert ^{14}C-tyrosine into catecholamines.[24] One hour after a single injection or at the end of a 1-hour infusion of ^{14}C-tyrosine, the amount of ^{14}C-catecholamines formed was slightly increased in the hearts and markedly increased in the adrenal medulla of hypertensive rats (Table 2). Since the endogenous norepinephrine and epinephrine levels were normal in the adrenal glands of hypertensive rats, the increase in the synthesis rate was probably accompanied by an increased liberation of catecholamines into the circulation.

TABLE 1.—*Effect of 1-Week Treatment with Doca and Sodium on Norepinephrine Storage*

	Systolic Blood Pressure (mm Hg)	*Endogenous Norepinephrine (ng per heart)*	*^{3}H-Norepinephrine (nCi per heart)*
Control	112±4.5	466±12	38±2.8
Doca and sodium (1 week)	120±2.5	449±29	28±4.0 *
Percentage change	+7.5	−3.5	−26

Based on data taken from de Champlain, J., Krakoff, L. R., and Axelrod, J.[25]
* $P < 0.05$
The treated group of rats was given one subcutaneous injection 10 mg of a suspension of Doca and a 1% solution of sodium chloride to drink at will. One week later, the animals were injected intravenously with 15 μCi of ^{3}H-norepinephrine and were killed 24 hours later. Each value is the mean ± SEM of 10 animals.

TABLE 2.—*Catecholamine Synthesis from ^{14}C-tyrosine in Heart and Adrenal Glands of Hypertensive Rats*

	Endogenous Norepinephrine (*μg per organ*)	*^{14}C-Catecholamine* (*counts per minute*)	
		After injection	*After infusion*
Heart (total organ)			
Control	0.844±0.050	110±15	75±12
Hypertensive	0.555±0.035 †	133±12	88±24
Percentage change	−34%	+20%	+19%
Adrenal glands (pair)			
Control	3.12±0.34	517±25	493±64
Hypertensive	2.94±0.63	1056±200 *	823±136 *
Percentage change	−6%	+105%	+67%

Based on data from de Champlain, J., Mueller, R. A., and Axelrod, J.[24]
* $P < 0.05$
† $P < 0.01$
The heart and adrenal glands were examined for ^{14}C-catecholamine either 1 hour after injection of 15 μCi of ^{14}C-tyrosine or after a 1-hour infusion of 20 μCi of ^{14}C-tyrosine. Groups of six or seven animals were used with either technique. The specific activity of tyrosine was similar in normotensive and hypertensive rats. The systolic blood pressure of hypertensive animals was 215 ± 7.5 mm Hg compared to 118 ± 1.5 mm Hg in normotensive rats.

When subcellular fractionation studies were made, it was found that the capacity of the storage vesicles of the heart of hypertensive rats to retain norepinephrine was markedly impaired.[19] Although the initial uptake capacity of these vesicles was normal, the storage vesicles of hypertensive animals lost 45 percent of their initial norepinephrine content within 4 hours after injection of tritiated norepinephrine, whereas the storage vesicles of normotensive animals merely lost 8 percent of their content during the same period. It appeared, therefore, that there was a defect in the binding mechanism of norepinephrine within the storage vesicles in hypertensive rats. Studies on the intraneuronal distribution of norepinephrine confirmed that the fraction of soluble or free norepinephrine was proportionally greater in the hearts of hypertensive animals than in the hearts of normotensive rats (Fig. 3). This abnormal distribution is probably due to a less efficient binding of norepinephrine into the storage vesicles and suggests that greater amounts of physiologically active norepinephrine are in the vicinity of receptors in this condition.[19]

Because of the increased norepinephrine turnover resulting in a larger proportion of soluble or free norepinephrine exposed to the action of intraneuronal monoamine oxidase and to the action of extraneuronal catechol-O-methyl transferase, the pattern of metabolites is markedly disturbed in hypertensive rats.[27] After injection of tritiated norepinephrine, the norepinephrine was utilized and excreted more rapidly in the hypertensive animals. In the urinary collections made 4 to 24 hours after injection, at a time when the tritiated compounds are derived exclusively from the tritiated norepinephrine which was initially taken up and stored in the sympathetic nerve fibers, the amount of tritiated amines and metabolites excreted in the urine of hypertensive rats was approximately twice that excreted in the urine of normotensive rats. The pattern of metabolites in the kidney and urine of hypertensive rats showed that norepinephrine, normetanephrine, deaminated catechols, vanillylmandelic acid (VMA), and 3-methoxy-4-hydroxyphenylglycol were all markedly and significantly increased (Table 3). The increment in the excretion of free norepinephrine and O-methylated metabolites suggests that a larger amount of physiologically active norepinephrine available to react with the receptors is

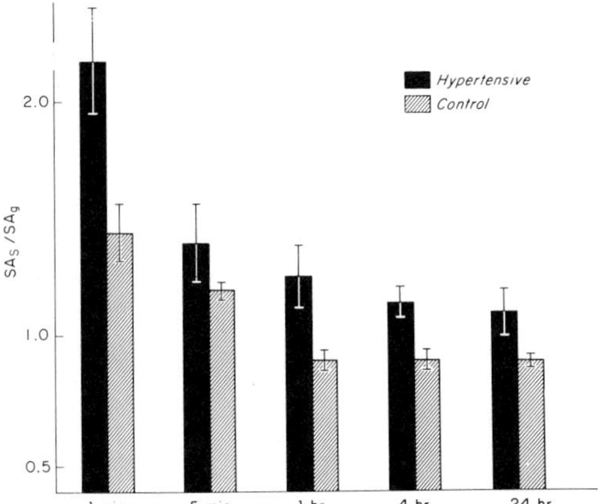

FIG. 3.—Subcellular distribution of norepinephrine in the hearts of hypertensive and normotensive rats at various intervals after the injection of 25 μCi of the tritiated amine. Groups of seven to 10 animals were used each time. The intraneuronal distribution of norepinephrine is expressed as the ratio of the specific activity of the supernatant fraction over the specific activity of the granular fraction (SAs/SAg). From 1 hour until 24 hours after the injection, this ratio remained constant in the hearts of control animals. In the hearts of the hypertensive rats, this ratio was always higher than that of the control animals and continued to decrease progressively during the first 24 hours after the injection. (From Krakoff, L. R., de Champlain, J., and Axelrod, J.: Abnormal storage of norepinephrine in experimental hypertension in the rat. Circ. Res. 21:583, 1967, by permission of The American Heart Association, Inc.)

TABLE 3.—*Excretion of Norepinephrine and Tritiated Metabolites in the Kidney and Urine of Doca-Hypertensive Rats*

	Kidney, 30 minutes after injection	*Urine, 4 to 24 hours after Injection*
Norepinephrine	+ 35%	+100%
Deaminated catechols	+137%	+ 35%
Normetanephrine	+193%†	+126%†
Vanillylmandelic acid	+119%†	+ 75%
3-methoxy-4-hydroxyphenylglycol	+124%†	+ 59%†

Based on data from de Champlain, J., Krakoff, L. R., and Axelrod, J.[27]

* $P < 0.05$

† $P < 0.01$

The results are expressed as the percentage of change from control values in normotensive rats. In the study on the kidney, the animals were injected with 25 μCi of tritiated norepinephrine and were killed 30 minutes later. For the urinary studies, rats were injected with 50 μCi and the urinary collection was made 4 to 24 hours after the injection.

coming out of the adrenergic nerve fibers of hypertensive rats.

To determine whether the abnormal norepinephrine metabolism in hypertensive animals was due to a local metabolic defect at the nerve ending or to an increased central sympathetic activity, the effect of ganglionic blockade on the norepinephrine storage was studied in these animals. After treatment of the hypertensive animals with a potent ganglion blocker, the blood pressure fell within the normal range and simultaneously the capacity of the hearts to retain norepinephrine was restored to normal (Fig. 4).

These results indicate that the neurogenic tone is increased in these animals and that the central vasomotor centers could be involved in the pathogenesis or the maintenance of hypertension. In support of a central neurogenic mechanism in this form of hypertension, recent findings have shown that the endogenous norepinephrine level is elevated and that the turnover rate is significantly reduced in the brainstem of hypertensive rats whereas the endogenous norepinephrine and turnover rates are normal in the spinal cord and in the telediencephalon (de Champlain, J., and Van Ameringen, M. R., unpublished data). Nakamura, Gerold and Thoenen[23] have also reported similar findings in Doca-hypertensive rats. Moreover, the endogenous norepinephrine content of the superior and stellate ganglion was found to be markedly increased in hypertensive rats (unpublished data).

Both the adrenal medulla and the peripheral sympathetic fibers are participating in the maintenance of elevated blood pressure in Doca-hypertensive rats. The use of 6-hydroxydopamine (6-OH-DA) to produce chemical sympathectomy in combination with bilateral adrenalectomy has permitted us to study more precisely the respective roles of the two components of the sympathetic system. In studies with electron microscopy[28] and with fluorescent histochemistry[29,30] this compound was found to selectively destroy the adrenergic terminal fibers without damaging the adrenal

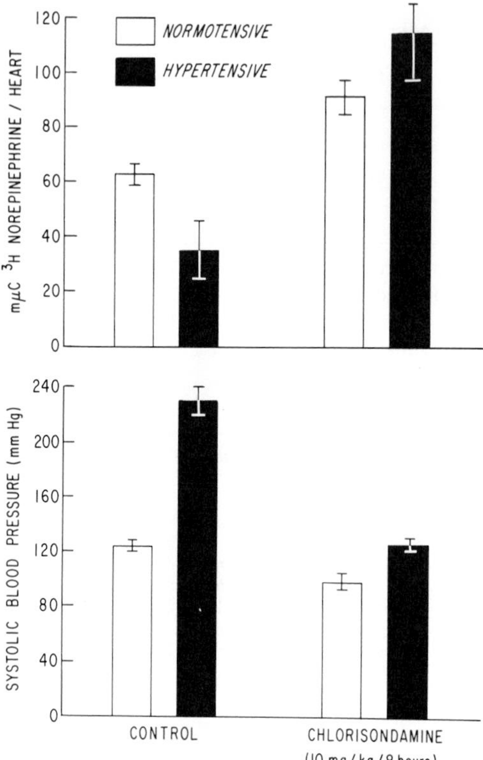

FIG. 4.—Effect of ganglionic blockade by chlorisondamine on norepinephrine storage and on systolic blood pressure in normotensive and hypertensive rats. The animals were first injected with 25 μCi of norepinephrine and 15 minutes later the treatment with chlorisondamine (10 mg per kilogram every 8 hours) was begun. The rats were killed 24 hours after beginning of the treatment. Each group contained seven to eight rats and the results are expressed as the mean ± SEM. This treatment lowered the blood pressure of the hypertensive animals to normotensive levels while it simultaneously restored the norepinephrine-storage capacity of the heart to normal within 24 hours after the start of the treatment. (From de Champlain, J., Krakoff, L. R., and Axelrod, J.: Relationship between sodium intake and norepinephrine storage during the development of experimental hypertension. Circ. Res. 23:479, 1968, by permission of The American Heart Association, Inc.)

medulla. Moreover, biochemical, pharmacologic, and physiologic studies have demonstrated that this drug can produce an efficient sympathectomy.[31] One week after bilateral adrenalectomy or sympathectomy by injection of 6-OH-DA (100 mg per kilogram), the systolic blood pressure was reduced by about 40 mm Hg in unanesthetized, hypertensive rats. In normotensive rats the blood pressure was decreased by about 30 mm Hg after sympathectomy but was decreased only slightly following adrenalectomy.[32] Although each procedure alone significantly reduced the blood pressure in hypertensive rats, the levels of systolic blood pressure remained at hypertensive levels. Neither the sympathetic nerve fibers of the vascular system nor the adrenal medulla alone can account entirely for the elevated blood pressure in unanesthetized rats. However, it seems that both components of the sympathetic system have a synergic influence on the maintenance of hypertension in these rats. The combination of both procedures in anesthetized animals reduces the blood pressure to an identical level in normotensive and hypertensive ani-

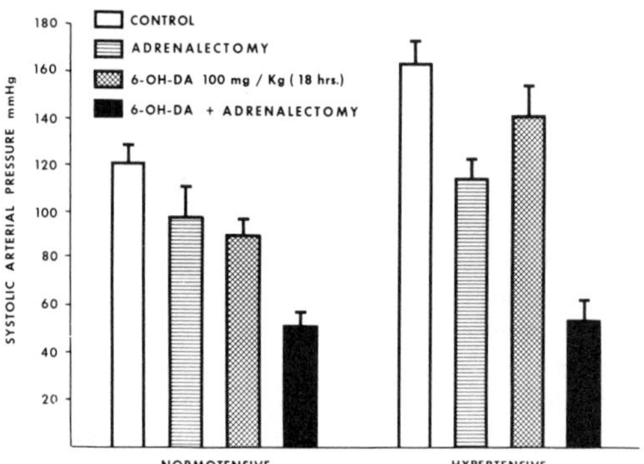

FIG. 5.—Hypotensive effects of chemical sympathectomy, bilateral adrenalectomy, and the combination of both procedures in groups of normotensive and hypertensive rats. The animals were anesthetized with sodium pentobarbital and blood pressure was recorded through the carotid artery. Bilateral adrenalectomy was performed during the anesthesia and the blood pressure reported is the level of blood pressure observed 1 hour after this procedure. Chemical sympathectomy was produced by treating the animals with intravenous injection of 6-OH-DA 18 hours previously. Each procedure decreased the systolic blood pressure 20 to 30 mm Hg in normotensive animals and 20 to 40 mm Hg in hypertensive rats. When bilateral adrenalectomy was performed in animals which had been previously treated with 6-OH-DA, the blood pressures fell rapidly and stabilized around 50 mm Hg in normotensive and hypertensive animals. (Reproduced from de Champlain, J., and Van Ameringen, M. R., unpublished data.)

mals, thus indicating that the basal blood pressure in both groups of animals is similar in the absence of the sympathetic system (Fig. 5). Therefore, the only factor which can account for the difference in blood pressures between hypertensive and normotensive rats with intact sympathetic systems is the level of activity of that system through the synergic effect of the sympathetic fibers and the adrenal medulla. It is also interesting to note that even normotensive animals fall into deep shock in the absence of both components of the sympathetic system, thus suggesting that the role of that system in the maintenance of normal blood pressure is more important than it was previously thought.

Moreover, it was also found that the sympathetic fibers are essential for the development of that form of hypertension. In animals sympathectomized from birth by weekly injections of 6-OH-DA, the treatment with Doca and sodium for 6 weeks did not increase the blood pressure above normotensive levels (Table 4). These findings are in agreement with those of Ayitey-Smith and Varma,[33] who have shown that Doca and sodium hypertension cannot be induced in totally immunosympathectomized animals.

TABLE 4.—*Effect of Sympathectomy on the Development of Doca Hypertension*

	Mean Arterial Pressure (mm Hg)	*Heart Rate (beats per minute)*
Control	124 ± 5	403 ± 10
Doca and sodium	154 ± 9 *	358 ± 25
6-OH-DA	80 ± 7 *	335 ± 18 *
6-OH-DA+Doca and sodium	115 ± 15	331 ± 25 *

From de Champlain, J., and Van Ameringen, M. R., unpublished data.

* $P < 0.05$

Animals treated with 6-OH-DA received a weekly dose of 100 mg per kilogram subcutaneously from the first day of birth for the following 13 weeks. When the animals weighed about 100 gm, they were uninephrectomized and two groups of them were given weekly subcutaneous injections of Doca (10 mg per week) and 1% saline to drink for 6 weeks. Because of the impossibility of measuring blood pressure by tail plethysmography in the 6-OH-DA-treated rats, the mean blood pressure was measured by a cannula through the carotid artery in anesthetized animals. A group of eight animals was studied and the results are expressed as the mean ± SEM.

Numerous experimental findings strongly support the participation of the sympathetic nervous system in the development and maintenance of hypertension in this form of experimental hypertension. The dysfunction of the sympathetic system in these animals is reflected in the periphery by an increased amount of physiologically active norepinephrine at the receptor site. This abnormality appears to result from hyperactivity of the sympathetic nervous fibers and adrenal medulla which is probably under the influence of the vasomotor centers localized in the brainstem.

RELATIONSHIP OF SODIUM INTAKE, BLOOD PRESSURE, AND NOREPINEPHRINE METABOLISM

Among the various factors which may contribute to the dysfunction of the sympathetic nervous system in Doca hypertensive rats, the sodium or related ions or both appear to be the most obvious choice. Since sodium and po-

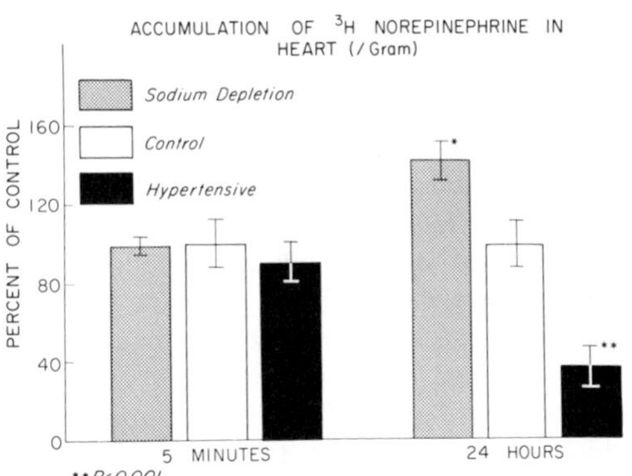

FIG. 6.—Uptake and retention of norepinephrine at 5 minutes and 24 hours after the injection of 20 μCi of tritiated norepinephrine in the hearts of control, sodium-depleted, and Doca-hypertensive rats. The results are expressed as the percentage of the values observed in control animals. Each bar represents the mean of six to 10 animals. Although the initial uptake (5 minutes) was normal in the hypertensive and sodium-depleted animals, the retention of norepinephrine (24 hours) was significantly increased during sodium depletion and markedly decreased in the hypertensive rats. (From de Champlain, J., Krakoff, L. R., and Axelrod, J.: Interrelationship of sodium intake, hypertension and norepinephrine storage in the rat. Circ. Res. 24–25(Suppl. 1):I-75, 1969, by permission of The American Heart Association, Inc.)

tassium are consistently found to be increased in vessels of Doca-hypertensive rats,[34–40] and since various functions of the adrenergic fibers are ion-dependent,[7–12] a closer look at the effect of sodium balance on norepinephrine metabolism was indicated.

Sodium restriction was produced in rats by giving them a synthetic sodium-deficient diet (Nutritional Biochemical Co.) and distilled water for a period of 2 weeks. A state of sodium depletion was induced by treating the sodium-restricted rats with subcutaneous injection of a natriuretic agent (meralluride 0.05 ml per kilogram) the first and third day after the start of the sodium restriction. Control animals received the same synthetic diet to which 22 gm of sodium chloride per kilogram of diet was added.[25,27]

During sodium depletion, a condition which is associated with a lowering of blood pressure, the retention of norepinephrine by the nerve endings was found increased in contrast to the findings in hypertensive animals (Fig. 6). As for the hypertensive animals, the uptake of norepinephrine was normal in the hearts of sodium-depleted animals but 24 hours later the norepinephrine levels remaining in the heart were significantly greater than in control rats, whereas these levels were markedly reduced in hypertensive rats. The decrease in norepinephrine turnover during sodium depletion could also be correlated with the changes in blood pressure, thus suggesting that these changes and those observed in Doca-hypertensive animals are probably part of the same mechanism which is influenced by the state of sodium balance. In various groups of rats receiving different sodium regimens the systolic blood pressure as well as the state of sodium balance could be inversely correlated with the capacity of the heart to retain tritiated norepinephrine (Fig. 7) or with the cardiac endogenous norepinephrine content (Fig. 8). The retention of tritiated norepinephrine and the endogenous norepinephrine content were highest during a state of negative sodium balance in sodium-depleted rats while they were lowest during a state of highly positive sodium balance in hypertensive rats.

The influence of sodium on the metabolism of norepinephrine and its importance in the pathogenesis of Doca hypertension is strongly suggested by the observation that the withdrawal of sodium from the diet of hypertensive rats results in the lowering of blood pressure within the normotensive range while simultaneously restoring to normal the endogenous storage capacity and the turnover rate (Fig. 9). Two weeks after the beginning of treatment with Doca and sodium, the animals were clearly hypertensive and the capacity of the

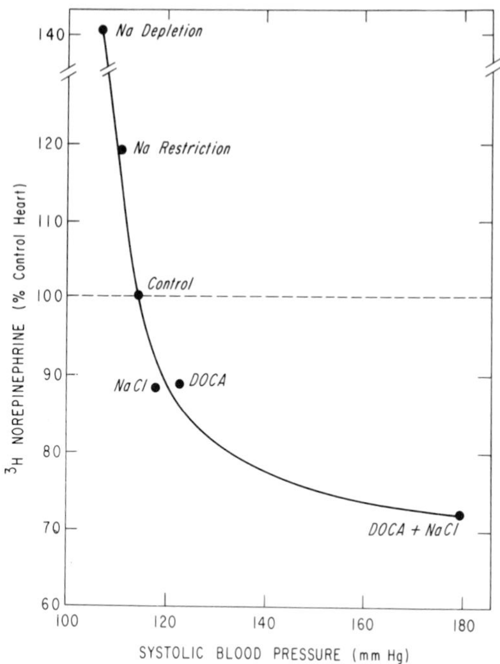

FIG. 7.—Relationship between systolic blood pressure and the capacity of the heart to retain tritiated norepinephrine in animals subjected to various sodium regimens for 6 weeks. NaCl refers to groups of rats given a solution of 1% sodium chloride to drink. Sodium restriction was produced by giving the animals a sodium-free diet and distilled water. Sodium depletion was produced by giving a natriuretic (chlorothiazide) on the first and third days of the sodium-free diet. The retention of norepinephrine was measured 1 hour after the intravenous injection of 25 μCi of tritiated norepinephrine. Each point is the mean of 7 to 18 individual values expressed as the percentage of the value for normotensive control rats. (From de Champlain, J., Krakoff, L. R., and Axelrod, J.: Relationship between sodium intake and norepinephrine storage during the development of experimental hypertension. Circ. Res. 23:479, 1968, by permission of The American Heart Association, Inc.)

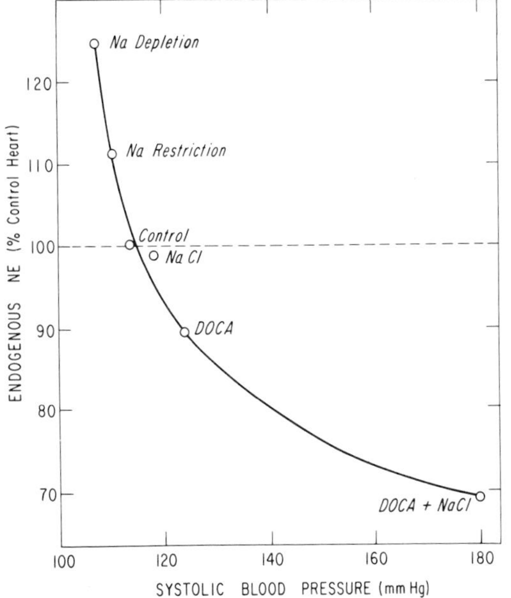

FIG. 8.—Relationship between systolic blood pressure and endogenous norepinephrine content of the hearts from the same groups of rats illustrated in Fig. 7. (Reproduced from de Champlain, J., Krakoff, L. R., and Axelrod, J.: Relationship between sodium intake and norepinephrine storage during the development of experimental hypertension. Circ. Res. 23:479, 1968, by permission of The American Heart Association, Inc.)

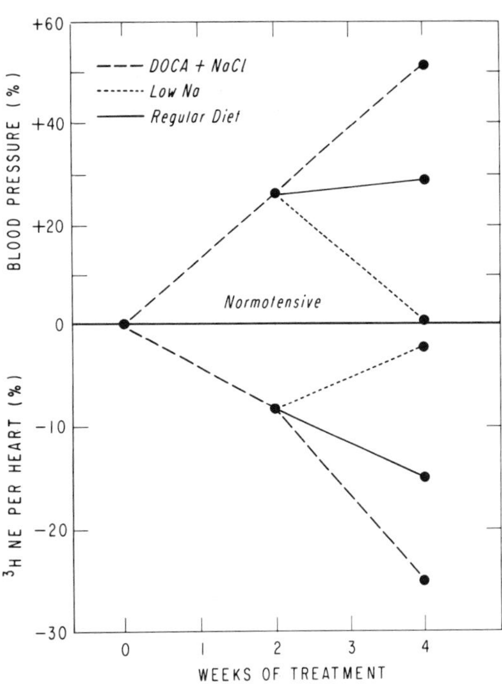

FIG. 9.—Comparative effects of sodium intake on blood pressure and on the capacity of the heart to retain norepinephrine. Each point is the mean of 6 to 8 values expressed as the percentage of increase or decrease compared to values in normotensive untreated animals. The upper part of the graph illustrates the changes in systolic blood pressure under treatment with various sodium regimens for 4 weeks. After 2 weeks of treatment with Doca and saline **(long dashed lines)**, the blood pressure was significantly increased. At this point, the rats were divided into three groups; one group continued to receive Doca and saline for the following 2 weeks and their blood pressures continued to rise progressively. In the other two groups, Doca and saline treatment ended. One of these groups was shifted to a normal laboratory diet **(full line)** and the blood pressure remained elevated at about the same level in the following 2 weeks. Finally, the other group of hypertensive rats was given a sodium-free diet **(short dashed lines)** and the blood pressure returned to normotensive levels within 2 weeks after the start of that diet. The lower part of the graph illustrates the retention of tritiated norepinephrine in the hearts of the same groups of animals 4 hours after intravenous injection of 25 μCi of the tritiated amine. The changes in the capacity to retain norepinephrine vary in the opposite direction to the changes in blood pressure. The retention capacity is the lowest when the blood pressure is the highest

heart to retain tritiated norepinephrine was reduced. When the treatment was continued for an additional 2 weeks, the blood pressure increased to higher levels and the norepinephrine retention was even more reduced. After the first 2 weeks of treatment with Doca and sodium, the change to a sodium-free diet for 2 weeks reduced the blood pressure to normotensive levels and restored the norepinephrine storage to normal. In another group of rats, the replacement of Doca and sodium by a normal laboratory diet for 2 weeks neither lowered the blood pressure nor changed the norepinephrine storage capacity. In the latter condition, it appeared that the sodium contained in a normal laboratory diet was sufficient to maintain the hypertension even in the absence of Doca.

The changes seen in the intraneuronal distribution of norepinephrine after sodium depletion are opposite to those observed during

and this abnormality can be restored to normal simultaneously with the blood pressure in hypertensive rats treated with a sodium-deficient diet for 2 weeks. (Based on data from de Champlain, J., Krakoff, L. R., and Axelrod, J.[25, 27])

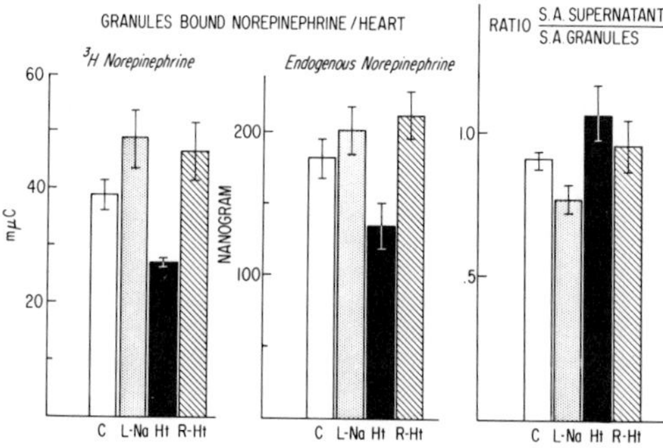

FIG. 10.—Subcellular distribution of exogenous and endogenous norepinephrine in the heart as seen in animals submitted to various sodium regimens. The letters under the bars identify the treatment: **C,** the control normotensive rats; **L-Na,** normotensive rats submitted to a low-sodium diet for 2 weeks; **Ht,** animals treated for 4 weeks with Doca and saline; **R-Ht,** animals treated for 2 weeks with Doca and saline, then a low-sodium diet for 2 weeks. The mean systolic blood pressure was 118 mm Hg for the normotensive rats **(C),** 109 mm Hg for the sodium-restricted rats **(L-Na),** 183 mm Hg for the Doca- and saline-treated rats **(Ht)** and 128 mm Hg for the hypertensive rats treated with a low-sodium diet **(R-Ht).** As shown, the endogenous and tritiated norepinephrine content (24 hours after intravenous injection of 25 μCi) of the heart granular fraction (105,000 g) were slightly higher in the sodium-restricted rats **(L-Na)** and markedly lower in Doca-hypertensive rats **(Ht).** The endogenous and tritiated norepinephrine content of the granular fraction was restored to normal in the hypertensive animals treated with low-sodium diets. The ratio of the specific activity of the supernatant over the specific activity of the granular fraction which was higher in hypertensive rats was lowered by treatment with low-sodium diet. In the normotensive rats treated with a low-sodium diet, this ratio was significantly lower. (Based on data from de Champlain, J., Krakoff, L. R., and Axelrod, J.[25,27])

Doca- and sodium-induced hypertension (Fig. 10). The endogenous norepinephrine levels of the storage granules, as well as their capacity to retain exogenous norepinephrine, were restored to normal simultaneously with the blood pressure in formerly hypertensive animals (R-HT) after 2 weeks of treatment with a sodium-free diet. Normotensive rats subjected to a low-sodium diet for 2 weeks (L-Na) showed a slightly greater retention of tritiated norepinephrine and slightly higher endogenous norepinephrine levels in the storage-granule fraction. Moreover, the ratio of the specific activity of the storage granules over the specific activity of the supernatant was significantly lower in the sodium-restricted, normotensive animals in contrast to the increased ratio observed in the hypertensive animals. In hypertensive rats subjected to sodium restriction for 2 weeks, the ratio of the specific activity of the granules over the specific activity of the supernatant was lowered toward the ratio found in normotensive animals. An increase in granule-bound norepinephrine was also observed after sodium depletion. In contrast to previous findings in hypertensive rats, sodium depletion or restriction seems to decrease the amount of free norepinephrine available to act at the receptor sites. This is probably due to a greater affinity of the amine for its storage sites. Again, the association of the changes in the subcellular distribution of norepinephrine with the variations of the systolic blood pressure in these animals strongly suggests that the effect of sodium balance on the blood pressure is mediated through the sympathetic nervous system. It is also possible that changes in the subcellular distribution of norepinephrine might explain the changes in vascular responsiveness to catecholamines. An increased sensitivity to catecholamines has been reported on isolated arteries of Doca-hypertensive rats[41,42] as well as on arteries of rats with other forms of experimental hypertension.[43–46] On the other hand, the vascular reactivity has been found in animals submitted to sodium deprivation[47,48] or after treatment with natriuretic agents.[49,50]

Whether the ionic disturbance affects the binding or the transport of amine locally at the site of the nerve ending or whether it influences the sympathetic activity through a direct or indirect action on the central nervous system is difficult to determine. The effect of sodium depletion is not exclusively related to the sympathetic nerve ending. A decrease in the catecholamine synthesis in the adrenal medulla was also observed in normotensive animals subjected to sodium depletion for 2 weeks (unpublished data). Moreover, the increased norepinephrine levels observed in the brainstem and in the superior sympathetic ganglia of hypertensive rats can be restored within normal limits simultaneously with the blood pressure when these animals are subjected to a period of sodium depletion for 3 weeks (Table 5). In the heart the opposite effect is observed and endogenous norepinephrine levels rise above the values of normotensive animals in treated hypertensive rats. These findings, in addition to the observation that elevated blood pressure and the reduced norepinephrine storage capacity can be restored to normal by an acute treatment with a ganglion blocker, suggest that the central sympathetic activity may be influenced directly or indirectly by variations of dietary sodium. The effect of sodium on the central or peripheral sympathetic system or both is probably a determinant factor in the development of this form of hypertension or in the hypotensive effect of sodium restriction or depletion.

The dysfunction of the sympathetic system is not exclusive of this form of experimental hypertension and abnormalities in the metabolism of norepinephrine have also been reported in other forms of experimental hypertension.

The turnover of norepinephrine was found to be increased in hearts of rats made hypertensive with renal artery stenosis for 5 weeks (Table 6). The uptake of norepinephrine was normal but the retention was significantly reduced 24 hours after injection of tritiated norepinephrine. In contrast to Doca-hypertensive rats, the endogenous norepinephrine levels were normal in renal hypertensive rats. An increased norepinephrine turnover rate was also observed in hearts of rats made hypertensive by renal encapsulation [51] or by renal infarction.[52]

In the New Zealand strain of genetically hypertensive animals, Phelan [53] has recently reported that the cardiac norepinephrine content is normal or increased in young hypertensive animals and decreased in older rats. Moreover, he also found that the uptake and turnover of norepinephrine is normal in the hearts of young hypertensive rats but that the turnover is decreased in older hypertensive rats thus indicating that the sympathetic activity is at least variable throughout the life span of these hypertensive rats. Nevertheless, the sympathetic fibers seem essential for the evolution of spontaneous hypertension since immunosympathectomy could prevent the development of hypertension in these animals.[54,55]

In the Japanese strain of genetically hypertensive rats there are several indications of a

TABLE 5.—*Effects of Sodium Depletion in Doca-Hypertensive Rats*

		Endogenous Norepinephrine		
	Blood Pressure (mm Hg)	*Heart (ng per total organ)*	*Superior Cervical Ganglion (ng per pair)*	*Brainstem (ng per gm)*
Normotensive	130 ± 2	373 ± 12	43	494 ± 27
Hypertensive	217 ± 2	242 ± 25	62	702 ± 76
Hypertensive plus sodium depletion	99 ± 5	563 ± 42	31	583 ± 56

From de Champlain, J., and Van Ameringen, M. R., unpublished data.

The hypertensive rats were treated for 6 weeks with Doca and sodium. Sodium depletion was obtained by giving the animals a sodium-free diet and distilled water to drink for a period of 3 weeks. Each group of animals contains six to eight animals and the results are expressed as the mean ± S.E. For the superior cervical ganglion all tissues from each group were pooled for greater accuracy of the values.

TABLE 6.—*Changes in Catecholamine Turnover in Experimental Renovascular Hypertension*

	Blood Pressure (mm Hg)	*Tritiated Norepinephrine (5 minutes)*	*nCi per Heart (24 hours)*
Control	110 ± 2.5	787 ± 47	249 ± 30
Sham-operated	109 ± 3.0	769 ± 131	227 ± 19
Hypertensive	185 ± 8.0 †	784 ± 87	167 ± 12*

From de Champlain, J., unpublished data.
* $P < 0.05$
† $P < 0.01$
The rats were made hypertensive by application of a silver clip on the left renal artery. Sham-operated animals had the same operation and the left renal pedicle was dissected. Eight weeks after this procedure, the animals were injected with 25 μCi of ^{3}H-norepinephrine via the tail vein and were killed 5 minutes and 24 hours later. Each group of rats contained eight to 10 animals and the results are expressed as the mean ± SEM.

dysfunction of the central vasomotor centers. Under the abnormal influence of the hypothalamus it has been proposed that the pressor centers of the medulla oblongata become hyperactive, thus increasing the activity of the peripheral sympathetic fibers and adrenal medulla.[56] The observation that endogenous norepinephrine levels and the activity of aromatic amino acid decarboxylase are both reduced in the brainstem and hypothalamus of hypertensive rats also gives support to the hypothesis of a dysfunction in the central vasomotor centers.[57] Fluorescent histochemical observations on the superior cervical ganglia and on the adrenergic fibers related to the arteries have indicated that the ganglion cells and terminal fibers of the sympathetic system are hyperactive in the spontaneously hypertensive rats.[58–60] Moreover, direct recording of the electrical activity of the left splanchnic sympathetic nerve of spontaneously hypertensive rats revealed that the peripheral sympathetic tone is markedly increased compared to control animals.[61] In the same strain of hypertensive animals, but using Wistar control rats of a different source, Louis and co-workers [22,62,63] have reported that the norepinephrine turnover and synthesis rates are decreased in the hearts of spontaneously hypertensive rats.

The norepinephrine turnover and synthesis rates were found to be increased in the heart and adrenal medulla of rabbits made hypertensive by sino-aortic denervation.[64] The sympathetic system seems therefore to contribute to the pathogenesis or to the maintenance of various forms of experimental hypertension. It is not known, however, whether the dysfunction of the sympathetic fibers can be influenced by sodium in these experimental conditions. It is nevertheless interesting to note that sodium and potassium are generally found increased in the vessels of renal hypertensive rats [35,37–39,65–70] and in aorta of rats with genetic hypertension.[70,71]

THE SYMPATHETIC SYSTEM IN HUMAN HYPERTENSION

The metabolism of sodium and other ions has been found to be abnormal in various forms of human and experimental hypertension.[6,72] The first indication that sodium could be associated with elevated blood pressure came from the observation that a low-sodium diet was efficient in lowering the blood pressure of hypertensive patients.[73,74] Other studies have shown that plasma sodium [75,76] and total exchangeable sodium [77–80] are both significantly increased in patients with essential hypertension. An epidemiologic study conducted among various populations has established a close correlation between the amount of sodium ingested in the diet and the incidence of hypertension in these populations.[61]

For many years, the sympathetic nervous system has been thought to play a role in the pathogenesis of human hypertension but until recently, direct evidence supporting that hypothesis was lacking. Hemodynamic studies have shown that the peripheral resistance is increased in all forms of human hypertension with the exception of labile hypertension [82] and that the cardiac output may be increased in the early phases of various forms of hypertension.[82,83] An increased activity of various autonomic functions, especially in regard to muscle-tone activity and basal metabolism, is also observed in patients with essential hypertension.[84] The existence of an important neurogenic component in the maintenance of elevated blood pressure is also indicated by the observation that most hypotensive drugs interfere in some way with the function of the sympathetic system and that they produce greater blood pressure falls in hypertensive than in normotensive patients.[15,16,85–87]

Initial attempts to investigate more directly the sympathetic system, by studying the urinary excretion of catecholamines and their metabolites in hypertensive patients, failed to reveal any indication of hyperfunction of the sympathetic system except for pheochromocytoma. Until 1964, in 16 out of 19 studies the excretion of norepinephrine, epinephrine, vanillylmandelic acid, and normetanephrine was found to be normal or decreased. Nevertheless, in some of these studies, a group of hypertensive patients (10 to 26%) excreted quantities of norepinephrine or catecholamines exceeding the upper range of control values. The negative findings and discrepancies reported in these various studies may be explained by a variety of factors. In many of these studies, the determinations were made with bioassay techniques which lacked the sensitivity and specificity of the more recently developed fluorometric methods. Also, many of these patients were receiving hypotensive medication or were submitted to low-sodium diets at the time of the investigation. Moreover, the degree of arteriosclerosis and the impairment of renal function were seldom evaluated in hypertensive patients although these factors could influence the pattern of urinary excretion since norepinephrine can be significantly reabsorbed by the renal tubule [88] and since norepinephrine excretion can be correlated with urinary flow or volume.[89–91] Ikoma [92] has shown the importance of evaluating renal function before interpreting urinary studies in hypertensive patients. He found that the excretion of catecholamines is significantly increased in essential hypertensive patients with normal renal function while it is decreased in those with impaired renal function. Since 1965, several other studies, carried out under more standardized conditions in unmedicated hypertensive patients with normal renal function, have reported increased urinary levels of norepinephrine,[92–96] vanillylmandelic acid, and normetanephrine [94,97,98] in many patients with essential hypertension. More recently, Engelman, Portnoy, and Sjoerdsma,[99] using a highly sensitive, double-isotope technique, reported that circulating catecholamine levels in essential hypertension were about twice those of normotensive subjects. Moreover, a highly significant correlation was found between the systolic or diastolic blood pressure and the levels of norepinephrine in the urine of normotensive and hypertensive patients.[92,94] This striking correlation between blood pressure and urinary catecholamines in humans is in accordance with the inverse relationship found between the turnover and storage of norepinephrine and the systolic blood pressure in Doca-hypertensive rats and in rats submitted to low-sodium diets.

To evaluate more specifically the activity of the cardiovascular adrenergic fibers, the fate of tritiated norepinephrine was studied in hypertensive patients. Gitlow and co-workers [100] suggested that the storage and binding of norepinephrine was reduced in the sympathetic fibers of patients with essential hypertension since tritiated norepinephrine declined more rapidly from their plasma after intravenous infusion. After one intravenous injection of norepinephrine the amount of tritiated norepinephrine and metabolites excreted in the urine during the following 24 hours was significantly greater in hypertensive patients, indicating again that the turnover of noradrenaline is probably increased in the vascular sympathetic fibers.[101] This abnormality in the pattern of excretion of tritiated norepinephrine and metabolites in hypertensive patients is strikingly similar to the pattern of urinary excretion in Doca-hypertensive rats after an identical treatment.[102] De Quattro and Sjoerdsma [95] failed to detect any abnormality in the rate of disappearance of ^{3}H-norepinephrine from the plasma of hypertensive patients after administration of tritiated dopa.

In contrast to the findings in hypertension, the urinary catecholamines and the synthesis of norepinephrine are both decreased in patients with postural hypertension.[103,104] Moreover, the lowering of blood pressure in hypertensive patients by treatment with hypotensive drugs or by a low-sodium diet is also accompanied by a reduction of norepinephrine excretion.[105,106]

Ganglion blockers which lower blood pressure have also been found to be natriuretic [107] and it is possible that part of the hypotensive effect of these drugs might occur through a change in the ionic content at the nerve ending. In humans the sympathetic fibers also seem to influence the metabolism of sodium. In man, the severity of sodium retention after infusion of saline or administration of desoxycorticosterone is markedly reduced during treatment with ganglion blockers.[107] Experimentally, it was also found that immunosympathectomy can prevent the increase in sodium concentration as well as the development of hypertension following a treatment with Doca and sodium.[33]

CONCLUSIONS

Several studies have revealed a dysfunction of the sympathetic nervous system in various forms of experimental hypertension. In Doca- and sodium-induced hypertension, hyperactivity of the sympathetic nervous system (sympathetic fibers and adrenal medulla) seems to contribute directly or indirectly to the pathogenesis and maintenance of hypertension.

Recent studies on human hypertension have also revealed signs of increased sympathetic activity. The abnormalities found in the metabolism of norepinephrine in patients with essential hypertension are strikingly similar to those reported in Doca- and sodium-induced hypertension. A highly significant, inverse relationship between the turnover of norepinephrine and the level of blood pressure was reported in humans as well as in experimental animals.

In experimental animals, the state of sodium balance appears to influence the blood pressure as well as the metabolism of norepinephrine. In rats made hypertensive with Doca and sodium, the observation that a low-sodium diet could correct the dysfunction of the sympathetic system while simultaneously rendering those rats normotensive suggests that changes in ionic concentration is a major factor in the abnormal sympathetic activity of this form of hypertension. Moreover, the hypotensive effect of sodium depletion or restriction in normotensive rats appears to be secondary to a decreased sympathetic activity. In these conditions, the variations of blood pressure from hypotension to hypertension, in association with various sodium intakes, are probably mediated through the same mechanism influencing the activity of the sympathetic nervous system. Whether other forms of experimental or human hypertension can be explained by the same mechanism is still unsettled. Nevertheless, abnormal ionic concentrations have been found in vascular tissues of experimental animals and hypertensive patients. The hypotensive effect of a low-sodium diet in some hypertensive conditions and the correlation between the incidence of hypertension and dietary sodium intake in various populations strongly suggest that the mechanism described in Doca-hypertensive rats could probably contribute to the pathogenesis and maintenance of other forms of hypertension.

Although sodium was more currently studied in hypertension, it is possible that changes in other ions might have a more important influence than sodium on adrenergic mechanisms. Recently, the calcium content was found to be increased in the heart of renal hypertensive rats [108] and in the tail artery of Doca-hypertensive rats.[40] The changes in calcium levels could be influenced by the sodium concentration through a sodium-calcium exchange pump.[109] Since calcium is important for the uptake and binding of norepinephrine in the nerve endings,[19,110] for catecholamine liberation from the nerve endings and adrenal medulla,[12,111] and for the effects of catecholamine on the effector cells [8] it is possible that sodium might influence the catecholamine metabolism through changes in calcium concentration. However, further studies on calcium and other ions are needed for a better understanding of the link between catecholamine ions and hypertensive diseases.

References

1. Guyton, A. C., Coleman, T. G., Fourcade, J. C., and Navar, L. G.: Physiologic control of arterial pressure. Bull. N.Y. Acad. Med. 45:811, 1969.
2. Page, I. H.: The nature of arterial hypertension. Arch. Intern. Med. 3:103, 1963.
3. Hollander, W., Kramsch, D. M., Farnelant, M., and Madoff, I. M.: Arterial wall metabolism in experimental hypertension of coarctation of the aorta of short duration. J. Clin. Invest. 47:1221, 1968.
4. Friedman, S. M., Nakashima, M., and Friedman, C. L.: Sodium, potassium and peripheral resistance in the rat. Circ. Res. 13: 223, 1963.
5. Bohr, D. F.: Electrolytes and smooth muscle contraction. Pharmacol. Rev. 16:85, 1964.
6. Raab, W.: Transmembrane cationic gradient and blood pressure regulation. Interaction of corticoids, catecholamines and electrolytes on vascular cells. Am. J. Cardiol. 4:752, 1959.
7. Bogdanski, D. F., and Brodie, B. B.: The effects of inorganic ions on the storage and uptake of H^3-norepinephrine by rat heart slices. J. Pharmacol. Exp. Ther. 165:181, 1969.
8. Daniel, E. E., Paton, D. M., Taylor, G. S., and Hodgson, B. J.: Adrenergic receptors for catecholamine effects on tissue electrolytes. Fed. Proc. 29:1410, 1970.
9. Gillis, C. N., and Paton, D. M.: Cation dependence of sympathetic transmitter retention by slices of rat ventricle. Br. J. Pharmacol. 29:309, 1967.
10. Horst, W. D., Kopin, I. J., and Ramey, E. R.: Influence of sodium and calcium on norepinephrine uptake by isolated perfused rat hearts. Am. J. Physiol. 215:817, 1968.
11. Iversen, L. L. and Kravitz, E. A.: Sodium dependence of transmitter uptake at adrenergic nerve terminals. Mol. Pharmacol. 2:360, 1966.
12. Keen, P. M., and Bogdanski, D. F.: Sodium and calcium ions in uptake and release of norepinephrine by nerve endings. Am. J. Physiol. 219:677, 1970.
13. Mendlowitz, M.: Vascular reactivity in essential and renal hypertension in man. Am. Heart J. 73:121, 1967.
14. Axelrod, J.: The fate of norepinephrine and the effect of drugs. Physiologist 11:63, 1968.
15. Carlsson, A.: Pharmacology of the sympathetic nervous system. *In* Gross, F. (Ed.): Antihypertensive Therapy. New York: Springer, 1966.
16. Abrams, W. B.: The mechanisms of action of antihypertensive drugs. Chest 55:148, 1969.
17. de Champlain, J., Krakoff, L. R., and Axelrod, J.: The metabolism of norepinephrine in experimental hypertension in rats. Circ. Res. 20:136, 1967.
18. de Champlain, J., Krakoff, L. R. and Axelrod, J.: A reduction in the accumulation of tritiated norepinephrine in experimental hypertension. Life Sci. 5:2283, 1966.
19. Krakoff, L. R., de Champlain, J., and Axelrod, J.: Abnormal storage of norepinephrine in experimental hypertension in the rat. Circ. Res. 21:583, 1967.
20. Doyle, A. E.: Endogenous catecholamine content of cardiac muscle in sodium-loaded and sodium-depleted rats. Lancet 1:1399, 1968.
21. Kazda, S., Pohlova, I., Bibr, B., and Kockova, J.: Norepinephrine content of tissues in Doca-hypertensive rats. Am. J. Physiol. 216:1472, 1969.
22. Louis, W. J., Kraus, K. R., Kopin, I. J., and Sjoerdsma, A.: Catecholamine metabolism in hypertensive rats. Circ. Res. 27:589, 1970.
23. Nakamura, K., Gerold, M., and Thoenen, H.: Experimental hypertension of the rat: Reciprocal changes of norepinephrine turnover in heart and brain-stem. Naunyn Schmiedebergs Arch. Pharmakol. 268:125, 1971.
24. de Champlain, J., Mueller, R. A., and Axelrod, J.: Turnover and synthesis of norepinephrine in experimental hypertension. Circ. Res. 25:285, 1969.
25. de Champlain, J., Krakoff, L. R., and Axelrod, J.: Relationship between sodium intake and norepinephrine storage during the development of experimental hypertension. Circ. Res. 23:479, 1968.
26. Udenfriend, S.: Tyrosine hydroxylase. Pharmacol. Rev. 18:43, 1966.
27. de Champlain, J., Krakoff, L. R., and Axelrod, J.: Interrelationship of sodium intake, hypertension and norepinephrine storage in the rat. Circ. Res. 24:I-75, 1969.
28. Tranzer, J. P., and Thoenen, H.: Ultramorphologische Veranderungen der sympathischen nerven digungen der Katze nach Vorbehandlung mit 5-und-6-Hydroxy-Dopamin. Arch. Exp. Path. Pharmakol. 257:343, 1967.
29. Malmfors, T., and Sachs, C.: Degeneration of adrenergic nerves produced by 6-hydroxydopamine. Eur. J. Pharmacol. 3:89, 1968.
30. de Champlain, J.: Degeneration and regrowth of adrenergic nerve fibers in the rat periph-

eral tissues after 6-hydroxydopamine. Can. J. Physiol. Pharmacol. 49:345, 1971.

31. de Champlain, J., and Nadeau, R.: 6-hydroxy dopamine, 6-hydroxy dopa and degeneration of adrenergic nerves. Fed. Proc. 30:877, 1971.
32. de Champlain, J.: The role of the sympathetic nervous system in experimental hypertension. *In* Barbeau, A. and McDowell, F. H. (Eds.): L-Dopa and Parkinsonism. Philadelphia: Davis, 1970, pp. 269–277.
33. Ayitey-Smith, E., and Varma, D. R.: An assessment of the role of the sympathetic nervous system in experimental hypertension using normal and immunosympathectomized rats. Br. J. Pharmacol. 40:175, 1970.
34. Tobian, L., and Binion, J.: Arterial wall electrolytes in renal and DOCA hypertension. J. Clin. Invest. 33:1407, 1954.
35. Daniel, E. E., and Dawkins, O.: Aorta and smooth muscle electrolytes during early and late hypertension. Am. J. Physiol. 190:71, 1957.
36. Gross, F., and Schmidt, H.: Natrium- und Kaliumgehalt von Plasma und Geweben beim cortexon—Hochdruck. Arch. Exp. Path. Pharmakol. 233:311, 1958.
37. Fukuchi, S., Hanata, M., Takahashi, H., Demura, H. and Torikai, T.: Renin-angiotensin and aldosterone in experimental hypertension. Tohoku J. Exp. Med. 84:125, 1964.
38. Cier, J. F., and Froment, A.: Le sodium dans les hypertensions expérimentales. Pathol. Biol. 13:1052, 1965.
39. Demura, H., Fukuchi, S., Takahashi, H., and Goto, K.: The vascular reactivity to vasoactive substances and the electrolyte contents in arterial walls. Tohoku J. Exp. Med. 86:366, 1965.
40. Hinke, J. A. M.: Effect of Ca^{++} upon contractility of small arteries from DOCA-hypertensive rats. Circ. Res. (suppl. I)18–19:23, 1966.
41. Hinke, J. A. M.: In vitro demonstration of vascular hyper-responsiveness in experimental hypertension. Circ. Res. 17:359, 1965.
42. Bohr, D. F. and Sitrin, M.: Regulation of vascular smooth muscle contraction: Changes in experimental hypertension. Circ. Res. (suppl. II)26–27:83, 1970.
43. McGregor, D. D., and Smirk, F. H.: Vascular responses in mesenteric arteries from genetic and renal hypertensive rats. Am. J. Physiol. 214:1429, 1968.
44. Moerman, E. J., Herman, A. G., Bogaert, M. G., and de Schaepdryver, A. F.: Noradrenergic vascular responsiveness in hypertensive dogs. Arch. Int. Pharmacodyn. 178:492, 1969.
45. Zimmerman, B. G., Rolewicz, T. F., Dunham, E. W., and Gisslen, J. L.: Transmitter release and vascular responses in skin and muscle of hypertensive dogs. Am. J. Physiol. 217:798, 1969.
46. Bandick, N. R., and Sparks, H. V.: Contractile response of vascular smooth muscle of renal hypertensive rats. Am. J. Physiol. 219: 340, 1970.
47. Raab, W., Humphreys, R. J., Makous, N., Degrandpre, R., and Gigee, W.: Pressor effects of epinephrine, norepinephrine and desoxycorticosterone acetate (DCA) weakened by sodium withdrawal. Circulation 6:373, 1952.
48. Blair-West, J. R., Coghlan, J. P., Denton, D. A., Goding, J. R., Munro, J. A., and Wright, R. D.: Reduction of the pressor action of angiotensin II in sodium deficient conscious sheep. Aust. J. Exp. Biol. Med. Sci. 41:369, 1963.
49. Bock, K. D., and Gross, F.: Abschwachung pressorisches Wirkungen durch Sali-Diuretica. Naunyn Schmiedebergs Arch. Pharmakol. 238:339, 1960.
50. Hollander, W., Chobonian, A. V., and Wilkins, R. W.: Role of diuretics in the management of hypertension. Ann. N.Y. Acad. Sci. 88:975, 1960.
51. Volicer, L., Scheer, E., Hilse, H., and Visweswaram, D.: Turnover of norepinephrine in the heart during experimental hypertension in rats. Life Sci. 7:525, 1968.
52. Henning, M.: Noradrenaline turnover in renal hypertensive rats. J. Pharm. Pharmacol. 21:61, 1969.
53. Phelan, E. L.: Genetic autonomic factors in inherited hypertension. Circ. Res. (suppl. II)26–27:65, 1970.
54. Clark, D. W. J.: Effects of immunosympathectomy on the blood pressure of genetically hypertensive rats. Proc. Univ. Otago Med. Sch. 49:42, 1969.
55. Smirk, F. H.: The neurogenically maintained component in hypertension. Circ. Res. (suppl. II)26–27:55, 1970.
56. Okamoto, K.: Spontaneous hypertension in rats. Int. Rev. Exp. Pathol. 7:227, 1969.
57. Yamori, Y., Lovenberg, W., and Sjoerdsma, A.: Norepinephrine metabolism in brainstem of spontaneously hypertensive rats. Science 170:544, 1970.
58. Haebara, H., Ichijima, K., Tetsuzo, M., and Okamoto, K.: Fluorescence microscopical studies on noradrenaline in the peripheral

blood vessels of spontaneously hypertensive rats. Jap. Circ. J. 32:1391, 1968.

59. Matsumoto, M.: Morphological studies on the autonomic nervous system of hypertensive rats. IV. Fluorescence microscopical observation on the superior cervical sympathetic ganglia of spontaneously hypertensive rats. Jap. Circ. J. 33:411, 1969.
60. Ichijima, K.: Morphological studies on the peripheral small arteries of spontaneously hypertensive rats. Jap. Circ. J. 33:785, 1969.
61. Okamoto, K., Nosaka, S., Yamori, Y., and Matsumoto, M.: Participation of neural factor in the pathogenesis of hypertension in the spontaneously hypertensive rat. Jap. Heart J. 8:168, 1967.
62. Louis, W. J., Spector, S., Tabei, R., and Sjoerdsma, A.: Synthesis and turnover of norepinephrine in the heart of the spontaneously hypertensive rat. Circ. Res. 24:85, 1969.
63. Louis, W. J.: Turnover of catecholamines in experimental hypertension. Circ. Res. (suppl. II)26–27:49, 1970.
64. DeQuattro, V., Nagatsu, T., Maronde, R., and Alexander, N.: Catecholamine synthesis in rabbits with neurogenic hypertension. Circ. Res. 24:545, 1969.
65. Tobian, L. and Redleaf, P. D.: Ionic composition of the aorta in renal and adrenal hypertension. Am. J. Physiol. 192:325, 1958.
66. Koletsky, S., Resnick, H., and Behrin, D.: Mesenteric artery electrolytes in experimental hypertension. Proc. Soc. Exp. Biol. Med. 102: 12, 1959.
67. Headings, V. E., and Rondell, P.: Changes in arterial ground substances electrolytes and water accompanying aging and hypertension. Univ. Mich. Med. Center J. 30:167, 1964.
68. Hagemeijer, F., Rorive, G., and Schoffeniels, E.: Composition cationique de différents tissus du rat au cours de l'hypertension artérielle expérimentale. Arch. Int. Physiol. 74: 807, 1966.
69. Van Cauwenberge, H., and Rorive, G.: Acquisitions récentes concernant la composition ionique des parois artérielles implication dans la pathogénie de l'hypertension artérielle. Acquis. Med. Recent., 1969, p. 219.
70. Phelan, E. L., and Wong, L. C. K.: Sodium, potassium and water in the tissues of rats with genetic hypertension and constricted renal artery hypertension. Clin. Sci. 35:487, 1968.
71. Nagaoka, A., Kikuchi, K., and Aramaki, Y.: Electrolyte pattern of the aorta in the spontaneously hypertensive rats. Jap. J. Pharmacol. 19:462, 1969.
72. Tobian, L.: Interrelationship of electrolytes, juxtaglomerular cells and hypertension. Physiol. Rev. 40:280, 1960.
73. Ambard, L., and Beauyard, E.: Causes de l'hypertension artérielle. Arch. Gen. Med. 1:520, 1904.
74. Allen, F. M., and Sherrill, J. W.: Treatment of arterial hypertension. J. Metabolic Res. 2:429, 1922.
75. Halley, H. L., Elliott, H. C., Jr., and Holland, C. M., Jr.: Serum sodium values in essential hypertension. Proc. Soc. Exp. Biol. Med. 77: 561, 1951.
76. Albert, D. G., Morita, Y., and Iseri, L. T.: Serum Mg and plasma Na in essential vascular hypertension. Circulation 12:761, 1958.
77. Ross, E. J.: Total exchangeable Na in hypertensive patients. Clin. Sci. 15:81, 1956.
78. Tominaga, T.: Total exchangeable sodium in human hypertension. J. Jap. Soc. Intern. Med. 50:560, 1961.
79. Dahl, L. K., Smilay, M. G., Silver, L., and Sparagen, S.: Evidence for prolonged biological half-life of ^{22}Na in patient with hypertension. Circ. Res. 10:313, 1962.
80. Hansen, J.: Blood volume and exchangeable sodium in essential hypertension. Acta Med. Scand. 184:517, 1968.
81. Knudsen, K. D., and Dahl, L. K.: Essential hypertension: Inborn error of sodium metabolism. Postgrad. Med. J. 42:148, 1966.
82. Frohlich, E. D., Tarazi, R. C., and Dustan, H. P.: Re-examination of the hemodynamics of hypertension. Am. J. Med. Sci. 257:9, 1969.
83. Finkielman, S., Worcel, M., and Agrest, A.: Hemodynamic patterns in essential hypertension. Circulation 31:356, 1965.
84. Von Eiff, A. W.: The role of the autonomic nerves system in the etiology and pathogenesis of essential hypertension. Jap. Circ. J. 34:147, 1970.
85. Doyle, A. E., and Smirk, F. H.: The neurogenic component in hypertension. Circulation 12:543, 1955.
86. Green, A. F.: Antihypertensive drugs. Advances Pharmacol. Chemother. I:161, 1962.
87. Lucchesi, B. R., and Whitsitt, L. S.: The pharmacology of beta-adrenergic blocking agents. Progr. Cardiovasc. Dis. 11:410, 1969.
88. Overy, H. R., Pfister, R., and Chidsey, C. A.: Studies on the renal excretion of norepinephrine. J. Clin. Invest. 46:482, 1967.

89. De Schaepdryver, A. F., and Leroy, J. G.: Urine volume and catecholamine excretion in man. Acta Cardiol. 16:631, 1961.

90. Dawson, J., and Bone, A.: The relationship between urine volume and urinary adrenaline and noradrenaline excretion in a group of psychotic patients. Br. J. Psychiat. 109: 629, 1963.

91. Hathaway, P. W., Brehm, M. L., Clapp, J. R., and Bogdonoff, M. D.: Urine flow, catecholamines, and blood pressure. The variability of response of normal human subjects in a relaxed laboratory setting. Psychosom. Med. 31:20, 1969.

92. Ikoma, T.: Studies on catechols with reference to hypertension. Jap. Circ. J. 29:1269, 1965.

93. Boak, W. C., and Riek, L. I.: Urinary excretion of catecholamines and metabolites in hypertensive and normotensive subjects. Clin. Res. 13:202, 1965.

94. Nestel, P. J., and Doyle, A. E.: Excretion of free noradrenaline and adrenaline by healthy young subjects and by patients with essential hypertension. Aust. Ann. Med. 17: 295, 1968.

95. De Quattro, V., and Sjoerdsma, A.: Catecholamine turnover in normotensive and hypertensive man: effects of anti-adrenergic drugs. J. Clin. Invest. 47:2359, 1968.

96. Küchel, O., Cuche, J. L., Barbeau, A., Brecht, M., Boucher, R., and Genest, J.: The role of dopamine, norepinephrine and epinephrine in the orthostatic regulation of renin in normotensive and hypertensive subjects. *In* Barbeau, A., and McDowell, F. H. (Eds.): D-DOPA and Parkinsonism. Philadelphia: Davis, 1970, pp. 293–305.

97. Wolf, R. L., Mendlowitz, M., Roboz, J., and Gitlow, S. E.: Simultaneous urinary assay for the combined metanephrines and 3-methoxy-4-hydroxy phenylglycol in patients with pheochromocytoma and primary hypertension. N. Engl. J. Med. 273:1459, 1965.

98. Stott, A. W., and Robinson, R.: Urinary NMN excretion in essential hypertension. Clin. Chim. Acta 16:249, 1967.

99. Engelman, K., Portnoy, B., and Sjoerdsma, A.: Plasma catecholamine concentrations in patients with hypertension. Circ. Res. (suppl. 1)26–27:141, 1970.

100. Gitlow, S. E., Mendlowitz, M., Wilk, E. K., Wilk, S., Wolf, R. L., and Naftchi, N. E.: Plasma clearance of *dl*-H^3-norepinephrine in normal human subjects and patients with essential hypertension. J. Clin. Invest. 43: 2009, 1964.

101. Gitlow, S. E., Mendlowitz, M., Bertani, L. M., Wilk, E. K., and Glabman, S.: Tritium excretion of normotensive subjects after administration of tritiated norepinephrine. J. Lab. Clin. Med. 73:129, 1969.

102. de Champlain, J.: Hypertension and the sympathetic nervous system. *In* Snyder, S. S. (Ed.): Perspectives in Neuropharmacology. Oxford: Oxford Univ. Press, 1972, pp. 215–265.

103. Goodall, Mc., Harlan, W. R., and Alton, H.: Decreased noradrenaline synthesis in neurogenic orthostatic hypotension. Circulation 38:592, 1968.

104. Hedeland, H., Dymling, J.-F., and Hokfelt, B.: Catecholamines, renin and aldosterone in postural hypotension. Acta Endocrinol. 62:399, 1969.

105. Ikoma, T.: Studies on catechols with reference to hypertension. Jap. Circ. J. 29:1279, 1965.

106. Serrano, P. A., Figueroa, G., Tores, M. Z., and Rominez del Angel, A.: Adrenaline, noradrenaline and dopamine excretion in patients with essential hypertension. Am. J. Cardiol. 13:484, 1964.

107. Gill, J. R., Mason, D. T., and Bartter, F. C.: Adrenergic nervous system in sodium metabolism: effect of guanethidine and sodium-retaining steroids in normal man. J. Clin. Invest. 43:117, 1964.

108. Tobian, L., and Duke, M.: Increased calcium and water concentrations in the left ventricle of hypertensive rats. Am. J. Physiol. 217: 522, 1969.

109. Baker, P. F., Blaustein, M. P., Hodgkin, A. L., and Steinhardt, R. A.: Influence of calcium on sodium efflux in squid axons. J. Physiol. (London)200:431, 1969.

110. Potter, L., and Axelrod, J.: Properties of norepinephrine storage particles of the rat heart. J. Pharmacol. Exp. Ther. 142:299, 1963.

111. Rubin, R. P.: The metabolic requirement for catecholamine release from the adrenal medulla. J. Physiol. 202:197, 1969.

Part IV. MANIFESTATIONS OF ESSENTIAL HYPERTENSION

Vascular Morphologic Changes in Essential Hypertension

By Sheldon C. Sommers, M.D. and Barbro Andersson

ESSENTIAL HYPERTENSION means elevated blood pressures without known cause. Aside from primary systemic hypertension, primary pulmonary and primary intracranial hypertensions have been described.[1,2] Doubtless hypertension is multifactoral and probably several types of primary systemic hypertension exist.[3–6] With epidemiologic, genetic, anthropometric, biochemical, physiologic, and pathologic analyses separate entities are being distinguished. For example, a genetic combination of obesity, diabetes mellitus, and hypertension [7] is well known, and another syndrome occurs in women with obesity, postmenopausal estrogen activity, and hypertension.[8] Four more recently recognized subgroups had other metabolic abnormalities: hyperuricemia with defective renotubular excretion of uric acid, affecting about half of hypertensive individuals; [9,10] low renin essential hypertension; [11] glucose-6-phosphate dehydrogenase (G-6-PD) deficiency in Negro men; [12] and one patient with hyperkalemia and defective renotubular potassium excretion.[13] Endocrine abnormalities that may accompany essential hypertension include adrenocortical hyperplasia,[14] deficient insulin, excessive estrogen,[8,15] and defective dehydroepiandrosterone excretion, the last possibly acting to inhibit renal G-6-PO.[16]

By studying the pathology of essential hypertension it is hoped to discover underlying mechanisms and identify the resulting morphologic changes in this disease. In this chapter, the vascular alterations associated with hypertension are considered, but not the local renal, retinal, and other changes, which will be reviewed by others.

At autopsy the vascular alterations in essential hypertension include an enlarged heart, particularly due to left ventricular myocardial hypertrophy. The aortic wall is thicker and less elastic than usual for the patient's age, particularly when due to intimal fibrosis; the media is stretched and also fibrotic.[15] The kidneys are shrunken and granular. Death often has occurred from ischemic damage with or without hemorrhage, necrosis, and fibrosis, affecting particularly the heart, brain, kidneys, or all three. Microscopically extensive tortuosity, thickening and narrowing of the systemic arterioles are found, especially in the kidneys, retroperitoneal periadrenal connective tissues, pancreas, retina, striated muscles, and gastrointestinal tract.

Aorta. Blood pressure is traditionally measured by inflating a cuff around the arm which causes compression of the brachial artery. Systolic hypertension so measured is mathematically related to the thickness of the aortic wall (Fig. 1).[15] With persistent hypertension aortic atherosclerosis is enhanced both in extent and severity. Increased intraluminal pressure forces additional plasma lipoproteins, lipids including cholesterol, and macromolecules such as fibrinogen through the aortic wall.[17]

In ranking the various factors that exaggerate aortic atherosclerosis in hypertension, the severity and duration of pressure elevation come first, and the related chronologic age is second. With age the aortic elastic tissue degenerates and fibrosis increases, producing relative rigidity, which is enhanced by chronic hypertension.[18] Individuals who are well or overnourished and sedentary are prone to abnormally increased blood concentrations of lipoproteins, lipids, and cholesterol, exaggerating the tendency for their intramural deposition. However, hypertension is not uniformly

From the Departments of Pathology of Columbia University College of Physicians and Surgeons and the Lenox Hill Hospital, New York City.

Supported by a grant from The Council for Tobacco Research, U.S.A.

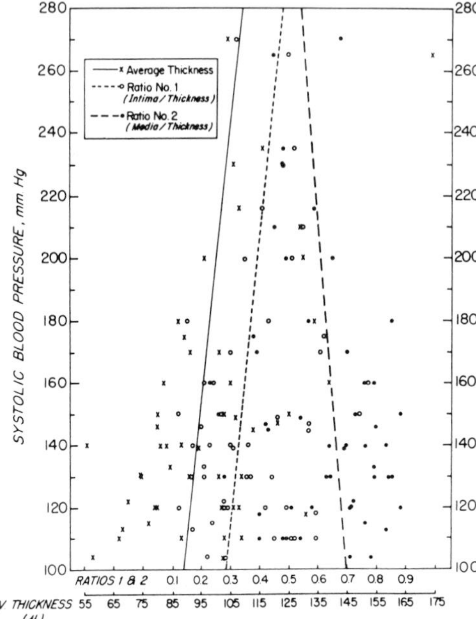

FIG. 1.—The linear relation between systolic blood pressure and the average aortic wall thickness indicates its increase from about 90 to 120 μ as the pressure rises from 120 to 270 mm Hg.

associated with significantly increased lipid accumulations,[19] and obesity by itself is not closely correlated with the aortic dry weight [20] or with the grade of atherosclerosis.[21]

Altered lipid metabolism in older men, predisposing to hypercholesterolemia and increased plasma lipoproteins, ranks third.[22–24] Increased aortic acid mucopolysaccharides [25] and decreased permeability of the hyalinized collagen [26] contribute to intramural lipid localization. Prolonged poor nutrition is accompanied by some resorption of the lipids and decreased severity of aortic atherosclerosis,[27] but malnutrition is not common among hypertensives.

Large Muscular Arteries. Although these are not often studied, it appears that systolic hypertension is correlated with the number of atherosclerotic plaques in the carotid and iliac arteries [28] and the quantity of lipid deposited in the femoral arteries.[19] In arteries of the extremities, degeneration of the intramural elastic tissue and medial fibrosis are considered to be responses to pressure and pulse stress.[29] Calcification of the internal elastic lamina is found to be age- but not pressure-related.[30] In hypertensive individuals tested in vivo the brachial artery showed a decreased distensibility compared to normotensive controls.[31]

Cerebral Arteries. Few quantitative investigations have been found but in endomorphs and mesomorphs with hypertension cerebral atherosclerosis often exceeds coronary disease in severity.[32] Both systolic and diastolic hypertension are statistically correlated with more severe sclerosis [33] and with increased intramural lipid.[19,34] Strokes are found significantly increased in persons with severe diastolic hypertension.[35]

Coronary Arteries. Clinically and pathologically the severity of coronary atherosclerotic lesions is related to hypertension, particularly in older men.[36] Intramural lipid is particularly increased in young hypertensive groups.[34] Although not conclusively demonstrated, it appears that enhanced human coronary atherosclerosis, like that in the aorta, is more closely related to the level of systolic rather than to diastolic hypertension (Figs. 2 through 4).[35] Coronary atherosclerosis is not correlated with the degree of aortic atherosclerosis.[21,36,38] Obesity and hypercholesterolemia contribute independently.[37] Endomorphy and mesomorphy with coronary disease are common [39] and are more significant predictors of coronary heart disease in men than either obesity or cholesterol levels.[40] Men who habitually performed light manual labor showed a

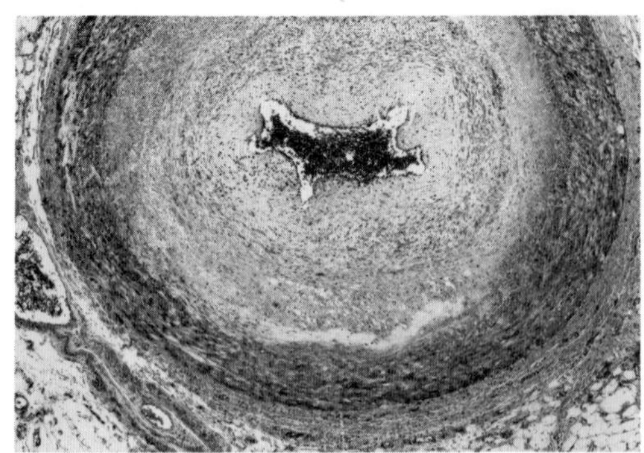

FIG. 2.—With hypertension some coronary artery branches, like the one shown here, with an outside diameter of 3 mm demonstrate marked intimal thickening and fibrosis, resembling the aortic atherosclerotic changes accompanying elevated systolic blood pressures. Masson, ×120.

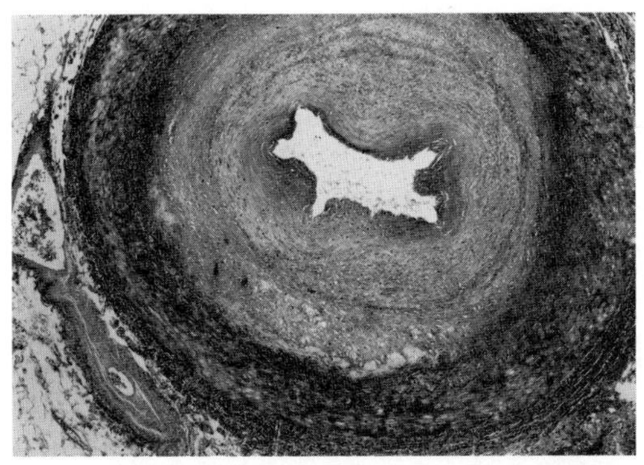

FIG. 3.—The same coronary artery as seen in Figure 2 has been stained for mucopolysaccharides, which are accumulated just beneath the endothelium, and for elastica and phospholipids, shown to be darkly stained in the media. Luxolfast blue-PAS, ×120.

closer relation between hypertension and clinical coronary sclerosis.[41] Increased coronary arteriosclerosis is more evident in sedentary hypertensive men than women, who in middle age lag about 20 years behind until after 70 years of life.[42]

A tentative ranking of factors responsible for coronary atherosclerosis places chronologic age first,[42–44] maleness second, and endomorphy-mesomorphy third.[40] Two genetic factors rank high. Obesity, hypercholesterolemia, serum lipoproteins, and systolic hypertension[33,45] are ranked fourth through seventh, followed by

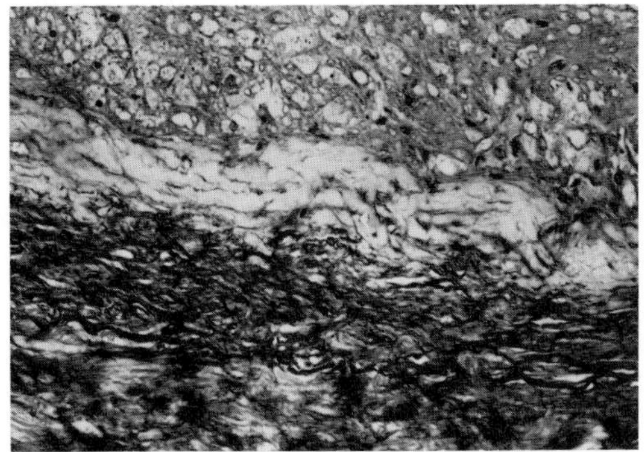

FIG. 4.—A higher-power detail of Figure 3 shows characteristic pooling of lipid near the top, hyaline deposition in the center, and fragmented elastica at the bottom. All three processes contribute to thickening the arterial wall and rendering it inelastic. Luxolfast blue-PAS, ×440.

diabetes mellitus and deficient ovarian function.[46]

Renal Arteries. No correlation is found between the severity of gross aortic and main renal arterial atherosclerosis.[38] Furthermore, the degree of main renal arterial atherosclerosis is not related to the severity of arteriolar nephrosclerosis.[47,48] Intrarenal arteriosclerosis, however, is correlated with the presence and severity of arteriolar nephrosclerosis.[47] Microscopically, renal artery elastosis and hyalinization were found to be exaggerated with hypertension.[49]

Mesenteric Arteries. In hypertension the superior mesenteric artery is hypertrophied, with an increased wall mass of the primary branch vessels about 5.0 mm in the outside diameter. Injected autopsy specimens showed the smallest mesenteric arteries and arterioles (30 to 300 μ in their outside diameters) to be constricted but not hypertrophied.[50]

Arterioles. Diastolic essential hypertension is closely correlated with increased wall-thickness/lumen-diameter ratios of the striated muscular, cutaneous, retinal, and renal arterioles.[51–54] Elevated pressures are present proximal to these and other narrowed systemic arterioles throughout much of their visceral distribution. Myocardial arterioles were thickened and narrowed in individuals with angina pectoris.[55] These arterioles and those from the pectoral muscles of hypertensive patients were both hypertrophied and hyperplastic, as judged by the numbers of intramural nuclei and muscle layers (Fig. 5).[51,55]

Biopsies and surgical specimens have provided information concerning earlier morphologic stages of the vascular changes in hypertension. Histologically, the initial alterations are focal and not diffuse in various tissues including the striated muscles and skin arterioles. The apparent sequence of changes includes arteriolar vasospasm, intramural edema, muscular hypertrophy, degeneration and intramural deposition of pooled ground substance, fragmented elastin, smooth muscle, and coagulated plasma proteins. Later intramural arteriolar fibrosis and hyaline degeneration follow. When essential hypertension becomes established the whole systemic circulation is not altered uniformly, except in the final and most severe stage. Fibrinoid arteriolar necrosis

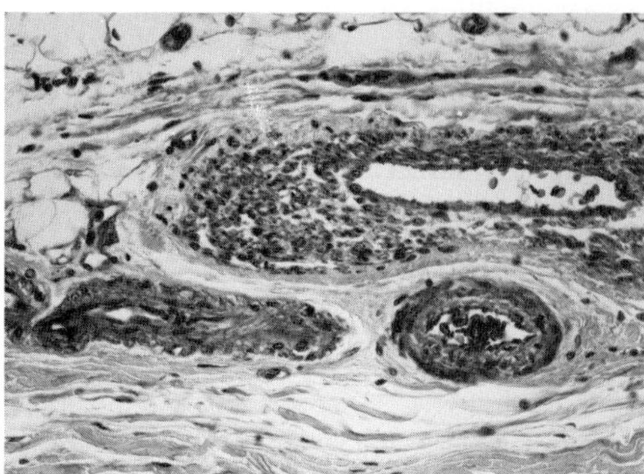

FIG. 5.—Hypertrophy and hyperplasia of the smooth muscle of an arteriole, shown just at the bottom edge of Figure 3. The larger parallel vessel is a vein. The arteriolar thickening and narrowing are moderate, corresponding to an average diastolic blood pressure of 110 mm Hg. Masson, ×440.

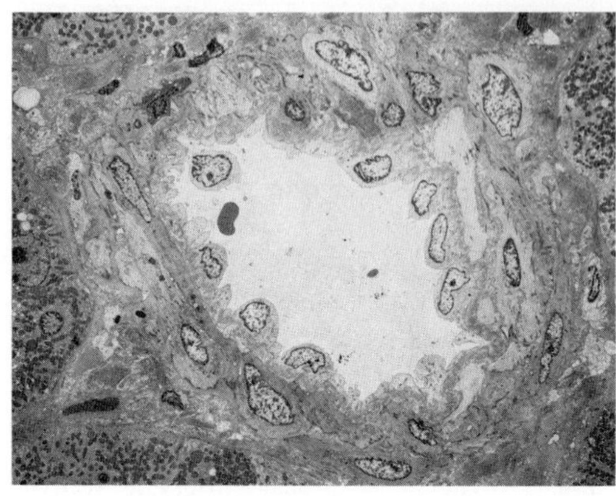

FIG. 6.—A slightly altered arteriole shows prominent endothelium with some pale-appearing hyaline deposits beneath it on the right side. The large intramural cell at the top with pale cytoplasm may be considered a facultative smooth-muscle or fibroblastic cell. ×1,450.

indicates an extremely increased local permeability, but in biopsies fibrinoid has not been correlated with clinically malignant hypertension or with a poor prognosis after definitive surgical or medical therapy.[56]

Biopsies also show certain instructive discrepancies with autopsy observations, apart from demonstrating that hypertension may precede any recognizable vascular lesions and that arteriolar sclerosis is not generalized in living hypertensive patients. In pancreas, salivary gland, and kidney there was a close correlation between increased arteriolar wall/lumen ratios and diastolic hypertension. While small arteries and arterioles of the gallbladder and gastrointestinal tract have been found constricted in autopsied hypertensive individuals,[50] our analysis of surgical material has showed no significant relation between the arteriolar wall/lumen ratios and systemic blood pressures in the gallbladder, stomach, small intestine, and colon.[56] Processes other than systemic hypertension may evidently lead to arteriolar sclerosis in the gallbladder, intestines, uterus, and ovaries.[57] Comparable situations include Bartter's syndrome, a rare condition with advanced arteriolar nephrosclerosis without hypertension, and renal biopsies of glomerulonephritis that show the same discrepancy.

Electron microscopy demonstrates in greater detail the arteriolar alterations already described in human and experimental hypertension. Endothelial crowding in vasospasm and subendothelial unspecialized multipotential cells are seen (Fig. 6).[58–61] The endothelial basement membrane and internal elastica manifest localized thickening, degeneration, and hyaline deposits. Muscular hypertrophy, degeneration, and fibrosis occur in the media (Figs. 7 through 9).[62–66] Intramural fibrin deposition is not regularly identified in long-standing hypertension, although found intramurally associated with increased vascular permeability in experimental acute hypertension.[67,68] Some smooth muscle persists, and its norepinephrine respon-

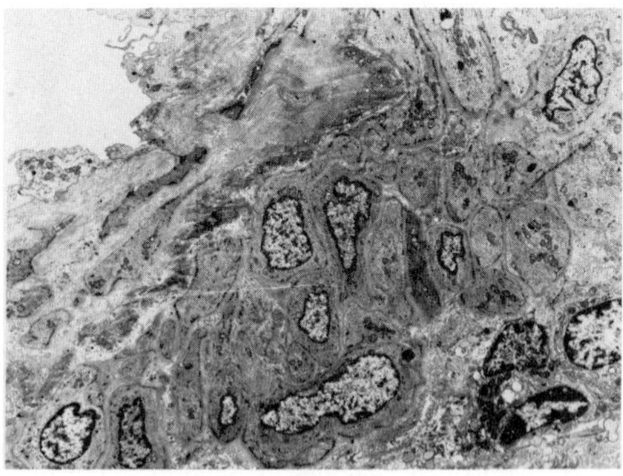

FIG. 7.—The arteriolar lumen is at the upper left, and the center is composed of crowded, hypertrophied and hyperplastic smooth-muscle cells. ×3,263.

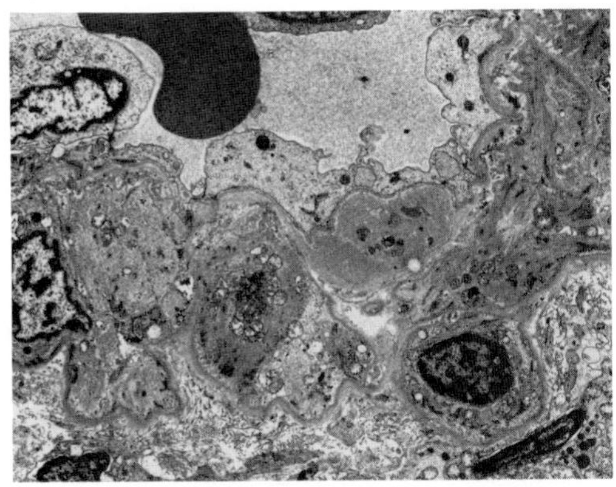

FIG. 8.—Arteriolosclerosis locally manifests hyaline degeneration, shown forming gray, rounded masses beneath the thin, wavy endothelial basement membrane in the center. At the left the basement membrane is split and reduplicated. Periarteriolar collagen fibers are dispersed along the bottom. ×5,100.

siveness could partly account for the persistent contracture of hypertensive arterioles.

The aorta, and large and small arteries are all less distensible in hypertensive individuals than in age-matched, normotensive controls. This is partly caused by increased intramural fibrosis and is partly attributed to a persistent hypertonic contracture. The increased resistance to blood flow is not of nervous origin [69]

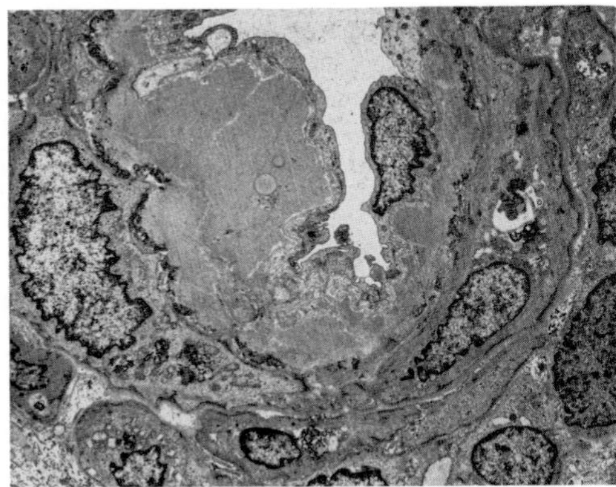

FIG. 9.—Nodular subendothelial deposits of hyaline material protrude partly into the arteriolar lumen. High-power magnification may demonstrate fibrin in such deposits. The smooth-muscle cells are somewhat swollen and degenerated. ×4,250.

and is demonstrable in the aorta,[70] and on the skin of arm or hand, and in the forearm muscles by injecting norepinephrine or angiotensin II.[71-73] The threshold of response to norepinephrine is normal in essential hypertension but the slope of the dose-response curve to graded injections is considerably increased.[73]

In addition, the minimal resistance in limb arteries and arterioles is increased in hypertension, and the arterioles are less distensible than normal,[74,75] except in the youngest group with essential hypertension.[76] Single rat arteriolar smooth-muscle cells were increased in thickness up to 70 percent after graded norepinephrine exposures.[77]

Increased arterial and arteriolar resistance and decreased distensibility in essential hypertension evidently reflect structural changes in these vessels, initially vasoconstrictive [78,79] but later involving hypertrophied smooth muscle with some encroachment on the vessel lumens even at maximal dilatation.[73] Structural contracture may predispose the smallest arterioles to develop hyaline sclerosis [80,81] and increased rigidity.[69] Sodium accumulation in arterial and arteriolar walls increases their vasoconstrictive responses, maintains diastolic hypertension, and enhances the vascular morphologic abnormalities in experimental animals and in human patients.[72,82,83]

Arterial and arteriolar changes in the intestine [56] and gallbladder [84] do not correlate with systemic hypertension in living patients, perhaps because these splanchnic vessels show an "autoregulatory escape" from vasomotor control which differs greatly from responses in skeletal muscle and skin.[85]

Shunt Vessels. Arteriovenous shunts occur in the skin, skeletal muscle,[85] coronary circulation,[86,87] and lung.[88] In pulmonary arterial hypertension the shunts open.[88] In the heart, norepinephrine increases the effective capillary flow relative to total coronary blood flow less than either isoproterenol or nicotine.[87] Coronary bypass vein grafts have developed intimal fibrous proliferation as a response to the arterial pressure.[89] Presumably in hypertension coronary collaterals may likewise become sclerotic, adversely affecting the myocardial nutritional blood flow.

Capillaries and Veins. Capillaries, venules, veins, and lymphatics have not often been investigated in essential hypertension. Poststenotic systemic capillary distension might theoretically be anticipated.[90] Capillaries lack smooth muscle, and increased capillary pressure is mainly associated with open-shunt vessels.[85,88] In chronic diastolic hypertension systemic capillary structural changes, if present, usually comprise ischemic degeneration and collagenous sclerosis.[15] No known venous abnormalities accompany essential hypertension.[76]

Diabetics with or without hypertension have ultrastructurally distinctive arteriolar and capillary basement membrane thickenings and reduplications, which may be considered as a different vascular abnormality from that of essential hypertension.[91,92] Muscular arterial changes in diabetics with or without hypertension are comparatively severe.[91,93] Other types of endocrine hypertension,[94] renovascular hypertension,[95] and toxemia of pregnancy[75] also may be superimposed on essential hypertension but show distinguishably different vascular abnormalities.

Summary

Vascular morphologic alterations in essential hypertension appear initially as systemic arteriolar vasoconstriction, followed by smooth-muscle hypertrophy and sequential degenerative changes, and ending with hyaline fibrosis. The lesions are focal until the last stages. Systolic hypertension is significantly correlated with (1) greater aortic wall thickness and fibrosis; (2) increased large muscular arterial plaques, degeneration, and fibrosis; and (3) cerebral atherosclerotic degeneration. But it is not closely related to the severity of coronary or main renal arterial atherosclerosis. Diastolic hypertension is significantly related to systemic arteriolar thickness expressed as wall/lumen ratios. Certain splanchnic arterioles appear spared. In established essential hypertension the aorta, systemic arteries and arterioles are characterized by decreased distensibility, partly attributable to intramural fibrosis and partly to smooth-muscle hypertrophy and contraction.

References

1. Walcott, G., Burchell, H. B., and Brown, A. L.: Primary pulmonary hypertension. Am. J. Med. 49:70, 1970.
2. Wilson, D. H., and Gardner, W. J.: Benign intracranial hypertension with particular reference to its occurrence in fat young women. Can. Med. Assoc. J. 95:102, 1966.
3. McMichael, J.: Reorientations in hypertensive disorders. Br. Med. J. 2:1239, 1310, 1961.
4. Page, I. H.: A story of hypertension. Fed. Proc. 23:693, 1964.
5. Corcoran, A. C.: Concepts of "primary hypertension" and their epidemiological significance. Am. Heart J. 69:137, 1965.
6. Evans, J. G., and Rose, G.: Hypertension. Br. Med. Bull. 27:37, 1971.
7. Thomas, C. B., and Cohen, B. H.: The familial occurrence of hypertension and coronary artery disease, with observations concerning obesity and diabetes. Ann. Intern. Med. 42:90, 1955.
8. Yin, P. H., and Sommers, S. C.: Some pathologic correlations of ovarian stromal hyperplasia. J. Clin. Endocrinol. Metab. 21:472, 1961.
9. Breckenridge, A.: Hypertension and hyperuricemia. Lancet 1:15, 1966.
10. Cannon, P. J., Stason, W. B., Demartini, F. E., Sommers, S. C., and Laragh, J. H.: Hyperuricemia in primary and renal hypertension. N. Engl. J. Med. 275:457, 1966.
11. Gruskin, A. B., Linshaw, M., Cote, M. L., and Fleisher, D.: Low-renin essential hypertension. Another form of childhood hypertension. J. Pediatr. 78:765, 1971.
12. Wiesenfeld, S. L., Petrakis, N. L., Sams, B. J., Collen, M. F., and Cutler, J. L.: Blood pressure, pulse and serum creatinine in G-6-PD deficiency. N. Engl. J. Med. 282:1001, 1970.
13. Arnold, J. E., and Healy, J. K.: Hyperkalemia, hypertension and systemic acidosis without renal failure associated with a tubular defect in potassium excretion. Am. J. Med. 47:461, 1969.
14. Wilens, S. L., and Plair, C. M.: The relationship between cortical hyperplasia of the adrenals and arteriosclerosis. Am. J. Pathol. 41:225, 1962.
15. Sommers, S. C.: Pathology of essential hypertension. *In* Cyclopedia of Medicine, vol. 4. Philadelphia: Davis, 1964, pp. 9–15.
16. Kölbel, F., Gregorová, I., and Šonka, J.: Hyperuricemia in hypertension. Lancet 1:519, 1965.
17. Waris, E.: Studies on serum lipids and lipoproteins in hypertension. Acta Med. Scand. 161 (Suppl. 337):1, 1958.
18. Burton, A. C.: On the physical equilibrium

of small blood vessels. Am. J. Physiol. 164: 319, 1951.

19. Paterson, J. C., Mills, J., and Lockwood, C. H.: The role of hypertension in the progression of atherosclerosis. Can. Med. Assoc. J. 82:65, 1970.
20. Faber, M. F., and Lund, F.: The human aorta. Arch. Pathol. 48:351, 1949.
21. Bjurulf, P.: Atherosclerosis and body-build with special reference to size and number of subcutaneous fat cells. Acta Med. Scand. Suppl. 349:99, 1959.
22. Corcoran, A. C., Page, I. H., Dustan, H. P., and Lewis, L. A.: Atherosclerotic complications of hypertensive disease: Relation to therapeutic response and to serum protein and to lipoprotein concentrations. Clev. Clin. Q. 23:115, 1956.
23. Malmros, H., Biörck, G., and Swahn, B.: Hypertension, atherosclerosis and the diet. Acta Med. Scand. 154 (Suppl. 312):71, 1956.
24. Bronte-Stewart, B.: Lipids and atherosclerosis. Fed. Proc. 20:127, 1961.
25. Fisher, E. R., and Tapper, E.: The effect of renal hypertension on cholesterol atherosclerosis in cortisone-treated rabbits. Am. J. Pathol. 37:713, 1960.
26. Weiss, D. L.: An approach to an atherogenetic factor. Mt. Sinai J. Med. N.Y. 24:1346, 1957.
27. Creed, D. L., Baird, W. F., and Fisher, E. R.: The severity of aortic arteriosclerosis in certain diseases. A necropsy study. Am. J. Med. Sci. 230:385, 1955.
28. Schwartz, C. J., Mitchell, J. R. A.: Observations on localization of arterial plaques. Circ. Res. 11:63, 1962.
29. Robertson, J. H.: The influence of mechanical factors on the structure of the peripheral arteries and the localization of atherosclerosis. J. Clin. Pathol. 13:199, 1960.
30. Wright, I.: The microscopical appearance of human peripheral arteries during growth and aging. J. Clin. Pathol. 16:499, 1963.
31. Greene, M. A., Friedlander, R., Boltax, A. J., Hadjigeorge, C. G., and Lustig, G. A.: Distensibility of arteries in human hypertension. Proc. Soc. Exp. Biol. Med. 121:580, 1968.
32. Wilens, S. L.: Orthostatic influences on the distribution of atheromatous lesions in the cerebral and other arteries. Arch. Intern. Med. 82:431, 1948.
33. Okinaka, S.: Macroscopic grading of severity of coronary sclerosis. Ann. N. Y. Acad. Sci. 79:920, 1963.
34. Giersten, J. C.: Atherosclerosis in an autopsy series. Relation of hypertension to atherosclerosis. Acta Pathol. Microbiol. Scand. [A] 66:331, 1966.
35. Dimond, G. E.: Hypertension, body weight and coronary heart disease. Arch. Intern. Med. 112:550, 1963.
36. Yater, W. M., Traum, A. H., Brown, W. G., Fitzgerald, R. P., Geisler, M. A., and Wilcox, B. B.: Coronary artery disease in men eighteen to thirty-nine years of age. Am. Heart J. 36:334; 481; 683; 1948.
37. Dawber, T. R., Moore, F. E., and Mann, G. V.: Coronary heart disease in the Framingham study. Am. J. Public Health 47 (Suppl.): 1957.
38. Glagov, S., Rowley, D. A., and Kohut, R. I.: Atherosclerosis of human aorta and the coronary and renal arteries. Arch. Pathol. 72: 558, 1961.
39. Thorne, M. C., Wing, A. L., and Paffenbarger, R. S., Jr.: Chronic disease in former college students. VII. Early precursors in nonfatal coronary heart disease. Am. J. Epidemiol. 87: 520, 1968.
40. Damon, A., Damon, S. T., Harpending, H. C., and Kannel, W. B.: Predicting coronary heart disease from body measurements of Framingham males. J. Chronic Dis. 21:781, 1969.
41. Morris, J. N.: Occupation and coronary heart disease. Arch. Intern. Med. 104:903, 1959.
42. Giersten, J.: Atherosclerosis in an autopsy study: Relation to age and sex. Acta Pathol. Microbiol. Scand. 65(V):1, 1965.
43. Neufeld, H. N., Wagenvoort, C. A., and Edwards, J. E.: Coronary arteries in fetuses, infants, juveniles, and young adults. Lab. Invest. 11:837, 1962.
44. Giersten, J.: Atherosclerosis in an autopsy series. Relation of nutritional state to atherosclerosis. General summary and conclusion. Acta Pathol. Microbiol. Scand. [A] 67:305, 1966.
45. Allison, R. B., Rodriguez, F. L., Higgins, E. A., Jr., Leddy, J. P., Abelmann, W. H., Ellis, L. B., and Robbins, S. L.: Clinicopathologic correlations in coronary atherosclerosis. Four hundred thirty patients studied with postmortem coronary angiography. Circulation 27:170, 1963.
46. Edwards, J. E.: An Atlas of Acquired Diseases of the Heart and Great Vessels, vols. 1–3. Philadelphia: Saunders, 1961.
47. Blackman, S. S., Jr.: Arteriosclerosis and partial obstruction of the main renal arteries in association with "essential" hypertension in man. Johns Hopkins Med. J. 65:353, 1939.
48. Williams, R. H., and Harrison, T. R.: A study of the renal arteries in relation to age

and to hypertension. Am. Heart J. 14:645, 1937.

49. Lendrum, A. C.: Structural results of hypertension. Br. J. Surg. 51:723, 1964.
50. Short, D.: The vascular fault in chronic hypertension. Lancet 1:1302, 1966.
51. Kernohan, J. W., Anderson, E. W., and Keith, N. M.: The arterioles in cases of hypertension. Arch. Intern. Med. 44:395, 1929.
52. Foa, P. O., Foa, N. Y., and Peet, M. M.: Arteriolar lesions in hypertension: A study of 350 consecutive cases treated surgically. J. Clin. Invest. 22:727, 1943.
53. Hines, E. A., Jr., and Farber, E. M.: The arterioles of the skin in essential hypertension. J. Lab. Clin. Med. 33:1486, 1948.
54. Sommers, S. C.: Pathology of the kidney and adrenal gland in relationship to hypertension. *In* Moyer, J. H. (Ed.): Hypertension. Philadelphia: Saunders, 1959, pp. 8–23.
55. More, B. M., and Sommers, S. C.: Status of the myocardial arterioles in angina pectoris. Am. Heart J. 64:323, 1962.
56. Sommers, S. C., McLaughlin, R. J., and McAuley, R. L.: Pathology of diastolic hypertension as a generalized vascular disease. Am. J. Cardiol. 9:653, 1962.
57. Reeves, G.: Specific stroma in the cortex and medulla of the ovary. Obstet. Gynecol. 37: 832, 1971.
58. Pease, D. C., and Molinari, S.: Electron microscopy of muscular arteries; pial vessels of the cat and monkey. J. Ultrastruct. Res. 3:447, 1960.
59. Haust, M. D., More, R. H., and Movat, H. F.: The role of smooth muscle cells in the fibrogenesis of arteriosclerosis. Am. J. Pathol. 37: 372, 1960.
60. Geer, J. C., McGill, H. C., Jr., and Strong, J. P.: The fine structure of human atherosclerotic lesions. Am. J. Pathol. 38:263, 1963.
61. Becker, C. G., and Murphy, G. E.: Demonstration of contractile protein in endothelium and cells of the heart valves, endocardium, intima, arteriosclerotic plaques, and Aschoff bodies of rheumatic heart disease. Am. J. Pathol. 55:1, 1969.
62. Parker, F.: An electron microscopic study of experimental atherosclerosis. Am. J. Pathol. 36:19, 1960.
63. McGee, W. G., and Ashworth, C. T.: Fine structure of chronic hypertensive arteriopathy. Am. J. Pathol. 43:273, 1963.
64. Fisher, E. R., Perez-Stable, E., and Pardo, V.: Ultrastructural studies in hypertension. I. Comparison of renal vascular and juxtaglomerular cell alterations in essential and renal hypertension in man. Lab. Invest. 15:1409, 1966.
65. Salgado, E. D.: Medial aortic lesions in rats with metacorticoid hypertension. Am. J. Pathol. 58:305, 1970.
66. Aikawa, M., and Koletsky, S.: Arteriosclerosis of the mesenteric arteries of rats with renal hypertension. Am. J. Pathol. 61:293, 1970.
67. Olsen, F.: Arteriolar permeability and destruction of elastic membrane in hypertension. Acta Pathol. Microbiol. Scand. [A] 75:527, 1969.
68. Hüttner, I., More, R. H., and Rona, G.: Fine structural evidence of specific mechanism for increased endothelial permeability in experimental hypertension. Am. J. Pathol. 61:395, 1970.
69. Coles, D. R., and Gough, K. R.: The critical closing pressure of blood vessels of the fingers in hypertensive and normal subjects. Clin. Sci. 19:587, 1960.
70. Greenfield, J. G., Jr., and Patel, D. J.: Relation between pressure and diameter in the ascending aorta of man. Circ. Res. 10:778, 1962.
71. Doyle, A. E., and Fraser, J. R. E.: Essential hypertension and inheritance of vascular reactivity. Lancet 2:509, 1961.
72. Mendlowitz, M., Naftchi, N. E., Gitlow, S. E., and Wolf, R. L.: Vascular responsiveness in hypertensive and hypotensive states. Geriatrics 20:797, 1965.
73. Silvertsson, R.: Hypertension, essential vascular changes. Acta Physiol. Scand. Suppl. 343:1, 1970.
74. Conway, J.: A vascular abnormality in hypertension. Circulation 37:520, 1963.
75. Ginsburg, J., and Duncan, S. L. B.: Peripheral blood flow in normal pregnancy. Cardiovasc. Res. 1:356, 1967.
76. Lund-Johansen, P.: Hemodynamics in early essential hypertension. Acta Med. Scand. 183(Suppl. 482):1, 1968.
77. Baez, S.: Vascular smooth muscle: Quantitation of cell thickness in the wall of arterioles in the living animal in situ. Science 159:537, 1968.
78. Bordley, J., III, and Eichna, L. W.: Hypertension, evolution of retinal lesions. Trans. Assoc. Am. Phys. 55:270, 1940.
79. Van Citters, R. L.: Architecture of small arteries during vasoconstriction. Circ. Res. 10:668, 1962.
80. Tracy, R. E., and Overll, E. O.: Arterioles of perfusion-fixed hypertensive and aged kidneys. Arch. Pathol. (Chicago) 82:526, 1966.

81. Editorial: Arterioles in hypertension. Lancet 1:966, 1966.
82. Koletsky, S.: Role of salt and renal mass in experimental hypertension. Arch. Pathol. 68:11, 1959.
83. Wulkinson, R., Scott, D. F., Uldall, P. R., Kerr, D. N. S., and Swinney, J.: Plasma renin and exchangeable sodium in the hypertension of chronic renal failure. Q. J. Med. 39:377, 1970.
84. More, B. M., Merdinger, W. F., and Sommers, S. C.: Cholecystitis and stenotic arteriosclerosis. Am. J. Clin. Pathol. 45:465, 1966.
85. Mellander, S., and Johansson, B.: Control of resistance, exchange, and capacitance functions in the peripheral circulation. Pharmacol. Rev. 20:117, 1968.
86. Blumgart, H. L., Schlesinger, M. J., and Davis, D.: Studies on the relation of the clinical manifestations of angina pectoris, coronary thrombosis, and myocardial infarction to the pathology findings. Am. Heart J. 19:1, 1940.
87. Tillich, G., Mendoza, L., and Bing, R. J.: Total and nutritional coronary flow. Circ. Res. 28:I, 1971.
88. Recavarren, S.: The preterminal arterioles in the pulmonary circulation of high-altitude natives. Circulation 33:177, 1966.
89. Vlodaver, F., and Edwards, J. E.: Pathologic changes in aortic-coronary arterial saphenous vein grafts. Circulation 44:719, 1971.
90. Rodbard, S.: Capillary control of blood flow and fluid exchange. Circ. Res. 28(Suppl. I):1, 1971.
91. Warren, S., LeCompte, P. M., and Legg, M. A.: *In* The Pathology of Diabetes Mellitus. Philadelphia: Lea & Febiger, 1966, pp. 310–332.
92. Vracko, R., and Benditt, E. P.: Capillary basal lamina thickening in diabetics. J. Cell Biol. 47:281, 1970.
93. Blumenthal, H. T., Alex, M., and Goldenberg, S.: A study of lesions of the intramural coronary artery branches in diabetes mellitus. Arch. Pathol. 70:13, 1960.
94. O'Neal, L. W., Kissane, J. M., and Hartroft, P. M.: The kidney in endocrine hypertension. Arch. Surg. 100:498, 1970.
95. Buda, J. A., McAllister, F. F., and Sommers, S. C.: Surgical treatment of renovascular hypertension. Am. J. Surg. 119:574, 1970.

Renal Morphologic Changes in Essential Hypertension

By Robert H. Heptinstall, M.D.

THE KIDNEY DAMAGE in essential hypertension is dependent on changes that take place in the arteries and arterioles. Various factors contribute to these vascular changes; chief among these are hypertension, aging, and arteriosclerosis. The amount of renal damage is proportional to the severity and duration of these changes.

In the benign phase of essential hypertension the appearance of the kidney is variable. In certain cases where the pressure has been modest and of short duration, and where generalized arteriosclerosis is minimal, the kidneys may show little gross change. In other cases the kidneys may be considerably reduced in size, with a finely granular surface. These reduced kidneys are usually found in patients who have been hypertensive for a long time and in whom there is much arteriosclerosis in the aorta and larger branches of the renal artery.

The first change is in the arterial tree, and in a patient with granular kidneys the afferent arterioles show thickening of the wall and reduction of the lumen. The wall is thickened by a process known as hyalinization. In its early stages this is a patchy change in which a certain length of artery shows an eosinophilic thickening of the wall, with intervening segments showing no change. The involved segment is frequently affected only in part of its circumference. The interlobular arteries show intimal thickening and this is brought about by an increase in elastic tissue (Fig. 1). Larger vessels may show fibrous intimal thickening. Arteriosclerotic changes may be found in the main renal artery. The consequence of this narrowing of arteries and arterioles is tubular atrophy and loss. Because the arterial changes are not uniform, certain parts of the parenchyma are affected less than others, and hypertrophy and dilatation of tubules may occur in these areas. It is the presence of such groups of tubules that causes the minute elevations on the subcapsular surface which, alternating with depressed scarred areas, give the finely granular appearance. The glomeruli may show little change, but usually many are sclerotic. This change is due to the glomeruli developing collagen-like material on the inside of Bowman's capsule. This material increases and at the same time the capillary tuft undergoes shrinkage (Fig. 2). Eventually all the capsular space is filled with this material and a solidified or hyalinized glomerulus is produced.

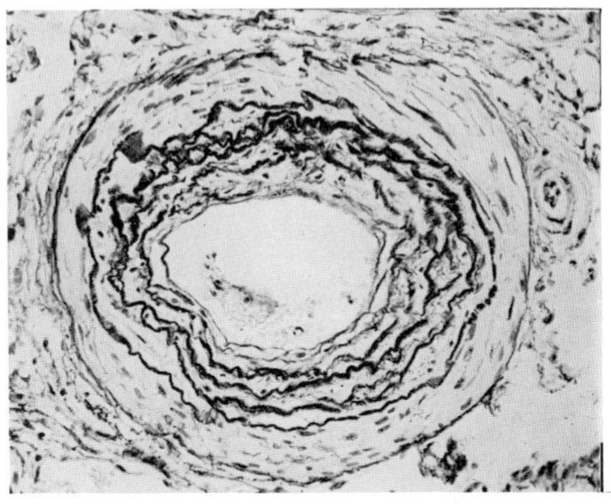

Fig. 1.—Increased elastic tissue is present in the thickened intima. The lumen is reduced. Elastic stain, ×300.

As seen by the naked eye the malignant phase may show the same spectrum of changes as the benign phase. Where there has been only a brief preceding benign phase there is little reduction in size, but where there has been a protracted benign phase there is shrinkage. Multiple petechial hemorrhages are frequently seen on the subcapsular surface. Histologically there are two characteristic vascular changes: First there is a fine, sometimes mucinous thickening of the intima of the interlobular arteries (Fig. 3); and secondly, there is fibrinoid necrosis of the afferent arterioles with a frequent

From the Department of Pathology, the Johns Hopkins University School of Medicine and Hospital, Baltimore, Maryland.

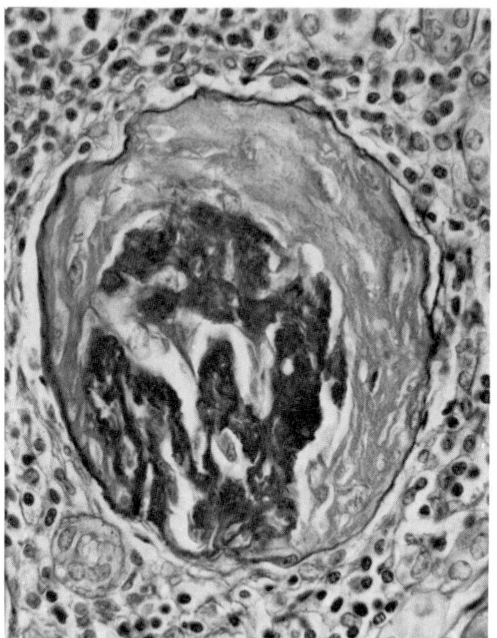

FIG. 2.—Ischemic glomerulus. Bowman's space is partially filled with material that has many of the features of collagen. The glomerular tuft is shrunken and more solid than usual. PAS, $\times 600$.

extension of the necrosis into the glomerular tuft (Fig. 4). Small microthrombi may be seen in the lumen of a necrotic arteriole or small artery (Fig. 5), and similar microthrombi can be seen in the glomerular capillaries. Apart from showing necroses and microthrombi, the

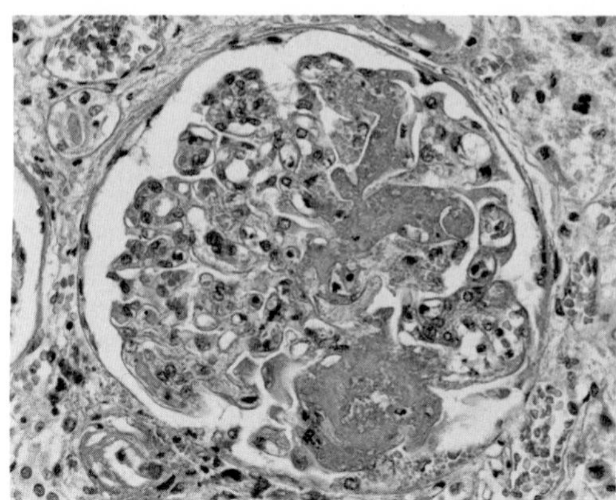

FIG. 4.—Glomerulus with necrosis which is also seen in the terminal part of the afferent arteriole. Hematoxylin and eosin, $\times 350$.

glomeruli may have areas of proliferation, collections of hyaline droplets, and sometimes epithelial crescents. Tubules show loss and atrophy, and hyaline droplets are frequently found in certain segments of proximal convoluted tubules.

Arterial and arteriolar changes have been studied in biopsy material and at autopsy. As a result there is a large amount of information available on the type and severity of arterial and arteriolar changes in patients with different levels of blood pressure and varying durations of hypertension. There is still disagreement over certain fundamental questions. Chief among these are: first, the order of events, whether hypertension produces the vascular

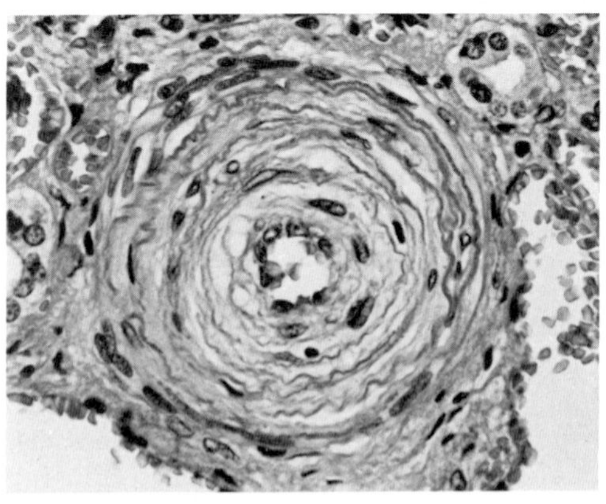

FIG. 3.—Interlobular artery shows fine intimal thickening with considerable reduction of lumen in malignant phase. Hematoxylin and eosin, $\times 600$.

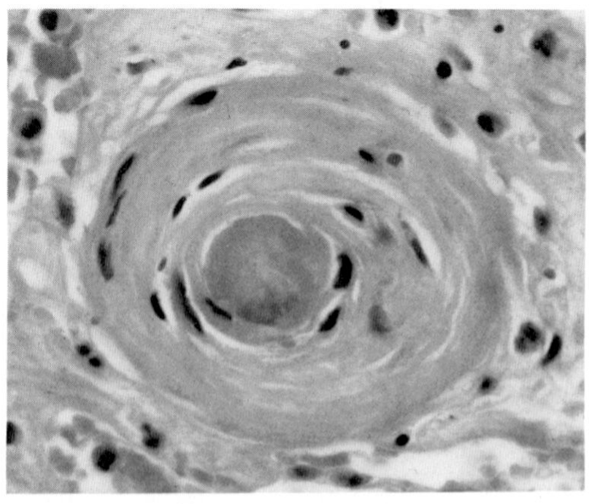

FIG. 5.—Small artery in kidney contains microthrombus. Hematoxylin and eosin, $\times 900$.

TABLE 1.—*Changes in Interlobular Arteries in Patients with Normal Blood Pressure and Benign Essential Hypertension*

	No. of Patients	*Grading of Changes (Percentage of Patients in Each Grade)*			
		0	*1*	*2*	*3*
Controls over 50 yr. of age	311	0	37.3	32.1	30.5
Hypertensive patients dying from heart failure	226	0.9	12.8	32.3	54.0
Hypertensive patients dying from cerebrovascular accidents	194	0	11.3	31.4	57.2

From Bell, E. T.: Renal Diseases, 2nd ed. Philadelphia: Lea & Febiger, 1950, p. 340.

changes or whether the vascular changes are the cause of the hypertension; and second, the contribution of arteriosclerotic and aging changes to the production of arterial changes. Moritz and Oldt,[1] after a study of vascular changes in the vessels of the kidney at autopsy, concluded that renal arteriolar disease was more likely to be the cause of hypertension than the consequence. This was based largely on their opinion that arteriolar hyalinization was the counterpart of arteriosclerosis, and the observation that it became more widespread with advancing years. On the other hand, as the result of a similar study, Bell [2] came to the following conclusions:

1. That intimal thickening (elastic reduplication) of interlobular arteries increases with age and is independent of hypertension. He felt it was likely to be accentuated by hypertension.

2. That arteriolar hyalinization increases with age and is never found except in association with intimal thickening of interlobular arteries.

3. That arteriolar hyalinization increases as the blood pressure rises (Tables 1 and 2).

Smith [3] came to conclusions similar to those of Bell, namely, that arteriolosclerosis, as hyalinization of arterioles is called, is an aging process that is made worse by hypertension. Bell felt that arteriolosclerosis did not cause hypertension.

Biopsy studies of the wedge type, done at a time when sympathectomy enjoyed a great vogue in the treatment of hypertension, also give little support to the notion that small-vessel changes produce the elevated pressure in essential hypertension. In the several studies it was noted that hypertension, often severe, could occur in the presence of normal or only mildly involved small arteries and arterioles.[4–7] The criticism of biopsy studies is that they provide only a small amount of tissue for study and that they allow no assessment of larger vessels. From the time of experiments by Goldblatt et al. in the 1930s [8] it has been accepted that vascular narrowing can cause hypertension.

TABLE 2.—*Changes in Afferent Arterioles in Patients with Normal Blood Pressure and Benign Essential Hypertension*

	No. of Patients	*Grading of Changes (Percentage of Patients in Each Grade)*			
		0	*1*	*2*	*3*
Controls over 50 yr. of age	312	61.5	35.5	2.6	0.3
Hypertensive patients dying from heart failure	226	26.5	33.6	19.5	20.4
Hypertensive patients dying from cerebrovascular accidents	194	16.5	30.4	20.6	32.5

Based on data from Bell, E. T.: Chapter 10. *In* Renal Diseases, 2nd ed. Philadelphia: Lea & Febiger, 1950, pp. 329-406.

Numerous cases in man have been described in which stenosis of the main renal artery, or even a segmental branch, can precipitate hypertension. Therefore, although we can conclude that small-vessel changes are not essential in the genesis of hypertension, it would be impossible to exclude the possibility that stenosis of a large artery has initiated the hypertensive process. I have on several occasions seen whole kidneys from patients in the benign phase of essential hypertension in which the main renal arteries, main divisions, and segmental branches have been free from stenotic changes of a degree that would be necessary to initiate hypertension. Further, studies of the renin-angiotensin system in the benign phase of essential hypertension give no support to the idea that larger-artery stenosis plays a role in the production of hypertension. In conclusion it can be said that there is little to commend the concept that arterial and arteriolar changes initiate hypertension in the benign forms of essential hypertension.

When the malignant phase is studied, necrosis of arterioles and small arteries is a prominent feature. There is good experimental and human evidence to show that such necroses are the consequence, rather than the cause, of the hypertension. The presence of arterial necroses in the contralateral kidney of rats in which hypertension has been produced by the application of a silver clip to one renal artery is a common finding.[9] In contrast is the almost invariable absence of necroses in the kidney whose renal artery has been occluded by the clip. The latter is considered to protect the vessels beyond from hypertensive changes.[9] The same findings have been encountered in man with severe hypertension brought about by stenosis of one renal artery. Thus, arteriolar necroses may be seen in the opposite kidney but not in the kidney with the stenotic renal artery. In DOCA-induced hypertension in the rat, necroses can be restricted to one kidney by the application of a silver clip to the opposite kidney.[10] Further evidence for arterial and arteriolar necrosis as being the consequence of hypertension is provided by examination of lungs from patients with pulmonary hypertension.[11–13] The fine intimal thickening of the interlobular arteries seen in the malignant phase is also considered to be the result of the hypertension, but the evidence for this is not so convincing. Moreover, the virtually identical changes seen in small arteries in the scleroderma kidney, which may not be associated with an elevated blood pressure, indicate that such changes can be produced by means other than hypertension. It is also of interest that hypertension may develop terminally in scleroderma, presumably brought about by ischemia consequent on this type of lesion in the interlobular artery. The explanation of the arteriolar necroses in patients with scleroderma and a normal blood pressure is likewise unexplained. A further example of the extreme intimal thickening of the type seen in malignant hypertension is provided by the end-stage kidneys of patients on chronic hemodialysis.[14] In these there may be virtual obliteration of the lumen. At the present time we regard these changes as being disuse endarteritis, the artificial kidney taking over the function of the patient's own damaged kidneys. In summary, while the arteriolar necrosis in the malignant phase is almost certainly the consequence of the high blood pressure, the same degree of probability cannot be applied to the fine intimal thickening of the interlobular arteries.

A change that has aroused interest in recent years is the presence in malignant hypertension of small thrombi in the lumen of afferent arterioles and in the capillary tuft of the glomerulus.[15–17] Similar changes in arterioles and small arteries may be seen in the myocardium. These small thrombi are similar to those seen in cases of thrombotic thrombocytopenic purpura and in the hemolytic uremic syndrome. Such cases invariably show abnormal red blood cells such as helmet and burr cells in the circulation; anemia is also a feature. It has been proposed that the abnormal red cell forms are produced by damage inflicted on red cells in their transit through damaged small blood vessels. It is felt that the thrombi form in areas of damage to the endothelium. The question must be raised whether these thrombi and the attending vascular changes may be responsible for accentuating hypertension in patients with malignant hypertension.[17] In cases of the hemolytic-uremic syndrome there is a possibility that the coagulation process and the microthrombi initiate hypertension.

References

1. Moritz, A. R., and Oldt, M. R.: Arteriolar sclerosis in hypertensive and non-hypertensive individuals. Am. J. Pathol. 13:679, 1937.
2. Bell, E. T.: Renal Diseases, 2nd ed. Philadelphia: Lea & Febiger, 1950.
3. Smith, J. P.: Hyaline arteriolosclerosis in the kidney. J. Pathol. Bacteriol. 69:147, 1955.
4. Castleman, B., and Smithwick, R. H.: The relation of vascular disease to the hypertensive state based on a study of renal biopsies from one hundred hypertensive patients. JAMA 121:1256, 1943.
5. Castleman, B., and Smithwick, R. H.: The relation of vascular disease to the hypertensive state: II. The adequacy of the renal biopsy as determined from a study of 500 patients. N. Engl. J. Med. 239:729, 1948.
6. Heptinstall, R. H.: Renal biopsies in hypertension. Br. Heart J. 15:133, 1954.
7. Sommers, S. C., Relman, A. S., and Smithwick, R. H.: Histologic studies of kidney biopsy specimens from patients with hypertension. Am. J. Pathol. 34:685, 1958.
8. Goldblatt, H., Lynch, J., Hanzal, R. F., and Summerville, W. W.: Studies on experimental hypertension: I. The production of persistent elevation of systolic blood pressure by means of renal ischemia. J. Exp. Med. 59:347, 1934.
9. Wilson, C., and Byrom, F. B.: The vicious circle in chronic Bright's disease: Experimental evidence from the hypertensive rat. Q. J. Med. 10:65, 1941.
10. Heptinstall, R. H., and Hill, G. S.: Steroid-induced hypertension in the rat. A study of the effects of renal artery constriction on hypertension caused by deoxycorticosterone. Lab. Invest. 16:751, 1967.
11. Old, J. W., and Russell, W. O.: Necrotizing pulmonary arteritis occurring with congenital heart disease (Eisenmenger complex): Report of case with necropsy. Am. J. Pathol. 26:789, 1950.
12. Symmers, W. St. C.: Necrotizing pulmonary arteriopathy associated with pulmonary hypertension. J. Clin. Pathol. 5:36, 1952.
13. Spencer, H.: Pulmonary lesions in polyarteritis nodosa. Br. J. Tuberc. 51:123, 1957.
14. Heptinstall, R. H.: Pathology of end-stage kidney disease. Am. J. Med. 44:656, 1968.
15. Brain, M. C., Dacie, J. V., and Hourihane, D. O'B.: Microangiopathic haemolytic anaemia: the possible role of vascular lesions in pathogenesis. Br. J. Haematol. 8:358, 1962.
16. Linton, A. L., Gavras, H., Gleadle, R. I., Hutchison, H. E., Lawson, D. H., Lever, A. F., McNicol, G. P., and Robertson, J. I. S.: Microangiopathic haemolytic anaemia and the pathogenesis of malignant hypertension. Lancet, 1:1227, 1969.
17. Gavras, H., Brown, W. C. B., Brown, J. J., Lever, A. F., Linton, A. L., MacAdam, R. F., McNicol, G. P., Robertson, J. I. S., and Wardrop, C.: Microangiopathic hemolytic anemia and the development of the malignant phase of hypertension. Circ. Res. (Suppl. II) 28–29: II-127, 1971.

Clinical-Physiologic Classification of Hypertensive Heart Disease in Essential Hypertension

By Edward D. Frohlich, M.D.

OVER THE PAST DECADE strong clinical evidence has confirmed [1,2] the initial clinical and epidemiologic projections [3–5] that antihypertensive drug therapy clearly reduces the cardiovascular morbidity and mortality from hypertensive cardiovascular disease. Little information is available, however, which details the clinical, physiologic, and pathologic changes associated with the development of hypertensive heart disease although clinical studies frequently refer to development of left ventricular hypertrophy and cardiac failure as the hallmarks of cardiac involvement in hypertension.[6] Equally as frequent in description are the other "complications" of hypertensive cardiovascular disease—angina pectoris and myocardial infarction.

Clearly, these two types of cardiac problems are expressions of two distinct pathophysiologic processes: hypertension, producing left ventricular hypertrophy and failure at one end of the spectrum; and atherosclerosis, producing ischemic heart disease, at the other. To be sure, hypertrophy and hypertension increase left ventricular work and oxygen demand [7] and hence aggravate already impaired myocardial oxygen delivery; they may even produce angina pectoris. However, as commonly used, "angina pectoris" is equated with atherosclerotic coronary arterial disease resulting from atherosclerosis, rather than chest pain provoked by increased myocardial demand resulting from increased intraventricular pressure and wall tension. In actuality and in clinical practicality both problems represent highly complex interrelated "diseases of disregulation" [8,9] and in both a clearer understanding of the pathophysiologic stages in their development is lacking.

From the Division of Hypertension, Department of Medicine, College of Medicine, the University of Oklahoma Health Sciences Center, Oklahoma City, Oklahoma.

Hemodynamic Concepts

Background. In this discussion we shall be concerned with the clinical and pathophysiologic correlates of developing *hypertensive* heart disease, and more specifically, in patients with hypertension of unknown cause—essential hypertension. Much of our previous understanding of the development of this clinical problem has been inferential, resulting from hemodynamic studies concerned with left ventricular hypertrophy and failure in patients having aortic valvular or subvalvular disease,[10] rheumatic heart disease,[11] aortic coarctation,[12,13] or from experimental animal models [14–16] which may not be at all analogous to hypertensive cardiac disease in the "usual" patient with essential hypertension. Moreover, those hemodynamic studies concerned with the hypertensive patient also have failed to differentiate or to consider the clinical, etiologic, or physiologic differences which exist in hypertensive patients (in general) with respect to the pressor mechanisms involved.[17,18]

Basic Considerations. Arterial pressure is the function of three major hemodynamic variables: the cardiac output; the "state of tone" of the blood vessels or the actual vascular resistance to the flow of blood; and the intrinsic viscous resistance offered by the fluid, the blood. The last factor, however, is so negligible and so similar to that in the normal subject that it can be discounted. The other two, however, are dependent upon a variety of physiologic variables including neural, chemical, hormonal, electrolytic, volume, osmotic, and autoregulatory factors (Table 1).

Because of this earlier "lumping" of all patients with hypertension into one unhomogeneous clinical grouping, it is no wonder that hypertension was considered a problem hemodynamically ascribed to increased vascular resistance; cardiac output on the average was normal and the elevated arterial pressure there-

TABLE 1.—*Factors Affecting Cardiac Output and Total Peripheral Resistance*

1. Neural
   - A. Innervation
     1. Adrenergic
     2. Dopaminergic
     3. Parasympathetic
   - B. Storage, release, and reuptake of the neurohumoral substance
   - C. Receptor site responsiveness (alpha, beta)
2. Chemical
   - A. Electrolytes—cations, anions
   - B. Metabolites—adenine nucleotides, Krebs intermediates
   - C. Naturally occurring vasoactive substances—histamines, serotonin, prostaglandins, angiotensin, kinins, vasopressin
   - D. Catecholamines—epinephrine, norepinephrine, dopamine
3. Hormonal
   - A. Thyroid
   - B. Parathyroid
   - C. Adrenocortical hormones including aldosterone
   - D. Vasopressin, ADH
4. Osmotic
   - A. Active receptors
   - B. Passive changes due to "waterlogging" or dehydration
5. "Autoregulatory" factors

fore was attributed to an increased total peripheral resistance.

Present Concepts. In recent years reports from laboratories from all areas of the globe have indicated that elevated peripheral resistance no longer should be considered the hemodynamic hallmark of hypertension (Table 2).[19] Thus, patients with labile (borderline) or mild essential hypertension may have an elevated cardiac output. In these individuals vascular resistance may be numerically normal (or slightly elevated); but this, however, is inappropriately so, since were cardiac output to be so increased in normotensive individuals the vascular resistance would be reduced. Similarly, patients with coarctation of the aorta also have an elevated cardiac output and a normal or increased vascular resistance. Those patients with renal arterial disease (of fibrosing as well as atherosclerotic causes) have elevated cardiac output and increased total peripheral resistance. Other patients with renal parenchymal disease (not in renal failure or anemic), primary aldosteronism, and pheochromocytoma have a normal cardiac output and increased vascular resistance; but clearly the pressor mechanisms whereby arteriolar smooth-muscle tone is increased in these highly different etiologic types of hypertension are distinctly different.[20,21]

Essential Hypertension. Our present considerations concern that very broad group of patients with hypertension of undetermined and, as yet, unknown causes, i.e., *essential hypertension.* In the following discussion the physiologic and hemodynamic characteristics will be correlated with the development of progressive cardiac involvement related to hypertension per se (e.g., left ventricular hypertrophy and later cardiac failure).

Clinical-Physiologic Correlations in Essential Hypertension

It should be acknowledged at the outset of this discussion that with the knowledge that antihypertensive drug therapy is necessary to prevent the development and progression of hypertensive cardiovascular disease, no patient was or could be followed longitudinally to test the progression of this concept of the pathogenetic development of the disease. However, in approximately 200 such essential hypertensive patients studied hemodynamically in our laboratory, all had been thoroughly investigated clinically to find a cause of the elevated arterial pressure; and these studies were all performed after all antihypertensive drugs, including diuretics, had been discontinued for at least one month. Measurements were performed when the patient was fasting in the early morning, without premedication, in a well-lit, quiet, and undisturbed setting. Details of the hemodynamic techniques and calculations have been described in detail;[19,22,23] but in general catheters were inserted percutaneously, by the Seldinger technique,[24] into a brachial artery and antecubital vein to the shoulder and central venous levels, respectively. Cardiac output was calculated from indocyanine green dye-dilution curves using a Gilford densitometer; the electrocardiogram was recorded continuously.

Classification of Patients. Essential hyper-

TABLE 2.—*Hemodynamic Characteristics of the Various Clinical Arterial Hypertensions*

Hypertension	*Heart Rate*	*Cardiac Output*	*Stroke Volume*	*Total Peripheral Resistance*
Labile (borderline, juvenile)	↑	↑	N	N, ↑
Essential				
Mild	↑	N, ↑	N or ↓	↑
Moderate	↑	N	N or ↓	↑↑
Severe	↑	↓	↓	↑↑↑
with congestive heart failure	↑	↓↓	↓↓	↑↑↑↑
Coarctation of aorta	↑	↑	N	↑
Renal arterial disease	↑	↑	N	↑↑
Renal parenchymal disease				
No anemia or renal failure	↑	N	↓	↑↑
Renal failure	↑	↑	N or ↓	↑↑
with anemia correction	↑	N	N	↑↑↑
Primary aldosteronism	↑	N	↓	↑
Pheochromocytoma	↑	N	↓	↑

Symbols and abbreviations: ↑, Increased; ↓, decreased; N, unchanged or normal.

tensive patients were subdivided into three *cardiac* severity groupings based upon specific and commonly used clinical roentgenographic and electrocardiographic criteria (Table 3). Hemodynamic indices characterizing each of these three clinical groups were compared with those of a group of volunteer subjects free of cardiovascular, renal, and hematologic disease. These findings are the subject of a previous report.[23]

TABLE 3.—*Criteria Used for Left Atrial and Left Ventricular Enlargement*

LEFT ATRIAL ENLARGEMENT

1. Terminal atrial forces in $V_1 \leq -0.04$ mm-sec [25]
2. Bipeak interval (of deeply notched P waves) ≥ 0.04 second [26]
3. Ratio of P-wave duration to P-R segment in Lead II ≥ 1.6 [27]
4. P wave in Lead II ≥ 0.3 mV or 0.12 second.[28]

LEFT VENTRICULAR ENLARGEMENT

1. Chest x-ray Ungerleider index $\geq +15$ percent [29]
2. Ungerleider index $\geq +10$ percent [30] plus electrocardiographic criteria:
   A. Precordial voltage (tallest R and deepest S waves) exceeding 4.5 mV [31]
   B. Left ventricular strain (QRS and T-wave vectors 180° apart) [32]
   C. Frontal plane QRS vector axis $\leq 0°$ [33]
3. All three (2A, B, and C) electrocardiographic criteria

Patients with essential hypertension were therefore categorized as having: no cardiac enlargement, on the basis of demonstrating no evidence of left atrial or ventricular enlargement; left atrial enlargement, by demonstrating at least two of four electrocardiographic criteria of left atrial abnormality (Table 3); or left ventricular enlargement, in which both roentgenographic and electrocardiographic criteria were employed. Thus, in this last group, left ventricular enlargement was diagnosed if the Ungerleider index was equal to, or greater, than 15 percent or if all three electrocardiographic criteria of left ventricular hypertrophy (Table 3) were present. A third criterion, using both clinical measurements, was used if the Ungerleider index was 10 percent and was also associated with at least two positive electrocardiographic criteria. In reality, if the Ungerleider index was 15 percent or all three electrocardiographic criteria were present, the third criterion (above) was usually satisfied. Patients with cardiac failure, or even those receiving digitalis were excluded from this classification.

Group Hemodynamic Characteristics. As severity of clinical hypertensive cardiovascular disease progressed in patients free of cardiac enlargement, and then, to left ventricular enlargement, so did the impairment of the hemodynamic measurements. Thus, arterial pressure and total peripheral resistance increased progressively and significantly from one group to the succeeding severity group (the level of statistical significance between successive groups was at least $p < 0.001$). Heart rate was significantly faster than normal in all hypertensive groups; but there were no significant differences among these hypertensive groups (Fig. 1). It should be emphasized that when we describe significant differences between groups (i.e., between the normal and a group of hypertensive patients) we are signaling statistically and physiologically significant *group* differences. Thus, no group of hypertensive patients demonstrates gross tachycardia or evidence of hyperkinesis such as that demonstrated by patients having thyrotoxicosis, arteriovenous fistulae, or beriberi. These physiologic differences are therefore significant in that they point up, in a sophisticated manner, differences in similar types of hypertensive patients in order to understand better those physiologic differences which exist between groups as hypertensive disease progresses.

Only with early development of cardiac involvement (left atrial enlargement) did left ventricular function become impaired (Fig. 2). Thus, even though the minute output from the heart was preserved at normal levels (cardiac output became reduced significantly only with evidence of ventricular hypertrophy), the rate of ejection of blood from the left ventricle was significantly reduced at this relatively early stage of cardiac involvement.

Since arterial pressure (systolic, diastolic, and mean) increased progressively from one hypertensive group to the succeeding severity group, left ventricular work and power neces-

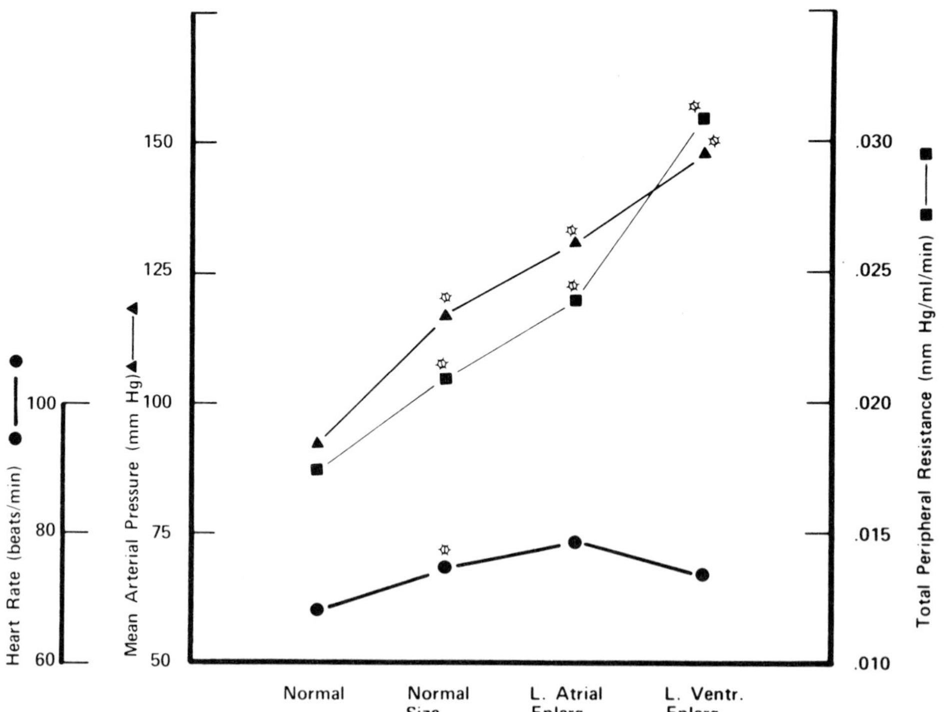

FIG. 1.—Comparison of heart rate, arterial pressure, and total peripheral resistance among the normotensive (**Normal**) and hypertensive (**Normal Size, L. Atrial Enlarg.,** and **L. Ventr. Enlarg.**) groups. Asterisk (*) denotes statistically significant difference from the preceding (severity) group.

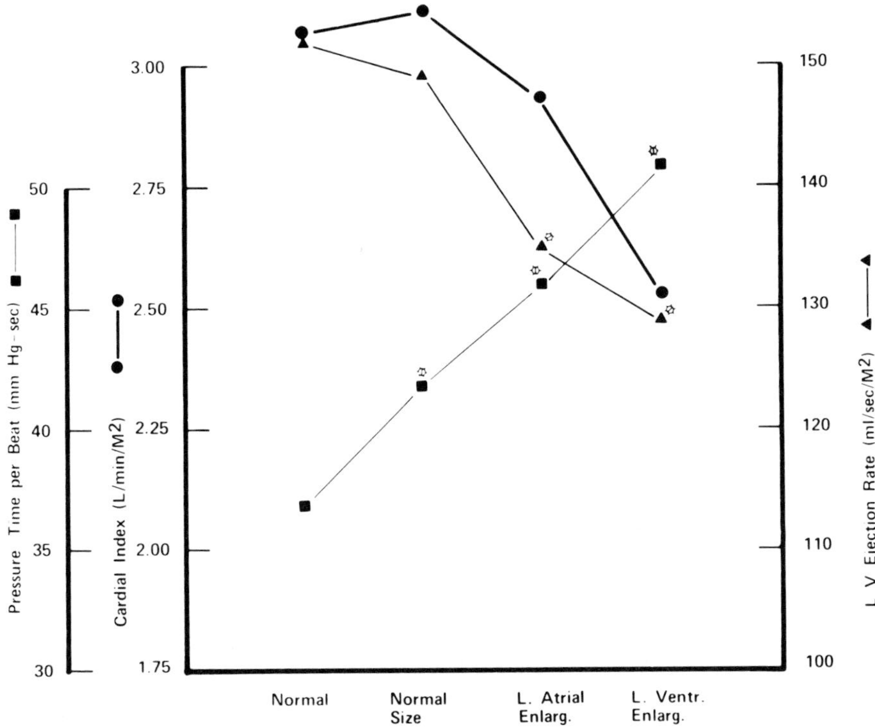

FIG. 2.—Comparison of cardiac index, left ventricular ejection rate index, and pressure-time per beat among the normotensive (**Normal**) and hypertensive (**Normal Size, L. Atrial Enlarg.,** and **L. Ventr. Enlarg.**) groups. Asterisk (*) denotes statistically significant difference from the preceding (severity) group.

sarily increased; one of the major determinants of these left ventricular functions is the mean systolic pressure. However, because the left ventricular stroke index progressively diminished (albeit insignificantly) with developing cardiac involvement, and heart rate decreased slightly with development of left ventricular hypertrophy, these ventricular functions, which reflect myocardial oxygen consumption, demonstrate the progressive myocardial involvement resulting from the unrelenting progression in vascular disease. And as total peripheral resistance significantly and progressively increased from one hypertensive severity group to the next (Fig. 1), pressure-time per beat also increased (Fig. 2). This latter estimation of ventricular function provides a valid and useful index of left ventricular oxygen consumption since it represents left ventricular tension without considering these insignificant, but measurable, group variations in heart rate.

Over twenty patients with essential hypertension underwent selective coronary arteriography because of chest-pain complaints suggesting coronary atherosclerosis. In these patients there was no evidence of occlusive coronary arterial disease and their "angina pectoris" remitted with reduction and control of arterial pressure. The hemodynamic data in these individuals were no different from the findings presented above and lend further credence that the hemodynamic alterations reflect progressive myocardial changes in response to hypertensive vascular disease rather than to coexistent myocardial impairment from associated coronary atherosclerosis.

Considerations and Discussion

These findings obtained in patients with untreated, cardiac-compensated, essential hypertension provide a new orientation to the development and progression of cardiac involvement resulting from hypertensive vascular disease. Thus, the original notion that the cardiac function in hypertension remains normal until left ventricular failure supervenes does not appear to be completely valid. Careful clinical evaluation of the hypertensive patient will permit a clinical and working classification of progressive secondary cardiac involvement from increasing severity of hypertensive vascular disease.

Thus, the earliest clinical evidence of ventricular involvement may be seen with evidence of left atrial enlargement. This abnormality can be detected with reasonable certainty with the appearance of at least two (of the four described) electrocardiographic criteria of left atrial abnormality.[34] In a large series of hypertensive patients who were matched with respect to age and sex with normal subjects, we have found that only the hypertensives demonstrated two or more of these criteria. We have also found that the existence of left atrial abnormality (in a hypertensive patient) is associated with higher systolic arterial pressures, greater frequency and incidence of arrhythmias, and is independent of coexisting occlusive coronary arterial disease.[34] A further study has shown that these electrocardiographic findings of left atrial enlargement are highly concordant with the atrial diastolic gallop rhythm (fourth heart sound).[35] Thus, there are two clinical findings (one electrocardiographic, the other auscultatory) which to the clinician should suggest developing ventricular involvement in hypertension. That these findings are related to atrial events should not indicate erroneously that the myocardial involvement first affects the left atrium. These atrial findings are only manifestations of a "hypertrophying" left ventricle and its associated decreased ventricular compliance.[36] Hence, the auscultatory event indicates that the atrium is ejecting its blood into a less compliant left ventricle;[37] and left atrial hypertrophy and abnormality detected electrocardiographically indicate the atrial response to ventricular disease. At this arbitrarily defined stage, ventricular function is already measurably impaired physiologically, as evidenced by the reduced left ventricular ejection rate and increased tension-time index and pressure-time per beat (Fig. 2). Perhaps the reason why cardiac output has not yet been reduced significantly is that the atrium is providing that augmenting "kick," as originally suggested by Braunwald and Frahm in other cardiac diseases.[38–40]

As ventricular hypertrophy develops further (as vascular disease progresses) it ultimately becomes clinically manifest by the criteria utilized (Table 3). That atrial hypertrophy already exists is demonstrated by the presence of this abnormality in all of the patients classified as having left ventricular hypertrophy. In addition, ventricular function has become further impaired so that the minute output of the left ventricle is significantly reduced, its rate of ejection is further decreased, and the work and tension developed with each beat are increased still further.[23] Although ventricular function is said to be impaired, the patients may still appear to be well compensated clinically by the adaptive hypertrophy.

This classification and delineation of patients by grouping was purely arbitrary; but it has been a useful means of identifying the physiologic progression of cardiac involvement at a time prior to development of obvious ventricular failure. Nevertheless, the stages seem to be clinically identifiable, and when so recognized should alert the physician to provide better control of arterial pressure before development of overt left ventricular failure.

Until now there have been no studies suggesting the development and progression of hypertensive heart disease in man. Studies in experimental models have included animals with banded aortas,[41] "clipped" renal arteries,[42] pretreatment with expanded intravascular volume,[43] or isoproterenol;[44] but none have been reported with chronically developing hypertension such as that found in man with essential hypertension. Physiologic or pathologic studies in man with left ventricular hypertrophy have been reported for patients with idiopathic hypertrophic subaortic stenosis,[10] aortic stenosis,[11] aortic coarctation, or in hypertensive patients who died from cardiac failure or myocardial infarction. Indeed, these clinical problems are entirely different from the circumstances associated with developing ventricular hypertrophy in man with *uncomplicated* essential hypertension. That these studies can be accomplished only by comparing group indices, renders solution of this problem even more difficult.[45] This is because morally and ethically, the clinical investigator is committed to treat his patient in order to prevent progression of the unrelenting hypertensive cardiovascular disease. Nevertheless, answers will be forthcoming from further studies similar to that reported herein or from a new animal model, the spontaneously hypertensive rat, very similar to essential hypertensive man.[46]

Speculations on the Developmental Pathophysiology in Essential Hypertension

As suggested, the phase of marked lability of arterial pressure may very well be a very early stage in the development of sustained diastolic hypertension.[47] At this stage the hyperkinetic circulatory findings might be the result of increased adrenergic cardiovascular outflow or adrenergic stimulation from modest increases in circulating angiotensin levels,[47] enhanced responses of adrenergic receptor sites,[48] other possibilities of autonomic imbalance, or a combination of any, all, or other factors. As a result, early in this "borderline" hypertension stage the increased adrenergic manifestations are reflected chronotropically by increased heart rate, inotropically by increased contractility (i.e., left ventricular ejection rate), and in the vessels by an "inappropriately" normal peripheral vascular resistance. As part of this last manifestation, peripheral venoconstriction redistributes the effective circulating intravascular volume to the central circulation, thereby further augmenting cardiac output and the hyperkinetic circulatory state.[49] As vascular involvement of progressing hypertension ensues, the further arteriolar and venular constriction promotes a progressive contraction of plasma volume [50] and a redistribution of fluid volumes to such an extent that the ratio between the plasma and the interstitial fluid compartments becomes reduced. Consequently, the augmented venous return effected by the redistribution of blood centrally in the labile and mild essential hypertensive phase, is no longer reflected in an augmented cardiac output.

Nevertheless, because of the unrelenting vascular involvement (in the untreated patient), peripheral resistance and arterial pressure increase further and plasma volume continues to contract. The latter effect (by decreasing venous return and "preload") is insufficient for the myocardium to cope with its increased work load; it must begin its adaptive hypertrophy, or "compensatory hyperfunction." [51] Because early hypertrophy is difficult to recognize (until gross measurable enlargement is apparent clinically) we have attempted to identify this early phase as the left atrial enlargement stage, possibly the early phase of "isometric hyperfunction" as described by Meerson.[51] At this stage myocardial force and velocity seem already reduced; and the myocardium can only adapt further by increasing its mass in an effort to restore function. However, even though ventricular tension increases (by greater cardiac diameter and systolic pressure) myocardial function becomes compromised (diminished rate of ejection). With development of clinically recognizable hypertrophy, function becomes further impaired, and cardiac output falls. The myocardial adaptability, at the stage of obvious clinical hypertrophy, no longer can withstand the ever-increasing peripheral resistance burden; the third stage of compensatory hypertrophy is achieved and only awaits such progressive deterioration of function (unless arterial pressure is reduced therapeutically) that cardiac failure becomes inevitable.

Thus, in severely essential hypertensive man without clinical congestive heart failure (but already with impaired myocardial function and reduced cardiac output) the already hypertrophied heart may no longer be able to adapt further by hypertrophy. How long this stable phase of hypertrophy lasts is a moot point. The myocardial work already has achieved its stage of physiologic failure, albeit it remains clinically compensated for the time being.

At this stage (clinically hypertrophied, but nonfailing) adrenergically mediated, reflexive responses become attenuated,[23] a response not unlike that of experimental studies of nonfailing hypertrophied myocardium in vitro [52] and in vivo.[53]

Summary and Conclusions

A concept of the hemodynamic characteristics of the various clinical hypertensions is presented with particular emphasis on that of essential hypertension. The concept is developed in the light of recent studies obtained in patients having various degrees of severity of hypertensive cardiac disease thereby providing validity to an arbitrary clinical classification of hypertensive heart disease (Table 4). Thus, early in hypertension when arterial pressure is elevated and there is no electrocardiographic or roentgenographic evidence of cardiac involvement (Stage I) the only cardiac effect is that of early isometric hyperfunction; these are patients with "normal-sized hearts" and increased left ventricular work. With progression of vascular disease and increasing vascular resistance the hypertrophying left ventricle is only detected electrocardiographically by the P-wave changes of left atrial abnormality and by auscultation, i.e., the fourth heart sound (Stage II). Physiologically, left ventricular function is already compromised, but resting cardiac output remains normal. Ultimately, left·ventricular hypertrophy can be detected electrocardiographically and by chest x-ray (Stage III), but by this time cardiac functional reserve is already impaired, since resting cardiac output is reduced with further deterioration of left ventricular function. Eventually, if uncorrected, the final phase (Stage IV) of hypertensive heart disease is reached with clinical evidence of left ventricular decompensation and cardiac failure. This classification is supported by a working hypothesis explaining the pathophysiologic cardiovascular mechanisms involved in the progression of hypertensive cardiovascular disease in man.

TABLE 4.—*Proposed Clinical-Physiologic Classification of Hypertensive Heart Disease*

Stage I.	Normal-sized heart with no evidence of cardiac involvement by ECG or chest x-ray
Stage II.	Early left ventricular hypertrophy as detected by left atrial abnormality (ECG) and fourth heart sound
Stage III.	Clinically evident left ventricular hypertrophy by chest x-ray and by ECG
Stage IV.	Left ventricular failure

ACKNOWLEDGMENT

Many of the studies referred to in this review were performed with the association and collaboration of my two good friends and colleagues of the Research Division, Cleveland Clinic, Doctors Harriet P. Dustan and Robert C. Tarazi, and I am indebted to them for their support, intellectual stimulation, and friendship.

REFERENCES

1. Veterans Administration Cooperative Study Group on Antihypertensive Agents. Effects of treatment on morbidity in hypertension. Results in patients with diastolic blood pressures averaging 115 through 129 mm Hg. JAMA 202:116, 1967.
2. Veterans Administration Cooperative Study Group on Antihypertensive Agents. Effects of treatment on morbidity in hypertension. Results in patients with diastolic blood pressures averaging 90 through 119 mm Hg. JAMA 213:1143, 1970.
3. Society of Actuaries. Build and Blood Pressure Study, vol. 1. Chicago: Society of Actuaries, 1959.
4. Metropolitan Life Insurance Company. Blood Pressure: Insurance Experience and Its Implications. New York: Metropolitan Life Insurance Company, 1961.
5. Pickering, G. W.: Prognosis. *In* High Blood Pressure, 2nd ed. New York: Grune & Stratton, 1968, p. 367.
6. Kirkendall, W. M.: The Heart and Hypertension. *In* Gross, F. (Ed.): Antihypertensive Therapy: Principles and Practice. New York: Springer, 1966, pp. 170–177.
7. Sarnoff, J. J., Braunwald, E., Welch, G. H., Jr., Case, R. B., Stainsby, W. N., and Marcruz, R.: Hemodynamic determinants of oxygen consumption of the heart with special reference to the tension-time index. Am. J. Physiol. 192:148, 1958.
8. Page, I. H.: The mosaic theory of arterial hypertension—its interpretation. Perspect. Biol. Med. 10:325, 1967.
9. Page, I. H.: Diet and exercise for prevention of atherosclerosis—both or neither? Mod. Med. 39:81, 1971.
10. Braunwald, E., Lambrew, C. T., Morrow, A. G., Rockoff, S.D., and Ross, J., Jr.: Idiopathic hypertrophic subaortic stenosis. Circulation 30 (Suppl. IV): 3, 1964.
11. Schlant, R. C.: Altered Cardiovascular Function of Rheumatic Heart Disease and Other Acquired Valvular Disease. *In* Hurst, J. W.,

and Logue, R. B. (Eds.): The Heart, Arteries, and Veins, 2nd ed. New York: McGraw-Hill, 1970, p. 751.
12. Gapta, T. C., and Wiggers, C. J.: Basic hemodynamic changes produced by aortic coarctation of different degrees. Circulation 3:17, 1951.
13. Werko, L., Ek, J., Bucht, H., and Karnell, J.: Cardiac output, blood pressures, and renal dynamics in coarctation of the aorta. Scand. J. Clin. Lab. Invest. 8:193, 1956.
14. Oscai, L. B., Mole, P. A., and Holloszy, J. O.: Effects of exercise on cardiac weight and mitochondria in male and female rats. Am. J. Physiol. 220:1944, 1971.
15. Spann, J. F., Jr.: Heart failure and ventricular hypertrophy, altered cardiac contractility and compensatory mechanisms. Am. J. Cardiol. 23:504, 1969.
16. Bing, O. H. L., Matsushita, S., Fanburg, B. L., and Levine, H. J.: Mechanical properties of rat cardiac muscle during experimental hypertrophy. Circ. Res. 28:234, 1971.
17. Page, I. H., and McCubbin, J. W.: Physiology of Arterial Hypertension. *In* Hamilton, W. F., and Dow, P. (Eds.): Handbook of Physiology, Section 2: Circulation, vol. 3. Washington, D.C.: American Physiological Society, 1966, pp. 2163–2208.
18. Freis, E. D.: Hemodynamics of hypertension. Physiol. Rev. 40:27, 1960.
19. Frohlich, E. D., Tarazi, R. C., and Dustan, H. P.: Re-evaluation of the hemodynamics of hypertension. Am. J. Med. Sci. 257:9, 1969.
20. Dustan, H. P., Tarazi, R. C., and Frohlich, E. D.: Pressor Mechanisms. *In* Frohlich, E. D. (Ed.): Pathophysiology: Altered Regulatory Mechanisms. Philadelphia: Lippincott, 1972, pp. 41–66.
21. Frohlich, E. D., Ulrych, M., Tarazi, R. C., Dustan, H. P., and Page, I. H.: Hemodynamics of renal arterial disease and hypertension. Am. J. Med. Sci. 255:29, 1968.
22. Frohlich, E. D., Ulrych, M., Tarazi, R. C., Dustan, H. P., and Page, I. H.: A hemodynamic comparison of essential and renovascular hypertension. Cardiac output and total peripheral resistance supine and tilted. Circulation 35:289, 1967.
23. Frohlich, E. D., Tarazi, R. C., and Dustan, H. P.: Clinical-physiological correlations in the development of hypertensive heart disease. Circulation 44:446, 1971.
24. Seldinger, S. I.: Catheter replacement of the needle in precutaneous arteriography. Acta Radiol. Scand. 15:368, 1960.
25. Morris, J. J., Jr., Estes, H. E., Jr., Whalen, R. E., Thompson, H. K., and McIntosh, H. D.: P-wave analysis in valvular heart disease. Circulation 29:242, 1964.
26. Thomas, P., and DeJong, D.: The P-wave in the electrocardiogram in the diagnosis of heart disease. Br. Heart J. 16:241, 1967.
27. Macruz, R., Perloff, J. K., and Case, R. B.: Method for the ECG recognition of atrial enlargement. Circulation 17:882, 1958.
28. Lamb, L. E.: Electrocardiography and Vectorcardiography: Instrumentation, Fundamentals, and Clinical Applications. Philadelphia: Saunders, 1965, p. 99.
29. Ungerleider, H. E.: Cardiac enlargement. Radiology 48:129, 1947.
30. Ungerleider, H. E., and Clark, C. P.: Study of the transverse diameter of the heart silhouette with prediction table based on the teleroentgenogram. Am. Heart J. 17:92, 1939.
31. McPhie, J.: Left ventricular hypertrophy: Electrocardiographic diagnosis. Australas. Ann. Med. 7:317, 1958.
32. Grant, R. P.: The Spatial Vector Approach: Clinical Electrocardiography. New York: McGraw-Hill, 1957.
33. Cumming, G. R., and Proudfit, W. L.: High-voltage QRS complexes in the absence of left ventricular hypertrophy. Circulation 19:406, 1959.
34. Tarazi, R. C., Miller, A., Frohlich, E. D., and Dustan, H. P.: Electrocardiographic changes reflecting left atrial abnormality in hypertension. Circulation 34:818, 1966.
35. Tarazi, R. C., Frohlich, E. D., and Dustan, H. P.: Left atrial abnormality and ventricular pre-ejection period in hypertension. Dis. Chest 55:214, 1969.
36. Stewart, S., Mason, D. T., and Braunwald, E.: Impaired rate of left ventricular filling in idiopathic hypertrophic subaortic stenosis and valvular aortic stenosis. Circulation 37:8, 1968.
37. Leonard, J. J., Weissler, A. M., and Warren, J. V.: Observations on the mechanisms of atrial gallop rhythm. Circulation 17:1007, 1958.
38. Braunwald, E., and Frahm, C. J.: Studies on Starling's law of the heart. IV. Observations on the hemodynamic functions of the left atrium in man. Circulation 24:633, 1961.
39. Braunwald, E.: Symposium on Cardiac Arrhythmias. Introduction: With comments on the hemodynamic significance of atrial systole. Am. J. Med. 37:665, 1964.
40. Heidenreich, F. P., Shaver, J. A., Thompson, M. E., and Leonard, J. J.: Left atrial booster

function in valvular heart disease. J. Clin. Invest. 49:1605, 1970.

41. Beznak, M.: Cardiac output in rats during the development of cardiac hypertrophy. Circ. Res. 6:207, 1958.
42. Ledingham, J. M., and Pelling, D.: Cardiac output and peripheral resistance in experimental renal hypertension. Circ. Res. 21 (Suppl. II):187, 1967.
43. Douglas, B. H., Guyton, A. C., Langston, J. B., and Bishop, V. S.: Hypertension caused by salt loading. II. Fluid volume and tissue pressure changes. Am. J. Physiol. 207:669, 1964.
44. Stanton, H. C., Brenner, G., and Mayfield, E. D., Jr.: Studies on isoproterenol induced cardiomegaly in rats. Am. Heart J. 77:72, 1969.
45. Sannersteadt, R., Bjure, J., and Varnauskas, E.: Correlation between electrocardiographic changes and systemic hemodynamics in human arterial hypertension. Am. J. Cardiol. 26:117, 1970.
46. Pfeffer, M. A., and Frohlich, E. D.: Electromagnetic flowmetry in anesthesized rats. J. Appl. Physiol. 33:137–140, 1972.
47. Frohlich, E. D., Tarazi, R. C., and Dustan, H. P.: Physiological comparison of labile and essential hypertension. Circ. Res. 18 (I):55, 1970.
48. Frohlich, E. D., Tarazi, R. C., and Dustan, H. P.: Hyperdynamic beta-adrenergic circulatory state: Increased beta receptor responsiveness. Arch. Intern. Med. 123:1, 1969.
49. Ulrych, M., Frohlich, E. D., Dustan, H. P., and Page, I. H.: Cardiac output and distribution of blood volume in central and peripheral circulations in hypertensive and normotensive man. Br. Heart J. 31:570, 1969.
50. Tarazi, R. C., Frohlich, E. D., and Dustan, H. P.: Plasma volume in men with essential hypertension. N. Engl. J. Med. 278:762, 1968.
51. Meerson, F. Z.: The myocardium in hyperfunction, hypertrophy and heart failure. Circ. Res. 25 (Suppl. II):1, 1969.
52. Spahn, J. R., Jr., Buccino, R. A., Sonnenblick, E. H., and Braunwald, E.: Contractile state of cardiac muscle obtained from cats with experimentally produced ventricular hypertrophy and heart failure. Circ. Res. 21: 341, 1967.
53. Spahn, J. F., Jr., Mason, D. T., and Zelis, R. F.: The altered performance of the hypertrophied and failing heart. Am. J. Med. Sci. 258:291, 1969.

Left Ventricular Function in Hypertensive Heart Disease

By Jay N. Cohn, M.D., Ernesto Rodriguera, M.D., and Nabil H. Guiha, M.D.

Considerable attention has been directed in recent years to the study of those factors which contribute to the genesis of hypertrophy in a ventricle chronically exposed to an increased work load.[1] Similarly, the contractile properties of the hypertrophied ventricle have been examined in a number of different ways in an attempt to resolve the conflict as to whether the hypertrophied muscle performs better than normal, normally, or less well than normal.[2–4] Little consideration has been given, however, to the reasons why symptomatic left ventricular failure develops in patients with hypertension.

Any analysis of the mechanism of congestive heart failure in hypertension must deal satisfactorily with several pertinent clinical observations. First of all, heart failure is not a predictable complication of hypertension. Some patients with severe hypertension for many years do not manifest signs of heart failure, but others seem to develop it as a relatively early complication of their disease. Indeed, the acute hypertension of glomerulonephritis and toxemia of pregnancy may be characterized by left ventricular failure even though the blood pressure is only moderately elevated. Furthermore, acute bouts of hypertension may induce left ventricular failure both in man and in experimental animals whereas gradually developing hypertension of greater severity may be tolerated without cardiac symptoms for years.[5]

The suggestion has been made frequently in the past that congestive heart failure in long-standing hypertension results from the superimposition of ischemic heart disease due to progressive coronary atherosclerosis.[6] Autopsy studies have confirmed that coronary artery disease is far more frequent in hypertensive patients dying with congestive heart failure than in those without cardiac symptoms.[7] Despite the circumstantial evidence favoring this view of the pathophysiology of hypertensive heart failure, an explanation must be provided for the usual absence in hypertensive heart failure of the symptoms and electrocardiographic signs associated with myocardial infarction or coronary insufficiency.

Some insight into the mechanism of hypertensive heart failure also may be provided by more recent studies in the area of effective drug therapy. Although earlier studies revealed an extremely poor prognosis in hypertensive patients who had exhibited signs of left ventricular failure with a mean survival of only 1.8 years,[8] recent data suggest that if blood pressure is controlled, long-term survival is possible and heart failure does not usually recur. If these observations are correct, it would seem less likely that severe coronary artery disease could be implicated as a dominant factor in the precipitation of left ventricular failure. Furthermore, these clinical observations tend to downgrade the importance of a depression in myocardial contractility in the genesis of hypertensive heart failure.[4]

To explore the mechanism of hypertensive heart failure, we have performed hemodynamic studies on two groups of male hypertensive patients.[9] One group consisted of patients with severe long-standing essential hypertension complicated by heart failure. Although one individual gave a history of angina on exertion, there was no clinical evidence of significant coronary arterial disease in the others. All had severe symptoms of left ventricular failure at the time of study. Three were studied before treatment was instituted and two were studied while they were receiving antihypertensive drugs which were not controlling their blood pressure. The other group consisted of patients of a similar age who had long-standing hypertension of similar severity but had never had

From the Veterans Administration Hospital and Georgetown University School of Medicine, Washington, D.C.

significant cardiorespiratory symptoms. Three subjects in this group had been treated with drugs which were discontinued 2 weeks prior to study. The other two had not been treated with antihypertensive agents (Table 1).

All subjects in both groups had electrocardiographic findings of left ventricular hypertrophy and x-ray findings of cardiomegaly with left ventricular prominence. Pulmonary venous engorgement was detected in all patients in the first group but none in the second.

Hemodynamic studies were performed in a catheterization laboratory with the patient resting supine in the postabsorptive state. Left ventricular filling pressure (LVFP) was assessed either by retrograde catheterization of the left ventricle or by measuring pulmonary artery wedge (pulmonary "capillary") pressure. Cardiac output was determined by the dye-dilution method and left ventricular volume was calculated from an ultrasonic measurement of left ventricular transverse internal diameter.[10]

TABLE 1.—*Clinical Data in 10 Male Hypertensive Patients Studied*

Patient	*Age (yr.)*	*Blood Pressure (mm Hg)*	*Clinical Heart Failure*
1	43	220/128	yes
2	43	212/140	yes
3	41	280/140	yes
4	51	186/130	yes
5	51	272/160	yes
6	40	248/124	no
7	48	204/110	no
8	35	192/124	no
9	44	240/130	no
10	48	243/138	no

During the control period (Fig. 1), the only striking hemodynamic difference between the two groups was that the patients with heart failure (indicated by hatched bars) all had significantly elevated LVFP whereas LVFP was normal in the nonfailure patients, despite simi-

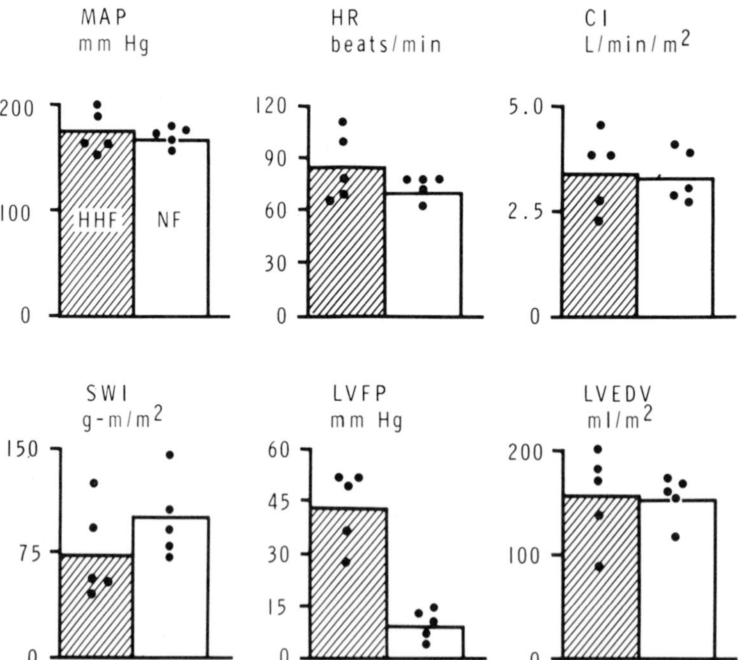

FIG. 1.—Control hemodynamics in patients with hypertensive heart failure **(HHF)** and those with severe hypertension without heart failure **(NF)**. **MAP,** mean arterial pressure; **HR,** heart rate; **CI,** cardiac index; **SWI,** stroke work index; **LVFP,** left ventricular filling pressure; **LVEDV,** left ventricular end-diastolic volume.

lar levels of arterial pressure, similar cardiac index, and a similar increase in left ventricular end-diastolic volume. Because of the increased end-diastolic volume, the ejection fraction was reduced in all these patients to an average of 0.30 in the heart failure group and 0.31 in the nonfailure group.

Thus, in this small group of patients hypertensive heart failure was not accompanied by a low cardiac output. Although other larger surveys have demonstrated a significant reduction in cardiac output in hypertensive patients with cardiac involvement, many of these latter patients may have been in an older age group with significant coronary artery disease contributing to the hemodynamic abnormality. The patients studied in the present series were younger and were selected specifically because of the severity of their hypertension and the severity of their coexistent heart failure. It is possible that the normal outputs represent a chance finding in a nonrepresentative small series, but it is also possible that in acute hypertensive heart failure of this severity the resting cardiac output remains within the normal range.

Another surprising finding in these studies is that the left ventricle was similarly dilated in all patients whereas the LVFP remained normal in the group without heart failure but was markedly elevated in the presence of heart failure. If these pressure-volume data are interpreted in terms of static diastolic compliance, one would conclude that compliance was increased in the hypertensive, nonfailing ventricle and decreased in the failing ventricle. However, the normal pressure in the dilated chamber chronically exposed to an increased work load might better be viewed as a manifestation of myocardial structural adaptation rather than increased distensibility.[11] Nonetheless, if it is assumed that the patients in the nonfailure group represent an earlier stage of the ventricular functional abnormality noted in the failure group, then the onset of failure could be viewed as a change in the ventricular pressure-volume relationship so that end-diastolic pressure rises with little or no further increase in end-diastolic volume (a decrease in compliance).

Such a thesis could be confirmed best by following a patient as he develops heart failure. Since treatment with antihypertensive drugs prevents the development of heart failure, we have not yet had the opportunity to make such observations. However, we have performed the reverse experiment by monitoring left ventricular function when arterial pressure was acutely reduced.

Intravenous infusion of sodium nitroprusside in the two groups of patients lowered arterial pressure to within or near the normotensive range within a few minutes (Fig. 2). The LVFP fell dramatically in the heart failure group from an average of 42 to 18 mm Hg, whereas in the nonfailure group the LVFP was reduced to a lower normal range. We could not detect a significant change in left ventricular end-diastolic volume during nitroprusside infusion in the nonfailure patients, but in the failure group end-diastolic volume actually rose acutely in response to the reduction in arterial pressure (Fig. 3). Therefore, an acute increase in compliance apparently occurred and the ventricle was able to accommodate a larger volume at a markedly lowered end-diastolic pressure. Furthermore, the increase in end-diastolic fiber length which must have accompanied the increase in end-diastolic volume contributed to a marked increase in stroke volume (Frank-Starling mechanism) during infusion of nitroprusside in the heart failure group. Such an increase in stroke volume was not noted in the nonfailure group, in whom no change in volume could be detected (Fig. 4). The high cardiac outputs noted in the heart failure group when arterial pressure was acutely reduced undoubtedly would have returned to normal with time as volume and vascular adjustment occurred, but studies were not continued long enough to determine the time course of these events.

As might be expected, right-sided heart pressures were elevated in the patients with heart failure but not in those without failure and these pressures also fell when arterial pressure was reduced. Since an abnormality in right ventricular compliance would be unlikely, the high pressures probably reflect an enlarged right atrial and right ventricular volume in these patients. It is therefore likely that further enlargement of the cardiac shadow noted when a hypertensive patient develops heart

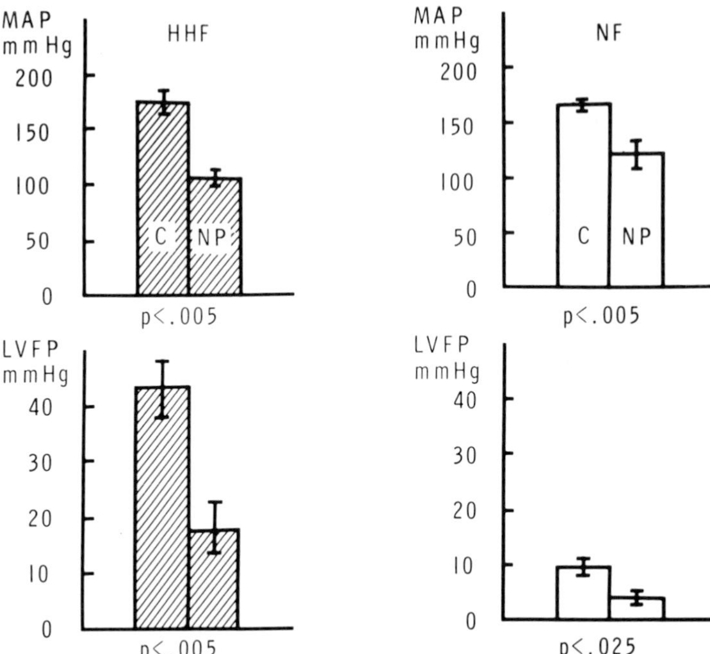

FIG. 2.—Effect of nitroprusside **(NP)** on mean arterial pressure **(MAP)** and left ventricular filling pressure **(LVFP)** in hypertensive patients with **(HHF)** and without **(NF)** heart failure. **Brackets** represent standard error of mean. **C,** control observations; **NP,** those during nitroprusside infusion.

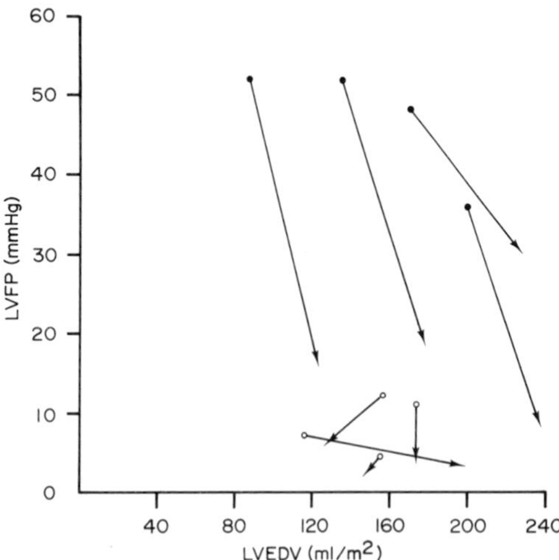

FIG. 3.—Effect of nitroprusside **(arrowheads)** on the relationship between left ventricular filling pressure **(LVFP)** and left ventricular end-diastolic volume **(LVEDV)** in patients with heart failure **(solid dots)** and patients without heart failure **(circles).**

failure may reflect enlargement of the right atrium, right ventricle, and left atrium, which dilate passively in response to the decrease in left ventricular compliance.

Although the results of these studies in the small group of patients certainly must be confirmed in a larger series, the consistency of the data makes it possible to use them in proposing a schema for the mechanism of hypertensive heart failure (Fig. 5). An increase in arterial pressure results in increased ventricular wall tension by increasing intraventricular pressure during ejection and by increasing the radius of the chamber (dilatation). This increase in wall tension, which would increase myocardial oxygen consumption,[12] is restored to normal by the development of left ventricular hypertrophy and increased wall thickness. This process of dilation and hypertrophy represents an asymptomatic phase which may continue for many years. So long as hypertrophy keeps pace with the increase in ventricular pressure or volume,

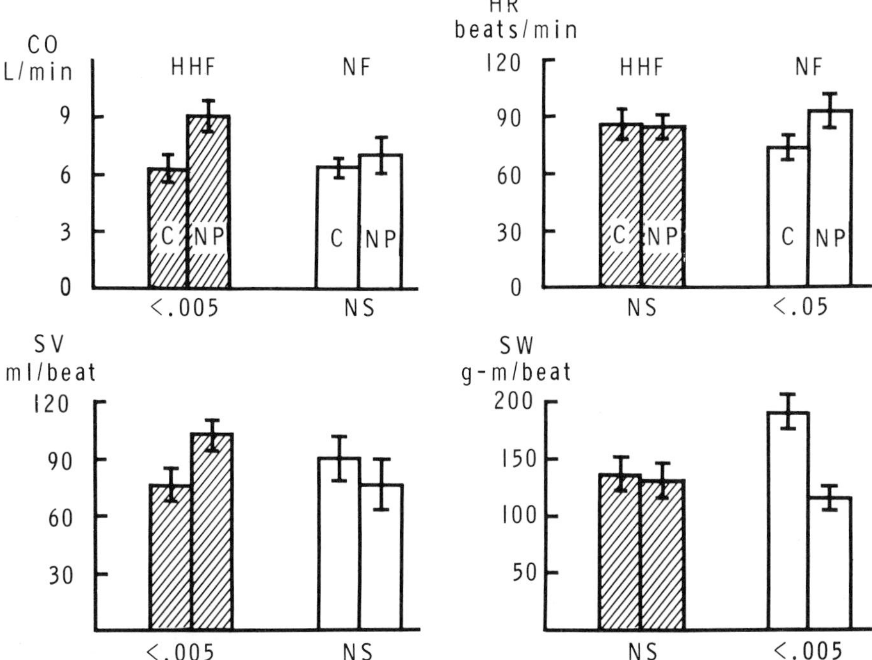

FIG. 4.—Effect of nitroprusside **(NP)** on cardiac output **(CO),** heart rate **(HR),** stroke volume **(SV),** and stroke work **(SW)** in the two groups of patients. **C,** control observations; **NP,** those during nitroprusside infusion.

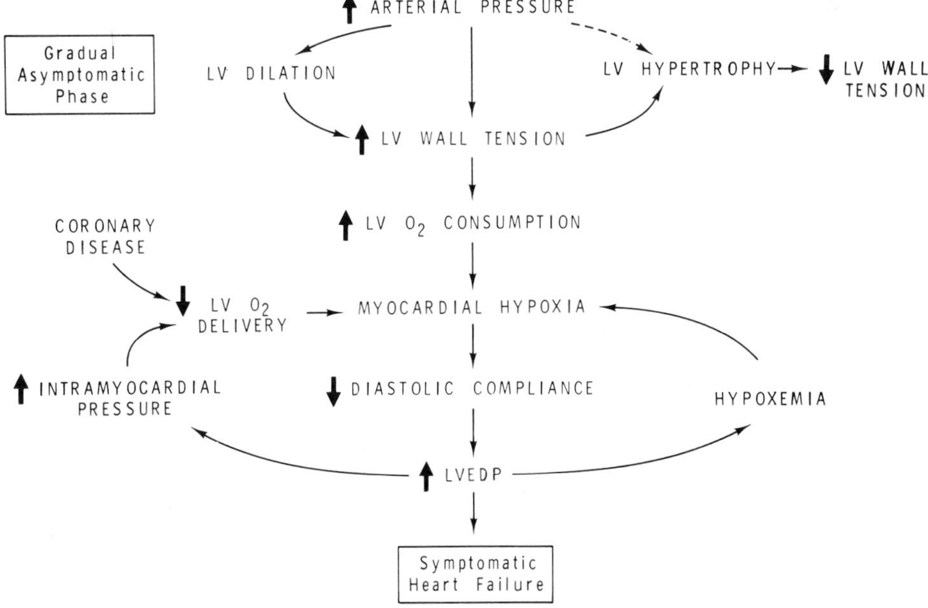

FIG. 5.—Schema showing possible mechanisms in the development of hypertensive heart failure. **LV,** left ventricular; **LVEDP,** left ventricular end-diastolic pressure.

wall tension will not rise and myocardial oxygen consumption (per tissue mass) will not be increased. However, sudden rises in arterial pressure or sudden dilation not accompanied by hypertrophy could increase myocardial oxygen consumption and induce myocardial hypoxia. Such an event might occur in glomerulonephritis or pheochromocytoma, when pressure rises suddenly in a nonhypertrophied ventricle. In the chronic hypertensive patient such an event may result from sudden acceleration of hypertension or from some limitation in the process of hypertrophy. An important contributing factor consonant with previous impressions might be the development of coronary artery disease, which would limit oxygen delivery to a ventricle with an increased oxygen requirement. Such a limitation of oxygen delivery might be most severe in the inner layers of the myocardium because of the increased intramyocardial pressure generated in this area as a result of the increased intraventricular systolic pressure.[13] Regardless of cause, however, the myocardial hypoxia would be expected to result in a decrease in diastolic compliance similar to the decreased compliance noted in acute myocardial infarction and angina pectoris.[14,15] A rise in left ventricular end-diastolic pressure would result and lead directly to pulmonary capillary hypertension, pulmonary congestion, arterial hypoxemia, and perhaps to further myocardial hypoxia. In addition, the increase in diastolic pressure in the left ventricle might aggravate the endocardial flow deficiency by impeding flow during diastole. The end result of these and other positive feedback mechanisms would be progressively severe left ventricular failure which can be relieved most effectively by lowering arterial pressure.

These studies in this highly selected group of hypertensive patients are not intended to provide a global view of heart failure occurring in the natural course of hypertension. Sodium retention with expansion of extracellular volume undoubtedly contributes to the rise in cardiac filling pressure. The sequence of the cardiac hemodynamic and renal excretory abnormalities is not known. Nonetheless, the increase in intravascular volume in the heart failure patient undoubtedly is an important factor contributing to the increased cardiac output when arterial pressure is acutely reduced. Although considerable left ventricular dilatation was detected in all these severely hypertensive patients, even in the absence of cardiac symptoms, an increase in ventricular volume may not always accompany long-standing hypertension. In patients with less severe chronic hypertension significant left ventricular dilatation may not occur until heart failure is precipitated by progressive coronary artery disease with loss of muscle mass or impairment in myocardial function. Such a sequence of events may be more common in patients whose blood pressure is partially or completely normalized with drug therapy. Furthermore, the left ventricular dilatation noted in the patients in this series need not be viewed as irreversible, even though it was not corrected by acute reduction in arterial pressure. More detailed sequential studies of left ventricular hemodynamics in hypertension are needed before the relationships between ventricular hypertrophy, ventricular dilatation, myocardial metabolism, and myocardial performance are understood.

In summary, symptomatic heart failure which develops in the patient with chronic severe hypertension appeared to be related to an acute, reversible reduction in left ventricular compliance which can be explained best as a response to myocardial hypoxia. Although impairment of myocardial contractility may accompany the ventricular hypertrophy, especially when significant ischemic heart disease coexists, the most effective therapy for hypertensive heart failure is to reduce myocardial oxygen consumption by lowering arterial pressure.

References

1. Meerson, F. Z.: The myocardium in hyperfunction, hypertrophy and heart failure. Circ. Res. 25 (Suppl. 2):1, 1969.
2. Alexander, N., Goldfarb, T., and Drury, D. R.: Cardiac performance of hypertensive aorta-constricted rabbits. Circ. Res. 10:11, 1962.
3. Geha, A. S., Duff, J. P., and Swan, H. J. C.: Relation of increase in muscle mass to performance of hypertrophied right ventricle in the dog. Circ. Res. 19:255, 1966.
4. Spann, J. F., Buccino, R. A., Sonnenblick, E. H., and Braunwald, E.: Contractile state of cardiac muscle obtained from cats with

experimentally produced ventricular hypertrophy and heart failure. Circ. Res. 21:341, 1967.

5. Pickering, G.: High Blood Pressure, 2nd ed. New York: Grune & Stratton, 1968, p. 359.
6. Fishberg, A. M.: Hypertension and Nephritis, 5th ed. Philadelphia: Lea & Febiger, 1954, p. 774.
7. Averbuck, S. H.: Heart failure in hypertension. Am. Heart J. 11:99, 1936.
8. Goldring, W., and Chasis, H.: Hypertension and Hypertensive Disease. New York: Commonwealth Fund, 1944.
9. Rodriguera, E., Guiha, N., and Cohn, J. N.: Left ventricular function in hypertensive heart failure (HHF). Circulation 44:476, 1971.
10. Popp, R. L., Wolfe, S. B., Hirata, T., and Feigenbaum, H.: Estimation of right and left ventricular size by ultrasound. A study of the echoes from the interventricular septum. Am. J. Cardiol. 24:523, 1969.
11. Linzbach, A. J.: Heart failure from the point of view of quantitative anatomy. Am. J. Cardiol. 5:370, 1960.
12. Sonnenblick, E. H., Ross, J., Jr., and Braunwald, E.: Oxygen consumption of the heart. Newer concepts of its multifactoral determination. Am. J. Cardiol. 22:328, 1968.
13. Kirk, E. S., and Honig, C. R.: Nonuniform distribution of blood flow and gradients of oxygen tension within the heart. Am. J. Physiol. 207:661, 1964.
14. Broder, M. I., Rodriguera, E., and Cohn, J. N.: Evolution of abnormalities in left ventricular function after acute myocardial infarction. Ann. Intern. Med. 74:817, 1971.
15. Dwyer, E. M., Jr.: Left ventricular pressure-volume alterations and regional disorders of contraction during myocardial ischemia induced by atrial pacing. Circulation 42:1111, 1970.

Retinopathy in Essential Hypertension

By Colin T. Dollery, M.B., and D. A. Archer, M.B.

COTTON-WOOL SPOTS and hemorrhages in the retinas of patients with severe hypertension were described within a few years of the invention of the ophthalmoscope although at that time they were linked with Bright's disease rather than with the level of blood pressure.[1] Bull, in 1886, pointed out that patients with neuroretinitis and Bright's disease had a poor prognosis.[2] Two-thirds of 87 patients he followed were dead within a year of the development of neuroretinitis. Bull anticipated the work of Keith, Wagener, and Barker at the Mayo Clinic more than 50 years later.[3] The work of Keith and his colleagues is still widely used as the basis for classification of the severity of hypertension and it is the purpose of this chapter to reconsider the usefulness of this classification in the light of recent work on the retinal circulation.

The grading system evolved by the Mayo Clinic group relied upon the presence of arterial changes to define the first two grades and hemorrhages, exudates, and papilledema to define the third and fourth. The pathologic changes underlying the first and second grades are very different and they will be discussed separately.

Arterial Changes (Keith-Wagener-Barker Grades I and II)

Features

In hypertensive patients the retinal arteries are often diffusely or irregularly narrowed, the vessel wall is less translucent than normal, and an increased reflection from it gives it a shiny appearance. Where the artery crosses a vein the darker venous blood column can no longer be seen through the artery and the caliber of the vein may be reduced at the crossing. If the "nip" is severe, the blood may be dammed back upstream ("banking") and severe crossing abnormalities sometimes form the origin of a branch retinal vein thrombosis.

The pathologic mechanisms underlying these changes in the appearance of the vessels are often misunderstood. Retinal arteries which vary in caliber from about 100 μ downward are too small to be involved by atheroma. Two processes are at work. The first is active vasoconstriction usually accompanied by smooth-muscle hypertrophy. This is the pathology which underlies the generalized vessel narrowing found in young patients with severe hypertension. If the blood pressure is lowered promptly the vessels may dilate and return to a nearly normal appearance.[4] The second process is diffuse fibrosis and hyalinization with the replacement of the smooth muscle. These changes are found in long-standing hypertension and their clinical counterpart is caliber irregularity, increased light reflex, and nipping of veins. These changes appear to be irreversible and when the blood pressure is lowered the larger vessel affected by them either does not change in caliber or becomes narrower.

Prognostic Significance

Keith, Wagener, and Barker[3] claimed that these features were of value in predicting the prognosis of patients with hypertension but this has been doubted in recent years for two main reasons. The first is that many patients with an elevated pressure do not have these features, and the second is recognition that they are common in normotensive elderly people.

Bechgaard, Kopp, and Nielsen[5] studied 500 patients with a blood pressure exceeding 160/100 mm Hg. Two-thirds of these patients were judged to have arteries with a normal caliber and just over half had a normal light reflex. Only 10 percent had very narrow arteries and 7 percent had major irregularities of vessel caliber. Van Buchem, Heuvel-Aghina, and Heuvel[6] have pointed out that arterial narrowing and an increased light reflex may be found in normotensive individuals. These workers

From the Department of Clinical Pharmacology, Royal Postgraduate Medical School, University of London, London, England.

This work was supported by the Medical Research Council and the Wellcome Trust.

also found that crossing changes were related to the patient's age. Only 13 percent of men aged 40 to 44 years had them compared with 43 percent in the 55 to 59 age group. Attempts to put arterial narrowing on a quantitative basis have been of little avail because of the variable branching pattern of the retinal vessels.[7] The most recent effort to quantitate the retinal vascular changes in hypertension was made by Kagan, Aurell, and Tibblin[8] as part of an epidemiologic study of men born in 1913 in Gothenburg, Sweden. They found that the arteries were on average narrower in hypertensive patients, but the overlap between groups was so great that the values were of little use in classification.

On the basis of these findings, we have argued that classification of hypertensive patients grounded on the basis of changes in the retinal arteries is of little or no value.[9]

Hemorrhages, Exudates, and Papilledema (Keith-Wagener-Barker Grades III and IV)

Bull's observation concerning the poor prognosis of patients with Bright's disease who develop neuroretinitis has been repeatedly confirmed. The presence of papilledema in a hypertensive patient indicates a very poor prognosis unless the blood pressure is lowered rapidly and effectively. Several large series of patients studied before effective antihypertensive medication became available showed that approximately 90 percent of such patients die within 1 year of the diagnosis being made.[3,10] The presence of hemorrhages and cotton-wool spots without papilledema also indicates a bad prognosis in the absence of treatment. In the series reported by Keith, Wagener, and Barker the mean survival time of such patients was only 15 months.

Features

The earliest features are the formation of fine linear hemorrhages lying radially among the nerve fibers accompanied by white spots varying from about 0.1 to 1 mm in diameter in the nerve-fiber layer. These white spots have been given various names, but the descriptive term "cotton-wool spot" is to be preferred to "soft exudate" because they are infarcts and not exudates.

Cotton-wool spots appear first as a grayish indistinct area in the retina which evolves in a day or two into a shiny white spot with frayed indistinct edges. Both cotton-wool spots and hemorrhages are most common around the main vessel groups within about 3 diam of the disc. Cotton-wool spots clear within 6 to 12 weeks and as they do so they become dull, white, and granular. Appearance of fresh cotton-wool spots is a danger signal indicating poor pressure control.

Hard fatty exudates appear as minute, clearly demarcated, white spots. They may not be present when a patient first presents with cotton-wool spots and hemorrhages, but they appear during treatment, and their appearance at this stage does not indicate ineffective therapy. If the patient has been left untreated for some time, all three features may coexist and the hard fatty exudates spreading radially like spokes of a wheel from the macula may form a macular star figure.

The first change in the optic disc is a pinkish coloration due to hyperemia. Later the disc margin becomes indistinct and the physiologic cup is filled in. Usually the patient is treated before papilledema becomes severe and with treatment papilledema regresses in a few weeks to a few months. It may increase in severity for a few days after hypotensive therapy has begun. Papilledema in hypertension is rarely unilateral, but it may be more prominent on one side than on the other. If a hypertensive patient develops papilledema without cotton-wool spots or hemorrhages in the retina, thought should be given to alternative causes such as a cerebral tumor.

The most important step in understanding the pathologic processes underlying the retinopathy of accelerated hypertension has come from a combination of fluorescence angiography and new experimental pathologic techniques. In particular, these have clarified the nature and significance of the cotton-wool spot.

The Cotton-Wool Spot

Fluorescence angiography in patients with accelerated hypertension shows that vascular lesions are commonly associated with cotton-wool spots (Figs. 1 through 3). The most common abnormality is aneurysmal dilatation of capillaries around the edge of the area occupied by the cotton-wool spot. These aneurysms sometimes form a complete ring around the white area.[11,12] The appearance on the fluorescence angiograms is very similar to that demonstrated in pathologic specimens by Ashton.[13,14] Fluorescein leaks from the aneurysms giving a ring-like appearance on photographs taken after the vascular bed has been emptied of dye. The central part of the cotton-wool spot often remains dark on fluorescence studies and this appearance suggests that the capillary bed is not perfused. As the spots fade, capillary perfusion is restored although sometimes a few aneurysms remain.

One of the most interesting findings in fluorescence angiograms of patients with accelerated hypertension is the points of dye leakage upon retinal arterioles of about 15 mμ-diameter.[11] These are found only in patients who have not been treated and are actively forming fresh cotton-wool spots. These leaking points most often lie upon the arteriole supplying an area of retina occupied by a cotton-wool spot or where one is soon to form. However, a few leaking points are not associated with cotton-wool spots or hemorrhages.

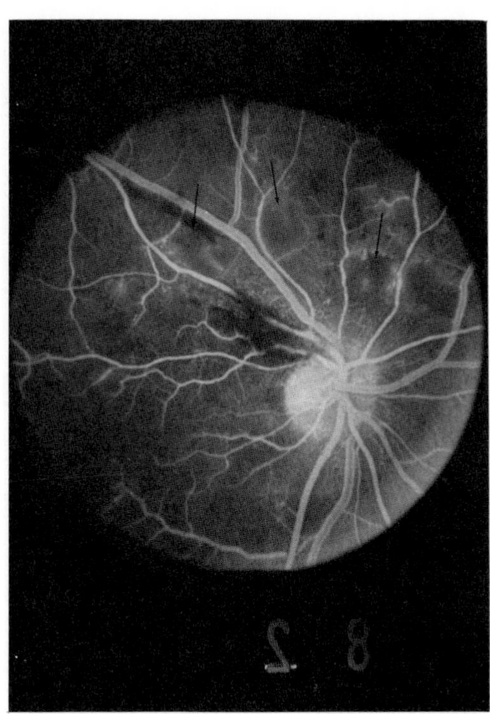

FIG. 2.—A capillary-phase fluorescence angiogram of the patient shown in Fig. 1. The capillary bed underlying the cotton-wool spots is not perfused **(arrows)**.

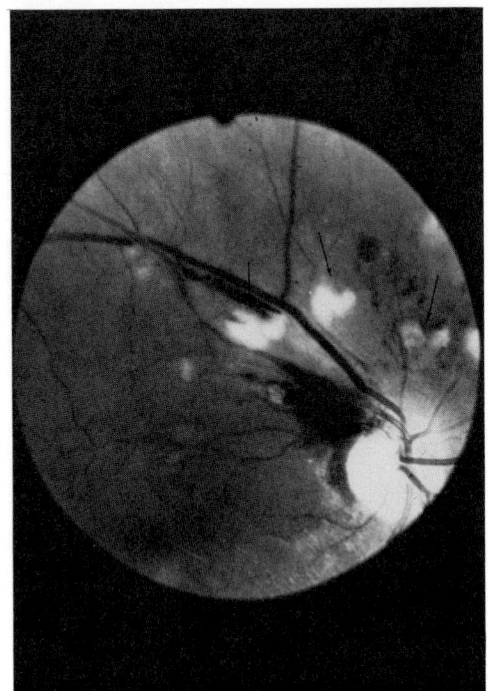

FIG. 1.—The retina of a patient with accelerated hypertension. Note numerous cotton-wool spots **(arrows)** and hemorrhages.

The finding of leaking points upon the feeding arterioles in untreated accelerated hypertension suggested that they must be related to the causation of the cotton-wool spots downstream, but further progress on this point had to await animal experiments.

Animal Studies

The pig retina provided the first satisfactory model of the formation of cotton-wool spots. The experiments were designed to study the circulatory changes that followed acute interruption of the arterial blood supply by embolizing the retinal vessels with glass microspheres. Two days later these animals had typical retinal cotton-wool spots in the territory

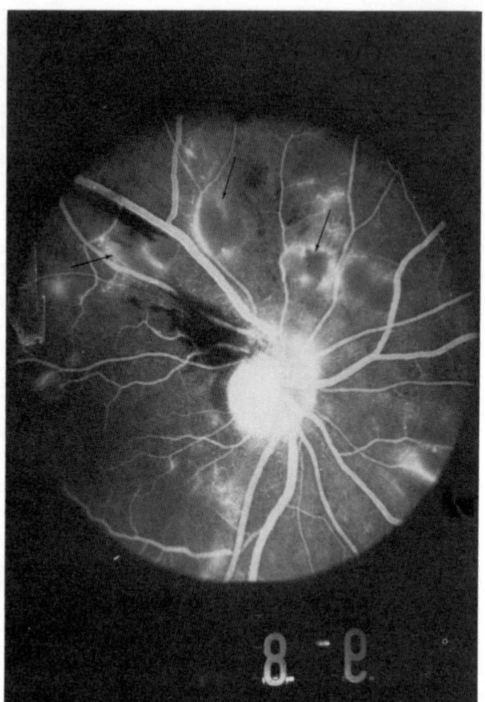

FIG. 3.—Appearance of patient in Fig. 2, taken 4 seconds later. Leakage of fluorescein is taking place from blood vessels around the edge of the cotton-wool spots **(arrows).**

of the embolized artery (Fig. 4). A further point of resemblance to the human lesions was that the point at which the embolus lodged often leaked fluorescein, and pathologic studies suggested that this occurred because of local trauma to the vessel which disrupted the continuity of the endothelium. Pathologic studies of the cotton-wool spots formed showed that they were identical to the human lesions and consisted of swollen axons some of which were broken and forming terminal swellings of Cajal. Later these terminal swellings accumulated cell organelles into a central mass or "pseudonucleus." These are the cytoid bodies, the typical pathologic feature of the cotton-wool spot. These studies settled beyond doubt that the cotton-wool spot was an infarct in the nerve-fiber layer. It formed as a result of ischemic damage to the axons and later resolved through phagocytosis by macrophages.[15] However, there are no glass-sphere emboli in accelerated hypertension and doubts remained about the precise mechanism involved in the formation of these lesions in hypertensive patients. These questions were answered by another animal model.

Retinopathy in animals with experimental hypertension has been reported by several authors. Keyes and Goldblatt[16] noted superficial retinal hemorrhages and retinal edema in animals with renal hypertension. Byrom[17] and Uyama[18] found that rats with hypertension originating from a renal artery developed both general and focal narrowing of their retinal arteries and this was reversible by removing the clip. Experimental hypertension in macaque monkeys causes a retinopathy which very closely resembles the fundus of humans with accelerated hypertension.[19] The retinal lesions include flame-shaped hemorrhages, cotton-wool spots, hard fatty exudates, and arterial changes. A conspicuous feature of fluorescein angiograms of these animals has been multiple leaking spots on small retinal arteries at an early stage of the development

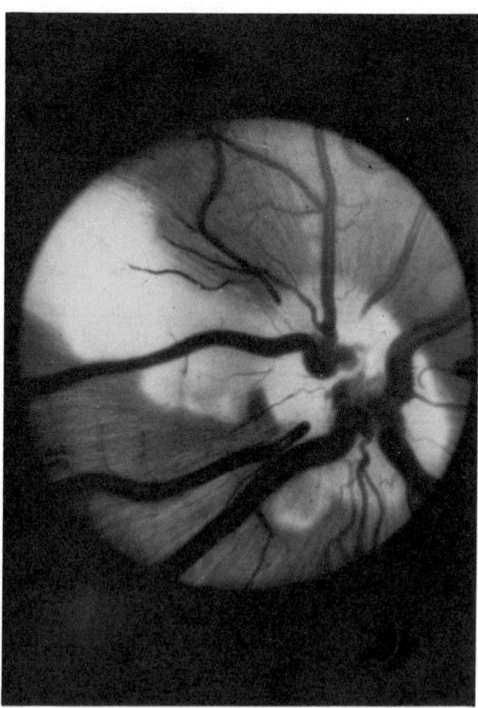

FIG. 4.—A hog retina taken 2 days after glass microspheres were injected into the carotid artery. Two cotton-wool spots have appeared at the edge of the optic disc. Glass spheres are visible in the lumen of the artery supplying the larger one.

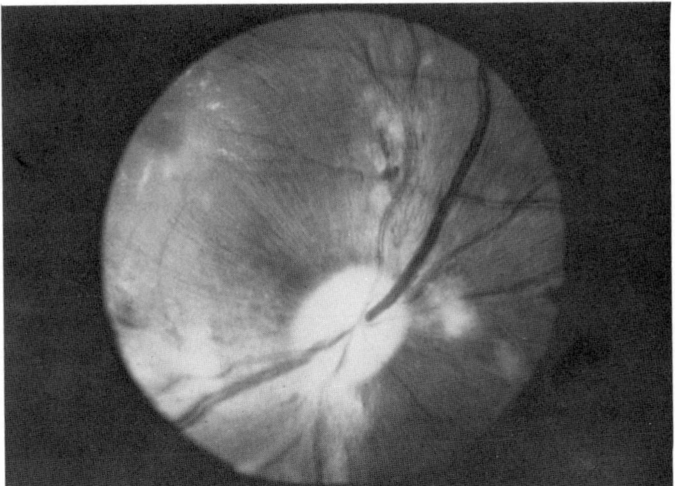

FIG. 5.—The retina of a macaque monkey with accelerated hypertension caused by renal encapsulation. There are several small cotton-wool spots and hemorrhages.

of hypertension (Figs. 5 and 6). These changes are very reminiscent of the leaking points found on human retinal arterioles in patients with untreated accelerated hypertension.[11] Pathologic investigations have shown that these vessels have leaked plasma into their walls with deposition of fibrin and necrosis of smooth-muscle cells. Thus the underlying pathologic lesion in accelerated hypertension is arteriolar necrosis, in the retina as it is elsewhere in the body.

The precise mechanism whereby severe hypertension causes focal damage to the arteriolar wall is unknown. In the kidney this lesion leads to nephron damage and ultimately to uremia. In the retina it causes infarction of small areas of the nerve-fiber layer and the appearance of cotton-wool spots. The presence of these lesions in the retina is a direct clinical indication that hypertension has entered a rapidly progressive phase in which the kidneys are liable to severe and irreversible damage. It

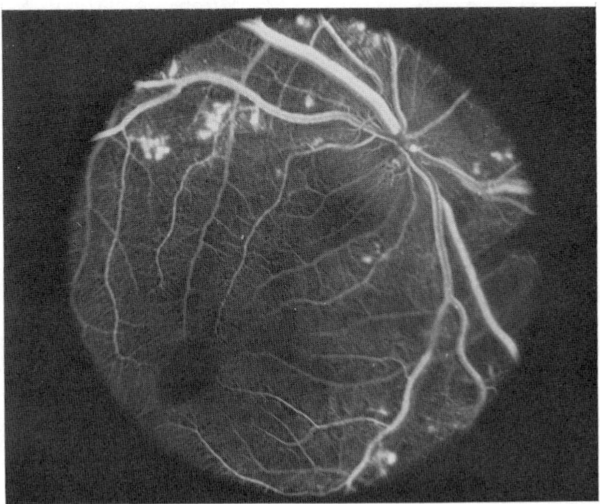

FIG. 6.—A capillary-phase fluorescence angiogram of the same area as seen in Fig. 5. There are numerous points of focal damage to small arterioles which leak fluorescein.

is vital to detect this clinical sign if present and to initiate blood pressure reduction as soon as possible.

Conclusions

There are several important distinctions to be made between the first two grades of the Keith-Wagener-Barker classification and the second two. The arterial changes are a graded characteristic prone to observer error and similar changes are found as a result of aging. In contrast, the clinical features of Grades III and IV are clear-cut and are not found in normal people. It is true that cotton-wool spots and hemorrhages are found in other conditions such as severe anemia, after severe hemorrhage, in diabetes, etc., but the differentiation between these conditions on other grounds is usually obvious. The first two grades have no specific pathology whereas the pathology underlying Grades III and IV is fibrinoid necrosis of the wall of small arterioles. In the absence of treatment, Grades III and IV have a fairly uniform and bad prognosis whereas Grades I and II are so heterogeneous as to be of little prognostic significance and should be discarded.

Retinopathy of Grades III and IV can conveniently be grouped together as the retinopathy of accelerated hypertension, since without treatment Grade III usually progresses to Grade IV. This condition is most often found in young and middle-aged patients with very high levels of pressure. The diastolic blood pressure often exceeds 140 mm Hg. Accelerated hypertension is uncommon in older people, although hypertension is very common among them. Leishman [20] suggested that this is because aging changes in blood vessels tended to protect them from the high pressure. He called this "defence by sclerosis." The retinal features of accelerated hypertension remain a most important clinical sign.

References

1. Liebreich, R.: Ophthalmoskopisher Befund bei Morbus Brightii. Graefe Arch. Ophthal. 5:265, 1859.
2. Bull, C. S.: Analysis of 103 cases of exudative neuroroetinitis associated with Bright's disease. Trans. Am. Ophthalmol. Soc. 4:184, 1886.
3. Keith, N. M., Wagener, H. P., and Barker, N. W.: Some different types of essential hypertension; their course and prognosis. Am. J. Med. Sci. 197:332, 1939.
4. Ramalho, P. S., and Dollery, C. T.: Hypertensive retinopathy. Calibre changes in retinal blood vessels following blood-pressure reduction and inhalation of oxygen. Circulation 37:580, 1968.
5. Bechgaard, P., Kopp, H., and Nielsen, J. H.: 1000 hypertensive patients followed from 16–22 years. Acta Med. Scand. 154(Supp. 312): 175, 1956.
6. van Buchem, F. S. P., von der Heuvel-Aghina, J. W. M., and von der Heuvel, J. E. A.: Hypertension and changes of the fundus oculi. Acta Med. Scand. 176:539, 1964.
7. Stokoe, W. L., and Turner, R. W.: Normal retinal vascular pattern. Arteriovenous ratio as a measure of arterial caliber. Br. J. Ophthalmol. 50:21, 1966.
8. Kagan, A., Aurell, E., and Tibblin, G.: Signs in the fundus oculi and arterial hypertension. Bull. WHO 36:231, 1967.
9. Wise, G. N., Dollery, C. T., and Henkind, P.: The Retinal Circulation. New York: Harper & Row, 1971.
10. Kincaid-Smith, P., McMichael, J., and Murray, E. A.: The clinical course and pathology of hypertension with papilloedema (malignant hypertension). Q. J. Med. 27:117, 1958.
11. Hodge, J. V., and Dollery, C. T.: Retinal soft exudates. A clinical study by colour and fluorescence photography. Q. J. Med. 33:117, 1964.
12. Mizobe, A., Murai, S., and Mizushima, N.: Fluorescein studies of hypertensive retinopathy. Jap. Circ. J. 31:789, 1967.
13. Ashton, N.: Retinal microaneurysms in the non-diabetic subject. Br. J. Ophthalmol. 35: 189, 1951.
14. Ashton, N.: Diabetic retinopathy. A new approach. Lancet 2:265, 1959.
15. Ashton, N., Dollery, C. T., Henkind, P., Hill, D. W., Paterson, J. W., Ramalho, P. S., and Shakib, M.: Focal retinal ischaemia: Ophthalmoscopic, circulatory and ultrastructural changes. Br. J. Ophthalmol. 50:281, 1966.
16. Keyes, J. E. L., and Goldblatt, H.: Experimental hypertension. IV. Clinical and pathological studies of the eyes. Arch. Ophthalmol. 17:1040, 1937.
17. Byrom, F. B.: The nature of malignancy in hypertensive disease. Evidence from the retina of the rat. Lancet 1:516, 1963.
18. Uyama, M.: A clinical observation of the rat

eye with experimental hypertension. Acta Soc. Ophthalmol. Jap. 70:1321, 1966.
19. Ashton, N., Peltier, S., and Garner, A.: Experimental hypertensive retinopathy in the monkey. Trans. Ophthalmol. Soc. U.K. 88: 167, 1968.
20. Leishman, R.: The eye in general vascular disease, hypertension and arteriosclerosis. Br. J. Ophthalmol. 41:641, 1957.

The Malignant Phase of Essential Hypertension

By Gaddo Onesti, M.D., Kwan Eun Kim, M.D.,
and Charles Swartz, M.D.

The characteristics of malignant hypertension were defined by Volhard and Fahr in 1914.[1] They included: (1) the presence of severe fixed hypertension; (2) the presence of severe retinopathy with exudates, hemorrhages, and papilledema; (3) a severe impairment of renal function; (4) a rapidly progressive clinical course terminating most frequently with death in uremia; and (5) from a histologic standpoint, the presence of diffuse vascular lesions affecting chiefly the kidney and taking the form of fibrinoid necrosis of the arterioles and intimal proliferation of the small-caliber arteries. These criteria continue to be valid and well accepted in their entirety a half-century later.

Objections, however, have been raised to papilledema as an essential sign of malignant hypertension by Perera.[2] Similarly, McMichael and Murphy [3] contended that renal failure was not always present in malignant hypertension. It is our opinion that the consideration of such objections is not helpful, as it is now apparent that we are dealing with the linear course of a dynamic entity in which manifestations may appear at varying time intervals.

In 1935, Derow and Altschule [4] made the important contribution that malignant hypertension is not a separate nosologic entity, but a clinical syndrome that may occur secondary to renal parenchymal disease, pheochromocytoma, and Cushing's disease as well as essential hypertension. Finally, in 1939 [5] Fishberg introduced the term "the malignant phase of essential hypertension," and implied that this was not a distinct disease entity but "an ominous form of that very common disease, essential hypertension."

It is well known that the malignant phase of essential hypertension, if untreated, terminates rapidly in the death of the patient [5–8] and that the most common cause of death is uremia due to extensive malignant nephrosclerosis.[5–9] A controversy has existed for many years as to whether the lesions of malignant nephrosclerosis represent the cause [10] or the effect of severe blood pressure elevation.[11] It is our opinion that the majority of experimental [11–13] and clinical [5,9,14,15] evidence indicates that the renal lesions are secondary to the hypertension and that, in fact, the kidney is the main target organ of this hypertensive process.

Volhard [16] considered the possibility that hypertension in the malignant phase might be due to the release of a vasopressor substance by the kidney initiated by arteriolar spasm; the arteriolar anatomical lesions were considered to be another consequence of this vascular spasm. Both arteriolar fibrinoid necrosis and arterial intimal proliferation would then lead to further release of vasopressor material by the kidney. Thus, a vicious circle would be established in the malignant phase of essential hypertension. Since 1966 we have had the opportunity to conduct serial hemodynamic observations in six patients with the "malignant phase of essential hypertension" and terminal uremia who underwent bilateral nephrectomy while on a maintenance hemodialysis program. The results of these studies have clarified the concept of the vicious circle suggested by Volhard.[16]

To draw valid pathophysiologic conclusions, it is necessary to establish the diagnosis of the "malignant phase of essential hypertension" without any evidence of primary renal disease. Such a diagnosis in our series was based on the following criteria:

1. No previous history of primary renal parenchymal disease
2. Absence of stenosis of renal arteries or branches demonstrated by renal angiography

---

From the Division of Nephrology and Hypertension, Department of Medicine, Hahnemann Medical College and Hospital, Philadelphia, Pennsylvania.

3. Definite family history of hypertension
4. Severe retinopathy with papilledema, hemorrhages, and exudates
5. Histologic diagnosis of malignant nephrosclerosis with no evidence of primary or interstitial renal disease.

In all the patients studied, mild or moderate diastolic hypertension had been present for 2 to 3 years before the onset of the malignant phase.

Bilateral nephrectomies were performed after 2 to 3 months of hemodialysis and after all standard treatment modalities for hypertension had failed.

Removal of both kidneys resulted in an immediate decrease in blood pressure in every instance. Figure 1 illustrates the effect of bilateral nephrectomy on the blood pressure of a patient in this series. There was a dramatic decrease in blood pressure. Sodium balance was kept constant before and after bilateral nephrectomy (total exchangeable sodium between 37 and 45 mEq per kilogram of body weight) by appropriate ultrafiltration dialysis. Thus, the decrease in blood pressure was not due to changes in sodium balance but to the removal, with the nephrectomy, of a "renal vasopressor factor" responsible for the malignant phase. Approximately 12 to 14 weeks after bilateral nephrectomy was performed, the retinal hemorrhages, exudates, and papilledema had cleared, leaving only a Grade II hypertensive retinopathy. Concomitantly there was a generalized clinical improvement characterized by better cerebration, increased appetite, and a better state of nutrition. It is apparent that the clinical features of the malignant phase of essential hypertension had been reversed by bilateral nephrectomy. It is also apparent (Fig. 1) that approximately 7 weeks after the nephrectomy, mild diastolic hypertension was again present (diastolic blood pressure between 110 and 120 mm Hg). This phenomenon was observed in all six patients studied, with a

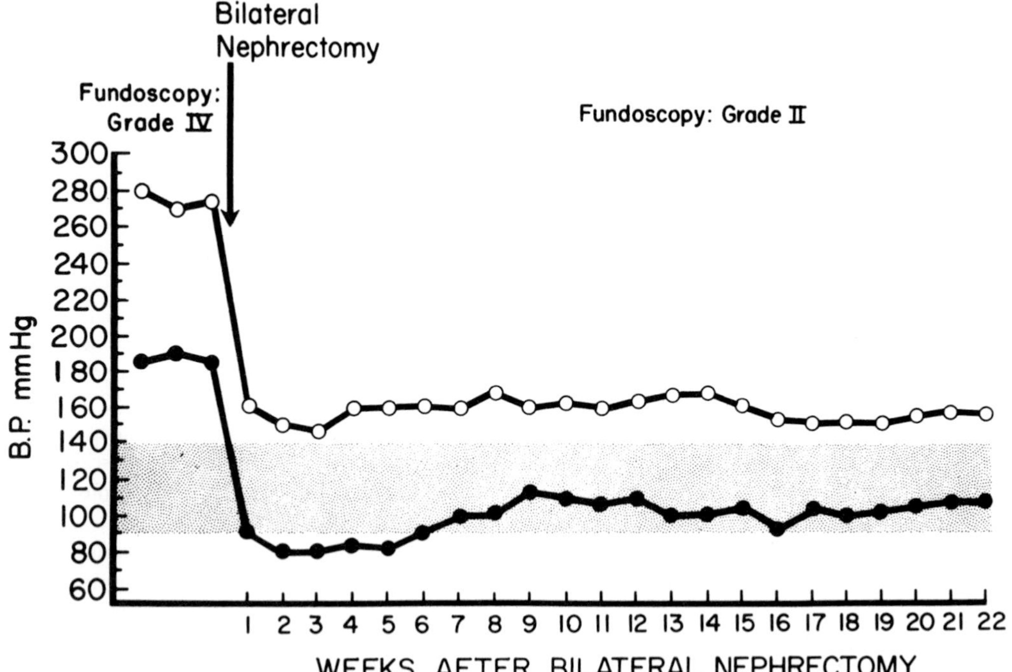

Fig. 1.—Effect of bilateral nephrectomy on the blood pressure of a 34-year-old female with essential hypertension in the malignant phase with terminal malignant nephrosclerosis and uremia. The patient was maintained on hemodialysis before and after bilateral nephrectomy. Salt and water balance was maintained constant by ultrafiltration dialysis.

follow-up period of from 6 months to 3 years. Our interpretation of these findings is that the persistent diastolic hypertension in the anephric state (without sodium chloride and water excess) represents the moderate essential hypertension that affected these patients prior to the onset of the malignant phase. The presence of a family history of hypertension in all these patients emphasizes again the importance of the genetic factor in essential hypertension (see Part III). Thus, essential hypertension appears to persist in the anephric state. Bilateral nephrectomy, however, reverses the malignant phase and the diastolic pressure remains significantly lower in the absence of the kidneys. Furthermore no retinal hemorrhages, exudates, or papilledema recur following nephrectomy. While bilateral nephrectomy exerted no effect on essential hypertension in this series of patients, it invariably reversed the malignant phase.

Figure 2 represents the effect of bilateral nephrectomy on mean arterial pressure, cardiac output (dye-dilution technique) and total peripheral resistance in the second patient of this series. Before bilateral nephrectomy, the mean arterial pressure was 190 mm Hg. This was associated with a very high total peripheral vascular resistance (4000 dynes per second per cm^{-5}). Bilateral nephrectomy resulted in an immediate decrease in mean arterial pressure from 190 to 90 mm Hg. At the same time, cardiac output increased progressively and total peripheral resistance decreased. Long-term hemodynamic follow-up (from 6 months to 3 years) has shown that this hemodynamic effect persists. Total peripheral resistance remains lower and cardiac output higher in the

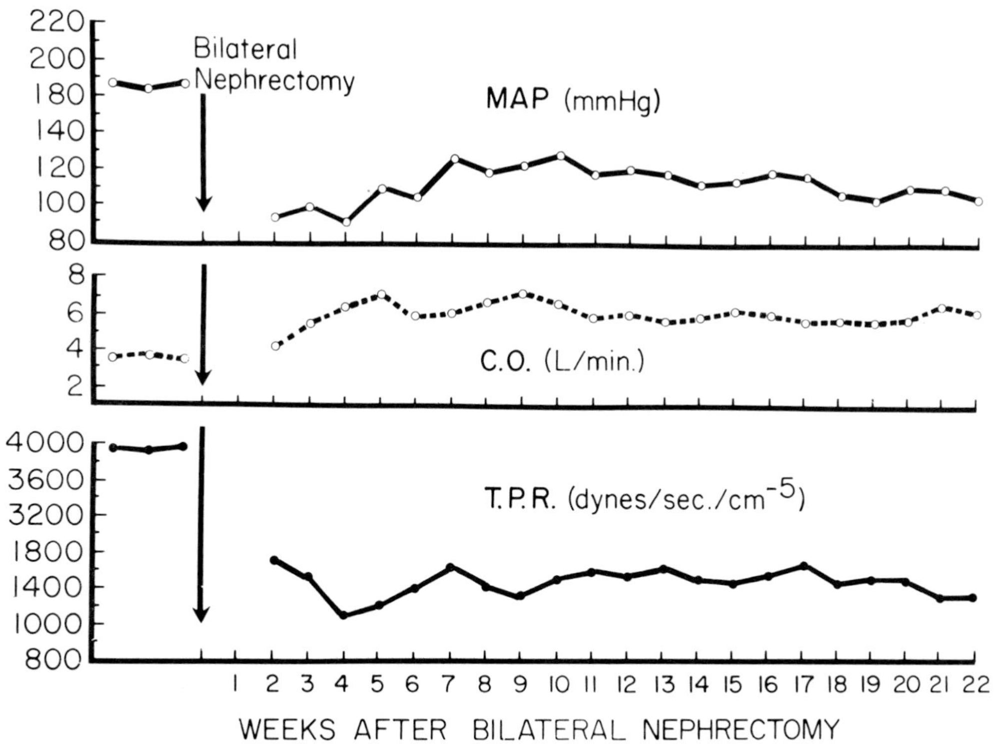

FIG. 2.—Hemodynamic effect of bilateral nephrectomy in a 37-year-old female with essential hypertension in the malignant phase with terminal malignant nephrosclerosis and uremia. The patient was maintained on hemodialysis before and after bilateral nephrectomy. Salt and water balance was maintained constant by ultrafiltration dialysis. **MAP,** mean arterial pressure; **C.O.,** cardiac output (in liters per minute); **T.P.R.,** total peripheral resistance (dynes per second per cm^{-5}).

absence of renal tissue. This hemodynamic pattern was recognized in all six patients studied.

The hemodynamic studies described indicate that, with the removal of the kidneys, a vasoconstrictor agent of renal origin has been removed. We therefore postulate that the severe blood pressure elevation of the "malignant phase of essential hypertension" is the result of renal vasopressor material that elevates the total peripheral resistance and depresses cardiac output.

In keeping with this concept, in 1964 Grollman [17] reported that the renal venous effluent in malignant hypertension contained a pressor substance similar to that secreted by the kidney in surgically remediable hypertension. The identity of this vasopressor factor is not clearly established. Renin, angiotensin, and aldosterone have been found to be elevated in the majority of patients with the malignant phase of essential hypertension.[18,19]

In our series, peripheral plasma renin activity [20] was studied before bilateral nephrectomy on a diet containing 10 mEq of sodium per day and subsequently on a diet containing 100 mEq of sodium per day. The results are shown in Table 1. The normal values for this laboratory are up to 1,600 ng per 100 ml. Peripheral plasma renin activity was significantly elevated in every patient on the 10 mEq-sodium diet, varying between 2,800 and 10,000 ng per 100 ml. Furthermore, it remained elevated on the higher sodium intake (100 mEq per day). It is therefore apparent not only that renin was elevated, but that it remained abnormally high even in the face of high salt intake.

TABLE 1.—*Peripheral Plasma Renin Activity Before Bilateral Nephrectomy in Six Patients with the Malignant Phase of Essential Hypertension and Uremia (Supine Position)*

Patient	*Diet: 10 mEq per day (in ng per 100 ml)*	*Diet: 100 mEq per day (in ng per 100 ml)*
1	4,300	3,600
2	10,000	6,000
3	4,600	4,200
4	10,000	3,600
5	3,600	3,800
6	2,800	3,000

The resolution of the malignant hypertension syndrome in our patients following bilateral nephrectomy indicates that the "malignant phase of essential hypertension" is renal in origin. The persistence of moderate diastolic hypertension in the anephric state, even in the absence of sodium chloride and water excess, suggests that essential hypertension continues to be present after removal of both kidneys.

The high values of peripheral plasma renin activity prior to bilateral nephrectomy in all of our patients, and the failure of high salt intake to suppress renin, suggest that inappropriate hypersecretion of renin may play a role in the pathophysiology of the malignant phase of essential hypertension.

A cause-and-effect relationship between renin and blood pressure elevation has, however, not been established.[21,22]

Regardless of the possible role of the renin-angiotensin system, the hemodynamic studies presented support the existence of a potent vasopressor function of the kidneys with malignant nephrosclerosis. Thus, the concept expressed by Volhard of a vicious circle [16] in the malignant phase of essential hypertension appears to be confirmed. According to this concept, the kidney is both the cause of the malignant phase and the target of it. The precise stimulus responsible for the secretion of vasopressor material by the kidney and the initiation of the malignant phase remains unknown.

REFERENCES

1. Volhard, F., and Fahr, K. T.: Die Brightsche Nierenkrankheit: Klinik, Pathologie und Atlas. Berlin: Springer, 1914.
2. Perera, G. A.: Hypertensive vascular disease; description and natural history. J. Chron. Dis. 1:33, 1955.
3. McMichael, J., and Murphy, E. A.: Methonium treatment of severe and malignant hypertension. J. Chron. Dis. 1:527, 1955.
4. Derow, H. A., and Altschule, M. D.: Malignant hypertension. N. Engl. J. Med. 213:951, 1935.
5. Fishberg, A. M.: Hypertension and Nephritis, 4th ed. Philadelphia: Lea & Febiger, 1939.
6. Kincaid-Smith, P., McMichael, J, and Murphy, E. A.: The clinical course and

pathology of hypertension with papilledema (malignant hypertension). Q. J. Med. 27:117, 1958.

7. Dustan, H. P., Schneckloth, R. E., Corcoran, A. C., and Page, I. H.: The effectiveness of long-term treatment of malignant hypertension. Circulation 18:644, 1958.
8. Moyer, J. H., Heider, C., Pevey, K., and Ford, R. V.: The effect of treatment on the vascular deterioration associated with hypertension with particular emphasis on renal function. Am. J. Med. 24:177, 1958.
9. McMahon, H. E., and Pratt, J. H.: Malignant nephrosclerosis (malignant hypertension). Am. J. Med. Sci. 189:221, 1935.
10. Montz, A. R., and Oldt, M. R.: Arteriolar sclerosis in hypertensive and non-hypertensive individuals. Am. J. Pathol. 13:679, 1937.
11. Wilson, C., and Byrom, F. B.: Renal changes in malignant hypertension; experimental evidence. Lancet 1:136, 1939.
12. Byrom, F. B., and Dodson, L. F.: The causation of acute arterial necrosis in hypertensive disease. J. Pathol. Bacteriol. 60:357, 1948.
13. Masson, G. M. C., Corcoran, A. C., and Page, I. H.: High arterial pressure as a primary cause of hypertensive vascular lesions. Cleve. Clin. Q. 26:24, 1959.
14. Heptinstall, R. H.: Renal biopsies in hypertension. Br. Heart J. 16:133, 1954.
15. McCormack, L. J., Beland, J. F., Schneckloth, R. E., and Corcoran, A. C.: Effect of antihypertensive treatment on the evolution of renal lesions in malignant nephrosclerosis. Am. J. Pathol. 34:1011, 1958.
16. Volhard, F.: Der arterielle Hochdruck. Verh. Dtsch. Ges. Inn. Med. 35:134, 1923.
17. Grollman, A.: Antihypertensive and pressor agents of renal origin. Can. Med. Assoc. J. 90:299, 1964.
18. Hollenberg, N. K., Epstein, M., Basch, R. I., Couch, N. P., Hickler, R. B., and Merrill, J. P.: Renin secretion in essential and accelerated hypertension. Am. J. Med. 47:855, 1969.
19. Creditor, M. C., and Loschky, U. K.: Plasma renin activity in hypertension. Am. J. Med. 43:371, 1967.
20. Boucher, R., Veyrat, R., de Champlain, J., and Genest, J.: New procedures for measurement of human plasma angiotensin and renin activity levels. Can. Med. Assoc. J. 90:194, 1964.
21. Macdonald, G. J., Lovis, W. J., Renzini, V., Boyd, G. W., and Peart, W. S.: Renal-clip hypertension in rabbits immunized against angiotensin II. Circ. Res. 27:197, 1970.
22. Reubi, F., and Hodler, J.: L'activité rénin au cours des néphropathies parenchymateuses avec ou sans hypertension. Actual. Nephrol. 9:221, 1968.

Hypertension: A Precursor of Arteriosclerosis

By Quentin B. Deming, M.D., Marie M. Daly, Ph.D., and Harvey Wolinsky, M.D., Ph.D.

Humans with above-average arterial blood pressure do not die of the pressure itself but of ischemic damage secondary to degenerative arterial disease which itself is secondary (at least in part) to the elevated blood pressure. Humans who die of the complications of degenerative arterial disease usually have had elevated blood pressure.

This degenerative disease of arteries is conventionally divided into categories which include atherosclerosis and arteriolosclerosis, as well as localized weakening of the vessel wall of different sorts and locations which result in dissections and aneurysms of both large and small vessels.

Atherosclerosis accounts for most coronary, aortic, and peripheral vascular disease, some renal disease, and perhaps 60 to 70 percent of stroke. Pickering [1] has emphasized that hemorrhagic stroke may result from rupture of Charcot-Bouchard aneurysms. (It may, of course, originate from the larger berry aneurysms of the circle of Willis.) He considers Charcot-Bouchard unrelated to atherosclerosis. Most pathologists consider arteriolosclerosis, which accounts for much of the renal disease, to be distinct from atherosclerosis. Whether the pathogeneses of these three lesions, each of which is blood-pressure-dependent, are, in fact, unrelated or have a common cause has not been demonstrated.

It may not be surprising that the end result of the same process looks different in an arteriole, which has negligible amounts of collagen and elastin and a narrow lumen, than it does in a major elastic vessel with a wide lumen. It may not be surprising that a lesion dependent on hemodynamic stresses has a different frequency in the coronaries which have no flow during systole and which are supported from the outside by the myocardium for much of their lengths.

The following facts have been established beyond a reasonable doubt. Morbidity and mortality from the major complications of arteriosclerosis: i.e., cerebral infarction (both thrombotic and hemorrhagic); cardiac infarction; renal failure; aortic dissection; and peripheral sclerosis are directly related to blood pressure.

This is true if one studies a population free of clinical evidence of vascular disease. The incidence of new cerebral, coronary, or peripheral vascular disease will be proportional to blood pressure.[2,3] It is equally true if one studies a population of those who have already manifested coronary or cerebral vascular disease.[4] The recurrence rate of cardiac infarction in those who have angina or have already experienced one infarction is much higher in hypertensives than in normotensives.[5]

This correlation between ischemic damage and blood pressure is more evident with systolic blood pressure than with diastolic.[4] The correlation holds down to and below levels of blood pressure usually accepted as normal.[2,3,6]

The correlation holds in both sexes and in all ages.[6]

The etiology of the elevation of blood pressure is irrelevant to its sequelae but the height and duration of elevation are relevant.

So far we have referred to a correlation between blood pressure and the results of arterial disease. There is very good evidence that the rate of development of degenerative arterial disease itself, including specifically (but not exclusively) the rate of atherogenesis, is directly related to the blood pressure. Again the correlation is closer with systolic than with diastolic blood pressure.[7–9]

The effect of systemic blood pressure elevation is not quantitatively identical in all arterial beds. It is, for example, greater in the cerebral than the coronary vasculature. The effect is

From the Departments of Medicine, Biochemistry, and Pathology, Albert Einstein College of Medicine, Bronx, New York.

local. The effect on the vessels is seen at sites where the pressure is high, not where it is not high. However, systemic lipid metabolism may be altered.[10]

Lowering an elevated blood pressure does affect the rate of atherogenesis favorably in animals [11] and also the incidence of at least some of the complications of arteriosclerosis in man.[12] Specifically it has been shown to decrease the occurrence or recurrence rate of stroke,[13] to decrease the occurrence or progression of dissection,[14] and to slow the progress of renal disease.[15] It also decreases angina and relieves heart failure.[1,16]

However, it is not yet clear what effect lowering blood pressure has on the progress of coronary disease. It is not certain whether the effect in stroke is as true for thrombotic as for hemorrhagic events. Some of the beneficial effects previously cited represent merely decreased metabolic demand in an underperfused tissue. Some may represent decreased stress on a damaged vessel wall, without necessarily representing a healing process. We do not know whether there is a decreased rate of vessel degeneration nor do we know if there is reversal of established vascular damage.

What accounts for the difference in response between the cerebral, coronary, and peripheral vascular beds? Does the vessel wall, altered by previous hypertension, continue as an atherogenic stimulus or does it heal? How soon in the course of hypertension must blood pressure be controlled? How important is blood pressure for the action of other "risk factors"? Are blood pressure and cholesterol truly independent variables? What is the effect of being male or female on the action of hypertension?

An approach to these questions requires an understanding of the pathogenesis of degenerative arterial disease and the role of blood pressure in it. We have no such understanding. The following is a review of some of the experimental observations which have so far been made in the field and a consideration of where they leave us at the moment.

First we will consider experimental atherosclerosis per se and cholesterol metabolism. We know that experimental hypertension, as produced by a variety of methods—renal, renovascular, adrenal, or genetic, increases the rate of development and the severity of dietary atherosclerosis. This has been shown in dogs,[17] rabbits,[18] and rats.[19] This is also true in humans.

We also know that if rats are made hypertensive and then their blood pressures are controlled pharmacologically the rate of atherogenesis is slower than if their blood pressures are not controlled.[10,11] In this study the animals had not been hypertensive very long before treatment was instituted so it is difficult to determine the relevancy of this to a human whose "hypertension" may be recognized at 35 but whose blood pressure may actually have been above the optimal for his age for 35 years.

Blood pressure affects cholesterol metabolism in the following manner:

1. Elevation of blood pressure increases the concentration of cholesterol in serum of rats [19] and dogs.[17] Data relevant to humans are conflicting. It has been shown that decreasing hypertension lowers serum cholesterol in man.[20–22]

2. Elevation of blood pressure increases the concentration and total content of cholesterol in the liver and in the whole body of rats.[19]

3. While it is not certain how these effects are produced it has been shown that: [10] (a) Hypertension does not decrease the rate of metabolism or excretion of labeled cholesterol; (b) hepatic cholesterol synthesis, as measured by incorporation of intraperitoneally injected acetate 1-C^{14}, is more rapid in hypertensive than in normotensive rats. The effect, if any, of hypertension on absorption of dietary cholesterol has not been established.

Elevation of blood pressure results in an increase in both concentration and total content of cholesterol in the arterial wall. Aortic cholesterol synthesis, as measured in vitro or in vivo by the incorporation of labeled acetate or mevalonate into cholesterol, is more rapid in aortas of hypertensive than of normotensive rats.[23]

The effect of blood pressure on aortic cholesterol concentration is independent of serum cholesterol concentration. Hypertension increases aortic cholesterol at any serum cholesterol concentration. Dietary hypercholesterolemia, on the other hand, may have comparatively little effect on cholesterol in the aortic wall in the absence of hypertension.[3]

The increased atherogenesis caused by hypertension is also independent of the effect on serum cholesterol.[10,19] The concentration of cholesterol in the sera of parabiotic twin rats is kept identical by the cross circulation but when one member of such a pair is made hypertensive it develops atherosclerosis more rapidly than its normotensive partner.[10,11]

The fact that arterial cholesterol metabolism is altered in vitro indicates that it results from some change which has been produced in the arterial wall by exposure to pressure rather than being a direct result of the intraluminal pressure itself. To look for the primary event we must consider what changes are produced in arteries by elevation of the blood pressure.

Both Karsner [24] and Wolinsky [28] have pointed out that many of the vascular changes seen with hypertension are similar to those we associate with aging. Changes which are common to both hypertension and aging include: thickening of the wall; dilation of the vessel (both lumen and wall); increase in muscle; increase in collagen; increase in elastin; increase in mucopolysaccharides; decrease in elasticity; and increase in metabolic rate or oxygen consumption.

The arteries dilate and the diameter of the lumen increases. The dilated wall is, of course, less distensible, more stiff, as Aars [25] has shown. We are used to seeing this in the aged. It occurs at an early age in the hypertensive.

Karsner [24] has suggested that hypertension produces accelerated aging of vessels. On the basis of calculated wall stresses in vessels of aged animals, we consider it more likely that the changes we associate with aging are the result of the stress of "normal" blood pressure operating over a longer period in a progressively dilating vessel.

Are, in fact, those who demonstrate aging changes, those whose blood pressures are or have been on the high side of normal? It is, of course, a self-intensifying process since as the lumen dilates, calculated tension on the wall increases even at a fixed intraluminal pressure (law of Laplace).

The result, so far as the wall is concerned, is that of hypertension even though the patient is normotensive. Furthermore, as the vessel dilates its increased stiffness raises the systolic pressure.

The arteries get bigger in the presence of hypertension. Enlargement of the ventricle in hypertension has been observed since Bright's initial observation and has been shown to be proportional to height and duration of elevation of blood pressure.[1] The same is true of arteries. It may be useful to think of arteries as being similar to the heart. Some of the same things happen to them. The weight of the aortas of hypertensive rats increases as much proportionately as the weight of the left ventricle.[26]

In aging normotensive humans the vessel wall thickens progressively until by the age of 60 it may have tripled in thickness. The vascular thickening associated with hypertension is therefore more easily appreciated in younger individuals and is partially obscured in the elderly by the similar change which would have occurred in the absence of hypertension.

The medial area on cross section is increased by hypertension.[27,28] (The medial area is a function of both diameter and wall thickness.) Wolinsky [29] has shown that the wall thickening results not from an increase in the number of medial lamellar units but from an increase in the thickness of individual lamellar units. Though normally in mammals the number of units is related predictably to the normal calculated tangential tension,[29] increased tension resulting from hypertension does not increase the number of these units. Tension per lamellar unit is therefore greatly elevated. Tension per unit of wall thickness (wall stress), however, normalizes with time because of the progressive wall thickening.

The media consists of three principal elements, smooth-muscle cells and the two structural proteins they secrete, collagen and elastin. In the presence of hypertension the absolute amounts of all three components increase.[30,31] A marked, disproportionate increase in alkali-soluble, noncollagenous protein is indicative of the increase in muscle mass which is evident on histologic inspection and there is a modest increase in DNA, suggesting the presence of hyperplasia. This increase in smooth muscle occurs within a few weeks after the induction of hypertension. An increase in collagen and elastin in the media does occur progressively but less rapidly than the increase in smooth muscle. That this increase is due to new synthesis is suggested by an increased lysine content of the elastin. The absolute amounts of both collagen and elastin which accumulate are proportional to the height and duration of the elevation of blood pressure.[32] Thus the ratio of muscle to fiber rises at first as muscle increases faster than fibrous proteins; then the ratio normalizes as the amount of fibrous protein increases greatly without much further increase in smooth muscle. All these changes tend to be more marked in male than in female animals.

If the hypertension is reversed in the non-growing female rat the thickness of the vessel wall decreases strikingly. This reversibility is not so evident in the continuously growing male rate. In animals of either sex the muscle mass decreases to that appropriate to the lower blood pressure within 2 months. However, the increased mass of collagen and elastin which has accumulated during the period of hypertension shows no decrease 3 months after lowering blood pressure in females and may even show some further increase in males. It is of some interest that estrogen treatment of hypertensive males has been shown to inhibit almost completely the accumulations of fibrous protein usually seen in the media. The increase in the cellular component is also decreased but not eliminated. Androgens have recently been shown to exert an opposite effect and one not merely reflecting an estrogen deficit.

Kajimahara and Ooneda [33] and Salgado [34] have demonstrated necrosis of muscle cells in the media of hypertensive arteries. In the smaller vessels, muscle is the principal support of the wall. In the larger vessels muscle cells provide some support themselves but more importantly they are the source of the fibrous proteins which provide the rest of the support. It seems conceivable that extensive necrosis of muscle cells in severe hypertension might be related to the pathogenesis of vascular aneurysms, whether located in the lenticulostriate vessels of man or the mesenteric arteries of the rat. Extensive cellular damage of this sort could also be related to the beginnings of atherosclerotic lesions.

Increased blood pressure produces another change in artery wall, a generally increased rate of metabolism with a marked increase in oxygen consumption.[30] This is not surprising since there is an increased mass of contractile muscle and an increased rate of synthesis of proteins. It was suggested by Daly that the simultaneous increase of oxygen demand and increase of the distance oxygen was required to diffuse because of the increase of wall thickness might lead to areas of relative anoxia and damage. This she thought might be a cause of degeneration and necrosis (as myocardial hypertrophy has been proposed as a cause of coronary insufficiency [35]). This postulate basically proposes that medial muscle hypertrophy in itself may be a cause of atherosclerosis.

To test this hypothesis we sought a way of producing increased muscle stress (as a stimulus to hypertrophy) without increased intraluminal pressure. We administered a lathyrogen, β-aminopropionitrile (BAPN), to growing rats, reasoning that if the development of the collagen and elastin structure of the arteries was impaired the muscle cells would be stressed by a greater proportion of the normal blood pressure and should hypertrophy. Exposure of such animals to an atherogenic diet demonstrated that BAPN, like hypertension, causes a marked acceleration of atherogenesis. Appropriately enough the distribution of the atherosclerosis is different in the two conditions. The atherosclerosis associated with hypertension in rats is most marked peripherally, where there is normally a higher proportion of muscle and less fibrous protein to share the load. The atherosclerosis associated with lathyrism is most marked proximally where there is normally a larger proportion of fibrous protein, which is now weakened.

The results fit the theory but, of course, they do not establish its validity. Muscular hypertrophy in these animals has been assumed but not established. The experiment may simply be another example of atherosclerosis occurring at any site of injury. This seems to happen whether the provoking agent is endogenous or exogenous.

Changes in the arteries caused by hypertension are, of course, not limited to the media. Still [36] has clearly demonstrated intimal changes including gaps in the internal elastic lamella and localized infiltration of mononuclear cells. There is intimal thickening. The farther peripherally one goes in the arterial tree the greater in proportion is the intimal change.

There are critically important questions about the relationship between hypertension and atherosclerosis which we are still unable to answer and which we may not be able to answer until we understand the pathogenesis of the relationship.

Why is the correlation between blood pressure and disease of the cerebral vessels closer than that between blood pressure and disease of the coronaries? Is this, as Sir George Pickering believes, only because part of the cerebral disease is represented by aneurysm formation? No, the correlation between blood pressure and atheroma of the cerebral vessels is also close. What is the relationship between blood pressure, age, aneurysm formation, and atherogenesis? Is the difference between the cerebral vessels and the coronaries a hemodynamic one related to the differences in anatomy and flow characteristics? There is good anatomic reason for assuming this may be part of it. What is the role of the sex hormones and what is the effect of these hormones at different ages? Are the indications for hormone replacement different in hypertensives from those in normotensives? Are the deleterious effects of hypertension reversible? Animal work suggests that they are to some extent. However, if dilation of a vessel, once produced, initiates a self-sustaining process resembling that of aging then the time of diagnosis and initiation of treatment may be important. If the effects of aging are the effects of lower blood pressures over longer periods of time, at how low a blood pressure should treatment be considered?

The information necessary to supply answers to these questions is still missing.

References

1. Pickering, G.: High Blood Pressure. New York: Grune & Stratton, 1968.
2. Kannel, W. B., Castelli, W. P., and McNamara, P. M.: The coronary profile: 12 year follow-up in the Framingham study. J. Occup. Med. 9:611, 1967.
3. Kannel, W. B., Dawber, T. R., and McNamara, P. M.: Vascular disease of the brain, epidemiologic aspects: The Framingham study. Am. J. Public Health 55:1355, 1965.
4. Deming, Q. B.: Blood pressure: Its relation to atherosclerotic disease of the coronaries. Bull. N.Y. Acad. Med. 44:968, 1968.
5. Weinblatt, E., Shapiro, S., Frank, C. W., and Sager, R. V.: Prognosis of men after first myocardial infarction: Mortality and first recurrence in relation to selected parameters. Am. J. Public Health 58:1329, 1968.
6. Lew, E. A.: Build and Blood Pressure Study, vols. 1 and 2. Chicago: Society of Actuaries, 1959.
7. Davis, D., and Klainer, M. J.: Studies in hypertensive heart disease. 1. The incidence of coronary atherosclerosis in cases of essential hypertension. Am. Heart J. 19:185, 1940.
8. Evans, P. H.: Relation of long-standing blood pressure levels to atherosclerosis. Lancet 1: 516, 1965.
9. Paterson, J. C., Mills, J., and Lockwood, C. H.: The role of hypertension in the progression of atherosclerosis. Can. Med. Assoc. J. 82:65, 1960.
10. Deming, Q. B.: Experimental atherosclerosis and hypertension. *In* Gross, F. (Ed.): Antihypertensive Therapy (Principles and Practice). Berlin: Springer, 1966, p. 111.
11. Deming, Q. B.: The effect of pharmacologic control of previously established hypertension on the development of dietary atherosclerosis in rats. *In* Brest, A. N. and Moyer, J. H. (Eds.): Hypertension: Recent Advances. Philadelphia: Lea & Febiger, 1961, p. 160.
12. Veterans Administration Cooperative Study Group on Antihypertensive Agents: Effects of treatment on morbidity in hypertension. II. Results in patients with diastolic blood pressure averaging 90 through 114 mm Hg. JAMA 213:1143, 1970.
13. Marshall, J.: A trial of long-term hypotensive therapy in cerebrovascular disease. Lancet 1:10, 1964.
14. Wheat, M. W., Palmer, R. F., Bartley, T. D., and Seelman, R. C.: Treatment of dissecting aneurysms of the aorta wtihout surgery. J. Thorac. Cardiovasc. Surg. 50:364, 1965.
15. Moyer, J. H., Heider, C., Pevey, K., and Ford, R. V.: The effect of treatment on the vascular deterioration associated with hypertension,

with particular emphasis on renal function. Am. J. Med. 24:177, 1958.

16. Smirk, F. H., Hamilton, M., Doyle, A. E., and McQueen, E. G.: The treatment of hypertensive heart failure and of hypertensive cardiac overload by blood pressure reduction. Am. J. Cardiol. 1:143, 1958.
17. Moss, W. G., Kelly, J. P., Neville, J. B., Bourque, J. E., and Wakerlin, G. E.: Effect of experimental renal hypertension on experimental cholesterol atherosclerosis. Fed. Proc. 10:94, 1951.
18. Bronte-Stewart, B., and Heptinstall, R. H.: The relationship between experimental hypertension and cholesterol induced atheroma in rabbits. J. Pathol. Bacteriol. 68:407, 1954.
19. Deming, Q. B., Mosbach, E. H., Bevans, M. D., Daly, M. M., Abell, L. L., Martin, E., Brun, L. M., Halpern, E., and Kaplan, R.: Blood pressure, cholesterol content of serum and tissues, and atherogenesis in the rat. J. Exp. Med. 107:581, 1958.
20. Deming, Q. B., Hodes, M., Baltazar, A., Edreira, J. G., and Torosday, S.: The changes in concentration of cholesterol in the serum of hypertensive patients during antihypertensive therapy. Am. J. Med. 24:882, 1958.
21. Perry, H. M., Jr., and Schroeder, H. A.: Depression of cholesterol levels in human plasma following ethylenediamine tetracetate and hydralazine. J. Chronic Dis. 2:520, 1955.
22. Orvis, H. G., Tamagna, J. G., and Evans, J. M.: The serum lipids in hypertensive patients treated with pentolinium. Clin. Res. Proc. 4:108, 1956.
23. Adel, H. N., Deming, Q. B., Daly, M. M., Raeff, V. M., and Brun, L. M.: The effect of experimental hypertension on cholesterol synthesis in the rat. J. Lab. Clin. Med. 66:571, 1965.
24. Karsner, H. T.: Thickness of aortic media in hypertension. Trans. Assoc. Am. Physicians 53:54, 1938.
25. Aars, H.: Static load-length characteristics of aortic strips from hypertensive rabbits. Acta Physiol. Scand. 73:101, 1968.
26. Daly, M. M., Deming, Q. B., Raeff, V., and Brun, L.: Cholesterol concentration and cholesterol synthesis in aortas of rats with renal hypertension. J. Clin. Invest. 42:1606, 1963.
27. Daly, M. M., and Raeff, V.: Effect of hypertension on lipid composition of rat aorta. Bull. N.Y. Acad. Med. 41:225, 1965.
28. Wolinsky, H.: Response of the rat aortic media to hypertension: morphological and chemical studies. Circ. Res. 26:507, 1970.
29. Wolinsky, H., and Glagov, S.: Comparison of abdominal and thoracic aortic medial structure in mammals: Deviation of man from the usual pattern. Circ. Res. 25:677, 1969.
30. Daly, M. M., and Gurpide, E. G.: The respiration and cytochrome oxidase activity of rat aorta in experimental hypertension. J. Exp. Med. 109:187, 1959.
31. Wolinsky, H.: Response of the rat aortic wall to hypertension. Importance of comparing absolute amounts of wall components. J. Atheroscler. Res. 11:251, 1970.
32. Wolinsky, H.: Effects of hypertension and its reversal on the thoracic aorta of male and female rats: Morphological and chemical studies. Circ. Res. 28:622, 1971.
33. Kajimahara, M., and Ooneda, G.: Electron microscope study on the middle cerebral artery lesions in kept rats. Acta Pathol. Jap. 20:399, 1970.
34. Salgado, E. D.: Medial aortic lesions in rats with metacortoid hypertension. Am. J. Pathol. 58:305, 1970.
35. Woods, J. D.: Relative ischaemia in the hypertrophied heart. Lancet 1:696, 1961.
36. Still, W. J. J.: Pathogenesis of the intimal thickenings produced by hypertension in large arteries in the rat. Lab. Invest. 19:84, 1968.

Natural History of Untreated Essential Hypertension

By Sir F. Horace Smirk, K.B.E., M.D., D.Sc.

Our group was exceedingly fortunate that about 1944, before effective hypotensive drugs became available, we began a deliberate prospective study in New Zealand of untreated hypertension.[1] When effective drugs became available we were most careful to arrange that our prospective study of treated hypertensives could be properly compared with the results on untreated patients.

In untreated hypertensives with retinal grade 4 or retinal grade 3 the results are so fully documented that a brief statement should suffice. With retinal grade-4 changes present, the average survival time is between 8 and 12 months. Under 10 percent of patients survive 2 years. In retinal grade-3 patients about 40 percent may survive 2 years.

Even at similar levels of the blood pressure the outlook is worse when these exudative changes are present in the retina. In general, however, casual blood pressures are higher in grade-3 and grade-4 patients than in those of retinal grades 1 or 2 and this contributes to the gloomy outlook of untreated cases. In our series the mean blood pressure of 28 otherwise uncomplicated, retinal grade-3 female patients aged 50 to 59 was 243/136 and in 40 females of the same age group with retinal gradings of 1 or 2, the mean blood pressure was 223/124.

Furthermore, when exudative retinal changes are present the basal blood pressure is usually raised disproportionately; there is a smaller fall of blood pressure under basal conditions than with retinal grade-1 or grade-2 patients. I matched 20 grade-3 and 20 grade-1 or grade-2 female patients aged 50 to 59 for equal casual blood pressures. The basal pressure of these grade-3 patients was 188/111 as against 170/104 for the retinal grade-1 or grade-2 patients.

From the Department of Medicine, Wellcome Medical Research Institute, University of Otago Medical School, Dunedin, New Zealand.

This work was supported by a grant from The Medical Research Council of New Zealand.

Irrespective of the presence or absence of retinopathy, the relationship between the 5- and 8-year mortality of untreated hypertensive patients to their casual, basal, and supplemental pressures is shown in Tables 1, 2, and 3.

As this chapter leads up to consideration of milder cases and the rationale of early treatment (see my chapter titled "Rationale for the Early Treatment of Hypertension") I shall confine myself in what follows to the natural history of patients with retinal grades 1 or 2.

Even among retinal grade-1 and grade-2 patients there is a wide mortality range. Reference will be made to four important factors which influence the mortality of untreated hypertensives, namely, sex, age, level of the blood pressure, and the number of substantial hypertensive disabilities or complications sustained at or before the start of the follow-up period. The hypertensive disabilities referred to are the presence of either congestive heart failure or left ventricular failure, of minor or major strokes, of impairment of the renal excretory function, or of coronary artery disease, either thrombosis or angina.

Before serious hypertensive disabilities have developed, before the blood pressure has risen to excessive heights, and before the occurrence of exudative retinopathy, electrocardiographic changes and x-ray evidence of cardiac enlargement provide evidence that for the untreated person a degree of cardiovascular deterioration has already occurred.

We have results on 198 untreated hypertensives, all of retinal grades 1 or 2. Brief mention will be made of 266 treated hypertensives also of retinal grades 1 or 2.[2,3]

The 198 untreated hypertensives can be subdivided into three groups or steps in terms of the number of disabilities: no disability is on the bottom step, one disability is one upward step in severity, and two disabilities are two upward steps in severity. Figure 1 shows the

TABLE 1.—*Casual Blood Pressures in Relation to Survivals, and to Deaths Due to or Accelerated by Hypertension*

	Dead within 8 years		*Alive 8 years or more*		*Dead within 5 years*		*Alive 5 years or more*	
Age	*No.*	*B.P. (mm Hg)*	*No.*	*B.P. (mm Hg)*	*No.*	*B.P. (mm Hg)*	*No.*	*B.P. (mm Hg)*
Males								
0–29	0	—	4	175.8/ 95.8	0	—	4	175.8/ 95.8
30–39	0	—	4	190.5/111.0	0	—	4	190.5/111.0
40–49	6	219.2/117.0	9	183.3/106.9	4	221.3/116.8	11	189.1/117.5
50–59	19	213.7/129.0	7	175.0/116.4	16	221.6/130.6	17	182.5/115.8
60–69	22	207.5/117.6	6	206.6/122.3	20	209.5/117.4	16	195.8/116.4
70+	11	202.9/118.0	1	168.0/ 86.0	9	203.9/118.2	3	188.7/106.7
Total	58		31		49		55	
Females								
0–29	0	—	4	195.0/126.3	0	—	4	195.0/128.8
30–39	2	227.0/139.0	10	189.1/110.0	0	—	17	193.7/114.6
40–49	4	260.0/147.0	21	193.7/112.6	3	260.0/147.7	28	199.6/115.1
50–59	21	235.3/131.6	13	221.1/127.9	15	244.8/133.5	39	210.3/122.6
60–69	18	236.9/126.0	17	214.6/120.2	16	243.3/126.3	26	216.0/119.0
70+	11	213.2/119.5	7	222.9/125.4	12	217.1/122.1	11	216.4/119.8
Total	56		72		46		125	
Grand Total Males and Females	114		103		95		180	

From Smirk, F. H., Veale, A. M. O., and Alstad, K.,[1] with permission.
Abbreviation used: B.P., blood pressure.

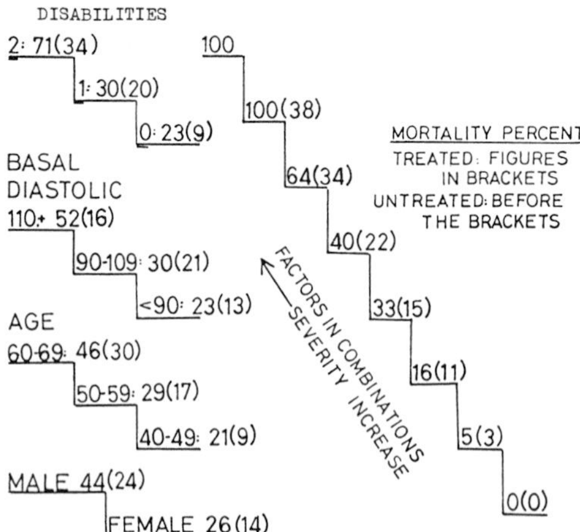

FIG. 1.—Some factors influencing mortality in hypertension. One hundred ninety-eight untreated hypertensives and 266 treated hypertensives are classified similarly in terms of increased severity at the outset of a 5-year follow-up period.

The upward steps to the left represent increases in severity in respect of the number of disabilities (0, 1, 2), the basal diastolic pressure (3 grades), age (3 decades), and sex. Each upward step is associated with an increase in the subsequent 5-year mortality. Thus, comparing patients with disabilities increasing in number from 0 to 1 to 2, the mortality rose from 23 to 30 to 71 percent in the untreated group and from 9 to 20 to 34 percent in the treated group. The maximum number of adverse upward steps which can be taken, combining all categories, is 7.

On the right is shown the effect on mortality of selecting the persons with various numbers of adverse factors. As the number of adverse factors represented by the number of upward steps rises from 0 to 7 the mortality rises from 0 to 5, 16, 33, 40, 64 to 100 percent in the untreated group.

In a corresponding treated group, the group mortality rises from 0 to 3, 11, 15, 22, 34, 38 percent as the number of adverse factors represented by upward steps rises from 0 to 6.

TABLE 2.—*Basal and Supplemental Blood Pressures in Relationship to 5-Year Survivals and to Deaths Due to or Accelerated by Hypertension*

	Basal Blood Pressure				*Supplemental Blood Pressure*			
	Dead within 5 years		*Alive 5 years or more*		*Dead within 5 years*		*Alive 5 years or more*	
Age	*No.*	*Mean B.B.P. (mm Hg)*	*No.*	*Mean B.B.P. (mm Hg)*	*No.*	*Mean S.B.P. (mm Hg)*	*No.*	*Mean S.B.P. (mm Hg)*
Males								
0–29	0	—	4	114.5/73.5	0	—	4	61.3/22.3
30–39	0	—	4	130.0/91.0	0	—	4	60.5/20.0
40–49	4	157.5/ 94.3	11	130.7/88.4	4	63.8/22.5	11	58.4/29.1
50–59	16	164.9/106.9	17	131.3/84.7	16	56.7/23.7	17	51.2/31.1
60–69	20	159.4/ 95.0	16	136.9/86.0	20	50.2/22.4	16	58.9/30.4
70+	9	159.3/ 94.0	3	132.0/81.3	9	44.6/24.2	3	56.7/25.3
Total	49		55		49		55	
Females								
0–29	0	—	4	141.5/94.5	0	—	4	53.5/34.3
30–39	0	—	17	149.1/98.4	0	—	17	44.6/16.2
40–49	3	202.0/132.0	28	148.9/98.2	3	58.0/15.7	28	50.7/16.9
50–59	15	183.2/113.7	39	154.9/97.6	15	61.6/19.7	39	55.4/25.0
60–69	16	185.3/105.1	26	158.5/95.4	16	58.1/21.1	26	57.5/23.6
70+	12	174.9/ 95.1	11	162.9/85.9	12	42.2/27.0	11	53.5/33.9
Total	46		125		46		125	
Grand Total Males and Females	95		180		95		180	

From Smirk, F. H., Veale, A. M. O., and Alstad, K.,[1] with permission.
Abbreviations used: B.B.P., basal blood pressure; S.B.P., supplemental blood pressure.

percentage mortalities of untreated hypertensives immediately before the percentage mortalities of the treated hypertensives, which are shown in brackets.

The rise in severity as we go from 0 to 1 to 2 disabilities is associated with a corresponding rise in mortality of the untreated hypertensives from 23 through 30 to 71 percent and of the treated from 9 through 20 to 34 percent.

Additionally we may subdivide the same 198 untreated hypertensives into three severity grades or steps by three levels of basal diastolic pressure, or by three age groups: 40 to 49, 50 to 59, and 60 to 69. There is also a rise in the expected risk and in the percentage mortality of males when compared with females.

Each upward step in severity in whatever category—disabilities, blood pressure, age, and male sex—is associated with an increase in mortality, of both the untreated and treated persons.

Let us now consider the effect of combining these various factors. Starting at the bottom of the ladder we have the mildest of the combinations: eight females in the 40 to 49 age group with a basal diastolic pressure under 90 mm Hg and with no disabilities. In this combination of the lowest severity there were eight females and no deaths in the 5-year follow-up period.

For the sake of simplicity, the results in the four categories are combined and represented qualitatively on a single ladder shown on the right. The percentage of mortality in both untreated and treated hypertensives is seen to be rising as the number of upward steps taken increases progressively from 0 to 7 steps, each upward step representing an increase in the severity grading of one of the various factors concerned.

TABLE 3.—*Basal and Supplemental Blood Pressures in Relationship to 8-Year Survivals and to Deaths Due to or Accelerated by Hypertension*

	Basal Blood Pressures				*Supplemental Blood Pressures*			
	Dead within 8 years		*Alive 8 years or more*		*Dead within 8 years*		*Alive 8 years or more*	
Age	*No.*	*Mean B.B.P. (mm Hg)*	*No.*	*Mean B.B.P. (mm Hg)*	*No.*	*Mean S.B.P. (mm Hg)*	*No.*	*Mean S.B.P. (mm Hg)*
Males								
0–29	0	—	4	114.5/ 73.5	0	—	4	61.3/22.3
30–39	0	—	4	130.0/ 91.0	0	—	4	60.5/20.0
40–49	6	153.3/ 96.8	9	129.1/ 80.2	6	63.8/20.2	9	54.2/26.7
50–59	19	162.2/104.9	7	124.0/ 82.0	19	51.5/24.0	7	51.0/34.4
60–69	22	156.0/ 93.6	6	146.3/ 93.0	22	51.5/24.0	6	60.3/29.3
70+	11	156.3/ 92.0	1	110.0/ 78.0	11	46.6/26.0	1	58.0/ 8.0
Total	58		31		58		31	
Females								
0–29	0	—	4	141.5/ 94.5	0	—	4	53.5/31.8
30–39	2	196.0/121.0	10	138.9/ 93.7	2	31.0/18.0	10	50.3/16.3
40–49	4	204.0/135.0	21	141.5/ 94.1	4	56.0/12.0	21	52.2/18.5
50–59	21	175.4/107.7	13	157.8/101.8	21	59.9/23.9	13	63.3/26.1
60–69	18	178.1/103.4	17	158.8/ 97.4	18	58.8/22.6	17	55.8/22.8
70+	11	164.4/ 92.5	7	164.3/ 86.7	11	48.8/27.0	7	58.6/38.7
Total	56		72		56		72	
Grand Total Males and Females	114		103		114		103	

From Smirk, F. H., Veale, A. M. O., and Alstad, K.,[1] with permission.
Abbreviations used: B.B.P., basal blood pressure; S.B.P., supplemental blood pressure.

If all the seven possible upward steps are taken we arrive at the top of each set of steps and reach the most severe combination. There was only one person with this combination of factors: a male in the 60 to 69 age group with a basal diastolic pressure of 110 mm Hg or more, who had already experienced two of the important hypertensive disabilities. He died within the 5-year follow-up period. If we select from the 198 untreated hypertensives those who are only one step below the most severe category, we still find 100 percent mortality. There were seven hypertensives in this category, and all died within the 5-year follow-up period.

The figures in brackets give the percentage mortalities for the 266 treated hypertensives subdivided in the same way. In all severity groups the mortality rate is less in the treated than in the untreated hypertensives.

The raw data from which these results have been derived are set out in Table 4, which contains the results on the 198 untreated and 266 treated hypertensives. All were of retinal grades 1 or 2; all were followed to the fifth anniversary of the initial investigation. In the 5-year follow-up, 33 percent of the untreated and 18 percent of the treated died.

In Table 4, results in females are listed in the top half and in males in the bottom half; the data on males and females are each subdivided into the three age groups, 60 to 69, 50 to 59, and 40 to 49. In the column to the left are those who have experienced none of the substantial hypertensive disabilities by the outset of the follow-up period, in the middle column they have had one disability, in the right-hand column, two disabilities. The hypertensives in any disability group are subdivided into the three categories of the basal diastolic

TABLE 4.—*The Mortality in Treated (T) and Untreated (U) Female and Male Patients in Relation to the Basal Diastolic Blood Pressure and Number of Specified Disabilities at the Outset of the Follow-up Period*

Basal Diastolic	0 Disability									1 Disability									2 Disabilities								
	110+			90-109			<90			110+			90-109			<90			110+			90-109			<90		
Female	D	N	%	D	N	%	D	N	%	D	N	%	D	N	%	D	N	%	D	N	%	D	N	%	D	N	%
60 T	0	1	0	1	5	20	0	2	0	2	6	33	2	8	25	2	5	40	1	4	25	4	7	57	1	4	25
		▲			▲						▲			●			▲			▲			▼			▲	
69 U	2	5	40	1	4	25	0	6	0	2	4	50	1	4	25	4	8	50	2	2	100	1	3	33	1	2	50
50 T	1	10	10	2	20	10	1	10	10	1	9	11	2	9	22	0	6	0	0	1	0	1	5	20	1	2	50
		▲			▲			▼			▲			●						▲			▲			▼	
59 U	1	3	33	3	11	27	0	5	0	2	7	29	2	9	22	0	8	0	4	4	100	1	1	100	0	1	0
40 T	1	10	10	0	17	0	0	1	0	0	8	0	0	8	0	0	6	0	1	4	25	0	4	0	1	2	50
		▲			▲																		▲				
49 U	2	6	33	1	10	10	0	8	0	0	2	0	0	5	0	0	2	0	0	0	0	1	1	100	0	0	0
40 T	2	21	10	3	42	7	1	13	8	3	23	13	4	25	16	2	17	12	2	9	22	5	16	31	3	8	38
69 U	5	14	36	5	25	20	0	19	0	4	13	31	3	18	17	4	18	22	6	6	100	3	5	60	1	3	33
Male																											
60 T	0	2	0	2	6	33	0	1	0	2	5	40	2	7	29	0	1	0	0	0	0	1	1	100	0	1	0
					▲			▲			▲			▲			▲						●			▲	
69 U	0	1	0	3	5	60	3	6	50	2	2	100	2	3	67	2	5	40	1	1	100	1	1	100	4	7	57
50 T	0	5	0	0	4	0	0	2	0	3	10	30	5	11	45	0	4	0	1	3	33	1	2	50	0	1	0
		▲			▲						▲			▼			▲			▲			▲			▲	
59 U	1	4	25	1	2	50	0	3	0	1	1	100	1	5	20	1	8	13	2	2	100	1	1	100	1	1	100
40 T	0	4	0	2	6	33	0	4	0	0	3	0	1	5	20	0	1	0	1	2	50	0	0	0	1	1	100
		▲			▼									▼			▲			▲							
49 U	2	3	67	1	6	17	0	3	0	0	0	0	0	1	0	2	4	50	1	1	100	1	1	100	0	0	0
40 T	0	11	0	4	16	25	0	7	0	5	18	28	8	23	35	0	6	0	2	5	40	2	3	67	1	3	33
69 U	3	8	38	5	13	38	3	12	25	3	3	100	3	9	33	5	17	29	4	4	100	3	3	100	5	8	63

Symbols and abbreviations used: ▲, indicates compartments in which the percentage mortality was less in the treated group; ▼, marks compartments with the mortality less in the untreated group; ●, compartments in which mortalities are equal; N, refers to number of patients in a compartment of the table; D, to the number who died; and % to the percentage mortality within the compartment.

blood pressure, namely, 110+ to the left, 90 to 109 in the middle, and under 90 to the right.

There are 54 combinations of the characteristics just mentioned and the results on untreated and treated persons with similar characteristics are set out in the 54 compartments of Table 4. Each compartment of the table contains matched cases. The mortality rates vary according to the characteristics of the persons within any particular compartment. Within any one of the 54 compartments of Table 4 the results recorded are on untreated and treated persons who, at the outset of the follow-up period were alike in respect to sex, age group, number of disabilities, and blood pressure range (casual or basal). Patients were all of retinal grades 1 or 2 and in all the result is recorded as dead or alive on the fifth anniversary of starting the follow-up period either as an untreated hypertensive or as one on treatment.

Table 4 is arranged to show at a glance the

result of comparing the mortality rates of treated and untreated persons. In compartments where the mortality was less in the treated group, there is a triangle with the apex above (▲) in that compartment of the table; when the mortality was greater in the treated than the untreated there is a triangle with apex down (▼), when the mortalities of treated and untreated were equal a large dot is the indication, and when no conclusion can be drawn there is neither triangle nor dot drawn within the compartment.

In Table 4 a count of the symbols referred to above indicates that in 30 of the compartments the percentage mortality of the treated persons was less than that of the untreated. In six of the compartments the percentage mortality was higher in the treated than in the untreated persons and in three the percentage mortalities were equal. The difference is highly significant and favorable to the conclusion that treatment was beneficial.

Lastly, may I refer very briefly to an interest I have in some epidemiologic data which relate to the natural history of hypertension. The point which has long attracted my interest is that populations exhibiting higher than average blood pressures usually had a higher incidence of essential hypertension and those with lower than average blood pressures usually had a lower incidence of essential hypertension.[4]

As is well known, the mean blood pressures, by age, of blacks in the United States is higher than that of whites and there is a higher incidence of frank hypertension.[5]

There appears to be no doubt that in some of the Pacific islands,[6,7] in New Guinea,[8] in Indians of low socioeconomic status,[9] and in some communities in Africa,[10,11] population groups are to be found with low mean blood pressures which rise very little with age, so that frank hypertension and hypertensive disease in such communities are unusual or even rare.

Many such low-blood-pressure groups when compared with European or Westernized communities are described as living in a primitive way; they often have lower body weights, and are less exposed to the stresses of a more complex, competitive way of life. Some low-blood-pressure communities have a low salt intake, e.g., the natives of the Pacific island of Pukapuka.[7]

Additionally, in several such communities, disorders may occur which, theoretically, might alter blood pressure levels. For example: ankylostomiasis, schistosomiasis, malaria, filariasis, yaws, various dysenteric infections, infestations with intestinal parasites, tuberculosis, and various forms of malnutrition. Such disorders may present themselves not one at a time but in combinations which are difficult to document and indeed may not have been ascertained by the local health services. In practice the health of such a community can rarely be fully evaluated even by the most industrious investigator.

Hence, it often happens that when attempts are made to explain even gross differences in the blood pressures of primitive groups which are considered to be racially similar, but living under different conditions, one cannot even distinguish between two possibilities: (1) that the lower blood pressure is the result of exposure to a factor or factors injurious to health, or (2) that the lower blood pressure is partly or entirely due to a factor or factors which are not injurious and may be beneficial to health.

Nevertheless, the low mean blood pressure is associated in almost all instances with a very low incidence of essential hypertension and of hypertensive disease. In several New Guinea [8,9] communities it appears that although some of the known health risks may be responsible for a degree of blood pressure reduction, it has been shown that physical fitness is not incompatible with low blood pressure levels and absence of the rise of blood pressure with age [9] characteristic of most European communities.

There are a few such low-blood-pressure communities which appear to be healthy and adequately nourished. A very full investigation of their way of life would, I believe, be an important contribution to the natural history of the disease.

Acknowledgment

I am indebted to Mrs. Joy Tomlin, who has been responsible for the secretarial work involved in the preparation of this paper, and to Professor F. O. Simpson for his helpful comments. I am grateful to Dr. John Hunter, Professor of Medicine in the Medical School, Dunedin, for generous facilities within the Wellcome Medical Research Institute.

References

1. Smirk, F. H., Veale, A. M. O., and Alstad, K.: Basal and supplemental blood pressures in relationship to life expectancy and hypertension symptomatology. N. Z. Med. J. 58: 711, 1959.
2. Smirk, F. H.: Observations on the mortality of 270 treated and 199 untreated retinal grade I and II hypertensive patients followed in all instances for five years. N. Z. Med. J. 63:413, 1964.
3. Smirk, F. H.: Prognosis in retinal grade I and II patients. *In* Gross, F. (Ed.): CIBA Symposium on Antihypertensive Therapy, Siena, Italy. Summit, N. J.: CIBA, 1965, pp. 355–369.
4. Smirk, F. H.: Pathogenesis of essential hypertension. Br. Med. J. 1:791, 1949.
5. Saunders, G. M., and Bancroft, H.: Blood pressure studies on Negro and white men and women living in the Virgin Islands of the United States. Am. Heart J. 23:410, 1942.
6. Maddocks, I.: Possible absence of essential hypertension in two complete Pacific island populations. Lancet 2:396, 1961.
7. Prior, I. A. M., and Evans, J. G.: Sodium intake and blood pressure in Pacific populations. *In* Eliakim, M. (Ed.): Proceedings of the Fourth Asian Pacific Congress of Cardiology. New York: Academic Press, 1968, pp. 166–169.
8. Maddocks, I.: Blood pressures in Melanesians. Med. J. Aust. 1:1123, 1967.
9. Whyte, H. M.: Body fat and blood pressure of natives in New Guinea; reflections on essential hypertension. Australas. Ann. Med. 7–8:36, 1958–1959.

Part V. PHARMACOLOGY AND THERAPY USING ESTABLISHED DRUGS

Hemodynamic Effects of Antihypertensive Agents

By Gaddo Onesti, M.D., Kwan Eun Kim, M.D.
Charles Swartz, M.D., and John H. Moyer, M.D.

Although the pathophysiology of essential hypertension remains unknown, extensive hemodynamic studies have now revealed its basic hemodynamic characteristics (see the chapters entitled "Hemodynamic Alterations in Essential Hypertension" and "Regional Blood Flow in Essential Hypertension"). Studies of the hypertensions of renal origin have also disclosed the basic hemodynamic derangements in some patients (see the chapters entitled "Hemodynamics of Renal Hypertension in Man" and "Hemodynamics of Hypertension in End-Stage Renal Parenchymal Disease").

We postulate that the desirable way of lowering blood pressure with pharmacologic agents is to correct the hemodynamic derangement characteristic of the individual hypertensive state being treated. Thus if the hemodynamic pattern of well-established essential hypertension is a normal cardiac output and an increased total peripheral resistance, therapeutic efforts should be directed, if possible, toward a normalization of the resistance. Contrariwise, in early essential hypertension, the reduction of the elevated cardiac output should be the purpose of therapy.

The hemodynamic effects of antihypertensive agents in man are complex and are the result of their multiple sites of actions as well as of the homeostatic circulatory responses that they may elicit.

In this book the hemodynamic effect of beta-adrenergic blockers, diuretics, clonidine, and diazoxide are presented in detail. In the present chapter the discussion will summarize the systemic and renal hemodynamic effects of reserpine, guanethidine, hydralazine, alpha-methyldopa, pargyline hydrochloride, and debrisosquine sulfate.

Reserpine

In normal dogs under general pentothal anesthesia, studied in our laboratory, intravenous administration of reserpine produced a significant decrease in blood pressure after a variable period of 1 to 2 hours. Associated with the reduction in blood pressure, the cardiac output was quite variable, occasionally decreasing slightly. The reduction in blood pressure, therefore, was caused primarily by a decrease in total peripheral vascular resistance.[1]

The acute systemic hemodynamic effects of intravenous administration of reserpine in one patient with essential hypertension are shown in Fig. 1. Three hours following reserpine administration the mean arterial pressure was decreased. No tangible change in cardiac output occurred. There was, however, a significant decrease in heart rate and a rise in stroke volume. As a consequence, the total peripheral vascular resistance decreased. No change in oxygen consumption was seen.

The acute hemodynamic studies in patients with essential hypertension by Reubi, Müller, and Stuck [2] are in agreement with our findings. Chronic oral administration of reserpine for several days, however, is reported to produce a moderate decrease in heart rate and cardiac output.[3]

From the Division of Nephrology and Hypertension, Department of Medicine, Hahnemann Medical College and Hospital, Philadelphia, Pennsylvania.

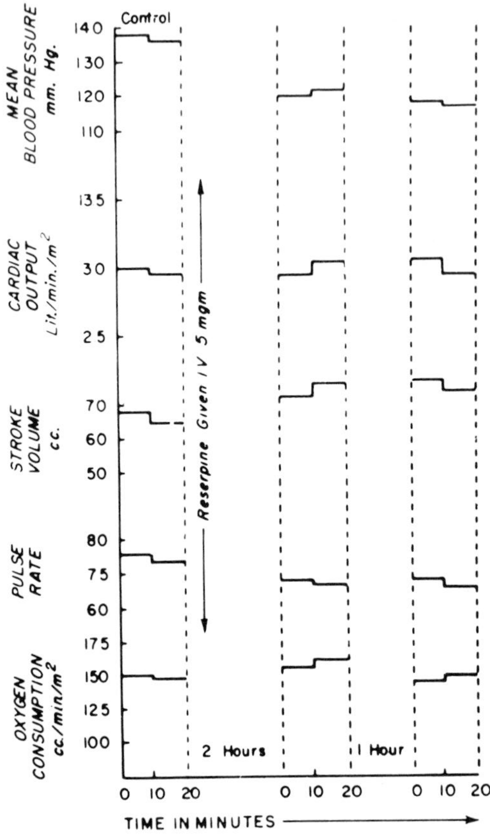

FIG. 1.—Acute systemic hemodynamic effects of reserpine in a patient with essential hypertension.

Observations on renal hemodynamics in six patients with essential hypertension who received 2 to 3 mg of reserpine intravenously are summarized in Fig. 2. The control values of renal blood flow and glomerular filtration rate were below normal because of nephroangiosclerosis usually associated with essential hypertension present for several years. After administration of reserpine, five of the six patients showed a slight reduction of glomerular filtration rate at the time of maximum decrease in blood pressure which occurred 2 to 3 hours after administration of the drug (Period D_1, Fig. 2). The sixth patient actually showed a sharp increase in glomerular filtration rate. One hour later, there was very little additional change in either blood pressure or glomerular filtration rate (Period D_2, Fig. 2). Concomitantly with the blood pressure reduction there was no major consistent change in renal blood flow. Renovascular resistance was therefore decreased. The renal hemodynamic effects of oral reserpine for 3 weeks in patients with essential hypertension were similar to the described acute effects. There was no decrease in renal blood flow nor glomerular filtration rate.

Human studies by Bock and Müller in 1956 have demonstrated that reserpine reduces the vascular resistance in both muscle and skin.[4] The cerebral blood flow in patients with essential hypertension was found to be unchanged following reserpine administration, while the cerebral vascular resistance was reduced.[5]

It may therefore be concluded that the fall in blood pressure produced by reserpine is due to vasodilation unaccompanied by reduction in cardiac performance. The vasodilation is apparent in all the segments of the circulations studied.

GUANETHIDINE

Maxwell and co-workers demonstrated in 1960 that intravenous administration of guanethidine in anesthetized normotensive dogs produced a triphasic blood pressure response.[6] An initial fall in blood pressure was followed by a period of moderate hypertension lasting approximately 45 minutes, followed in turn by a gradual progressive decline. The hypotensive response was sustained for several hours of observation. Although the hemodynamics of both the initial hypotensive and hypertensive effects have been studied, the present discussion will include primarily the hemodynamic effects of sustained blood pressure reduction.

In unanesthetized normotensive dogs the sustained decrease in blood pressure produced by 15 mg of guanethidine per kilogram of body weight, given intravenously, was found to be associated with a reduction in cardiac output and an inconsistent increase in total peripheral vascular resistance.[6]

Figure 3 shows the hemodynamic effects observed during the hypotensive response that followed acute intravenous administration of guanethidine in 10 patients with essential hypertension studied in the supine position. The dose used was 0.25 mg per kilogram of body weight. The patients were studied in the supine

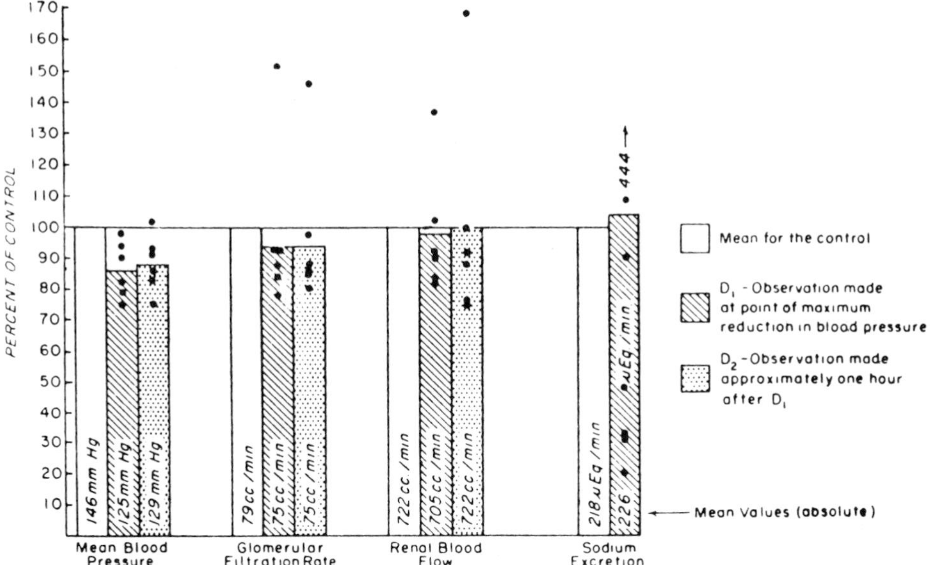

FIG. 2.—Acute renal hemodynamic response to an intravenously administered 3-mg dose of reserpine in six patients with essential hypertension.

position. There was a 35 percent fall in mean arterial pressure. Cardiac output decreased significantly from an average of 5.40 liters per minute to an average of 3.80 liters per minute (30%). The decrease in cardiac output was associated with both a decrease in heart rate and a decrease in stroke volume. Heart rate diminished from 86 beats per minute to 71 beats per minute (13%) and stroke volume from 63 to 54 ml per beat. Since the changes

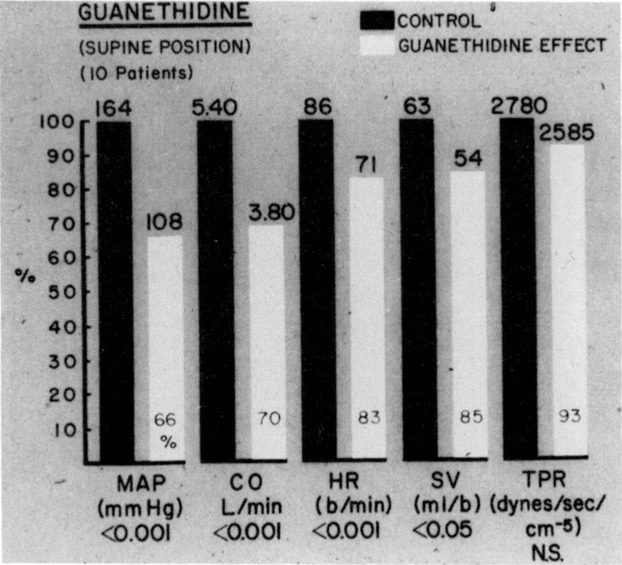

FIG. 3.—Systemic hemodynamic effects during the hypotensive response following intravenous administration of guanethidine in 10 patients with essential hypertension. **MAP,** mean arterial pressure; **CO,** cardiac output; **HR,** heart rate; **SV,** stroke volume; **TPR,** total peripheral resistance.

in blood pressure and cardiac output were in the same direction, the calculated total peripheral resistance was unchanged.

Systemic hemodynamic studies in patients with essential hypertension after 5 to 7 days of oral administration of guanethidine were conducted by Richardson and co-workers.[7] The hemodynamic effects were the same as in our acute study. Blood pressure reduction was associated with a drop in cardiac output and no changes in total peripheral resistance.

The decrease in cardiac output could be attributed either to a direct cardiac effect of the drug or to a decreased venous return to the right heart caused by pooling of blood in the capacitance vessels. This distinction is important in view of the reduced catecholamine content in the heart demonstrated after treatment with guanethidine.[8] The available experimental [9] evidence supports the contention that the decrease in cardiac output is due primarily to pooling of blood in the capacitance vessels. This is due, in turn, to a decrease in venous tone mediated by the sympathetic inhibition exerted by guanethidine.

The renal hemodynamic effects occurring during the sustained antihypertensive response that followed intravenous guanethidine in seven patients with essential hypertension are shown in Fig. 4. The studies were conducted between 30 and 60 minutes following drug administration. With the seven patients in supine position, the decrease in mean arterial pressure was from an average of 138 mm Hg to an average of 121 mm Hg. The renal plasma flow, renal blood flow, and glomerular filtration rate were significantly decreased. The renal vascular resistance increased in every patient from an average of 275 dynes per second per $cm^{-5} \times 10^3$ to an average of 330 dynes per second per $cm^{-5} \times 10^3$.

Richardson and co-workers [7] studied the renal hemodynamic effects of oral guanethidine administration for 1 to 2 weeks in 11 patients with essential hypertension. The degree of renal function impairment due to the nephroangiosclerosis in their patients was similar to that observed in the patients of our acute study. Daily administration of guanethidine resulted in a reduction of blood pressure, glomerular filtration rate, and renal plasma flow.

Thus the hemodynamic effect of guanethidine in essential hypertension is that of a predominant decrease in cardiac output whereas

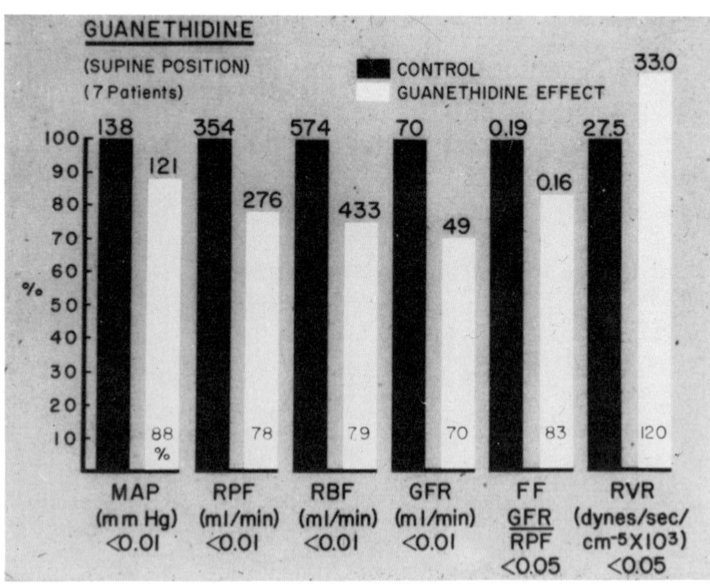

FIG. 4.—Renal hemodynamic effects during the hypotensive response following intravenously administered guanethidine in seven patients with essential hypertension. **MAP,** mean arterial pressure; **RPF,** renal plasma flow; **RBF,** renal blood flow; **GFR,** glomerular filtration rate: **FF,** filtration fraction; **RVR,** renal vascular resistance.

the total peripheral resistance is not significantly effective. It is of interest to note that studies of ganglionic blockers (e.g., hexamethonium) have yielded similar results both quantitatively and qualitatively.[10]

It is therefore postulated that guanethidine exerts a more potent inhibition of the sympathetic stimuli to the "capacitance vessels": this results in venous pooling of blood which in turn results in decreased venous return. It should also be noted, however, that peripheral resistance ought to rise in response to drug-induced reduction in cardiac output.[11] This expected compensatory increase in resistance appears to be blocked by guanethidine.

The systemic hemodynamic effects of guanethidine are the same following acute intravenous administration and after 1- to 2-week oral administration. Thus the sequence of hemodynamic events described for the diuretic agents[12] has not been recorded with guanethidine. The initial decrease in cardiac output is not followed by a decrease in resistance. The chronic hemodynamic studies of Richardson and co-workers, however, did not go beyond 2 weeks.[7] It is therefore not excluded that resistance changes might be recorded after more prolonged administration.

Hydralazine

Although hydralazine has been demonstrated to have a central (vasomotor center) site of action, its most important pharmacologic effect peripherally is on the arteriolar smooth muscle.[13,14] This results in prolonged dilation of arteriolar vessels.

The acute cardiac effects of intravenous hydralazine in five dogs studied in our laboratory under pentothal anesthesia are shown in Table 1. There is an immediate decrease in the systolic, diastolic, and mean blood pressures. The average heart rate is increased from 111 beats per minute to 203 beats per minute. Cardiac output is increased from an average of 2.58 liters per minute to an average of 4.74 liters per minute while the stroke volume remains unchanged. Total peripheral resistance is significantly decreased.

This represents the hemodynamic pattern of acute vasodilation where the increase in cardiac output is represented primarily by tachycardia.

Table 1.—*Acute Cardiovascular Effects of Intravenously Administered Hydralazine in Five Dogs Under Pentothal Anesthesia*

	Control	*Hydralazine (1 mg per kg)*
Blood pressure (mm Hg)		
Systolic	138	120
Diastolic	101	78
Mean	113	92
Heart rate (beats per minute)	111	203
Cardiac output (liters per minute)	2.58	4.74
Stroke volume (milliliters per beat)	23	23
Total peripheral vascular resistance (dynes per second per cm^{-5})	3,500	1,551

Figure 5 shows the acute effects of orally administered hydralazine on blood pressure and cardiac output in a patient with essential hypertension. Hydralazine in a 100-mg dose produced a prompt decrease in systolic and diastolic blood pressure. This is associated with increased cardiac output and tachycardia.

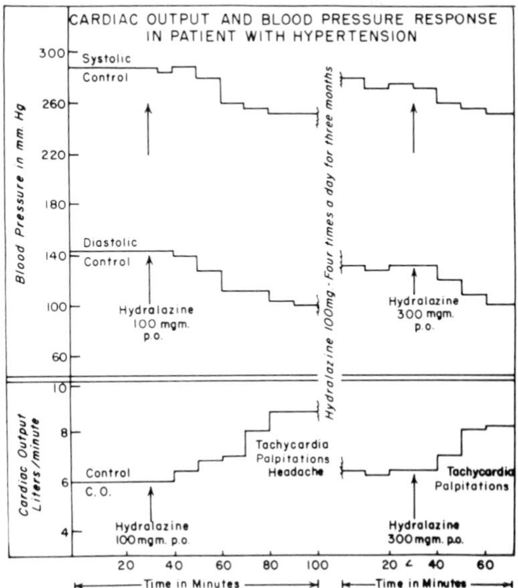

Fig. 5.—Acute effects of orally administered hydralazine.

Headaches and palpitation are the common side effects of acute administration.

In 1950 when the pharmacologic properties of hydralazine were studied in the rabbit by Gross, Drevy, and Meier,[15] it was immediately noted that the antihypertensive effect was accompanied by an increase in heart rate and renal blood flow. The latter observation was soon confirmed by acute studies in man. Reubi demonstrated that subcutaneous administration of hydralazine in patients produced an average increase of 38.6 percent in renal plasma flow, while the glomerular filtration rate was not significantly changed.[16] Wilkinson, Backman, and Hecht [17] noted that the percentage increase in cardiac output produced by hydralazine exceeded the percentage increase in renal blood flow. This indicates that the renal fraction of cardiac output is not augmented. In addition, it should be noted that direct injection of hydralazine into the renal artery of the dog produces an immediate decrease in renal blood flow; and only after hydralazine reaches the systemic circulation is an increase in renal blood flow in the contralateral side observed.[18] These studies demonstrate that although the acute renal effect of hydralazine is an increase in renal blood flow there is no effect on the glomerular filtration rate and that the "renal hyperemia" is secondary to an increase in cardiac output. In addition, it is also noteworthy that studies of Vanderkolk, Dontas, and Hoobler [19] showed that the acute enhancement of renal blood flow is subsequently lost in chronic prolonged oral administration of hydralazine.

Alpha-Methyldopa

In 1963 we conducted studies on the systemic and renal hemodynamic effects of alpha-methyldopa in patients with essential hypertension.[20] After the control hemodynamic evaluation was made with the patients in supine and tilted positions, alpha-methyldopa was administered intravenously in 2- to 2.5-gm doses to 11 hospitalized patients with essential hypertension. The maximum hypotensive response occurred within 10 to 20 hours after administration of the drug, and the cardiac and renal hemodynamic studies were repeated at this time, again with the subjects in both the supine and tilted positions.

The systemic hemodynamic effects in the supine position are reported in Fig. 6*A*. A significant reduction in mean arterial pressure (24%) was observed after drug administration, but there were no consistent effects on heart rate. At the time of the maximum antihypertensive response, cardiac output was not significantly changed, while total peripheral vascular resistance decreased (26%). The systemic hemodynamic effects in the erect position are shown in Fig. 6*B*. During the hypotensive response the cardiac output was again not significantly affected while an even greater decrease in total peripheral resistance (32%) and in mean arterial pressure (35%) occurred.

Similar hemodynamic studies at rest and in the sitting position were conducted by Sannerstedt, Varnauskas, and Werkö [21] following prolonged oral administration of the drug. The systemic hemodynamic effects described were entirely similar to those observed in our laboratory. Furthermore, these investigators showed that the reduction of arterial pressure produced by alpha-methyldopa in resting patients not only persisted during exercise, but was even augmented without unfavorable effects on cardiac performance. Thus, the hypertensive patients showed a normal blood pressure response during exercise under treatment with alpha-methyldopa. There was no tendency to postexercise hypotension.[21] Exercise under alpha-methyldopa treatment produced a normal rise in cardiac output with less increase in heart rate as compared to control performance before therapy. As a consequence, there was an increase in stroke volume.[21]

Figure 7 shows the renal hemodynamic effects of intravenous alpha-methyldopa in 11 patients with essential hypertension. During the hypotensive response to alpha-methyldopa, renal blood flow and the glomerular filtration rate did not show any significant changes. In each instance, however, the renal vascular resistance was significantly reduced, both in the supine and in the tilted position. In 1963 Sannerstedt and co-workers [22] reported the effects of more prolonged oral administration of alpha-methyldopa on renal function in patients with essential hypertension. As ob-

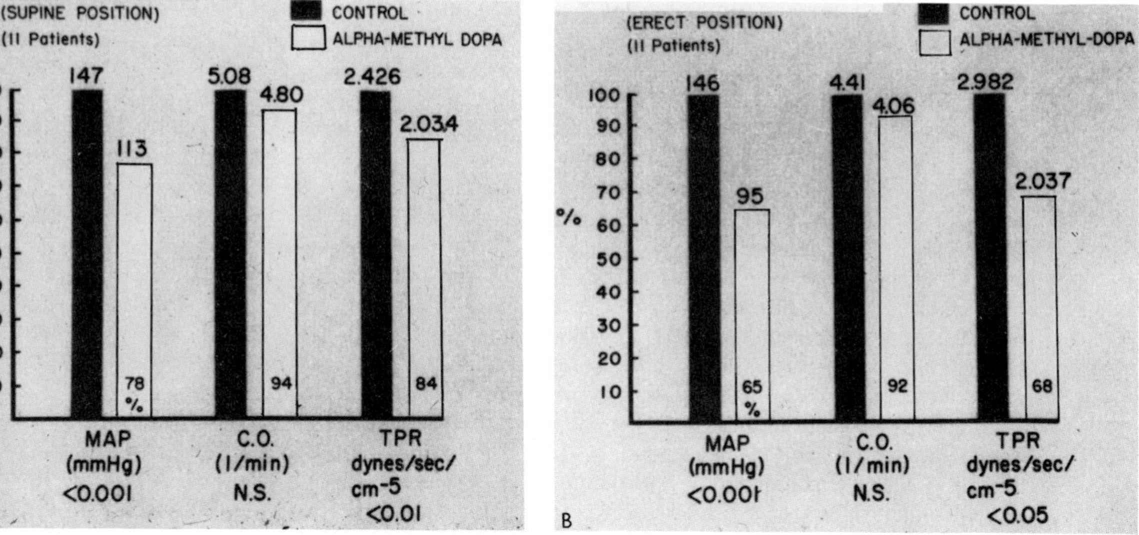

FIG. 6.—Systemic hemodynamic effects of alpha-methyldopa in 11 patients with essential hypertension. (A) supine position; (B) erect position. **MAP,** mean arterial pressure; **CO,** cardiac output; **TPR,** total peripheral resistance.

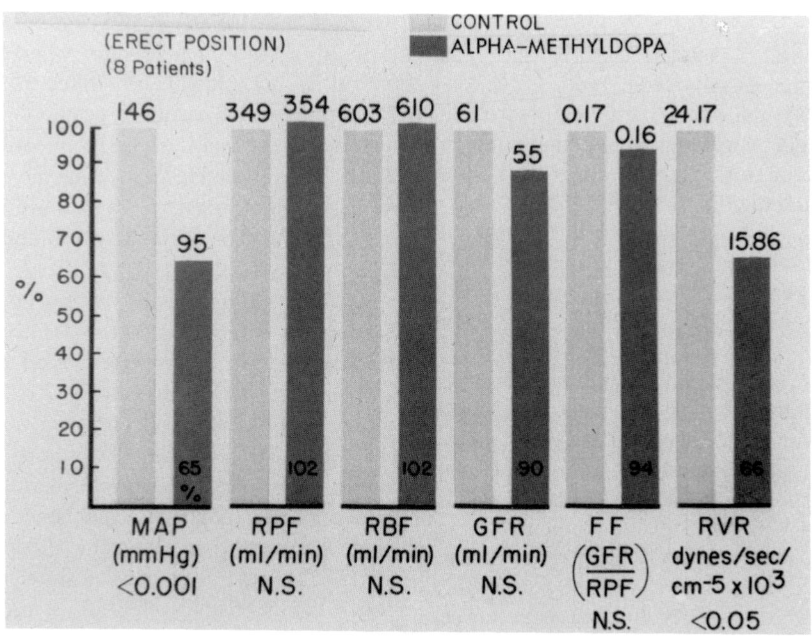

FIG. 7.—Renal hemodynamic effects of alpha-methyldopa in 11 patients with essential hypertension studied in the erect position. **MAP,** mean arterial pressure; **RPF,** renal plasma flow; **RBF,** renal blood flow; **GFR,** glomerular filtration rate; **FF,** filtration fraction; **RVR,** renal vascular resistance.

served in our laboratory, the decrease in blood pressure produced by alpha-methyldopa was not accompanied by significant changes in the glomerular filtration rate and renal plasma flow. The renal vascular resistance was consistently decreased and the renal fraction of cardiac output was found to be increased.

Also in 1963 Weil, Barbour, and Chesne [23] studied the administration of alpha-methyldopa for 8 to 24 days and described no change in renal blood flow, but an actual increase in creatinine clearance when the blood pressure was reduced. A decrease in blood pressure by alpha-methyldopa without a decrease in renal blood flow and glomerular filtration rate was also confirmed by Cannon and Laragh.[24] In 1968 Mohammed and co-workers also found that alpha-methyldopa decreased renal vascular resistance in hypertensive patients in the supine position.[25] The hemodynamic studies described suggest that the drug lowers blood pressure primarily by peripheral arteriolar relaxation. The renal circulation participates in the general decrease in total peripheral resistance.

Pargyline

In 1964 we studied the cardiac and renal hemodynamic effects of the monoamine oxidase (MAO) inhibitor, pargyline hydrochloride, in eight hospitalized patients with essential hypertension who were observed in both the supine and tilted positions.[26]

After the control study, the drug was administered orally in dosages ranging from 75 to 200 mg per day. The maximum antihypertensive response occurred within 10 to 28 days after the initiation of drug therapy, and the cardiac and renal hemodynamic studies were repeated at this time.

The systemic hemodynamic effects of pargyline in the supine position are depicted in Fig. 8*A*. There was an average reduction in mean arterial pressure of 26 percent. There was no consistent change in heart rate. Cardiac output and stroke volume were not significantly altered. There was a consistent reduction in total peripheral resistance in all patients from an average of 2451 to 1913 dynes per second per cm^{-5}.

The systemic hemodynamic effects of pargyline in the erect position are presented in Fig. 8*B*. There was an average blood pressure reduction of 31 percent. Cardiac output and stroke volume were not substantially altered. In contrast, total peripheral resistance was consistently reduced in all patients from an average of 2872 to 2000 dynes per second per cm^{-5}.

The renal hemodynamic effects of pargyline in the supine position are shown in Fig. 9*A*. During the antihypertensive response, renal blood flow did not change significantly. In contrast, the glomerular filtration rate decreased in all cases (13%) with a decrease of the filtration fraction. Changes in renal vascular resistance were inconsistent.

The renal hemodynamic effects of pargyline in the erect position are shown in Fig. 9*B*. With a greater reduction in mean arterial pressure (31%) there were no significant changes in renal blood flow. The glomerular filtration rate decreased sharply (36%) with again a decrease of the filtration fraction. Renal vascular resistance did not show a consistent trend.

Our hemodynamic studies demonstrate that oral administration of pargyline for 10 to 20 days in hospitalized patients with essential hypertension lowers the blood pressure by decreasing vascular resistance, whereas cardiac output is not significantly affected either in the supine or the standing position. The antihypertensive effects are predominantly orthostatic. This systemic hemodynamic pattern is similar to that reported by Maxwell and co-workers [27] with another MAO inhibitor, OR4-1038.

At some variance with our results, in 1967 Sannerstedt [28] reported that oral administration of pargyline for an average period of 5 days lowered the blood pressure at rest, in the sitting position, with a decrease in cardiac output while total peripheral resistance remained almost unchanged. The shorter period of treatment in the patients of Sannerstedt may possibly account in part for the differences. If this is the case, we may postulate that the initial hemodynamic effect of pargyline is a decrease in cardiac output and that a decrease in resistance, with return of cardiac output to control levels, follows. This sequence of hemodynamic events has been recorded with diuretic agents [12] and has been considered to be in

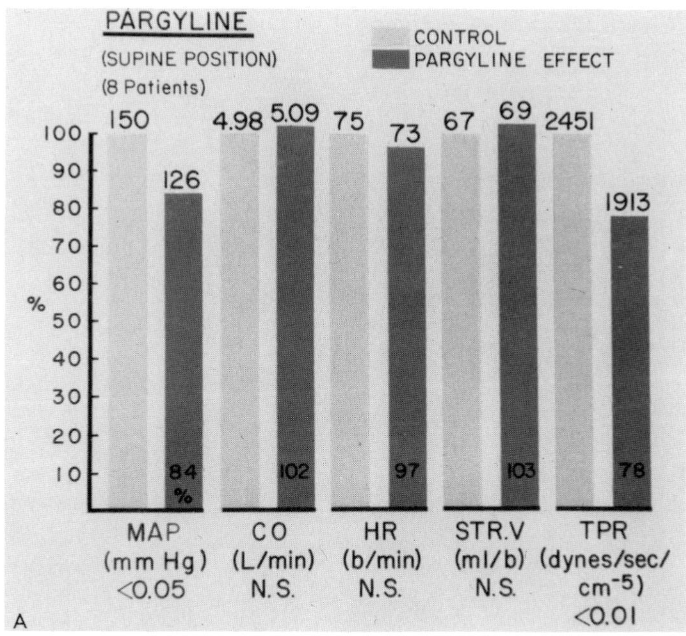

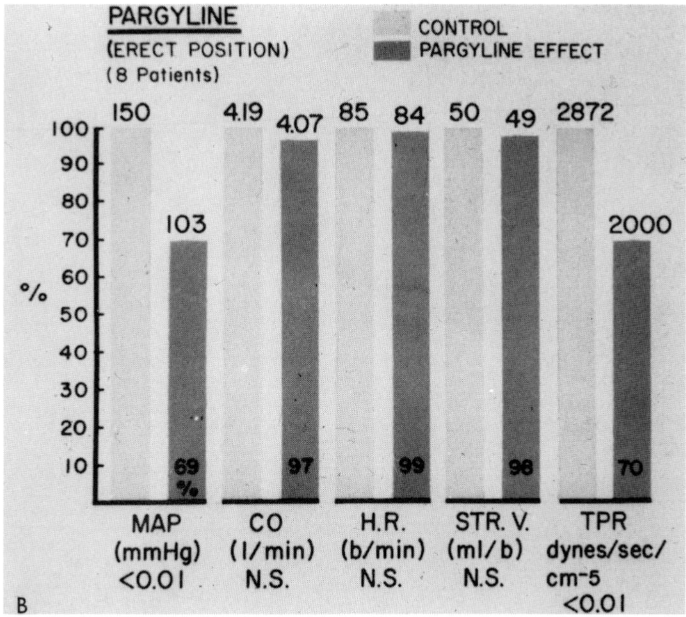

FIG. 8.—Systemic hemodynamic effects of prolonged oral administration of pargyline in eight patients with essential hypertension: (A) supine position; (B) erect position. **MAP,** mean arterial pressure; **CO,** cardiac output; **HR,** heart rate; **STR. V.,** stroke volume; **TPR,** total peripheral resistance.

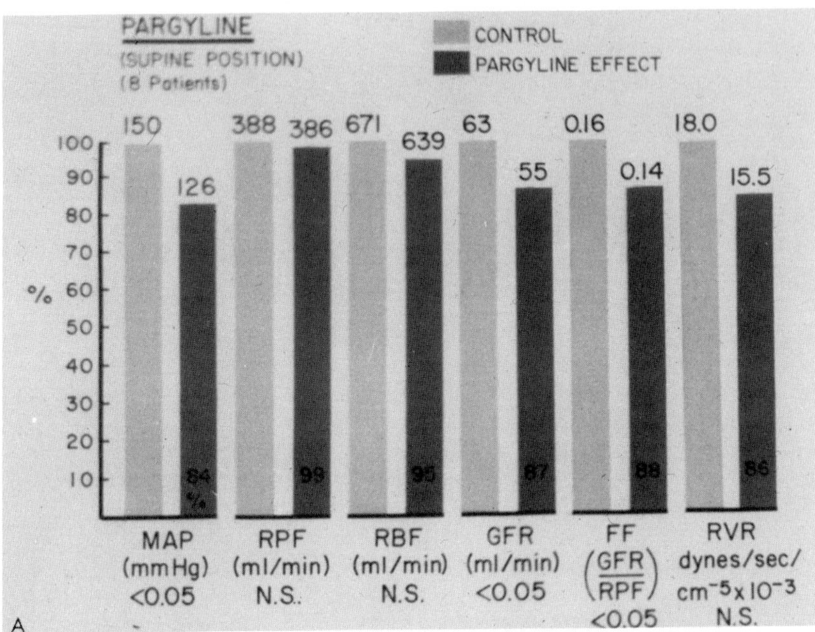

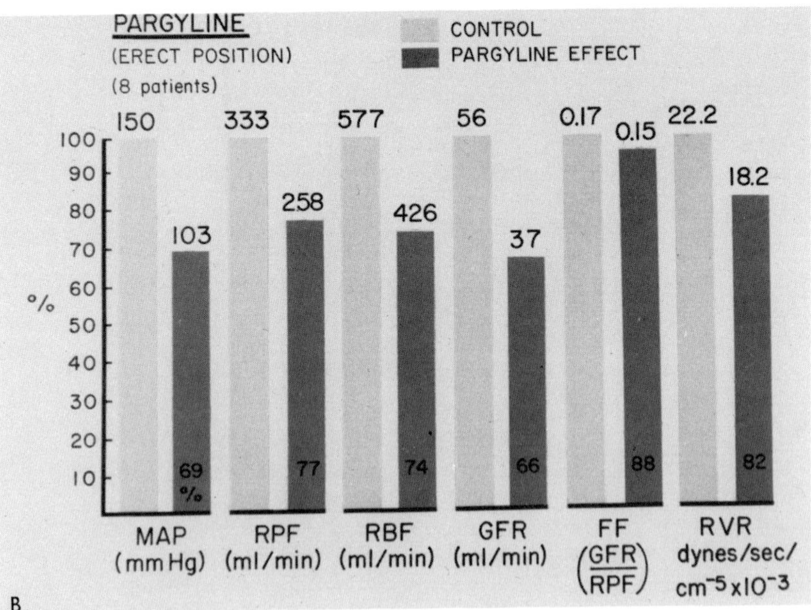

FIG. 9.—Renal hemodynamic effects of prolonged oral administration of pargyline in eight patients with essential hypertension. (A) Supine position; (B) erect position.

TABLE 2.—*Systemic and Renal Hemodynamic Effects of Debrisoquine Sulfate in Eight Patients with Essential Hypertension*

A. Supine Position

	MAP		*CO*		*HR*		*SV*		*TPR*		*RBF*		*GFR*		*RVR*	
	C	*R*	*C*	*R*	*C*	*R*	*C*	*R*	*C*	*R*	*C*	*R*	*C*	*R*	*C*	*R*
Average	141	122	7.65	4.55	71	62	110	84	1554	2023	624	595	89	27	18.07	16.56
% Control		86		76		87		87		—		98		98		92
P Value <		0.01		0.01		0.01		N.S.		N.S.		N.S.		N.S.		N.S.

B. Erect Position

	MAP		*CO*		*HR*		*SV*		*TPR*		*RBF*		*GFR*		*RVR*	
	C	*R*	*C*	*R*	*C*	*R*	*C*	*R*	*C*	*R*	*C*	*R*	*C*	*R*	*C*	*R*
Average	145	112	5.79	3.46	74	66	80	59	2169	2451	580	441	81	59	21.57	18.72
% Control		77		60		89		73		113		77		85		80
P Value <		0.01		0.02		0.05		N.S.		N.S.		0.01		N.S.		0.05

Abbreviations: C = control; R = response to debrisoquine sulfate; MAP = mean arterial pressure (mm Hg); CO = cardiac output (liters per minute); HR = heart rate (beats per minute); SV = stroke volume (milliliters per beat); TPR = total peripheral vascular resistance (dynes per second per cm^{-5}); RBF = renal blood flow (milliliters per minute); GFR = glomerular filtration rate (milliliters per minute); RVR = renal vascular resistance (dynes per second per $cm^{-5} \times 10^3$).

keeping with the theory of myogenic autoregulation.[29]

Sannerstedt also reported that during exercise, with pargyline therapy, there was less increase in heart rate than during the control period. Brachial artery pressure was also lower.[28]

Our renal hemodynamic study shows that renal blood flow is not significantly decreased despite the decrease in systemic arterial pressure. The preservation of cardiac output is probably responsible for maintaining renal blood flow during the hypotensive response. With the decrease in renal perfusion pressure, however, the glomerular filtration rate was decreased with a decrease in filtration fraction. This renal hemodynamic effect is in keeping with a predominant dilatation of the efferent arteriole and consequent decrease in the glomerular filtration pressure.

Debrisoquine Sulfate

In 1966, we conducted studies on the cardiac and renal hemodynamic effects of debrisoquine sulfate in eight hospitalized patients with essential hypertension.[20] After the control study, 3,4-dihydro-2(1H)-isoquinolinecarboxamide sulfate (debrisoquine sulfate) was administered orally in dosages ranging from 60 to 160 mg daily. The maximum antihypertensive response occurred within 5 to 20 days after initiation of drug therapy. At that time, the cardiac and renal hemodynamic studies were repeated.

The hemodynamic effects of drug administration in the supine position are summarized in Table 2*A*. A modest blood pressure reduction was observed in every patient (14%). Cardiac output decreased an average of 24 percent. Since cardiac output and heart rate both decreased, there was no significant change in stroke volume. Similarly, total peripheral vascular resistance did not change. During the antihypertensive response, changes in renal blood flow and the glomerular filtration rate were not significant.

The hemodynamic effect of drug administration in the erect position is recorded in Table 2*B*. The blood pressure decreased in every patient, the average reduction being 23 percent. There was a consistent reduction in heart rate. Cardiac output decreased an average of 40 percent. There was no significant variation in stroke volume. Again, total peripheral resistance did not change. Renal blood flow decreased in seven of the eight patients, the average reduction being 23 percent. The glomerular filtration rate decreased in every instance, averaging a 15 percent reduction.

Thus it is concluded that oral administration of debrisoquine sulfate exerts a moderate antihypertensive effect which lowers the blood pressure primarily by reducing cardiac output whereas arteriolar tone is not reduced. The decrease in cardiac output is associated with a reduction in heart rate in both the supine and standing positions. The mechanism responsible for cardiac output was not elucidated by our studies. It is perhaps noteworthy in this regard that biochemical studies in rats have demonstrated that the drug does not decrease the level of serotonin and norepinephrine in the myocardium.[31] The modest blood pressure reduction (14%) produced in the supine position was not accompanied by any significant decrease in renal hemodynamics. However, in the erect position, the more marked reduction in mean arterial blood pressure was associated with significant reduction in renal blood flow.

References

1. Moyer, J. H., Hughes, W., and Huggins, R. A.: The cardiovascular and renal hemodynamic response to the administration of reserpine (Serpasil). Am. J. Med. Sci. 227: 640, 1354.
2. Reubi, F., Müller, P., and Stuck, P.: Effets circulatoires de la réserpine (Serpasil). Helv. Med. Acta 21:493, 1954.
3. Shumann, H.: Die Veränderung von Schlagvolumen und gefässwiderstand unter dem Einfluss blutdrucksenkender Stoffe beim Hochdruckkranken. II. Reserpin (Serpasil-Ciba) seine Kombination mit Nepresol. Klin. Wochenschr. 32:220, 1954.
4. Bock, K. D., and Müller, H.: Die Wirkung von Reserpin auf die Haut—und Muskeldurchblutung bei gesunden Menschen und Hochdruckkranken. Klin. Wochenschr. 34: 318, 1956.

5. Hafkenschiel, J. H., Sellers, A. M., King, G. A., and Thorner, M. W.: Preliminary observations on the effects of parenteral reserpine on cerebral blood flow, oxygen and glucose metabolism and electroencephalogram in patients with essential hypertension. Ann. N.Y. Acad. Sci. 61:78, 1955.
6. Maxwell, R. A., Plummer, A. J., Schneider, F., Povalski, H., and Daniel, A. I.: Pharmacology of [2-(octahydro-1-azocinyl-ethyl]-guanidine sulfate (SU-3864). J. Pharmacol. Exp. Ther. 123:128, 1958.
7. Richardson, D. W., Wyso, E. M., Magee, J. H., and Cavell, G. G.: Circulatory effects of guanethidine. Clinical, renal and cardiac responses to treatment with a novel antihypertensive drug. Circulation 22:184, 1960.
8. Cass, R., Kuntzman, R., and Brodie, B. B.: Norepinephrine depletion as a possible mechanism of action of guanethidine (SU 5864), a new hypotensive agent. Proc. Soc. Exp. Biol. 103:871, 1960.
9. Gaffney, T. E., Bryant, W. H., and Braunwald, E.: Effects of reserpine and guanethidine on venous reflexes. Circ. Res. 11:889, 1962.
10. Freis, E. D., Rose, J. D., Partenope, E. A., Higgins, T. F., Kelley, R. T., Schnaper, H. W., and Johnson, R. L.: The hemodynamic effects of hypotensive agents in man. III. Hexamethonium. J. Clin. Invest. 32:1285, 1953.
11. Trapold, J. H.: Role of venous return in the cardiovascular response following injection of ganglion-blocking agents. Circ. Res. 5:444, 1957.
12. Villarreal, H., Exaire, J. E., Revollo, A., and Soni, J.: Effects of chlorothiazide on systemic hemodynamics in essential hypertension. Circulation 26:405, 1962.
13. Craver, B. N., Barrett, W., Cameron, A., and Yonkman, F. F.: Activities of 1-hydrazinophthalazine (BA-5968), a hypotensive agent. J. Am. Pharm. Assoc. (Sci. Ed.) 40: 559, 1951.
14. Schroeder, H. A.: Pharmacology of hydralazine. *In* Moyer, J. H. (Ed.): Hypertension: The First Hahnemann Symposium on Hypertensive Disease. Philadelphia: Saunders, 1959, pp. 332–344.
15. Gross, F., Drevy, J., and Meier, D.: Eine neues Gruppe Blutdrucksenkender Substanzen von besonderem Wirkungschataker. Experientia 6:19, 1950.
16. Reubi, F. C.: Renal hyperemia induced in man by a new phthalazine derivative (17591). Proc. Soc. Exp. Biol. Med. 73:102, 1950.
17. Wilkinson, E. L., Backman, H., and Hecht, H. H.: Cardiovascular and renal adjustments to hypotensive agent (1-hydrazinophthalazine: CIBA Ba-5968—Apresoline). J. Clin. Invest. 31:872, 1952.
18. Moyer, J. H.: Discussion. *In* Brest, A. N. and Moyer, J. H. (Eds.): Hypertension: Recent Advances. The Second Hahnemann Symposium on Hypertensive Disease. Philadelphia: Lea & Febiger, 1961, p. 309.
19. Vanderkolk, K., Dontas, A. S., and Hoobler, S. W.: Renal and hypotensive effects of acute and chronic oral administration with 1-hydrazinophthalazine (Apresoline) in hypertension. Am. Heart J. 48:95, 1954.
20. Onesti, G., Brest, A. N., Novack, P., Kasparian, H., and Moyer, J. H.: Pharmacodynamic effects of alpha-methyl-dopa in hypertensive subjects. Am. Heart J. 67:32, 1964.
21. Sannerstedt, R., Varnauskas, E., and Werkö, L.: Hemodynamic effects of methyl dopa (Aldomet) at rest and during exercise in patients with arterial hypertension. Acta Med. Scand. 171:75, 1961.
22. Sannerstedt, R., Bojs, G., Varnauskas, E., and Werkö, L.: Alpha-methyl-dopa in arterial hypertension. Clinical, renal and hemodynamic studies. Acta Med. Scand. 174:53, 1963.
23. Weil, M. H., Barbour, B. H., and Chesne, R. B.: Alpha-methyl-dopa for the treatment of hypertension. Clinical and pharmacodynamic studies. Circulation 28:165, 1963.
24. Cannon, P. J., and Laragh, J. H.: Treatment of hypertension with alpha-methyl-dopa. Pharmakotherapia 1:171, 1963.
25. Mohammed, S., Hanenson, I. B., Magenheim, H. G., and Gaffney, T. E.: Effects of alpha-methyl-dopa on renal function in hypertensive patients. Am. Heart J. 76:21, 1968.
26. Onesti, G., Novack, P., Ramirez, O., Brest, A. N., and Moyer, J. H.: Hemodynamic effects of pargyline in hypertensive patients. Circulation 30:830, 1964.
27. Maxwell, M. H., Gonick, H. C., Scaduto, L., Pearce, M. L., and Kleeman, C. R.: Hemodynamic studies of a monoamine oxidase inhibitor, DL-serine-N^2-isopropylhydrazide (RO 4-1038). Mechanism of hypotensive action. Circulation 26:1279, 1962.
28. Sannerstedt, R.: Hemodynamic effects of pargyline hydrochloride at rest and during exercise in hypertension. Acta Med. Scand. 181:699, 1967.
29. Coleman, T. G., Granger, H. J., and Guyton, A. C.: Whole-body circulatory autoregulation

and hypertension. Circ. Res. 29(Suppl. II): 76, 1971.

30. Onesti, G., La Schiazza, D., Brest, A. N., and Moyer, J. H.: Cardiac and renal hemodynamic effects of debrisoquine sulfate in hypertensive patients. Clin. Pharmacol. Ther. 7:17, 1966.

31. Moe, R. A., Bates, H. M., Palkoski, Z. M., and Banziger, R.: Cardiovascular effects of 3,4-dihydro-2(1H)-isoquinolinecarboxamidine (Declinax). Curr. Ther. Res. 6:299, 1964.

Effects of Antihypertensive Agents on Skin and Muscle Blood Flow in Man

By Peter Merguet, M.D. and Klaus D. Bock, M.D.

In this chapter we will discuss our studies on the effects of commonly used antihypertensive agents on skin and muscle blood flow in man. Reserpine, hydralazine, alpha-methyldopa, clonidine, and guanethidine will be discussed. The studies were performed with the purpose of determining whether the peripheral actions of these drugs in therapeutic dosage contribute to the blood pressure lowering effect, or whether the vascular beds of skin and muscle are only passively involved.

Methods

The most important methods for measuring peripheral blood flow in acute experiments in man are summarized below:

1. Quantitative
   a. Venous occlusion plethysmography
2. Semiquantitative
   a. Heat clearance device
      Skin
      Muscle
   b. Isotope clearance

Venous occlusion plethysmography gives fairly exact quantitative data, but it has the disadvantage of not differentiating between skin blood flow and muscle blood flow. In contrast the heat-clearance devices allow a separate and simultaneous estimation of skin and muscle blood flow; the procedure, however, is difficult and sometimes time-consuming. The calibration is performed in a percentage of resting blood flow, using complete arterial occlusion to estimate the zero blood flow. The tissue clearance of isotopes also permits a separate estimation of skin and muscle blood flow. Rapid changes, however, are detected with insufficient accuracy, and the duration of the observation is limited. For these reasons, in our studies we have combined occlusion plethysmography with heat-clearance devices for skin and muscle blood flow evaluation.

Figure 1A shows different types of heat-conductivity probes. Method details have been reported elsewhere.[1] The probe at the right demonstrates a recently developed model which contains an additional injection cannula. Through the cannula, small amounts of drugs can be injected locally into the muscle, within the area in which the muscle blood flow is measured. Figure 1B shows the heat-clearance device for the skin.

Figure 2 shows a comparative estimate of hand blood flow by means of plethysmography and of skin blood flow by means of the heat-clearance device before and after the injection of 0.15 mg of clonidine. The good agreement of the two methods is evident.

Figure 3 shows the effects of clonidine on the blood flow in different areas measured by different methods. In the skin of the hand the reduction of blood flow is of short duration whereas the skin blood flow in the calf remains reduced for a longer period of time. This is evident in this example that the reduction of skin blood flow are different in different areas of the body and that the blood flow of the hand and of the foot is not representative for the skin as a whole. Furthermore, total blood flow in the forearm decreases, whereas the muscle blood flow in the calf remains unchanged after an initial minimal increase. It is evident in this example that the reduction of forearm blood flow, which usually is considered to represent mainly muscle blood flow, is caused by the decrease in skin blood flow.

The technique for the evaluation of local effects of drugs is shown in Fig. 4. For local administration of the test substances a very small "injection system" is inserted into the skin. The heat-clearance device, for the measurement of skin blood flow, is fixed directly above the injection cannula. The administra-

From the Division for Renal and Hypertensive Disease, Medizinische Klinik, Klinikum der Ruhruniversitaet, Essen, West Germany.

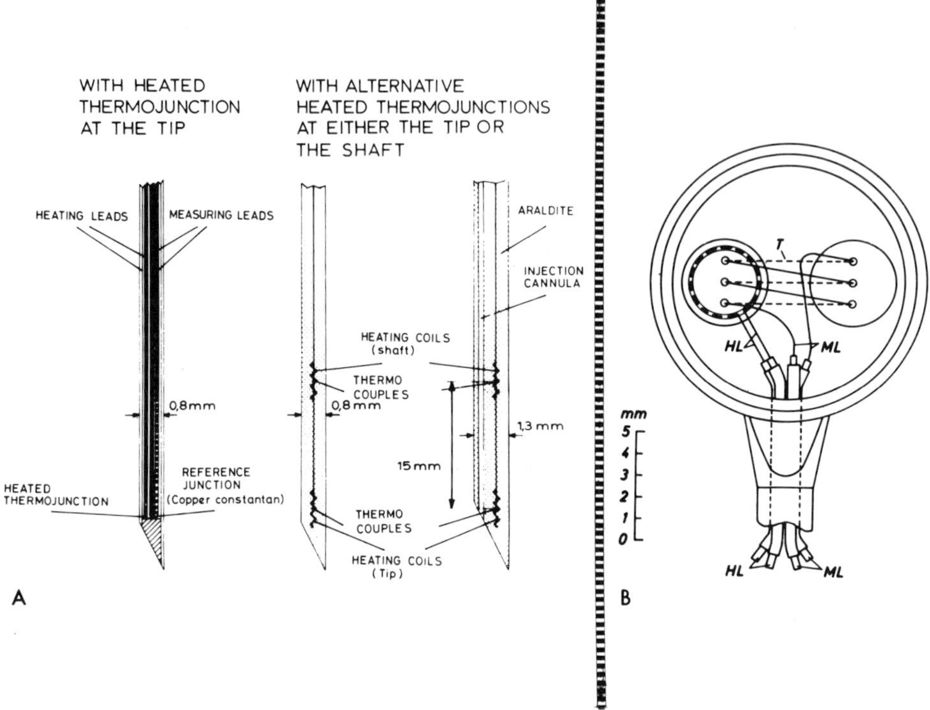

FIG. 1.—(A) Three different types of heat-conductivity probes for measurements of muscle blood flow. Note the injection system in the probe at the right for local administration of drugs. (B) Heat-clearance device for measurement of skin blood flow. **T,** thermo battery; **HL,** heating leads; **ML,** measuring leads.

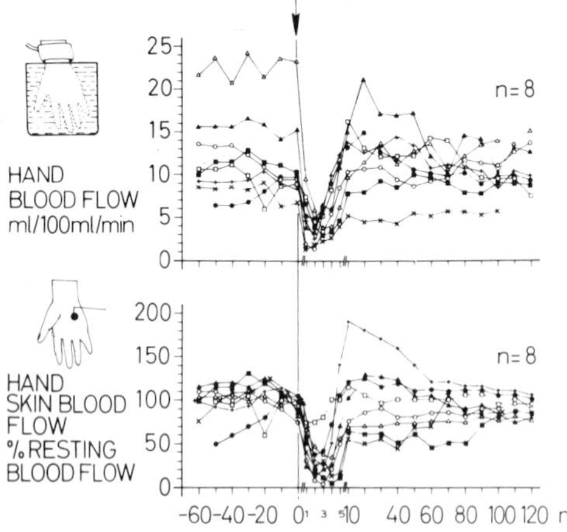

FIG. 2.—Comparison of skin blood flow, determined by a heat-clearance device at the palmar surface, with total blood flow of the hand determined by venous-occlusion plethysmography. Observations in eight normotensive subjects after intravenous administration of 0.15 mg of clonidine.

tion of drugs into the muscle is performed through a heat-conductivity probe containing an additional "injection system."

Figure 5 is an original tracing obtained with this method after local application of hydralazine into skin and muscle. The injection is usually followed by a short deflection of the recording system due to local temperature and pressure changes. Local application of hydralazine causes an increase of both skin and muscle blood flow indicating a direct vasodilating action of the drug on these vascular beds. Intra-arterial injections of hydralazine had similar effects. The results of a series of studies with hydralazine are summarized in Fig. 6.

Using the experimental setting, depicted in Fig. 7, we investigated the effects of the abovementioned five antihypertensive agents in both normotensive and hypertensive subjects. Although some minor differences between normotensives and hypertensives were observed, only

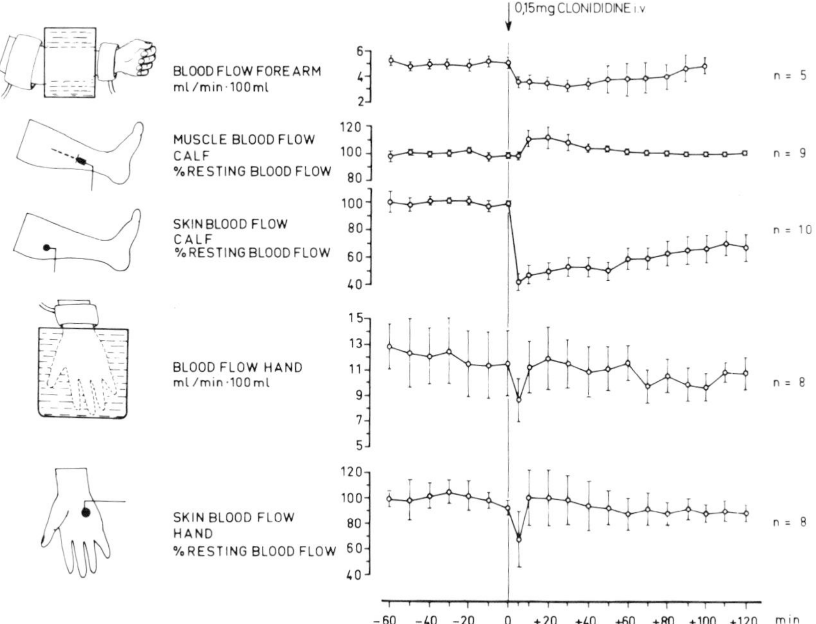

FIG. 3.—Comparison of blood flow measurements in different regions and with different techniques. From above: Occlusion plethysmography, forearm; heat-conductivity probe, calf; heat-clearance device for skin at the calf; occlusion-plethysmography, hand; heat-clearance device at the skin of the palmar surface. Number of observations is indicated by **n.**

the results of the hypertensive group will be reported in detail.

Reserpine

Reserpine (Fig. 8) in a 1-mg dose given intravenously causes a slow decrease of blood pressure and a slight fall in heart rate by about 6 to 10 beats per minute. Total blood flow of the forearm and of the hand, and skin blood flow in the calf increased distinctly. Muscle blood flow in the calf, however, remained unchanged. It can be concluded, therefore, that the increase of total blood flow in the forearm is due to the increase of skin blood flow. These observations are in accordance with earlier findings of others [2,3] with the

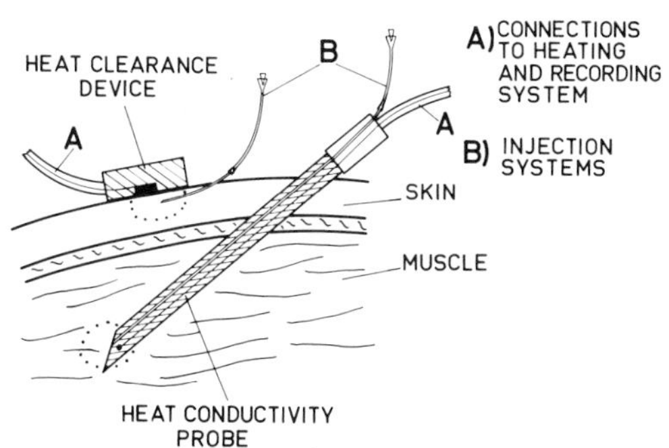

FIG. 4.—Method for measurements of skin and muscle blood flow demonstrating the position of the injection systems for local administration of drugs.

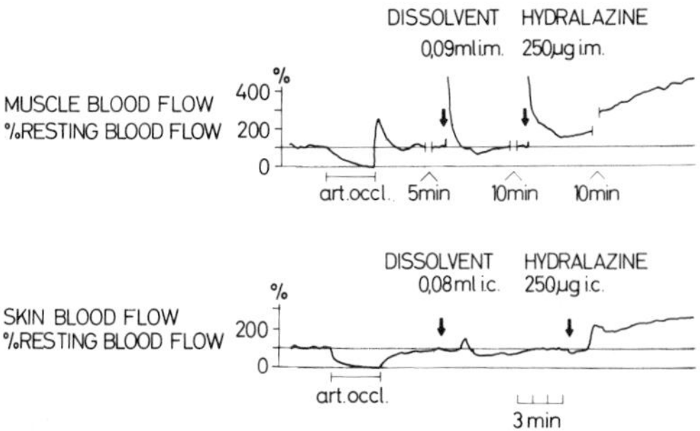

FIG. 5.—Local effects of hydralazine and its dissolvent on muscle and skin blood flow. Original record; **art. occl.,** arterial occlusion.

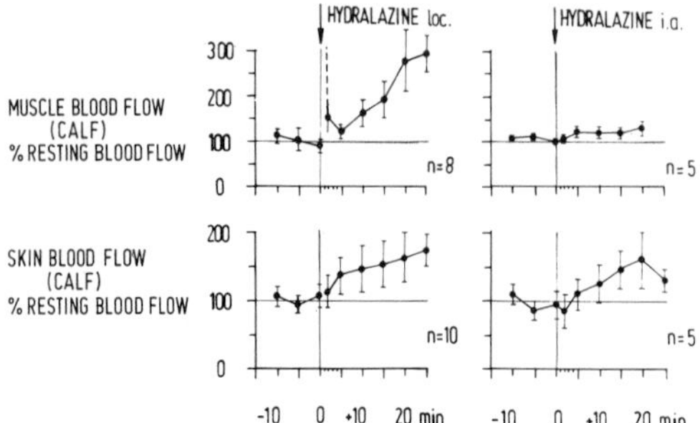

FIG. 6.—Mean values (± SD) of the effects of hydralazine on muscle and skin blood flow after (left) local (0.25-mg dose) and (right) intra-arterial (1.25-mg dose) administration. Number of experiments is indicated by **n.**

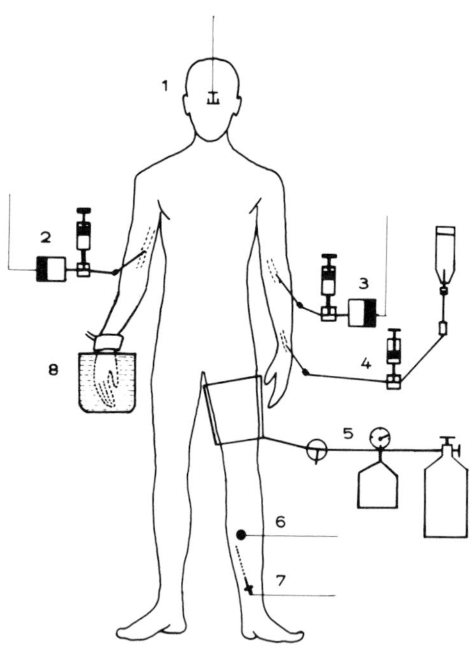

FIG. 7.—Methods used in the acute experiments described in the text. (1) Respiration rate by means of a thermistor in the nostril. (2, 3) Venous and arterial pressure directly with Statham elements. (4) Injection system, invisible to the subject. (5) Arterial occlusion system for repeated calibrations of heat-clearance devices. (6) Heat-clearance device for skin (can be attached to any other region). (7) Heat-conductivity probe. (8) Water-filled (34°C), venous-occlusion plethysmograph (alternatively or simultaneously applied at the calf or at the forearm).

exception of Åblad [4] and of Freis and Ari.[5] Others [6–8] who measured total blood flow of the forearm and the hand after intra-arterial application of reserpine concluded that the drug exerts a direct vasodilating effect. Our own studies with local administration of reserpine revealed a very slight increase in muscle blood flow.

Hydralazine

Hydralazine (Fig. 9), given intravenously as dihydralazine in a 12.5-mg. dose, elicited, within 5 to 10 minutes after injection, a marked fall of systolic and diastolic blood pressure, resulting in a decrease of mean arterial pressure of 25 mm Hg. The heart rate increased by about 25 to 30 beats per minute. Total blood flow of the forearm was not measured in hypertensive patients. In normotensive subjects, however, a slight increase of blood flow in the forearm was observed. Total blood flow of the hand increased markedly. The skin blood flow in the calf also rose, but to a lesser degree. This indicates again the different behavior of the vascular bed of the skin in different regions. The muscle blood flow in the calf did not show any remarkable change. Our observations are in accordance with the extensive experimental work of Åblad and coworkers.[9–11] These investigators also demonstrated an increase of total blood flow in the forearm and the hand after intra-arterial infusion of hydralazine; this finding led them to conclude that hydralazine acts directly on the vascular smooth muscle. Our studies with local administration of hydralazine into muscle and skin (Figs. 5 and 6) are in complete agreement with these findings. We emphasize, however, that even the small, 12.5-mg dose of dihydralazine produced extremely unpleasant side effects, including palpitations, a sensation of "pressure to the head," a migraine-type headache, and occasionally nausea and vomiting.

Alpha-methyldopa

Alpha-methyldopa (Fig. 10) in a 1-gm dose, given intravenously, produced essentially no change of any of the measured parameters within an observation time of 2 hours after injection, and in some patients within 160 minutes. The complete lack of a methyldopa-

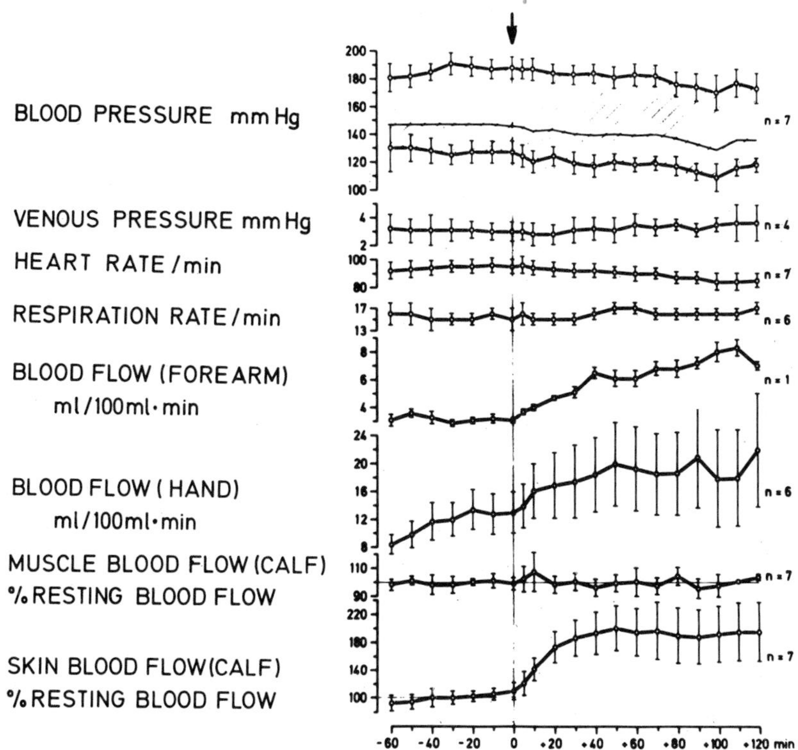

FIG. 8.—Circulatory reactions elicited by a 1-mg dose of reserpine, given intravenously to hypertensive subjects. Mean values (± mean error of the mean); number of subjects studied is indicated by **n.**

induced effect in our study may be due to two reasons: (1) We used the drug in the commercially available form, as the ethyl-ester; and (2) the observation time might have been too short. The published reports on the effects of parenterally given alpha-methyldopa show different results.[12–16] The onset of a drop in blood pressure varied from 30 minutes up to 4 hours after administration. One group who measured the blood pressure directly described a decrease 3 hours after injection.[17]

Clonidine

Clonidine (Fig. 11) in a 0.15-mg dose, given intravenously, lowered both systolic and diastolic blood pressure in all hypertensive patients studied. As has been shown earlier,[18–27] immediately after intravenous injection a brief, transitory, initial blood pressure rise occurred. Heart rate decreased slightly (5 to 7 beats per minute). The total blood flow of the forearm decreased due to the definite decrease in skin blood flow (Figs. 2 and 3). Muscle blood flow remained unchanged after a short-lasting, slight initial increase. Local administration of clonidine into the muscle caused no change of muscle blood flow, whereas local application into the skin resulted in a marked decrease of blood flow indicating a peripheral vasoconstrictor action in the skin. (For further details see the chapter entitled, "Effects of Clonidine on Regional Blood Flow and Its Use in the Treatment of Hypertension.")

Guanethidine

Guanethidine (Fig. 12) in a 20-mg dose, given intravenously, lowered both systolic and diastolic blood pressure. In some patients the decrease in blood pressure lasted only a short time, i.e., from 5 to 15 minutes. To our surprise, in none of eight studies in hypertensive patients was the initial transitory pressor phase[28–38] observed. In 17 acute experiments on normotensive subjects, we observed

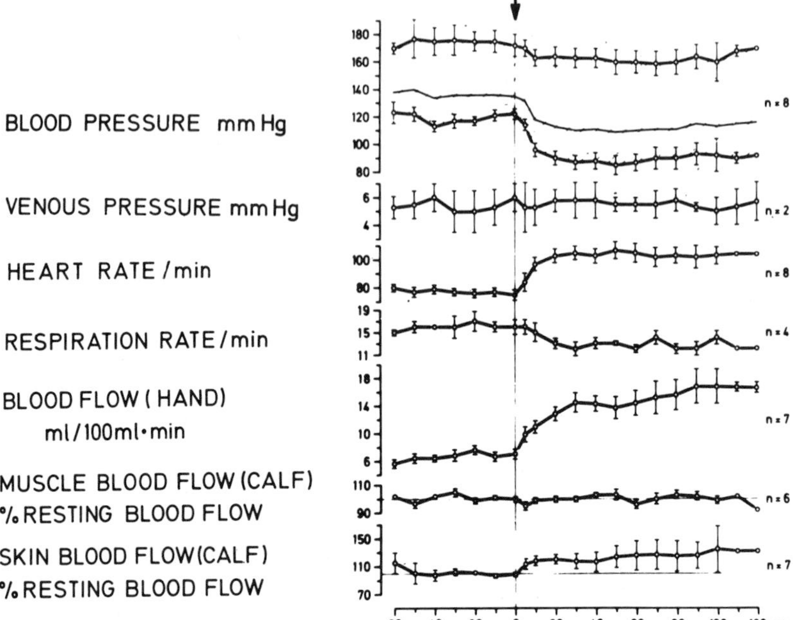

FIG. 9.—Circulatory reactions elicited by a 12.5-mg dose of hydralazine, given intravenously to hypertensive subjects. (See Fig. 8.)

an initial blood pressure increase only on three occasions. Heart rate decreased slightly (by 6 to 8 beats per minute). Total blood flow in the forearm and in the hand remained almost unchanged or increased slightly with time. Skin blood flow in the calf also had a slight tendency to rise whereas muscle blood flow remained unaltered. Others have reported similar results with regard to forearm blood flow.[8,39–41] After local administration of guanethidine a slight increase of muscle and skin blood flow was seen.

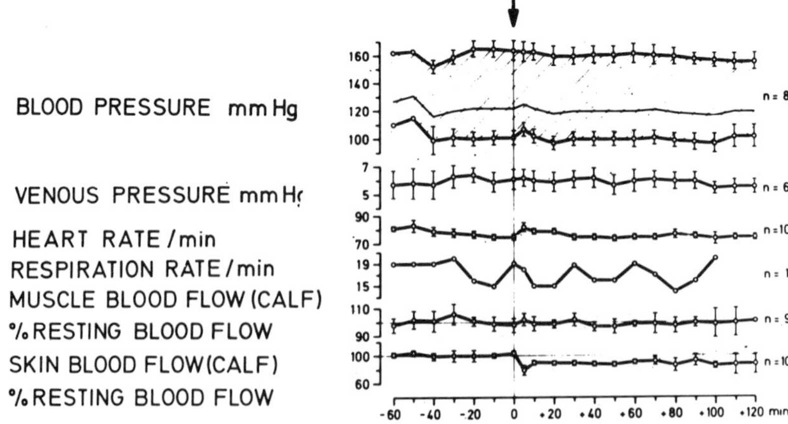

FIG. 10.—Circulatory reactions elicited by a 1-gm dose of alpha-methyldopa, given intravenously to hypertensive subjects. (See Fig. 8.)

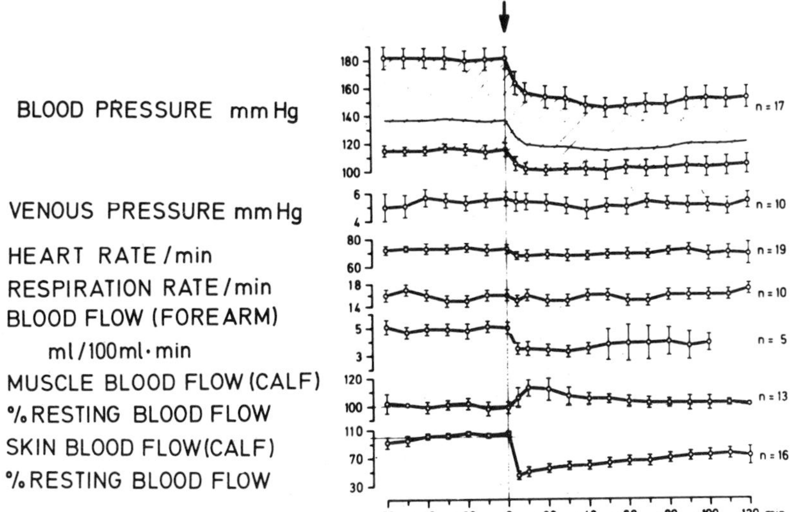

Fig. 11.—Circulatory reactions elicited by a 0.15-mg dose of clonidine given intravenously to hypertensive subjects. (See Fig. 8.)

Discussion

Table 1 gives a summary of our results including those which have not been described in the foregoing text for reasons of space. With the exception of a slight increase of muscle blood flow in some normotensive subjects after guanethidine administration, it is evident that none of the tested antihypertensive agents alters muscle blood flow significantly when given intravenously, regardless of whether a fall in blood pressure occurs. A decrease in blood

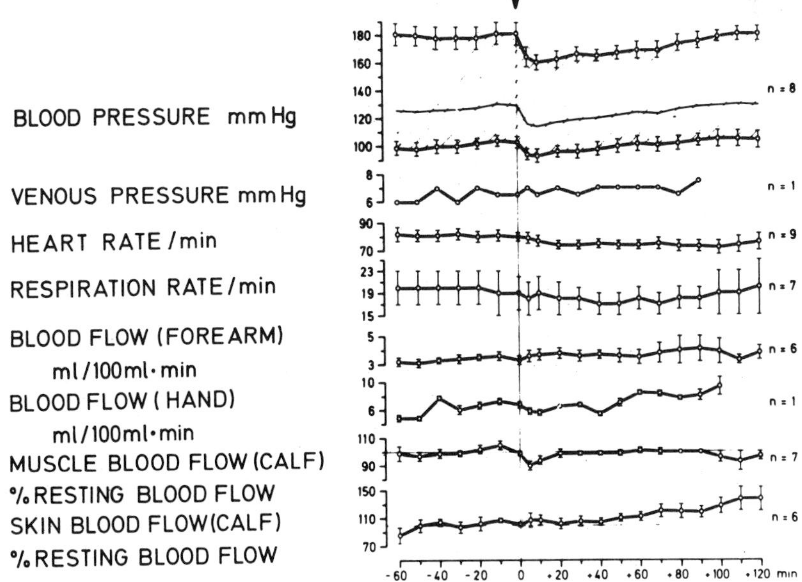

Fig. 12.—Circulatory reactions elicited by a 20-mg dose of guanethidine, given intravenously to hypertensive subjects. (See Fig. 8.)

TABLE 1.—*Effects of Various Antihypertensive Agents on Blood Pressure, Muscle and Skin Blood Flow in Man*

Agent	*Patient*	*Blood Pressure*	*Muscle Blood Flow*		*Skin Blood Flow*	
			i.v.	*loc.*	*i.v.*	*loc.*
Reserpine	N	— or 0	0	+ or 0	+	+ or 0
	H	—	0		+	
Hydralazine	N	0	0	+	+	+
	H	—	0		+	
Guanethidine	N	0	+ or 0	+ or 0	0	+ or 0
	H	—	0		+ or 0	
Clonidine	N	— or 0	0	0	—	—
	H	—	0		—	

Abbreviations and symbols used: i.v. = intravenous administration; loc. = local administration; N = normotensives; H =hypertensives; + = increase; — = decrease; 0 = no change.

pressure, together with an unchanged muscle blood flow, indicates that a vasodilatation in the muscular vascular bed has taken place. This vasodilatation in the muscle could be due to a local drug effect; if so, this local effect would contribute to the fall in blood pressure. A direct, local drug action on muscle vessels was demonstrable only with hydralazine and, to a very small extent, with reserpine and guanethidine; an indirect effect, e.g., via the central sympathetic nervous system, cannot be excluded or proved with our experimental design. Another possible explanation for the constant muscle blood flow is that local blood flow regulation may compensate immediately for each change in pressure. A definite answer, however, cannot be obtained in the present experimental setting.

Skin blood flow, on the other hand, increases or decreases regardless of whether the blood pressure falls. A direct, local action on skin vessels was demonstrated for hydralazine (vasodilatation), for clonidine (vasoconstriction), and to a small extent for guanethidine (vasodilation). These local drug effects, together with the others mediated through the sympathetic nervous system, appear to be responsible for the changes of blood flow in the skin. The lack of correlation between blood pressure alterations and skin blood flow changes indicates that the cutaneous vascular bed is not involved to an important extent in blood pressure regulation during treatment with antihypertensive agents under resting conditions. From a teleologic point of view this seems to be understandable if one considers the prominent role of skin blood flow in heat regulation.

SUMMARY

In acute experiments on normotensive and hypertensive men the effects of reserpine, hydralazine, alpha-methyldopa, clonidine, and guanethidine on arterial and venous blood pressure (directly recorded), heart rate, respiration rate, and peripheral blood flow were investigated. Total blood flow in the forearm or in the hand was measured by venous-occlusion plethysmography, muscle and skin blood flow in the calf or in the hand by heat-clearance devices. In special experiments the local vascular effects of the drugs after intramuscular and intracutaneous injection were investigated. After intravenous administration of drugs in hypertensives the following results were obtained: The arterial blood pressure was lowered by reserpine, hydralazine, clonidine and guanethidine. Skin blood flow was increased by reserpine, hydralazine, and guanethidine, and was reduced by clonidine. Muscle blood flow was not altered by any of the agents. By this, the alterations of total blood flow corresponded to the changes of skin blood flow. Alpha-methyldopa had no effects at all within 2 hours. Local effects on skin vessels occurred with hydralazine, guanethidine (both vasodilatation), and clonidine (vasoconstriction), on muscle vessels with reserpine, hydralazine, and guanethidine (vasodilatation). It is assumed under these conditions that the skin vessels play no important role in blood pressure regulation. In contrast, the unchanged muscle blood flow during the fall in blood pressure indicates vasodilatation in the muscle which may be drug-induced or the result of local flow regulation.

References

1. Golenhofen, K., Hensel, H., and Hildebrandt, G.: Durchblutungsmessung mit Wärmeleitelementen. Stuttgart: Thieme, 1963.
2. Bock, K. D., and Müller, H.: Die Wirkung von Reserpin auf die Haut- und Muskeldurchblutung bei gesunden Menschen und Hochdruckkranken. Klin. Wochenschr. 34:318, 1956.
3. Moore, J .G., Singh, B. P., Herzig, D., and Assali, N. S.: Hemodynamic effects of Rauwolfia alkaloid (reserpine) in human pregnancy. Results of intravenous administration. Am. J. Obstet. Gynec. 71:237, 1956.
4. Åblad, B.: Adrenergic block by reserpine in man. Acta Pharmacol. 13:213, 1957.
5. Freis, E. D., and Ari, R.: Clinical and experimental effects of reserpine in patients with essential hypertension. Ann. N.Y. Acad. Sci. 59:45, 1954.
6. de la Lande, I. S., Parks, V. J., Sandison, A. G., Skinner, S. L., and Whelan, R. F.: The peripheral dilator action of reserpine in man. Aust. J. Exp. Biol. Med. Sci. 38:313, 1960.
7. Parks, V. J., Sandison, A. G., Skinner, S. L., and Whelan, R. F.: The mechanism of the vasodilator action of reserpine in man. Clin. Sci. 20:289, 1961.
8. Whelan, R. F.: Control of the peripheral circulation in man. Springfield, Ill.: Thomas, 1967.
9. Åblad, B., Johnsson, G., and Henning, M.: The effect of intra-arterially administered hydralazine on blood flow in the forearm and hand. Acta Pharmacol. 18:191, 1961.
10. Åblad, B., Johnsson, G., and Henning, M.: The effects of hydralazine administered into the brachial artery on adrenergic vasoconstrictor stimuli in the hand. Acta Pharmacol. 19:166, 1962.
11. Åblad, B.: A study of the mechanism of the hemodynamic effects of hydralazine in man. Acta Pharmacol. 20 (Suppl. 1):1, 1963.
12. Dollery, C. T., Harington, M., and Hodge, J. V.: Haemodynamic studies with methyldopa: Effect on cardiac output and response to pressor amines. Br. Heart J. 25:670, 1963.
13. Schaub, F., Nager, F., Schaer, H., Ziegler, W., and Lichtlen, P.: Alpha-methyl-dopa: Therapeutische Erfahrungen bei Hypertonie und biochemische Untersuchungen zu seiner Wirkungsweise. Schweiz. Med. Wochenschr. 92: 620, 1962.
14. Gillespie, L., Jr., Oates, J. A., Crout, J. R., and Sjoerdsma, A.: Clinical and chemical studies with alpha-methyl-dopa in patients with hypertension. Circulation 25:281, 1962.
15. Götze, H.: Erfahrungen mit Alpha-Methyl-Dopa bei renal bedingten Hypertonien. *In* Heilmeyer, L., and Holtmeier, H. J. (Eds.): Therapie des Bluthochdrucks, Medizinische Klausurgespräche 2. Berlin-Freiburg: Verlag für Gesamtmedizin, 1963.
16. Kuschke, H. J., Wölfer, H. J., Igata, A., and Becker, G.: Die Behandlung der Hypertonie mit α-Methyl-dopa; klinische und hämodynamische Untersuchungen. Munch. Med. Wochenschr. 105:1305, 1963.
17. Wilson, W. R., Fisher, F. D., and Kirkendall, W. M.: The acute hemodynamic effects of α-methyldopa in man. J. Chronic Dis. 15:907, 1961.
18. Bock, K. D., Heimsoth, V., Merguet, P., and Schönermark, J.: Klinische und klinisch-experimentelle Untersuchungen mit einer neuen blutdrucksenkenden Substanz: Dichlorphenylaminoimidazolin. Deutsch. Med. Wochenschr. 91:1761, 1966.
19. Bock, K. D., Merguet, P., Murata, T., and Heimsoth, V.: Klinisch-experimentelle Untersuchungen über die Wirkungen von Dichlorphenylaminoimidazolin. *In* Heilmeyer, L. and Holtmeier, H. J. (Eds.): Hochdrucktherapie. Symposion über 2-(2,6-Dichlorphenylamino)-2-imidazolinhydrochlorid in Ulm 20./21.10. 1967. Stuttgart: Thieme, 1968, p. 28.
20. Merguet, P., Heimsoth, V., Murata, T., and Bock, K. D.: Experimental study on the circulatory effects of 2-(2,6-dichlorophenylamino)-2-imidazolinehydrochloride in man. Pharmacol. Clin. 1:30, 1968.
21. Merguet, P., Brandt, T., Murata, T., and Bock, K. D.: Vergleich der akuten blutdrucksenkenden Wirkung von parenteral verabreichten Antihypertensiva bei Normotonikern und Hypertonikern. Verh. Dtsch. Ges. Inn. Med. 75:166, 1969.

22. Barnett, A. J., and Cantor, S.: Observations on the hypotensive action of "Catapres" (St 155) in man. Med. J. Aust. 55:87, 1968.
23. Kühns, K., Oloffs, J., and Pohlmann, F.: Über die Blutdruckwirkung von Dichloraminoimidazolin bei intravenöser Anwendung. Dtsch. Med. Wochenschr. 93:438, 1968.
24. Muir, A. L., and Burton, J. L.: Circulatory effects at rest and exercise of clonidine, an imidazoline derivative with hypotensive properties. Lancet 2:181, 1969.
25. Pozenel, H.: Das Verhalten hämodynamischer Größen von Hypertonikern unter Therapie mit Dichlorphenylamino-Imidazolinhydrochlorid. Wien. Klin. Wochenschr. 81:187, 1969.
26. Vorburger, C., Butikofer, E., and Reubi, F.: Die akute Wirkung von St-155 auf die cardiale und renale Hämodynamik. *In* Heilmeyer, L., and Holtmeier, H. J.: Hochdrucktherapie. Symposion über 2-(2,6-Dichlorphenylamino)-2-imidazolinhydrochlorid in Ulm 20./21.10. 1967. Stuttgart: Thieme, 1968, p. 86.
27. Onesti, G., Bock, K. D., Heimsoth, V., Kim, K. E., and Merguet, P.: Clonidine: A new antihypertensive agent. Am. J. Cardiol. 28: 74, 1971.
28. Page, I. H., and Dustan, H. P.: A new, potent antihypertensive drug. Preliminary study of [(2-(octahydro-1-azocinyl)-ethyl)]-guanidine sulfate (guanethidine). JAMA 170:1265, 1959.
29. Page, I. H., Hurley, R. E., and Dustan, H. P.: The prolonged treatment of hypertension with guanethidine. JAMA 175:543, 1961.
30. Imhof, P. R., Lewis, R. C., Page, I. H., and Dustan, H. P.: Effects of guanethidine on arterial pressure and vasomotor reflexes. *In* Symposium on Guanethedine (Ismelin), sponsored by The University of Tennessee College of Medicine, Memphis, Tennessee, April 22, 1960. Summit, N. J.: CIBA, 1960, pp. 24–29.
31. Lichtlen, P., Bühlmann, A., and Schaub, F.: Zum Mechanismus der blutdrucksenkenden Wirkung von intravenös verabreichtem Guanethidin. Cardiologia 38:197, 1961.
32. Abrahamsen, A. M., Humerfelt, S., and Sigstad, E.: Combined guanethidine and hydrochlorothiazide therapy in hypertension. Acta Med. Scand. 173:155, 1963.
33. Cohn, J. N., Liptak, T. E., and Freis, E. D.: Hemodynamic effects of guanethidine in man. Circ. Res. 12:298, 1963.
34. Dollery, C. T., Emslie-Smith, D., and Shillingford, J. P.: Haemodynamic effects of guanethidine. Lancet 2:331, 1961.
35. Finnerty, F. A., Jr., Chupkovich, V., and Merendino, J.: Preliminary observations on parenterally administered guanethidine in patients with severe hypertension. *In* Symposium on Guanethidine (Ismelin), sponsored by The University of Tennessee College of Medicine, Memphis, Tennessee, April 22, 1960. Summit, N.J.: CIBA, 1960, pp. 96–102.
36. Pigeon, G., Davignon, J., Biron, P., Trudel, J., Dufault, G., and Genest, J.: Guanethidine administration in 28 hypertensive patients. Can. Med. Assoc. J. 83:690, 1960.
37. Richardson, D. W., and Wyso, E. M.: Human pharmacology of guanethidine. Ann. N.Y. Acad. Sci. 88:944, 1960.
38. Nickerson, M.: Drugs inhibiting adrenergic nerves and structures innervated by them; and antihypertensive agents and the drug therapy of hypertension. *In* Goodman, L. S., and Gilman, A. (Eds.): The Pharmacological Basis of Therapeutics, 4th ed. London: Macmillan, 1970.
39. Abboud, F. M., Eckstein, J. W., and Wendling, M. G.: Early potentiation of the vasoconstrictor action of norepinephrine by guanethidine. Proc. Soc. Exp. Biol. Med. 110:489, 1962.
40. Cooper, C. J., Fewings, J. D., Hodge, R. L., and Whelan, R. F.: Effects of bretylium and guanethidine on human hand and forearm vessels and on their sensitivity to noradrenaline. Br. J. Pharmacol. 21:165, 1963.
41. Abramson, D. I.: Circulation in the Extremities. New York: Academic Press, 1967.

Diuretic Drugs: Mechanisms of Antihypertensive Action

By Robert C. Tarazi, M.D.

As in all basically unsolved problems, opinions regarding the mechanism(s) underlying the antihypertensive effects of diuretic drugs have swung between opposite extremes ranging from a "simple sequela of blood volume reduction" to some ill-defined "peripheral vascular effect." Although a definite answer is not yet available, a more balanced evaluation of the problem has been made possible by recent work on blood and extracellular fluid volumes and on the intricate effects of variations in blood flow on vascular resistance. Study of diuretic agents with differing chemical structure and physiologic action has helped to determine the common factors of their antipressor effect, and the more precise characterization of various types of hypertension is leading to more discriminate assessment of therapy.

Basic Considerations

Direct Vasodilator Action

A direct vasodilator action of the diuretic agent per se is improbable [1,2] because of the number of chemically unrelated drugs that share the same hypotensive characteristics, and the fact that they all lower arterial pressure in hypertensive but not in normotensive subjects. These antipressor effects can be nullified by a high-sodium intake [3–5] or mimicked by low-sodium diets which also produce the same negative sodium and water balance as diuretics. Intra-arterial injections of chlorothiazide under controlled steady-flow conditions leave vascular resistance unchanged although diminishing vascular responsiveness to norepinephrine.[6]

From the Research Division of The Cleveland Clinic Foundation and The Cleveland Clinic Educational Foundation, Cleveland, Ohio.

This study was supported in part by grants from the National Heart and Lung Institute, PHS (HE-6835) and from the American Heart Association (70–960).

The importance of diuresis for the antipressor action of thiazides is nevertheless sometimes questioned because of the direct vasodilator effect of diazoxide, a closely related compound with strong sodium-retaining properties. However, diazoxide reduces arterial pressure even in normotensive subjects [7] and whereas it immediately lowers peripheral resistance and increases cardiac output,[7] the thiazides initially reduce output and increase peripheral resistance.[8–10] Furthermore, the time course of the antihypertensive action of the two drugs is different.

Correlation Between Diuretic and Antihypertensive Effects

In contrast with the direct vasodilator action, this correlation seems well established. Thiazides lower arterial pressure only as effective saluresis is established; [1,11–13] in the experience of most investigators the decline in pressure does not precede the diuretic effect. Spironolactone takes a longer time to achieve the full potential of its natriuretic effect,[14] and the onset of its hypotensive action is also more gradual than chlorothiazide.[15] By the same token, in our experience, the main value of furosemide for antihypertensive treatment derives from its wide dosage range and its ability to induce diuresis in the face of relatively diminished glomerular filtration rate.

This correlation between diuresis and antihypertensive effect holds true for the time sequence of the two effects but it does not necessarily mean that effective natriuresis will lower arterial pressure in all subjects indiscriminately. Thiazides will not, for instance, reduce blood pressure in normotensive subjects despite significant weight loss and extracellular fluid depletion; [11, 15–17] this is also true for spironolactone.[15] The hypotensive effect of diuretics thus depends on whether the subject is normotensive or hypertensive and also on the type of hypertension. Certainly not all hypertensive patients respond to a low-sodium diet [18] nor do all forms of hypertension share the same hemodynamic [19] or volume-pressure [20] characteristics. It is not surprising therefore that in unselected groups, the antihypertensive effect of thiazides or spironolactone did not relate in magnitude to the diuretic response.[21] This relationship can, however, be shown by study of more homogeneous groups; thus we found that in volume-dependent hypertensions, arterial pressure reduction correlated significantly ($r = 0.613$) with plasma volume contraction achieved by long-term thiazide and/or spironolactone treatment.[22] McQueen and Morrison [23] also found that the early hypotensive effects of chlorothiazide, hydrochlorothiazide, and mersalyl correlated directly with extracellular fluid though not with plasma volume losses.

Mathematical correlations, however, do not mean a causal association and the significant values reported do not necessarily indicate that pressure reduction was due to volume contraction per se. Changes in sodium balance or its selective redistribution may be as important as or may play a more important role than the associated volume alterations. Most studies have not revealed any significant reduction of total exchangeable sodium following long-term diuretic therapy [15,16,24] except for a more recent report by Hansen.[25] The observation of unchanged total exchangeable sodium during treatment does not rule out the possibility of chronic extracellular fluid volume contraction; in the face of a stable or slightly reduced serum sodium, it may only indicate an intracellular diffusion of sodium.[1] Since Tobian et al.[26,27] have demonstrated an increased sodium content in arterial walls in human and experimental hypertension, it was attractive to hypothesize that thiazides specifically corrected this abnormality. However, repeated studies from different groups [28–30] found no evidence for a reduction of arterial sodium by diuretic agents. The absence of absolute changes does not negate the possibility or the importance of variations in ionic gradients, as dynamic relationships between intra- and extracellular ions, both sodium and potassium, determine smooth-muscle tone to a large extent.[31] However, studies in man have not provided evidence for or against changes in sodium gradient across cell membrane, although the possibility of their occurrence must be taken into account in all reactivity studies.[31]

Evidently more complex factors than simple volume contraction underlie the reduction in arterial pressure. Indeed, there was at one time a tendency to discount completely its importance in long-term diuretic therapy because of reports that plasma and extracellular fluid volume returned to normal with protracted treatment.[15,16,24,32,33] This will be discussed in more detail in a later section. Concomitantly a change in hemodynamic pattern was described with maintained thiazide treatment; Conway and Lauwers [10] reported that the reduction in cardiac output responsible for the early decrease in arterial pressure was later replaced by a reduction in peripheral resistance as output was restored to normal. Thus it appeared as if thiazides lowered blood pressure at first by one mechanism and then later by an entirely different one, a hypothesis that Freis et al. legitimately found difficult to accept.[17]

Sympathetic Reflexes and Diuretic Therapy

Both acute and chronic treatment with thiazides diminishes vasoconstrictor response to norepinephrine [1–6,34] and most investigators suggested that their diuretic action was somehow necessary for that effect.[1,2,5,11,35] A series of investigations by Eckstein and co-workers [36–38] showed that thiazides not only reversed the peripheral vasoconstrictor effect of norepinephrine but also blunted the effectiveness of cardioinhibitory reflexes. Preziosi et al.[39] and Aoki and Brody [40] suggested that thiazides reduced the amount of norepinephrine released with each sympathetic nerve impulse. This could be overcome by an increased nerve impulse traffic so that the arterial pressure of their treated animals was not necessarily affected, nor was their responsiveness to carotid occlusion. Thus the background was laid for a possible interference by sodium depletion with the neurogenic control of blood pressure and with the organism's capacity for adaptation to intravascular volume changes.

Reevaluation of Volume Alterations by Long-term Diuretic Therapy

In contrast to earlier reports,[15,32,33] recent studies have shown that treatment with thiazides is associated with sustained reductions in plasma volume and extracellular fluid. The conflicting results of earlier observations were partly due to difficulties in technique [1] but also possibly to insufficient appreciation of the importance of subtle changes in volume.[20,41,42] Other problems in evaluating these results stemmed from natural dietary variations over prolonged periods of time and from the possibility of alterations in severity of the hypertensive disease [5] with consequent new cardiovascular equilibria. To obviate some of these difficulties we investigated plasma and extracellular fluid volume changes over a month following cessation of long-term thiazide therapy (Fig. 1).[43] Peripheral plasma renin activity was also determined at the time of volume measurements. When hydrochlorothiazide therapy was discontinued, fluid retention and volume expansion occurred promptly with marked reduction of plasma renin activity. Plasma volume then gradually declined to plateau at levels above those obtained during treatment. There was no evidence during these variations for any redistribution of fluid between the plasma and interstitial components of extracellular fluid as the PV:IF ratio was unchanged during and after therapy (Table 1). On the other hand, arterial pressure rose slowly so that its maximum lagged behind the peak of volume expansion. Our conclusions regarding the persistence of plasma volume contraction with thiazide therapy thus agreed with those of Hansen [25] and were subsequently confirmed by a careful prospective study of Leth.[44]

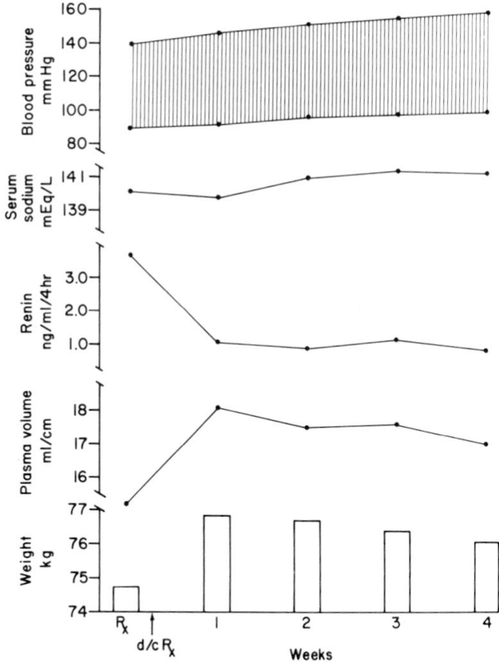

Fig. 1.—Sequential changes in blood pressure, serum sodium, peripheral plasma renin activity, plasma volume, and body weight before and following discontinuance of thiazide diuretics. (From Tarazi, R. C., Dustan, H. P., and Frohlich, E. D.: Long-term thiazide therapy in essential hypertension. Circulation 41:709, 1970, by permission of the American Heart Association.)

As noted by the latter,[44] the impressive feature in the majority of reports including studies of the subject is the consistency with which persistent plasma volume contraction (of slight or of major degree) was found during long-term thiazide therapy, rather than the level of statistical significance achieved by a particular series. In contrast to statistical significance, the biologic importance of even minor extracellular volume changes was underlined by the variations we found in plasma renin activity following cessation of therapy.[43] Its persistent elevation during treatment and prompt reduction within the first week of discontinuance reflected the relevance of measured volume changes to the body's economy, especially as serum sodium concentration was not appreciably altered in that study (Fig. 1). The partial restoration of plasma and extracellular fluid volume during therapy [32] has been ascribed to secondary aldosteronism, which may also be responsible in part for the associated hypokalemia. Along the same lines Tobian et al.[28] had also noted significantly higher juxtaglomerular counts in rats given thiazides for 5 weeks. These different indications of chronic activation of the renin system thus suggest that some volume deficit persists during diuretic therapy and that whatever its actual degree, it is indeed physiologically significant.

TABLE 1.—*Effect of Discontinuing Chronic Thiazide Therapy on Extracellular Water Volume*

Patient	Before Discontinuing Treatment			Following Cessation of Treatment: First Week			Following Cessation of Treatment: Fourth Week		
	Weight (kg)	ECW (liters)	PV/IF * Ratio	Weight (kg)	ECW (liters)	PV/IF Ratio	Weight (kg)	ECW (liters)	PV/IF Ratio
C. W.	64.1	14.3	0.179	—	—	—	65.9	16.1	0.177
F. H.	88.6	16.02	0.185	90.9	18.87	0.187	90.5	18.6	0.181
S. G.	88.4	17.7	0.189	91.4	20.6	0.206	—	—	—
J. S.	97.5	20.6	0.243	98.8	22.4	0.225	96.4	20.8	0.234
A.B.	56.4	11.1	0.236	57.4	11.9	0.255	57.3	12.2	0.256
AVERAGE CHANGE				+1.9	+2.3	+0.005	+1.95	+1.42	+0.002

* Abbreviations used: ECW, extracellular water; PV/IF, ratio of plasma to interstitial fluid volume.
From Tarazi, R. C., Dustan, H. P., and Frohlich, E. D.: Long-term thiazide therapy in essential hypertension. Circulation 41:709, 1970, by permission of The American Heart Association.

Similar long-term plasma volume contraction and elevation of plasma renin activity were found in a group of 14 hypertensive patients effectively treated with spironolactone alone for a median duration of 5 months (Table 2). The main difference between the two diuretics related to serum potassium levels. Essentially similar results for shorter periods of treatment (4 weeks) were also reported by Winer, Lubbe, and Colton.[45] As noted above, arterial pressure reduction by spironolactone in responsive patients was related to plasma volume contraction.[22] Neither Crane and Harris[46] nor we[47] have found any evidence for a "diagnostic" arterial pressure response to spironolactone as Spark and Melby have described.[48] Its antihypertensive effect, like that of other diuretics, depends on adequate plasma and/or extracellular fluid volume depletion in a volume-dependent type of hypertension; primary aldosteronism is only one of such types.[20,22]

In short, it seems no longer possible to discount persistent fluid depletion as a significant factor in arterial pressure lowering by chronic diuretic therapy. Whether the significant index here is intravascular or interstitial volume[43,49] is not completely settled; however, under ordinary conditions diuretics did not seem to influence the volume partition ratio of plasma to interstitial fluid.[43]

TABLE 2.—*Hydrochlorothiazide and Spironolactone Treatment * in Patients with Essential Hypertension*

Treatment (no. of patients)	Arterial Pressure (mm Hg)	Plasma Volume ml per cm	Renin Activity ng per ml	Serum Na (mEq per liter)	Serum K (mEq per liter)
Hydrochlorothiazide (12)					
Before	175/106	18.2	0.7	141	4.0
During	151/94	16.1	3.2	139	3.6
SED †	2.8	0.4	1.1	0.5	0.02
Spironolactone (14)					
Before	165/109	18.0	0.8	142	3.9
During	144/97	16.2	3.7	137	4.6
SED †	1.6	0.28	0.37	0.6	0.06

* Duration of treatment ranged from one to 12 months (median $>$ 4 months) in both groups. All differences between control and treatment values were significant ($p < .001$) in both treatment groups.
† SED: standard error of difference; for arterial pressure, this represents SED for diastolic pressure only.

Type of Hypertension and Arterial Pressure Response to Diuretics

Not all hypertensive patients and not all types of experimental hypertension are equally responsive to volume depletion. Some of the types of hypertension that are particularly sensitive to volume depletion include renoprival hypertension,[50] that associated with renal parenchymal disease,[20,50–52] some forms of steroid hypertension,[22,46] and some subgroups of essential hypertension.[20,47]

During the early days of low-sodium diets, it was rapidly recognized that a minority (about 20 to 25%) of "essential" hypertensive patients responded dramatically to chronic sodium depletion.[18] Despite some attempts to do so,[53] no specific clinical characteristics could be defined for that group. More recently comparable observations were again reported using different approaches. Woods described a group with higher exchangeable sodium than hypertensive controls and with a specific responsiveness to aminoglutethimide;[54] others have reported that spironolactone seemed specific antihypertensive therapy for some essential hypertensives.[46] Nontumorous, hypertensive adrenocortical disorders stemming from subtle enzymatic defects have been described.[55] We have reported a subgroup of patients with seeming "essential" hypertension characterized by inappropriately expanded plasma volume and a remarkable arterial pressure responsiveness to thiazide and spironolactone therapy.[20] Thus, the types of hypertension responding to volume depletion are varied and probably of different etiologies (renal parenchymal disease, steroid abnormalities, "low renin" hypertension, etc.). In some patients, a steroid abnormality may be at fault, but possibly in others a subtle neurogenic dysfunction renders some hypertensive patients particularly sensitive to volume manipulations. In fact, hypervolemia does not seem an indispensable prerequisite for pressure responsiveness to sodium depletion. Dustan, Bravo, and Tarazi[22] have recently reported a small group of patients with low plasma volume and paradoxically low peripheral plasma renin activity whose arterial pressure was normalized by just 4 days of sodium depletion. Volume-dependent hypertensions thus include various types that must be carefully differentiated when evaluating the hypotensive effects of diuretic treatment.

Hemodynamic Relationship of Volume to Arterial Pressure Variations (Fig. 2)

The recognition of persistent volume reduction by long-term therapy does not necessarily mean that it is alone responsible for the lowering of arterial pressure. Its magnitude in some cases is such that it does not seem adequate for the hypotensive effect noticed. Further, the rise in arterial pressure following cessation of therapy lags behind the "rebound volume expansion" (Fig. 1), and though saline or sodium-free infusions during diuretic treatment raise arterial pressure,[3,4,11] the latter does not always return to control values.[4]

Acute reductions in blood volume[56] or in cardiac output[57] do not necessarily lead to hypotension. Venoconstriction demonstrable even in large veins such as the inferior vena cava[56] "takes the slack" in the circulation, while arteriolar constriction can adequately compensate for reductions in cardiac output of

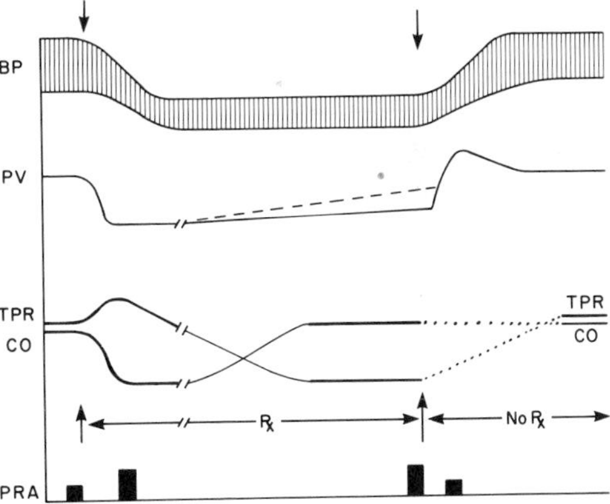

Fig. 2.—Diagram shows changes in blood pressure **(BP)**, plasma volume **(PV)**, cardiac output **(CO)**, total peripheral resistance **(TPR)**, and peripheral plasma renin activity **(PRA)** during various stages of diuretic therapy and in the early weeks following its discontinuance. Magnitude of changes depicted is diagrammatic, not quantitative; thin and dotted lines **(CO** and **TPR)** represent theoretic (nondocumented) links between generally accepted (thicker lines) concepts.[10] Different stages of plasma volume changes during treatment indicate varying degrees of volume restoration in different patients.[32,43,44]

the same magnitude as that noted with diuretic therapy. The importance of intact neural function for these compensatory mechanisms was underlined by Freis's demonstration of the exquisite sensitivity of patients with ganglion-blockade or peripheral adrenergic inhibition to slight degrees of volume loss.[41] Dustan et al. showed that potentiation of the hypotensive effect of neuroplegic drugs by diuretics was due to the relative unavailability of neurogenic vasoconstriction when called for by volume depletion.[8] One of the functions of an intact sympathetic system obviously is to maintain arterial pressure despite variations in the volume filling the vascular tree. When its functions are interfered with, intravascular volume and arterial pressure become direct correlates [42] reversing their original independence or even negative relationship with each other.[20]

Logically, therefore, sodium depletion by either thiazides, spironolactone, mercurials, low-sodium diets, or other agents must somehow interfere with autonomic function to account for the sequence of hemodynamic events produced by these various measures. The relationships discussed above regarding diuretics and the sympathetic nervous system might provide some clues for the mechanism of that interference. Recent studies by de Champlain, Krakoff, and Axelrod [58] suggest that norepinephrine storage and its subcellular distribution are affected by sodium balance, in agreement with the conclusion of Aoki and Brody [40] on diminished norepinephrine release by sympathetic nerve stimulation in rats during thiazide administration. The final answer is, obviously, not yet available.

Whatever the actual mechanism, its result is an inadequate venoconstriction to compensate for a diminished intravascular volume, hence a lowered cardiac output, and an inadequate increase of peripheral resistance to compensate for the fall in output, hence the arterial pressure reduction. This inadequacy of the peripheral resistance response is not necessarily a late manifestation. Despite the fact that resistance does increase during the first few weeks of thiazide treatment [8–10] it can be argued that its rise was not sufficient to counter the reduction in cardiac output. Further, under stress, as by exercise, the inadequacy of vasoconstriction is uncovered, as for a given increase in output, peripheral resistance falls more during thiazide therapy than in the control stage.[59] Thus, just as volume depletion was found to play a role all through diuretic therapy (early and late), interference with vascular adaptation to the reduced volume can be detected from the first days of effective diuresis. Arterial pressure reduction by diuretic agents is thus not achieved at first by one mechanism alone and then by another later on, but is rather the result of the interplay between the same two mechanisms at all phases of therapy (Fig. 3). A different rate of dissipation of the various effects of sodium depletion might help explain the lag of pressure rise behind volume expansion which follows cessation of diuretic therapy. This possibility is suggested by the lingering effects of thiazides on forearm vascular reactivity.[37]

The important role ascribed to subtle autonomic dysfunction and altered reactivity does not mean that other mechanisms cannot slowly develop during therapy. The actual lowering of peripheral resistance following months of continued therapy and persistent reduction in intravascular volume may suggest some form of "autoregulation." Though this term means different things to different people, it is used here in a nonspecific sense meaning a secondary lowering of resistance as flow is chronically diminished and a secondary increase in resistance as flow is chronically increased, whatever the way(s) mediating this response. Its main value is that of a working hypothesis that might link such disparate observations as the late rise in resistance in experimental renovascular hypertension [60] or the late reduction of peripheral resistance following cardiac output depression by propranolol [61] or, for that matter, by diuretics. The greater or lesser alteration of any individual physiologic function by these different agents would depend, of course, on the many conditions peculiar to each of them. Another possibility is that following prolonged therapy with maintained good arterial pressure control, severity of the hypertensive disease may be altered [5] and this may account in some patients for normalization of cardiac output. The prolonged periods of normotension following discontinuance of treat-

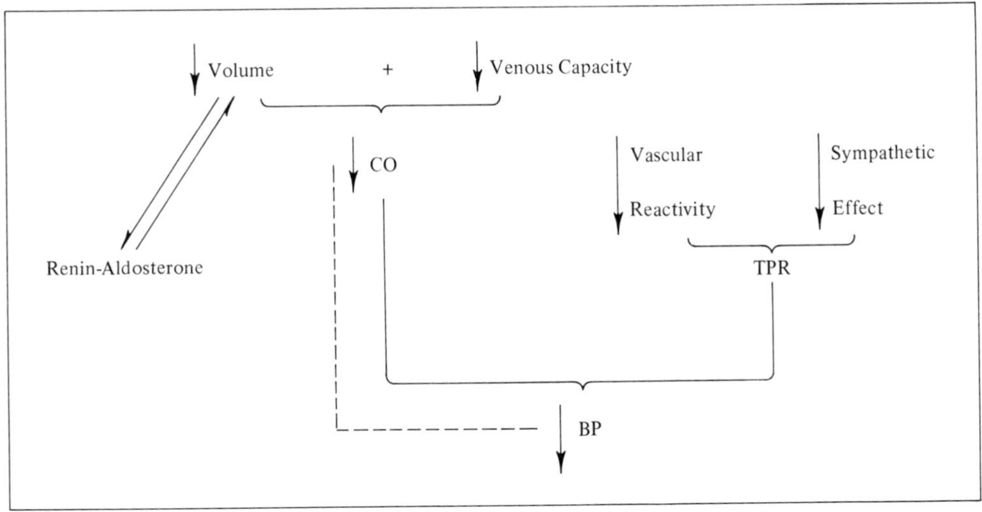

FIG. 3.—Diuretic therapy in hypertension. Tentative outline of interrelations between different factors contributing to hypotensive effect of diuretic agents (see text). Another linking "diminished BP" to cardiac output is meant to indicate that lowering of blood pressure would tend to restore output to normal. Similarly activation of renin-aldosterone system by volume contraction would also tend to restore volume partly to normal. **BP,** blood pressure; **CO,** cardiac output; **TPR,** total peripheral resistance.

ment in some patients[62] suggest that such alterations of the disease may indeed occur.

SUMMARY

The antihypertensive action of diuretic agents seems linked to the interplay of two factors throughout the duration of treatment, a mild to moderate volume contraction and an inadequate cardiovascular compensation for that contraction. There appears to be no evidence for a direct vasodilator effect of these drugs nor for any specific antipressor effect peculiar to a particular diuretic agent. Effective diuresis leads to plasma and extracellular fluid volume contraction which is probably maintained throughout the duration of therapy, although its actual magnitude may vary with time. This volume reduction accounts for the marked sensitivity of treated patients to neuroplegic drugs; its physiologic importance is indicated by available evidence suggesting persistent activation of the renin-aldosterone system; and its therapeutic relevance is underlined by the direct correlation between arterial pressure and intravascular volume during treatment of volume-dependent types of hypertension.

As sodium depletion or altered distribution alters vascular reactivity and blunts the effectiveness of sympathetic reflexes, cardiovascular compensation for modest volume reduction may not be adequate and arterial pressure is then reduced. The relative participation of these various factors may naturally vary from case to case and from time to time. Other factors may also interfere with the hemodynamic pattern of responses. Thus, the gradual lowering of peripheral resistance with long-term treatment might be linked to developing autoregulation and possibly in some instances to altered severity of hypertensive disease.

It must be stressed that not all types of hypertension are equally sensitive to volume depletion and therefore that diuretic and antipressor effects may not be quantitatively related in inhomogeneous groups. The exact definition of volume-dependent hypertensions, we hope, will gradually help to identify other pressor mechanisms at work in different cases.

ACKNOWLEDGMENT

This presentation is based on work done in close and continued collaboration with Dr. H. P. Dustan, and the author gratefully acknowledges his indebtedness to her.

REFERENCES

1. Freis, E. D.: Mechanism of hypotensive action of saluretics. *In* Bock, K. D., and Cottier, P. T. (Eds.): Essential Hypertension: An International Symposium. Berlin: Springer, 1960, pp. 179–191.
2. Tobian, L.: Why do thiazide diuretics lower blood pressure in essential hypertension? Ann. Rev. Pharmacol. 7:399, 1967.
3. Winer, B. M.: The antihypertensive action of benzothiadiazines. Circulation 23:211, 1961.
4. Winer, B. M.: The antihypertensive mechanisms of salt depletion induced by hydrochlorothiazide. Circulation 24:788, 1961.
5. Freis, E. D.: The effects of salt and extracellular fluid depletion on vascular responsiveness with particular reference to chlorothiazide. *In* Skelton, F. R. (Ed.): Proceedings, Council on High Blood Pressure Research, Cleveland, Ohio, November, 1958. New York: American Heart Association, 1959, pp. 6–21.
6. Gillenwater, J. Y., Scott, J. B., Frohlich, E. D.: Effect of chlorothiazide upon the response of the renal bed to vasoactive substances. Circ. Res. 11:283, 1962.
7. Wilson, W. R., and Okun, R.: Acute hemodynamic effects of diazoxide in man. Circulation 28:89, 1963.
8. Dustan, H. P., Cumming, G. R., Corcoran, A. C., and Page, I. H.: A mechanism of chlorothiazide-enhanced effectiveness of antihypertensive ganglioplegic drugs. Circulation 19:360, 1959.
9. Frohlich, E. D., Schnaper, H. W., Wilson, I. M., and Freis, E. D.: Hemodynamic alterations in hypertensive patients due to chlorothiazide. N. Engl. J. Med. 262:1261, 1960.
10. Conway, J., and Lauwers, P.: Hemodynamic and hypotensive effects of long-term therapy with chlorothiazide. Circulation 21:21, 1960.
11. Freis, E. D., Wanko, A., Wilson, I. M., and Parrish, A. E.: Chlorothiazide in hypertensive and normotensive patients. Ann. N.Y. Acad. Sci. 71:450, 1958.
12. Aleksandrow, D., Wysznacka, W., and Gajewski, J.: Studies on mechanism of hypertensive action of chlorothiazide. N. Engl. J. Med. 260:51, 1959.
13. Dollery, C. T., Harington, M., and Kaufman, G.: The mode of action of chlorothiazide in hypertension: With special reference to potentiation of ganglion-blocking agents. Lancet 1:1215, 1959.
14. Laragh, J. H.: The proper use of newer diuretics. Ann. Intern. Med. 67:606, 1967.
15. Hollander, W., Chobanian, A. V., and Wilkins, R. W.: The role of diuretics in the management of hypertension. Ann. N.Y. Acad. Sci. 88:975, 1960.
16. Wilkins, R. W., Hollander, W., and Chobanian, A. V.: Chlorothiazide in hypertension: Studies on its mode of action. Ann. N.Y. Acad. Sci. 71:465, 1958.
17. Freis, E. D., Wanko, A., Schnaper, H. W., and Frohlich, E. D.: Mechanism of the altered blood pressure responsiveness produced by chlorothiazide. J. Clin. Invest. 39:1277, 1960.
18. Corcoran, A. C., Taylor, R. C., and Page, I. H.: Controlled observations on the effect of low-sodium dietotherapy in essential hypertension. Circulation 3:1, 1951.
19. Frohlich, E. D., Tarazi, R. C., and Dustan, H. P.: Re-examination of the hemodynamics of hypertension. Am. J. Med. Sci. 257:9, 1969.
20. Tarazi, R. C., Dustan, H. P., Frohlich, E. D., Gifford, R. W., Jr., and Hoffman, G. C.: Plasma volume and chronic hypertension. Arch. Intern. Med. 125:835, 1970.
21. Conway, J., and Palmero, H.: The vascular effect of the thiazide diuretics. Arch. Intern. Med. 111:203, 1963.
22. Dustan, H. P., Bravo, E. L., and Tarazi, R. C.: Volume-dependent essential and steroid hypertensions. J. Lab. Clin. Med. 44:18, 1971.
23. McQueen, E. G., and Morrison, R. B. I.: The hypotensive action of diuretic agents. Lancet 1:1209, 1960.
24. Gifford, R. W., Mattox, V. R., Orvis, A. L., Sones, D. A., and Rosevear, J. W.: Effect of thiazide diuretics on plasma volume, body electrolytes and excretion of aldosterone in hypertension. Circulation 24:1197, 1961.
25. Hansen, J.: Hydrochlorothiazide in the treatment of hypertension. Acta Med. Scand. 183:317, 1968.
26. Tobian, L., and Binion, J. T.: Tissue cations and water in arterial hypertension. Circulation 5:754, 1952.
27. Tobian, L., Janecek, J., Tomboulian, A., and Ferreira, D.: Sodium and potassium in the walls of arterioles in experimental renal hypertension. J. Clin. Invest. 40:1922, 1961.
28. Tobian, L., Janecek, J., Foker, J., and Ferreira, D.: Effect of chlorothiazide on renal juxtaglomerular cells and tissue electrolytes. Am. J. Physiol. 202:905, 1962.
29. Daniel, E. E.: On the mechanism of antihypertensive action of hydrochlorothiazide in rats. Circ. Res. 11:941, 1962.

30. Weller, J. M., and Haight, A. S.: Effect of chlorothiazide on blood pressure and electrolytes of normotensive and hypertensive rats. Proc. Soc. Exp. Biol. Med. 112:820, 1963.
31. Friedman, S. M., Nakashima, M., and Friedman, C. L.: Relation of saluretic and hypotensive effects of hydrochlorothiazide in the rat. Am. J. Physiol. 198:148, 1960.
32. Wilson, I. M., and Freis, E. D.: Relationship between plasma and extracellular fluid volume depletion and the antihypertensive effect of chlorothiazide. Circulation 20:1028, 1959.
33. Lauwers, P., and Conway, J.: Effect of long-term treatment with chlorothiazide on body fluids, serum electrolytes and exchangeable sodium in hypertensive patients. J. Lab. Clin. Med. 56:401, 1960.
34. Mendlowitz, M., Naftchi, N., Gitlow, S. E., Weinreb, H. L., and Wolf, R. L.: The effect of chlorothiazide and its congeners on the digital circulation in normotensive subjects and in patients with essential hypertension. Ann. N.Y. Acad. Sci. 88:964, 1960.
35. Aleksandrow, D., Wysznacka, W., and Gajewski, J.: Influence of chlorothiazide upon arterial responsiveness to norepinephrine in hypertensive subjects. N. Engl. J. Med. 261: 1052, 1959.
36. Eckstein, J. W., Abboud, F. M., and Pereda, S. A.: The effect of norepinephrine on cardiac output, arterial blood pressure and heart rate in dogs treated with chlorothiazide. J. Clin. Invest. 41:1578, 1962.
37. Feisal, K. A., Eckstein, J. W., Horsley, A. W., and Keasling, H. H.: Effects of chlorothiazide on forearm vascular responses to norepinephrine. J. Appl. Physiol. 16:549, 1961.
38. Eckstein, J. W., Wendling, M. G., and Abboud, F. M.: Circulatory responses to norepinephrine after prolonged treatment with chlorothiazide. Circ. Res. 18 (Suppl. 1):48, 1966.
39. Preziosi, P., Schaepdryver, de A. F., Marmo, E., and Miele, E.: On the mechanism of the anti-hypertensive effect of hydrochlorothiazide. Arch. Int. Pharmacodyn. Ther. 131:209, 1961.
40. Aoki, V. S., and Brody, M. J.: The effect of thiazide on the sympathetic nervous system of hypertensive rats. Arch. Int. Pharmacodyn. Ther. 177:423, 1969.
41. Freis, E. D., Stanton, J. F., Finnerty, F. A., Jr., Schnaper, H. W., Johnson, R. L., Rath, C. E., and Wilkins, R. W.: The collapse produced by venous congestion of the extremities or by venesection following certain hypotensive agents. J. Clin. Invest. 30:435, 1951.
42. Dustan, H. P., Tarazi, R. C., and Bravo, E. L.: Dependence of arterial pressure on intravascular volume in treated hypertensive patients. N. Engl. J. Med. 286:861, 1972.
43. Tarazi, R. C., Dustan, H. P., and Frohlich, E. D.: Long-term thiazide therapy in essential hypertension. Circulation 41:709, 1970.
44. Leth, A.: Changes in plasma and extracellular fluid volumes in patients with essential hypertension during long-term treatment with hydrochlorothiazide. Circulation 42:479, 1970.
45. Winer, B. M., Lubbe, W. F., and Colton, T.: Antihypertensive actions of diuretics. JAMA 204:775, 1968.
46. Crane, M. G., and Harris, J. J.: Effect of spironolactone in hypertensive patients. Am. J. Med. Sci. 260:311, 1970.
47. Bravo, E. L., Dustan, H. P., and Tarazi, R. C.: Specific and non-specific effects of spironolactone in the treatment of primary aldosteronism. (Unpublished observations.)
48. Spark, R. F., and Melby, J. C. Aldosteronism in hypertension. The spironolactone response test. Ann. Intern. Med. 69:685, 1968.
49. Davidov, M., Gavrilovich, L., Mroczek, W., and Finnerty, F. A., Jr.: Relation of extracellular fluid volume to arterial pressure during drug-induced saluresis. Circulation 40: 349, 1969.
50. Dustan, H. P., and Page, I. H.: Some factors in renal and renoprival hypertension. J. Lab. Clin. Med. 64:948, 1964.
51. Planque, de B. A., Mulder, E., and Mees, E. J. D.: The behaviour of blood and extracellular volume in hypertensive patients with renal insufficiency. Acta Med. Scand. 186:75, 1969.
52. Blumberg, A., Nelp, W. B., Hegstrom, R. M., and Scribner, B. H.: Extracellular volume in patients with chronic renal disease treated for hypertension by sodium restriction. Lancet 2:69, 1967.
53. Schroeder, H. A.: Hypertensive Diseases, Causes and Control. Philadelphia: Lea & Febiger, 1948, p. 295.
54. Woods, J. W., Liddle, G. W., Stant, E. G., Jr., Michelakis, A. M., and Brill, A. B.: Effect of an adrenal inhibitor in hypertensive patients with suppressed renin. Arch. Intern. Med. 123:366, 1969.
55. Salti, I. S., Stiefel, M., Ruse, J. L., and Laidlaw, J. C.: Non-tumorous "primary" aldo-

steronism: I. Type relieved by glucocorticoid. Can. Med. Assoc. J. 101:1, 1969. II. Type not relieved by glucocorticoid. Can. Med. Assoc. J. 101:11, 1969.

56. Dow, R. W., and Fry, W. J.: Venous compensatory mechanisms in acute hypovolemia. Surgery 125:511, 1967.

57. Ulrych, M., Frohlich, E. D., Dustan, H. P., and Page, I. H.: Immediate hemodynamic effects of beta-adrenergic blockade with propranolol in normotensive and hypertensive man. Circulation 37:411, 1968.

58. de Champlain, J., Krakoff, L., and Axelrod, J.: Interrelationships of sodium intake, hypertension, and norepinephrine storage in the rat. Circ. Res. (Suppl. 1) 24–25:I–75, 1969.

59. Varnauskas, E., Cramer, G., Malmcrona, R., Werkö, L.: Effect of chlorothiazide on blood pressure and blood flow at rest and on exercise in patients with arterial hypertension. Clin. Sci. 20:407, 1961.

60. Ferrario, C. M., Page, I. H., and McCubbin, J. W.: Increased cardiac output as a contributory factor in experimental renal hypertension in dogs. Circ. Res. 27:799, 1970.

61. Tarazi, R. C., and Dustan, H. P.: Beta-adrenergic blockade in hypertension: Practical and theoretical implications of long-term hemodynamic variations. Am. J. Cardiol. 29:633, 1972.

62. Dustan, H. P., Page, I. H., Tarazi, R. C., and Frohlich, E. D.: Arterial pressure responses to discontinuing antihypertensive drugs. Circulation 37:370, 1968.

Clinical Use of Diuretics in Hypertension

By Paul J. Cannon, M.D.

During the past three decades a variety of potent pharmacologic agents have been developed which promote diuresis and a negative sodium balance by inhibiting the renotubular reabsorption of sodium. Use of these compounds has constituted a significant therapeutic advance in the treatment of congestive heart failure and other forms of edema. Diuretic agents differ significantly in chemical structure (Fig. 1). Each class of diuretics exerts characteristic pharmacologic effects upon the transport processes whereby the renotubular cells reabsorb sodium, chloride, bicarbonate, and water from the glomerular filtrate and simultaneously eliminate potassium and hydrogen ions. Each class of drugs also differs in its major sites of action within the nephron, i.e., proximal tubules, loops of Henle, distal tubules, and collecting ducts.

Hypotensive Action of Diuretics

Many diuretic drugs have been found to significantly lower the elevated arterial blood pressure of hypertensive patients (Table 1). When administered chronically, they are without effect upon the blood pressures of normotensive subjects. The mechanisms which mediate the antihypertensive action of diuretic drugs are unclear, however.

After acute administration of a diuretic, plasma volume and cardiac output fall as diuresis ensues, and there is a reduction in the level of arterial pressure.[1–4] The contraction of plasma volume consequent to natriuresis does not appear to be solely responsible for the fall in pressure, however. Several studies have indicated that reexpansion of plasma volume to normal after acute diuretic administration, e.g., by infusions of salt-free dextran, did not return blood pressure to control levels.[5–8] In addition, plasma volume and cardiac output have returned to normal during chronic thiazide treatment even though an antihypertensive effect persisted.[6]

Nor has the antihypertensive action of diuretics been adequately explained by alteration of total-body sodium stores. Total exchangeable sodium has returned to control levels during prolonged diuretic therapy despite maintenance of a lowered blood pressure level.[9] Hollander and Chobanian found that administration of large amounts of sodium, sufficient to induce positive sodium balance, to patients receiving mercurial or thiazide diuretics, did not restore the blood pressure to previous hypertensive levels.[10] Lastly, diazoxide, a drug with chemical similarities to thiazide diuretics, induces significant renal sodium retention while causing dramatic reductions of blood pressure.[11] Theories that diuretic drugs lower arterial pressure by (1) altering the sodium and water content of arterial smooth muscle;[12,13] (2) influencing the response of vascular beds to catecholamines;[14–16] or (3) modifying vascular receptors and the responsiveness of arterioles to the circulating pressor polypeptide angiotensin II[17] have been reviewed in the chapter entitled "Diuretic Drugs: Mechanisms of Antihypertensive Action."

The physician's choice of drugs in the treatment of hypertensive patients is conditioned by his therapeutic aims. In most patients, one aims to normalize the blood pressure in an attempt to prevent or to reduce the symptoms, the complications (cerebral, ocular, cardiac, and renal), and the increased mortality associated with prolonged diastolic hypertension. In other patients, however, this aim may be tempered. It may be desirable to reduce the

Table 1.—*Diuretics with Significant Antihypertensive Properties*

Organomercurials
Thiazides
Spironolactone
Furosemide
Ethacrynic acid

From the Department of Medicine, College of Physicians and Surgeons of Columbia University, New York, New York.

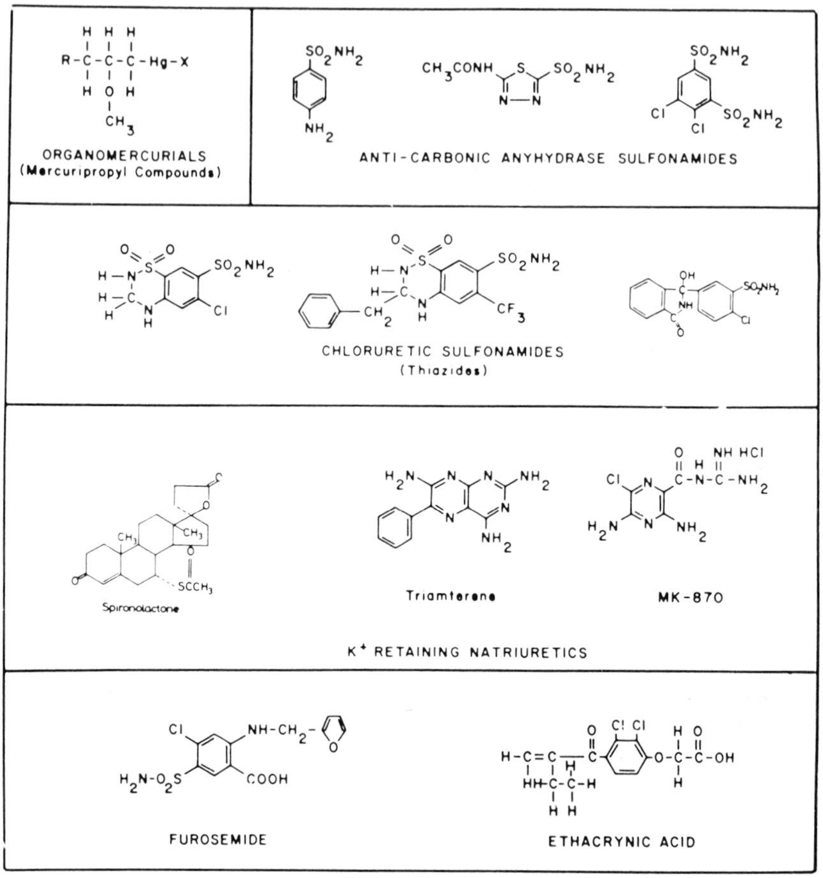

ORGANOMERCURIALS (Mercuripropyl Compounds)

ANTI-CARBONIC ANYHYDRASE SULFONAMIDES

CHLORURETIC SULFONAMIDES (Thiazides)

Spironolactone

Triamterene

MK-870

K^+ RETAINING NATRIURETICS

FUROSEMIDE

ETHACRYNIC ACID

FIG. 1.—Chemical structures of five classes of diuretics.

diastolic pressure only partially, if more extensive lowering of the arterial pressure aggravates angina pectoris, induces or increases transient cerebral ischemic attacks, or is associated with a significant deterioration of renal function. In both situations the beneficial effects expected from pharmacologic therapy must be weighed against the expense, discomfort, and toxicity of the drugs used.

PURPOSES OF DIURETIC THERAPY IN HYPERTENSIVE DISEASE

The principal uses of diuretic drugs in the treatment of hypertensive patients are four:

1. Diuretics may be administered continuously as primary antihypertensive therapy for patients with mild degrees of hypertension.
2. Diuretics may be combined with other classes of antihypertensive drugs to enhance blood pressure lowering in patients with more advanced hypertensive disease.
3. Diuretics may be administered to prevent the renal salt retention which may accompany blood pressure reduction with the use of more powerful antihypertensive drugs.
4. Diuretics may be used, as in treatment of other forms of edema, to mobilize extracellular fluid surpluses from hypertensive patients with congestive heart failure.

In addition, there are several specialized uses:

1. Thiazides or other kaliuretic diuretics may be administered to hypertensives as a provocative test to uncover the renal potassium wastage and hypokalemia of patients with primary hyperaldosteronism.
2. The aldosterone antagonist spironolactone may be given diagnostically in an attempt to

detect patients with mineralocorticoid hypertension.

3. The property of large doses of furosemide or ethacrynic acid to produce renal vasodilatation may be used to counteract the fall in renal blood flow which accompanies lowering of arterial pressure with intravenous diazoxide.

4. Finally, a combination therapy which includes a diuretic along with one or more other antihypertensive drugs may be required to produce slow gradual blood pressure reduction without orthostasis in patients with hypertension and cerebrovascular disease in whom abrupt depression of blood pressure by stronger antihypertensive drugs is undesirable or dangerous.

Pharmacology of the Major Classes of Diuretics

Diuretic therapy in the treatment of edema or hypertensive disease should be individualized for each patient and based upon a sound understanding of the pharmacologic actions of the drugs employed. Table 2 summarizes the principal sites of action in the nephron and the major physiologic effects of the most commonly used diuretic agents. An understanding of diuretic action upon tubular transport processes enables the physician to use combination diuretic therapy more effectively. It also allows him to forestall some of the disturbances of electrolyte or acid-base balance which may occur, not as toxic effects, but as direct consequences of the diuretics' pharmacologic actions upon ion transport within the nephron.

Organomercurials

The organomercurial diuretics are the oldest and remain among the most effective natriuretic drugs. Studies in the 1950s indicated that administration of this class of compounds exerts a significant antihypertensive effect in patients with essential hypertension.[10] Because the drugs must be administered intramuscularly, their use as antihypertensives has been replaced by the oral diuretic agents. Mercurials are used intermittently, however, to counteract sodium retention induced by other antihypertensive drugs, and in the treatment of hypertensive patients with edema.

Compounds such as meralluride produce a sustained diuresis lasting for 12 to 24 hours after intramuscular injection. This agent exerts little effect upon renal blood flow or glomerular filtration rate, but it significantly inhibits the tubular reabsorption of sodium, chloride, and water.[18] The precise site of action of mercurial diuretics in the nephron is unclear.[18–21] Many mercurials appear to act in the loop of Henle and/or the distal nephron.[21,22] Meralluride, which contains theophylline, may have a proximal action; delivery of rejected sodium from the proximal tubule to the distal nephron enhances urinary dilution.[1] This makes meralluride a useful drug in therapy of patients with dilutional hyponatremia.

Mercurial diuretics partially inhibit the distal tubular mechanism by which sodium reabsorption is coupled with potassium secretion into the urine. Despite this effect, potassium depletion may occur during a mercurial diuresis, because increased delivery of sodium to the distal nephron accelerates the Na^+-K^+ and Na^+-H^+ ion-exchange mechanisms located in this region. Urinary hydrogen ion excretion (titratable acidity and ammonium minus bicarbonate) also rises during a mercurial diuresis. During sustained therapy, therefore, the patient may develop a hypokalemic alkalosis at which time the renal tubules become unresponsive to the natriuretic effects of a mercurial. Pretreatment of the patient with a compound (e.g., ammonium chloride) which induces hyperchloremia and metabolic acidosis restores responsiveness and may even potentiate a mercurial diuresis.

Because some patients exhibit hypersensitivity to mercurials, a test dose is advisable before first administration. Large doses of mercury are nephrotoxic, and acute tubular necrosis has been reported in some patients with renal disease who had received large or frequent injections of mercurial diuretics.[23] The presence of renal functional impairment is not an absolute contraindication to mercurial therapy in a hypertensive patient. Nevertheless, in patients with significant renal damage, it is advisable to administer either lower doses of a mercurial or another diuretic such as furosemide to mobilize edematous fluid.

Carbonic Anhydrase Inhibitors

Carbonic anhydrase inhibitors were the first effective oral diuretic agents.[24] These drugs,

TABLE 2.—*Physiologic Effects of Diuretics*

Agents	*Route of Administration*	*Major Sites of Diuretic Action*	*Relative Diuretic Potency*	*Relative Antihypertensive Action*	*Effect on Glomerular Filtration Rate*	*Effect on Urinary Potassium Excretion*	*Effect on Urinary Hydrogen Ion Excretion*	*Effect on Urinary Dilution*
Mercurials								
e.g., meralluride	Intramuscular	Proximal and/or distal tubules	++++	+	Little	↓ or ↑	↑	↑
Carbonic anhydrase inhibitors								
e.g., acetazolamide	Oral	Proximal tubules	++	−	Little	↑	↓	↑
Thiazide								
e.g., chlorothiazide	Oral	Loops of Henle and distal tubules within the renal cortex	+++	+	↓	↑	Little	↓
K^+-retaining agents,								
e.g., spironolactone,	Oral	Distal tubules and collecting ducts	+	+	0 or ↓	↓	↓	↓
triamterene	Oral		+	−	↓	↓	↓	↓
"Loop of Henle" diuretics								
e.g., ethacrynic acid	Oral or intravenous	Proximal tubules and ascending limbs of Henle's loop	+++++	+	0 or ↑	↑	↑	↓
and furosemide			+++++	+	0 or ↑	↑	↑	↓

acetazolamide and dichlorphenamide (Daranide), are weak natriuretic agents which are rarely used as primary diuretics in treatment of edema. Micropuncture studies have clearly indicated that carbonic anhydrase inhibitors reduce sodium reabsorption in proximal tubules.[25] Therefore, coadministration of these drugs increases or potentiates the natriuresis produced by other diuretics, such as furosemide or thiazides, which block sodium reabsorption more distally in the nephron. Because the drugs result in a bicarbonate diuresis, they are occasionally administered to correct a metabolic alkalosis induced by another diuretic (e.g., a thiazide). There is no conclusive evidence that carbonic anhydrase inhibitors have significant antihypertensive properties; hence, they are not used to lower blood pressure of hypertensive patients.

Thiazide Diuretics

Chlorothiazide and its many derivative compounds are among the most effective and widely used oral diuretics.[9] Thiazides have been demonstrated to significantly reduce the blood pressure of hypertensive patients.[26–28] The antihypertensive effect of chronic therapy is sustained, and drug intolerance is rare. Normotension (e.g., blood pressure $<140/90$ mm Hg) is achieved for the most part in patients with milder degrees of hypertension (diastolic <110 mm Hg). In patients with higher levels of diastolic pressure some antihypertensive effect is generally observed, even though a normal blood pressure is less commonly attained. In this situation, thiazide diuretics have been successfully combined with other drugs such as hydralazine, alpha-methyldopa, or guanethidine to attain the desired degree of blood pressure reduction.[28]

In contrast to their uses intermittently to mobilize edema fluid, thiazides are administered daily in the treatment of hypertension. Antihypertensive effects of peak doses of the various thiazide derivatives are comparable; the different preparations differ mainly in their natriuretic effects on a weight basis and in their duration of action. The names of various thiazide-derivative diuretics and of the other oral diuretic agents with antihypertensive properties are listed in Table 3, along with customary antihypertensive doses.

The prototype thiazide diuretic, chlorothiazide, when administered intravenously, may produce an abrupt 15 to 20 percent reduction of renal blood flow and glomerular filtration rate.[2,18] This effect may induce a reversible increase in blood urea nitrogen after oral administration, particularly in patients with renal parenchymal disease. Although thiazides possess a slight ability to inhibit carbonic anhydrase, their prime action is to inhibit tubular reabsorption of sodium, chloride, and water in the loop of Henle and in the diluting segment of distal tubule located in the renal cortex.[9,18] Because of their action to impede urinary dilution, thiazides may contribute to the production of dilutional hyponatremia in edematous patients whose water intake is large. Thiazides do not impair renal concentrating ability.[29]

During diuresis with a thiazide, potassium excretion increases as increased amounts of sodium are presented to the more distal Na^+-K^+ ion exchange mechanisms. Claims that one or another thiazide derivative induces greater or lesser degrees of kaliuresis or a more favorable Na:K ratio in the urine are not convincing. Recent studies[47–49] have indicated that the magnitude of kaliuresis observed after diuretic administration is influenced by a number of factors. These include: drug dosage, the magnitude of induced natriuresis, the anion composition of the glomerular filtrate, the state of potassium and of acid-base balance (alkalosis favors kaliuresis), and the circulating level of aldosterone. When other factors are held constant, the degree of potassium excretion induced by a diuretic varies directly with the circulating aldosterone level of the patient. For this reason thiazides or other diuretics such as furosemide or ethacrynic acid are more likely to induce potassium depletion and hypokalemia in patients with primary hyperaldosteronism, in patients with severe or malignant hypertension and secondary hyperaldosteronism, and in patients on low-sodium diets than in patients with mild essential hypertension or normal subjects who ingest normal sodium diets and have normal aldosterone secretion rates.[30] The clinical manifestations of potassium depletion include muscular weakness, or-

TABLE 3.—*Oral Diuretics Used in Management of Hypertension*

Agent	*Approximate Range of Oral Antihypertensive Doses (in mg)*	*Frequency*
Thiazides and Related Agents		
Bendroflumethiazide (Naturetin)	5–15	daily
Benzthiazide (Aquatag, ExNa)	25–75	twice daily
Chlorothiazide (Diuril)	500	one to three times daily
Cyclothiazide (Anhydron)	2–4	daily
Hydrochlorothiazide (Esidrex Diuril)	25–100	once or twice daily
Hydroflumethiazide (Saluron)	50–100	one or twice daily
Methyclothiazide (Enduron)	2.5–15	daily
Polythiazide (Renese)	1–8	daily
Trichlormethiazide (Metahydrin, Naqua)	2–8	daily
Others		
Chlorthalidone, a phthalimidine derivative (Hygroton)	50–100	daily
Quinethazone, a quinazoline derivative (Hydromox)	50–75	once or twice daily
Ethacrynic acid, a phenoxyacetic acid derivative (Edecrin)	50	one to four times daily
Furosemide, an anthranilic acid derivative (Lasix)	40	one to four times daily
Spironolactone, an aldosterone antagonist (Aldactone)	25–100	one to four times daily

thostatic hypotension, paralytic ileus, and the development of digitalis toxicity in patients who are receiving maintenance doses of glycoside. These complications can be prevented or reversed by administration of potassium as the chloride salt (in liquid solution to avoid jejunal or ileal ulcerations). When potassium salts are given as alkaline salts, the ingested potassium is excreted rapidly and almost quantitatively into the urine. Potassium depletion may also be prevented or corrected by administration of a potassium-sparing diuretic such as spironolactone, amiloride, or triamterene.

During initial therapy with thiazides, hydrogen ion balance is not altered significantly because the tendency of these agents to increase excretion of titratable acid and ammonium is offset by their action to inhibit carbonic anhydrase.[31] The metabolic alkalosis which may develop during thiazide therapy appears to be related to the induced potassium depletion and also to chloride depletion.[31,32] Large intravenous doses of thiazides are uricosuric whereas urate excretion falls during chronic oral administration of lower doses.[33] Hyperuricemia and gouty arthritis may be precipitated by thiazide therapy. Urate is filtered and both reabsorbed and secreted by the renal tubules. It has been proposed that large doses of thiazides inhibit urate reabsorption whereas lower doses inhibit secretion.[33] Other recent studies have indicated that during extracellular fluid volume depletion, induced either by thiazide diuretics or by dietary sodium restriction, there is an increased reabsorption of sodium by the proximal tubules. Increased proximal sodium reabsorption is accompanied by increased reabsorption of water, urea, Ca^{++}, and urate. Thiazide-induced hyperuricemia in normal subjects has been reversed by oral salt-loading despite continuance of the drug.[34]

Aldosterone Antagonists

Spironolactone is a competitive inhibitor of aldosterone at its renal sites of action.[35,36] The drug has little effect upon renal blood flow or glomerular filtration rate. It inhibits tubular reabsorption of sodium and chloride largely at distal sites in the nephron, and it impedes distal sodium-potassium and sodium-hydrogen ion-exchange mechanisms. Spironolactone has no diuretic action in adrenalectomized subjects.[37] It is most effective in the therapy of edematous patients with marked hypersecretion of aldosterone (e.g., cirrhosis with ascites). Because aldosterone accounts for only 1 to 2 percent of tubular sodium reabsorption, spironolactone is regarded as a mild diuretic agent; however, the cumulative effects of a 25- to 100-mg dose by mouth given one to four times daily in patients with excessive circulating aldosterone may be impressive. The drug is usually combined with other diuretic agents which block sodium reabsorption in more proximal segments of the nephron; such combination therapy not only increases sodium excretion but also reduces the rise in potassium and hydrogen ion excretion induced by mercurials, thiazides, ethacrynic acid, or furosemide.

When used in treatment of essential hypertension, spironolactone has been found to have an antihypertensive potency comparable to thiazide diuretics.[38,39] In patients who develop potassium depletion on thiazides, use of spironolactone offers a distinct advantage. Recent studies have indicated that only 40 to 60 percent of patients with primary hyperaldosteronism may be rendered normotensive by adrenalectomy;[40] persistent hypertension is most common in those who at operation were found to have bilateral adrenal nodular hyperplasia rather than adrenal adenoma.[41] Spark and Melby[42] have claimed that the probability of finding an adenoma at operation is greater if the hypokalemic patient's blood pressure is returned to normal by preoperative therapy with spironolactone (400 mg per day) for 3 to 6 weeks. They have advocated this as a screening test for patients with an aldosterone-secreting adenoma. A partial reduction in blood pressure was found in hypokalemic patients with nodular hyperplasia. The other claim of these workers that the blood pressure response to spironolactone treatment is useful as a screening test for other forms of mineralocorticoid hypertension in normokalemic patients with suppressed renin levels awaits confirmation by other groups.[43]

The most important side effect of spironolactone therapy which is related to the drug's mechanism of action is hyperkalemia. This is an uncommon complication because spironolactone administration tends to elevate aldosterone secretion which diminishes the drug effect. Nevertheless, dangerous levels of hyperkalemia may be induced in patients with renal disease and in those with a large potassium intake. Deterioration of renal function or acidosis may also be seen when large doses of spironolactone are administered to hypertensives with significant azotemia.

Triamterene and amiloride are two diuretic compounds which also depress distal tubular sodium chloride reabsorption and inhibit Na^+-K^+ and Na^+-H^+ exchange mechanisms.[44,45] Although both compounds can block the renal effects of an aldosterone infusion, they are not competitive inhibitors of the hormone since both induce the characteristic changes in urinary electrolyte excretion when administered to adrenalectomized patients. They are mild diuretics and are primarily used in therapy of edema to augment natriuresis and to reduce the potassium and hydrogen in excretion induced by other diuretics. Both drugs may depress the glomerular filtration rate and elevate the level of blood urea nitrogen, particularly in patients with renal disease. In the latter, these drugs have been reported to occasionally produce hyperkalemia and also acidosis as a consequence of their actions to depress urinary potassium and hydrogen ion excretion rates. For these reasons triamterene and amiloride are not generally used as antihypertensive drugs.

Diuretics Which Inhibit Sodium Transport in the Ascending Limb of Henle's Loop

Ethacrynic acid and furosemide are two newer diuretics which may be administered either intravenously or by mouth. Although the drugs have different chemical formulas (Fig. 1), their physiologic properties are quite similar.[46] The drugs are distinguished from other diuretics by their greater natriuretic potency and by the fact that they produce a major inhibition of sodium reabsorption in the ascending limb of Henle's loop.[22,47–49]

In therapeutic doses, ethacrynic acid and furosemide have little effect on the glomerular filtration rate in man; larger doses may induce renal vasodilatation. Studies in animals have suggested that the drugs may produce selective increases in blood flow to the superficial renal cortex.[50] Both of the diuretics inhibit the tubular reabsorption of sodium together with chloride in proximal tubules and also in the ascending limb of Henle's loop. The latter action impairs the kidney's ability to dilute or to concentrate the urine. Potassium excretion and hydrogen ion excretion increase during their action. These combined effects may tend to produce potassium depletion and alkalosis. Uric acid excretion rises when large doses of either drug are given by vein; urate retention and hyperuricemia may result with oral therapy using lower dosage levels.

As a consequence of their strong action to block tubular sodium chloride reabsorption, up to 25 to 40 percent of the glomerular filtrate may be delivered into the urine after intravenous administration of furosemide or ethacrynic acid. The natriuretic potency of the compounds permits mobilization of edema from patients with azotemia or disturbances of electrolytes or acid-base disturbances. Because the drugs do not depress renal blood flow they are the drugs of choice to mobilize edema from hypertensive patients who have a significant degree of renal failure. Intermittent administration of oral furosemide (40 to 80 mg given one to four times daily), or ethacrynic acid (50 mg given one to four times daily) for 1 to 3 days may prove efficacious in this situation.

Muth [51] and Berman and Ebrahimi [52] have reported successful management of edema in patients with renal disease complicated by significant azotemia by using a regimen consisting of very high doses of furosemide administered orally or intravenously. Similar results in patients with renal failure have been reported by Maher and Schreiner using ethacrynic acid.[53]

Intravenous administration of ethacrynic acid (0.5 to 1.0 mg per kilogram of body weight) or of furosemide (20 to 100 mg) results in a prompt increase in urinary output within 15 minutes. Natriuresis peaks at 0.5 to 1.5 hours and lasts 2 to 6 hours. The magnitude and rapidity of diuresis have made these drugs important adjuncts in the treatment of acute pulmonary edema secondary to left ventricular failure in the hypertensive patient.[47,49,54,55] Diuresis with either drug results in a prompt diminution in extracellular fluid and blood volume, with a consequent fall in venous return and cardiac output.[56,57] These hemodynamic consequences of diuresis are also useful in the management of patients who appear to have developed tolerance to their antihypertensive drug regimen. Successful antihypertensive therapy with the more potent drugs such as alpha-methyldopa or guanethidine is accompanied by a subtle degree of renal sodium retention in many patients. This probably results as a consequence of hemodynamic changes in the peritubular capillaries which modulate net proximal tubular sodium reabsorption.[58] The retained sodium and water may not be obvious as rales or edema, but may be detected from a gain in weight or a rise in blood pressure. Intermittent administration of a diuretic, such as furosemide, to return sodium balance to zero in this situation frequently restores the desired degree of blood pressure control. Kakaviatos and co-workers [11] have administered furosemide intravenously together with diazoxide in treating hypertensive emergencies, because furosemide counteracts both the renal vasoconstriction and the sodium induced by this powerful antihypertensive drug.

Ethacrynic acid and furosemide also exert an antihypertensive action which is independent of the acute hemodynamic consequences of diuresis.[3,47,49,59] The magnitude of this effect appears to be comparable to that produced by thiazide diuretics irrespective of whether the drugs are used singly in treating mild hypertension or are combined with other drugs to treat more advanced cases. Because the hazards of inducing either true sodium chloride depletion or hypokalemia and metabolic alkalosis by chronic antihypertensive treatment are significant, these drugs have not replaced the thiazides or aldosterone antagonists in most clinics.

Complications of Diuretic Therapy

Complications of diuretic therapy can be divided into toxic or idiosyncratic reactions to the drugs and those disturbances of fluid, electrolyte, and acid-base balance which may arise as consequences of the pharmacologic effects of the drugs upon tubular transport processes.

Toxic and Idiosyncratic Reactions

In patients with renal disease, acute renal failure has occurred after administration of mercurial diuretics;[23] hence it is advisable to pretest for hypersensitivity by a small test injection of the organomercurial. Large doses of mercurial diuretics should be avoided in the presence of significant azotemia because of mercurial nephrotoxicity. Rashes or blood dyscrasias (anemia, leukopenia, thrombocytopenia) may occur with any diuretic, but are more commonly observed with thiazides and other sulfonamide derivatives.[9] The thiazides and furosemide may impair the carbohydrate tolerance of some patients;[9,60] pancreatitis has been observed occasionally after administration of thiazides. Administration of ethacrynic acid, amiloride, or triamterene may be associated with gastric irritations, nausea, vomiting, or abdominal pain. Both ethacrynic acid and furosemide have produced hearing loss, particularly in patients with renal disease who received large doses.[46,61] Administration of spironolactone may induce a reversible painful gynecomastia, menstrual irregularity, or impotence.

Side Effects Related to Pharmacologic Actions

Depletion of extracellular fluid volume by excessive diuresis has several clinical manifestations. Orthostatic hypotension, tachycardia, or even shock may occur after a large rapid diuresis induced by a mercurial, ethacrynic acid, or furosemide. When extracellular fluid volume depletion occurs because of a chronically negative sodium balance due to diuretic administration, the patient complains of lethargy and weakness and frequently exhibits orthostatic hypotension and poor tissue turgor. As a consequence of the contraction of blood volume there may be either a fall in renal perfusion pressure or secondary renal vasoconstriction or both. This may result in a fall in the glomerular filtration rate and a rise in serum creatinine concentration. In addition, the serum concentrations of urea, calcium, urate, and phosphorus may also increase, probably as a consequence of a hemodynamically mediated increase in proximal tubular reabsorption of sodium, water, and other ions. Because sodium chloride balance has been negative, but water balance normal, the serum sodium and chloride concentrations may be depressed in such edema-free patients. (The coexistence of potassium depletion and alkalosis provides a clue that hyponatremia is related to diuretic therapy.)

Azotemia which is not associated with extracellular fluid volume depletion may result from direct pharmacologic effects of thiazides, spironolactone, triamterene, and amiloride. This deterioration of renal function is reversible and is observed most frequently in patients with underlying kidney damage. In edematous hypertensives whose daily water intake is large, the administration of diuretics such as the thiazides or spironolactone, which inhibit sodium reabsorption in the loop of Henle and distal diluting segments of the nephron, may be a contributing factor in the production of "dilutional" hyponatremia (i.e., the situation in which increased body sodium stores are accompanied by proportionally greater surpluses of body water). Potassium losses into the urine which occur during therapy with mercurials, carbonic anhydrase inhibitors, thiazides, ethacrynic acid, and furosemide may be associated with weakness, hyporeflexia, or development of digitalis toxicity. This complication may be avoided or prevented by administration of fruit juices, oral potassium chloride solutions, or coadministration of an aldosterone antagonist.

Urinary losses of hydrogen during diuresis with mercurials, ethacrynic acid, and furosemide may contribute to development of a metabolic alkalosis.[46] Hypochloremia induced by any of these agents or the thiazide diuretics may perpetuate alkalosis in salt-restricted patients by inducing inappropriate H^+ elimination and bicarbonate retention by the kidney.[32] Provision of chloride as dietary salt, potassium chloride or ammonium chloride facilitates correction of this acid-base disturbance.[62] Potassium retention and hyperkalemia may occur in patients with renal disease as a consequence of the diuretic action of spironolactone, triamterene, and amiloride; metabolic acidosis may occur with the same drugs due to depression of urinary titratable acid and ammonium excretion.

Hyperuricemia is observed particularly in patients receiving chronic oral doses of thiazides, ethacrynic acid, or furosemide. Renal urate retention and hyperuricemia may also occur as a nonspecific reaction to extracellular fluid depletion after diuresis with any diuretic agent.[34] (It must be realized, however, that a large percentage of untreated hypertensive patients exhibit hyperuricemia [63] probably because of renal urate retention due to functional changes in their renal circulation.) Attacks of gout may be prevented by prophylaxis with colchicine. Serum urate levels can be lowered by stopping the diuretic or by administration of allopurinol. There is suggestive but not conclusive evidence that marked elevations of urate (>10 mg per 100 cc) in hypertensive patients may contribute to renal deterioration by precipitating in the renal medulla.[63,64] Administration of allopurinol may be beneficial in this situation but it has not been advocated for lesser asymptomatic elevations.

Conclusions

Diuretics have an established position in current antihypertensive therapy. Although the variety of compounds available today permits the physician to selectively modify various ion transport processes in the renal tubules, the biochemical bases for these diuretic effects remain largely obscure, and even less is known concerning the mechanisms by which these varied compounds act to lower arterial pressure. Further investigation into their modes of action may provide important insights into the pathogenesis of the hypertensive process.

References

1. Freis, E. D.: Acute antihypertensive effects of chlorothiazide. Am. J. Cardiol. 8:880, 1961.
2. Crosley, A. P., Jr., Cullen, R. C., White, D., Freeman, J. F., Castillo, C. A., and Rose, G. G.: Studies of the mechanism of action of chlorothiazide in cardiac and renal diseases. I. Acute effects on renal and systemic hemodynamics and metabolism. J. Lab. Clin. Med. 55:182, 1960.
3. Davidov, M., Kakaviatos, N., and Finnerty, F. A., Jr.: Diuretic and antihypertensive properties of furosemide. J. New Drugs 6: 123, 1966.
4. Conway, J., and Leonetti, G.: Hypotensive effect of ethacrynic acid. Circulation 31:661, 1965.
5. Conway, J., and Lauwers, P.: Mode of action of chlorothiazide in the reduction of blood pressure in hypertension. Am. J. Cardiol. 8: 884, 1961.
6. Conway, J., and Lauwers, P.: Hemodynamic hypotensive effects of long-term therapy with chlorothiazide. Circulation 21:21, 1960.
7. Finnerty, F. A., Jr., Davidov, M., and Kakaviatos, N.: Relation of sodium balance to arterial pressure during drug-induced saluresis. Circulation 37:175, 1968.
8. Wilson, I. M., and Freis, E. D.: Relationship between plasma and extracellular fluid volume depletion and antihypertensive effect of chlorothiazide. Circulation 20:1028, 1959.
9. Laragh, J. H.: Mode of action and use of chlorothiazide and related compounds. Circulation 26:121, 1962.
10. Hollander, W., and Chobanian, A. V.: Mode of action of chlorothiazide and mercurial diuretics as antihypertensive agents. J. Clin. Invest. 37:907, 1958.
11. Kakaviatos, N., Davidov, M., Gavrilovich, L., and Finnerty, F. A., Jr.: Letter to the Editor: Diazoxide and furosemide in hypertension. Lancet 2:725, 1967.
12. Tobian, L., Jr., and Binion, J. T.: Tissue cations and water in arterial hypertension. Circulation 5:754 ,1952.
13. Winer, B. M.: Antihypertensive mechanisms of salt depletion induced by hydrochlorothiazide. Circulation 24:788, 1961.
14. Dollery, C. T., Harington, M., and Kaufmann, G.: Mode of action of chlorothiazide in hypertension with special reference to potentiation of ganglion-blocking agents. Lancet 1:1215, 1959.
15. Feisel, K. A., Eckstein, J. W., Horsley, A. W., and Keasling, H. H.: Effects of chlorothiazide on forearm vascular responses to norepinephrine. J. Appl. Physiol. 16:549, 1961.
16. Freis, E. D., Wanko, W., Schnaper, H. W., and Frohlich, E. D.: Mechanism of the altered blood pressure responsiveness produced by chlorothiazide. J. Clin. Invest. 39: 1277, 1960.
17. Laragh, J. H., Cannon, P. J., and Ames, R. P.: Interaction between aldosterone secretion, sodium and potassium balance, and angiotensin activity in man: Studies in hypertension and cirrhosis. Can. Med. Assoc. J. 90:248, 1964.
18. Heinemann, H. O., Demartini, F. E., and Laragh, J. H.: The effect of chlorothiazide on renal excretion of electrolytes and free water. Am. J. Med. 26:853, 1959.
19. Goldstein, M. H., Levitt, M. F., Hauser, A. D., and Polimeros, D.: Effect of meralluride on solute and water excretion in hydrated man: Comments on site of action. J. Clin. Invest. 40:731, 1961.

20. Porush, J. G., Goldstein, M. G., Eisner, G. M., and Levitt, M. F.: Effect of organomercurials on the renal concentrating operation in hydropenic man: Comments on site of action. J. Clin. Invest. 40:1475, 1961.
21. Levitt, M. F., Goldstein, M. H., Lenz, P. R., and Wedeen, R.: Mercurial diuretics. Ann. N.Y. Acad. Sci. 139:375, 1966.
22. Seldin, D. W., Eknoyan, G., Suki, W. N., and Rector, F. C., Jr.: Localization of diuretic action from the pattern of water and electrolyte excretion. Ann. N.Y. Acad. Sci. 139:328, 1966.
23. Freeman, R. B., Maher, J. F., Schreiner, G. E., and Mostofii, F. K.: Renal tubular necrosis due to nephrotoxicity of organic mercurial diuretics. Ann. Intern. Med. 57:34, 1962.
24. Berliner, R. W.: Carbonic anhydrase inhibitors. Pharmacol. Rev. 8:137, 1956.
25. Dirks, J. H., Cirksena, W. J., and Berliner, R. W.: Micropuncture study of the effect of various diuretics on sodium reabsorption by the proximal tubule of the dog. J. Clin. Invest. 45:1875, 1967.
26. Wilkins, R. W.: New drugs for hypertension with special reference to chlorothiazide. N. Engl. J. Med. 257:1026, 1957.
27. Hollander, W., and Wilkins, R.: Chlorothiazide: A new type of drug for treatment of arterial hypertension. Boston Med. Q. 8:69, 1957.
28. Freis, E. D., Wanko, A., Wilson, I. M., and Parrish, A. E.: Treatment of essential hypertension with chlorothiazide (Diuril): Its use alone and combined with other antihypertensive agents. JAMA 166:137, 1958.
29. Earley, L. E., Kahn, M., and Orloff, J.: Effects of infusions of chlorothiazide on urinary dilution and concentration in the dog. J. Clin. Invest. 40:857, 1961.
30. Laragh, J. H., Sealey, J. E., Sommers, S. C.: Patterns of adrenal secretion and urinary excretion of aldosterone and plasma renin activity in normal and hypertensive subjects. Circ. Res. 18:158, 1966.
31. Goldring, R. M., Cannon, P. J., Heinemann, H. O., and Fishman, A. P.: Respiratory adjustment to chronic metabolic alkalosis in man. J. Clin. Invest. 47:188, 1968.
32. Schwartz, W. B., Van Ypersele de Strihou, C., and Kassirer, J. P.: Role of anions in metabolic alkalosis and potassium deficiency. N. Engl. J. Med. 279:630, 1968.
33. Demartini, F. E., Wheaton, E. A., Healy, L. A., and Laragh, J. H.: Effect of chlorothiazide on renal excretion of uric acid. Am. J. Med. 32:572, 1962.
34. Hull, A. R., Suki, W. N., Rector, F. C., Jr., and Seldin, D. W.: Mechanism of diuretic-induced hyperuricemia. Abstracts of the First Annual Meeting of the American Society of Nephrology, Washington, D.C., November 1967, p. 13.
35. Bartter, F. C., (Ed.): The Clinical Use of Aldosterone Antagonist. Springfield, Ill.: Thomas, 1960.
36. Coppage, W. S., Jr., and Liddle, G. W.: Mode of action and clinical usefulness of aldosterone antagonists. Ann. N.Y. Acad. Sci. 88:815, 1960.
37. Liddle, G. W.: Specific and nonspecific inhibition of mineralocorticoid activity. Metabolism 10:1021, 1961.
38. Johnston, L. C., and Greible, H. G.: Treatment of arterial hypertensive disease with diuretics. V. Spironolactone, an aldosterone antagonist. Arch. Intern. Med. 119:225, 1967.
39. Crane, M. G., and Harris, J. J.: Effect of spironolactone in hypertensive patients. Am. J. Med. Sci. 260:311, 1970.
40. Biglieri, E. G., Schambelan, M., Slaton, P. E., and Stockigt, J. R.: The intercurrent hypertension of primary aldosteronism. Circ. Res. 26 and 27 (Suppl. I):I–195, 1970.
41. Baer, L., Sommers, S. C., Krakoff, L. R., Newton, M. A., and Laragh, J. H.: Pseudoprimary aldosteronism. Circ. Res. 26 and 27 (Suppl. I):I–203, 1970.
42. Spark, R. F., and Melby, J. C.: Aldosteronism in hypertension: The spironolactone response test. Ann. Intern. Med. 69:685, 1698.
43. Spark, R. F., and Melby, J. C.: Hypertension and low plasma renin activity: Presumptive evidence for mineralocorticoid excess. Ann. Intern. Med. 75:831, 1971.
44. Crosley, A. P., Jr., Ronquillo, L. M., Strickland, W. H., and Alexander, F.: "Triamterene," a natriuretic agent. Preliminary observations in man. Ann. Intern. Med. 56:241, 1962.
45. Bull, M. D., and Laragh, J. H.: "Amiloride": A potassium-sparing natriuretic agent. Circulation 37:45, 1968.
46. Cannon, P. J., and Kilcoyne, M. M.: Ethacrynic acid and furosemide: Renal pharmacology and clinical use. Progr. Cardiovasc. Dis. 12:99, 1969.
47. Cannon, P. J., Heinemann, H. O., Stason, W. B., and Laragh, J. H.: Ethacrynic acid: Effectiveness and mode of diuretic action in man. Circulation 31:5, 1965.
48. Goldberg, M., McCurdy, D. K., Foltz, E. L., and Bluemle, L. W., Jr.: Effects of ethacrynic acid (a new saluretic agent) on renal diluting and concentrating mechanisms: Evidence for

site of action in the loop of Henle. J. Clin. Invest. 43:201, 1964.
49. Stason, W. B., Cannon, P. J., Heinemann, H. O., and Laragh, J. H.: Furosemide, a clinical evaluation of its diuretic action. Circulation 34:910, 1966.
50. Birtch, A. G., Zakheim, R. M., Jones, L. G., and Barger, A. C.: Redistribution of renal blood flow produced by furosemide and ethacrynic acid. Circ. Res. 21:869, 1967.
51. Muth, R. G.: Diuretic response to furosemide in the presence of renal insufficiency. JAMA 195:1066, 1966.
52. Berman, L. B., and Ebrahimi, A.: Experiences with furosemide in renal disease. Proc. Soc. Exp. Biol. Med. 118:333, 1965.
53. Maher, J. F., and Schreiner, G. F.: Studies on ethacrynic acid in patients with refractory edema. Ann. Intern. Med. 62:15, 1965.
54. Davidov, M., Kakaviatos, N., and Finnerty, F. A., Jr.: Intravenous administration of furosemide in heart failure. JAMA 200:824, 1967.
55. Ledingham, J. G. G.: Ethacrynic acid parenterally in treatment and prevention of pulmonary edema. N. Engl. J. Med. 273:583, 1965.
56. Davidov, M., Kakaviatos, N., and Finnerty, F. A., Jr.: Antihypertensive properties of furosemide. Circulation 36:125, 1967.
57. Nash, H. L., Fitz, A. E., Wilson, W., Kirkendall, W. M., and Kioschos, J. M.: Cardiorenal hemodynamic effects of ethacrynic acid. Am. Heart J. 71:153, 1966.
58. Schrier, R. W., and de Wardener, H. E.: Tubular reabsorption of sodium ion. N. Engl. J. Med. 285:1231, 1292, 1971.
59. Wolfer, H. J., Schneider, K. W., Gattenlohner, W., and Gunther, J.: Behandlung der arteriellen Hypertonie mit Fursemid. Munch. Med. Wochenschr. 106:1767, 1964.
60. Breckenridge, A., Welbern, T. A., Dollery, C. T., and Fraser, T. R.: Glucose tolerance in hypertensive patients on long-term diuretic therapy. Lancet 1:61, 1967.
61. Schneider, W. J., and Becker, E. L.: Acute transient hearing loss after ethacrynic acid therapy. Arch. Intern. Med. 117:715, 1966.
62. Kassirer, J. P., Berkman, P. M., Lawrenz, D. R., and Schwartz, W. B.: Critical role of chloride in the correction of hypokalemic alkalosis in man. Am. J. Med. 38:172, 1965.
63. Cannon, P. J., Stason, W. B., Demartini, F. E., Sommers, S. C., and Laragh, J. H.: Hyperuricemia in primary and renal hypertension. N. Engl. J. Med. 275:457, 1966.
64. Cannon, P. J., Symchych, P. S., and Demartini, F. E.: The distribution of urate in human and primate kidney. Proc. Soc. Exp. Biol. Med. 129:278, 1968.

Long-term Use of Furosemide Alone in Hypertension

By Leland L. Atkins, M.D.

THE ROUTINE TREATMENT of hypertension has been greatly simplified by the advent of the oral diuretic agents, either used alone or in combination with other agents. Blood pressure generally is not reduced by these drugs in normotensive subjects; therefore the oral saluretics should be considered antihypertensive rather than hypotensive agents. Although their precise mechanism of action in hypertension has not been clearly defined, the fall in blood pressure is associated with enhancement of salt excretion and diuresis, so that equivalent doses of the various thiazides exert equivalent effects on blood pressure and water excretion.[1,2]

It is essential to differentiate between acute and chronic changes produced by saluretics in hypertensive subjects. In the acute phase, in addition to the drop in blood pressure, a negative sodium balance is established and body weight is reduced as a result of fluid loss associated with reduction in plasma volume.[3,4] These changes are reversed usually within a week. The reduction of blood pressure in the acute phase may be due to the decrease in plasma volume and cardiac output.[5] The increase in peripheral resistance which can result may be regarded as an attempt by the organism to restore the blood pressure.

In responsive patients, chronic thiazide therapy results in sustained and more consistent reduction in blood pressure. A new equilibrium in plasma and extracellular fluid volume usually is established in about 3 to 4 weeks after starting treatment.[4] During long-term administration, the blood pressure-lowering action of saluretics is considered to be due primarily to the decreased peripheral resistance associated with changes in arteriolar responsiveness.[6,7]

The diuretics can be expected to produce some reduction in blood pressure in about two-thirds of hypertensive subjects and the decrease achieved with diuretic antihypertensive agents may be related to the initial blood pressure level. It has been estimated that approximately 30 to 40 percent of patients with mild or moderate hypertension can be satisfactorily maintained with the use of oral saluretics alone.[8,9] In responsive subjects, mean arterial pressure is reduced by about 15 percent, averaging 20 to 30 mm Hg systolic and 10 to 20 mm Hg diastolic.

The newer diuretics, furosemide and ethacrynic acid, are more effective than the thiazides in promoting salt and water excretion and could therefore be of special interest in treating hypertension.

Furosemide is distinguished from the thiazides by its chemical structure (Fig. 1) and the greater natriuretic and diuretic effect which it can produce. It has a more rapid onset and relatively brief duration of diuretic action and its effectiveness is not limited by depression of glomerular filtration rate, renal blood flow, or changes in acid-base balance.

In both acute and chronic studies, furosemide manifested antihypertensive properties and hemodynamic alterations similar to those of another oral saluretic.[10–14]

In hypertensive subjects a measurable reduction in blood pressure occurs usually in the second hour after intravenous administration of 20 to 40 mg of furosemide. After an oral dose of 80 mg, reduction in the elevated blood pressure appears after 2 hours and lasts for approximately 24 hours. In most patients with mild or moderate essential hypertension, the optimal dosage for long-term oral therapy is from 40 to 80 mg per day. In nonedematous hypertensive patients, diuresis was evident only during the first 24 to 48 hours of treatment while blood pressure reduction had not yet reached a maximum in most patients. Thus it would appear that diuretic and antihypertensive effects of the drug are separate.

We previously reported on the use of furosemide in edematous subjects and on its acute

From the Medical Associates Clinic, Memphis, Tennessee.

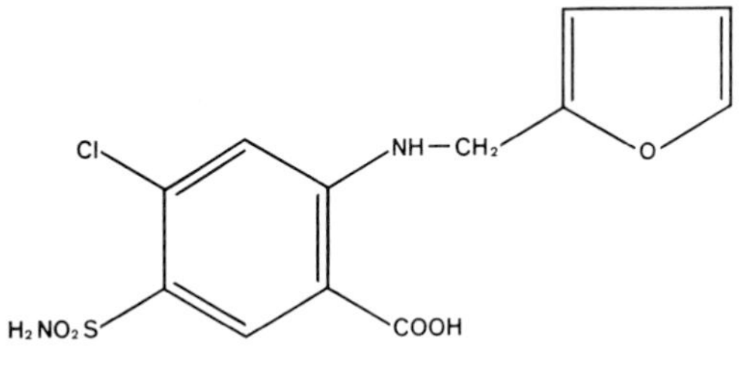

4-Chloro-N-furfuryl-5-sulfamoylanthranilic acid.

FIG. 1.—Structural formula of furosemide.

antihypertensive effect following parenteral administration.[15,16] Single intramuscular injections of 20 or 40 mg of furosemide had no appreciable effect on blood pressures in normotensive subjects, but in patients with hypertension a dose-related reduction in both systolic and diastolic pressures could readily be demonstrated (Fig. 2). Similarly, when weekly injections of furosemide were administered to hypertensive patients maintained on daily oral doses of 50 mg of hydrochlorothiazide, additional and statistically significant decreases in blood pressure consistently occurred (Fig. 3).

Treatment of hypertension is generally prolonged and it is therefore important that therapy be continuous and properly supervised.

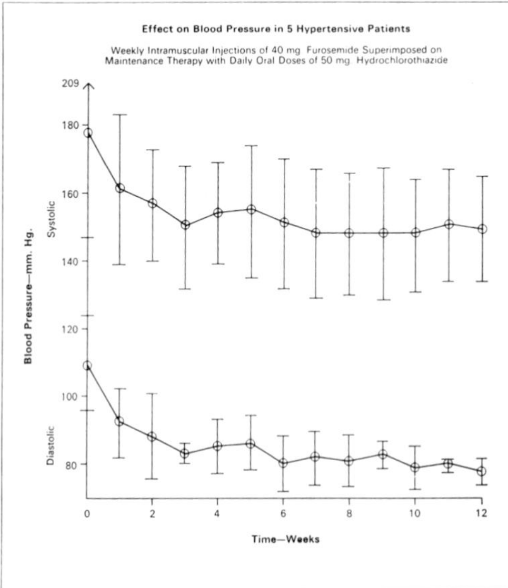

FIG. 2.—Average blood pressure changes (mm Hg) after single intramuscular injections of furosemide. (From Atkins,[16] with permission.)

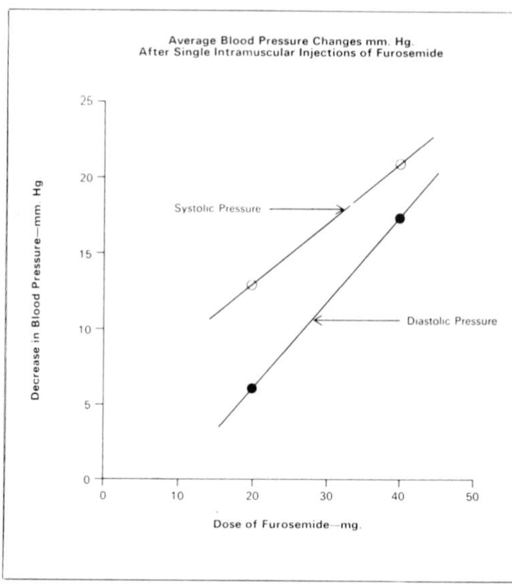

FIG. 3.—Effect of furosemide on blood pressure in five hypertensive patients. Weekly intramuscular injections of 40 mg of furosemide superimposed on maintenance therapy with daily oral doses of 50 mg of hydrochlorothiazide. (From Atkins,[16] with permission.)

Patients attending the Medical Associates Clinic are well suited for the assessment of long-term therapeutic results. Compared with the typical outpatient, who attends a hypertension clinic in a large city hospital, our patients appear to be better motivated and more likely to follow instructions. This impression is supported by the relatively low rate of loss of patients to follow-up resulting from inability or unwillingness to continue treatment.

PATIENTS AND METHODS

At present, furosemide is part of the standard regimen of approximately 200 hypertensive subjects regularly attending our clinic. The majority of these were given combination therapy from the start because their hypertension was judged to be above our criteria for moderate hypertension, i.e., a diastolic pressure of at least 120 mm Hg and/or significant changes in the optic fundi.

Ninety patients, however, with mild to moderate hypertension were started with furosemide alone. Of these, 24 patients could not be adequately controlled with furosemide alone and after variable periods of time received furosemide in combination with other antihypertensive agents.

The remaining 66 patients with mild to moderate hypertension were further analyzed to provide more detailed information on the control of elevated blood pressure with the use of furosemide alone. These patients have been maintained on continuous, uninterrupted furosemide therapy for 4 to 37 months, the average length of therapy being 20 months.

Hypertension was diagnosed in most patients during routine examination. At the initial visit, a complete history is taken. Each patient is given a complete physical examination and screened with the following tests to diagnose secondary or potentially curable hypertension: complete blood count, urinalysis, examination of the optic fundi, chest x-ray, and electrocardiogram. An intravenous pyelogram is taken or other special tests are done if indicated. The workup also includes determination of serum sodium, chloride, potassium and uric acid, fasting blood sugar and blood urea nitrogen. Multiple blood pressure readings are obtained with the patient in the supine, sitting, and erect positions.

Patients usually are seen at weekly or biweekly intervals on three or four occasions. Blood pressure is taken in the sitting position several times at about 2-minute intervals and the lowest value obtained is recorded on the chart. If these repeat visits reveal a persistent elevation of systolic and/or diastolic blood pressure, the patient is started on oral furosemide. He is given a month's supply of tablets and is told to return for reexamination after this period.

Clinical Evaluation of the Results

For evaluation of the efficacy of treatment, the 66 patients in this series were divided into two groups. Group I consisted of 40 patients who received a single 40-mg dose of furosemide daily, and Group II consisted of 26 patients who were given 40 mg of furosemide twice daily.

The blood pressures recorded at the monthly follow-up visits were averaged for each patient for the first year of treatment and again for the remainder of the treatment period. These averaged values were compared with the baseline blood pressure. Thus each patient served as his own control. It was felt that this method of handling blood pressure values for each patient would tend to cancel out nonspecific alterations in blood pressure due to emotions, exercise, seasonal changes, etc. Blood chemistries were determined repeatedly throughout the period of treatment at 4- to 6-month intervals or more frequently if indicated. Dietary sodium was not restricted but patients were advised to refrain from adding excessive salt to prepared foods and to use potassium-rich fruits, fruit juices, vegetables, etc.

Statistical Analysis

For each patient, the mean arterial pressure was calculated as diastolic pressure plus one-third of the pulse pressure. This was done from the baseline blood pressure, from the first-year average blood pressure and from the beyond-1-year average blood pressure. Using the t-test for paired observations, the mean of the differences in the mean arterial pressures between the first-year average value and the baseline value was tested for significance for Group I and Group II. The correlation between the difference in the mean arterial pressure and the baseline value was also calculated. Additionally, for males, females, and all patients combined, the correlation between the baseline diastolic blood pressure and age and baseline body weight was examined.

Results

Most of the patients in the series would appear to fit the WHO classification of Stage I hypertension, i.e., high blood pressure without clinical symptoms or obvious signs of organic changes in the cardiovascular system.[17] The remainder could be classified under Stage II hypertension, i.e., high blood pressure with only electrocardiographic or roentgenographic evidence of cardiac hypertrophy or strain and/or symptoms such as headache, dizziness, and fatigue. None of the patients had evidence of significant renal insufficiency.

Some characteristics of the sample population are presented in Table 1. All of the patients in this study are black. About one-third of the 40 patients in Group I and 10 of

TABLE 1.—*Frequency Distribution of Age and Weight by Sex*

Age and Weight	No. of Patients: Group I—40 mg of Furosemide Daily, Female	Group I, Male	Group II—40 mg of Furosemide Twice Daily, Female	Group II, Male
Age (yr)				
less than 40	1	0	0	2
40–49	3	3	4	2
50–59	9	1	5	2
60–69	8	3	6	4
70–79	6	6	0	0
80–85	0	0	1	0
TOTAL	27	13	16	10
Weight (lb)				
less than 124	5	1	0	0
125–149	4	3	3	1
150–174	9	4	5	2
175–199	7	4	4	1
200–224	2	0	1	2
225–249	1	0	0	3
250 or greater	0	1	3	1
TOTAL	28	13	16	10

the 26 patients in Group II are males. The age of 63 of the 66 patients ranges from 40 to 85 years; and three patients (one female) are less than 40 years old. Approximately 45 percent of the females and 55 percent of the males are in the 60- to 79-year age group. Initial body weights ranged from less than 100 to more than 250 pounds; a large percentage of patients are obese (Table 2). Coincidental organic disorders are also listed in Table 2. Approximately 20 percent of the patients in Group II had a history of (mild) congestive heart failure. No patients in Group II had a history of cerebrovascular episodes or myocardial infarction. Four patients in Group I and 2 in Group II are diabetic.

The duration of treatment is shown in Table 3. Fifty-three of the 66 patients were treated for periods greater than 1 year (up to 37 months).

Examination of the relationship between initial diastolic blood pressure levels and age, sex, and body weight of the patients reveals

TABLE 2.—*Diagnosis of Organic Disorders in 66 Patients with Essential Hypertension*

Disease	No. of Patients *: Group I †—40 mg of Furosemide Daily	Group II ††—40 mg of Furosemide Twice Daily
None	20	8
Diabetes mellitus	4	2
Previous myocardial infarction	1	0
Previous cerebrovascular accident	2	0
Chronic pulmonary insufficiency	1	0
Previous congestive heart failure	0	5
Atrial fibrillation	1	1
Obesity	11	14

* Some patients had more than one disorder.
† Forty patients.
†† Twenty-six patients.

a negative correlation between advancing age and baseline diastolic blood pressure which is statistically significant for males and for females ($p < 0.05$) and for the entire group of 66 patients ($p < 0.01$). There is a significant positive correlation ($p < 0.05$) between initial diastolic blood pressure and body weights for the 66 patients (Table 4).

At the final evaluation, body weights de-

TABLE 3.—*Duration of Treatment*

Months	No. of Patients: Group I †—40 mg of Furosemide Daily	Group II ††—40 mg of Furosemide Twice Daily
4–12	6	7
13–18	8	3
19–24	20	3
25–30	5	8
31–37	1	5

† Forty patients.
†† Twenty-six patients.

TABLE 4.—*Relationship of Baseline Diastolic Blood Pressure to Age and Body Weight by Sex*

Sex	*No. of Patients*	*Correlation Age*	*Coefficient (r) Weight*
Males	23	−0.496 *	0.367
Females	43	−0.324 *	0.240
TOTAL	66	−0.397 †	0.298 *

* $p < 0.05$.
† $p < 0.01$.

creased in 57.5 percent of the patients in Group I and in 77 percent in Group II. The decrease ranged from 1 to 33 pounds (mean of 9.7 pounds). The largest loss, 33 pounds, occurred over a period of 31 months of treatment (from 241 to 208 pounds). Weight gain was observed in 42.5 percent in Group I and in 12 percent in Group II (average about 5 pounds). Eleven percent of Group II showed no change in body weight.

The results of treatment on mean arterial pressures are tabulated in Tables 5 and 6, where the patients are stratified into four groups according to initial mean arterial pressure levels of increasing severity. Table 7 shows the initial levels and mean changes in systolic and diastolic pressures.

The baseline mean arterial pressure in Group I (Table 5) ranged from 123.3 to 146.7 mm Hg (average 133.6 mm Hg); the average decrease was 19.7 mm Hg (14.6%) during the first year of treatment. In the 34 patients who continued on furosemide for as long as 37 months, an additional modest fall in average mean arterial pressure of 5.8 mm Hg (4.8%) occurred. The average change in mean arterial pressure between the baseline value and the first-year value was statistically significant ($p < 0.0001$).

The baseline systolic pressure in Group I ranged from 170 to 210 mm Hg (mean of 190.3); the average drop was 31.3 mm Hg (16.4%) during the first year of continuous treatment. An additional drop of 5.8 mm Hg (3.6%) occurred in the 34 patients treated for more than 1 year (Table 7). The baseline diastolic pressure ranged from 100 to 120 mm Hg (mean of 105.2 mm Hg); the average decrease during the first year amounted to 11 mm Hg (9.1%) with a further decrease of 4.0 mm Hg (3.6%) on continued treatment (Table 7).

TABLE 5.—*Results of Treatment with Furosemide on Mean Arterial Pressure in Group I (40 mg/day)*

Baseline Mean Arterial Pressure (mm Hg)	*Average Change in Mean Arterial Pressure (mm Hg)*			
	First Year (from Baseline)		*Beyond First Year (from First Year)*	
	No. of Patients	*Mean (Range)*	*No. of Patients*	*Mean (Range)*
120–124	1	+1.0	1	−4.3
125–129	4	−13.8 (−2.0 to −27.3)	4	−6.2 (+2.0 to −11.8)
130–134	19	−15.0 (−4.7 to −29.0)	16	−7.7 (+5.4 to −18.7)
135–139	14	−27.9 (−15.3 to −42.3)	11	−4.1 (+4.7 to −18.0)
140–147	2	−28.4 (−26.7 to −30.0)	2	0.0 (+0.3 to −0.3)
x=133.6 (123.3 to 146.7)	40	x=−19.7 (+1.0 to −42.3)	34	x=−5.8 (+5.4 to −18.7)

TABLE 6.—*Results of Treatment with Furosemide on Mean Arterial Pressure in Group II (40 mg twice a day)*

Baseline Mean Arterial Pressure (mm Hg)	*Average Change in Mean Arterial Pressure (mm Hg)*			
	First Year (from Baseline)		*Beyond First Year (from First Year)*	
	No. of Patients	*Mean (Range)*	*No. of Patients*	*Mean (Range)*
130–134	6	−17.3 (−3.3 to −32.0)	5	−7.3 (+1.6 to −17.6)
135–139	7	−19.2 (−13.3 to −26.7)	6	−5.1 (+5.0 to −16.5)
140–144	8	−25.0 (−10.3 to −35.7)	4	+0.8 (+23.3 to −10.2)
145–149	1	−36.0	—	—
150–154	2	−24.6 (−23.3 to −26.0)	2	−15.2 (−11.0 to −19.5)
155–165	2	−38.4 (−35.7 to −40.0)	2	−8.4 (−7.1 to −9.8)
141.2 (132.7 to 163.3)	26	−23.1 (−3.3 to −40.0)	19	−5.9 (+23.3 to −19.5)

Blood pressure changes of similar magnitude were observed in Group II patients who received 40 mg of furosemide twice daily (Table 6). The mean arterial pressure in this group ranged from 132.7 to 163.3 mm Hg (mean of 141.2 mm Hg); the average fall during the first year was 23.1 mm Hg (16.2%) and a further average decrease of 5.9 mm Hg (4.6%) was noted in the 19 patients who continued treatment for up to 3 years.

There was a noticeable trend for greater blood pressure reduction in patients with higher baseline blood pressures (Tables 5 and 6). This is also shown in Figure 4 for calculated

TABLE 7.—*Average Changes in Systolic and Diastolic Blood Pressures Following Treatment with Furosemide in Groups I and II*

Blood Pressure by Group	*Baseline BP (mm Hg) Mean (Range)*	*Average Change in Blood Pressure (mm Hg)*			
		First Year (from Baseline)		*Beyond First Year (from First Year)*	
		No. of Patients	*Mean (Range)*	*No. of Patients*	*Mean (Range)*
Group I (40 mg/day)					
Systolic	190.3 (170–210)	40	−31.2 (+5.0 to −58.0)	34	−5.8 (+12.0 to −44.7)
Diastolic	105.2 (100–120)	40	−13.9 (+2.0 to −46.0)	34	−4.0 (+5.0 to −19.0)
Group II (40 mg twice a day)					
Systolic	193.5 (170–230)	26	−29.1 (+10.0 to −58.0)	19	−5.4 (+50.0 to −29.5)
Diastolic	115.1 (104–130)	26	−20.1 (−4.0 to −36.0)	19	−6.1 (+10.0 to −16.7)

mean arterial pressure. The correlation coefficient between the change in mean arterial pressure (difference between first-year average and baseline value) and the baseline mean arterial pressure is —0.92 for the entire series of 66 patients.

An analysis of the percentage of all patients responding with specific percentage changes in blood pressure are shown in Figures 5 to 7. Figure 5 gives the percentage distribution of patients at various levels of mean arterial pressure. A total of 76 percent of the patients had

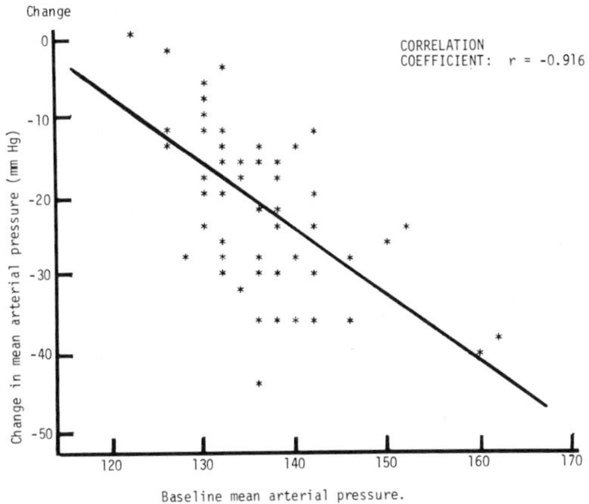

FIG. 4.—Change in mean arterial pressure (from baseline to ≦ 1-year average) versus baseline mean arterial pressure.

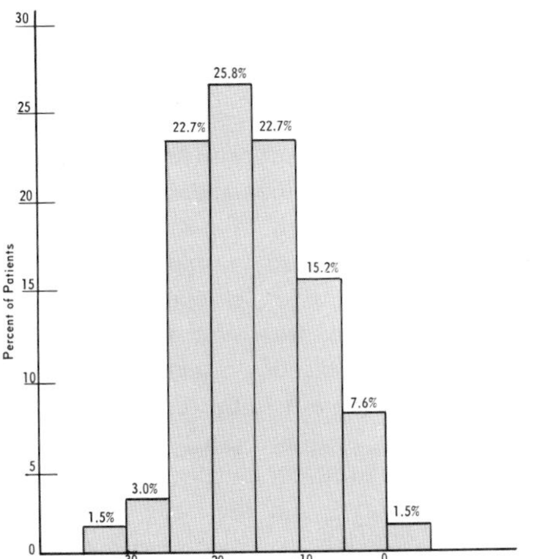

FIG. 5.—Frequency distribution of percentage change in mean arterial pressure from baseline to ≦ 1-year average.

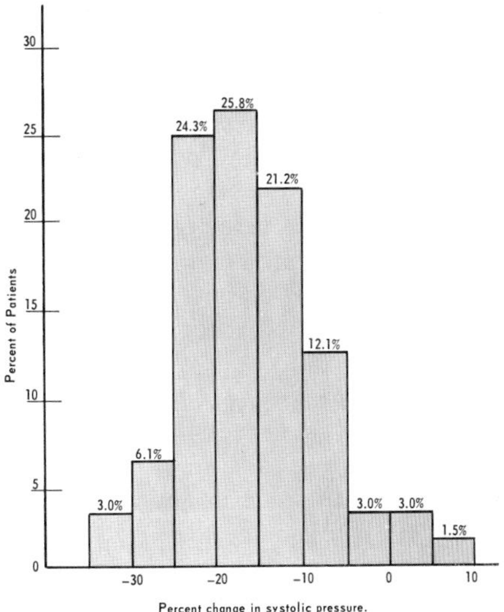

FIG. 6.—Frequency distribution of percentage change in systolic pressure from baseline to ≦ 1-year average.

a reduction in mean arterial pressure between 10 and 31 percent. Figures 6 and 7 show a similar distribution of patients responding at various levels of changes in systolic and diastolic pressures. Figures at the top of each column are the percentages of patients responding with that particular change in blood pressure.

Improvement in clinical symptoms paralleled the reduction and stabilization of blood pressure. Headache, dizziness, weakness, and fa-

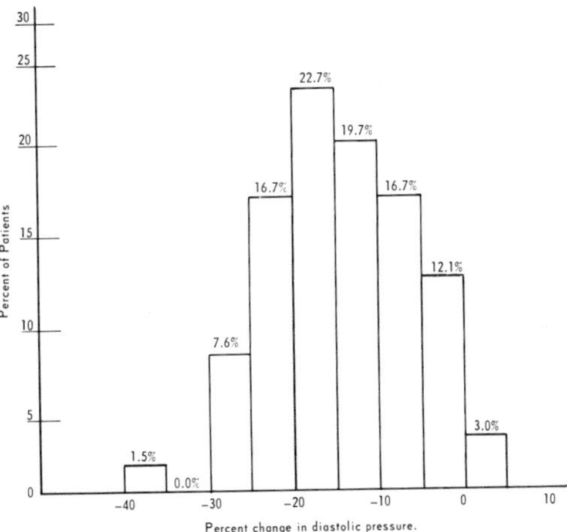

FIG. 7.—Frequency distribution of percentage change in diastolic pressure from baseline to ≦ 1-year average.

tigue, when present initially, usually disappeared.

Repeated blood chemistries revealed minor fluctuations particularly of serum potassium and uric acid, but abnormal values were very rare and comparisons of average pretreatment and posttreatment levels revealed no significant differences in any of the parameters tested. There was no evidence of gout in any of the patients treated with furosemide.

Discussion

Within the limits of this study, the results leave no doubt that long-term antihypertensive treatment with furosemide in responsive patients with mild or moderate essential hypertension can be maintained for indefinite periods with apparently minimal risk of undesirable effects. It should be emphasized that this report deals with a selected population in which effectiveness and safety of a single drug have been assessed.

About 70 percent of male and 60 percent of female patients in our study fell in the age group of 60 to 79 years, which would seem to agree with the results of the U.S.P.H.S. report released in 1964 [19]: the number of hypertensive subjects rises with advancing age, so that in the 64- to 74-year age group 16.3 percent of white men and 50.2 percent of black men were found to have elevated blood pressures. The proportion in this age group was, respectively, 37.5 percent for white women and 66.4 percent for black women. The prevalence of cardiac, cerebral, and renal complications was increased proportionately.

The apparent negative correlation of diastolic blood pressure with advancing age found in our study is supported by other epidemiologic studies, in which a trend of declining relative importance of diastolic pressure with age and a corresponding increase in the importance of systolic pressure was recorded.[20] On the third examination cycle in the Framingham study, 2.6 percent of men, 35 to 39 years old, had systolic pressures of 160 mm Hg or greater and 9.8 percent had diastolic pressures of 95 mm Hg or greater. By the ages of 70 to 74 years the situation was reversed: The percentages for men (on the seventh examination cycle) were, respectively, 26.8 percent with systolic pressure of 160 mm Hg or more and 11.3 percent with a diastolic pressure of 95 mm Hg or more.[20]

The apparent correlation of pretreatment diastolic pressure with increasing weight also agrees with results reported in other studies [21] which indicated an obvious and consistent increase in the frequency of higher levels of diastolic pressure with increasing relative weight (ratio of actual weight to recommended weight of the Metropolitan Life Insurance Company, 1959).

Essential hypertension generally is asymptomatic for many years before signs of cardiovascular impairment become manifest, followed in subsequent years by damage to the cerebral and renal vessels. Because of the variable and unpredictable course of so-called "benign essential hypertension," it is recognized that even 3 years of follow-up may be too brief a period to attempt to judge the usefulness of treatment on the progression of cardiovascular or other sequelae. Final judgment on the potential benefits of drug therapy in mild or moderate hypertension must await the completion of long-term studies.

At our clinic we endeavor to treat sustained hypertension in all patients unless specific contraindications are present such as the risk of aggravating the condition of elderly arteriosclerotic hypertensives. Our selection of patients to be treated is based on sensible therapeutic assessment of what is practicable. In some instances we prefer limited effectiveness to use of more potent hypotensive drugs and the risk of troublesome side effects or toxicity. We are particularly concerned with selecting a simple and relatively inexpensive regimen that will maintain and stabilize the blood pressure as close to normal levels as possible.

The results of this study would seem to indicate that oral furosemide is a relatively safe and effective medication with the important additional characteristic of patient acceptance. Another advantage which the drug may offer is its reported safety and effectiveness in patients with depressed renal function. Numerous reports indicate that the drug appears to be safe and effective in patients with reduced renal blood flow and filtration rate.[22,23] From the standpoint of efficacy and convenience, furosemide can provide long-term therapy for large numbers of patients with mild or moderate essential hypertension.

References

1. Freis, E. D.: Antihypertensive action of benzothiadiazines. N. Y. State J. Med. 68: 259, 1968.
2. Cranston, W. I., Juel-Jensen, B. E., Semmence, A. M., Jones, R. P. C. H., Forbes, J. A., and Mutch, L. M. M.: Effect of oral diuretics on raised arterial pressure. Lancet 2:966, 1963.
3. Gifford, R. W.: Use of diuretics in hypertension. JAMA 177:70, 1961.
4. Hansen, J.: Hydrochlorothiazide in the treatment of hypertension. Acta Med. Scand. 183: 317, 1968.
5. Rowe, G. G., Castillo, C. A., Crosley, A. P., Maxwell, G. M., and Crumpton, C. W.: Acute systemic and coronary hemodynamic effects of chlorothiazide in subjects with systemic arterial hypertension. Am. J. Cardiol. 10:183, 1962.
6. Lund-Johansen, P.: Hemodynamic changes in long-term diuretic therapy of essential hypertension. A comparative study of chlorthalidone, polythiazide and hydrochlorothiazide. Acta Med. Scand. 187:509, 1970.
7. Tobian, L.: Why do thiazide diuretics lower blood pressure in essential hypertension? Ann. Rev. Pharmacol. 7:399, 1967.
8. Schwid, S. A., and Gifford, R. W.: The use and abuse of antihypertensive drugs in the aged. Geriatrics 22:172, 1967.
9. Singer, P., Gawellek, F., and Faulhaber, H. D.: Treatment of hypertension. II. Characteristics of the action of saluretics in the treatment of hypertension. Dtsch. Gesundheitsw. 23:1729, 1968.
10. Bracharz, H., and Laas, H.: Comparative studies on the hypotensive effect of furosemide and hydrochlorothiazide. Geriat. Dig. 6:33, 1969.
11. Finnerty, F. A., Jr., Davidov, M., and Kakaviatos, N.: Relation of sodium balance to arterial pressure during drug-induced saluresis. Circulation 37:175, 1968.
12. Weidling, I.: Comparative investigations of the effects of furosemide and hydrochlorothiazide on blood pressure and diuresis in clinical studies. Thesis, University of Wurzburg, 1969.
13. Wertheimer, L., Finnerty, F. A., Jr., Bercu, B. A., and Hall, R. H.: Furosemide in essential hypertension. A statistical analysis of three double blind studies. Arch. Intern. Med. 127:934, 1971.
14. Wolfer, H. J., Schneider, K. W., Gattenlohner, W., and Gunther, J.: Treatment of arterial hypertension with furosemide. Munch. Med. Wochenschr. 106:1767, 1964.
15. Atkins, L. L.: Furosemide in the treatment of geriatric patients. Geriatrics 21:143, 1966.
16. Atkins, L. L.: Experience with furosemide injection. Clin. Med. 76:30, 1969.
17. WHO Expert Committee: Arterial hypertension and ischaemic heart disease. Preventive aspects. WHO Tech. Rep. Ser. 231:3, 1962.
18. Smith, W. M., Damato, A. N., Galluziz, N. J., Garfield, C. F., Hanowell, E. G., Stimson, W. H., Thurm, R. H., Walsh, J. J., and Bromer, L.: The evaluation of antihypertensive therapy. Cooperative clinical trial method. Ann. Intern. Med. 61:829, 1964.
19. Gordon, T.: Heart disease in adults. U.S. Public Health Service Publication, No. 1000, Series 11, No. 6:1, 1964.
20. Kannel, W. B., Gordon, T., and Schwartz, M. J.: Systolic versus diastolic blood pressure and risk of coronary heart disease. The Framingham study. Am. J. Cardiol. 27:335, 1971.
21. Veterans Administration Cooperative Study Group: Effects of treatment on morbidity in hypertension. JAMA 213:1143, 1970.
22. Mroczek, W. I., Davidov, J., Gavrilovich, L., and Finnerty, F. A., Jr.: The value of aggressive therapy in the hypertensive patient with azotemia. Circulation 40:893, 1969.
23. Stone, A. M., and Stahl, W. M.: Effect of ethacrynic acid and furosemide on renal function in hypovolemia. Ann. Surg. 174:1, 1971.

The Pharmacology of Reserpine and Guanethidine

By Vincent J. Zarro, M.D., Ph.D.

Reserpine was introduced into Western medicine in 1953 and has since enjoyed widespread clinical use. It remains one of the most important drugs in experimental adrenergic pharmacology. Guanethidine, introduced in 1959, is one of the most valuable drugs in the treatment of severe hypertension. The purpose of this discussion is to review some aspects of the basic pharmacology of these two interesting agents. First we will briefly consider the structure of the adrenergic nerve ending.

The Adrenergic Nerve Ending

The study of the adrenergic nervous system dates back to the start of modern pharmacology. Indeed some very accurate experiments with adrenergic agents were carried out in the early 1900s. The discovery of von Euler that norepinephrine is the sole mediator at the postganglionic sympathetic nerve ending and the introduction of an accurate assay for norepinephrine led the way to a critical analysis of adrenergic transmission. Classically, pharmacologists have studied the peripheral parts of the autonomic nervous system, that is, they consider only the two neuron efferent fibers, essentially the preganglionic and the postganglionic fiber, the ganglia and the receptors. It should be remembered that there are central autonomic nervous centers that are more complex than originally imagined, and that they also may be affected by drugs.

Hundreds of experiments utilizing, among other techniques, denervated structures and reserpine pretreatment have permitted the construction of a model of an adrenergic nerve ending. A simplified version is illustrated in Fig. 1. The synthesis of norepinephrine takes place in the axon up to the dopamine step. Dopamine then enters the granules, where the synthesis to norepinephrine is completed. The intragranular norepinephrine is bound to adenosine triphosphate (ATP) in a four-to-one molar ratio and serves as a never-ending supply to the available pool. When the nerve is stimulated norepinephrine is released from the available pool into the synaptic space, where it is free to unite with the adrenergic receptor. Once the receptor is triggered there is an active uptake of the norepinephrine back into the nerve ending, terminating its action. There is no enzyme in the synaptic space which rapidly inactivates norepinephrine. This is different from cholinergic action which is terminated by the rapid cleavage of acetylcholine by acetylcholinesterase.

Norepinephrine that spills into the bloodstream, or injected circulating norepinephrine is metabolized by catechol-o-methyltransferase. Finally, it is important to note that monoamine oxidase (MAO) is present in the cytoplasm of the adrenergic nerve ending. This enzyme slowly metabolizes intraneuronal norepinephrine which is not bound in the granule.

One may construct a more complicated scheme which subdivides the pool sites but for purposes of this discussion the above outline is complete enough. By referring to Fig. 1 it is easy to see the ways that the adrenergic nerve ending may be blocked.

Interference with Synthesis of Norepinephrine

It is now established that the total content of norepinephrine in the nerve ending can be decreased only by interfering with the rate-limiting step in the synthetic scheme, namely, the conversion of tyrosine to dihydroxyphenylalanine. This step requires the enzyme tyrosine hydroxylase.

Interference with Storage of Norepinephrine in the Granules

When norepinephrine is bound to ATP inside the granules it cannot be broken down by MAO. If the granules of the bound storage site

From the Departments of Pharmacology and Medicine, Hahnemann Medical College and Hospital, Philadelphia, Pennsylvania.

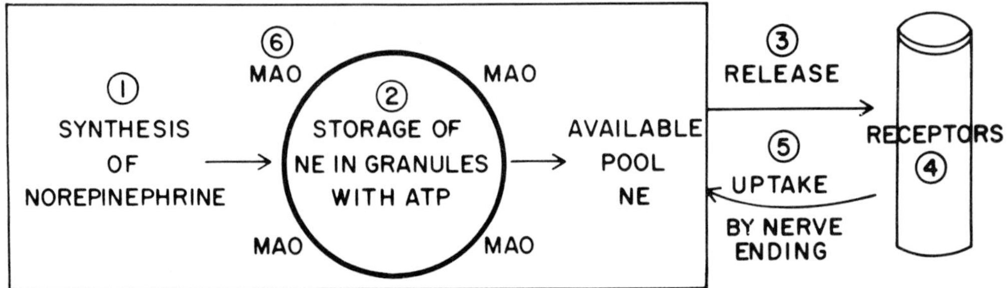

FIG. 1.—The adrenergic nerve ending. (See text for details.)

are altered so as to release (or not take up) norepinephrine, the free norepinephrine in the cytoplasm of the axon will be slowly metabolized, with a resultant decrease in total norepinephrine content in the nerve ending.

Blockade of the Release of Available Pool

An agent that blocks the release of norepinephrine from the available pool will decrease sympathetic tone. Since this is believed to be the principal mechanism of action of bretylium it has been referred to as a "bretylium-like action," even when referring to other drugs working through this mechanism.

Receptor Blockade

This is the classic way of blocking the action of administered drugs or endogenous mediators. The alpha- and beta-receptor blockers work at this site.

Agents that block adrenergic transmission by interfering with the storage or release of norepinephrine by the adrenergic nerve ending are known as neuronal blocking agents.

RESERPINE

Mechanism of Action

A great many studies are now available dealing with virtually every aspect of the action of reserpine. Much of the argument about the intimate mechanism of action, especially on acute administration, seems to arise from differences in dosage, method of administration, and species differences. For a more intimate discussion of a particular aspect, one of the many reviews and references should be consulted.[1–3]

The reader should recall that sympathomimetic amines may be divided into direct, indirect, and mixed acting. A direct-acting adrenergic agent has the ability to directly trigger the receptor; it does not require the presence of a nerve ending (Fig. 1, number 4). Norepinephrine is such a drug. Tyramine requires the presence of an intact adrenergic nerve ending to produce its effect and is acting consequently by releasing endogenous norepinephrine (Fig. 1, number 3). Tyramine, therefore, is an indirect-acting sympathomimetic amine. If one cuts the postganglionic adrenergic nerve to a sympathetically innervated organ (such as the nictitating membrane of the cat), the action of tyramine is sharply reduced.

A mixed-acting adrenergic agent has components of both direct and indirect action, that is, some of its action is mediated through release of endogenous norepinephrine and some by directly triggering the receptor.

When reserpine is administered 24 hours before an experiment there is a depletion of norepinephrine from the adrenergic nerve ending which results in a decreased sympathetic tone. If tyramine is given before and after reserpine pretreatment, the dose-response curve is shifted down and to the right (Fig. 2). If reserpine is administered intravenously there is a minimal rise in blood pressure, serving to illustrate that the available pool is not liberated by reserpine. Some studies do show an acute sympathomimetic effect of reserpine but certainly the pressor response is not nearly so great as that seen with tyramine.

The above facts are best explained by assuming that reserpine is acting at the bound storage site of norepinephrine, perhaps on the granular membrane. Work on isolated granules

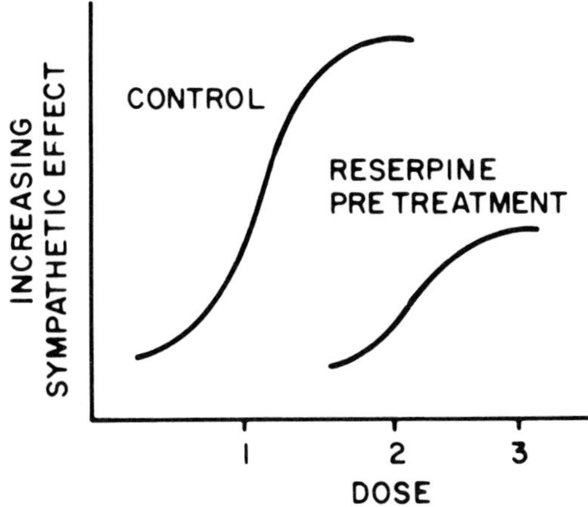

FIG. 2.—Dose-response curves for an indirect-acting sympathomimetic drug. After reserpine pretreatment the curve is shifted downward and to the right indicating that in the intact animal the drug is acting by releasing endogenous norepinephrine.

favors the hypothesis that there is an active transport of norepinephrine across the granular membrane so as to establish a dynamic equilibrium between bound and free amine. The norepinephrine outside the granule is metabolized by MAO in the neuron which over a period of time will decrease the total norepinephrine content. Other explanations of course are possible.[4]

Besides norepinephrine, reserpine also depletes the tissues of epinephrine and serotonin. A decrease in the level of epinephrine in chromaffin tissue may play a role in reduced sympathetic tone. The reduction of serotonin instead of norepinephrine in the brain was at first thought to explain the sedative action of reserpine; however, the biochemical changes produced by reserpine in the brain are complex and no good single hypothesis is available to explain the mechanism of sedation.[5,6]

It must be stressed that experiments in animals showing large reductions in catecholamine content in various organs have been carried out with large doses of reserpine (1 to 2 mg per kilogram of body weight in dogs, 3 to 5 mg per kilogram in cats). This would be equivalent to much larger doses than are used clinically in man; however, decreased catecholamine content in human tissue has been shown.[7]

Effect on Organ Systems

When reserpine is administered intravenously to an animal or human there is a latency of about 1 hour and the effect persists for 24 to 48 hours. This is best explained by the fact that the effect of reserpine must await the relatively slow breakdown of the norepinephrine. The action terminates when the level of amine builds up again. This is also a slow process. Reserpine itself is metabolized before its full effect is seen and for this reason has been called a "hit-and-run" drug.

Reserpine acts in the central nervous system (CNS) to cause sedation. The sedation is more like the effect of the phenothiazines than that of the barbiturates, and it is therefore a tranquilizer. It has no direct effect on the EEG and is not anticonvulsant. In fact in higher doses it may precipitate seizures; also, in higher doses it usually causes extrapyramidal effects and may lower body temperature.

The cardiovascular effects of reserpine are essentially a consequence of interfering with the effects of the sympathetic nervous system and the consequent overtone of the parasympathetic system. Therefore bradycardia is seen, with hypotension and a decrease in peripheral resistance. In animals given high doses sympathetic reflexes are depressed but in man this is not prominent. On chronic administration in man the cardiac output may be decreased and reflex increase may be altered.

Toxicity

Several adverse effects, some of which are quite serious, have been reported. Bradycardia, flushing, nasal congestion, salivation, and diarrhea are consequences of parasympathetic overtone. Activation of a peptic ulcer, and an increase in gastric acidity or gastric bleeding have been reported and may be serious. Severe mental depression, seizures, and drug-induced parkinsonism may occur as manifestations of CNS toxicity.

GUANETHIDINE

Interest in another category of neuronal-blocking agents started with the introduction of choline 2:6 xylyl ether (TM 10). This was followed by the introduction of bretylium and guanethidine. As a group these agents block the effects of adrenergic-nerve stimulation but do not block the effects of injected norepinephrine. TM 10 and bretylium have other effects which limit their use. Choline 2:6 xylyl ether has cholinergic effects and tolerance to bretylium develops on chronic administration. Neither of these drugs is available for general clinical use.[5,8–11]

Mechanism of Action

Guanethidine is a strongly basic compound having the following chemical structure:

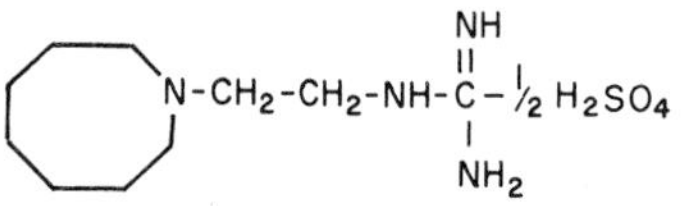

$$\text{(cyclooctyl)}\,N\text{-}CH_2\text{-}CH_2\text{-}NH\text{-}\underset{\displaystyle NH_2}{\overset{\displaystyle NH}{\overset{\|}{C}}}\text{-}\tfrac{1}{2}\,H_2SO_4$$

This drug is poorly soluble in lipids and does not cross the blood-brain barrier in any appreciable amount.

Guanethidine has a complex pharmacology.[11–16] The effect on the sympathetic nervous system is best described by considering that it occurs in three steps. Immediately after intravenous injection there is a block of adrenergic transmission with a drop in blood pressure. This is followed rapidly by a sympathomimetic response with cardioacceleration, hypertension, contraction of the nictitating membrane, piloerection, etc. This sympathetic stimulation lasts a few minutes to 1 hour depending on the dose. Finally there is a prolonged sympathetic blockade with reduction of blood pressure lasting 24 hours. Many experiments have been carried out to elucidate this triphasic response.

The first phase of sympathetic blockade can be demonstrated on the nictitating membrane of the cat. When guanethidine is administered and the adrenergic nerve to the nictitating membrane is stimulated there is no response. The drug acts by blocking the release of norepinephrine from the available pool. As mentioned above this is referred to as a bretylium-like action.

The next response, the sympathomimetic effect, is probably due to a direct release of the available pool and prevention of uptake of norepinephrine which as mentioned above is the mechanism for terminating sympathetic action.[11,15] This sympathomimetic effect is of significance only when guanethidine is administered intravenously.

The final phase, that of sympathetic blockade lasting over 24 hours, is due to depletion of norepinephrine from the adrenergic nerve ending. In this phase the action of guanethidine resembles reserpine. Norepinephrine depletion has been shown to occur in the heart, aorta, and spleen.[17] Unlike reserpine, guanethidine does not lower the epinephrine content of chromaffin tissue.

On chronic oral administration the main mechanism of action is sympathetic blockade and is no doubt related to the depletion of norepinephrine.[18]

Most of the side effects of guanethidine are exaggerations of its pharmacologic effect. Orthostatic hypotension is common. As with other sympathetic blockers, diarrhea and failure of ejaculation may occur. Skeletal muscle weakness may be seen but the mechanism is unknown. Tolerance to guanethidine is not significant and people have continued to respond to its hypotensive effect after years of use.

Effect on Organ Systems and Toxicities

For reasons given above guanethidine is devoid of CNS effects. It decreases heart rate and lowers blood pressure especially when it is elevated above normal. Sympathetic blockade may give rise to parotid pain but this is seen more frequently with bretylium than with guanethidine. It may cause diarrhea due to parasympathetic overtone and may inhibit ejaculation without affecting potency.

If guanethidine is administered intravenously, it would be contraindicated whenever a sympathomimetic response would be dangerous, such as the presence of a pheochromocytoma. No parenteral preparations, however, are available for clinical use. The oral dose is incompletely (about 40 percent) but predictably absorbed.

References

1. Schlittler, E., and Bein, H. J.: *Rauwolfia* alkaloids. *In* Schlittler, E. (Ed.): Antihypertensive Agents. New York: Academic Press, 1967, pp. 191–221.
2. Alper, M. H., Flacke, W., and Krayer, O.: Pharmacology of reserpine and its implications for anesthesia. Anesthesiology 24:524, 1963.

3. Bein, H. J.: The pharmacology of *Rauwolfia*. Pharmacol. Rev. 8:435, 1956.
4. von Euler, U. S., Stjarne, L., and Lishajko, F.: Effects of reserpine, segontin and phenoxybenzamine on the catecholamines and ATP of isolated nerve and adrenomedullary storage granules. Life Sci. 3:35, 1964.
5. Maxwell, R. A.: Adrenergic blocking drugs. In Di Palma, J. R. (Ed.): Drill's Pharmacology in Medicine. New York: McGraw-Hill, 1971, pp. 675–707.
6. Nickerson, M.: Drugs inhibiting adrenergic nerves and structures innervated by them. *In* Goodman, L. S., and Gilman, A. (Eds.): The Pharmacological Basis of Therapeutics. New York: Macmillan, 1970, pp. 549–584.
7. Chidsey, C. A., Braunwald, E., Morrow, A. G., and Mason, D. T.: Myocardial norepinephrine concentration in man. N. Engl. J. Med. 269:653, 1963.
8. Shore, P. A.: Release of serotonin and catecholamines by drugs. Pharmacol. Rev. 14: 531, 1962.
9. Malmfors, T.: Studies on adrenergic nerves. Acta Physiol. Scand. 64(Supp. 248):1, 1965.
10. Maxwell, R. A., Mull, R. P., and Plummer, A. J.: [2-(Octahydro-1-azocinyl) ethyl]guanidine sulfate (CIBA 5864-SU), a new synthetic antihypertensive agent. Experientia 15: 267, 1959.
11. Mull, R. P., and Maxwell, R. A.: Guanethidine and related adrenergic neuronal blocking agents. *In* Schlittler, E. (Ed.): Antihypertensive Agents. New York: Academic Press, 1967, pp. 115–149.
12. Boura, A. L. A., and Green, A. F.: Adrenergic neuron blocking agents. Annu. Rev. Pharmacol. 5:183, 1965.
13. Pardo, E. G., Vargas, R., and Vidrio, H.: Antihypertensive drug action. Annu. Rev. Pharmacol. 5:77, 1965.
14. Furst, C. I.: The biochemistry of guanethidine. Adv. Drug Res. 4:133, 1967.
15. Green, A. F.: Antihypertensive drugs. Adv. Pharmacol. 1:161, 1962.
16. Boura, A. L. A., Copp, F. C., and Green, A. F.: New antiadrenergic compounds. Nature 184:70, 1959.
17. Cass, R., Kuntzman, R., and Brodie, B. B.: Norepinephrine depletion as a possible mechanism of action of guanethidine. Proc. Soc. Exp. Biol. Med. 103:871, 1960.
18. Dollery, C. T., Emslie-Smith, D., and Milne, M. D.: Clinical and pharmacological studies with guanethidine in the treatment of hypertension. Lancet 2:381, 1960.

The Multiple Sites of Action of Methyldopa

By Thomas E. Gaffney, M.D., Philip J. Privitera, Ph.D., and Shakil Mohammed, M.D., Ph.D.

Although methyldopa is similar to guanethidine in terms of its hypotensive efficacy (Fig. 1),[1] its effects differ from those of guanethidine: There appear to be at least three patterns of response in hypotensive patients treated with this drug.[1] Some patients show only postural hypotension similar to that seen during treatment with guanethidine. Others show either no decline in pressure or only a transient hypotensive effect, i.e., "resistance" and "tolerance" respectively. Finally, other patients exhibit a simultaneous and nearly equal decline in supine and standing arterial pressures. These varied patterns of hypotension seen during treatment with methyldopa may be related to the multiple sites of action of this drug, i.e., the peripheral adrenergic neuron, the central nervous system (CNS), and the effect on the release of renin from the kidney.

Effects on the Peripheral Adrenergic Neuron

In contrast to classic adrenergic neuronal-blocking drugs such as guanethidine which can easily be shown to produce adrenergic nerve blockade,[2] methyldopa does not usually block and only under special circumstances has it been shown to reduce the response to sympathetic nerve stimulation. For example, the intravenous injection of a single large dose of methyldopa attenuates but does not block the cat nictitating membrane response to direct sympathetic nerve stimulation (Fig. 2).[3] Similarly, the heart rate response to cardioaccelerator nerve stimulation in dogs is impaired but not blocked.[4] In contrast to the attenuated response seen after a single intravenous dose, the repeated administration of large doses of methyldopa on each of several days fails to produce a measurable impairment in the response to sympathetic nerve stimulation in heart,[4,5] limb resistance vessels,[6] and the nictitating membrane.[7]

In those patients who show postural hypotension, and in those laboratory situations in which an impaired response to sympathetic nerve stimulation is found, the underlying mechanism appears to be the substitution of methyldopa for dopa as a substrate for transmitter synthesis, with the ultimate substitution of methylnorepinephrine for norepinephrine as the sympathetic transmitter.[8,9] Day and Rand postulated that this substitution accounted for impaired peripheral sympathetic neuronal function because the false transmitter, methylnorepinephrine, was less potent as a pressor substance than norepinephrine.[3,10] Although reports vary on the relative potency of methylnorepinephrine and norepinephrine in laboratory preparations,[3,7,11] Mueller and Horwitz [12] have reported that intravenously administered methylnorepinephrine is less potent as a pressor amine than norepinephrine in normotensive subjects; there is a need for confirmation of these results. The development of supersensitivity to norepinephrine (Fig. 3) and/or methylnorepinephrine during prolonged treatment with methyldopa in man [13,14] and in laboratory animals [4,7,15] may counteract the lowered potency of neuronally released methylnorepinephrine. In some patients, this supersensitivity to the transmitter may account for normal or nearly normal peripheral sympathetic reflex control despite continued treatment with methyldopa. The development of supersensitivity may also account for the development of tolerance to the hypotensive effects of methyldopa.[14,16] In any event, the false-transmitter hypothesis of Day and Rand is an acceptable explanation for the postural hypotension observed in some patients treated with methyldopa.

It is less clear how methyldopa decreases

From the Division of Clinical Pharmacology, Departments of Medicine and Pharmacology, University of Cincinnati College of Medicine, Cincinnati, Ohio.

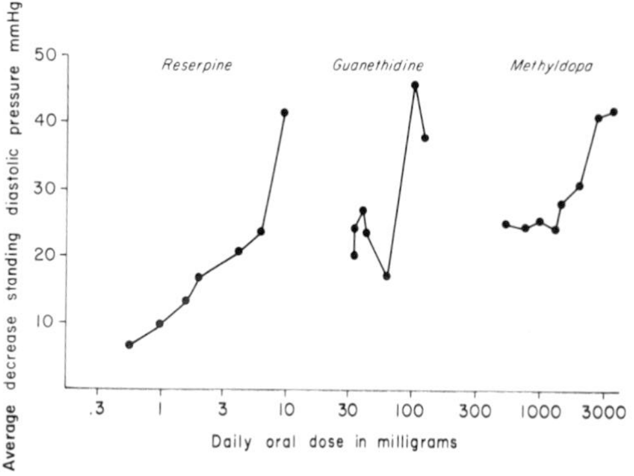

FIG. 1.—The relative antihypertensive efficacy and potency of oral reserpine, guanethidine and methyldopa. (From Gaffney et al.,[1] with permission.)

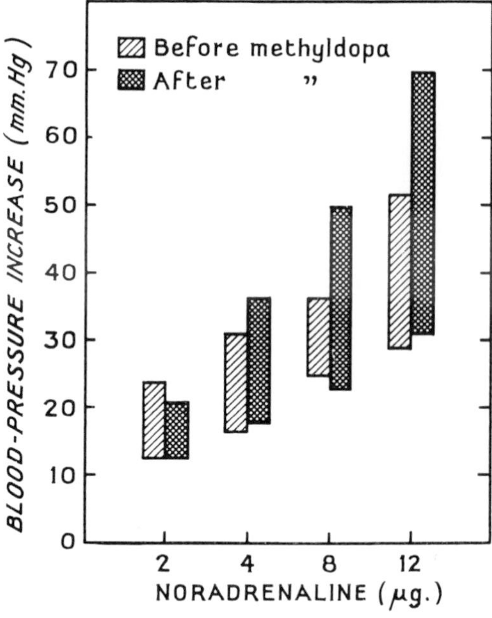

FIG. 3.—The increases in blood pressure in man, read from intra-arterial pressure records, after graded doses of noradrenaline were administered intravenously. The columns show the increase in systolic and diastolic pressure before treatment, and after 4 days' treatment with 2 gm of methyldopa daily. (From Dollery and Harington,[14] with permission.)

arterial pressure in those patients in whom supine (Fig. 4) and standing pressures are decreased to the same extent, or in those animal preparations in which vascular resistance is decreased without evidence of impaired sympathetic function. A number of investigators have emphasized that methyldopa decreases arterial pressure in the supine as well as standing position.[13,17–20] Similarly, Moham-

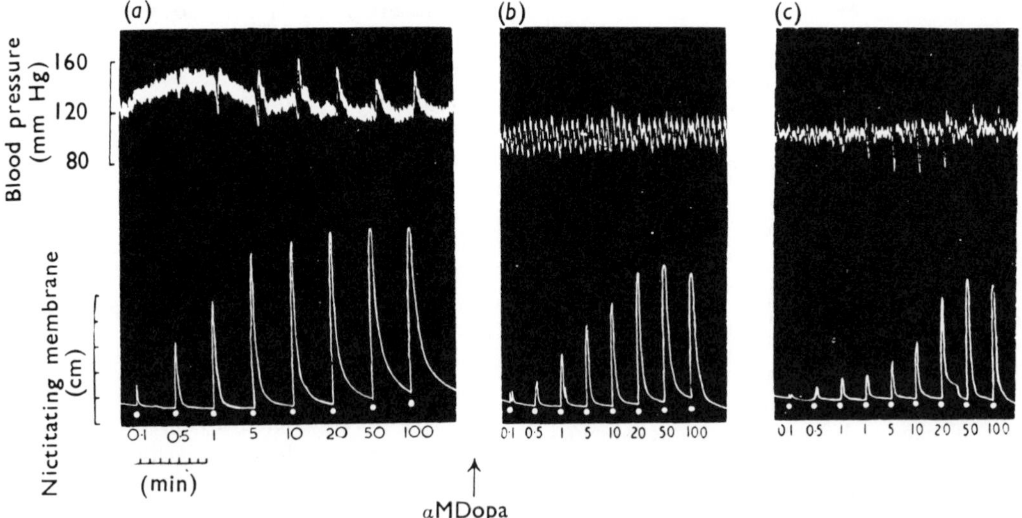

FIG. 2.—Record from an experiment with a cat. Top record: blood pressure; lower record: responses of nictitating membrane to stimulation of postganglionic sympathetic nerves. Methyldopa (200 mg per kilogram) was injected intravenously, between panels (a) and (b). Panel (b) was recorded 2 hours and panel (c) 5 hours after the injection. (From Day and Rand,[3] with permission.)

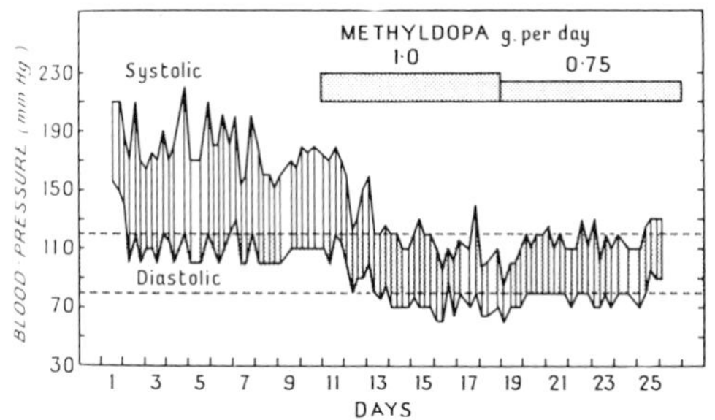

FIG. 4.—Supine blood pressure before and during treatment with methyldopa in one hypertensive patient. (From Bayliss and Harvey-Smith,[20] with permission.)

med et al.[6] have shown that methyldopa decreases vascular resistance in the innervated hindlimb of the dog without producing a measurable impairment of postganglionic sympathetic neuron function (Fig. 5). Reduced sympathetic outflow from the CNS could account for some of these effects of methyldopa.

EFFECTS ON THE CNS

Methyldopa injected into the cerebral circulation of laboratory animals will reduce systemic arterial pressure; the same dose injected

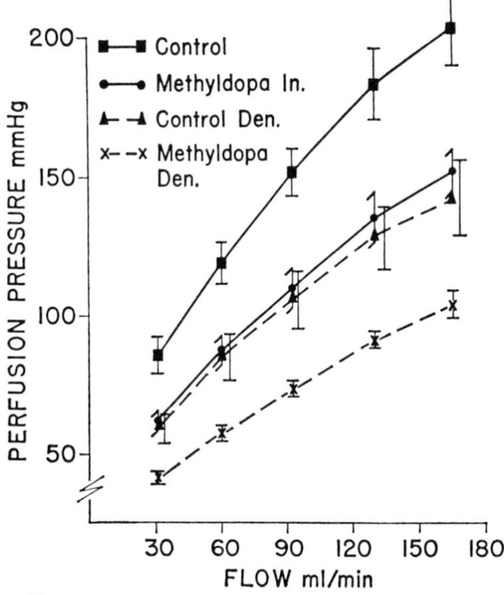

FIG. 5.—Notice the decrease in perfusion pressure in the innervated **(In.)** and denervated **(Den.)** hindlimbs of dogs after chronic treatment with methyldopa. (From Mohammed et al.,[6] with permission.)

intravenously in the systemic circulation does not regularly lower arterial pressure (Fig. 6).[21,22] Henning and Rubenson[23,24] have shown that the hypotensive effect produced by the injection of methyldopa into the vertebral artery can be prevented by prior treatment with a dopa-decarboxylase or beta-hydroxylase inhibitor that enters the brain. In contrast, prior treatment with a dopa-decarboxylase inhibitor that does not enter the brain does not prevent the hypotension. Carlsson and Lindqvist[8] had shown earlier that methyldopa is converted to methylnorepinephrine in the brain. These results[8,21,23,24] have led to the suggestion that the hypotensive effects of methyldopa may partly result from the formation of methylnorepinephrine in the brain with a resultant displacement of the more potent, natural transmitter norepinephrine. Evidence in man pertinent to this hypothesis is the report by Sjoerdsma, Vendsalu, and Engelman,[25] who found that prior treatment with MK485, a dopa-decarboxylase inhibitor which does not enter the brain, failed to prevent the hypotensive effect of orally administered methyldopa in patients with hypertension (Fig. 7). This finding is consistent with a centrally mediated, hypotensive effect of methyldopa in man.

Replacement of norepinephrine by methylnorepinephrine in the brain could result in a lowered outflow of sympathetic activity from the CNS with a resultant decline in peripheral vascular resistance. The possibility that methyldopa decreases arterial pressure by reducing sympathetic outflow from the CNS is an attractive hypothesis to explain some of the varied patterns of hypotension seen during treatment with methyldopa.

THE EFFECT ON RENIN RELEASE

Methyldopa lowers plasma renin activity and it is possible that this effect may contribute to the hypotensive effect of the drug in some patients. In contrast to such antihypertensive drugs as reserpine,[26] hydralazine,[27] nitroprusside,[28] and chlorothiazide,[29] methyldopa has been shown to decrease plasma renin activity in man (Fig. 8).[30] Methyldopa has also been shown to decrease plasma renin activity in a child with Bartter's syndrome (Fig. 9)[31] and in patients with renal failure and uncontrollable hypertension.[32] Methyldopa decreased plasma

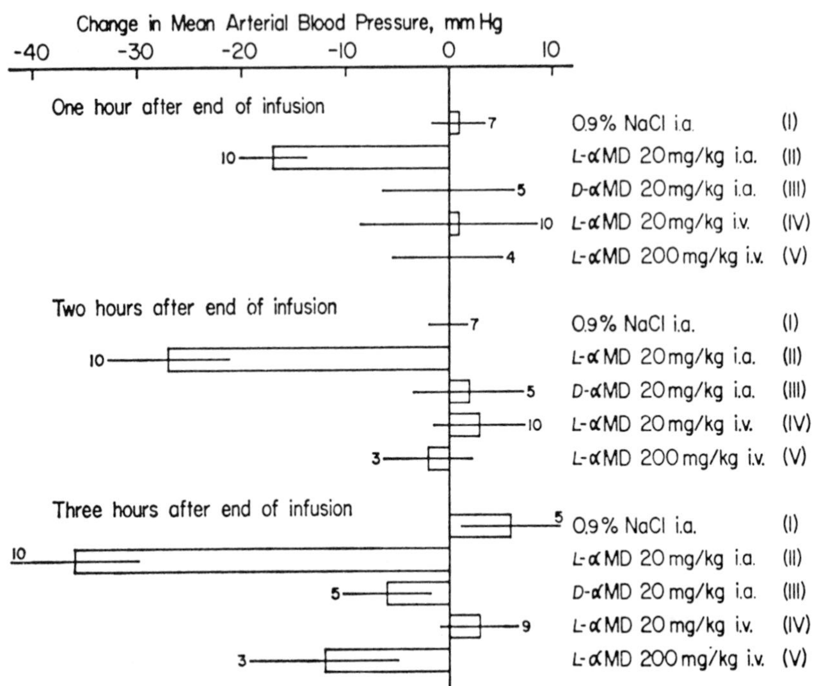

FIG. 6—Changes in mean arterial blood pressure after infusion of saline or methyldopa intra-arterially **(i.a.)** into the left vertebral artery or intravenously **(i.v.)** into the femoral vein of anesthetized cats. The number of experiments is indicated by the arabic numbers. (From Henning and Van Zwieten,[21] with permission.)

renin activity in normotensive subjects and in a child with Bartter's syndrome despite the fact that it decreased arterial pressure, a known stimulus to renin release.

These findings in humans have been corroborated by studies in dogs.[33] Oral treatment with methyldopa for 7 to 10 days decreased plasma renin activity from 13 ± 2 to 7 ± 1 ng per milliliter ($p < .05$) of formed angiotensin II. This decrease in plasma renin activity may explain the development of supersensitivity to injected angiotensin observed by Privitera and Mohammed[34] in dogs chronically treated with methyldopa (Fig. 10). In other experiments with dogs[35] it was observed that methyldopa abolished the release of renin seen in response to renal sympathetic nerve stimulation (Fig. 11) without impairing the renal vasoconstrictor effect of such stimulation. These findings suggest that methyldopa's suppressive effect on plasma renin activity is mediated through an effect of the drug on the postganglionic sympathetic neuron. Privitera and Mohammed[35] have also observed that although infusions of norepinephrine and methylnorepinephrine both increase plasma renin activity, methylnorepinephrine is only one-third as potent as norepinephrine for this effect. These observations suggest that the suppressive effect of methyldopa on plasma renin activity is related to the displacement of norepinephrine in the renal sympathetic nerves by methylnorepinephrine, a less potent false transmitter which is formed from methyldopa. These studies do not eliminate the possibility that methyldopa may also affect plasma renin activity through an effect on the CNS. Although methyldopa appears to have a predictable suppressive effect on plasma renin activity, Cannon et al.[36] have reported that methyldopa does not influence electrolyte balance or aldosterone secretion rate in patients with hypertension.

Since the role of the renin-angiotensin system in the regulation of arterial pressure is unclear in normotensive and most hypertensive patients, the clinical significance of the renin-

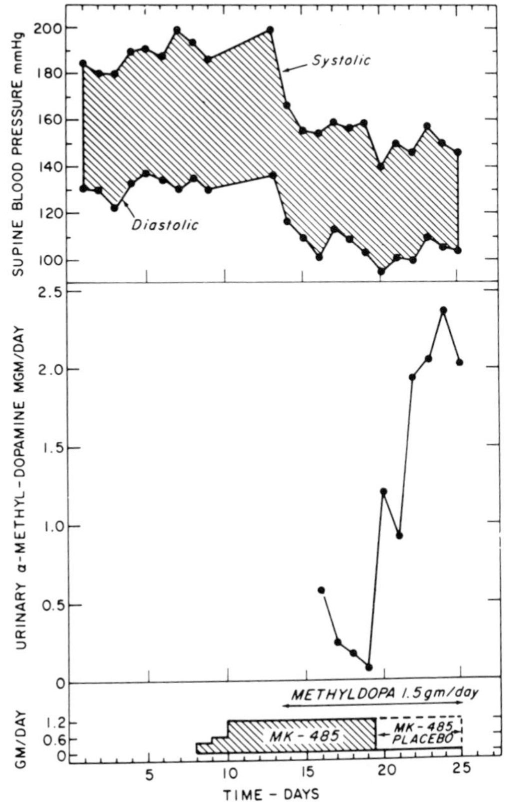

FIG. 7.—Failure of α-methyldopa hydrazine (MK485) to alter the blood pressure response to methyldopa despite apparent inhibition of decarboxylation to urinary α-methyldopamine in a single hypertensive patient. (From Sjoerdsma, Vendsalu, and Engelman,[25] with permission.)

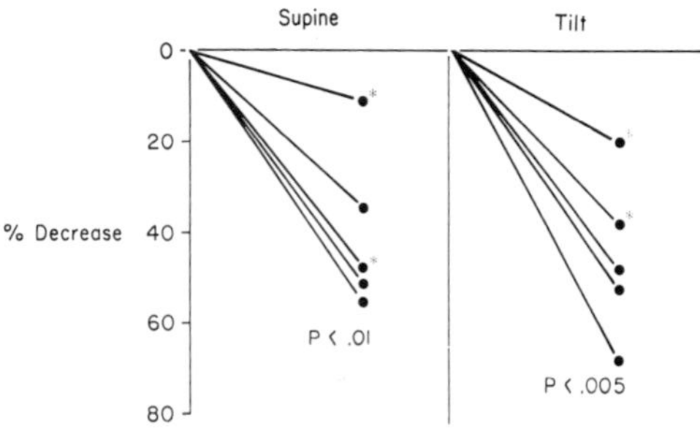

FIG. 8.—The effect of oral methyldopa on plasma renin activity in one hypertensive and four normotensive subjects in supine and tilted positions. (From Mohammed, et al.,[30] with permission.)

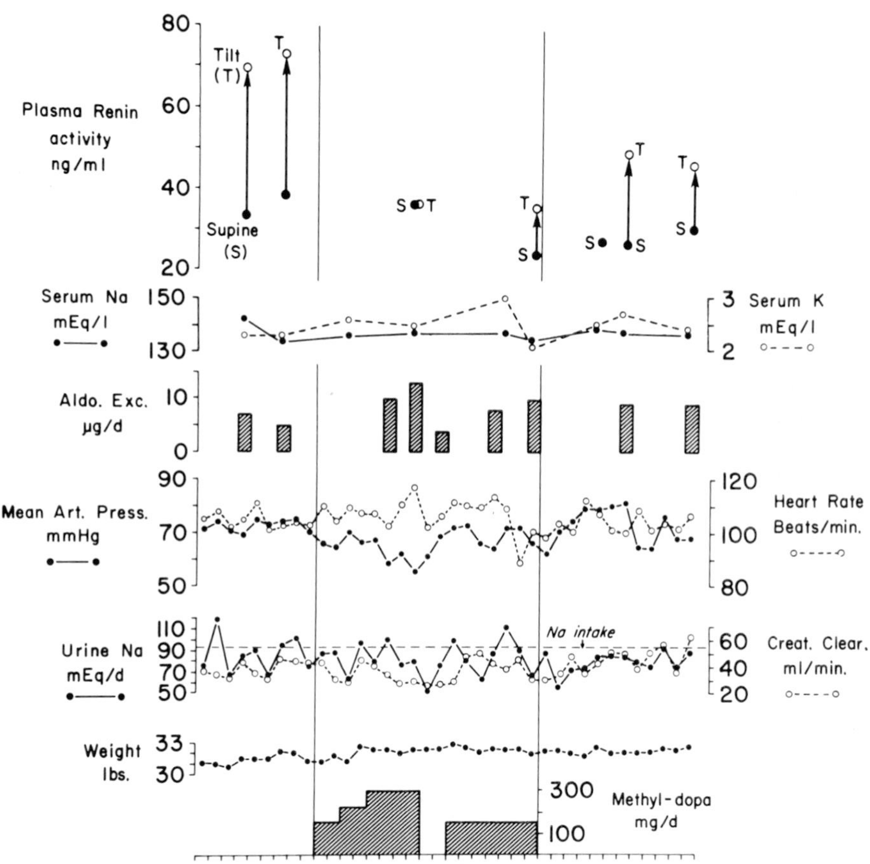

FIG. 9.—The effect of methyldopa on plasma renin activity, serum sodium, potassium, and aldosterone excretion, daily average arterial pressure and heart rate in the standing position, urine sodium excretion, creatinine clearance, and body weight in a child with Bartter's syndrome. (From Strauss et al.,[31] with permission.)

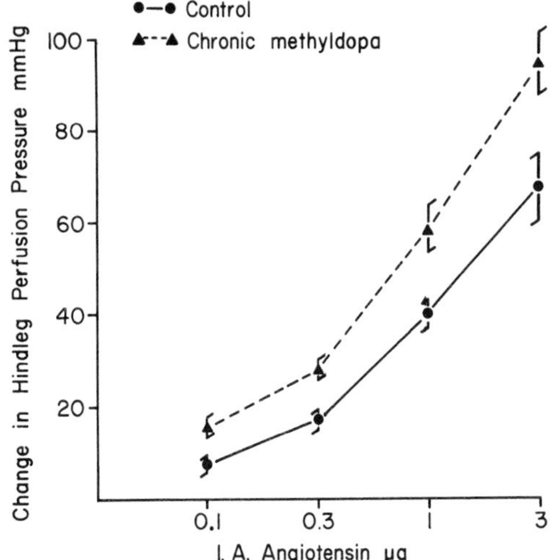

FIG. 10.—Notice the increased pressor responses to intra-arterially (**i.a.**) administered angiotensin in the denervated hindlegs of dogs after chronic treatment with methyldopa (150 mg per kilogram per day, intravenously administered for 4 to 7 days).

suppressive effect of methyldopa remains to be determined.

METABOLISM AND EXCRETION

Methyldopa is distributed to adrenergic neurons throughout the body, where less than 10 percent of the drug undergoes subsequent metabolic conversion to pharmacologically active metabolites. Methyldopa enters the same neuronal metabolic pathways utilized by L-dopa. Methyldopamine is formed by decarboxylation of methyldopa and is then converted to methylnorepinephrine by beta-hydroxylase in the amine storage granules of the sympathetic neurons. The newly formed methylnorepinephrine is stored in these granules until it is released into the synaptic cleft by a postganglionic action potential.[9]

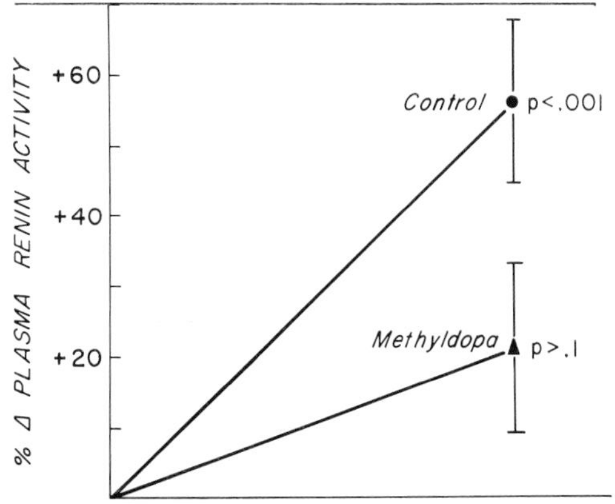

FIG. 11.—Effect of renal nerve stimulation on plasma renin activity in control and methyldopa-treated dogs.

Less than 10 percent of a single oral dose of methyldopa is converted to methyldopamine and methylnorepinephrine. Ninety percent of the administered dose is excreted in the urine as either free methyldopa or its ether sulfate conjugate.[37,38] Since methylnorepinephrine is not a substrate for monoamine oxidase (MAO) it is excreted as methylnorepinephrine and its inactive 3-methoxy-methylnorepinephrine metabolite.[39] Treatment with methyldopa is therefore associated with the appearance of methylnorepinephrine in the urine in microgram amounts with a reciprocal and nearly equal decrease in the excretion of norepinephrine.[40] Exercise in normal adult volunteers and in one patient with hypertension under treatment with methyldopa augmented the urinary excretion of norepinephrine and methylnorepinephrine about equally, suggesting that these two amines are released from sympathetic neurons in roughly equivalent amounts during treatment with methyldopa.

The urinary excretion of total metanephrines is almost double during treatment with methyldopa.[40] This is probably accounted for by the conversion of methylnorepinephrine to 3-methoxy-methylnorepinephrine by catechol-o-methyl transferase. Vanillylmandelic acid excretion is not affected by treatment with methyldopa.[36]

The observation that less than 10 percent of methyldopa is converted to metabolites which are responsible for the hypotensive effects of the drug emphasizes the need to be alert to the significance of small metabolic pathways of drugs. The pharmacologic significance of a metabolite is determined primarily by its potency, anatomic site(s) of formation, and tissue distribution.

SUMMARY

Methyldopa appears to affect the peripheral adrenergic neuron, the CNS, and, under certain circumstances, the release of renin from the kidney. The extent to which each of these effects occurs in a given patient may help explain the patterns of the hypotensive response observed.

References

1. Gaffney, T. E., Sigell, L. T., Mohammed, S., and Atkinson, A. J.: The clinical pharmacology of antihypertensive drugs. Progr. Cardiovasc. Dis. 12:52, 1969.
2. Maxwell, R. A., Plummer, A. J., Schneider, F., Povalski, H., and Daniel, A. I.: Pharmacology of [2-(octahydro-1-azocinyl)-ethyl]-guanidine sulfate (SU-5864). J. Pharmacol. Exp. Ther. 128:22, 1960.
3. Day, M. D., and Rand, M. I.: Some observations on the pharmacology of α-methyldopa. Br. J. Pharmacol. 22:72, 1964.
4. Sugarman, S. R., Margolius, H. S., Gaffney, T. E., and Mohammed, S.: Effect of methyldopa on chronotropic responses to cardioaccelerator nerve stimulation in dogs. J. Pharmacol. Exp. Ther. 162:115, 1968.
5. Varma, D. R., and Benfey, B. G.: Antagonism of reserpine-induced subsensitivity to tyramine by methyldopa. J. Pharmacol. Exp. Ther. 141:310, 1963.
6. Mohammed, S., Gaffney, T. E., Yard, A. C., and Gomez, H.: Effect of methyldopa, reserpine and guanethidine on hindleg vascular resistance. J. Pharmacol. Exp. Ther. 160:300, 1968.
7. Haefely, W., Hurlimann, A., and Thoenen, H.: The effect of stimulation of sympathetic nerves in the cat treated with reserpine, α-methyldopa and α-methylmetatyrosine. Br. J. Pharmacol. 26:172, 1966.
8. Carlsson, A., and Lindqvist, M.: In-vivo decarboxylation of α-methyldopa and α-methyl metatyrosine. Acta Physiol. Scand. 54:87, 1962.
9. Muscholl, E., and Maitre, L.: Release by sympathetic stimulation of α-methylnoradrenaline stored in the heart after administration of α-methyldopa. Experientia 19:658, 1963.
10. Day, M. D., and Rand, M. J.: A hypothesis for the mode of action of α-methyldopa in relieving hypertension. J. Pharm. Pharmacol. 15:221, 1963.
11. Conradi, E. C., Gaffney, T. E., Fink, D. A., and Vangrow, J. S.: Reversal of sympathetic nerve blockade: A comparison of dopa, dopamine, and norepinephrine with their α-methylated analogues. J. Pharmacol. Exp. Ther. 150:26, 1965.
12. Mueller, P. S., and Horwitz, D.: Plasma free fatty acid and blood glucose responses to analogues of norepinephrine in man. J. Lipid Res. 3:251, 1962.
13. Dollery, C. T., Harington, M., and Hodge, J. V.: Haemodynamic studies with methyldopa. Effect on cardiac output and response to pressor amines. Br. Heart J. 25:670, 1963.
14. Dollery, C. T., and Harington, M.: Methyldopa in hypertension: Clinical and pharmacological studies. Lancet 1:759, 1962.
15. Brunner, H., Hedwall, P. R., Maitre, L., and Meier, M.: Antihypertensive effects of alpha-methylated catecholamine analogues in the rat. Br. J. Pharmacol. 30:108, 1967.
16. Okun, R., Roth, S. E., Gordon, A., and Maxwell, M. H.: The long-term effectiveness of methyldopa in hypertension. Calif. Med. 104:46, 1966.
17. Oates, J. A., Gillespie, L., Udenfriend, S., and Sjoerdsma, A.: Decarboxylase inhibition and blood pressure reduction by α-methyl-3,4-dihydroxy-DL-phenylalanine. Science 131:1890, 1960.
18. Sannerstedt, R., Varnauskas, E., and Werkö, L.: Hemodynamic effects of methyldopa (Aldomet) at rest and during exercise in patients with arterial hypertension. Acta Med. Scand. 171:75, 1962.
19. Mohammed, S., Hanenson, I. B., Magenheim, H. G., and Gaffney, T. E.: The effects of alpha-methyldopa on renal function in hypertensive patients. Am. Heart J. 76:21, 1968.
20. Bayliss, R. I. S., and Harvey-Smith, E. A.: Methyldopa in the treatment of hypertension. Lancet 1:763, 1962.
21. Henning, M., and Van Zwieten, P. A.: Central hypotensive effect of α-methyldopa. J. Pharm. Pharmacol. 20:409, 1968.
22. Ingenito, A. J., Barrett, J. P., and Procita, L.: A centrally mediated peripheral hypotensive effect of α-methyldopa. J. Pharmacol. Exp. Ther. 175:593, 1970.
23. Henning, M.: Studies on the mode of action of α-methyldopa. Acta Physiol. Scand. Suppl. 322:1, 1969.
24. Henning, M., and Rubenson, A.: Evidence that the hypotensive action of methyldopa is mediated by central actions of methylnoradrenaline. J. Pharm. Pharmacol. 23:407, 1971.
25. Sjoerdsma, A., Vendsalu, A., and Engelman, K.: Studies on the metabolism and mechanism of action of methyldopa. Circulation 28:492, 1963.
26. Ayers, C. R., Harris, R. H., and Lefer, L. G.: Control of renin release in experimental hypertension. Circ. Res. 24(Suppl. I):103, 1969.

27. Ueda, H., Yagi, S., and Kaneko, Y.: Hydralazine and plasma renin activity. Arch. Intern. Med. 122:387, 1968.
28. Kaneko, Y., Ikeda, T., Takeda, T., and Ueda, H.: Renin release during acute reduction of arterial pressure in normotensive subjects and patients with renovascular hypertension. J. Clin. Invest. 46:705, 1967.
29. Catt, K. J., Cain, M. D., Coghlan, J. P., Zimmet, P. Z., Cran, E., and Best, J. B.: Metabolism and blood levels of angiotensin II in normal subjects, renal disease, and essential hypertension. Circ. Res. 27(Suppl. II): 177, 1970.
30. Mohammed, S., Fasola, A. F., Privitera, P. J., Lipicky, R., Martz, B. L., and Gaffney, T. E.: Effect of methyldopa on plasma renin activity in man. Circ. Res. 25:543, 1969.
31. Strauss, R. G., Mohammed, S., Loggie, J. M. H., Schubert, W. K., Fasola, A. F., and Gaffney, T. E.: The effect of methyldopa on plasma renin activity in a child with Bartter's syndrome. J. Pediat. 77:1071, 1970.
32. Weidmann, P., Maxwell, M. H., Lupu, A. N., Lewin, A. J., and Massry, S. G.: Plasma renin activity and blood pressure in terminal renal failure. N. Engl. J. Med. 285:757, 1971.
33. Mohammed, S., and Privitera, P. J.: Effect of methyldopa on plasma renin activity in dogs. Clin. Res. 19:329, 1971. (Abstract)
34. Privitera, P. J., and Mohammed, S.: Potentiation by alpha-methyldopa of pressor responses to angiotensin. Proc. Soc. Exp. Biol. Med. 133:1358, 1970.
35. Privitera, P. J., and Mohammed, S.: Studies on the mechanism of renin suppression by alpha-methyldopa. *In* Assaykeen, T. A. (Ed.): Advances in Experimental Medicine and Biology: Control of Renin Secretion. New York: Plenum Press, 1972, pp. 93–101.
36. Cannon, P. J., Whitlock, R. T., Morris, R. C., Angers, M., and Laragh, J. H.: Effect of alpha-methyl dopa in severe and malignant hypertension. JAMA 179:673, 1962.
37. Buhs, R. P., Beck, J. L., Speth, O. C., Smith, J. L., Trenner, N. R., Cannon, P. J., and Laragh, J. H.: The metabolism of methyldopa in hypertensive human subjects. J. Pharmacol. Exp. Ther. 143:205, 1964.
38. Prescott, L. R., Buhs, R. P., Beattie, J. O., Speth, O. C., Trenner, N. R., and Lasagna, L.: Combined clinical and metabolic study of the effects of alpha-methyldopa on hypertensive patients. Circulation 34:308, 1966.
39. Stott, A. W., Robinson, R., and Smith, P.: Total metadrenaline excretion in patients treated with α-methyldopa. Lancet 1:266, 1963.
40. Lindmar, R., Muscholl, E., and Rahn, K. H.: Effects of rest and physical activity on the urinary excretion of noradrenaline and α-methylnoradrenaline in human subjects treated with α-methyldopa. Eur. J. Pharmacol. 2:317, 1968.

Alpha-Methyldopa in the Treatment of Hypertension: Long-term Experience

By Colin T. Dollery, M.B., and C. J. Bulpitt, M.B.

Treatment with antihypertensive drugs has to be continued indefinitely in most patients. Hopes that it might prove possible to discontinue treatment without a rise in pressure, after several years of good pressure control, have not been sustained.[1,2]

The long-term efficacy and safety of drugs used to treat hypertension have, therefore, become of prime importance. Published clinical trials rarely extend for more than 2 years and often most of the patients have been treated for only a few weeks or months. Very little information has been published concerning long-term use of individual antihypertensive drugs.

Epidemiologic surveys of untreated hypertension show that pressure levels rise with age and that the rate of rise in pressure is highest in those individuals in whom pressure is already elevated.[3]

Thus, even if the efficacy of the drugs used remains constant throughout a period of time, it is conceivable that the pressure control would become progressively worse because the underlying disease had changed. On the other hand, resetting of the baroreceptors and possibly other pressure-control mechanisms may tend to make long-term control easier.

As there is so little information on these points, we have carried out a study of a random sample of patients from the Hammersmith Hospital Hypertension Clinic who have been treated with methyldopa over a period of 5 to 11 years. We have also included data on the side effects and toxicity of methyldopa gathered from a survey at the same clinic.

The Blood Pressure Survey

All patients registered at Hammersmith Hospital are given a serial number in order of accession. Three digits between 0 and 9 were selected from a table of random numbers and the records of all clinic patients whose number ended in these digits were included in the survey. The criteria for selection were: (1) that the patient had been on methyldopa therapy for more than 5 years of continuous treatment; and (2) that he was on no other antihypertensive drugs save a diuretic.

As a result of this procedure 31 sets of case papers were available for analysis. All blood pressure readings with the dates they were recorded were abstracted and a note was also made of the dose changes with their dates, and if a diuretic was added.

The average dose of methyldopa immediately following the initial stabilization was 1,090 mg per day and at that time 13 patients were taking a diuretic. The average final dose was 1,470 mg per day and 23 patients were taking a diuretic.

The method of study adopted will tend to bias the results in favor of the drug because patients who could not tolerate it or be controlled by it would have been switched to an alternative regimen before 5 years were up. Most such alterations take place early in the course of treatment and the present data do provide useful evidence about the long-term efficacy of methyldopa.

Analysis of Blood Pressure Readings

All of the patients studied have attended the same hypertension clinic at regular intervals throughout their treatment. Blood pressures are recorded in the clinic with standard sphygmomanometers using phase 4 as the diastolic pressure. Throughout the period of study, standing pressures have been measured after the patient has been upright for 10 to 30 seconds. In the period 1966–1971 pressures have also been recorded with the patient lying flat but prior to this date the pressure in the sitting position was used instead. Thus the number of readings in recumbency is fewer in the earlier years of treatment.

From the Department of Clinical Pharmacology, Royal Postgraduate Medical School, University of London, London, England.

Once patients have been stabilized on antihypertensive drugs, which is usually carried out in hospital, they are seen at approximately 3-month intervals. Data tapes were punched containing all the readings from the case notes with their dates. Thus, in a patient followed for 11 years, there were 50 sets of dated readings. In all there were 971 sets of readings available, covering 231 patient years. These values were averaged year by year by a computer to give the systolic and diastolic pressure standing and lying for each year of follow-up for that patient. The computer then averaged the readings for each patient for each year of follow-up. Thus the years averaged are not the same in each patient. Year 1 in one patient might be 1961, while in another it might be 1965.

Because of the criteria of selection, the number of patients in the first 5 years of analysis was always the same for the standing readings (the whole group of 31) but by the tenth and eleventh years the numbers were small, six and three patients respectively (Table 1). The most striking feature of the data is that relatively good pressure control was achieved throughout the period of follow-up. The pressure control in years 6 to 9 inclusive was on average slightly better than in the first 5 years of treatment although these patients had on the average higher blood pressures before treatment was begun than those followed for shorter periods. The average blood pressures were higher again in years 10 and 11 but the number of patients included was small and the significance of this finding will have to be reassessed when there are more data available. It is also noteworthy that the difference between lying and standing pressures was relatively small. In years 6 to 9 this difference averaged only 11.9/418 mm Hg although in the same period the average reduction in recumbent pressure from the pretreatment value was 73.5/38.2 mm Hg. This shows the relatively small postural effect of methyldopa. Prichard et al.[4] in a crossover study comparing different antihypertensive drugs found an average difference between lying and standing pressures of 30/11 with methyldopa, 47/21 with bethanidine, and 40/15 mm Hg with guanethidine. It is of interest that the change in pressure with posture was less in this long-term study than was observed by Prichard et al. in a 3-month period of treatment. It raises the possibility that long-continued treatment allows some resetting of pressure-control mechanism.[1]

The Symptom Survey

Patients attending the clinic over a 3-month period were sent a postal questionnaire the week before their next visit was due. There were 24 questions in the basic questionnaire and three additional ones for male patients alone. The response was good as 477 forms were completed out of 572 dispatched. Of

Table 1.—*Average Blood Pressures on Treatment and Before Treatment for Patients Tested with Methyldopa for 1 to 11 Years*

	Lying Blood Pressure			*Standing Blood Pressure*			*Pretreatment*	
Year	*Systolic*	*Diastolic*	*N*	*Systolic*	*Diastolic*	*N*	*Systolic*	*Diastolic*
1	170.5	102.7	11	150.6	95.9	31	201.4	122.3
2	169.4	101.7	18	152.6	96.4	31	212.5	123.9
3	158.8	97.0	20	149.1	93.0	31	210.2	124.7
4	160.6	96.4	25	149.4	91.1	31	214.2	125.8
5	159.5	94.9	28	145.6	90.2	31	219.8	149.2
6	157.1	99.2	31	142.5	88.7	31	221.1	127.3
7	152.9	89.9	24	142.7	87.3	24	228.7	129.2
8	153.9	89.9	18	143.3	86.2	18	230.6	130.3
9	160.3	89.6	12	148.0	87.1	12	237.5	135.0
10	168.4	95.1	6	158.3	89.1	6	244.2	130.8
11	180.0	92.2	3	158.3	87.8	3	260.0	131.7

Abbreviation: N, the number of patients averaged for each set of blood pressure readings.

these 288 patients were taking methyldopa either alone or in combination with other drugs. Of the remainder there were 188 not taking methyldopa and two in whom there was doubt about the precise therapeutic regimen being followed. Patients were asked to give details of symptoms they had suffered since their last visit to the clinic because of doubts about the accuracy of recall for longer periods. The results of this survey will be reported in more detail elsewhere but some of the more important results concerned with methyldopa are included here with data about patients taking diuretics alone, for comparison.

The questionnaire covered symptoms attributed to various antihypertensive drugs such as postural hypotension, sedation, fatigue, exertional dyspnea, headaches, blurred vision, depression, loose stools, nocturia, dry mouth, and sexual problems in men. It would have been of interest to ask for much more detailed information upon many points but the questionnaire was already long enough to daunt some of our patients.

Dry Mouth

Patients were asked the following questions:

21. Do you suffer from a dry mouth?

If YES,

22. Does the dry mouth interfere with talking or eating?

The results were scored as follows:

If the answer to Q.21 was NO, score 0.
If the answer to Q.21 was YES, but to Q.22 was NO, score 1.
If the answer to both Q.21 and 22 was YES, score 2.

The average score of 42 patients on diuretic alone was 43; that of 34 patients on methyldopa alone was 35, and of 123 on methyldopa plus a diuretic it was 53. The relatively high incidence of dry mouth in patients taking diuretics and the lower value in patients taking methyldopa alone was unexpected although the dose of methyldopa used in the patients who were also using diuretics was higher than in those using methyldopa alone.

Sedation and Depression

The patients were asked the following questions:

8. Since your last visit have you felt sleepy during the day?

16. Have you, since your last visit, been depressed?

If YES to Q.16

17. Did you consult a doctor about your depression?

The patients taking methyldopa complained of sleepiness significantly more often ($p = 0.02$) than those using a diuretic alone, and they slept longer (Table 2) although this difference was not significant.

The depression results were scored as follows:

If the answer to Q.16 was NO, score 0.
If the answer to Q.16 was YES, but to Q.17 it was NO, score 1.
If the answer to both Q.16 and 17 was YES, score 2.

The average score of each drug-treated group is referred to as a "depression index" in Table 2 purely to facilitate comparisons.

Patients taking methyldopa complained of depression less often than those using a diuretic alone, although this difference was not significant. It has been suggested that methyldopa

TABLE 2.—*Symptoms of Patients on Long-Term Antihypertensive Therapy*

	Diuretic Alone	*Methyldopa Alone*	*Methyldopa and Diuretic*
Number of patients	49	50	160
Sleepy during the day	39%	51%	59%
Hours of sleep	7.2	7.6	7.5
Depression index	0.52	0.32	0.36
Loose or liquid stools	37%	31%	26%
Bowel actions per day	1.2	1.4	1.2

may cause depression, but these data do not provide much support for this view. It is also noteworthy that there was no difference in the methyldopa dosages of those who were not depressed (1,329 mg per day) compared with those who were sufficiently depressed to consult a doctor (1,350 mg per day).

Bowel Habit

The number of patients complaining of occasional loose or liquid stools was much the same irrespective of the drug regimen (Table 2). The average daily frequency of bowel actions was just over one on each regimen.

Effect upon Male Sexual Function

Failure of ejaculation is a common complaint among young men treated with adrenergic neuronal-blocking drugs and they may refuse to continue treatment for this reason. Methyldopa appears to be less troublesome in this respect and this result is borne out by the survey.

Male patients were asked the following questions:

During sexual intercourse are you:

25. Troubled by failure to maintain an erection?
26. Troubled by failure to pass semen?
27. How often do you have sexual intercourse?

Times per week
Times per month
Times per year

Patients who found these questions difficult to answer were given further explanations when they attended the clinic.

Difficulty with ejaculation was uncommon in patients taking methyldopa alone (5%), more common in those taking diuretics alone (14%), and in those using both drugs (24%). A low incidence of failure of ejaculation with methyldopa was reported by Prichard et al.[4] (14%) and a much higher figure for guanethidine (79%) and bethanidine (70%).

An interesting and unexpected finding was the substantial proportion of patients reporting difficulty in maintaining an erection. About one-third of patients taking a diuretic alone, a diuretic plus methyldopa, and methyldopa alone, complained of this problem (Table 3). The frequency of sexual intercourse was low and this appeared to be strongly correlated with the patient's age. Patients taking methyldopa had sexual intercourse slightly less often than those taking a diuretic alone.

Toxicity

The two main toxic effects of methyldopa are fever and a positive direct antiglobulin test.

Fever

The incidence of a drug-induced fever with methyldopa appears to be about 1 percent of all patients treated with the drug. The fever may be high, with values of up to 104°F having been reported.[5] Fever usually appears 10 to 20 days after initiating treatment. The patient has an illness resembling influenza with malaise and fever. These symptoms usually persist if the drug is continued and return if the patient is rechallenged with the drug[6] after stopping it. Once it has been established that the drug is responsible, it is probably best not to treat the patient with methyldopa again.

Positive Direct Antiglobulin (Coombs') Test

Up to 20 percent of patients treated with methyldopa develop a positive direct anti-

TABLE 3.—*Sexual Patterns in Men on Long-Term Antihypertensive Therapy*

Complaint	*Diuretic Alone*		*Methyldopa Alone*		*Methyldopa and Diuretic*	
Difficulty with erection	32%	(22)	32%	(22)	37%	(59)
Difficulty with ejaculation	14%	(22)	5%	(22)	24%	(59)
Frequency of sexual intercourse (times per year)	42	(20)	26	(26)	27	(65)

The figures in brackets represent the number of individuals affected in each group.

globulin test upon their red cells.[7] The proportion who do so is related to the dose, rising from 11 percent on 1 gm or less a day to 36 percent on more than 2 gm daily. The test does not become positive until the patient has been treated for a minimum of 4 months. Some patients with mildly positive tests may fluctuate between a positive and negative test but in the great majority it remains positive so long as the drug is continued. If the drug is stopped the test slowly becomes negative, but it may take many months to do so.[8] About 15 percent of patients treated with methyldopa also develop a positive antinuclear factor but there is no correlation between this and the positive direct antiglobulin tests.

By itself, a positive direct antiglobulin test is not a hazard, except if rapid crossmatching of blood for transfusion is necessary. However, some patients with a positive antiglobulin test develop an autoimmune hemolytic anemia, and a few deaths have been reported as a complication of the hemolytic anemia. The anemia responds rapidly to withdrawal of the drug and treatment with corticosteroids.[9] A number of patients followed for 5 to 11 years have a positive antiglobulin test and there is little doubt that it has been positive throughout this period. They do not appear to have come to any harm and we do not consider a positive test requires a change in treatment unless a hemolytic anemia develops.

It has been suggested that there is a correlation between development of a positive direct antiglobulin test to methyldopa and the lupus erythematosus-like syndrome in patients treated with hydralazine. Patients who develop hydralazine toxicity are almost always slow acetylators and so have a higher plasma concentration of the drug. Methyldopa is not acetylated and in a small sample of patients with a positive antiglobulin test there were both slow and fast acetylators (Ellard, personal communication).

Discussion

More than 10 years' experience with methyldopa has not greatly altered the conclusions drawn from its use for much shorter periods.[10–13] It is an effective drug that lowers the blood pressure in both the recumbent and upright positions. The effect is maintained over periods of 10 years or more with only a moderate increase in the average dose needed. If anything, blood pressure control is better in the second 5-year period on the drug than it is in the first, although self-selection of good responders may influence this result.

Many patients on the drug complained of symptoms but as the incidence of most of them is the same or greater in patients treated with diuretics alone, they are probably not related to any particular therapeutic regimen. Use of a questionnaire to elicit symptoms invites a high proportion of positive responses. The only symptom that stands out to a significant extent is sedation. In patients who have to do brain work, this can be a problem, although most find it no more than an inconvenience. Methyldopa causes a much smaller incidence of failure of ejaculation in men than do bethanidine and guanethidine, but they cause less sedation.

The main toxic effects are fever and a positive direct antiglobulin test upon red cells which, rarely, leads to a hemolytic anemia. Fever and hemolytic anemia are indications to stop treatment with the drug, but a positive antiglobulin test is not.

Methyldopa is undoubtedly one of the most useful antihypertensive agents available, and experience over more than a decade confirms its value.

References

1. Page, I. H., and Dustan, H. P.: Persistence of normal blood pressure after discontinuing treatment in hypertensive patients. Circulation 25:443, 1962.
2. Pickering, G. W.: High Blood Pressure. London: Churchill, 1968.
3. Miall, W. E., and Lovell, H. G.: Relation between change of blood pressure and age. Br. Med. J. 2:660, 1967.
4. Prichard, B. N. C., Johnston, A. W., Hill, I. D., and Rosenheim, M. L.: Bethanidine, guanethidine, and methyldopa in treatment of hypertension: A within-patient comparison. Br. Med. J. 1:135, 1968.
5. Tallgren, L. G., and Servo, C.: Hypertension in association with administration of L-alpha-methyldopa. Acta Med. Scand. 186:213, 1969.

6. Dollery, C. T.: Alpha-methyldopa in the treatment of hypertension. Med. Clin. North Am. 48:335, 1964.
7. Carstairs, K. C., Breckenridge, A., Dollery, C. T., and Worledge, S. M.: Incidence of a positive direct Coombs test in patients on L-methyldopa. Lancet 2:133, 1966.
8. Breckenridge, A., Dollery, C. T., Worledge, S. M., Holborow, E. J., and Johnson, G. D.: Positive direct Coombs' tests and antinuclear factor in patients treated with methyldopa. Lancet 2:1265, 1967.
9. Worledge, S. M.: Autoimmune haemolytic anaemia associated with L-methyldopa therapy. Lancet 2:135, 1966.
10. Oateis, J. A., Gillespie, L., Udenfriend, S., and Sjoerdsma, A.: Decarboxylase inhibition and blood pressure reduction by α-methyl-3,4-dihydroxy-DL-phenylalanine. Science 131: 1890, 1960.
11. Gillespie, L., Oates, J. A., Crout, J. R., and Sjoerdsma, A.: Clinical and chemical studies with alpha-methyldopa in patients with hypertension. Circulation 25:281, 1962.
12. Dollery, C. T., and Harington, M.: Methyldopa in hypertension. Clinical and pharmacological studies. Lancet 1:759, 1962.
13. Dollery, C. T.: Methyldopa in the treatment of hypertension. Progr. Cardiovasc. Dis. 8: 278, 1965.

Reserpine and Guanethidine in the Treatment of Hypertension

By Ray W. Gifford, Jr., M.D.

While reserpine and guanethidine selectively inhibit the sympathetic nervous system and both have a long duration of action, their roles in the clinical management of hypertension are dissimilar.

Guanethidine is one of the most potent antihypertensive agents presently available, while reserpine, the most active purified alkaloid derived from *Rauwolfia serpentina,* is one of the least potent. Both reserpine and guanethidine promote fluid and sodium retention which blunt their antihypertensive effect and may lead to apparent drug resistance. Consequently an oral diuretic should nearly always be incorporated in the regimen with either of these drugs in order to augment the hypotensive response, thereby permitting control of hypertension with lesser dosages.

The popularity of reserpine is waning since the advent of methyldopa which is at least equally potent and produces fewer annoying untoward effects. Guanethidine remains the mainstay of therapy for severe hypertension.

Dosage and Method of Administration

Reserpine (Eskaserp, Reserpoid, Sandril, Serpasil). The usual oral dose of reserpine is 0.25 mg daily (Table 1). As little as 0.1 mg daily is sometimes effective and some clinicians use as much as 1.0 mg daily, although untoward effects seem to be dose-related and are more frequent and annoying with larger doses. Because of its long duration of action, reserpine should be given once daily for convenience. Some clinicians advocate starting therapy with a priming dose of 1.0 mg daily for a week, following which a maintenance dose of 0.1 or 0.25 mg daily is prescribed. I have seen no particular virtue in this regimen. Parenteral administration will be discussed in the chapter on "Treatment of Hypertensive Emergencies."

From the Department of Hypertension and Nephrology, The Cleveland Clinic Foundation, Cleveland. Ohio.

Guanethidine (Ismelin). Oral therapy with guanethidine must be started with a low dose to prevent severe orthostatic hypotension and the dosage should not be increased more often than once every 4 or 5 days to prevent cumulative effect, unless the patient is under observation in the hospital. The average initial dose is 10 mg, given once daily, preferably at the same time each day (Table 1). For patients with coronary or cerebrovascular disease in which orthostatic hypotension might be particularly hazardous, as little as 5 mg daily should be given initially, and increments should be made at intervals of no less than once a week. For patients with hypertension severe enough to imminently threaten the integrity of the cardiovascular system (e.g., diastolic blood pressure > 120 mm Hg or malignant hypertension) the initial daily dose may be 25 mg or even 50 mg and the frequency of increments may be increased to every 3 days provided the patient is under surveillance in the hospital. There is no maximal dose of guanethidine, the dosage being increased in stepwise fashion until the desired hypotensive effect is obtained or until untoward effects preclude further increments in dosage. In particularly resistant cases it may be necessary to use as much as 150 mg or more of guanethidine daily. Few patients can tolerate doses of this magnitude, however.

Indications for Use

Reserpine. This drug should be used for mild or moderate hypertension when an oral diuretic alone has failed to control the blood pressure adequately (Table 1). Reserpine should be added to the diuretic, not substituted for it. In my opinion, methyldopa is now the drug of choice in this role because it produces fewer unpleasant side effects than reserpine and is probably a more potent agent when administered with an oral diuretic. The comparative disadvantages of methyldopa are its shorter duration of action necessitating 2 to 4 doses daily and its higher cost.

TABLE 1.—*Reserpine and Guanethidine: Their Dosage, Methods of Administration, and Indications and Contraindications*

	Reserpine	*Guanethidine*
Tablet size	0.1, 0.25, and 1.0 mg	10 and 25 mg
Dosage and method of administration	Oral: 0.1–1.0 mg daily, in single dose I.M.: 0.5–5.0 mg	Oral: 10–150+ mg daily, in single dose
Indications	Oral: Mild or moderate hypertension. usually in conjunction with an oral diuretic; may also be used in same regimen with hydralazine I.M.: Certain hypertensive emergencies *	Oral: Severe or resistant hypertension, usually in conjunction with an oral diuretic; may also be used in same regimen with methyldopa and hydralazine
Contraindications	Depression, active peptic ulcer, parkinsonian states, drug sensitivity (rare)	Drug sensitivity (rare), pheochromocytoma; do not use in conjunction with a monoamine oxidase inhibitor. *Warning:* Concomitant use of a tricyclic antidepressant or amphetamines will block antihypertensive effect of guanethidine.

Abbreviation used: I.M., intramuscularly.
* See chapter entitled "Treatment of Hypertensive Emergencies."

Because of its bradycrotic effect, reserpine is particularly indicated for the mildly hypertensive patient who has tachycardia and palpitations ("hyperdynamic circulation"). It is also useful to prevent the reflex tachycardia and palpitations induced by therapy with hydralazine. To accomplish this, it is usually desirable to delay the start of hydralazine therapy until the patient has received reserpine for at least a week. Even its role as a bradycrotic agent is being usurped by propranolol, which seems to be better tolerated and is a more effective antihypertensive agent than reserpine in patients with hyperdynamic circulation or in conjunction with hydralazine. In my experience the combination of an oral diuretic, propranolol, and hydralazine is comparable in its hypotensive effect to that of an oral diuretic and guanethidine.

When the combination of an oral diuretic and reserpine fails to control hypertension adequately, hydralazine should be added to the regimen, or methyldopa should be substituted for the reserpine.

Reserpine administered orally has no place in the management of severe hypertension.

Guanethidine. The principal indication for guanethidine is in the management of severe hypertension (Table 1). When diastolic blood pressure is greater than 120 mm Hg, or when complications are present or impending, or when Group III or IV changes are present in the retina, it is imperative to reduce blood pressure promptly and oral therapy should be started with a diuretic and guanethidine simultaneously. The dosage and frequency of increments should be determined by the severity of hypertension and the presence or absence of complications (see previous section). Guanethidine has a slow onset of action (48 to 72 hours) and consequently it may require several days of dosage adjustments before the hypertension can be adequately controlled on the oral regimen. During this interval it is sometimes prudent to reduce blood pressure promptly by using parenteral agents until the oral regimen becomes effective.

The addition of methlydopa to a regimen consisting of an oral diuretic and guanethidine will often permit better control of severe hypertension with a lesser dose of guanethidine, thereby minimizing untoward effects.[1] Frequently it is advantageous to initiate therapy with all three drugs simultaneously for patients with severe hypertension.

Occasionally guanethidine is indicated for

patients with mild or moderate hypertension that is resistant to combinations of less potent drugs, or for patients who for any reason cannot tolerate effective doses of less potent agents. Under these circumstances the dose of guanethidine is usually less than prescribed for severe hypertension and consequently untoward effects are less likely to be troublesome.

One of the disadvantages of guanethidine is the postural hypotension which it characteristically induces. Frequently this is more marked when the patient first gets up after being recumbent all night. Often this morning orthostatism precludes adequate control of supine blood pressure throughout the entire 24-hour period.[2] The addition of methyldopa to the regimen tends to smooth out this diurnal variation in blood pressure but seldom eliminates it entirely.[1] In my opinion, measurement of blood pressure by the patient or a member of his family in the home is indispensable to the good management of hypertension when orthostatism is a problem. Blood pressure should be measured in the supine and standing positions when the patient first awakens in the morning and again in the evening. The dosage of guanethidine should be adjusted to keep the morning standing blood pressure as low as possible without inducing incapacitating symptoms. All patients receiving guanethidine should be warned about orthostatic hypotension and advised not to arise suddenly from the recumbent or seated posture.

Contraindications to Use

There are few absolute contraindications to antipressor drugs. In each instance the physician must weigh the anticipated benefits of treatment against the potential hazards. Rarely, if ever, is reserpine indispensable to the regimen as there are satisfactory alternatives and consequently the contraindications to this drug assume greater relative importance. The same is not true for guanethidine, which may be the only effective drug in managing severe hypertension. Usually it is safer to employ guanethidine cautiously in the face of relative contraindications than it is to let uncontrolled hypertension take its toll.

Reserpine. This drug should be avoided in patients known to be sensitive to it and in patients who are, have been, or tend to be depressed (Table 1).[3] Likewise, active or recurrent peptic ulcer constitutes an absolute contraindication because reserpine increases gastric acidity. Parkinsonian states may also be aggravated by reserpine. Although there is experimental evidence that depletion of myocardial stores of catecholamine by therapy with reserpine may precipitate or aggravate congestive heart failure, this has not been a problem clinically, possibly because reserpine is almost always administered in conjunction with an oral diuretic.

Contrary to popular belief, it is not necessary to stop therapy with reserpine several days before elective surgery, provided the anesthesiologist and the surgeon are aware that the patient is receiving it. Inhibition of the sympathetic nervous system by reserpine will make the patient more susceptible to hypotension from blood loss, and care must be exercised to replace plasma volume rapidly and liberally in case of excessive bleeding. If hypotension occurs it will respond to plasma volume expansion (by whole blood or appropriate fluid replacement) and administration of a direct-acting sympathomimetic agent such as levarterenol. Indirect-acting sympathomimetic agents such as tyramine, ephedrine, and mephentermine will not be effective because tissue stores of norepinephrine have been depleted by reserpine.

Renal failure and symptomatic coronary or cerebrovascular disease are not contraindications to therapy with reserpine.

Guanethidine. Drug sensitivity is the only absolute contraindication to therapy with guanethidine (Table 1). While it is desirable, if possible, to control hypertension complicated by renal insufficiency or manifestations of cerebrovascular disease with agents that do not cause orthostatic hypotension, it is better to use guanethidine cautiously with an oral diuretic (preferably furosemide if renal insufficiency is present) and either hydralazine or methyldopa than to permit the hypertension to remain uncontrolled. In such cases therapy should be started with small doses (e.g., 5 mg daily) of guanethidine and patients should be particularly warned about orthostatic hypotension and they should take their blood pressures at home. For patients with renal insufficiency, determinations of blood urea nitrogen and serum creatinine should be made at least once a week until the blood pressure has been stabilized. More often than not, blood pressure control can be achieved in this manner without aggravating symptoms of cerebral ischemia or worsening of renal function.

While similar precautions are warranted for patients with angina pectoris who require guanethidine in their antipressor regimens, it has been my experience that they tolerate blood pressure reduction surprisingly well, and in most cases angina has improved when hypertension is controlled.

Guanethidine should not be used in the same regimen with a monoamine oxidase (MAO) inhibitor because of the danger of precipitating a hypertensive crisis.

Amphetamines and tricyclic antidepressants [4] attenuate or abolish the antihypertensive effect of guanethidine because they prevent guanethidine from gaining access to the nerve terminal of the sympathetic fiber, a position it must occupy to be effective.

Remarks concerning reserpine and congestive heart failure or elective anesthesia are equally pertinent to guanethidine.

Untoward Effects

Although reserpine and guanethidine both inhibit the sympathetic nervous system and deplete tissue stores of catecholamines, their untoward pharmacologic effects differ qualitatively and quantitatively (Table 2). The high incidence of depression, lassitude, lethargy, and somnolence induced by reserpine can be explained by the fact that it depletes catecholamine and serotonin stores in the CNS, while guanethidine does not. It is these CNS effects that are most troublesome in patients taking reserpine and make it a less desirable agent than methyldopa. Nasal congestion is a frequent and annoying untoward effect of reserpine, but it is less troublesome and frequent during therapy with guanethidine. The effects on the gastrointestinal tract can be explained by relative overactivity of the uninhibited parasympathetic nervous system, yet even these are different. Reserpine seems to have a greater propensity to increase gastric acidity while guanethidine has a greater tendency to increase motility of the bowel thereby producing diarrhea which is particularly troublesome after meals.

Bradycardia is somewhat more pronounced during therapy with guanethidine than with reserpine although the difference is neither great nor consistent. When patients are also receiving digitalis, it is often difficult to determine which drug is responsible for the bradycardia.

Orthostatic hypotension, especially in the morning and during exercise, is a frequent pharmacologic effect of guanethidine but is uncommon with reserpine.

TABLE 2.—*Untoward Effects of Reserpine and Guanethidine Therapy*

Untoward Effects	*Reserpine*	*Guanethidine*
Depression	Common	Rare
Bizarre dreams; nightmares	Common	Not reported
Lassitude, lethargy, somnolence	Common	Not reported
Nasal congestion	Common	Occasionally
Activation of peptic ulcer	Common	Rare
Diarrhea	Occasionally	Common
Bradycardia	Common	Common
Orthostatic hypotension (especially upon arising in A.M.)	Rare	Common
Exertional hypotension	Rare	Common
Parkinsonian state	Sometimes	Not reported
Impotence	Occasionally	Occasionally
Loss of ejaculation without true impotence	Rare	Common

The parkinsonian state is sometimes an untoward effect of reserpine, especially in older patients, but it is rarely, if ever, encountered during therapy with guanethidine.

Sexual problems in the male are more frequently associated with guanethidine than with reserpine. Both drugs occasionally interfere with obtaining and maintaining penile erection, but unlike reserpine, guanethidine frequently inhibits ejaculation without preventing erection and orgasm.

Comments

Reserpine and guanethidine are hypotensive drugs which selectively inhibit the sympathetic system but their clinical application is at opposite ends of the hypertensive spectrum. Reserpine is a mildly hypotensive agent which is used for managing mild or moderate hypertension and is not indispensable to the antihypertensive armamentarium because there are satisfactory alternatives. Guanethidine is a potent agent which should be reserved for severe or resistant hypertension, in which role it has no peer.

While I have expressed definite personal preferences for certain antihypertensive agents in this discourse, in the final analysis I am more concerned that hypertension be adequately treated than I am about the choice of drugs to accomplish this. A satisfactory regimen is one that keeps blood pressure within normal limits with a minimum of inconvenience and annoying untoward effects.

References

1. Leonard, J. W., Gifford, R. W., Jr., and Humphrey, D. C.: Treatment of hypertension with methyldopa alone or combined with diuretics and/or guanethidine. A report of 63 cases. Am. Heart J. 69:610, 1965.
2. Schirger, A., and Gifford, R. W., Jr.: Guanethidine, a new antihypertensive agent: Experience in the treatment of 36 patients with severe hypertension. Mayo Clin. Proc. 37: 100, 1962.
3. Quetsch, R. M., Achor, R. W. P., Litin, E. M., and Faucett, R. L.: Depressive reactions in hypertensive patients; comparison with those treated with Rauwolfia and those receiving no specific antihypertensive treatment. Circulation 19:366, 1959.
4. Mitchell, J. R., Arias, L., and Oates, J. A.: Antagonism of the antihypertensive action of guanethidine sulfate by desipramine hydrochloride. JAMA 202:973, 1967.

Monoamine Oxidase Inhibitors: Their Pharmacology and Place in Hypertension

By William B. Abrams, M.D.

MONOAMINE OXIDASES (MAO) are enzymes responsible for the oxidative deamination of a wide variety of amines, the best known of which are serotonin and the catecholamines dopamine, norepinephrine and epinephrine. This reaction applies to blood pressure regulation in that MAO is the principal intraneuronal inactivator of norepinephrine, the sympathetic neurohumoral transmitting agent. Norepinephrine gains access to sympathetic neurones by biosynthesis from the amino acid tyrosine through dopa and dopamine. In the postganglionic sympathetic neurone, norepinephrine is stored in granules which protect it from MAO in the mitochondria. The granules are the sites from which norepinephrine is released into the synaptic clefts in response to nerve stimuli. Norepinephrine is inactivated extraneuronally by reuptake into the neurone, and by the enzyme catechol-O-methyl transferase. Within the neurone, as mentioned, MAO metabolizes any norepinephrine which escapes the storage granules.[1] Thus MAO serves the function of regulating the content of norepinephrine in sympathetic neurones.[1,2] The main end-product of norepinephrine metabolism, by the action of the two enzymes, is vanillylmandelic acid (VMA).

MAO inhibitors are substances of diverse chemical structures capable of blocking or reducing the activity of MAO. The common biochemical property of MAO inhibition confers certain pharmacologic actions on these substances. Potentiation of indirect-acting amines such as amphetamine and tyramine, and reversal of the norepinephrine-depleting effects of reserpine and tetrabenazine in animals, have been associated with the antidepressant effects of these drugs in man. These same biochemical and pharmacologic properties, however, are also associated with adverse interactions with a variety of drugs and foodstuffs. During early clinical trials of MAO inhibitors as antidepressants, postural hypotension was encountered as a common but inconsistent side effect. A large number of MAO inhibitors were then prepared and studied specifically as antihypertensive agents. Of these, only pargyline is available today for use in hypertension.

Classification

MAO inhibitors may be classified by chemistry, enzyme kinetics, and tissue selectivity (Table 1). In the chemical classification, it has been traditional to divide MAO inhibitors into hydrazines and nonhydrazines [3] (Fig. 1). The first widely used MAO inhibitor, iproniazid, is in the former category. A hydrazine derivative has the diamine unit -NH-NH- in its structure. The clinical significance of this division is that hydrazine MAO inhibitors have been associated with a higher incidence of liver toxicity than their nonhydrazine counterparts. This apparent toxicity is the reason iproniazid was withdrawn from the market. There is some evidence that this reputation is not entirely deserved, since iproniazid is still available in England for the treatment of depression and its use has not been associated with an undue incidence of liver toxicity. It is also true, however, that the hydrazines are more likely than the nonhydrazine inhibitors to affect enzymes other than MAO.[4] Of the hydrazine MAO inhibitors, isocarboxazid, phenelzine, and nialamide are clinically available for use in the treatment of depression, but none are recommended for treatment of hypertension. All are general, irreversible enzyme inhibitors and are therefore capable of producing the adverse food and drug interactions characteristic of most MAO inhibitors. In addition, some agents have produced toxic reactions that appear unique to their chemical structures, as listed in Table 1.

There are several groups of nonhydrazine MAO inhibitors (Table 1; Fig. 1). These are represented in the clinic by the antidepressant

---

From Ayerst Laboratories and the Department of Medicine, College of Medicine and Dentistry of New Jersey, Newark, New Jersey.

TABLE 1.—*Monoamine Oxidase Inhibitors*

Chemistry	*Enzyme Kinetics*	*Selectivity*	*Clinical Use*	*Principal Toxicity*
Hydrazines Iproniazid *Isocarboxazid* Pheniprazine *Phenelzine* *Nialamide* Tersavid	Irreversible, long-acting	All tissues	Antidepressants, antihypertensives, angina pectoris	Food and drug interactions Hepatitis Amblyopia Hepatitis
Harmala alkaloids	Reversible, short duration	All tissues	Antihypertensive, angina pectoris, parkinsonism	Visual, neurologic
Tryptamine derivatives Etryptamine	Reversible	All tissues	Antidepressant	Agranulocytosis
Cyclopropylamines *Tranylcypromine*	Irreversible †	All tissues	Antidepressant	Hypertension, food and drug interactions
Propynylamines *Pargyline*	Irreversible, long-acting	All tissues	Antihypertensive (antidepressant)	Food and drug interactions
Guanidines and related drugs Debrisoquin Bethanidine Bretylium *	Reversible, short-acting	Adrenergic neurones	Antihypertensives	Drug interactions

Drug names in italics are marketed in the United States.
* Benzyl quaternary ammonium derivative.
† Most substrates.

tranylcypromine (Parnate) and the antihypertensive pargyline (Eutonyl, Eutron). Bretylium, bethanidine, and debrisoquin are postganglionic sympathetic-blocking agents which are enjoying considerable utility elsewhere for the treatment of hypertension, but have not been approved for marketing in the United States. The nonhydrazine MAO inhibitors are quite diverse in their characteristics. Tranylcypromine (most substrates) and pargyline are irreversible enzyme inhibitors and are distributed to all sites of MAO. The guanidines and bretylium, on the other hand, are reversible, short-acting inhibitors and have selective access to the MAO in peripheral adrenergic neurone.[5–7] The *harmala* alkaloids and tryptamine derivatives displayed unique forms of toxicity which proscribed their clinical use.

CLINICAL PHARMACOLOGY

MAO inhibitors encompass a wide variety of chemical structures and, similarly, display a wide range of pharmacologic activities. However, three general types of properties seem to have relevance to their clinical activity: reserpine reversal, potentiation of indirect-acting pressor amines, and inhibition of sympathetic nerve function. These properties are readily demonstrable in animals and man.

It is now well known that the norepinephrine in postganglionic sympathetic nerve fibers is highly concentrated in storage granules in terminal varicosities.[8] Figure 2 is a fluorescent photomicrograph of a stretch preparation of albino rat iris prepared by the method of Falck, Hillarp et al.[9] In this method, catecholamines in tissues form an intensely fluorescent product when exposed to formaldehyde.[10] The intensity of the fluorescence is proportional to the concentration of catecholamine.[8] Although the rat iris is a convenient tissue to work with, similar preparations can be made from any sympathetically innervated organ. Reserpine depletes norepinephrine from sympathetic neurones by impairing the storage mechanism at the granule level.[11] This action of reserpine can be dem-

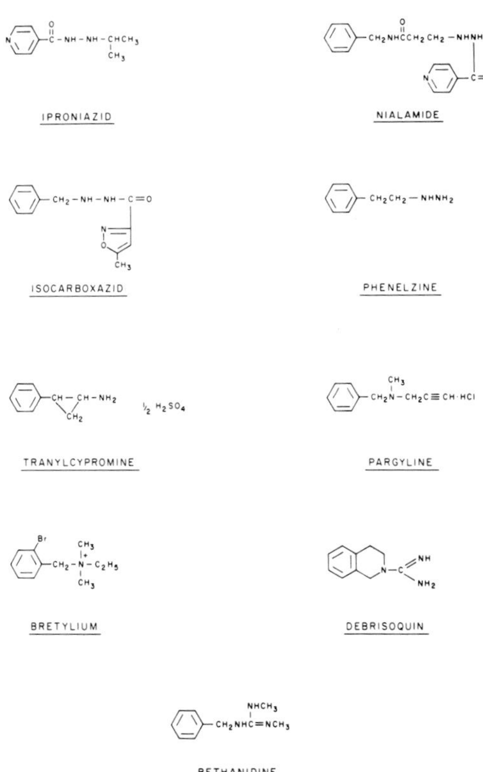

FIG. 1. Chemical structures of representative MAO inhibitors.

onstrated histochemically and pharmacologically. Figure 3 is a rat iris prepared as in Fig. 2 from an animal given 2.5 mg per kilogram of body weight of reserpine 4 hours before sacrifice. Note the near-total absence of fluorescent material, i.e. norepinephrine. The fluorescence cannot be restored even if norepinephrine is given 15 minutes before sacrifice.[8] If, however, the animal is given a MAO inhibitor after the reserpine, the norepinephrine content of the adrenergic nerve terminals is restored (Fig. 4). The effect is similar if the MAO inhibitor is given before the reserpine.[8] In other words, MAO inhibitor is capable of reversing the effects of reserpine.

Catecholamine depletion, repletion, and accumulation have significant pharmacologic and clinical consequences. Figure 5 shows the blood pressure responses to graded intravenous doses of tyramine administered to a patient with mild hypertension. Tyramine raises blood pressure only by releasing norepinephrine from sympathetic neurones, therefore the degree of blood pressure elevation reflects the content of norepinephrine in these nerve cells. The control responses are on the left. The curves in the center show that the blood pressure responses to the same doses of tyramine are

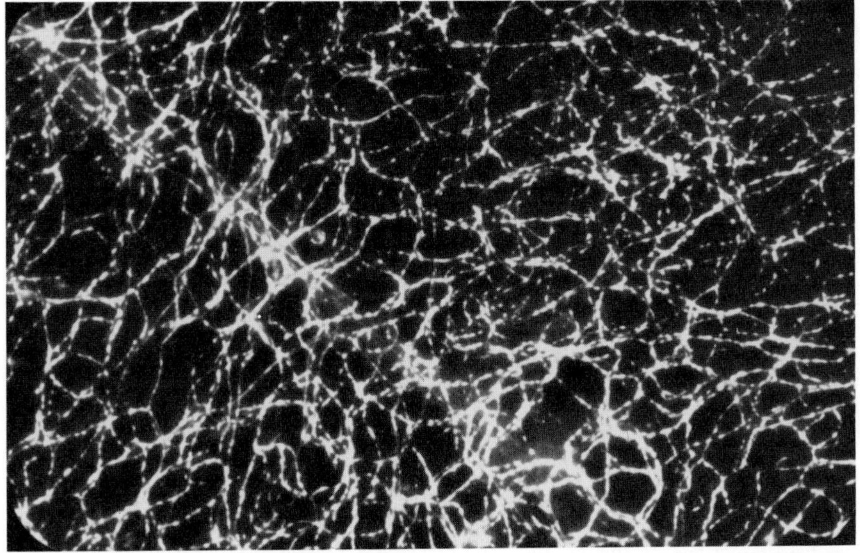

FIG. 2.—Fluorescent photomicrograph of a stretch preparation of albino rat iris prepared by the method of Falck and Hillarp from an untreated animal. The adrenergic ground plexuses of varicose terminals are readily seen. A few less fluorescent, smooth nonterminal axons are also present. ×250. (From Malmfors, and Abrams,[8] with permission.)

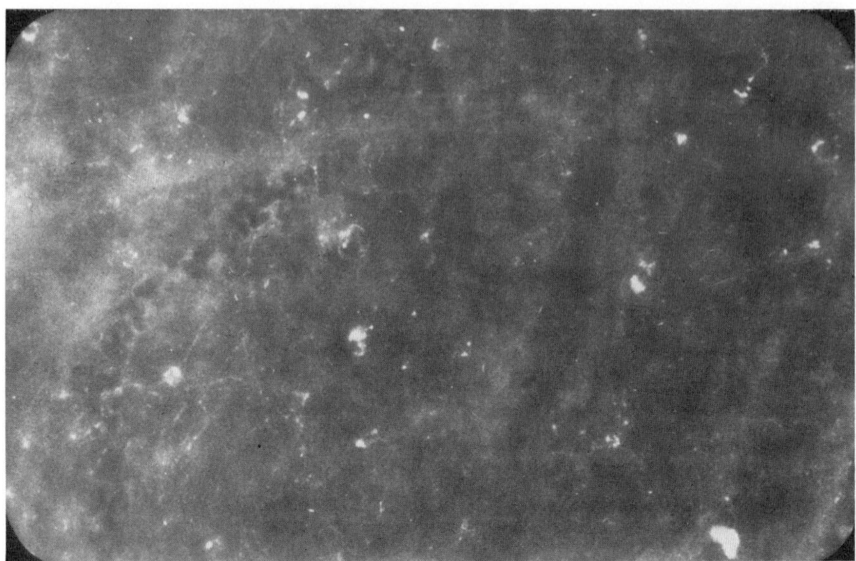

FIG. 3.—Rat iris prepared as in Fig. 2 from an animal given 2.5 mg of reserpine per kilogram of body weight, 4 hours before sacrifice. Only faint rests of the adrenergic terminals can now be seen. ×250. (From Malmfors, and Abrams,[8] with permission.)

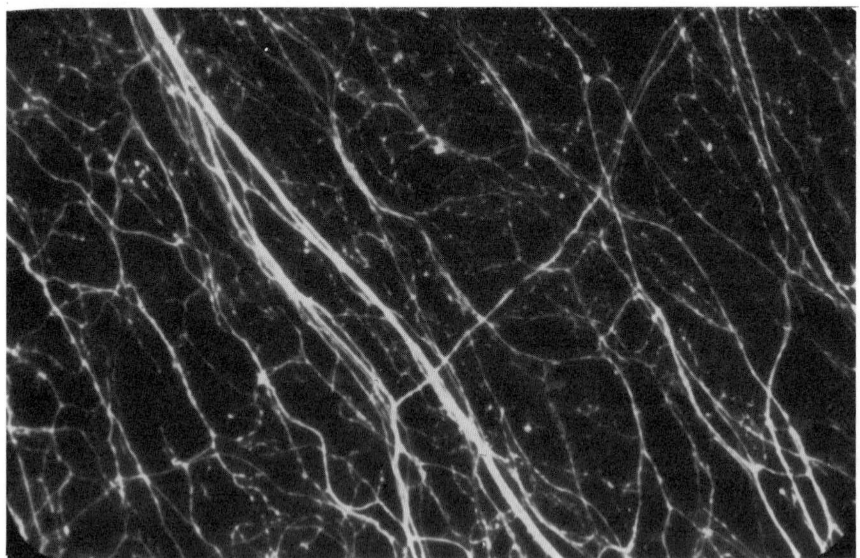

FIG. 4.—Rat iris prepared as in Fig. 2 from an animal given 10 mg of reserpine per kilogram of body weight, 16 hours before sacrifice; 2 mg of debrisoquin per kilogram of body weight, 1 hour before sacrifice; and 0.1 of norepinephrine per kilogram of body weight, 15 minutes before sacrifice. In this photomicrograph, the adrenergic nerve terminals are smoother than in the untreated animal (Fig. 2) and the nonterminal axons are more pronounced. The same effect is produced if 10 mg of bretylium per kilogram of body weight, or 20 mg of nialamide per kilogram of body weight is given in place of the debrisoquin. ×250. (From Malmfors, T., and Abrams, W. B.,[8] with permission.)

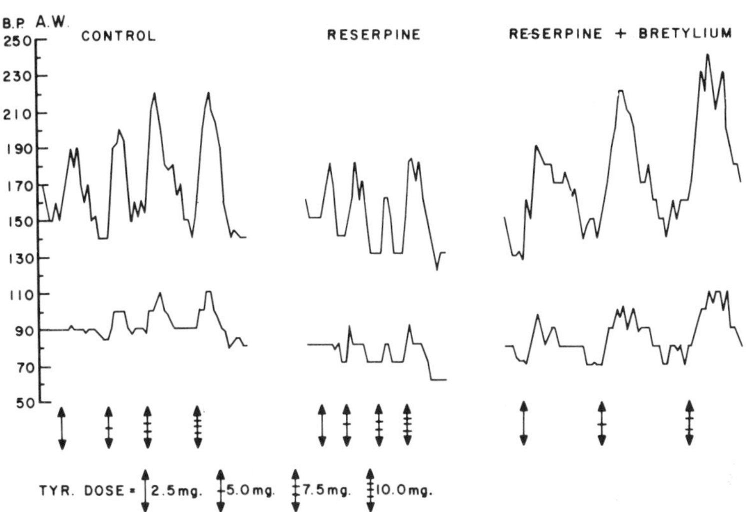

FIG. 5.—Blood pressure responses to graded doses of tyramine administered intravenously. Left: control; center, after 4 days of treatment with 2.5 mg of reserpine given twice daily by mouth. Right, after 4 days of treatment with 200 mg of bretylium given twice daily by mouth, in addition to the reserpine.

substantially reduced after the individual was treated with a 2.5-mg dose of reserpine, given orally, twice daily for 4 days. This is the pharmacologic counterpart of the histochemical evidence of norepinephrine depletion by reserpine. The curves on the right of Fig. 5 are the pharmacologic counterpart of the histochemical evidence of reserpine reversal by a MAO inhibitor. These blood pressure responses to tyramine were obtained after 200-mg of bretylium, given orally twice a day, was *added* to the reserpine treatment. Note that the pressor responses to the same doses of tyramine are not only restored, but exceed control levels. This suggests that norepinephrine was actually present in excess. Indeed, it has been demonstrated repeatedly that MAO inhibitors cause accumulation of catecholamines in sympathetic tissues.[4,12] Figure 5 was taken from a study of antihypertensive mechanisms, so bretylium was the drug employed, but the same effect could be produced with any MAO inhibitor.[13,14]

The pressor response to tyramine and the biochemical consequencs of MAO inhibition can be used to investigate the relationship of MAO inhibition to the blood pressure-lowering effects of this group of drugs. Figure 6 charts the mean daily supine and erect blood pressure values, the systolic pressor responses to tyramine and norepinephrine, and the urinary excretion of tryptamine obtained from a patient given 100 mg of pargyline daily for 10 days. Tryptamine is a ubiquitous monoamine dietary amino acid. When MAO is inhibited, it escapes deamination and large quantities appear in the urine. It can be seen that the onset of orthostatic hypotension was chronologically related to a sharp increase in the pressor response to tyramine and the urinary excretion of tryptamine. There was no significant change in the pressor response to norepinephrine. The failure of MAO inhibitors to influence the actions of direct-acting sympathomimetic amines such as norepinephrine has been repeatedly observed.[15] The disappearance of orthostatism, some 12 days after the pargyline was stopped, was also associated with definite reductions in the pharmacologic and biochemical indicators of MAO inhibition. Note, however, the increased pressor response to tyramine was still present 24 days after discontinuance. In another subject, an exaggerated pressor response to tyramine persisted 42 days after the drug was stopped. The long-lasting effect of par-

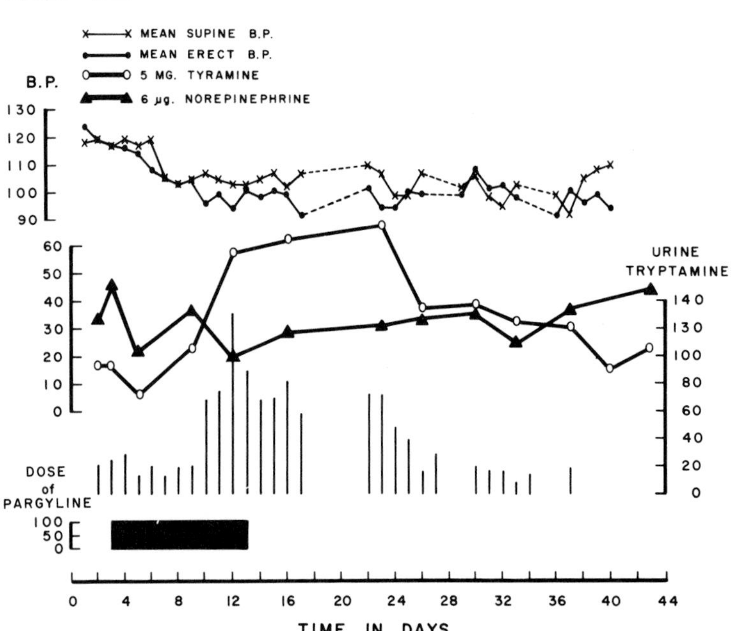

FIG. 6.—The effect of pargyline on blood pressure, systolic blood pressure response to tyramine, and urinary excretion of tryptamine. The blood pressure value for each day is the mean of four determinations, supine (x) and erect (●). The open circles are the systolic blood pressure responses to 5 mg of tyramine, given intravenously, and the closed triangles are the systolic pressure responses to 6 μg of norepinephrine, given intravenously. The vertical bars represent the urinary excretion levels of tryptamine in micrograms per 24-hour period (scale on right). The days and dose of treatment with pargyline are shown at the bottom.

gyline is important to keep in mind when this drug is stopped in anticipation of treatment with other, possibly interacting, drugs.

Clinical pharmacologic studies with an investigational agent provided an opportunity to examine more precisely the relationship between MAO inhibition and blood pressure-lowering.[16] Ro 5-7957 (4-methyl-N-propyl-S-oxazole-carbamic acid ethyl ester), a potent MAO inhibitor in animals and in vitro, was administered to a group of patients with mild essential hypertension. Measurements included supine and erect blood pressure determinations four times daily, pressor responses to tyramine and daily urinary excretion levels of tryptamine, normetanephrine, and vanillylmandelic acid (VMA). Normetanephrine and VMA levels reflect MAO activity in sympathetic neurones, whereas tryptamine excretion depends on MAO in other tissues. Normetanephrine is formed from norepinephrine by the action of catechol-O-methyl transferase. The conversion of normetanephrine to VMA requires MAO. MAO inhibition in sympathetic neurones, therefore, causes an increase of normetanephrine and a decrease in VMA excretion. Figure 7 shows the results from a representative subject. Orthostatism is represented as the difference between the patient's mean supine and mean erect blood pressure values. Thus orthostatic hypotension is present when the curve becomes negative. Drug administration in increasing doses is shown at the bottom. The pressor response to tyramine is recorded as the least dose which caused a 30-mm Hg rise in systolic blood pressure. The smaller the dose of tyramine, therefore, the greater the sensitivity to this indirect-acting sympathomimetic amine. It can be seen that intraneuronal MAO inhibition (increase in normetanephrine; decrease in VMA), catecholamine accumulation in adrenergic neurones (increased tyramine sensitivity), and MAO inhibition in other tissues (increased

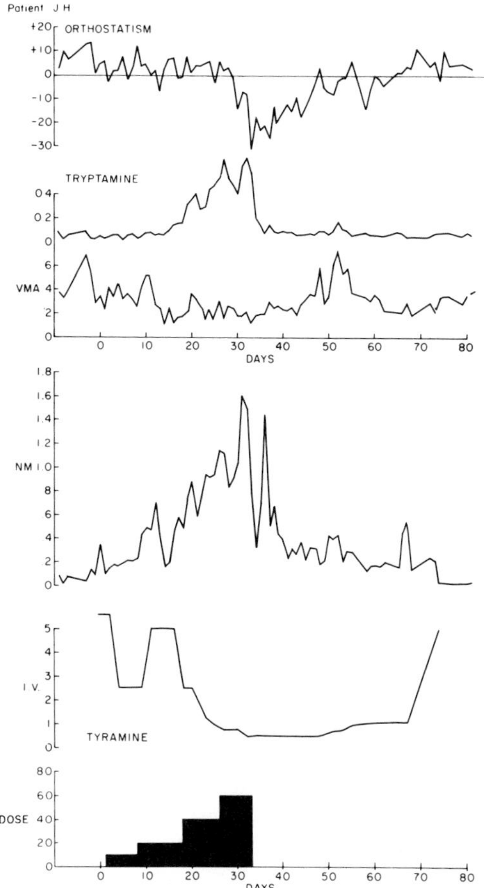

FIG. 7.—The effect of Ro 5-7957 on blood pressure, urinary amine excretion, and pressor response to tyramine. Orthostatism is recorded as the difference between the mean erect and mean supine daily blood pressure values. A negative value indicates the erect blood pressure is lower than the supine. The tryptamine and normetanephrine values are expressed as micrograms per gram of creatinine and VMA is expressed as milligram per gram of creatinine. The tyramine pressor response is expressed as the least dose which caused a 30-mm Hg rise in systolic blood pressure. The days and dose of treatment with Ro 5-7957 are shown at bottom.

tryptamine excretion) preceded the onset of orthostatic hypotension by some days. The peak effects, however, seemed to coincide. The prolonged, increased sensitivity to tyramine indicates this agent is also a long-lasting inhibitor.

The studies described thus far involved general, irreversible MAO inhibitors. Bretylium, bethanidine, and debrisoquin are weak, reversible MAO inhibitors in vitro, but achieve concentrations adequate to affect this enzyme in the body by virtue of their selective accumulation by adrenergic neurones.[6–8,17] The different profile of effects of these drugs is demonstrated in Figs. 8 and 9 from a study with debrisoquin.[7] The pressor sensitivities to oral and intravenous tyramine and intravenous norepinephrine are expressed as the ratio of the control to the treatment dose required to produce a 30-mm Hg rise in systolic blood pressure. The administration of debrisoquin was associated with a definite increase in the pressor sensitivity to tyramine administered

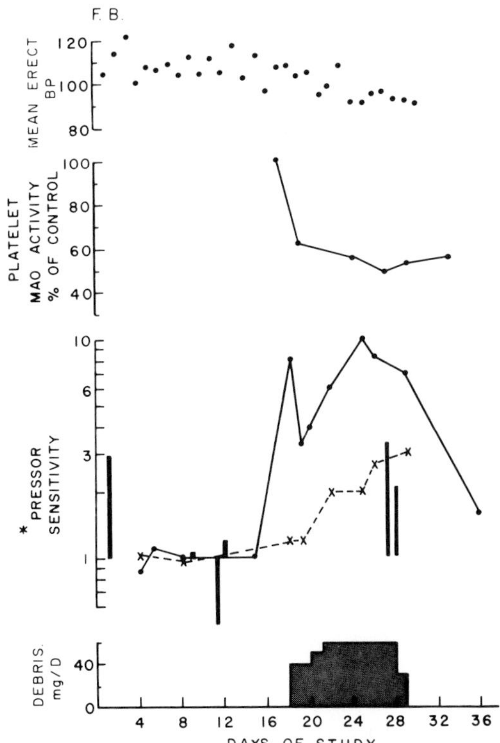

FIG. 8.—The effect of debrisoquin on mean erect blood pressure, platelet MAO activity, and pressor sensitivity to intravenous tyramine (●—●), oral tyramine (**vertical bars**), and intravenous norepinephrine (**x - - - x**). Pressor sensitivity is expressed as the ratio of the control to the treatment dose required to produce a 30-mm Hg rise in systolic blood pressure. The days and dose of treatment with debrisoquin are shown at the bottom. (From Pettinger, W. A., et al.,[7] with permission.)

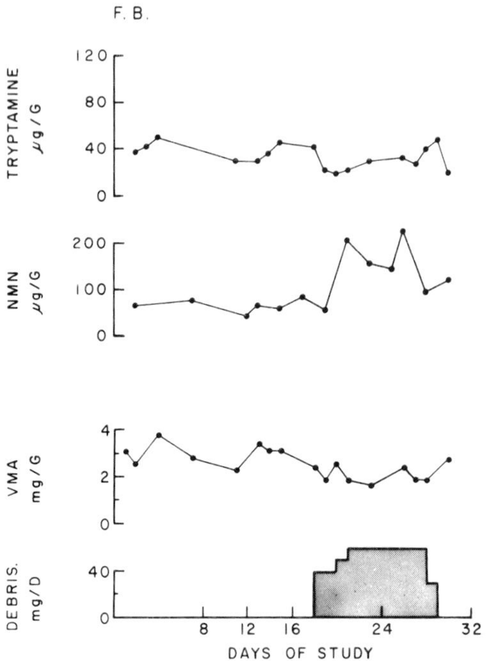

FIG. 9.—The effect of debrisoquin on the urinary excretion of tryptamine, normetanephrine (NMN) and VMA. Values expressed as microgram or milligram per gram of creatinine. The days and dose of treatment with debrisoquin are shown at the bottom. (From Pettinger, W. A., et al.,[7] with permission.)

intravenously, but only a moderate and variable increase in the pressor sensitivity to oral tyramine. In contrast to the general MAO inhibitors, pressor sensitivity to norepinephrine rose. This occurred because debrisoquin and related drugs are primarily adrenergic neurone-blocking agents, and increased norepinephrine responsiveness is characteristic of adrenergic neurone blockade, even with non-MAO inhibitors such as reserpine and guanethidine.[18] As expected, there was a fall in the mean erect blood pressure values. There was also a fall in platelet MAO activity. The platelet has been shown to imitate the adrenergic neurone under some circumstances.[19] The selective nature of the MAO inhibition is clearly demonstrated in Fig. 9 from the same subject. The urinary excretions of normetanephrine increased and VMA decreased as would be expected for intraneuronal MAO inhibition. However, the urinary excretion of tryptamine was unchanged, indicating no MAO inhibition in other tissues. It was also demonstrated in this study that urinary excretion of tyramine and gastrointestinal MAO activity was unaffected by debrisoquin administration.[7]

These studies, plus evidence provided by others,[20] would appear to suggest that MAO inhibition is related to the blood pressure effects of these drugs. Furthermore, the orthostatic nature of the blood pressure fall indicates that interference with sympathetic nerve transmission is at least part of the mechanism of action. The causal interrelationships between MAO inhibition, catecholamine accumulation and blood pressure-lowering are far from clear. Some investigators have been unable to correlate increased urinary excretion of tryptamine with blood pressure-lowering during administration of several MAO inhibitors.[21–23] However, these investigators did not attempt to establish the time course of events, as in the present studies. On the other hand, it is also true that certain potent MAO inhibitors failed to produce hypotensive effects in man.[24,25]

Regardless of whether or how MAO inhibition, per se, is involved in the blood pressure effects, it does seem to be basically a sympatholytic action. The site of this effect is also not established. Some years ago, it was proposed that MAO inhibitors were slow-acting, ganglion-blocking agents,[26] and this proposal found support in certain pharmacologic observations.[27] However, the subsequent failure to correlate MAO inhibition with ganglionic blockade in animals,[28–30] and the lack of parasympatholytic side effects in man,[31] make the autonomic ganglia unlikely sites of action for the sympatholytic effects of these drugs.

Most laboratory and clinical data point to the postganglionic sympathetic nerve terminal as the principal site of action for the blood pressure effects of MAO inhibitors. Several hypotheses have been proposed to explain the apparent paradox of catecholamine accumulation and impaired transmission in these nerves.[3,4] One such hypothesis is that catecholamine accumulation causes an end-product, feedback inhibition of norepinephrine biosynthesis, and this interferes with sympathetic nerve function.[32] The most recent theory, proposed independently by Day and Rand [33] and Kopin and associates,[34] suggests that MAO inhibition is associated with the replacement of at least some of the norepinephrine in sympathetic nerves by less active amines. This hypothesis is based on the observation that among the catecholamines accumulated in sympathetically innervated tissues by the administration of a MAO inhibitor, is the weak agonist octopamine.[34,35] Sympathetic nerve activity would be expected to release octopamine along with norephinephrine, but since octopamine has only 1 percent of the activity of norepinephrine at the receptor level,[36] the net effect is reduced transmission. This action would be similar to the "false-transmitter" mechanism of methyldopa.[37] Methyldopa is, of course, not a MAO inhibitor. This hypothesis was proposed to explain the general MAO inhibitors. Its application to the selective MAO inhibitors bretylium, bethanidine, and debrisoquin lacks experimental evidence.

Clinical Use

As mentioned, the only MAO inhibitor approved for use in the treatment of hypertension in the United States is pargyline. The clinical, hemodynamic and toxicologic characteristics of this agent are quite predictable from its pharmacologic properties. They may be considered in three general categories: (1) inhibition of sympathetic nerve function, (2) catecholamine accumulation, and (3) central nervous system (CNS) stimulation.

Inhibition of efferent sympathetic nerve function explains the predominantly orthostatic nature of the blood pressure-lowering.[38] It also explains the decrease in peripheral resistance [38] and the reduction in blood pressure and cardiac output in response to exercise.[39] The most frequently occurring side effects are those associated with excessive orthostatic hypotension, namely, dizziness, weakness, palpitation, and fainting. Inhibition of sympathetic nerve function is probably also responsible for the mild constipation, difficulty in micturition, delayed ejaculation, and fluid retention occasionally encountered with this agent. Any drug which reduces the level of sympathetic nerve activity in the heart is capable of precipitating congestive heart failure in individuals with severely compromised cardiac function. Pargyline is excreted primarily in the urine; therefore impaired renal function may lead to accumulation and excessive drug effect.

Under carefully controlled experimental conditions, the pressor response to tyramine is a useful tool to measure the intraneuronal catecholamine accumulation produced by MAO inhibition. However, tyramine and other pressor substances in certain foods, drinks, and medications may lead to serious hypertensive crises in patients on pargyline and other general MAO inhibitors.[13] These crises may be manifested by headache, chest pain, sweating, cardiac arrhythmias, visual disturbances, coma, or stroke. Foodstuffs rich in tyramine include Cheddar, Camembert and Stilton cheese, pickled herring, Chianti wine, and chicken liver. Similar complications may occur if other catecholamine-releasing drugs such as reserpine or guanethidine are used concomitantly. Amphetamine, ephedrine, phenylephrine, and similar monoamines may produce excessive sympathomimetic reactions in MAO-inhibitor treated patients, so anorexiant and cold remedies containing such drugs must be avoided.

CNS stimulation may produce desirable antidepressant effects, but may also produce undesirable hyperexcitability, nightmares, confusion, agitation, and disorientation. In susceptible individuals, a severe psychotic reaction with hallucinations and paranoid delusions may occur. The adverse interactions which have been reported with tricyclic antidepressants such as imipramine, desipramine, and amitriptyline may be associated with catecholamine accumulation or CNS stimulation or both. The reaction includes vascular collapse and hyperthermia.

The selective MAO inhibitors are not liable to CNS side effects or adverse interactions with tyramine-rich foods.[7] However, drugs capable of releasing intraneuronal catecholamine stores could possibly cause hypertensive reactions in patients treated with these drugs.[7]

As mentioned, pargyline is an irreversible, long-lasting enzyme inhibitor, therefore the onset of action is slow (days or weeks) and its effects are persistent after administration is stopped. It need be given only once daily. It is a potent drug, thus is recommended for use only in patients with moderate to severe hypertension. The concomitant use of an oral diuretic increases the supine response and tends to reduce the dose needed to accomplish blood pressure control. The reduced dose decreases the incidence of side effects. The usual starting dose is 25 mg per day and this is increased in 10-mg increments at weekly intervals until the desired effect is obtained or intolerable side effects are encountered.

REFERENCES

1. Kopin, I. J., and Axelrod, J.: The role of monoamine oxidase in the release and metabolism of norepinephrine. Ann. N.Y. Acad. Sci. 107:848, 1963.
2. Brodie, B. B., Spector, S., and Shore, P. A.: Interaction of drugs with norepinephrine in the brain. Pharmacol. Rev. 11:548, 1959.
3. Schoepke, H. G., and Swett, L. R.: Chemistry and pharmacology of monoamine oxidase inhibitors. *In* Schlittler, E. (Ed.): Antihypertensive Agents. New York: Academic Press, 1967, pp. 393–428.
4. Pletscher, A.: Monoamine oxidase inhibitors. Pharmacol. Rev. 18:121, 1966.
5. Kuntzman, R., and Jacobson, M. M.: The inhibition of monoamine oxidase by benzyl and phenethylguanidines related to bretylium and guanethidine. Ann. N.Y. Acad. Sci. 107: 945, 1963.
6. Medina, M. A., Giachetti, A., and Shore, P. A.: On the physiological disposition and possible mechanism of the antihypertensive action of debrisoquin. Biochem. Pharmacol. 18:891, 1969.
7. Pettinger, W. A., Korn, A., Spiegel, H., Solomon, H. M., Pocelinko, R., and Abrams, W. B.: Debrisoquin, a selective inhibitor of intraneuronal monoamine oxidase in man. Clin. Pharmacol. Ther. 10:667, 1969.
8. Malmfors, T., and Abrams, W. B.: The effects of debrisoquin and bretylium on adrenergic nerves as revealed by fluorescence histochemistry. J. Pharmacol. Exp. Ther. 174:99, 1970.
9. Falck, B., Hillarp, N.-A., Thieme, G., and Thorpe, A.: Fluorescence of catecholamines and related compounds by a fluorescence method. J. Histochem. Cytochem. 10:348, 1962.
10. Corrodi, H., and Jonsson, G.: The formaldehyde fluorescence method for the histochemical demonstration of biogenic monoamines. J. Histochem. Cytochem. 15:65, 1967.
11. von Euler, U. S., and Lishajko, F.: Mechanism of drug-induced catecholamine release from adrenergic nerve granules. Circ. Res. 21 (Suppl. III):63, 1967.
12. Schoepke, H. G., and Wiegand, R. G.: Relation between norepinephrine accumulation or depletion and blood pressure responses in the cat and rat following pargyline administration. Ann. N.Y. Acad. Sci. 107:924, 1963.
13. Horwitz, D., Lovenberg, W., Engelman, K., and Sjoerdsma, A.: Monoamine oxidase inhibitors, tyramine and cheese. JAMA 188: 1108, 1964.
14. Pettinger, W. A., and Oates, J. A.: Supersensitivity to tyramine during monoamine oxidase inhibition in man. Mechanism at the level of the adrenergic neuron. Clin. Pharmacol. Ther. 9:341, 1968.
15. Rand, M. J., and Trinker, F. R.: The mechanism of the augmentation of responses to indirectly acting sympathomimetic amines by monoamine oxidase inhibitors. Br. J. Pharmacol. 33:287, 1968.
16. Leon, A. S., Abrams, W. B., Maynard, D., and Markowitz, M.: Correlation of clinical, biochemical and pharmacologic effects of a monoamine oxidase inhibitor. Clin. Res. 16: 237, 1968.
17. Brodie, B. B., Chang, C. C., and Costa, E.: On the mechanism of action of guanethidine and bretylium. Br. J. Pharmacol. 25:171, 1965.
18. Abrams, W. B., Moe, R. A., Bates, H., Wallen, M., Odze, M., Crews, A., and Pocelinko, R.: Adrenergic mechanisms in the treatment of essential hypertension. Am. J. Cardiol. 12: 711, 1963.
19. Solomon, H. M., Ashley, C., Spirt, N., and Abrams, W. B.: The influence of debrisoquin on the accumulation and metabolism of biogenic amines by the human platelet, in vivo and in vitro. Clin. Pharmacol. Ther. 10:229, 1969.
20. Orvis, H. H., Tamagna, I. G., Horwitz, D., and Thomas, R.: Correlation of hypotensive effects and urinary tryptamine levels during pargyline therapy. Ann. N.Y. Acad. Sci. 107:958, 1963.
21. Gillespie, L., Terry, L. L., and Sjoerdsma, A.: The application of a monoamine-oxidase inhibitor, 1-phenyl-2-hydrazinopropane (JB-516), to the treatment of primary hypertension. Am. Heart J. 58:1, 1959.
22. Maxwell, M. H.: Observations pertinent to antihypertensive mechanisms of MAO inhibitors using *dl*-serine isopropylhydrazine. Ann. N.Y. Acad. Sci. 107:993, 1963.
23. Winsor, T.: Pargyline hydrochloride, hyper-

tension, urinary tryptamine and vascular reflexes. Geriatrics 19:598, 1964.
24. Bryant, J. M., Schvartz, N., Torosdag, S., Fertig, H., Fletcher, L., Jr., Schwartz, M. S., and Quan, R. B. F.: Long-term antihypertensive effect of pargyline HCl with and without diuretic sulfonamides. Ann. N.Y. Acad. Sci. 107:1023, 1963.
25. Everett, G. M., Wiegand, R. G., and Rinaldi, F. U.: Pharmacologic studies of some nonhydrazine MAO inhibitors. Ann. N.Y. Acad. Sci. 107:1068, 1963.
26. Hollander, W., and Wilkins, R. W.: *In* Moyer, J. (Ed.): Hypertension: First Hahnemann Symposium on Hypertensive Disease. Philadelphia: Saunders, 1959, p. 399.
27. Gertner, S. B.: The effects of monoamine oxidase inhibitors on ganglionic transmission. J. Pharmacol. Exp. Ther. 131:223, 1961.
28. Davey, M. J., Farmer, J. B., and Reinert, H.: Hypotension and monoamine oxidase inhibitors. Chemotherapia 4:314, 1962.
29. Levine, R. J.: Inhibition of monoamine activity in sympathetic ganglia of the cat. Biochem. Pharmacol. 11:395, 1962.
30. Urquiaga, X., Villarreal, J., Alonso de Florida, F., and Pardo, E. G.: On the ganglionic actions of certain anti-depressant drugs. Arch. Int. Pharmacodyn. Ther. 146:126, 1963.
31. Brest, A. N., Kodama, R., Dreifus, L., Weber, A., and Moyer, J. H.: Nialamide alone and in combination with thiazide derivatives in the treatment of essential hypertension. Am. J. Med. Sci. 241:199, 1961.
32. Spector, S., Gordon, R., Sjoerdsma, A., and Udenfriend, S.: End-product inhibition of tyrosine hydroxylase as a possible mechanism for regulation of norepinephrine synthesis. Mol. Pharmacol. 3:549, 1967.
33. Day, M. D., and Rand, M. J.: Tachyphylaxis to some sympathomimetic amines in relation to monoamine oxidase. Br. J. Pharmacol. 21: 84, 1963.
34. Kopin, I. J., Fischer, J. E., Musacchio, J. M., Horst, W. D., and Weise, V. K.: "False neurochemical transmitters" and the mechanism of sympathetic blockade by monoamine oxidase inhibitors. J. Pharmacol. Exp. Ther. 147:186, 1965.
35. Kakimoto, Y., and Armstrong, M. D.: On the identification of octopamine in mammals. J. Biol. Chem. 37:422, 1962.
36. Lands, A. M., and Grant, J. I.: Vasopressor action and toxicity of cyclohexylethylamine derivatives. J. Pharmacol. Exp. Ther. 106: 341, 1952.
37. Day, M. D., and Rand, M. J.: A hypothesis for the mode of action of alpha methyldopa in relieving hypertension. J. Pharm. Pharmacol. 15:221, 1963.
38. Onesti, G., Novack, P., Ramirez, O., Brest, A. N., and Moyer, J. H.: Hemodynamic effects of pargyline in hypertensive patients. Circulation 30:830, 1964.
39. Goldberg, L. I., Horwitz, D., and Sjoerdsma, A.: Attenuation of cardiovascular responses to exercise as a possible basis for the effectiveness of monoamine oxidase inhibitors in angina pectoris. J. Pharmacol. Exp. Ther. 137: 39, 1962.

PHARMACOLOGY AND CLINICAL USE OF BRETYLIUM AND BETHANIDINE IN HYPERTENSION

By SIR F. HORACE SMIRK, K.B.E., M.D.

BRETYLIUM TOSYLATE

BRETYLIUM TOSYLATE (*N*-ethyl-*N*-*o*-bromobenzyl-*N*, *N*-dimethylammonium tosylate) was first described by Boura et al.[1] It is rarely used now to reduce the blood pressure, but it represented a notable pharmacologic advance and when given intramuscularly, in recent years its antiarrhythmic action has found useful employment. Isotope studies show that it accumulates selectively in sympathetic neurones with adrenergic transmission, and in organs mainly innervated by the sympathetic system. It acts postganglionically, chiefly at sympathetic nerve endings. It blocks release of norepinephrine from the nerve endings, but it does not stop the action of norepinephrine. The pressor responses to tyramine and ephedrine are unaffected thus providing indirect evidence that bretylium does not deplete catecholamines from nerve endings. In this it differs, on similar evidence, from guanethidine.

Conway,[2] Kirkendall and Wilson,[3] and Freis, Sugiura, and Liptak[4] showed that bretylium reduces or abolishes the post-Valsalva hypertensive overshoot and Freis and his colleagues have reported that it decreases reactions to the cold pressor test. As with most drugs reducing sympathetic activity, there is a fall in cardiac output, probably due to dilatation of veins, causing a fall of pressure in the venous reservoir.

The great interest of bretylium at the time of its introduction was that unlike the ganglion blockers it did not affect the parasympathetic nervous system and thereby did not cause dry mouth, seriously blurred vision, constipation or paralytic ileus. It has been replaced by such drugs as bethanidine and debrisoquine, which for the reduction of blood pressure are vastly superior. At the time it was introduced and by skillful combination with other drugs advantage could be taken of its pharmacologic properties and patients thereby made more comfortable. Bretylium had a peculiar side effect, namely, in some patients it produced parotid pain, which sometimes did not disappear for as much as a year or more after withdrawal of the drug.

In the treatment of hypertension by orally administered bretylium Smirk and Hodge[5] reported that single effective doses are seldom as low as 100 mg and may exceed 600 mg. Drug toleration makes it necessary to raise the dosage periodically until full toleration has developed, and in exceptional instances as much as 2,800 mg daily was needed to maintain effective blood pressure reduction. Unexpectedly large variations of response occur on large oral doses.

Leveque[6] described an antiarrhythmic action of bretylium in 1965 and Bacaner and Schreinemachers[7,8] noted that bretylium decreased the vulnerability of the heart to experimental ventricular fibrillation, induced electrically or by hypothermia, and that when administered intramuscularly, bretylium decreased the spontaneous occurrence of ventricular fibrillation in humans, more particularly in the ventricular fibrillation associated with coronary artery disease. The substance also has a positive inotropic effect and is therefore not contraindicated when shock and heart failure are present. This observation on an antiarrhythmic effect may be connected with the blocking of sympathetic nerve endings in the heart, altering the responsiveness to various fibrillatory stimuli. It is unlikely to be related to any catecholamine depletion affecting the heart. It could be that the reduction

---

From Department of Medicine, Wellcome Medical Research Institute, University of Otago Medical School, Dunedin, New Zealand.

This work was supported by a grant from The Medical Research Council of New Zealand.

in sympathetic stimulation alters the responsiveness of the cardiac muscle.

There is a great deal more to be said about the pharmacology and about the clinical problems associated with bretylium and it will be of great interest to know whether bretylium itself or some better substance with similar properties can be used for the prevention as distinct from the treatment of arrhythmias. There are important reasons why this should be reconsidered because in our clinic and in some others coronary artery disease (e.g., sudden death, probably but not proved to be due to coronary disease) has become the main cause of death in treated hypertensives; actually in 42 percent of such deaths.[9] Many of these coronary deaths were sudden and any substances preventing the occurrence of sudden death, presumably by ventricular fibrillation, would appreciably reduce the mortality from hypertensive disease. These deaths involve hypertensive patients who otherwise have been doing well and showed no sign of an impending catastrophe.

While there appears to be no doubt about the action of bretylium when administered intramuscularly, I have seen no reports of an antifibrillatory action when the drug is administered by mouth. I examined the records of some half-dozen hypertensives, treated by orally administered bretylium, who had previous electrocardiograms with frequent premature systoles and was unable to find evidence of a substantial diminution in these.

BETHANIDINE

Soon after Boura et al.[10,11] described bethanidine (*N*-benzyl-N′, N″-dimethylguanidine; Esbatal) it became evident that this substance represented a major clinical as well as a pharmacologic advance. Superficially its mode of action appears to resemble that of bretylium, in that it blocks the endings of sympathetic nerves and prevents the release of the neurotransmitter; as for example, during stimulation of the splenic nerve of cats. Far from preventing the response of smooth muscle to epinephrine and norepinephrine, it increases the response, and also increases the response to doses of tyramine, thus indicating that there is no important depletion of catecholamines. Very industrious long-term administration of bethanidine did depress the pressor amine content of heart and spleen but this action does not appear to be important clinically.

Administered intravenously, it resembles bretylium in causing a temporary rise in blood pressure. An important pharmacologic difference between guanethidine and bethanidine is that guanethidine definitely depletes sympathetic amines and causes an enhancement of the responses to pressor amines in man. This can be a source of considerable danger if a patient with pheochromocytoma is by mischance treated with guanethidine. Like bretylium, bethanidine reduces the Valsalva overshoot.

Clinically bethanidine is a powerful and useful hypotensive agent,[12–14] certainly one of the most valuable of the strong drugs. It differs from guanethidine in having a shorter period of action, so that two or more, usually three, doses a day are advisable. But this can be an advantage in that, by adjusting the night dose, it is usually possible to avoid the symptom of morning hypotension. It has a more rapid action than guanethidine and does not produce diarrhea. Its rapid action is particularly valuable in malignant hypertension, where the blood pressure can be brought under control within 1 day by a combination of nursing in the upright sitting posture and rapid escalation of the dose of bethanidine. When the blood pressure has fallen to about 160 mm Hg systolic, further falls can be prevented or controlled by alteration of the posture. When the patient's reaction to blood pressure reduction has become apparent, further but slower reduction to a more satisfactory level can be undertaken.

Where there is no urgency, 10 mg is a suitable initial single dose and this may be raised as required by 5-mg increments. In malignant hypertension one may give an initial dose of even 30 mg followed by 10-mg increments every 2 hours until the pressure is approaching 160 mm Hg systolic in the sitting posture. The maximum fall in blood pressure with an effective dose usually occurs between 4 and 5 hours after administration, and a fully effective dose may reduce the blood pressure for approximately 12 hours. Ordinarily a dose is given about 8 A.M. and at bedtime but often it is necessary to give a supplementary dose about 2 P.M. to prevent a rise of blood pressure in the afternoon and early evening.

I had experience with about 200 patients taking bethanidine and many more patients have now been treated in our Dunedin clinic by Professor Simpson and his colleagues. A systematic study of bethanidine was made in 56 of the patients.[15] Later results on a larger number of patients did not differ in any important way. It was found that approximately one-third of the patients could be well managed on bethanidine alone, but a combination with a thiazide diuretic made it possible to reduce the dose of bethanidine and, on the whole, better results were obtained with the combination. The daily mean dose of bethanidine was about 65 mg.

The average casual blood pressure of our patients before the drug was 214.9/123.0. Using bethanidine alone, 26 out of 56 had standing blood pressures mostly below 150/95, nine had several readings of 160/95 or more, and 18 were usually above 160/95. In general a combination with thiazides gave a better blood pressure control. The pulse rate was not significantly affected by bethanidine.

It is desirable to regulate the magnitude of the two or three daily doses individually in order to obtain maximal control over the blood pressure throughout the 24-hour day.

Side Effects

Regarding side effects [15,16] there is, of course, postural hypotension as with all drugs impairing sympathetic nervous activity. Failure of ejaculation may occur and sometimes impotence, especially in older persons. Diarrhea is most unusual and no instances of jaw pain have been encountered as with bretylium.

Drug toleration occurs, and the average increase in the dose is to about twice the initial effective dose. This degree of drug toleration is rarely sufficient to interfere with the conduct of treatment. In the course of the initial study we found an example of mild thrombocytopenia [14] but we subsequently obtained information that the thrombocytopenia had been present before the administration of bethanidine. One other example of mild thrombocytopenia occurred which cleared up on stopping the drug. Since then no further example has been encountered nor so far as we know reported, and the relationship may well have been coincidental but we felt we had to report it.

Side effects can be reduced and improved blood-pressure control obtained by various combinations of bethanidine and other drugs which have been discussed in detail by Simpson and Hodge.[17,18]

ACKNOWLEDGMENT

I am indebted to Mrs. Joy Tomlin for her secretarial help in the preparation of this chapter and to Professor F. O. Simpson, who has been most helpful to me in the discussion of problems in the field of hypertension. I am grateful to Dr. John Hunter, professor of medicine in the Medical School, Dunedin, for generous facilities within the Wellcome Medical Research Institute.

REFERENCES

1. Boura, A. L. A., Green, A. F., McCoubrey, A., Laurence, D. R., Moulton, R., and Rosenheim, M. L.: Darenthin: hypotensive agent of new type. Lancet 2:17, 1959.
2. Conway, J.: Clinical pharmacology of bretylium tosylate: Preliminary observations. Ann. New York Acad. Sci. 88:956, 1960.
3. Kirkendall, W. M., and Wilson, W. R.: Pharmacodynamics and clinical use of guanethidine, bretylium and methyldopa. Am. J. Cardiol. 9:107, 1962.
4. Freis, E. D., Sugiura, T., and Liptak, D.: Selective inhibition of the sympathetic nervous system in man with bretylium tosylate, a new antihypertensive agent. Circulation 22:191, 1960.
5. Smirk, F. H., and Hodge, J. V.: Hypotensive action of bretylium tosylate. Lancet 2:673, 1959.
6. Leveque, P. E.: Anti-arrhythmic action of bretylium. Nature 207:203, 1965.
7. Bacaner, M. B.: Bretylium tosylate for suppression of induced ventricular fibrillation. Am. J. Cardiol. 17:528, 1966.
8. Bacaner, M., and Schreinemachers, D.: Bretylium tosylate for suppression of ventricular fibrillation after experimental myocardial infarction. Nature 220:494, 1968.
9. Smirk, F. H., and Hodge, J. V.: Causes of death in treated hypertensive patients. Br. Med. J. 2:1221, 1963.
10. Boura, A. L. A., Copp, F. C., Green, A. F.,

Hodson, H. F., Ruffell, G. K., Sim, M. F., Walton, E., and Grivsky, E. M.: Adrenergic neurone-blocking agents related to choline 2,6-xylyl ether bromide (TM 10), bretylium and guanethidine. Nature 191:1312, 1961.
11. Boura, A. L. A., and Green, A. F.: Adrenergic neurone blockade and other acute effects caused by *N*-benzyl-*N'N''*-dimethylguanidine and its ortho-chloro derivative. Br. J. Pharmacol. 20:36, 1963.
12. Montuschi, E., and Pickens, P. T.: A clinical trial of two related adrenergic-neurone-blocking agents—B.W. 392C60 and B.W. 467C60. Lancet 2:897, 1962.
13. Johnston, A. W., Prichard, B. N. C., and Rosenheim, M. L.: Adrenergic neurone-blocking agents. Lancet 2:996, 1962.
14. Smirk, F. H.: Hypotensive action of 467C60: A drug which blocks sympathetic neurones at a peripheral site. N. Z. Med. J. 61:608, 1962.
15. Smirk, F. H.: The hypotensive action of B.W. 467C60. Lancet 1:743, 1963.
16. Prichard, B. N., Johnston, A. W., Hill, I. D., and Rosenheim, M. L.: Bethanidine, guanethidine and methyldopa in treatment of hypertension: A within-patient comparison. Br. Med. J. 1:135, 1968.
17. Simpson, F. O., and Hodge, J. V.: Use of antihypertensive drugs in combination. *In* Schlittler, E. (Ed.): Antihypertensive agents. New York: Academic Press, 1967, pp. 459–482.
18. Simpson, F. O.: Combination antihypertensive therapy. Int. Cardiol. 2:38, 1970.

Management of the Ambulatory Patient with Uncomplicated Hypertension

By Kwan Eun Kim, M.D., Gaddo Onesti, M.D., and Charles Swartz, M.D.

WITH THE EXCEPTION of hypertensive emergencies and of the malignant phase of hypertension, the great majority of hypertensive patients are treated on an ambulatory basis in outpatient facilities. For this reason an outline of a comprehensive therapeutic regimen for the ambulatory patient with uncomplicated hypertension is included. The individual pharmacologic and clinical characteristics of the available antihypertensive drugs are discussed in detail elsewhere in this section of this book. In the present chapter the general therapeutic measures and the combination of drugs will be described. The therapeutic approach outlined has been used in the Hypertension Clinic of the Hahnemann Medical College and Hospital for several years.

General Considerations

The most recent Veterans Administration Cooperative Study [1] has demonstrated that active antihypertensive treatment significantly reduced morbidity and mortality in male hypertensive patients with diastolic pressure averaging 90 through 114 mm Hg. In this study, the difference in the incidence of morbid events between control and treated groups was significant in the subgroups with diastolic levels averaging 105 through 114 mm Hg and was favorable toward treatment, although not statistically significant in those entering with diastolic levels of 90 through 104 mm Hg.

While similar controlled studies are not available for female patients with mild hypertension, it is our opinion that blood pressure elevation, even if mild, is detrimental to the cardiovascular system and that therapy will be beneficial over the long term. It is our policy to treat all patients with sustained diastolic blood pressures above 90 mmHg. It therefore follows that we attempt to maintain the blood pressure of all patients below this level.

As the majority of the patients with mild or moderate hypertension are asymptomatic, it is our experience that they may be reluctant to remain on daily drug therapy for the rest of their lives. For this reason one of the most important steps in antihypertensive therapy is to explain to the patient the necessity of indefinite (lifetime) therapy in order to prevent serious cardiovascular complications and to prolong life. It is in fact well known that permanent remission of hypertension, following treatment, is extremely rare.[2] We emphasize the protective value of maintaining normal blood pressure and remind the patient that the absence of symptoms does not assure him of a normal blood pressure.

The majority of hypertensive patients without cardiac or cerebral complications do not need any restriction of activity. In fact not only is there no evidence of harmful effects of exercise in hypertensive patients, but it has been suggested that appropriately scheduled regular exercise may be beneficial.[3]

Obesity predisposes to blood pressure elevation,[4] and weight reduction of obese hypertensive patients significantly lowers blood pressure.[5] For this reason it is important that the overweight patient reduce his weight by an appropriate low-calorie diet.

It is well known that dietary restriction of sodium significantly reduces hypertension.[6,7] To achieve clinically meaningful results, the restriction must be below 500 mg sodium per day.[7] Such a restriction is extremely difficult for the ambulatory patient who continues his normal daily activities. For this reason the availability of the oral diuretics has been a

---

From the Division of Nephrology and Hypertension, Department of Medicine, The Hahnemann Medical College and Hospital, Philadelphia, Pennsylvania.

Supported in part by National Institutes of Health Grant No. T-12-HE-05878.

most important contribution to our present antihypertensive management. With the use of diuretics, dietary restriction of salt has become less important. We now advise the patient to avoid the saltier foods such as salt pork, potato chips and pretzels and not to add salt to table food. Some salt restriction is still required because it has been demonstrated that the antihypertensive efficacy of the oral diuretics may be significantly reduced by the concomitant administration of high-salt diet.[8]

Because of the vasoconstrictor effect of nicotine and of the harmful effects of smoking on coronary artery disease, we invariably discourage smoking.

The frequency of control visits for the hypertensive patient varies depending on the severity of hypertension and of its complications. A patient without complications should probably return for control visits every week until his hypertension is controlled and the dosage of his medications is titrated. He should subsequently be seen biweekly, and when the blood pressure is well controlled these visits can be reduced to one a month and then one every 2 to 4 months. Obviously the patient with severe hypertension may require visits weekly or even twice a week.

Home blood pressure recording is not routinely recommended. A small portion of our hypertensive patients who have intermittent orthostatic hypotension, or malignant phase of hypertension, record their pressures at home between office visits. They have been advised to adjust dosage of drugs at home by telephone calls between office visits.

After the preliminary steps and the instructions are completed, the hypertensive patient is placed into an arbitrary classification based on the level of diastolic pressure. Such a classification, although entirely arbitrary, has been a most useful guide for prescribing antihypertensive drug therapy for the individual patient. "Mild" hypertension is defined as diastolic pressure from 90 to 114 mm Hg. "Moderately severe" hypertension is defined as diastolic between 115 and 129 mm Hg and "severe" hypertension in any patient with a diastolic pressure greater than 130 mm Hg. This classification is based on at least three consecutive visits before therapy is started.

Therapeutic Principles

Three classes of antihypertensive drugs are currently used in our program for the management of the ambulatory patients: (1) oral diuretics; (2) sympathetic blockers; (3) direct peripheral vasodilators.

Diuretics

Of the various groups of antihypertensive drugs the oral diuretics have the greatest overall clinical usefulness (benzothiadiazines, phthalimidines, quinazoline, spironolactone, ethacrynic acid, furosemide). It is our policy to use one of the oral diuretics as initial and basic therapy because of the following reasons: (1) they lower the blood pressure in both supine and erect positions; (2) their antihypertensive effect is sustained despite prolonged administration; (3) they potentiate or enhance the effectiveness of all the other antihypertensive agents; (4) they have a low overall incidence of side effects.

Antihypertensive effects of benzothiadiazines (thiazides), phthalimidines (chlorthalidone), quinazoline (quinethazone), furosemide, and ethacrynic acid are comparable.[9–13] The antihypertensive effect of spironolactone in essential hypertension is comparable to[14] or less[15,16] than that of thiazides or chlorthalidone. It also has been shown that high doses of spironolactone are highly effective in lowering blood pressure in patients with primary aldosteronism[17] and in patients with essential hypertension who have a low plasma renin activity and a low aldosterone secretory rate.[18]

Sympathetic-Blocking Drugs

The sympathetic-blocking drugs commonly used in our therapeutic program include: alpha-methyldopa, guanethidine, *Rauwolfia* compounds, and pargyline. At this time our preference is to start with alpha-methyldopa. Other clinicians prefer to start with reserpine or guanethidine. The use of pargyline is rare in our program and reserved for those patients who cannot tolerate other drugs. As a group, the sympathetic-blocking drugs, with the exception of the orally administered *Rauwolfia,* produce an accentuated orthostatic antihypertensive effect. Now that we have become aware that the different sympathetic-blocking agents act by different mechanisms at different sites in the sympathetic nervous system, we have taken to adding a second sympathetic-blocking agent even when one is already in use. We have commonly added guanethidine to alpha-methyldopa with additive therapeutic effect.

Peripheral Vasodilators

Only hydralazine is currently available. It is our policy to use hydralazine only when a diuretic and a sympathetic blocker are present. The concomitant administration of a sympathetic blocker, in effective doses, prevents the reflex tachycardia produced by hydralazine and minimizes the complaints of palpitation, flushing, and headache.

MANAGEMENT OF MILD HYPERTENSION

A comprehensive therapeutic regimen for all ambulatory hypertensive patients is shown in Table 1.

For the mildly hypertensive patient it is our policy to start with one of the oral diuretics. Hydrochlorothiazide given in a 50-mg dose twice a day or chlorthalidone given in a 100-mg dose once a day are most commonly used. Other diuretics may be used with similar antihypertensive effects. Spironolactone may be successfully used when metabolic complications (diabetes, gout, etc.) or other side effects prevent the use of the other diuretic compounds.

Alpha-methyldopa should be added to the diuretic in starting dose of 250 mg to be given twice a day with a 250-mg increase at every office visit until a maximum of 3 gm daily has been prescribed or a satisfactory decrease in blood pressure obtained. In the majority of the mildly hypertensive patients a satisfactory response can be obtained with a diuretic plus alpha-methyldopa less than 1.0 gm daily. If the patient develops orthostatic hypotension with uncontrolled supine blood pressure, the dosage of alpha-methyldopa should be reduced and hydralazine should be added. The initial dose of hydralazine is 10 mg given four times a day. If an adequate response has not been obtained after an initial dose, the dosage of hydralazine should be increased over a 2-week period by increments of 25 mg every 3 to 4 days until a total of 100 mg administered four times a day is reached or an adequate blood pressure decrease is achieved. Hydralazine should be used cautiously for patients who have overt coronary artery disease and congestive heart

TABLE 1.—*Comprehensive Antihypertensive Regimen for Ambulatory Patients with Hypertension*

Severity of Hypertension	*Initial Therapy*	*First Adjunctive Therapy When Initial Therapy is Inadequate*	*Second Adjunctive Therapy When the First Adjunctive Therapy is Inadequate*
Mild: Diastolic blood pressure greater than 90 mm Hg but less than 115 mm Hg	Diuretic	Alpha-methyldopa or *Rauwolfia*	Hydralazine
Moderately severe: Diastolic blood pressure greater than 115 mm Hg but less than 130 mm Hg	Diuretic and alpha-methyldopa or diuretic and *Rauwolfia*	Hydralazine	Guanethidine
Severe: Diastolic blood pressure greater than 130 mm Hg	Diuretic and alpha-methyldopa or diuretic and guanethidine (alternatively diuretic and pargyline may be used in patients not tolerating other drugs)	Hydralazine	Guanethidine or alpha-methyldopa (whichever is not used in initial therapy)

failure because hydralazine increases cardiac output and heart rate.

An alternative antihypertensive drug to alpha-methyldopa in mildly hypertensive patients is one of the *Rauwolfia* compounds. A number of preparations of *Rauwolfia* compounds are currently available, including the single pure alkaloids of *Rauwolfia serpentina* (deserpidine, rescinnamine, and reserpine), various preparations containing multiple active alkaloids (alseroxylon and whole root) and synthetic reserpine-like analogues (syrosingopine). There is little difference in the antihypertensive responses obtained with these various derivatives.[19]

Reserpine in a 0.25-mg dose, given twice a day, or the equivalent dose of a *Rauwolfia* compound should be added to the diuretic. If an adequate response has not been achieved with a diuretic and *Rauwolfia,* hydralazine should be added as described above.

Management of Moderately Severe Hypertension

The principle in management of moderately severe hypertension is essentially the same as that of mildly hypertensive patients. However, we start the double-drug regimen as an initial therapy and treat more aggressively and use a four-drug regimen if necessary. One of the thiazide diuretics such as hydrochlorothiazide given in a 50-mg dose twice a day and alpha-methyldopa given in a 250-mg dose twice a day are the initial treatment (Table 1). If a satisfactory response is not obtained, the dosage of alpha-methyldopa should be increased by increments of 250 mg to 500 mg at every office visit until a satisfactory response is obtained or a maximum of 3 gm daily has been prescribed. If a satisfactory response is not obtained, hydralazine should be added as described above. By adding hydralazine, the dosage of alpha-methyldopa may be reduced, and a satisfactory control of supine pressure and a reversal of orthostatic hypotension may be achieved.

If a satisfactory response is not obtained with a three-drug regimen (thiazide, alpha-methyldopa, and hydralazine), guanethidine may be added. It should be given as a single morning dose of 10 mg, increased at weekly intervals by 10 mg until the desired blood pressure is obtained. Guanethidine usually reduces blood pressure more in the standing than in the supine position. Both supine and standing pressure must be taken in those patients who are taking alpha-methyldopa, guanethidine, or other antihypertensive drugs which induce orthostatic hypotension.

Alternative initial double-drug regimen of a diuretic and alpha-methyldopa in moderately severe hypertension consists of a diuretic and a *Rauwolfia* compound (Table 1). If a desirable response has not been achieved with these, hydralazine should be added as described above. Guanethidine may be added if a satisfactory response has not been obtained with these three-drug regimens.

Management of Severe Hypertension

For the management of the patient with severe hypertension (diastolic blood pressure greater than 130 mm Hg) it is necessary to start with the more potent drugs from the beginning. The oral diuretic is used as a general background therapy. Alpha-methyldopa is the drug most commonly used with the diuretic in our program. The dosage of the latter should be increased more rapidly until satisfactory blood pressure is observed or the side effects become prohibitive. Maximum doses of alpha-methyldopa used are 3 gm per day. An alternative potent sympathetic inhibitor to be used in combination with the diuretic is guanethidine, in a 20-to 25-mg dose per day with careful dose titration. Although rarely used, pargyline is available, and represents a useful alternative for the patient who cannot tolerate other sympathetic-blocking drugs. Because of their limited antihypertensive potency the *Rauwolfia* compounds are not employed for the treatment of severe hypertension in our program.

If the desirable response is not observed, a three-drug regimen should be used and hydralazine is then added. Hydralazine is prescribed in increasing doses from 25 mg, given four times a day, to 100 mg given four times a day.

The next step is a four-drug regimen: a diuretic, alpha-methyldopa, hydralazine, and guanethidine.

A more potent diuretic such as furosemide or ethacrynic acid may be used instead of the thiazide derivatives in patients with impairment of renal function or congestive heart failure. Furosemide or ethacrynic acid may be combined with spironolactone for potentiating effect and for reestablishing potassium balance.

Advantages and Disadvantages of Combined Drug Therapy

Appropriate combinations of antihypertensive agents result in additive antihypertensive effects in many instances. True potentiation may be achieved by combining drugs with different sites of action. Combination of drugs makes it possible to reduce the individual drug dosage with possible decreased incidence of severe side effects. In addition the pharmacologic effect of one drug may correct the side effects of another: e.g., the sympathetic-inhibiting effect of *Rauwolfia* or alpha-methyldopa or guanethidine prevents the reflex tachycardia produced by hydralazine. The addition of hydralazine to guanethidine or alpha-methyldopa allows a decrease of dosage of the sympathetic inhibitors and minimizes their orthostatic antihypertensive effect. The net result is a better overall control of supine and erect blood pressures. In patients in whom potassium losses are of immediate clinical importance the administration of oral diuretics may represent a potential danger. In that situation the combination of a thiazide diuretic or ethacrynic acid or furosemide with spironolactone or triamterene is probably the best therapeutic maneuver to minimize potassium imbalance.

Inappropriate combinations of drugs may actually worsen side effects and may even aggravate hypertension. The combination of *Rauwolfia* and alpha-methyldopa may aggravate drowsiness and fatigue. Since guanethidine, alpha-methyldopa, and reserpine all may initially release norepinephrine from adrenergic neurons, there exists the theoretical possibility that they might produce paradoxical hypertension in a patient already taking a MAO inhibitor.[20–23] We have not given any of these agents to patients already on pargyline.

Despite our extensive use of combined drug therapy, we do not routinely employ combination tablets nor do we recommend them. In fact, combination tablets make it difficult to adjust the dosage of one agent without simultaneously changing the others. In addition when the patient develops an adverse reaction to the drug, the physician does not know which of the combination is the offending agent and therefore has to stop the combination tablet and find a new drug regimen for the patient.

Conclusions

Although we have outlined a comprehensive drug regimen for the ambulatory hypertensive patient, depending primarily on severity of hypertension, this regimen is not rigidly fixed. The ideal regimen for hypertension is the one that produces sustained normal blood pressure without any adverse reaction. The physician must therefore select the ideal drug or combination of drugs for the individual clinical situation.

While the search for the ideal antihypertensive drug continues (see Part VI of this book) the combinations of drugs described above will control the blood pressure of the majority of ambulatory hypertensive patients. In addition to the introduction of new drugs, the acquisition of knowledge of combined drug therapy has been one of the most significant contributions to drug therapy of hypertension in the last decade.

References

1. Veterans Administration Cooperative Study Group on Antihypertensive Agents: Effects of treatment on morbidity in hypertension. II. Results in patients with diastolic blood pressure averaging 90 through 114 mm Hg. JAMA 213:1143, 1970.
2. Dustan, H. P., Page, I. H., Tarazi, R. C., and Frohlich, E. D.: Arterial pressure responses to discontinuing antihypertensive drugs. Circulation 37:370, 1968.
3. Boyer, J. L., and Kosch, F. W.: Exercise therapy in hypertensive men. JAMA 211: 1668, 1970.
4. Kannel, W. B., Brand, N., Skinner, J. J., Jr., Dawber, T. R., and McNamara, P. M.: The relation of adiposity to blood pressure and development of hypertension. The Framingham Study. Ann. Intern. Med. 67:48, 1967.

5. Fletcher, A. P.: The effect of weight reduction upon the blood pressure of obese hypertensive women. Q. J. Med. 23:331, 1954.
6. Grollman, A., Harrison, T. R., Mason, M. F., Baxter, J., Crampton, J., and Reichman, F.: Sodium restriction in the diet for hypertension. JAMA 129:533, 1945.
7. Corcoran, A. C., Tyler, R. D., and Page, I. H.: Controlled observations on the effect of low sodium diet therapy in essential hypertension. Circulation 3:1, 1951.
8. Weiner, B. M.: Electrolyte alteration during diuretic therapy. Desirable and undesirable effects. *In* Brest, A. N., and Moyer, J. H. (Eds.): Hypertension: Recent Advances. Philadelphia: Lea & Febiger, 1961, pp. 274–282.
9. Wertheimer, L., Finnerty, F. A., Jr., Bercu, B. A., and Hall, R. H.: Furosemide in essential hypertension. A statistical analysis of three double-blind studies. Arch. Intern. Med. 127:934, 1971.
10. Russell, R. P., Lindeman, R. D., and Prescott, L. F.: Metabolic and hypotensive effects of ethacrynic acid. Comparative study with hydrochlorothiazide. JAMA 205:81, 1968.
11. Brest, A. N., and Moyer, J. H.: Clinical use of diuretics in hypertension. *In* Brest, A. N., and Moyer, J. H. (Eds.): Hypertension: Recent Advances. Philadelphia: Lea & Febiger, 1961, pp. 250–255.
12. Brest, A. N., Onesti, G., Seller, R., Ramirez, O., Heider, C., and Moyer, J. H.: Pharmacodynamic effects of a new diuretic drug, ethacrynic acid. Am. J. Cardiol. 16:99, 1965.
13. Kim, K. E., Onesti, G., Moyer, J. H., and Swartz, C.: Ethacrynic acid and furosemide. Diuretic and hemodynamic effects and clinical uses. Am. J. Cardiol. 27:407, 1971.
14. Winer, B. M., Lubbe, W. F., and Colton, T.: Antihypertensive actions of diuretics. Comparative study of an aldosterone antagonist and a thiazide, alone and together. JAMA 204:117, 1968.
15. Friis, T. H., Lintrup, J., and Nissen, N. I.: Comparative studies on spironolactone (Aldactone) and chlorthalidone (Hygroton) in the treatment of arterial hypertension. Acta Med. Scand. 179:371, 1966.
16. Johnson, L. C., and Grieble, H. G.: Treatment of arterial hypertensive disease with diuretics. V. Spironolactone, an aldosterone antagonist. Arch. Intern. Med. 119:225, 1967.
17. Spark, R. F., and Melby, J. C.: Aldosteronism in hypertension. The spironolactone response test. Ann. Intern. Med. 69:685, 1968.
18. Spark, R. F., and Melby, J. C.: Hypertension and low plasma renin activity: Presumptive evidence for mineralocorticoid excess. Ann. Intern. Med. 75:831, 1971.
19. Moyer, J. H., Dennis, E., and Ford, R. V.: Drug therapy (*Rauwolfia*) of hypertension. Arch. Intern. Med. 96:530, 1955.
20. Van Rossum, J. M.: Potential dangers of monoamine oxidase inhibitors and α-methyldopa. Lancet 1:950, 1963.
21. Natarajan, S.: Potential danger of monoamine oxidase inhibitors and α-methyldopa. Lancet 1:1330, 1964.
22. Solomon, H. W.: Clinical disorders of drug interaction. Adv. Intern. Med. 16:285, 1970.
23. Brest, A. N.: Clinical pharmacology of antihypertensive drugs. Cardiovasc. Clin. 1:196, 1969.

Part VI. RECENT ADVANCES IN DRUG THERAPY

The Use of Beta-Adrenergic Blockade in Hypertension

By Edward D. Frohlich, M.D.

IN THE QUARTER-CENTURY that has elapsed since the advent of modern drug therapy for hypertension, it has become possible to effectively maintain arterial pressure at normal levels and thereby significantly reduce the morbidity and mortality from hypertensive cardiac and vascular disease.[1–3] These antihypertensive drugs reduce arterial pressure by three means: relaxation of arterial smooth muscle (principally in arterioles); inhibition of the adrenergic nervous system; and, with diuretics, by virtue of their natriuretic and volume-depleting properties as well as by additional, possibly direct vascular factors (yet to be identified precisely).

With respect to the array of the last two classes of drugs it has become possible to dissect the autonomic nervous system pharmacologically, and to inhibit renal function at a variety of levels in the nephron. Thus, with respect to autonomic-inhibiting drugs one may suppress cerebral, hypothalamic, ganglionic, adrenergic, parasympathetic, or receptor-site action; and with the variety of diuretics one can augment glomerular filtration or inhibit proximal and distal tubular sodium reabsorption or reabsorption at the loop of Henle (Table 1).

Such sophistication of pharmacologic tools has demanded a definite clinical price (over and above the material cost at the drug store). These agents have become more potent, and they are associated with potentially hazardous situations if the physician does not fully understand the mechanism of the drug action and the pathophysiologic circumstances for which the agent is prescribed.

From the Departments of Medicine and of Physiology and Biophysics, College of Medicine, University of Oklahoma Health Sciences Center, Oklahoma City, Oklahoma.

Pharmacology

With release of the neurotransmitter effector substances (i.e., for the most part, norepinephrine) two receptor sites on vascular smooth muscle or myocardial muscle membrane are stimulated. Langley[4] and Dale[5] initially described these effector sites as vasoexcitatory or inhibitory; but more recently, in 1948, Alquist suggested the current terminology of the alpha- or beta-adrenotropic receptors.[6]

Thus, with the release of norepinephrine from the nerve ending (or with the administration of sympathomimetic drugs) either alpha- or beta-adrenergic receptor sites will be stimulated. Alpha-receptor stimulation will produce arteriolar or venular constriction;[7] and those few alpha-adrenergic receptor sites in the myocardium will produce a positive inotropic effect.[8] In contrast, following beta-adrenergic stimulation there are arteriolar dilation, possible venodilation,[9] and increased myocardial inotropic, chronotropic, and metabolic activity.[7] Conversely, those agents which inhibit alpha-adrenergic activity will promote primarily vasodilatation; and those which inhibit beta-adrenergic activity will decrease cardiac rate and myocardial contractility and promote a mild degree of vasoconstriction. The most specific alpha-adrenergic agonists are methoxamine or phenylephrine, and the most specific beta-adrenergic agonist is isoproterenol. The two most commonly used alpha-adrenergic antagonists (or "blockers") are phentolamine and phenoxybenzamine; the most commonly used beta-adrenergic antagonist, and the only one presently commercially available in the United States is propranolol (Table 1).

There may be more than one type of beta-adrenergic receptor site since a newly synthesized congener of propranolol has been shown to selectively inhibit only the myocardial

TABLE 1.—*Autonomic-Inhibiting and Natriuretic Drugs*

Autonomic-Inhibiting Drugs			*Diuretics and Natriuretics*	
Level	*Stimulant*	*Inhibitor*	*Level*	*Example*
Cerebral-hypothalamic	Amphetamines	Barbiturates; antidepressants	Renal blood flow	Digitalis; xanthines; aminophylline
Medulla	Pentylenemetrazol; ethamivan	Phenothiazines	Glomerulus (filtration rate)	Water load; osmotic diuresis
Ganglion	Tetraethylammonium; nicotine; dimethylphenylpiperazinium	Hexamethonium; pentolinium; trimethaphan	Proximal tubule	Mercurials; thiazide congeners
Parasympathetic	Acetylcholine; choline esters	Atropine	Loop of Henle	Furosemide; ethacrynic acid
Adrenergic post-ganglionic neuron	Tyramine; ephedrine; cocaine	Reserpine; alpha-methyldopa; guanethidine; bethanidine	Distal tubule	Thiazide congeners; spironolactone; triamterene; carbonic anhydrase inhibitors (all different action)
Alpha-adrenergic receptor	Phenylephrine; methoxamine	Phentolamine; phenoxybenzamine		
Beta-adrenergic receptor	Isoproterenol	Propranolol; practolol		

It is now possible, with the variety of autonomic-inhibiting and natriuretic drugs, to dissect pharmacologically every level of the autonomic nervous system or of the fuctioning nephron, respectively. The above-listed agents best exemplify these functions, although the reader is cautioned that no drug has but one action.

beta-adrenergic receptor sites, leaving the other beta-adrenergic receptor sites in the bronchi and vascular smooth muscle free to be stimulated.[10] The nature of the beta-adrenergic receptor still must be described more completely; nevertheless, current belief is that it involves the adenyl cyclase 3′,5′-cyclic adenosine monophosphate system.[11,12]

As indicated, a number of compounds capable of inhibiting beta-adrenergic receptors have been synthesized. The first was pronethalol; but because it was found to have oncogenic effects in mice its clinical use soon was discontinued.[13] Nevertheless, this compound reportedly reduced arterial pressure in hypertensive man.[14] Its successor, propranolol, has been used clinically since 1964 as an antihypertensive agent [15] but to date its clinical usefulness has been approved by the United States Food and Drug Administration only for cardiac arrhythmias, idiopathic hypertrophic subaortic stenosis, and pheochromocytoma.[16] At present many other beta-adrenergic blocking drugs are under laboratory and clinical investigation; and these compounds, including propranolol, are also being evaluated for other cardiovascular conditions including hypertension (other than pheochromocytoma), angina pectoris from coronary arterial (atherosclerotic) disease, and the cardiovascular manifestations of thyrotoxicosis.

For the past 6 years we have been investigating the effects of the beta-adrenergic blocking drugs in patients with a wide variety of forms of hypertension. Because propranolol has been the most widely studied, this discussion concerning the effects of beta-adrenergic blockade in hypertension will be confined to this one agent when used alone without the additional effects from other antihypertensive or diuretic agents.

Hyperdynamic Beta-adrenergic Circulatory State

One of the first types of hypertension, for which we found beta-adrenergic blocking therapy extremely helpful, was in a group of patients who had, as their primary complaint, an unrelenting and disturbing cardiac awareness manifested by an intolerably rapid and forceful cardiac action.[17] Usually, these individuals were confined to bed (or extremely restricted in their daily activities) because even minimal exertion or upright posture so augmented heart rate and force of ventricular contraction that these routine functions seemed intolerable. In fact, even the supine, resting heart rate was more rapid than that of an otherwise normal group of age-matched subjects. In addition, when these individuals were studied hemodynamically, they had evidence of a hyperkinetic circulation, i.e., increased cardiac output, left ventricular ejection rate, and heart rate (Fig. 1). Other patients have reported a persistent exercise tachycardia and palpitations remaining inordinately long after cessation of even mild exercise. Some patients demonstrate a systolic ejection-type murmur, a finding which together with the hemodynamic studies, was not unlike the hyperkinetic heart syndrome described by Gorlin.[18] Whereas the chest radiograph may be normal, the electrocardiogram can show sinus tachycardia, ST-segment and minor T-wave changes, and even premature atrial beats. Some patients had low-grade temperature elevations. When the beta-adrenergic agonist isoproterenol was infused intravenously these patients had an inappropriate and exaggerated cardioacceleration, in addition to an unusual emotional response (often frank hysteria).[17,19] Since these patients demonstrated a hyperkinetic circulation and were able to have their symptoms provoked and mimicked by beta-adrenergic receptor-site stimulation (with isoproterenol), both of which were prevented with beta-adrenergic blocking drugs (with return of the patient to gainful activity), we referred to this syndrome as a "hyperdynamic beta-adrenergic circulatory state."

We have not suggested that this is a new disease; nor have we believed it to be a separate and discrete form of hypertension.[20] It merely has been a convenient way of categorizing certain hypertensive patients according to the presence of one predominant pressor mechanism, i.e., a hyperkinetic circulation manifested by increased responsiveness of the beta-adrenergic nervous component. Included among the clinical types of hypertension have been patients with labile or "borderline" hypertension, mild and moderately severe essential hypertension (we have deliberately excluded

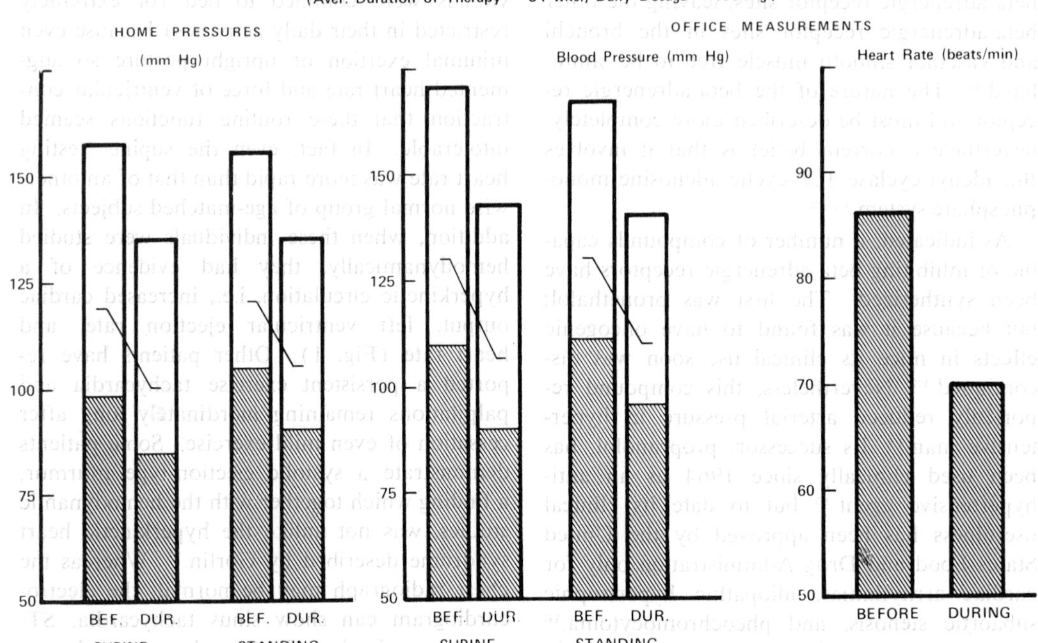

FIG. 1.—Response of long-term propranolol therapy in hypertensive patients. Home measurements represent the averages obtained from 39 patients who took their own pressures at home twice daily for an average of 54 weeks; only two failed to demonstrate a reduction in pressure. Office measurements represent the average for the 43 patients studied; and all had a fall in pressure. The **diagonal lines** represent the reduction in mean arterial pressure, represented by **horizontal lines** in the vertical bars.

patients with history of cardiac failure, reduced cardiac output, and severe disease from treatment with beta-adrenergic blocking drugs), and patients with renal arterial disease. We have also observed this syndrome in normotensive individuals.[17] The diagnosis, therefore, does not presume to ascribe an etiology for the hypertension; it merely indicates those specific pressor mechanisms which seem to participate in an exaggerated fashion in certain hypertensive patients. It should be emphasized that these neural functions operate in otherwise normal individuals to maintain normal cardiovascular function; however, in these patients the fine balance of the myriad of interrelating pressor mechanisms has been disrupted, and the resulting hypertension is but one manifestation of this loss of homeostasis. Indeed, this symptom complex seems quite similar to other imprecisely defined diagnoses, including neurocirculatory asthenia, functional disorder of the heart, irritable heart syndrome, cardiac neurosis, disordered action of the heart, soldier's heart, and effort syndrome, among many others.

In summary, patients displaying findings of this syndrome have the following characteristics in common: complaints of persistently disturbing cardiac awareness; hyperkinetic circulation; provocation of these symptoms by either physiologic (e.g., upright posture, exercise) or pharmacologic (e.g., isoproterenol) stimulation; inappropriate emotional response to isoproterenol infusion (but not when heart rate is increased by other mechanisms, e.g., atropine); and remission of all findings with beta-adrenergic blocking therapy.

Other Hypertensive Patients

Having demonstrated that beta-adrenergic mechanisms seem to participate more in certain hypertensive patients than others, and having indicated that there are certain clinical, physiologic, and pharmacologic characteristics of hypertensive patients which might render them more amenable to antihypertensive drug therapy with beta-adrenergic blocking drugs, we outlined certain criteria for preselection of hypertensive patients for beta-adrenergic blocking therapy.[21,22] We believed that with the inherent dangers of this new form of therapy in hypertension this cautious beginning might obviate many potential complications. From the general hypertensive population, 28 patients were selected for propranolol therapy using three criteria: symptoms of cardiac awareness; hemodynamic characteristics of hyperkinetic circulation; and an exaggerated cardioaccelerator response to isoproterenol infusion.[21] On the basis of these criteria 22 of the 28 patients responded to propranolol. Moreover, using these preselection criteria we have not yet observed any of the expected "side" or "adverse" effects in any of our patients to date. However, we have noted in two patients having a history of Raynaud's phenomenon signs of impending digital gangrene;[23] we have subsequently added this contraindication to our preselection of patients.

In the past several years we have had the opportunity to evaluate and treat 43 additional hypertensive patients (Table 2), and with these preselection criteria only two patients failed to respond to this treatment program. Included in this more recent group are 18 men and 25 women; 34 have either mild or moderately severe essential hypertension and nine have renal arterial disease. Their average age was 40 years (range: 17 to 55 years old).

TABLE 2.—*Clinical Characteristics of 43 Hypertensive Patients Treated with Propranolol*

Number of patients	43
Age (years)	
Average	40
Range	17 to 55
Sex	
Men	18
Women	25
Diagnosis	
Essential hypertension	34
Renal arterial disease	9
Propranolol therapy	
Average duration	54 weeks
Average daily dose	160 mg

TABLE 3.—*Physiologic Characteristics of Patients Treated with Propranolol*

Physiologic Characteristic	*Patients*	*Normal*
Pressures (mm Hg)		
Systolic arterial	166	under 140
Diastolic arterial	98	under 90
Mean arterial	121	under 100
Heart rate (beats per minute)	83	68 ± 2
Cardiac index (milliliters per minute per M^2)	3565	3048 ± 92
Left ventricular ejection rate index (milliliters per second per M^2)	158	151 ± 3.1
Isoproterenol cardioacceleration (beats per minute)	36	12 ± 4

Not all of these patients received pretreatment isoproterenol infusion either because of the presence of frequent premature atrial contractions, already existing tachycardia, or the patient's refusal to accept hemodynamic and/or isoproterenol-infusion studies. Nevertheless, isoproterenol was infused intravenously in sequentially increasing dosages of 0.01, 0.02, and 0.03 μg per kilogram of body weight per minute in 25 patients. The infusion was discontinued prematurely only if we believed that inappropriately exaggerated cardioacceleration had been demonstrated; if further increase in heart rate would not be to the patient's advantage; or if the patient was so disturbed by the infusion that its discontinuance was deemed mandatory. At the highest rate of infusion, heart rate increased an average of 36 beats per minute, a degree much greater than that of an otherwise normal population.[20]

The pretreatment hemodynamic characteristics of these patients are presented in Table 3. Associated with the increased arterial pressures (systolic 166, diastolic 98, and mean 121 mm Hg) was an increased resting, supine cardiac index (3.6 liters per minute per M^2), heart rate (83 beats per minute), and a left ventricular ejection rate index at the upper limits of normal (158 ml per second per M^2). Whereas most of the patients treated with propranolol demonstrated evidence of a hyperkinetic circulation and an exaggerated cardioaccelerator response to isoproterenol, only 12 were categorized as demonstrating all of the characteristics of the hyperdynamic beta-adrenergic circulatory state. These 43 patients have been treated an average of 54 weeks (range: 4 to 120 weeks) using only one drug, propranolol; the average daily dose was 160 mg.

On this treatment program systolic and diastolic arterial pressures were reduced in all 43 hypertensive patients on the basis of resting, sitting, and standing pressures taken in the physician's office, and in 37 of the 39 patients who obtained records of their blood pressures at home (twice daily in the supine and standing positions). Pretreatment and treatment values for these home blood pressure measurements are defined as the average of the most recent week just before propranolol therapy was begun, and the average of the most recent week during propranolol therapy, respectively. Office measurements for these two periods are defined as those sitting and standing pressures and heart rates obtained for the most recent pretreatment and treatment visits, respectively.

Office pressures were reduced in each of the 43 patients treated with propranolol (Table 4). Thus, pretreatment sitting and standing pressures were 171/109 and 167/111 mmHg, respectively (mean arterial pressures: 130 and 130 mmHg, respectively). With propranolol, these pressures were reduced approximately 15 to 18 percent (Table 3) to 143/89 and 141/95 mmHg in the sitting and standing positions (mean arterial pressure: 107 and 110 mmHg, respectively). But, despite a 20-percent reduction in heart rate in both positions, reflexive increases in heart rate were observed with upright posture. Hence, orthostatic hypotension was not observed during beta-adrenergic inhibition.

Response of arterial pressure to upright posture was similar in the patients in whom home arterial pressure records were obtained. However, two of the 39 patients who obtained home pressures failed to demonstrate a reduction in home pressures (Table 4). In

TABLE 4.—*Response of Home and Office Arterial Pressures to Long-Term Propranolol Therapy*

	Before Propranolol		*During Propranolol*		*Percentage of Change*	
Measurement	*Supine*	*Standing*	*Supine*	*Standing*	*Supine*	*Standing*
Office Measurements:						
Systolic pressure (mm Hg)	171	167	143	141	16	16
Diastolic pressure (mm Hg)	109	111	89	95	18	15
Mean arterial pressure (mm Hg)	130	130	107	110	18	15
Heart rate (beats per minute)	86	100	70	80	19	20
Home Measurements:						
Systolic pressure (mm Hg)	157	156	135	136	14	13
Diastolic pressure (mm Hg)	98	104	89	90	14	13
Mean arterial pressure (mm Hg)	118	121	101	105	9	13

Home pressures represent the average of the most recent week of placebo therapy prior to initiation of active propranolol (also average of the most recent week). Office pressures and heart rate represent the most recent week during placebo and active therapy.

general, these patients had higher arterial pressures in the physician's office than at home. Thus, sitting pretreatment office pressures averaged 171/109 mm Hg and supine home pretreatment pressures averaged 157/98 mm Hg; standing pretreatment pressures averaged 167/111 and 156/104 mm Hg at office and home, respectively. With treatment systolic and diastolic arterial home pressures were reduced by 14 percent so that supine and standing pressures were 135/89 and 136/90 mm Hg, respectively.

Discussion

The results of these studies indicate that beta-adrenergic blocking therapy is both effective and safe in selected hypertensive patients. Having followed a relatively large number of hypertensive patients of varied clinical types for many years, one may select those who will most likely respond to beta-adrenergic suppressive therapy. The present study is concerned with 41 patients, followed an average of 1 year; all responded with reduction of office pressures. However, two patients failed to demonstrate any reduction in arterial pressure in daily home pressure readings (weekly averages).

The most valuable criterion for preselection of these patients seems to be the clinical symptom of cardiac awareness. These complaints are those of awareness of increased heart rate and contractions in the absence of roentgenographic and electrocardiographic evidence of cardiac enlargement. In addition, these individuals report increased awareness of cardiac action following mild exercise or emotionally stimulating episodes which persist much longer than would be expected in otherwise normal individuals. These patients report that if they are able to obtain their own blood pressure measurements under such circumstances arterial pressure remains elevated for inordinately long periods of time. In addition to these clinical (and admittedly subjective criteria) we have utilized more physiologic and pharmacologic criteria: the supine resting hemodynamic indices and the response of heart rate to the intravenous infusion of isoproterenol. Both of these latter criteria have been useful in selecting patients.

By employing these preselection criteria we do not exclude the very real possibility that other hypertensive patients not demonstrating these findings might also respond to beta-adrenergic blocking antihypertensive therapy. Many studies involving larger numbers of hypertensive patients have demonstrated significant reduction in arterial pressure using propranolol as well as other beta-adrenergic blocking drugs.[14,15,24–29] These studies have indicated that arterial pressure can be reduced in hypertensive patients with or without evidence of a hyperkinetic circulation. In fact, this type of therapy has been shown to be of value alone as well as in conjunction with other forms of antihypertensive therapy including diuretics, vasodilating drugs, and sympatholytic agents.[30,31] We have also found that propranolol has been of value even in patients with malignant hypertension (without cardiomegaly or left ventricular failure).

Nevertheless, this report indicates that, in a controlled trial in hypertensive patients of varied clinical types, the use of propranolol as the sole antihypertensive agent is of value in reducing arterial pressure. That these findings have been extended in other studies to demonstrate the value of beta-adrenergic blocking therapy in hypertension in conjunction with other more conventional forms of antihypertensive therapy, only underscores the potential value of this form of therapy in hypertension. Furthermore, these findings in no way should be construed to indicate that beta-adrenergic blocking therapy need be used alone or restricted to only the less severe degrees of hypertensive cardiovascular disease. However, by using propranolol alone in preselected patients for prolonged treatment of hypertension (excluding those with history of cardiac and renal failure, cardiac enlargement, and severe vascular disease) we have obviated therapeutic complications and adverse effects.

An intriguing speculative point concerns the mechanism of the antihypertensive action of the beta-adrenergic blocking drugs. We have shown in earlier studies that following the intravenous administration of propranolol there is no immediate fall in arterial pressure.[32] However, within hours or days of long-term propranolol therapy, arterial pressure becomes reduced to those levels observed in the present study.[20–22,28,32,33] Prichard and Gillam have noted that prolonged therapy is necessary for demonstration of the antihypertensive effect of beta-adrenergic blocking drugs;[34] however, we differ in the degree of time necessary for the onset of action. We believe arterial pressure becomes reduced more rapidly (within days); perhaps because our patients obtain continuous home pressure recordings. At any rate, Prichard and Gillam suggest that with prolonged therapy there is a continuous and progressive downward resetting of the baroreceptors.[34] This mechanism seems unlikely since baroreceptor adjustment does not respond to changes in flow or cardiac output but to changes in pressure. Moreover, reduction of arterial pressure in hypertensive patients treated with propranolol is related to a reduction in cardiac output[28] rather than a reduction in peripheral vascular resistance; and with downward resetting of baroreceptors peripheral resistance will decrease, not increase. Were a resetting mechanism operative, it would seem more reasonable that with the prolonged reduction of cardiac output with propranolol, a reversal of the Bayliss mechanism[35] might occur. Under these circumstances, as described by Bayliss, with increasing blood flow rates the arterial smooth muscle responds by greater degrees of constriction. Conversely, with prolonged reduction of cardiac output it seems possible that arterial smooth muscle responds with relaxation. Under these circumstances there should be a progressive fall in vascular resistance with propranolol therapy; this does not seem to occur. Nevertheless, with a reduction in arterial pressure and a fall in output and possibly vascular resistance, some adaptation of the peripheral circulation seems to be likely.

A final and intriguing possibility invokes a decrease in the release of renin from the kidney. Thus, under these circumstances with inhibition of beta-adrenergic receptors there is reduced neural stimulation for renin release; this results in diminished generation of angiotensin and less stimulation of the medullary centers by angiotensin. In addition, there would be less stimulation of aldosterone production by the generated angiotensin and a consequent reduction in sodium retention and intravascular volume. Evidence supporting this line of reasoning seems to be at hand; but, admittedly, they are all inferential. Thus, evidence is accumulating that adrenergic-like stimulation by intra-arterial infusion of the beta-adrenergic agonist (isoproterenol), epinephrine, norepinephrine, and cyclic AMP promotes renin release.[36–43]

Conversely, this release can be blocked by pretreatment with propranolol.[42,43] Many studies have demonstrated that even subpressor doses of angiotensin will stimulate certain medullary centers;[44–49] and these responses mimic the hemodynamic characteristics observed in renovascular hypertensive man with hyperkinetic circulation.[50,51] Finally, in support of the possible secondary decrease in aldosterone production and the resultant contracted intravascular volume, we have recently reported that propranolol, unlike any other antihypertensive agent (except the diuretics), is associated with unchanged or reduced intravascular volume (rather than an expanded volume).[52]

Conclusions

The effect of prolonged (average, 1 year) antihypertensive therapy with propranolol as the sole antihypertensive agent has been studied in 43 patients with uncomplicated hypertension of varied clinical types. These patients were preselected with respect to certain clinical, hemodynamic, and pharmacologic criteria. All 43 patients had a reduction in arterial pressures (average, 18 percent) on the basis of office pressures; however, two of the 39 patients who obtained home blood pressure recordings failed to show a fall of arterial pressure. The reduction in arterial pressure was associated with a preservation of the normal response of pressure in the upright posture. Since with prolonged treatment arterial pressure reduction is associated with a fall in cardiac output and an increase in total peripheral resistance, a mechanism postulated on resetting of baroreceptors seems unlikely. A mechanism likened to the reverse of the Bayliss myogenic response might be possible if vascular resistance were to fall thereby providing an adaptation of the peripheral circulation. Also possible is a mechanism invoking an attenuated release of renin, resulting in reduced generation of angiotensin, reduced release of aldosterone, natriuresis, and contracted intravascular volume.

ACKNOWLEDGMENT

The author deeply appreciates the technical support of Miss Kay Cheadle, the secretarial assistance of Mrs. Irene Smith, and the supplies of propranolol generously provided by Dr. William B. Abrams of Ayerst Laboratories.

REFERENCES

1. Veterans Administration Cooperative Study Group on Antihypertensive Agents: Effects of treatment on morbidity in hypertension. Results in patients with diastolic blood pressures averaging 115 through 129 mm Hg. JAMA 202:116, 1967.
2. Veterans Administrative Cooperative Study Group on Antihypertensive Agents: Effect of treatment on morbidity in hypertension. Results in patients with diastolic blood pressures averaging 90 through 114 mm Hg. JAMA 213:1143, 1970.
3. Wolff, F. W., and Lindeman, R. D.: Effects of treatment in hypertension. Results of a controlled study. J. Chronic Dis. 19:227, 1966.
4. Langley, J. N.: On the reaction of cells and of nerve-endings to certain poisons, chiefly as regards the reaction of striated muscles to nicotine and curare. J. Physiol. 33:374, 1905.
5. Dale, H. H.: On some physiological actions of ergot. J. Physiol. 34:163, 1906.
6. Alquist, R. P.: A study of the adrenotropic receptors. Am. J. Physiol. 153:586, 1948.
7. Moran, N. C.: Adrenergic receptors, drugs, and the cardiovascular system. (2 parts) Mod. Conc. Cardiovasc. Dis. 35:93, 1966.
8. Govier, W. C., Mosal, N. C., Whittington, P., and Broom, A. H.: Myocardial alpha- and beta-adrenergic receptors as demonstrated by atrial functional refractory-period changes. J. Pharmacol. Exp. Ther. 154:255, 1966.
9. Abboud, F. M., Eckstein, J. W., and Zimmerman, B. G.: Venous and arterial responses to stimulation of beta-adrenergic receptors. Am. J. Physiol. 209:383, 1965.
10. Dunlop, D., and Shanks, R. G.: Selective blockade of adrenoreceptive beta receptors in the heart. Br. J. Pharmacol. 32:201, 1968.
11. Robison, G. A., and Butcher, R. W.: Some aspects of the biological role of cyclic AMP. Circulation 37:279, 1968.
12. Robison, G. A., and Sutherland, E. W.: Sympathin E, sympathin I, and the intracellular level of cyclic AMP. Circ. Res. 27 (Suppl. I):147, 1970.
13. Paget, G. E.: Carcinogenic action of pronethalol. Br. Med. J. 2:1266, 1963.
14. Prichard, B. N. C.: Hypotensive action of pronethalol. Br. Med. J. 1:1227, 1964.
15. Prichard, B. N. C., and Gillam, P. M. S.: Use of propranolol in the treatment of hypertension. Br. Med. J. 2:725, 1964.
16. Braunwald, E. (Ed.): Symposium on beta-adrenergic receptor blockade. Am. J. Cardiol. 18:303, 1966.
17. Frohlich, E. D., Dustan, H. P., and Page, I. H.: Hyperdynamic beta-adrenergic circulatory state. Arch. Intern. Med. 117:614, 1966.
18. Gorlin, R.: The hyperkinetic heart syndrome. JAMA 182:823, 1962.
19. Frohlich, E. D., Tarazi, R. C., and Dustan, H. P.: Hyperdynamic beta-adrenergic circulatory state. Increased beta-receptor responsiveness. Arch. Intern. Med. 123:1, 1969.
20. Frohlich, E. D., Dustan, H. P., and Tarazi, R. C.: Hyperdynamic beta-adrenergic circulatory state. An overview. Arch. Intern. Med. 126:1068, 1970.
21. Frohlich, E. D., Tarazi, R. C., and Dustan, H. P.: Beta-adrenergic blocking therapy in hypertension: Selection of patients. Int. J. Pharmacol. Ther. Toxicol. 4:151, 1970.
22. Frohlich, E. D., Tarazi, R. C., and Dustan, H. P.: Use of beta-adrenergic blockade in hypertensive disease. *In* Kattus, A. A., Ross, G., and Hall, V. (Eds.): Cardiovascular Beta-Adrenergic Responses. UCLA Forum in Medical Sciences, Number 13. Los Angeles: Univ. of California Press, 1970, pp. 223.
23. Frohlich, E. D., Tarazi, R. C., and Dustan, H. P.: Peripheral arterial insufficiency: A complication of beta-adrenergic blocking therapy. JAMA 208:2471, 1969.
24. Patterson, J. W., and Dollery, C. T.: Effect of propranolol in mild hypertension. Lancet 2:1148, 1966.
25. Waal, H. J.: Hypotensive action of propranolol. Clin. Pharmacol. Ther. 7:588, 1966.
26. Dorph, S., and Binder, C.: Evaluation of the hypertensive effect of beta-adrenergic blockade in hypertension. Acta Med. Scand. 185: 443, 1969.
27. Furberg, C., and Michaelson, J.: Effect of Aptin, a beta-adrenergic blocking agent, in arterial hypertension. Acta Med. Scand. 186: 447, 1969.
28. Frohlich, E. D., Tarazi, R. C., Dustan, H. P., and Page, I. H.: The paradox of beta-adren-

ergic blockade in hypertension. Circulation 37:417, 1968.
29. Török, E., Matos, L., Rausch, J., and Simenyi, J.: The effects of propranolol in essential circulatory hyperkinesis. Int. J. Clin. Pharmacol. 2:246, 1969.
30. Prichard, B. N. C.: The treatment of hypertension by beta-adrenergic blocking drugs. Angiologica 3:318, 1966.
31. Gilmore, E., Weil, J., and Chidsey, C.: Treatment of essential hypertension with a new vasodilator in combination with beta-adrenergic blockade. N. Engl. J. Med. 282:521, 1970.
32. Ulrych, M., Frohlich, E. D., Dustan, H. P., and Page, I. H.: Immediate hemodynamic effects of beta-adrenergic blockade with propranolol in normotensive and hypertensive man. Circulation 37:411, 1968.
33. Frohlich, E. D.: Beta-adrenergic inhibition in hypertension associated with renal arterial disease. *In* Fisher, J. W., and Cafrung, E. J. (Eds.): Renal Pharmacology. New York: Appleton-Century-Crofts, 1971, pp. 241–266.
34. Prichard, B. N. C., and Gillam, P. M. S.: Treatment of hypertension with propranolol. Br. Med. J. 1:7, 1969.
35. Bayliss, W. M.: On the local reactions of the arterial wall to changes of internal pressure. J. Physiol. 28:220, 1902.
36. Ayers, C. R., Harris, R. H., Jr., and Lefer, L. G.: Control of renin release in experimental hypertension. Circ. Res. 24(Suppl. I): 103, 1969.
37. Cohen, E. L., Rooner, D. R., and Conn, J. W.: Postural augmentation of plasma renin activity. JAMA 197:973, 1966.
38. Brown, J. J., Davies, D. L., Lever, A. F., McPherson, D., and Robertson, J. I. S.: Plasma renin concentration in relation to changes in posture. Clin. Sci. 30:279, 1966.
39. Bunag, R. D., Page, I. H., and McCubbin, J. W.: Neural stimulation of release of renin. Circ. Res. 19:851, 1966.
40. Nash, F. D., Rostorfer, H. H., Bailie, M. D., Wathen, R. L., and Schneider, E. G.: Renin release. Relation to renal sodium load and dissociation from hemodynamic changes. Circ. Res. 22:473, 1968.
41. Gordon, R. D., Kuchel, O., Liddel, G. W., and Island, D. P.: Role of the sympathetic nervous system in regulating renin and aldosterone production in man. J. Clin. Invest. 46:599, 1967.
42. Winer, N., Chokski, D. S., Yoon, M. S., and Freedman, A. D.: Adrenergic receptor mediation of renin secretion. J. Clin. Endocrinol. 29:1168, 1969.
43. Winer, N., Chokski, D. S., and Walkenhorst, W. G.: Effects of cyclic AMP, sympathomimetic amines, and adrenergic receptor antagonists on renin secretion. Circ. Res. 29: 239, 1971.
44. Bickerton, R. K., and Buckley, J. P.: Evidence for a central mechanism in angiotensin induced hypertension. Proc. Soc. Exp. Biol. Med. 106:834, 1961.
45. Yu, R., and Dickinson, C. J.: Neurogenic effects of angiotensin. Lancet 2:1276, 1965.
46. Scroop, G. C., and Whelan, R. F.: A central vasomotor action of angiotensin in man. Clin. Sci. 30:79, 1966.
47. Scroop, G. C., and Lowe, R. D.: Central pressor effect of angiotensin mediated by the parasympathetic nervous system. Nature 220: 1331, 1968.
48. Ferrario, C. M., Dickinson, C. J., and McCubbin, J. W.: Central vasomotor stimulation by angiotensin. Clin. Sci. 39:239, 1970.
49. Fukiyama, K., McCubbin, J. W., and Page, I. H.: Chronic hypertension elicited by infusion of angiotensin into vertebral arteries of unanesthetized dogs. Clin. Sci. 40:283, 1971.
50. Frohlich, E. D., Ulrych, M., Tarazi, R. C., Dustan, H. P., and Page, I. H.: Hemodynamics of renal arterial disease and hypertension. Am. J. Med. Sci. 255:29, 1968.
51. Frohlich, E. D., Tarazi, R. C., and Dustan, H. P.: Re-evaluation of the hemodynamics of hypertension. Am. J. Med. Sci. 257:9, 1969.
52. Tarazi, R. C., Frohlich, E. D., and Dustan, H. P.: Plasma volume changes with long-term beta-adrenergic blockade. Am. Heart J. 82:770, 1971.

Long-term Hemodynamic Effects of Beta-adrenergic Blockade in Hypertension

By Robert C. Tarazi, M.D.

THERE EXISTS a striking contrast between the immediate [1] and long-term [2–4] hemodynamic effects of beta-adrenergic blockade. Whereas cardiac output is depressed to the same extent by acute intravenous and chronic oral administration of propranolol, arterial pressure is reduced only with long-term treatment. This change in pressure response to the same drug suggested to us a varying adaptation in time of total peripheral resistance to cardiac output changes.[5] The question then naturally arose whether patients whose hypertension is not controlled by propranolol fail to respond because for some reason the initial reduction in output is not maintained or because of some altered behavior of peripheral resistance.

These hemodynamic considerations carry important practical implications. If reduction of cardiac output was the only factor responsible for control of hypertension, then it would follow that the selection of patients for propranolol therapy would depend on their hemodynamic characteristics. Further, since transient hypertensive responses to emotional stresses, office visits, pain, or similar stimuli, are usually thought to result from increased cardiac output,[6,7] beta-adrenergic blockade would be particularly suited for "apprehensive or tense" subjects. If, however, the control of hypertension involved more than reduction in output, then the implications of arterial pressure responses would be much less clear-cut.

Initial studies,[8–10] mainly of hypertensive patients who had responded to propranolol therapy, suggested that arterial pressure reduction was indeed correlated with the level of pretreatment cardiac output. However, as experience accumulated, a number of patients with high cardiac indices were encountered whose pressure did not respond to propranolol therapy. A review of our whole experience with responders and nonresponders to beta-adrenergic blockade was therefore undertaken to determine the hemodynamic background of different responses to the drug.[5] Repeated hemodynamic investigations were performed in patients given propranolol as the sole antihypertensive agent. Dosage used was 40 to 80 mg per day, and in all cases, efficacy of beta-adrenergic blockade was demonstrated during the studies by inhibition of chronotropic responses to a previously effective infusion of isoproterenol (0.03 μg per kilogram of body weight per minute).

Of the 52 patients studied, 42 had essential hypertension and 10, renal arterial disease. The latter did not differ from essential hypertensives either in blood pressure responsiveness to propranolol or in its alteration of hemodynamic patterns. This similarity which was noted before [8] allowed consideration of both types of hypertension together. For ease of handling data, blood pressure response was determined by comparing pretreatment mean arterial pressure (defined as the average for 1 month on "placebo" immediately before propranolol was begun) with average mean pressure during the third month on "active" therapy. This decision was based on previous demonstrations that the hypotensive effects of propranolol seem to increase over a period of 2 months with no further drop later.[11,12]

Four patients developed troublesome side effects necessitating early interruption of treatment so that their blood pressure response could not be adequately assessed. Among the remaining 48, reduction in mean arterial pressure by more than 10 mm Hg defined a group of 26 "responders." In 14 patients, mean arterial pressure was not affected and eight showed borderline changes (mean arterial pres-

---

From the Research Division, The Cleveland Clinic Foundation and the Cleveland Clinic Educational Foundation, Cleveland, Ohio.

This study was supported in part by grants from the National Heart and Lung Institute, PHS (HE-6835) and from the American Heart Association (70–960).

TABLE 1.—*Blood Pressure and Heart-Rate Response to Propranolol Therapy in 48 Hypertensive Patients*

Response	*Responders*	*Nonresponders*	*p*
Mean arterial pressure (mm Hg)			
Control home average	115	113	ns
Office reading	130	126	ns
Third month of treatment:			
Home average	99 (−13.9%)	111 (1.8%)	< .001
Office reading	114 (−12.3%)	123 (2.4%)	< .001
Heart rate (beats per minute)			
Control	83	85	ns
Third month of treatment	67 (−19%)	70 (−18%)	ns

Abbreviations used: p, statistical significance of difference between responders and nonresponders (see text for definition of these two groups); ns, not significant.

sure reduced by 5 to 8 mm Hg); these 22 patients were classified together as "nonresponders" (Table 1). The daily propranolol dose was practically equal in both groups, averaging 180 mg for responders and 200 mg for nonresponders. Heart-rate slowing occurred earlier than blood pressure reduction and was equal in both groups (Table 1). Once established, the hypotensive effect of propranolol persisted on prolonged follow-up in 23 of 26 responders; in two it appeared to diminish during the sixth month and in the third, pressure averages fluctuated towards higher levels after 18 months of uninterrupted treatment.

HEMODYNAMIC INVESTIGATIONS

Pretreatment Hemodynamic Studies

Pretreatment hemodynamic studies were performed in 41 of the 48 patients, 22 of the 26 responders and 19 of the 22 nonresponders. Apart from a somewhat higher incidence of increased cardiac index among responders, there was no significant hemodynamic difference between the two groups (Table 2). No significant correlation was found between pretreatment cardiac index and arterial pressure response to propranolol ($r = -0.049$). This was mainly due to a number of patients who did not respond to propranolol despite a high initial cardiac index.

Repeat Hemodynamic Studies

Repeated hemodynamic studies were obtained at various times during treatment in 22 patients; in 12 of them, the immediate effects of intravenous propranolol (10 mg) had also been determined before beginning oral therapy.[1] The 22 patients investigated include 21 studied within 1 year of beginning treatment and one studied after 18 months; repeat hemodynamic studies could be performed again in

TABLE 2.—*Initial Hemodynamic Characteristics and Response to Propranolol Therapy*

	Responders	*Nonresponders*
No. of patients	22	19
Basal heart rate	83	75
Cardiac index (liters per minute per M^2)		
Average *	3.30	3.10
> 3.3 (incidence) †	59% (13/22)	37% (7/19)
< 2.7 (incidence) †	14% (3/22)	37% (7/19)

* None of these differences was significant at the 5-percent level of confidence.

† Responders included 18 patients with essential hypertension and four with renal arterial disease; the nonresponders included 16 essential hypertensives and three with renal arterial disease.

TABLE 3.—*Hemodynamic Variations with Long-term Propranolol Therapy (Expressed as Percentage Change from Pretreatment Values ± 1 Standard Error of the Mean)*

	Time of Study Relative to Therapy	
	Within 1 Year	*Longer than 1 Year*
No. of patients	21	13
Duration of treatment (months)	7.2 (0.9)	19.9 (1.7)
Mean arterial pressure	−11.1 (2.3)	−18.6 (2.8)
Cardiac index	−19.4 (3.8)	−17.3 (4.2)
Heart rate	−25.6 (2.5)	−25.6 (2.6)
Total peripheral resistance	+14.5 (5.5)	−2.2 (4.4)

12 of 21. Changes observed at different periods of treatment (Table 3) were expressed as percentage variations from control studies to compensate for differing baseline values.[14,15] The more accentuated fall in arterial pressure (and total resistance) in the second study during therapy is due to the naturally greater number of responders maintained on propranolol alone. Cardiac output was reduced by propranolol in all patients but three: increasing in two (one responder and one nonresponder) and remaining practically unchanged (+4 to +6%) in the third. The main factor underlying blood pressure reduction was therefore not a depression in output alone since this occurred irrespective of arterial pressure response (Table 4). Variations in pressure during treatment were significantly related to change in peripheral resistance, i.e., $r = 0.737$, $p < .001$ (Fig. 1), not to changes in output ($r = 0.067$). Heart rate was slowed equally in all patients, with either intravenous or oral administration, during office visits or under basal conditions, in patients with pressure reduction or in nonresponders. A longitudinal study of variations in 10 patients, who were followed from inception of therapy on, showed a prompt reduction of cardiac output with intravenous propranolol that was maintained for the period of follow-up regardless of changes in arterial pressure; in contrast, peripheral resistance increased immediately and then gradually returned towards untreated control levels (Fig. 2).

Transient Hypertensive Episodes

Four patients whose home blood pressure responded remarkably and steadily to propranolol showed a transient marked increase in mean arterial pressure over home levels during one hemodynamic study but not during

TABLE 4.—*Comparison of Cardiac Output and Blood Pressure Effects of Oral Propranolol (Expressed as Percentage Change from Pretreatment Value ± 1 Standard Error of Mean)*

	MAP Reduced	*MAP Unchanged*	*p*
Number of patients	13	9	—
Duration of therapy: median (range) months	8 (3–12)	5 (2–11)	
MAP	−19.9 (2.1)	−1.2 (1.0)	< .001
Cardiac index	−18.2 (3.7)	−15.7 (6.5)	ns
Heart rate	−26.1 (3.3)	−22.2 (3.2)	ns
Total peripheral resistance	+0.6 (5.5)	+22.4 (8.6)	< .05

Abbreviations used: p, statistical significance of difference between the two groups in the table; MAP, mean arterial pressure; ns, not significant.

Groups defined on basis of MAP during first hemodynamic study with propranolol treatment, compared with MAP during pretreatment study.

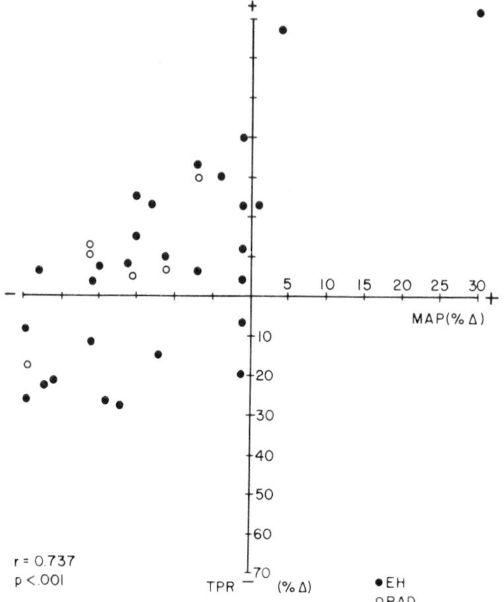

FIG. 1.—Relation between change in mean arterial pressure **(MAP)** and change in total peripheral resistance **(TPR)** during oral propranolol therapy; change expressed as the percentage variation from pretreatment value. (From Tarazi, R. C., and Dustan, H. P.,[5] with permission.)

another. This rise was not associated with an escape from the effect of propranolol; isoproterenol infusion demonstrated adequate beta-adrenergic blockade, and resting cardiac output and heart rate were similar on both occasions. This transient rise of pressure, which was observed five times in four patients, was associated in all instances with increased peripheral resistance, not output, so that the change in resistance was significant despite the small number of observations (Table 5).

DISCUSSION

In general, propranolol appeared an effective and relatively safe antihypertensive agent[11–13] in mild and moderate cases.[2,10] When effective, it lowered arterial pressure gradually during the first 2 months of therapy and the response was maintained for over a year in the majority of patients. The absence of "false tolerance" might be due to the fact that propranolol, in contradistinction to other neural-blocking agents, does not lead to plasma volume expansion and actually lowers it in some.[16] Its ability to reduce cardiac output during long-term therapy[2–4] was again confirmed. However, arterial pressure reduction by propranolol was not a simple or necessary consequence of the depression in output.

Initial reports on the antihypertensive effect of beta-adrenergic blockade stressed the unusual finding of chronic reduction in cardiac output with unchanged total peripheral resistance.[2–4] However, it seems that more is involved in the antihypertensive effect of propranolol than simple reduction in output: (1) its intravenous administration did not reduce arterial pressure (Fig. 2) despite a significant reduction of output; (2) patients whose pressures were not lowered had the same fall in output and the same bradycardia with propranolol as responders (Table 4). Previous conclusions relating the hypotensive effect of propranolol to reduced output alone were probably due to lack of adequate hemodynamic information on nonresponders. Reduction in cardiac output might well have been

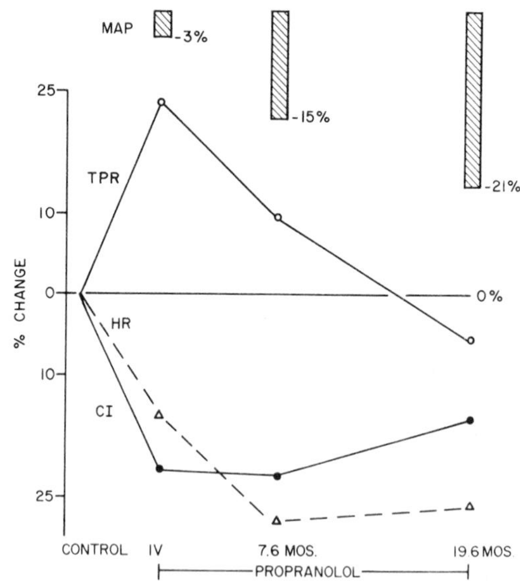

FIG. 2.—Sequential changes with intravenous and long-term (7.6 and 19.6 months) propranolol therapy in 10 hypertensive patients; changes in cardiac index **(CI)**, total peripheral resistance **(TPR)**, and heart rate **(HR)** as well as reduction of mean arterial pressure **(MAP)** are all expressed as the percentage of pretreatment value. (From Tarazi, R. C., and Dustan, H. P.,[5] with permission.)

TABLE 5.—*Transient Pressor Episodes Associated with Hemodynamic Studies During Propranolol Therapy*

		Propranolol Therapy	
	Pretreatment	*Concordant MAP*	*Discordant MAP*
MAP (mm Hg)			
Home average	120	108	104
During study	124	112	142
Heart rate	78	61	59
Cardiac index (liter per minute per M^2)	3.18	2.56	2.35
TPR (units)	39.0	43.5	61.0

Abbreviations used: MAP, mean arterial pressure; concordant and discordant refer to comparison of blood pressure during study with home blood pressure average at that time (see text); TPR, total peripheral resistance; the increase above pretreatment values was significantly higher in the discordant than in the concordant studies, averaging +46% with a standard error of difference = 11.5 (paired t test = 4.00, $p < .05$).

the initiating factor in the chain of events leading to lowering of arterial pressure but it was not per se solely responsible for that effect. The main difference in arterial pressure responses to beta-adrenergic blockade was related to the adaptability in time of total peripheral resistance to long-term reduction in flow. Following intravenous propranolol, an increase in calculated resistance compensated for the acute reduction in output; those who maintained the same increase in resistance during chronic therapy showed no fall in blood pressure, whereas responders demonstrated a gradual reduction of resistance from the high levels attained with intravenous propranolol toward pretreatment levels. Comparing total peripheral resistance during oral therapy with its level following intravenous propranolol, difference was significant in responders ($p <$ .005) and insignificant in the nonresponders ($p > 0.10$) (Fig. 3). That resistance was not significantly lowered below pretreatment levels, or was even higher in some patients, does not mean that readaptation did not occur.

The factors underlying this difference in behavior of peripheral resistance between different patients are not evident. In fact, the mechanism responsible for the reduction in resistance with maintained decrease in output is itself purely speculative. It might be related to some form of autoregulation,[17] an analogic counterpart to the increase in resistance following sustained increases in flow.[18,19] The hypothesis of a resetting of baroceptors [12,13] is difficult to accept as initial changes are those of blood flow not of pressure. On the other hand, a central action of propranolol cannot be excluded.[20] Still not fully clarified is the possible role of propranolol effects on renin release; responders to the drug tended to have higher pretreatment levels of plasma renin activity than nonresponders. However, there was no consistent relationship in this group of patients with moderate hypertension between reduction in plasma renin activity and changes in mean arterial pressure with treatment.[25]

As the lowering of pressure is not a simple or a necessary consequence of the depression in output, it is not surprising that no correlation was found between pretreatment cardiac index and blood pressure reduction by the drug.[5,21] Some hypertensive patients with inappropriate tachycardia and elevated cardiac output will report a marked quietening of their hearts with propranolol without concomitant control of their hypertension. Increased cardiac output was certainly found more frequently among responders (59%) than nonresponders (37%) (Table 1) but the difference was not significant and the exceptions were too frequent to allow an accurate guessing of responders. Birkenhäger et al.[21] also could not relate blood pressure change with propranolol treatment to either age, cardiac output, lability of arterial pressure, or blood volume.

A corollary of these observations is that the

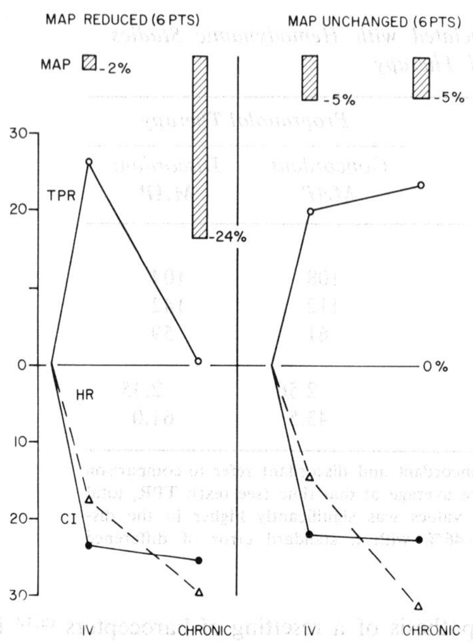

FIG. 3.—Comparison of hemodynamic indices between six patients who responded and six who did not respond to oral propranolol therapy; reduction of resistance (from intravenous to oral study) was significant in the first group ($p < .005$) but not in the second. All changes expressed in percentage of pretreatment value. **CI,** changes in cardiac index; **TPR,** total peripheral resistance; **HR,** heart rate; **MAP,** mean arterial pressure. (From Tarazi, R. C., and Dustan, H. P.,[5] with permission.)

hypotensive effect of propranolol cannot be used with confidence as an index of cardiac participation in hypertension. The immediate heart-rate response and output reduction might be some measure of beta-adrenergic influence on systemic hemodynamic balance in the patients investigated,[1,22] but long-term blood pressure reduction is a more complex effect precluding firm conclusions.

Transient rises in blood pressure during office visits or with similar emotional stimuli have been usually attributed to increased cardiac action,[7,23] hence the use of propranolol to minimize such reactions was a logical step. Unfortunately, however, its effectiveness for that purpose was not substantiated by this study; transient spontaneous hypertensive responses were still noted in spite of therapy during some office visits or hemodynamic investigations. They occurred even though neither cardiac output nor heart rate was increased; the only significant change during these episodes was a marked rise in peripheral resistance (Table 5). Similar observations with propranolol in hypertensive patients were reported with other stimuli than the unspecified "stress" associated with medical investigations. Responses investigated were those to pain,[6] mental arithmetic,[7] and static exercise.[24] In none of these studies was the hypertensive response to "stress" prevented or even blunted by propranolol despite its maintenance of flow at a reduced level. The therapeutic implication is obvious: hypertensive responses to this type of stimuli may still occur despite apparently effective propranolol therapy, only their hemodynamic mechanism will be altered.

ACKNOWLEDGMENT

This is a welcome opportunity to acknowledge the contribution of Dr. E. D. Frohlich to the initial studies underlying this report. The Inderal used was generously supplied by the Ayerst Laboratories.

REFERENCES

1. Ulrych, M., Frohlich, E. D., Dustan, H. P., and Page, I. H.: Immediate hemodynamic effects of beta-adrenergic blockade with propranolol in normotensive and hypertensive man. Circulation 37:411, 1968.
2. Frohlich, E. D., Tarazi, R. C., Dustan, H. P., and Page, I. H.: The paradox of beta-adrenergic blockade in hypertension. Circulation 37:417, 1968.
3. Wilson, D. F., Watson, O. F., Piel, J. S., Langley, R. B., and Turner, A. S.: Some hemodynamic effects of Trasicor (Ciba 39089/Ba). N. Z. Med. J. 68:145, 1968.
4. Prichard, B. N. C., Shinebourne, E., Fleming, J., and Hamer, J.: Hemodynamic studies in hypertensive patients on oral propranolol. Br. Heart J. 32:236, 1970.
5. Tarazi, R. C., and Dustan, H. P.: Beta-adrenergic blockade in hypertension: Practical and theoretical implications of long-term hemodynamic variations. Am. J. Cardiol. 29: 633, 1972.
6. Nicotero, J. A., Beamer, V., Moutsos, S. E., and Shapiro, A. P.: Effects of propranolol on pressor responses to noxious stimuli in hypertensive patients. Am. J. Cardiol. 22:657, 1968.
7. Ulrych, M.: Changes of general haemodynamics during stressful mental arithmetic and

non-stressing quiet conversation and modification of the latter by beta-adrenergic blockade. Clin. Sci. 36:453, 1969.

8. Frohlich, E. D.: Beta-adrenergic inhibition in hypertension associated with renal arterial disease. *In* Fisher, J. W., and Cafruny, E. J. (Eds.): Renal Pharmacology. New York: Appleton-Century-Crofts, 1971, pp. 241–266.
9. Frohlich, E. D., Kozul, V., Tarazi, R. C., and Dustan, H. P.: Physiological comparison of labile and essential hypertension. Circ. Res. 26–27 (Suppl. I):55, 1970.
10. Dorph, S., and Binder, C.: Evaluation of the hypotensive effect of beta-adrenergic blockade in hypertension. Acta Med. Scand. 185:443, 1969.
11. Prichard, B. N. C., and Gillam, P. M. S.: Use of propranolol in treatment of hypertension. Br. Med. J. 2:725, 1964.
12. Prichard, B. N. C.: Propranolol as an antihypertensive agent. Am. Heart J. 79:128, 1970.
13. Prichard, B. N. C., and Gillam, P. M. S.: Treatment of hypertension with propranolol. Br. Med. J. 1:7, 1969.
14. Pickering, G. W.: High Blood Pressure, 2nd Edition. New York: Grune & Stratton, 1968.
15. Tarazi, R. C., and Dustan, H. P.: Studies on neurogenic participation in hypertension. (Unpublished observations.)
16. Tarazi, R. C., Frohlich, E. D., and Dustan, H. P.: Plasma volume changes with long-term beta-adrenergic blockade. Am. Heart J. 82: 770, 1971.
17. Guyton, A. C., and Coleman, T. G.: Quantitative analysis of the pathophysiology of hypertension. Circ. Res. 24(Suppl. I):1, 1969.
18. Ferrario, C. M., Page, I. H., and McCubbin, J. W.: Increased cardiac output in experimental renal hypertension. Circ. Res. 27:799, 1970.
19. Conway, J.: Hemodynamic consequences of induced changes in blood volume. Circ. Res. 18:190, 1966.
20. Murmann, W., Almirante, L., and Saccani-Guelfi, M.: Central nervous system effects of four adrenergic blocking agents. J. Pharm. Pharmacol. 18:317, 1966.
21. Birkenhäger, W. H., Krauss, X. H., Schalekamp, M. A. D. H., Kolsters, G., and Kroon, B. J. M.: Antihypertensive effects of propranolol. Folia Med. Neerl. 14:67, 1971.
22. Sannerstedt, R., Julius, S., and Conway, J.: Hemodynamic responses to tilt and beta-adrenergic blockade in young patients with borderline hypertension. Circulation 42:1057, 1970.
23. Lund-Johansen, P.: Hemodynamics in early essential hypertension. Acta Med. Scand. Suppl. 482:44, 1967.
24. Tarazi, R. C., and Dustan, H. P.: Beta-adrenergic blockade and response to exercise. Clin. Pharmacol. Ther. 12:303, 1971.
25. Tarazi, R. C., Dustan, H. P., Frohlich, E. D., and Bravo, E. L.: Plasma renin activity and arterial pressure response to propranolol. (Unpublished observations.)

Guancydine, a New Vasodilator: Comparison with Hydralazine in a Regimen Including Propranolol and Quinethazone

By Niroo Gupta, M.D., and Leon I. Goldberg, Ph.D., M.D.

Maximum use of vasodilator therapy for the treatment of hypertension has not been possible because of unavailability of a potent, nontoxic drug acting by this mechanism. Hydralazine is not a very effective antihypertensive agent and can produce serious adverse effects when given in large doses.[1,2] Accordingly, it is important to investigate other potentially more suitable vasodilating agents.

Guancydine (1-cyano-3-*tert*-amylguanidine) (Fig. 1) was first studied as one of a series of novel synthetic cyanoguanidines and found to exhibit hypotensive activity in experimental animals by Gadekar, Nibi, and Cohen.[3] Cummings et al.[4,5] extensively investigated the pharmacologic actions of guancydine and found that the drug lowered blood pressure in both normotensive and hypertensive animals. The hypotension was dose-related and occurred without interruption of sympathetic adrenergic mechanisms or depression of myocardial function. Vasodilation of the mesenteric, renal, and cranial vascular beds was demonstrated.

Freis and Hammer [6] first investigated guancydine in 11 hospitalized patients. Reduction of blood pressure was observed in doses between 250 and 750 mg. Heart rate was increased moderately. Following a single oral dose of guancydine, the blood pressure reduction occurred within 30 minutes and the peak effect was obtained 1 to 3 hours after the drug was administered. Duration of the antihypertensive effect varied between 4 and 8 hours. Significant orthostasis did not occur and sympathetic vasoconstrictor responses evoked by the Valsalva maneuver and cold-pressor test were not inhibited.

Hemodynamic studies by Hammer, Ulrych, and Freis,[7] and Stenberg, Sannerstedt, and Werko,[8] demonstrated that the hypotensive action of guancydine was due to a marked reduction in systemic resistance. Guancydine,[7-10] as with other drugs acting by this mechanism,[1,11] causes reflex increases in cardiac output, heart rate and contractility, and sodium retention. Accordingly, Hammer and his colleagues [7] administered reserpine and the diuretic quinethazone concomitantly with guancydine and reduced the increased heart rate and eliminated edema and signs of congestive heart failure which occurred when guancydine was administered alone. Fourteen patients with an average supine blood pressure of 185/119 mm Hg were treated with guancydine (750 to 1,500 mg per day), reserpine (0.3 mg per day), and quinethazone (100 mg per day). With this regimen, blood pressure was reduced by 40/31 mm Hg in the supine position, by 40/34 mm Hg in the sitting position, and by 42/35 mm Hg in the erect position. When hydralazine, in 25-mg doses given three times daily, was substituted for guancydine, blood pressure in the sitting position increased by 6/13 mm Hg.

In a previous investigation in our clinic, Clark and Goldberg [12] administered guancydine in doses ranging from 500 to 1,500 mg per day to 10 patients already treated with guanethidine (average dose, 49 mg per day) and the diuretic quinethazone (100 mg per day). The addition of guancydine resulted in an additional reduction of blood pressure of 33/27 mm Hg in the supine position and 20/

From the Department of Medicine (Clinical Pharmacology), Emory University School of Medicine, Atlanta, Georgia.

Supported in part by Grants GM-14270, HE-06491 and FR-39 from the National Institutes of Health, and by a grant from Lederle Laboratories, Inc. Dr. Gupta was supported by a training grant from the National Institute of General Medical Sciences (GM-1543).

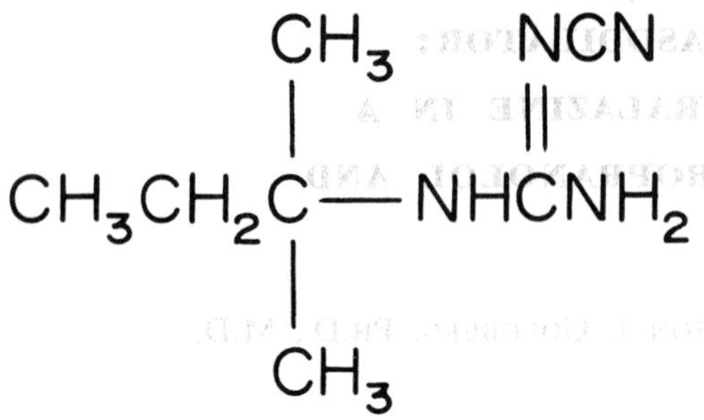

$$\begin{array}{c} \quad\quad CH_3 \quad\quad NCN \\ \quad\quad | \quad\quad\quad \| \\ CH_3CH_2C-NHCNH_2 \\ \quad | \\ \quad CH_3 \end{array}$$

FIG. 1.—Structural formula of guancydine.

48 mm Hg in the standing position. When guancydine was administered to eight patients with more severe hypertension (average dose: guanethidine, 234 mg per day; quinethazone, 100 mg per day), blood pressure decreased in the supine position by an average of 49/25 mm Hg and in the erect position by an average of 47/23 mm Hg.

Although blood pressure was adequately lowered with the above regimen, orthostasis and increased heart rate occurred in some patients. Accordingly, propranolol, in a dose of 20 mg, given four times a day, was substituted for guanethidine in five of the latter patients. Average blood pressure and heart rate when treated with guanethidine and quinethazone alone was 230/141 mm Hg and 71 beats per min in the supine position, and 201/135 mm Hg and 78 beats per min in the erect position. When guancydine was added in doses ranging from 1,000 to 2,000 mg per day, blood pressure in the supine position fell to 150/100 mm Hg and in the erect position to 127/85 mm Hg. Heart rate was 71 and 86 beats per minute, supine and standing respectively. When propranolol was substituted for guanethidine, average blood pressure in the supine position was 162/98 mm Hg, and 165/100 mm Hg in the erect position. Heart rate was 65 beats per min supine and 67 beats per min erect. Thus, the substitution of propranolol resulted in similar lowering of blood pressure in the supine position as occurred with guanethidine, but an orthostatic effect was not apparent and there was no increase in heart rate.

The present study is an extension of the investigation of Clark and Goldberg,[12] and was designed to determine whether hydralazine could be substituted for guancydine in patients previously treated with guancydine, propranolol, and quinethazone.

METHODS

Six patients with moderate or severe essential hypertension were observed in a hypertension clinic at intervals of 1 week to 1 month. All patients had left ventricular hypertrophy verified by chest x-ray and electrocardiogram, and grade II hypertensive retinopathy. Written consent of each patient was obtained prior to study. Other pertinent data are shown in Table 1. All patients were extensively evaluated to exclude curable causes of hypertension. Blood pressure and heart rate were recorded with the patient in the supine position and after standing for 3 minutes. A checklist was utilized to record subjective side effects. Extensive laboratory studies were obtained at biweekly to monthly intervals to detect any evidence of toxicity. Electrocardiograms, chest x-ray, and funduscopic examinations were obtained initially and repeated at monthly intervals.

Each patient had previously received guanethidine and a diuretic without adequate blood pressure control (Table 1) and was subsequently treated with propranolol, guancydine, and quinethazone for periods ranging from 6 to 18 months. After volunteering for the present investigation, the patients were asked to return to the clinic at 1- to 2-week intervals. Doses of guancydine, propranolol, and quinethazone previously used were maintained (Table 2). Blood pressure and heart rate recordings obtained during two consecutive visits were averaged and included as the first guancydine period (Table 2). Hydralazine was then added to the regimen in dosages beginning with 25 or 50 mg, given four times a day. The dose was gradually increased until each patient was receiving 100 mg four times daily. Guancydine was concomitantly withdrawn. The patients were treated with 100 mg of hydralazine, four times daily, for a period of 3 to 6 weeks, depending upon adequacy of control. The averages of the blood pressure recordings obtained during this time are recorded in Table 2. Hydralazine was then withdrawn and guancydine again administered. After the maximum tolerated dose of guancydine was achieved, blood pressure and heart-rate recordings obtained

TABLE 1.—*Patient Data and Previous Therapy*

Patient	Age	Sex	Serum Creatinine (mg/100 ml)	Previous Antihypertensive therapy (mg/day)		Blood Pressure (mm Hg)	
						Supine	Erect
S.C.	33	M	2.8	Guanethidine	150	192/137	145/115
				Bendroflumethiazide	10		
G.C.	57	F	1.7	Guanethidine	450	210/114	205/114
				Quinethazone	100		
C.C.	41	M	2.4	Quinethazone	100	183/123	125/96
				Guanethidine	100		
M.F.	48	F	2.4	Guanethidine	250	238/139	230/105
				Quinethazone	100		
I.H.	49	F	1.8	Guanethidine	350	232/145	196/134
				Quinethazone	100		
M.H.	30	F	1.1	Guanethidine	150	191/127	129/94
				Bendroflumethiazide	10		
Average						208/131	172/110

during two consecutive visits were averaged and included as the second guancydine period. Accordingly, a comparison between guancydine and hydralazine can be made, both before and after the period of hydralazine administration. The paired t-test was used for statistical comparisons.

RESULTS

Results of the comparative study are shown in Table 2. Average blood pressures of three patients were clearly lower during both guancydine periods than during the intervening hydralazine period. In two patients, average blood pressure during the guancydine and hydralazine periods was similar. In one patient (I.H.) higher blood pressures were recorded during the first than during the second guancydine period. Average blood pressure during the two guancydine periods was not significantly different. Statistical comparison of the combined guancydine periods with the hydralazine period indicated that the diastolic pressures in both positions were significantly lower with guancydine therapy, whereas the heart rate was significantly lower with hydralazine. The difference in rate can be explained by a greater reduction in blood pressure with guancydine in the presence of the competitive type of beta-adrenergic block produced by propranolol.

Figure 2 illustrates the markedly elevated blood pressure which occurred in patient G.C. when guancydine was entirely withdrawn and the patient was receiving 100 mg of hydralazine, four times a day; 40 mg of propranolol, four times a day; and 50 mg of quinethazone, twice daily. Because of the extreme elevation in blood pressure, it was necessary to add guancydine to the regimen after only 3 weeks of hydralazine treatment. When the full guancydine dose, 375 mg given four times

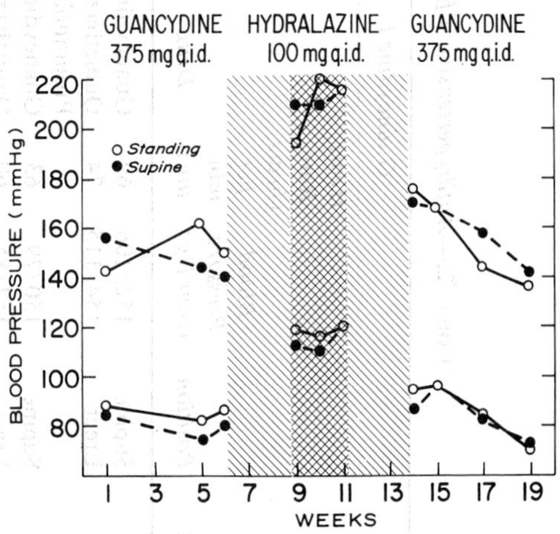

FIG. 2.—Effects of guancydine and hydralazine on blood pressure of patient G.C. **Slanted lines** denote periods of dosage adjustment.

TABLE 2.—*Antihypertensive Effects of Guancydine and Hydralazine with Quinethazone and Propranolol*

		Guancydine I				*Hydralazine*				*Guancydine II*			
Patient	*Position*	*Blood Pressure (mm Hg)*	*Heart Rate (beats per minute)*	*Drug*	*Dosage (mg per day)*	*Blood Pressure (mm Hg)*	*Heart Rate (beats per minute)*	*Drug*	*Dosage (mg per day)*	*Blood Pressure (mm Hg)*	*Heart Rate (beats per minute)*	*Drug*	*Dosage (mg per day)*
S.C.	Supine	152/106	69	Guancydine*	1500	151/112	70	Hydralazine	400	160/110	72	Guancydine	1125
	Erect	154/115	74	Quinethazone†	100	151/116	75	Quinethazone	100	144/112	78	Quinethazone	100
				Propranolol*	160			Propranolol	160			Propranolol	160
G.C.	Supine	150/79	63	Guancydine	1500	212/114	59	Hydralazine	400	150/77	68	Guancydine	1500
	Erect	152/85	60	Quinethazone	100	210/118	59	Quinethazone	100	140/77	68	Quinethazone	100
				Propranolol	80			Propranolol	80			Propranolol	80
C.C.	Supine	173/105	67	Guancydine	2000	167/107	54	Hydralazine	400	175/111	60	Guancydine	2000
	Erect	155/107	77	Quinethazone	100	167/112	56	Quinethazone	100	155/111	63	Quinethazone	100
				Propranolol	80			Propranolol	80			Propranolol	80
M.F.	Supine	136/82	67	Guancydine	1500	172/107	58	Hydralazine	400	147/87	59	Guancydine	1500
	Erect	152/97	75	Quinethazone	100	178/120	61	Quinethazone	100	155/99	63	Quinethazone	100
				Propranolol	80			Propranolol	80			Propranolol	80
I.H.	Supine	189/118	76	Guancydine	1500	179/111	71	Hydralazine	400	133/89	80	Guancydine	1500
	Erect	200/125	83	Quinethazone	100	187/122	75	Quinethazone	100	158/99	76	Quinethazone	100
				Propranolol	80			Propranolol	80			Propranolol	80
M.H.	Supine	130/90	79	Guancydine	1500	165/116	75	Hydralazine	400	136/97	79	Guancydine	1500
	Erect	124/92	82	Quinethazone	100	149/118	81	Quinethazone	100	120/93	84	Quinethazone	100
				Propranolol	120			Propranolol	120			Propranolol	120
Average	Supine	155/97	70			171/113†	61‡			150/95	70		
Average	Erect	156/103	75			174/118†	68†			145/98	72		

* Divided in 4 doses per day; † divided in 2 doses per day; ‡ $p < 0.05$; § $p < 0.01$ as compared to average of guancydine periods I and II.

daily, was attained, blood pressure was again well controlled. A different response occurred when hydralazine was administered to M.H. (Fig. 3). Blood pressure decreased during the first 3 weeks of hydralazine treatment, but again increased on the fourth week and reached very high levels on the fifth week, requiring reinstitution of guancydine therapy for effective control of blood pressure. In the other four patients, higher levels of blood pressure were also recorded at the end of the hydralazine period than during the beginning, suggesting a type of tolerance. Less pronounced fluctuations were occasionally observed during guancydine therapy, especially in I.H.

Side Effects

Subjective side effects reported during both guancydine and hydralazine periods included headache, nervousness, palpitation, vague chest pain, dizziness, and ankle swelling. None of these were severe and disappeared on continuous administration. Objective signs of edema were not seen.

One patient (C.S.) experienced restlessness, anxiety, and a feeling of drunkenness during initial administration of guancydine requiring temporary reduction in dosage. The drug was tolerated when the dose was increased gradually. Administration of hydralazine in a dose of 25-mg given four times a day caused anorexia, nausea, and vomiting in one patient

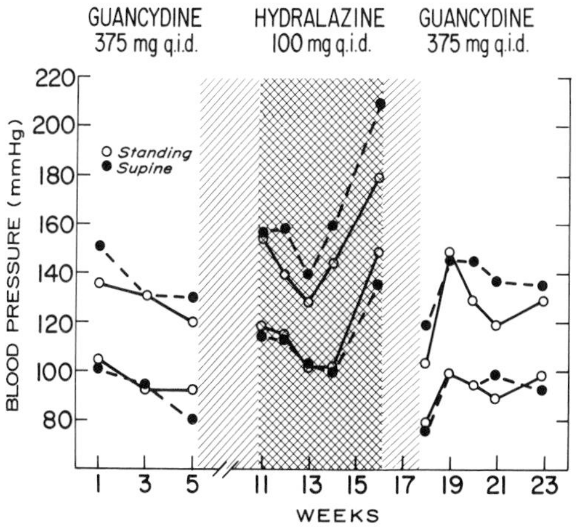

FIG. 3.—Effects of guancydine and hydralazine on blood pressure of patient M.H. **Slanted lines** denote periods of dosage adjustment.

(C.C.). These effects disappeared on reducing the dose to 10 mg. With small weekly increments, the dose of hydralazine was increased to the 400-mg daily level without significant side effects.

No significant alteration of laboratory values, chest x-ray, or electrocardiogram occurred during the course of this investigation.

Discussion

This study has demonstrated that hydralazine and guancydine, when used with propranolol and quinethazone, can lower blood pressure of patients previously inadequately treated with guanethidine and a diuretic. As in previous investigations,[12,13] the antihypertensive effect occurred without orthostasis, and, in fact, some of the patients experienced a higher blood pressure when erect than when supine. Propranolol, in four daily doses of 20 to 40 mg per kilogram of body weight, was effective in reducing reflex increase in heart rate, and 100 mg of quinethazone given daily prevented edema. Guancydine (1,500 to 2,000 mg per day) was more consistently effective than hydralazine (400 mg per day). It is possible that a higher dose of hydralazine might have demonstrated greater efficacy, but because of the lupus-erythematosus-like syndrome occurring with larger doses of this drug, higher doses were not used.

Guancydine and hydralazine produce a number of similar side effects, probably as common manifestations of vasodilation.[1,2,7–10] For example, each drug causes headache, palpitation, and central nervous system (CNS) excitation.[12,14] Thus far, the lupus-erythematosus-like syndrome observed with large doses of hydralazine has not been reported with guancydine. On the other hand, three males developed gynecomastia with guancydine therapy, and one female developed galactorrhea.[12] Both changes regressed when guancydine was discontinued. The mechanism responsible for these abnormalities has not been determined.

The present investigation supports the conclusion of Gilmore, Weil, and Chidsey[11] that administration of vasodilators in combination with a beta-adrenergic blocking agent and a diuretic represents a new type of antihypertensive therapy. Indeed, the more selective action of propranolol should obviate not only the orthostasis produced by drugs which indiscriminately reduce sympathetic function, but should also eliminate other side effects such as inability to ejaculate.[15] Gilmore and his colleagues[11] studied another potent vasodilating agent, minoxidil (PDP), which appears to be similar to guancydine in both mechanisms of action and efficacy. Recently, Gottlieb and Chidsey[16] reported that combined treatment with minoxidil, propranolol, and hydrochlorothiazide is more effective than the combination of hydralazine, propranolol, and hydrochlorothiazide.

Thus, it appears that although hydralazine may adequately lower blood pressure in some patients when used in combination with propranolol and a diuretic,[13] others do not respond to this regimen and require minoxidil or guancydine. These initial investigations clearly call for additional comparative studies of the three vasodilators to determine their relative efficacy and safety during long-term therapy.

Acknowledgment

We wish to thank Dr. Dwight Clark, Dr. Susan Fellner, Miss Marjorie A. Hewett, R.N., and Mrs. Mabel Moorhead, R.N., for assistance in these studies; Dr. Hugh McDonald, Lederle Laboratories, Inc., for the supplies of guancydine; and Dr. William E. Wagner, Ciba Pharmaceutical Company, for the hydralazine.

References

1. Nickerson, M.: Antihypertensive agents and the drug therapy of hypertension. *In* Goodman, L. S., and Gilman, A. (Eds.): The Pharmacological Basis of Therapeutics, 4th ed. New York: Macmillan, 1970, pp. 728–744.
2. Bendersky, G., and Ramirez, C.: Hydralazine poisoning. JAMA 173:1789, 1960.
3. Gadekar, S. M., Nibi, S., and Cohen, E.: Hypotensive activity of some cyanoguanidines. J. Med. Chem. 11:811, 1968.
4. Cummings, J. R., Welter, A. N., Grace, J. L., Jr., and Gray, W. D.: Angiotensin blocking actions of guancydine. J. Pharmacol. Exp. Ther. 170:334, 1969.
5. Cummings, J. R., Welter, A. N., Grace, J. L., Jr., and Lipchuck, L. M.: Cardiovascular actions of guancydine in normotensive and hypertensive animals. J. Pharmacol. Exp. Ther. 161:88, 1968.
6. Freis, E. D., and Hammer, J.: Guancydine, a new type of antihypertensive agent. Med. Ann. D.C. 38:69, 1969.
7. Hammer, J., Ulrych, M., and Freis, E. D.: Hemodynamic and therapeutic effects of guancydine in hypertension. Clin. Pharmacol. Ther. 12:78, 1971.
8. Stenberg, R., Sannerstedt, R., and Werko, L.: Haemodynamic studies on the antihypertensive effect of guancydine. Eur. J. Clin. Pharmacol. 3:63, 1971.
9. Werning, C., Schweikert, H. U., Stiel, D., Vetter, W., and Siegenthaler, W.: Erste Erfahrungen in der Langzeitbehandlung mit dem Antihypertensivum Guancydin. Dtsch. Med. Wochenschr. 95:1756, 1970.
10. Villarreal, H., and Arcila, H.: The effect of guancydine on systemic and renal hemodynamics in arterial hypertension. Clin. Pharmacol. Ther. 12:838, 1971.
11. Gilmore, E., Weil, J., and Chidsey, C.: Treatment of essential hypertension with a new vasodilator in combination with beta-adrenergic blockade. N. Engl. J. Med. 282:521, 1970.
12. Clark, D. W., and Goldberg, L. I.: Guancydine: A new antihypertensive agent. Use with quinethazone and guanethidine or propranolol. Ann. Intern. Med. 76:579, 1972.
13. Zacest, R., Gilmore, E., and Koch-Weser, J.: Treatment of essential hypertension by combined vasodilatation and beta adrenergic blockade. Clin. Pharmacol. Ther. 12:305, 1971.
14. Moser, M., Syner, J., Malitz, S., and Mattingly, T. W.: Acute psychosis as a complication of hydralazine therapy in essential hypertension. JAMA 152:1329, 1953.
15. Fox, C. A.: Reduction in the rise of systolic blood pressure during human coitus by the β-adrenergic blocking agent, propranolol. J. Reprod. Fertil. 22:587, 1970.
16. Gottlieb, T., and Chidsey, C.: Vasodilators in hypertension: A comparative evaluation of minoxidil and hydralazine. Circulation 43-44: II–129, 1971.

The Use of Vasodilators and Beta-adrenergic Blockade in Hypertension

By Charles A. Chidsey, M.D., Thomas B. Gottlieb, M.D., Richard G. Pluss, M.D., James C. Orcutt and John V. Weil, M.D.

In the modern era of therapy of hypertensive disease, antiadrenergic agents have an established and essential position among the available drugs. However, adequate therapy of hypertension requires long-term control of the blood pressure, and patient cooperation is an absolute necessity for pharmacotherapy. Such cooperation will be dependent on the patient's acceptance and tolerance of the administered drugs. It is the goal of any chronic therapeutic regimen to reduce both the frequency of medication and the side effects of the drugs in order to increase patient acceptance and the potential for long-term maintenance of drug therapy. Although the antiadrenergic drugs usually provide sufficient pharmacologic power to control even marked degrees of blood pressure elevation, their pharmacodynamic effect is such that the therapeutic response to these drugs is necessarily coupled with a high incidence of side effects. A recent study has defined the variety and frequency of these side effects for alphamethyldopa, guanethidine, and pargyline and has suggested that side effects occur with equal frequency with all of these drugs at equihypotensive doses.[1] It is possible that pharmacologic refinements may diminish the number of such side effects as more specific antiadrenergic drugs are developed, but a certain residual incidence can be expected to continue as the result of the basic activity of this type of drug, interference with physiologic activity of the adrenergic nervous system. Thus, postural and exertional hypotension with attendant fatigue and related symptomatology will remain a problem in the patient receiving drugs of this type on a chronic basis. Since the patient with high blood pressure who requires therapy is often totally asymptomatic, the production of symptomatology, such as dizziness on standing or easy fatigue on exertion, does not encourage the patient to accept chronic therapy. Because of these considerations we were led to pursue an alternate approach to drug therapy of the hypertensive patient.

The primary hemodynamic abnormality in sustained and uncomplicated hypertension appears to be an elevated vascular resistance,[2] and a direct approach to therapy could involve the use of arterial vasodilators which would reverse this hemodynamic abnormality. However, vasodilators have been difficult to use generally because of the problem of an associated reflex stimulation of the heart by cardiac adrenergic nerves. The increase in cardiac rate and contractility may lead to angina and even to myocardial infarction in patients with underlying coronary artery disease.[3] Therefore, vasodilators such as hydralazine have been used for chronic therapy only in combination with drugs inhibiting total adrenergic function with the side effects related thereto. In addition, hydralazine, the only vasodilator available for chronic therapy, is recognized to have limited pharmacologic power and to be associated with the occurrence of tachyphylaxis on chronic administration. The development of a new direct vasodilator, minoxidil (Fig. 1), with apparently greater pharmacologic power and no potential for tachyphylaxis provided a compound which might be useful in therapy.[4] In addition, the availability of beta-adrenergic antagonists, such as propranolol, suggested a means of attenuating reflexly mediated stimulation of cardiac function occurring with arterial vasodilator therapy without the undesired side effect of interference with total adrenergic

From the Departments of Medicine and Pharmacology, University of Colorado Medical Center, Denver, Colorado.

This work was supported by grants from the National Institutes of Health (HE 09932, HE 05722, and FR 00051), and from The Upjohn Company.

NH2

HO-N

HN=

N

N

MINOXIDIL

(6-amino-1,2-dihydro-1-hydroxy-2-imino-4-piperidino pyrimidine)

FIG. 1.—The chemical structure of minoxidil, a new direct-acting arterial vasodilator.

function. Thus, the use of minoxidil combined with propranolol offered a new therapeutic approach to hypertension. It might be possible to lower blood pressure without interfering with those peripheral adrenergic reflexes which are responsible for the maintenance of perfusion pressure during the potential cardiovascular stress of standing and exertion; with this approach we hoped to be able to reduce blood pressure and minimize the side effects thereby increasing the potential for patient acceptance of therapy. This report reviews evidence that minoxidil is indeed a hypotensive agent which promises to provide more effective antihypertensive therapy than currently available drugs.

PHARMACOLOGY OF MINOXIDIL IN EXPERIMENTAL ANIMALS

The vasodilator activity of minoxidil appears to result from the direct effect of this compound on arterial smooth muscle. Studies in experimental animals have shown that the decline in blood pressure resulting from administration of minoxidil is not associated with a significant interference with basal adrenergic tone or with cardiovascular reflexes mediated by the adrenergic nerves.[4] The hypotensive response to a single parenteral dose persisted for at least 24 hours in both the rat and dog although the drug was rapidly cleared from the body with over 80 percent of the dose recovered in the urine as drug or its metabolites in that period of time.[5] We were interested in determining whether the persistent hypotensive activity was due to retention of small but pharmacologically important quantities of minoxidil in the arterial vasculature. Normotensive rats received 10 mg of radiolabeled minoxidil intraperitoneally during carotid arterial blood pressure monitoring.[6] They were sacrificed at various times thereafter up to 12 hours and tissues removed for determination of total radioactivity (minoxidil and its metabolites) and for minoxidil itself. The blood pressure fell promptly after administration of the drug and was reduced significantly at 12 hours (Fig. 2). There was a rapid decline of minoxidil in the plasma with less than 1 percent of the peak levels measured at 0.5 hours persisting at 12 hours. A similar decline occurred in spleen and myocardium, but the disappearance of minoxidil from arterial tissue was delayed resulting in apparent retention of the drug at these sites after 2 hours, with as much as an eight-fold concentration of the

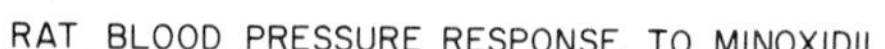

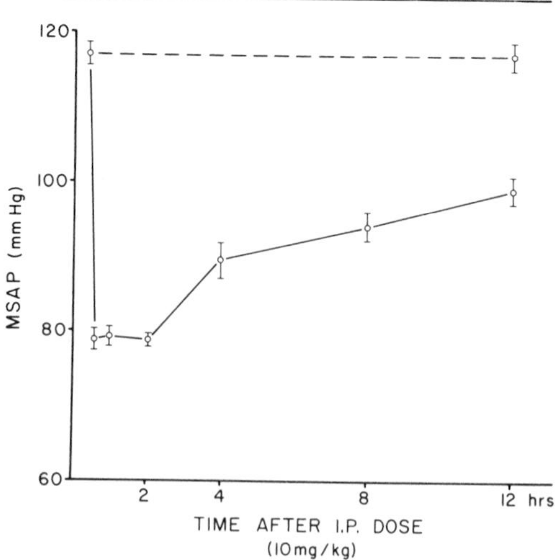

FIG. 2.—The response of mean systemic arterial pressure **(MSAP)** of rats to the intraperitoneal administration of 10 mg of minoxidil per kilogram of body weight is shown by the **solid line** through values of the mean with its standard error. The **broken line** shows the control data. (From Pluss, Orcutt, and Chidsey,[6] with permission.)

drug in femoral artery over the plasma at 12 hours (Fig. 3). These data suggest that accumulation of minoxidil at vascular receptor sites may be responsible for its prolonged activity.

Clinical Pharmacology of Minoxidil

Minoxidil has been evaluated in two groups of hypertensive patients.[7,8] The first evaluation was undertaken to determine therapeutic efficacy and to examine the extent of reflex activation of cardiac activity which occurred with arterial vasodilation and the capacity of propranolol to inhibit this activation. In 11 patients all therapy was discontinued 2 weeks before admission to the Clinical Research Center of the University of Colorado Medical Center, where the patients received a constant dietary intake of sodium (75 to 142 mEq per day). After a control period we administered either minoxidil alone incrementally to an adequate hypotensive dose (15 to 80 mg per day) and then added propranolol (80 to 240 mg per day) or we gave propranolol first (80 to 160 mg per day) and then added minoxidil (20 to 80 mg per day). The decrease in blood pressure with minoxidil was notable, occurred without postural hypotension, and was significantly greater with the addition of propranolol (Fig. 4). The supine blood pressure fell from an average of 188/124 to 159/108 mm Hg on minoxidil alone and to 134/86 mm Hg with the addition of propranolol with a consistent increase in pressure on standing (Table 1). The increase in heart rate observed with minoxidil alone, from 75 to 80 minutes^{-1}, was reversed with the addition of propranolol or prevented by pretreatment with such beta-adrenergic blockade.

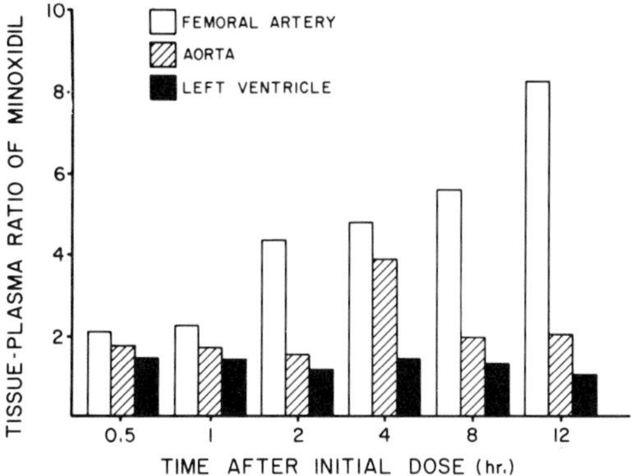

Fig. 3.—The ratio of ^{14}C-labeled minoxidil in tissue compared to plasma is shown over 12 hours following intraperitoneal injection of 10 mg per kilogram of body weight. (From Pluss, Orcutt, and Chidsey,[6] with permission.)

The hemodynamic changes induced during minoxidil administration and the role of beta-blockade were evaluated by measuring cardiac output and forearm vascular resistance in these patients. Cardiac index increased from 2.75 to 4.04 liters per minute/M^{-2} on minoxidil alone and propranolol (0.1 mg per kilogram intravenously) reduced this value to the control level (Fig. 5). Concordant increases in stroke volume and heart rate produced by minoxidil were also reversed by propranolol. The decrease in systemic vascular resistance produced by minoxidil was somewhat attenuated by the acutely induced beta-adrenergic blockade probably as a result of a compensatory increase of adrenergic activity in response to the blockade. This increased adrenergic drive was capable of producing vasoconstriction via uninhibited alpha-receptors. In the second group of patients, those pretreated with propranolol, although the increase in cardiac dynamics produced by minoxidil was not eliminated, this response was certainly attenuated. Forearm hemodynamic studies during minoxidil therapy showed that an increase in blood flow, from 3.02 to 4.54 ml per 100 ml per minute, occurred together with a decrease in vascular resistance, from 49.7 to 26.9 PRU, in this vascular bed with little change in venous compliance (Fig. 6). Propranolol alone tended to diminish flow and increase resistance, but these changes were reversed when minoxidil was added to beta-blockade.

The side effects from minoxidil observed in these patients were clinical evidence of myocardial ischemia and sodium retention with minimal edema. T-wave inversion on the ECG or transient chest pain occurred in the patients on minoxidil alone. Although sodium accumulation occurred consistently and averaged 44 mEq per day, it was of consequence in only one patient who developed left ventricular failure on propranolol which responded promptly to diuretic therapy. The signs of myocardial ischemia were attributed to reflexly

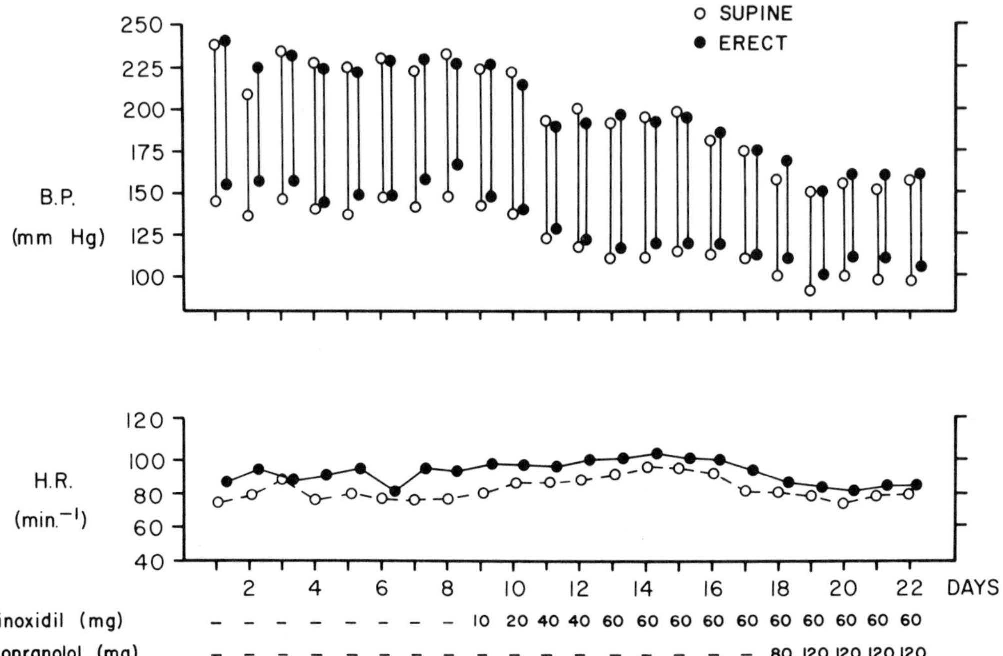

FIG. 4.—Blood pressure and heart-rate measurements during 3 weeks of hospitalization show the initial control values, the response to minoxidil alone, and the further response to addition of propranolol.

TABLE 1.—*Blood Pressure and Heart Rate Data Before and During Minoxidil Therapy*

	Blood Pressure (mm Hg)		*Heart Rate (minute⁻¹)*	
	Supine	*Erect*	*Supine*	*Erect*
Group 1 *				
Control	188/124	182/134	75	92
	± 21/4	± 12/6	± 5	± 3
Minoxidil	159/108 †	164/112 †	90 †	102 †
	± 16/12	± 9/3	± 6	± 4
Minoxidil and propranolol	134/86 ‡	142/99 ‡	79 ‡	84 ‡
	± 12/9	± 9/5	± 4	± 3
Group 2				
Control	170/116	165/124	76	89
	± 11/6	± 5/5	± 1	± 4
Propranolol	166/108	160/119	66	75
	± 12/7	± 4/5	± 2	± 4
Propranolol and minoxidil	135/89 †	135/99 †	80	84
	± 8/4	± 4/5	± 5	± 4

* The values given are the mean ± standard error of the mean.
† Mean value is different from control ($p < .01$).
‡ Mean value is different from minoxidil alone ($p < .01$).

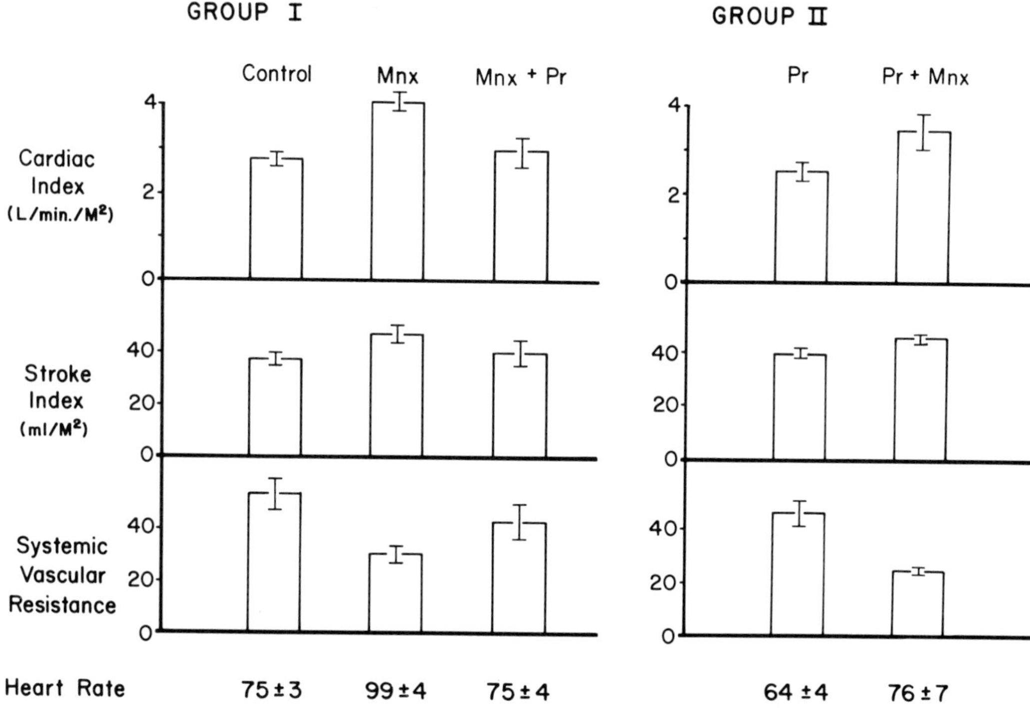

FIG. 5.—Hemodynamic data showing the effects of minoxidil **(Mnx)** and of propranolol **(Pr)** in hypertensive patients. In Group I, after control measurements, minoxidil was given orally for 6 to 7 days and the measurements were repeated. The propranolol was administered intravenously during the second study (0.1 mg per kilogram of body weight). In Group II the initial measurements were made while the patients received propranolol and the second study was carried out after oral administration of minoxidil for 7 days. (From Gilmore, Weil, and Chidsey,[7] with permission.)

induced increases of adrenergic activity based on the response to beta-blockade (Table 1; Fig. 5), as well as to the finding of a notably increased urinary excretion of norepinephrine and vanillylmandelic acid (VMA) (Fig. 7). Sodium retention could not be so easily explained since there was neither any consistent change in renal clearance of inulin or para-aminohippuric acid (PAH) nor a consistently increased aldosterone excretion. Although aldosterone excretion rose moderately with minoxidil alone from 13.4 ± 1.2 to 19.6 ± 3.0 μg per day, the addition of propranolol resulted in a lowering of aldosterone excretion to values unchanged from control in spite of persistent sodium retention. Thus, enhanced aldosterone-mediated, distal tubular reabsorption of sodium cannot be evoked to explain the sodium retention and it seems more likely that a proximal tubular change may be involved in this phenomenon.[9]

Since sodium retention appeared to be the main complication of the use of minoxidil and propranolol in the treatment of hypertension, we were interested in determining whether this complication could be eliminated by concurrent treatment with a diuretic. Accordingly, a second study was undertaken to answer this question, to compare the therapeutic efficacy of minoxidil with that of hydralazine, and to determine the fate and disposition of this drug in patients with hypertension.[8] This study involved 11 hypertensive patients hospitalized in the Clinical Research Center. The patients were selected for the study if they had been refractory to conventional antihypertensive therapy either because of side effects or because of lack of adequate hypotensive response on maximal therapy. Drugs were usually withdrawn several weeks before admission to the study but in four patients this was not possible because of the

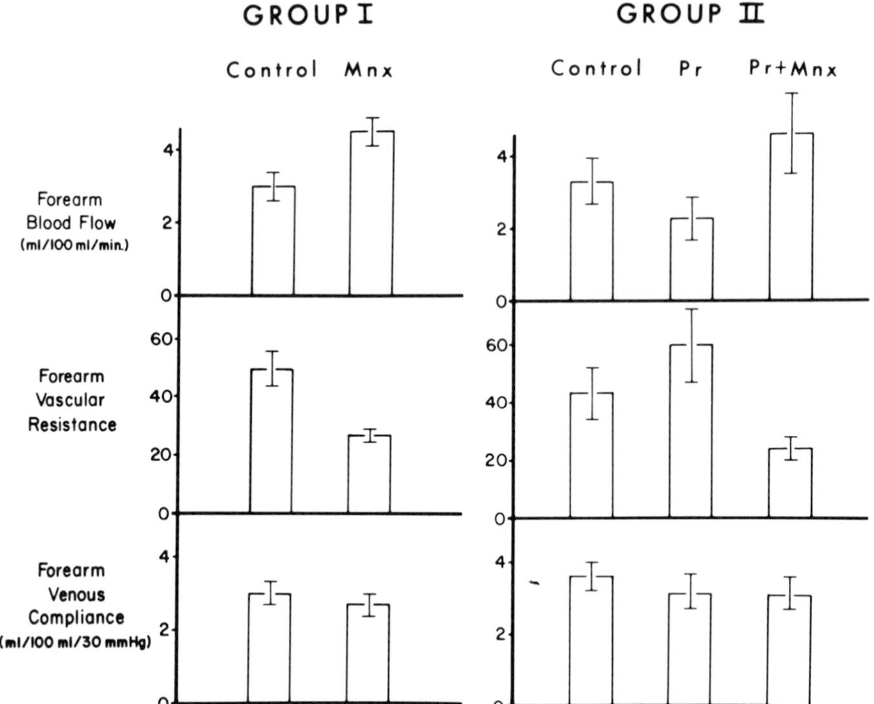

FIG. 6.—Forearm hemodynamic data showing the effects of minoxidil **(Mnx)** and propranolol **(Pr)** in hypertensive patients. Group I were studied only before and during oral minoxidil while Group II were studied during a control period, an oral propranolol period, and a period of minoxidil added to propranolol. (From Gilmore, Weil, and Chidsey,[7] with permission.)

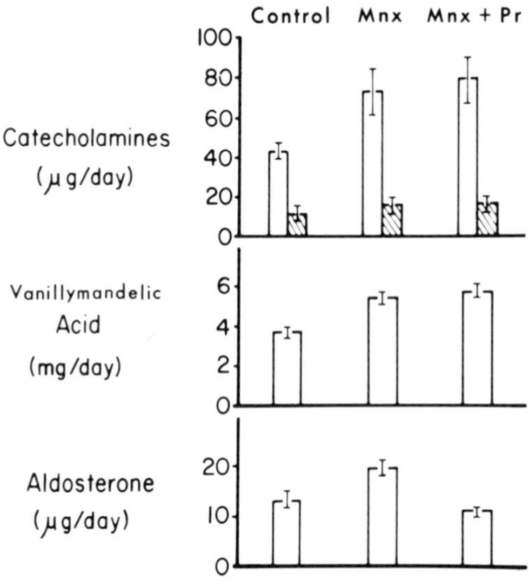

FIG. 7.—Endocrine responses to oral minoxidil and to propranolol added to minoxidil.

severity of the hypertensive cardiovascular disease; these patients were admitted directly to the study at which time their previous drugs were discontinued (alpha-methyldopa and guanethidine). During study all patients received propranolol (40 to 160 mg per day) and hydrochlorothiazide (50 to 200 mg per day) continually during control, hydralazine (200 to 800 mg per day), and minoxidil (2 to 30 mg per day) periods.

The therapeutic response to minoxidil was greater than that to hydralazine (Table 2). The average supine blood pressure falling from 191/128 mm Hg in the control period, on hydrochlorothiazide and propranolol to 169/108 mm Hg with the additions of hydralazine, and to 142/92 mm Hg with minoxidil. More notable than the average blood pressure changes were the observations that in four patients the hypertensive response to hydralazine was in-

TABLE 2.—*Comparison of Therapeutic Responses to Minoxidil and Hydralazine*

	Blood Pressure (mm Hg)		*Heart Rate (minute⁻¹)*	
	Supine	*Erect*	*Supine*	*Erect*
Control *	191/128 ± 7/5	166/125 ± 8/6	72 ± 3	82 ± 4
Hydralazine	169/108 † ± 6/6	148/108 † ± 7/5	74 ± 2	82 ± 3
Minoxidil	142/92 ‡ ± 4/2	131/95 ‡ ± 5/4	78 ± 2	84 ± 3

* Values represent the mean ± standard error of the mean.
† Mean value is different from control ($p < .01$).
‡ Mean value is different from hydralazine ($p < .01$).

adequate in spite of doses of 600 to 800 mg per day, whereas in these patients substitution of minoxidil resulted in a substantially greater hypotensive effect. Thus, these data indicate that minoxidil has both therapeutic potency and efficacy which are much greater than those of hydralazine. There was essentially no change in heart rate with either hydralazine or minoxidil. However, it was necessary to increase the amount of propranolol in five patients either to maintain a constant heart rate or because of the development of angina which occurred transiently in three patients as minoxidil was begun. There was no recurrence of the angina once the maximum hypotensive response to minoxidil had been achieved. In one patient we demonstrated the continued importance of beta-adrenergic blockade after 7 days of blood pressure reduction with vasodilator therapy (Fig. 8). The discontinuation of propranolol in this patient resulted in a prompt increase in heart rate to more than 110 minute^{-1} and an obvious rise in blood pressure. This patient was a young woman who could tolerate this increased cardiac activity without difficulty. However, in the presence of underlying coronary artery disease it is unlikely that this response would develop without clear evidence of myocardial ischemia such as angina, ECG changes, or myocardial infarction.

Sodium retention was not a problem in this study and we detected no increase in weight or decrease in sodium excretion on constant

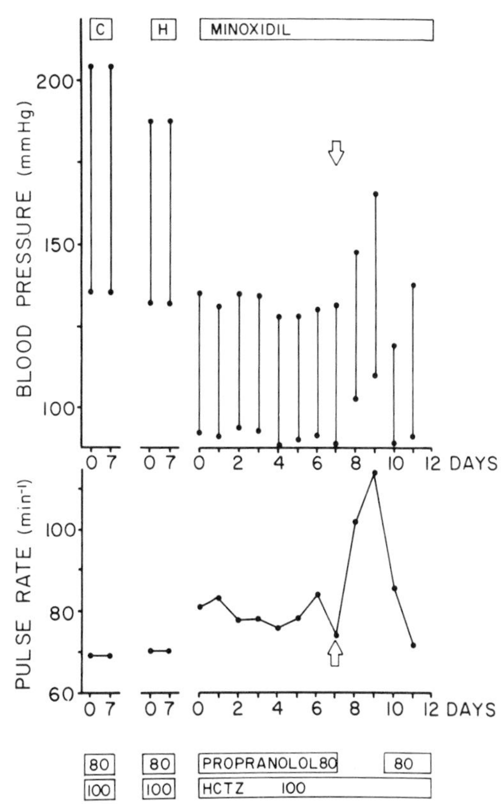

FIG. 8.—Blood pressure and pulse rates in an initial control period of 7 days followed by 7 days of hydralazine and 11 days of minoxidil therapy. Hydrochlorothiazide was given continuously as was propranolol except for the temporary discontinuation of the latter during days 7, 8, and 9. (From Gottlieb, Katz, and Chidsey,[8] with permission.)

dietary intakes. In three patients it was necessary to increase the amount of diuretic to prevent sodium accumulation. There was no significant change in renal clearance during the hypotension induced by either vasodilator. In reevaluating the question of the mechanism of the potential for enhanced sodium retention with vasodilator therapy, we measured plasma renin activity and aldosterone in these patients during both hydralazine- and minoxidil-induced hypotension. Measurements were made with the patients in both supine and erect positions. There was an increase in plasma renin activity during hypotension induced by either drug but the levels reached tended to be higher in the initial hydralazine period than in the later minoxidil periods, in spite of the greater hypotensive response in the latter period (Fig. 9). Individual patient responses of plasma renin activity were not uniformly compatible with existing concepts of renin secretion.[10] Thus, changes in plasma renin activity could not be correlated with individual hypotensive responses nor with changes in sodium excretion. One important pharmacologic factor in the renin response of this group of patients may be that of propranolol. This drug has been suggested to interfere with renin release[11] and this factor may have played a role in the present observations. The lack of increase of aldosterone levels as the renin values increased was an unexpected finding in view of the well-established relationship between plasma renin activity and both aldosterone secretion and excretion rates.[12] However, these findings are consistent with our previous measurements of aldosterone excretion in the first study quoted above which demonstrated that it was unchanged in patients treated with minoxidil when they received propranolol concurrently. The explanation of the failure to increase aldosterone secretion as indicated by the plasma aldosterone concentration, in the face of significant increases in plasma renin, is not readily apparent. It is interesting to speculate that propranolol may not only interfere with renin release,[11] but may alter the effect of the renin stimulus on the secretion of aldosterone, either by inhibition of angiotensin-I conversion, or by direct effect on the adrenal cortical response to angiotensin II.

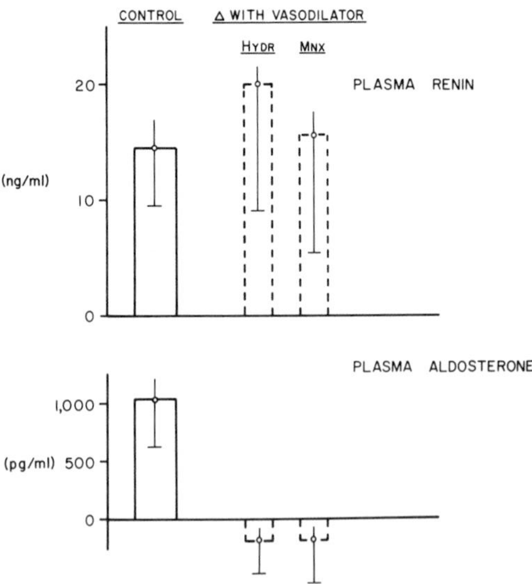

FIG. 9.—The plasma renin activity and aldosterone concentration before vasodilator therapy and the change in each with the vasodilator (Δ with vasodilator). These are the mean values with their standard errors obtained in seven patients studied under all three conditions and receiving diuretics and propranolol.

The hypotensive activity of minoxidil together with the minimal side effects found in this short-term study using propranolol and diuretics encouraged us to examine the long-term activity in nine patients in whom blood pressure control could not be achieved by other conventional drug therapy. We have been able effectively to control blood pressure in these patients with minoxidil (5 to 30 mg per day) over a period as long as 18 months and we have observed no evidence that tachyphylaxis has developed in any patient. The side effects of therapy have been only two: hirsutism and difficulty with sodium retention. Hirsutism has developed regularly in patients on more than 10 mg of minoxidil per day for more than 1 month, is confined to the malar and upper truncal areas, and is unassociated with detectable alteration of adrenal or gonadal physiology. Sodium retention presents a problem in some patients, namely those with diminished renal function, and we have had to employ both limitation of sodium intake and the addition of substantial quantities of furosemide to prevent edema and evidence of vascular congestion. However, left ventricular failure has not developed in any of these patients to date.

A notable characteristic, which is predictable from the experimental animal studies quoted above, is its apparent duration of action which seems greatly to exceed 24 hours. In one patient we discontinued minoxidil after having established satisfactory therapeutic blood pressure control with it in combination with propranolol and furosemide (Fig. 10). The blood pressure did not rise toward pretreatment levels for 3 days whereas on readministration of a single dose the blood pressure required 12 hours to demonstrate a maximum therapeutic response. Although the rate at which controlled blood pressure values will return to a hypertensive level when therapy is stopped may be extremely variable, it is generally the experience that the more severely hypertensive patients tended to revert more rapidly to their pretreatment levels.[13] These observations would suggest that the duration of the vasodilator activity of minoxidil greatly exceeds that of other arterial dilators such as diazoxide.[14]

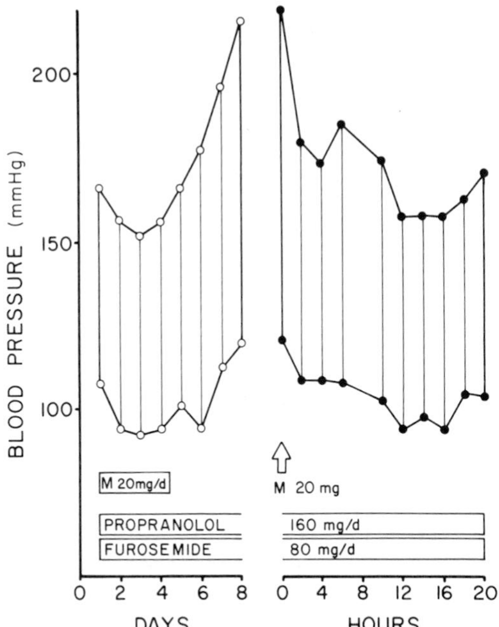

Fig. 10.—The blood pressure response to stopping minoxidil after 6 days of blood pressure control together with the initial blood pressure response to a single oral dose. (From Gottlieb, Katz, and Chidsey,[8] with permission.)

This prolonged duration of action may have important therapeutic implications in the chronic medication of the hypertensive patient by providing a powerful antihypertensive drug which may require but a single dose.

The prolonged hypotensive activity is inconsistent with a rapid disposition of the drug which has been found both in man[15] and in experimental animals.[5,6] We have found that the plasma half-life averaged 4.2 hours and that the drug is cleared primarily by metabolism with a 588 ml per minute clearance from a volume of distribution exceeding that of body water, 200 liters. When ^{14}C-minoxidil was given orally to patients after achieving blood pressure reduction with nonlabeled drug, we were able to recover all of the ^{14}C-label in the urine. However, only 10 percent of the dose appeared there unchanged and the remainder was excreted in the form of metabolites (Fig. 11). We have found that there are three major metabolites and one of these has been identified as a glucuronide conjugate. The glucuronide appears with minoxidil as the predominant metabolite early after drug administration (Fig. 12). Two other metabolites are the dominant metabolites later, but these represent a smaller portion of the total elimination of the drug than does the glucuronide.

These observations provide no pharmacokinetic basis for the prolonged action of minoxidil since it is obvious that the drug cannot

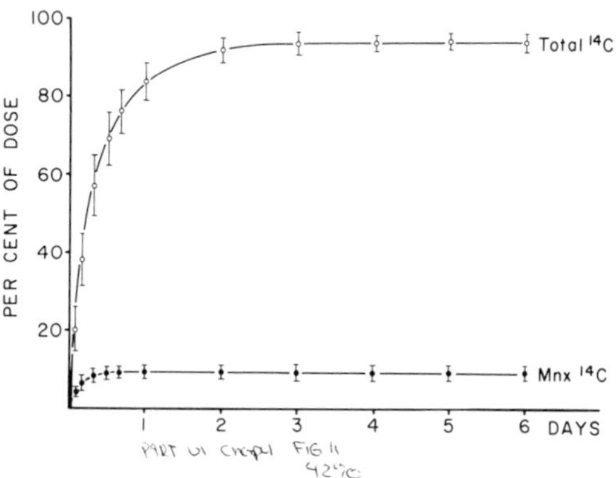

Fig. 11.—The cumulative urinary excretion of minoxidil (**Mnx ^{14}C**) over 6 days following its oral administration. (From Gottlieb, Thomas, and Chidsey,[15] with permission.)

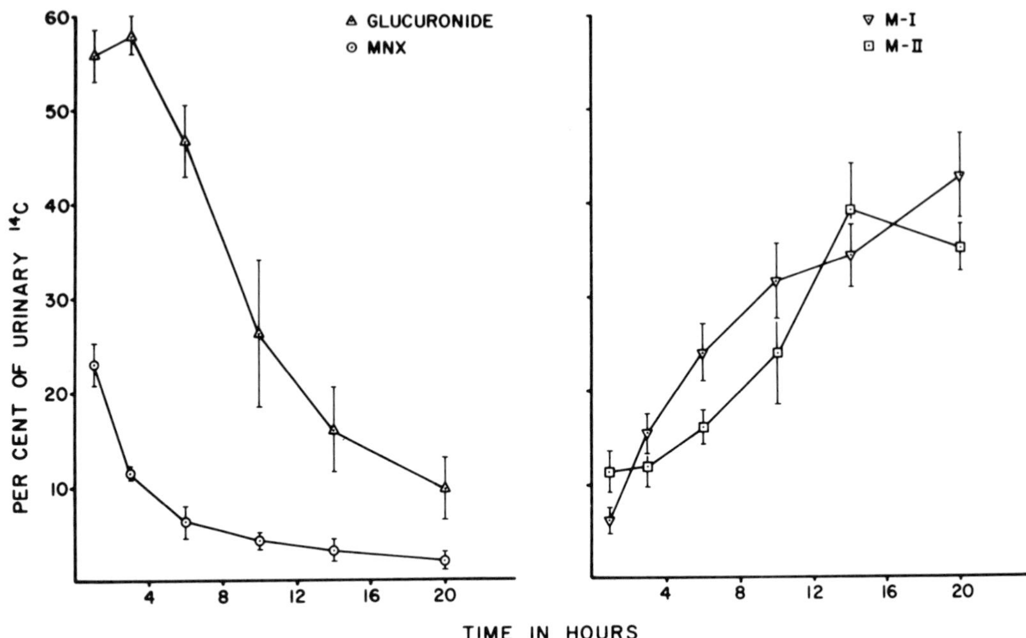

FIG. 12.—The fraction of urinary ^{14}C-activity as minoxidil **(Mnx),** its glucuronide, and M-I and M-II appearing in urine samples during 24 hours after an oral dose of ^{14}C-minoxidil. (From Gottlieb, Thomas, and Chidsey,[15] with permission.)

accumulate in the blood nor persist there in order to account for the prolonged action. One may speculate that the duration of action results from the fact that the drug is either retained at vascular receptor sites or produces a change in the functional state of the smooth muscle which requires a prolonged period for recovery. The former hypothesis has been proposed based on evidence in experimental animals that drug can be shown to be retained specifically in vascular tissues.[6] Further studies are in progress to evaluate critically the cellular basis for this important pharmacodynamic activity of minoxidil.

SUMMARY

The treatment of arterial hypertension is difficult because it involves protracted pharmacotherapy in a group of largely asymptomatic patients using drugs which frequently produce troublesome side effects. We have proposed a different pharmacologic approach to therapy which utilizes a new powerful vasodilator drug, minoxidil, in combination with beta-adrenergic blockade and diuretic therapy. We have shown that this approach is effective. Minoxidil has greater therapeutic efficacy than another available vasodilator, hydralazine: Blood pressure has lowered in a group of hypertensive patients from a control value of 191/128 to 142/92 mm Hg with minoxidil compared to 169/108 mm Hg with hydralazine. The side effects were minimal in comparison to those seen with existing powerful antihypertensive drugs. Although sodium retention and adrenergically induced stimulation of the heart with myocardial ischemia can occur, these side effects appear to be prevented by effective use of diuretics and propranolol. An additional advantage of minoxidil appears to be its prolonged activity which may extend for several days. This duration of effect contrasts to a rapid disposition of the drug from blood by metabolic transformation with a half-life in blood of only 4.2 hours.

REFERENCES

1. Oates, J. A., Seligman, A. W., Clark, M. A., Rousseau, P., and Lee, R. E.: The relative efficacy of guanethidine, Aldomet and pargy-

line as antihypertensive agents. N. Engl. J. Med. 273:729, 1965.

2. Hickam, J. B., and Cargill, W. H.: Effect of exercise on cardiac output and pulmonary artery pressure in normal persons and in patients with cardiovascular disease and pulmonary emphysema. J. Clin. Invest. 27:10, 1948.
3. Nickerson, M.: Antihypertensive agents and the drug therapy of hypertension. *In* Goodman, L. S., and Gilman, A. (Eds.): Pharmacological Basis of Therapeutics. New York: Macmillan, 1970, pp. 716–735.
4. Freyburger, W. F., DuCharme, D. W., and Zins, G. R.: Unpublished data.
5. Thomas, R. C.: Unpublished data.
6. Pluss, R. G., Orcutt, J., and Chidsey, C. A.: Tissue distribution and hypotensive effects of a new vasodilator, minoxidil. J. Lab. Clin. Med. 79:639, 1972.
7. Gilmore, E., Weil, J., and Chidsey, C.: Treatment of essential hypertension with a new vasodilator in combination with beta adrenergic blockade. N. Engl. J. Med. 282:521, 1970.
8. Gottlieb, T. B., Katz, F. H., and Chidsey, C. A.: Combined therapy with vasodilator drugs and beta adrenergic blockade in hypertension: A comparative study of minoxidil and hydralazine. Circulation 45:571, 1972.
9. Zins, G. R., Shoemaker, R. J., and Walk, R. A.: Characteristics of the antinatriuretic effect of the direct acting peripheral vasodilator. Fourth International Congress of Nephrology, Stockholm, Sweden, June 22–27, 1969, p. 442.
10. Davis, J. O.: What signals the kidney to release renin? Circ. Res. 28:301, 1971.
11. Winer, N., Chokshi, D. S., Yoon, M. S., and Freedman, A. D.: Adrenergic receptor mediation of renin secretion. J. Clin. Endocrinol. 29:1168, 1969.
12. Laragh, J., Sealy, J. E., and Sommers, S. C.: Adrenal secretion and urinary excretion of aldosterone and plasma renin activity in normal and hypertensive subjects. Circ. Res. 28, Suppl. I:158, 1966.
13. Dustan, H. P., Page, I. H., Tarazi, R. C., and Frohlich, E. D.: Arterial pressure response to discontinuing antihypertensive drugs. Circulation 37:370, 1968.
14. Powell, J., Green, R. M., Whiting, R. B., and Sanders, C. A.: Action of diazoxide on skeletal muscle vascular resistance. Circ. Res. 28: 167, 1971.
15. Gottlieb, T. B., Thomas, R. C., and Chidsey, C. A.: Pharmacokinetic studies of minoxidil, a new antihypertensive drug. Clin. Pharmacol. Ther. 13:436, 1972.

Pharmacologic Basis of the Cardiovascular Actions of Clonidine

By Walter Kobinger, M.D.

In 1962 Dr. Stähle synthesized an imidazoline derivative, clonidine * (Fig. 1), and submitted a 0.3% solution to the medical department of his pharmaceutical company for an evaluation of its nasal decongestive properties. Dr. M. Wolf, a physician of the trial group, administered to himself a few drops (approximately 1 to 2 mg) and immediately discovered the sedative, bradycardic, and hypotensive effects of the substance.[1] Detailed pharmacologic studies revealed a great number of activities (Table 1). However, the cardiovascular actions of the drug elicited the greatest interest, especially because they could be demonstrated with minute doses. Only the cardiovascular effects of clonidine will be considered in this chapter. Rapid intravenous injections of clonidine, in doses between 5 and 500 μg per kilogram of body weight, into anesthetized as well as conscious animals, invariably led to the typical reactions indicated in Fig. 2: A transient blood pressure increase is followed by a long-lasting hypotension, with a bradycardia accompanying both phases. The hypertensive phase was not observed if the drug was infused slowly intravenously.[2]

Initial Hypertensive Effect of Clonidine

There is little doubt that the hypertensive component of the action of clonidine is due to a direct alpha-sympathomimetic vasoconstricting action. The hypertension was antagonized by alpha-adrenergic blocking drugs (phentolamine, phenoxybenzamine.) [2-7] Clonidine elicited sympathomimetic effects, such as long-lasting contraction of the nictitating membrane (Fig. 2),[3,5,6,8] decrease in spleen volume and increase in hematocrit [8] in various animal species. Pupillary dilatation, however, occurred only in cats [9] and rats,[10] but not in dogs [10] or humans.[11-13] Alpha-sympathomimetic activities of clonidine were revealed in isolated preparations causing contraction of the seminal vesicle,[5] vas deferens,[14] aortic and popliteal venous strips,[4,5] and vascular constriction in the isolated perfused rabbit ear.[5,8] Intra-arterial injection of clonidine was followed by vasoconstriction of the resistance as well as of capacitance vessels in hindlimbs of cats [3,15] and in pump-perfused forelimbs of dogs.[4] Intra-arterial clonidine also decreased blood flow in human leg and foot.[16]

The sympathomimetic actions of clonidine are due to a direct action of the drug upon adrenergic receptors: A full or even exaggerated hypertensive response or nictitating membrane contraction was recorded after depletion of catecholamine stores (reserpine pretreatment),[2,3,5,7] treatment with cocaine [6] 1 week after denervation of the nictitating membrane,[6] or in immunosympathectomized rats.[17] This specific, direct stimulating effect of clonidine upon adrenergic alpha-receptors is very similar to that reported for other imidazolines such as naphazoline, tetrahydrozoline, and others.[18] Clonidine did not exert beta-adrenergic stimulating properties as no tachycardia was observed in isolated or in situ hearts.[3,4,8,19,20] Similarly there was no vasodilatation in those experiments where the drug was administered intra-arterially. In two studies with more complicated experimental approaches the involvement of beta-adrenergic activities of clonidine has been postulated.[21,22]

Acute Hypotensive Effect of Clonidine

The Cardiovascular Reaction Pattern of Clonidine

The typical clonidine effects of hypotension, bradycardia, fall in cardiac output,[2-4,8,9,23-25] and, in some reports, decrease in total periph-

From the Pharmacology Department of the Arzneimittelforschung Ges.m.b.H., Vienna, Austria.

* C. H. Boehringer Sohn, Ingelheim am Rhein.

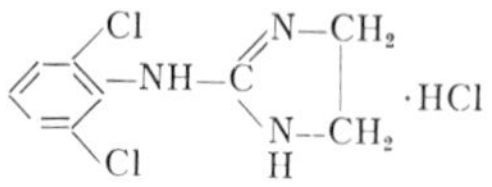

Cl N—CH_2 —NH—C ·HCl N—CH_2 Cl H

FIG. 1.—Clonidine (Catapresan; Catapresan St 155; 2-(2,6-dichlorphenylamino-)-2-imidazoline hydrochloride).

eral resistance,[4,23] were shown in various animal species and in humans.[23,25] This pattern is similar to that previously observed with older drugs which are known to exert their antihypertensive effect via a decrease in sympathetic activity: ganglionic-blocking agents, reserpine, guanethidine, bretylium, and possibly alpha-methyldopa.[26] The distribution of sympathetic tone seems to determine whether the decrease in cardiac output or in total peripheral resistance is preferably responsible for the hypotension; this has been demonstrated in tilting experiments in humans treated with clonidine,[27] alpha-methyldopa, or guanethidine.[28]

Possible Mechanisms of Action

Effect on Myocardial Function. A direct impairment of myocardial function was rejected by most of the investigators. In concentrations comparable to hypotensive doses in vivo no decrease in cardiac output, contractile force, or heart rate was observed in the heart-lung preparations of dogs,[8] in isolated perfused hearts of cats,[4] dogs,[20] rabbits, and rats [19] or in isolated auricle or papillary muscle preparations.[8,19] A direct-depressing action of clonidine upon pacemaker activity had been suggested [2] but this hypothesis was rejected later on the basis of additional results from the same laboratory.[19] These included experiments with dogs after cardiac transplantation, where injection of 1 mg of clonidine per kilogram of body weight did not significantly change the heart rate.[19] Injections of small doses of clonidine (0.1 μg) into the sinus node artery of dogs slowed the heart rate, an effect which was ascribed to a peripheral sympathetic-blocking action and was assumed to be of primary importance for the bradycardic effect of the drug.[29] It seems obvious, however, that this effect of clonidine is due to its alpha-adrenergic action: Several substances of this type were able to depress heart rate when injected into the sinus node artery.[30]

Peripheral Myogenic Vasodilatation. The

TABLE 1.—*Pharmacologic Actions of Clonidine (Noncardiovascular, Not Described in the Text)*

Object	*Effect*	*Species*	*References*
Isolated ileum	Contraction	Guinea pigs	8
	Adrenolytic	Humans	45
Local anesthesia	Positive	Guinea pigs	8
Sensory neurons	Action potential modified *	Crayfishes	47
Gastric secretion	Decrease	Mice, rats, guinea pigs	8, 58, 72, 73
	Increase	Rats	74
Blood glucose	Rise	Rabbits, rats, cats, dogs	8, 58, 75–77, 78
Saluresis	Increased	Rats	8
	No change	Dogs	8
Free water clearance	Increased	Dogs	79
Behavior	Sedation	Mice, rats, cats, dogs, chicks	8, 17, 65, 66, 80
	Aggression	Mice, rats	63, 81 †
	Tremor	Mice, dogs	8, 82
Conditioned salivation	Suppressed	Dogs	10, 83

* Similar to procaine.
† Chronic treatment.

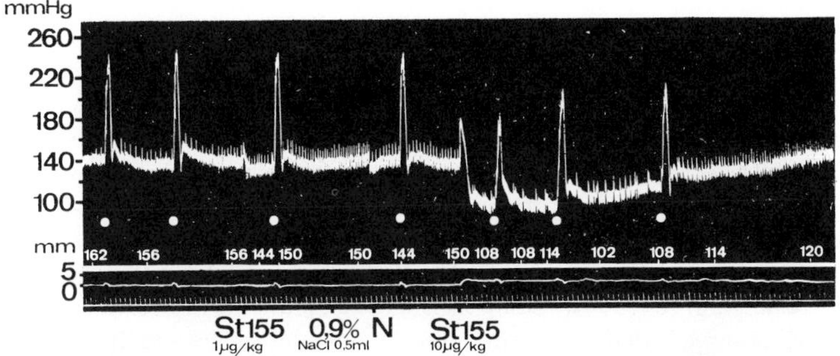

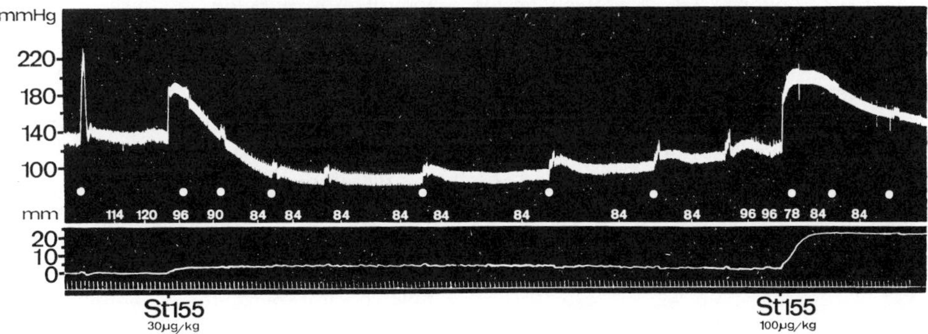

FIG. 2.—Results in a dog after vagus nerves were sectioned and pentobarbital was administered. Upper curve, blood pressure; middle curve, tension of nictitating membrane; lower curve, time in minutes; numbers, heart rate in beats per minute; circle, carotid sinus occlusion for 1 minute. Intravenous injection of clonidine (St 155). N, pentobarbital injection. (From Hoefke, W., and Kobinger, W.,[8] with permission.)

cardiovascular pattern of clonidine (see above) does not support the possibility of a peripheral myogenic vasodilatation. Primary vasodilatation elicits reflex tachycardia and an increase in cardiac output, as described for hydralazine.[31] No vasodilatation was demonstrated in isolated perfused vascular sections or with close arterial injection or infusion of clonidine within wide dose ranges.[3–5,8,15,16]

Effect in Spinal Animals and after Complete Autonomic Block. In spinal cats and rats (destruction of the whole brain including the medulla) clonidine (5 to 100 µg per kilogram of body weight) elicited no hypotension.[3,4,6,15,32] There was either no change in heart rate or a bradycardia which was definitely of less magnitude and duration than that in intact animals.[3,4] In spinal dogs, however, a bradycardia was observed; this finding was considered to indicate a direct effect of the drug upon cardiac pacemaker.[2,29] No hypotensive effect was observed in pithed rats.[5,7,33] Clonidine exerted no hypotensive effect following pretreatment with ganglionic-blocking agents.[2,5,21,34]

The lack of a blood pressure fall in "decentralized" or ganglionic-blocked animals seems to exclude peripheral effects of clonidine. The vascular tone and the blood pressure of these animals are, however, very low. Under these conditions the alpha-adrenergic, vasoconstrictor effect of clonidine becomes prevalent[35] and may mask a weak vasodilator action of the drug. In one report, in unanesthetized rabbits, pretreated with a combination of phenoxybenzamine, propranolol, and atropine ("postsynaptic autonomic block"), clonidine produced hypotension and a fall in total vascular resistance (increased cardiac output, no change in heart rate). These results were interpreted as a peripheral vasodilating action of the drug, becoming prominent after decrease in autonomic activities.[22]

Activation of the Vagus System. Clonidine did not potentiate the hypotensive effect of injected acetylcholine, nor the effect of stimulation of the peripheral end of the vagus nerve.[15,33,36] Following vagotomy or treatment with atropine, clonidine still elicited a profound decrease in blood pressure, heart rate, and cardiac output in dogs, cats, rabbits, and rats.[2,3,7,8,33,35,37–39] Therefore, most of the investigators agree that an activation of the vagus nerve cannot be the reason for the cardiovascular depressant effect of clonidine. It was, however, observed that vagotomy or atropine somewhat attenuated the bradycardic effect of clonidine [3,5,38,39a] as well as the fall in cardiac output.[3] In one experimental series, vagal inhibition abolished the bradycardic effect of clonidine and reduced the hypotensive effect.[17] It must be considered that the initial blood pressure rise after intravenous injection of clonidine will in any case elicit a bradycardia via baroreceptor reflexes and the efferent vagus nerve.[3,6] An additional vagal effect of the drug will be discussed below.

Action of Clonidine in "Debuffered" Animals. These experiments were planned in order to investigate whether clonidine facilitates afferent "depressor nerve" activities, decreasing blood pressure and heart rate, via a reflex similar to the one elicited by veratrum alkaloids.[40] In various species clonidine lowered blood pressure and heart rate after section of the carotid sinus nerves and laryngeal nerves or extirpation of the nodose ganglia,[7,34,41] or after section of sinus and vagus nerves.[42] Following sinus and aortic nerve section in cats and rabbits the hypotensive effect of clonidine was faster and shorter than in control,[33] and more pronounced.[22] This indicates that the real effect of the drug is modified by normal buffer mechanisms. Zaimis [17] recorded afferent impulses from single fibers of the vagus nerve in dogs, and could not find increased impulse discharges.

Ganglionic-Blocking Properties. A ganglionic-blocking effect has not been reported for clonidine.[6,8,37] An antagonism against the effect of muscarinic drugs but not against nicotinic ganglionic-stimulating drugs was reported by one group.[29]

Effect of Clonidine after Adrenergic Blockade. These experiments were conducted on the assumption that after adrenergic blockade clonidine would not show any hypotensive effect, if its action was due to inhibition of the sympathetic system. Interpretations of such experiments, however, have the same limitations as for spinal animals: Due to the pretreatment, the initial blood pressure of these animals is low, and may mask the hypotensive effect and facilitate the hypertensive property of clonidine. Pretreatment with reserpine,[2,3] guanethidine,[6,36] and bretylium [2,34] as well as with an alpha- plus beta-adrenergic blocker [43] abolished or markedly diminished the hypotensive effect of clonidine. Clonidine produced a mild bradycardia, even following guanethidine,[6,36] reserpine,[3] or an alpha- plus beta-adrenergic receptor blocker.[43] Atropine, however, abolished this effect.[6,22,36] The bradycardia was therefore interpreted as a reflex increase in vagal activity, in response to the initially elevated blood pressure.[3,6,36] Pretreatment with alpha-receptor blocking agents (phentolamine, phenoxybenzamine) diminished the hypotensive effect of clonidine.[2,3,5,17,43] Beta-adrenergic blockade either abolished or shortened the bradycardic effect of clonidine [3,6,43]; no change by beta-adrenergic blockade was observed in one report.[35] The hypotensive effect of clonidine was either diminished [3,43] or not changed [2,6] by this pretreatment. Excision of both stellate ganglia [34] or the dissection of one accelerans nerve [37] abolished or reduced the bradycardic effect of clonidine respectively.

The great majority of experimental results summarized above led to the conclusion that the hypotensive effect of clonidine is due to decreased sympathetic activity. Thereafter most experiments were carried on in this direction. The final results were reached through the investigational steps listed below.

Inhibitory Effects Within the Peripheral Sympathetic System

Adrenergic-receptor Inhibition. Clonidine exerted some alpha-adrenergic receptor blocking effects only in higher [5,8] dosages (>100 μg per kilogram of body weight).[5,6,34] In various isolated organs the effect of noradrenaline was reduced by clonidine: vas deferens of rats [33]; perfused ear artery of rabbits [33]; perfused mesenteric arteries of rats [44]; aortic strips of rabbits [4]; isolated ileum of rabbits [6] and of humans.[15] However, considering the drug concentrations used, most of the investigators did not consider this action to be relevant for the hypotensive effect. No beta-adrenergic blocking properties were reported.[5,6,29,34]

Adrenergic Neurone-blocking Effects. In various experiments sympathetic nerves were electrically stimulated and responses of the corresponding effector organs were recorded. In the following systems no blocking effect of clonidine was reported: cervical sympathetic nerve (pre- and postganglionic)—nictitating membrane [4–6,8]; hypogastric nerve (preganglionic)—vas deferens in vivo [37]; stellate ganglion—heart rate.[6] A decreased response was reported for sympathetic nerve—isolated ileum [6]; hypogastric nerve (preganglionic)—vas deferens in vitro [33]; periarterial nerve plexus (postganglionic)—isolated mesenteric artery perfusion.[44] A diminished response to low- but not to high-frequency stimulation was reported: inferior cardiac nerve (postganglionic)—heart rate [29,37] and periarterial nerve plexus—perfusion pressure of rabbit ears.[5] In isolated, perfused rabbit hearts clonidine diminished the positive inotropic and chronotropic effects as well as the release of noradrenaline following electrical stimulation of the sympathetic cardiac nerves.[46] Tetracaine had similar effects, although much higher concentrations were necessary. Obviously under some experimental conditions clonidine exerts inhibitory properties upon the transmission between nerves and organs, which may partly be explained by local anesthetic [8,47] or by alpha-adrenolytic (see above) effects of the drug. Some of the foregoing experiments have also been interpreted as revealing a specific adrenergic neurone-inhibiting property of clonidine which may explain the bradycardic and hypotensive effect of the drug in vivo.[29,39a,46] In those experiments where clonidine and "established" adrenergic neurone-blocking agents were compared, however, the differences became obvious: the latter drugs blocked electrical nerve stimulation completely and in all tested frequency ranges. Even in high doses clonidine inhibited the effects to a limited extent and only in the low-frequency stimulation range.[5,37] Moreover, vasopressor reflex activities, which presumably use physiologic stimulation frequencies along the peripheral sympathetic system, were completely blocked by reserpine, guanethidine, or bretylium, but not by clonidine [47a,48] (see section entitled "Cardiovascular Reflexes and Reactions"). We may therefore conclude that peripherally acting, adrenergic-inhibitory effects of clonidine are of little importance for the cardiovascular effects in intact animals.*

Effect on Biogenic Amines. High doses of clonidine did not affect the concentrations of endogenous noradrenaline, dopamine and their metabolites, as well as 5-hydroxytryptamine (5-HT) in heart [8] and brain [44] of rats, but they increased brain catecholamines in guinea pigs.[44] Chronic treatment with clonidine reduced the urinary output of catecholamines and their metabolites as well as the plasma renin level and aldosterone production.[27,49–52] Following inhibition of noradrenaline synthesis by α-methyl-tyrosine-methylester, clonidine retarded the expected depletion of noradrenaline and 5-HT in brain and spinal cord of rats (chemical and histochemical fluorescence methods)[53]; this effect was antagonized by alpha-adrenergic receptor inhibition.[53] The interpretation of these results is outlined in the section entitled "Mode of Central Action of Clonidine."

Administration of Clonidine into the Central Nervous System

In these experiments, small doses of clonidine produced a cardiovascular response similar to higher doses given systemically. Injection of 1 μg of clonidine per kilogram of body weight into the cisterna cerebellomedullaris (magna) of cats produced significantly greater hypotension and bradycardia than the same dose given intravenously.[37] In dogs, intracisternal injection of 1 μg of clonidine per kilogram of body weight resulted in about the same fall in blood pressure, heart rate, and cardiac output as seen after intravenous injection of 30 μg per kilogram of body weight.[9,15,27,41] The initial

* After completion of this manuscript Farnebo and Hamberger [48a] reported some evidence that stimulation or inhibition of alpha-adrenoreceptors regulate the release of noradrenaline from nerve endings, probably via feedback mechanisms. In their experiments clonidine decreased the stimulation-induced release of noradrenaline.

increase in blood pressure and total peripheral resistance was not observed after intracisternal injection as it was after intravenous injection. It may be pointed out that intracisternal injections of equieffective pressor or local anesthetic doses of noradrenaline or procaine did not affect blood pressure and heart rate.[9,37] Blood pressure, heart rate, and vascular resistance in hindlimbs decreased when small doses of clonidine were injected into the vertebral artery of cats [54] and dogs.[4] Blood pressure and heart rate were decreased by retrograde injection of 0.5 μg per kilogram of body weight into the common carotid artery of rats, where the axillary artery had been occluded.[7] In cross-circulation experiments, only the recipient dogs had nerve connections between head and body.[55] Injection of 10 and 20 μg of clonidine per kilogram of body weight into the donors, which reached the recipient's head, lowered heart rate and blood pressure in the recipient's body.[55] The same results were obtained after section of vagus and sinus nerves. All the above-mentioned results were interpreted as unequivocal evidence of an effect of clonidine upon the brain. Clonidine decreased the vascular resistance in isolated, perfused hindlimbs of rats [44] and cats [56] when injected into the upper part of the animals. The drug therefore was considered to act either at the CNS or the ganglionic level.

Decrease of Electrical Activity in Sympathetic Nerves

As first demonstrated by Schmitt et al.,[38] clonidine, in intravenously administered doses of 3 to 30 μg per kilogram of body weight, reduced or abolished the spontaneous discharges in preganglionic (sympathetic chain, splanchnic nerve) and postganglionic (inferior cardiac nerve, renal nerves) sympathetic fibers.[41,42,57,58a] This effect occurred 15 to 20 seconds after the injection, slightly before the onset of changes in blood pressure and heart rate.[41] The recovery paralleled the cardiovascular parameters.[57] Klupp et al.[58a] calculated a linear dependency between the log dose of clonidine and $\sqrt{\%}$ inhibition of spontaneous discharges: 50 percent inhibition was achieved with intravenous administration of 10.5 μg per kilogram of body weight (fiducial limits: 4.2; 20.0 μg per kilogram of body weight). Clonidine reduced discharges from splanchnic nerve > accelerans nerve > cervical sympathetic chain in descending order, indicating the pharmacologic heterogeneity of sympathetic centers.[57] The decrease in activity of sympathetic nerves was also observed after dissection of vagus, carotid sinus nerves, and the nodose ganglion, i.e., elimination of the main afferent cardiovascular reflex pathways.[41,42] After injection of 1 to 2 μg clonidine per kilogram of body weight into the cisterna magna, the third cerebral ventricle, or one lateral ventricle the splanchnic discharges gradually decreased.[32] Onset and development were delayed as compared with intravenous injection: 1 to 5 minutes were required for the maximal effect following intracisternal injection. Hukuhara et al.[42] registered the spontaneous spike discharges of vasomotor reticular neurones in immobilized cats and found that clonidine, in a 20- to 200-μg dose per kilogram of body weight, reduced the discharge frequency in 50 percent of the neurones under investigation.

Localization of the Effect Within the CNS

The successful use of small doses of clonidine and the short latent period (0.5 to 2 minutes) after intracisternal injection suggested an action upon sympathetic cardiovascular regulatory centers in the medulla oblongata.[9,32,37] This assumption was confirmed by experiments showing that clonidine still decreased blood pressure and sympathetic nerve activity after transection at the following brain levels rostrad to the medulla: mesencephalon,[32,58b] pons,[32,42] border between pons and medulla.[32] The actions were abolished after transection caudal of the medulla [32] (see also the section entitled "Effect in Spinal Animals and after Complete Autonomic Block"). An additional action of the drug at the diencephalic cardiovascular centers has been proposed, as the cardiovascular effects of clonidine were not identical in "pontine" rabbits (mesencephalic transection) and in control rabbits.[58b] Clonidine also exerts effects on sympathetic centers in the spinal cord. In spinal cats the electrical activity in renal nerves was decreased, albeit less and of shorter duration than in intact animals.[42] It may be mentioned that clonidine increased the flexor reflex in spinal rats, obviously by a direct-stimulating effect on central noradrenaline receptors [53] (see section entitled "Mode of Central Action of Clonidine").

Cardiovascular Reflexes and Reactions

Clonidine (>5 μg per kilogram of body weight) depressed the reflex increase in blood pressure, following occlusion of the common carotid arteries in dogs,[8,41] in most experiments on cats [6,48,54] but not in rats.[33] The chemoreceptor components seemed to be more affected than those of the baroreceptors.[54] Orthostatic hypotension, provoked by tilting of anesthetized animals, was enhanced by clonidine in doses higher than 8 μg per kilogram of body weight given intravenously.[4,58] Lower doses did not reveal this effect in spite of a decrease in the resting level of blood pressure and heart rate.[4] In isolated, perfused hindquarters of cats a reflex vasoconstriction was elicited by injection of histamine into the jugular vein. Clonidine injected into the inferior jugular vein did not depress but augmented this vasoconstrictor reflex,[48,56] while guanethidine and reserpine abolished it.[48] In conscious ducks, the diving reflex strongly reduces cardiac rate and output at a normal mean blood pressure, the latter being preserved by an intense sympathetic vasoconstriction.[58c] The mean blood pressure during experimental diving fell to low levels after treatment with reserpine or guanethidine, but not after clonidine in spite of a decreased resting blood pressure.[47a] Clonidine reduced the spontaneous electrical discharges in sympathetic nerves more effectively than those evoked by chemoreceptor-stimulating drugs, asphyxia, or electrical stimulation of hypothalamic and medullary pressor areas.[41,58a] A differentiation between reactions to mild and strong reflex stimuli has been demonstrated in experiments in unanesthetized, midbrain-sectioned rabbits (pontine preparations).[58b] The increase in blood pressure and total vascular resistance by lowering the arterial oxygen tension to 50 mm Hg (mild hypoxia) was abolished or significantly reduced by clonidine; the reaction to severe hypoxia, however (an oxygen tension of 30 mm Hg), was only partially antagonized. The hypertensive reaction to intravenous injection of physostigmine in rats was antagonized by clonidine.[33,41] (An increase in a cardiodepressor-reflex activity is discussed in the next section.) In conclusion, in several experiments clonidine was demonstrated to decrease the resting tone of the sympathetic nervous system, without completely blocking it for responses to urgent reflex circulatory adjustments.

Facilitation of Vagally Mediated Reflexes

In the previous sections of this chapter evidence has been presented that clonidine induces bradycardia by (1) a decrease in central sympathetic tone, and (2) a vagally mediated reflex in response to the initial hypertension. Robson et al. have proposed a third mechanism: an enhancement of pressor-sensitive cardiodepressor reflexes.[43] Following blockade of the sympathetic innervation of the heart (beta-adrenergic receptor block by guanethidine) clonidine increased the reflex bradycardia elicited by the injection of blood pressure-raising catecholamines.[36,43,59] It was recently shown that this effect is due to a specific and direct effect of clonidine upon the CNS: 0.5 to 1.0 μg of clonidine per kilogram of body weight injected into the cisterna of dogs effectively enhanced the vagally mediated bradycardia elicited by intravenously administered angiotensin or noradrenaline. The same dose of clonidine given intravenously was ineffective, as was 1 μg of naphazoline per kilogram of body weight injected intracisternally.[59,60] The sympathetic and the vagus systems are reciprocally related in reflex changes of the heart rate.[61] CNS connections between autonomic centers may "switch" the vagus to higher reflex activity as soon as sympathetic centers are depressed either by physiologic or by pharmacologic stimuli.[59]

Considering the results with clonidine in vagotomized animals (see section entitled "Activation of the Vagus System"), this activation of the vagus reflex system may play a partial role in the bradycardic effect of clonidine, but seems of minor significance with respect to the hypotensive effect.

Cardiovascular Effects after Chronic Treatment with Clonidine

The reactions of the blood pressure and femoral arterial blood flow to vasoconstricting (catecholamines and angiotensin) and vasodilating (isoprenaline) substances were tested in anesthetized rats, following chronic subcutaneous administration of clonidine (20 μg per kilogram per day for 7 days)[62] as well as in anesthetized cats (orally administered, 10 μg per kilogram of body weight per day, for 4 weeks or 20 μg per kilogram of body weight per day for 7 days).[17] Both studies reported a decreased vascular response. The conclusion was drawn that the chronic effect of clonidine made the vascular smooth muscle less responsive to constriction and dilatation.[17] Daily treatment with 1 mg of clonidine per kilogram of body weight, given orally for 17 to 19 days, did not lead to tolerance against the bradycardia in unanesthetized rats and dogs,[10] but a mild reduction of the hypotensive properties has been reported in a small number of rats.[63]

Mode of Central Action of Clonidine

Evidence is accumulating that clonidine exerts its actions upon the CNS by a direct stimulation of alpha-adrenergic receptors. Andén et al. demonstrated with clonidine a facilitation of the flexor reflex in spinal rats, similar to what was observed with dopa and amphetamine.[53,64] This effect was antagonized by alpha-adrenergic blocking substances and was demonstrated in spite of depletion of noradrenaline stores and blockade of noradrenaline synthesis in rats. No stimulation of central 5-HT or dopamine receptors was found in those studies. The reduced turnover rates of noradrenaline and 5-HT in brain and spinal cord (see section entitled "Effect on Biogenic Amines") were antagonized by alpha-adrenergic-receptor inhibition. These biochemical findings were explained by a negative feedback mechanism, evoked by the central adrenergic-receptor stimulation of clonidine.[53] In young chickens (3 to 10 days old) intravenous injection of 0.02 μg of clonidine per gram of body weight produced sleep, as does adrenaline (0.4 μg per gram of body weight). In older chicks clonidine, but not adrenaline, was still effective, indicating that clonidine penetrates the adult blood-brain barrier.[17,65] This effect of clonidine was antagonized by alpha-adrenergic-blocking drugs.[66] Clonidine had the same effect as noradrenaline, acting as a general inhibitor of thermoregulatory processes, decreasing heat loss at high and heat production at low temperatures. These experiments were done in unanesthetized sheep and one goat, the drugs being injected into the lateral cerebral ventricle. The doses of clonidine required (about 0.1 μg per kilogram of body weight) were about 50 to 100 times smaller than those of noradrenaline.[67] The facilitation of the vagally mediated cardiodepressor reflex by clonidine (see section entitled "Facilitation of Vagally Mediated Reflexes") was effectively blocked by alpha-adrenergic-receptor inhibitors, following intracisternal injection of these drugs in small doses.[68] These results demonstrate the role of central adrenergic stimulation by clonidine, and indicate the involvement of adrenergic receptors and neurones in the central transmission of vagus reflexes.[69] Although tolazoline and some alpha-receptor-blocking drugs were reported to antagonize the blood pressure-lowering effect of clonidine,[1,70–72a] there is no complete agreement on this point.[68] In 1933 experiments of Heller [72b] revealed hypotension after intracisternal injection of high doses of adrenalin. The results of this section lend support to the working hypothesis that clonidine exerts its typical cardiovascular effect by acting in the CNS by means of a "non-specific" alpha-adrenergic stimulation. The drug has, however, a "specific" ability to cross the blood-brain barrier (and the cerebrospinal liquor-brain barrier), thereby reaching the points of action.

Summary

The majority of experiments described have been interpreted as demonstrating that the hypotensive effect of clonidine is due to a centrally mediated decrease in the tone of the sympathetic system. This conclusion has been primarily based on the cardiovascular reaction pattern of the drug and on the exclusion of other possible mechanisms of action. The exclusion of a peripheral hypotensive component has not been unanimous and nonspecific actions of the drug (adrenolytic, local anesthetic, alpha-adrenergic) make the final interpretation difficult. The hypothesis of a central inhibition of the sympathetic system has been strongly confirmed (1) by experiments in which minute amounts of clonidine, injected into the CNS elicited the typical cardiovascular response of the drug; (2) by the demonstration of decreased spontaneous activity in presynaptic sympathetic nerves; and (3) by the preservation of circulatory reflexes. These findings are in contrast with the effects of peripherally acting hypotensive drugs. The specific stimulating effect of clonidine upon CNS-adrenergic receptors makes the substance a valuable tool for investigations concerning central regulatory systems.

REFERENCES

1. Graubner, W., and Wolf, M.: Kritische Betrachtungen zum Wirkungsmechanismus des 2-(2,6-Dichlorphenylamino)-2-Imidazolinhydrochlorids. Arzneim. Forsch. 16:1055, 1966.
2. Nayler, W. G., Price, J. M., Swann, J. B., McInnes, I., Race, D., and Lowe, T. E.: Effect of the hypotensive drug St 155 (Catapres) on the heart and peripheral circulation. J. Pharmacol. Exp. Ther. 164:45, 1968.
3. Kobinger, W., and Walland, A.: Kreislaufuntersuchungen mit 2-(2,6-Dichlorphenylamino)-2-Imidazolinhydrochlorid. Arzneim. Forsch. 17:292, 1967.
4. Constantine, J. W., and McShane, W. K.: Analysis of the cardiovascular effects of 2-(2,6-dichlorphenylamino)-2-imidazoline hydrochloride (Catapres). Eur. J. Pharmacol. 4:109, 1968.
5. Boissier, J. R., Giudicelli, J. F., Fichelle, J., Schmitt, H., and Schmitt, H.: Cardiovascular effects of 2-(2,6-dichlorphenylamino)-2-imidazoline hydrochloride (St 155). I. Peripheral sympathetic system. Eur. J. Pharmacol. 2: 333, 1968.
6. Rand, M. J., and Wilson, J.: Mechanisms of the pressor and depressor actions of St 155 (2–(2,6-dichlorphenylamino)-2-imidazoline-hydrochloride, Catapresan). Eur. J. Pharm. 3:27, 1968.
7. Hughes, I. E.: Acute actions of 2-(2,6-dichlorphenylamino)-2-imidazoline hydrochloride (St 155) in the rat. Aust. J. Exp. Biol. Med. Sci. 46:747, 1968.
8. Hoefke, W., and Kobinger, W.: Pharmakologische Wirkung des 2-(2,6-Dichlorphenylamino)-2-Imidazolinhydrochlorids, einer neuen, antihypertensiven Substanz. Arzneim. Forsch. 16:1038, 1966.
9. Kobinger, W., and Walland, A.: Investigations into the mechanism of the hypotensive effect of 2-(2,6-dichlorphenylamino)-2-imidazoline-HCl. Eur. J. Pharmacol. 2:155, 1967.
10. Wolland, A., and Kobinger, W.: On the problem of tolerance of 2-(2,6-dichlorphenylamino)-2-imidazoline. Arzneim. Forsch. 21: 61, 1971.
11. Makabe, R.: Ophthalmologische Untersuchungen mit Dichlorphenylamino-Imidazolin unter besonderer Berücksichtigung des Einflußes auf den intraokularen Druck. Dtsch. Med. Wochenschr. 91:1686, 1966.
12. Hasslinger, C.: Catapresan (2-(2,6-Dichlorphenylamino)-2-Imidazolin-Hydrochlorid), ein neues augendrucksenkendes Medikament. Klin. Monatsbl. Augenheilkd. 154:95, 1969.
13. Juenemann, G., und Schmidt, G.: Zur Catapresanwirkung am glaukomatösen Auge. Klin. Monatsbl. Augenheilkd. 157:193, 1970.
14. Brugger, A., Cliver, R., and Salva, J. A.: Accion del clorhidrato de 2-(2,6-dichlorofenilamino)-2-inidazolina sobre la terminacion adrenergica. Rev. Esp. Fisiol. 26:131, 1970.
15. Kobinger, W., and Hoefke, W.: Pharmakologische Untersuchungen über Angriffspunkt und Wirkungsmechanismus eines neuen Hochdruckmittels. *In* Heilmeyer, L., Holtmeier, H. J., and Pfeiffer, E. F. (Eds.): Hochdrucktherapie. Stuttgart: Georg Thieme, 1968, pp. 4–17.
16. Ehringer, H.: Die Wirkung von 2-(2,6-Dichlorphenylamino)-2-Imidazolinhydrochlorid auf die Extremitaetendurchblutung, den Blutdruck und die Venenkapazität bei Normotonikern. Arzneim. Forsch. 16:1165, 1966.
17. Zaimis, E.: On the pharmacology of Catapres (St 155). *In* Conolly, M. E. (Ed.): Catapres in Hypertension. London: Butterworth, 1970, pp. 9–22.
18. Mujic, M., and van Rossum, J. M.: Comparative pharmacodynamics of sympathomimetic imidazolines: Studies on intestinal smooth muscle of the rabbit and the cardiovascular system of the cat. Arch. Int. Pharmacodyn. 155:432, 1965.
19. Nyler, W. G., Price, J. M., Stone, J., and Lowe, T. E.: Further observations on the cardiovascular effects of St 155 (Catapres). J. Pharmacol. Exp. Ther. 166:364, 1969.
20. Kaplan, H. R., La Sala, S. A., Simon, A., and Robson, R. D.: St 55 induced cardiac slowing in dogs. Eur. J. Pharmacol. 6:193, 1969.
21. Nayler, W. G., Rosenbaum, M., McInnes, I., and Lowe, T. E.: Effect of a new hypotensive drug, St 155, on the systemic circulation. Am. Heart J. 72:764, 1966.

22. Shaw, J., Hunyor, S. N., and Korner, P. I.: The peripheral circulatory effects of clonidine and their role in the production of arterial hypotension. Eur. J. Pharmacol. 14:101, 1971.
23. Onesti, G., Schwartz, A. B., Kim, K. E., Swartz, C., and Brest, A. N.: Pharmacodynamic effects of a new antihypertensive drug, Catapres (St 155). Circulation 39:219, 1969.
24. Maxwell, G. M.: The effects of 2-(2,6-dichlorphenylamino)-2-imidazoline hydrochloride (Catapres) upon the systemic and coronary haemodynamics and metabolism of intact dogs. Arch. Int. Pharmacodyn. Ther. 181:7, 1969.
25. Grabner, G., Michalek, P., Pokorny, D., and Vormittag, E.: Klinische und experimentelle Untersuchungen mit der neuen blutdrucksenkenden Substanz 2-(2,6-Dichlorphenylamino)-2-Imidazolinhydrochlorid. Arzneim. Forsch. 16:1174, 1966.
26. Goodman, L. S., and Gilman, A.: The Pharmacological Basis of Therapeutics, 8th ed. London: Macmillan, 1970.
27. Onesti, G., Schwartz, A. B., Kim, K. E., Paz-Martinez, V., and Swartz, C.: Antihypertensive effect of clonidine. Circ. Res. 28 (Suppl. 2):53, 1971.
28. Chamberlain, D. A., and Howard, J.: Guanethidine and methyldopa: A haemodynamic study. Br. Heart J. 26:528, 1964.
29. Scriabine, A., Stavorski, J., Wenger, H. C., Torchiana, M. L., and Stone, C. A.: Cardiac slowing effects of clonidine (St 155) in dogs. J. Pharmacol. Exp. Ther. 171:256, 1970.
30. James, T. N., Bear, E. S., Lang, K. F., and Green, E. W.: Evidence for adrenergic alpha-receptor depressant activity in the heart. Am. J. Physiol. 215:1366, 1968.
31. Schroeder, H. A.: The pharmacology of hydralazine. *In* Moyer, J. H. (Ed.): Hypertension: The First Hahnemann Symposium on Hypertensive Disease. Philadelphia: Saunders, 1959, pp. 332–344.
32. Schmitt, H., and Schmitt, H.: Localization of the hypotensive effect of 2-(2,6-dichlorphenylamino)-2-imidazoline hydrochloride (St 155, Catapresan). Eur. J. Pharmacol. 6:8, 1969.
33. Bentley, G. A., and Li, D. M. F.: Studies of the new hypotensive drug St 155. Eur. J. Pharmacol. 4:124, 1968.
34. Magus, R. D., and Long, J. P.: Mechanism of hypotensive action of 2-(2,6-dichlorphenylamino)-2-imidazoline hydrochloride (St 155) in the cat. J. Pharm. Sci. 57:594, 1968.
35. Kündig, H., Monnier, H., Levin, N. W., and Charlton, R. W.: Mechanism of action of St 155 on the blood pressure in rats. Arzneim. Forsch. 17:1440, 1967.
36. Robson, R. D., and Kaplan, H. R.: An involvement of St 155 (2-(2,6-dichlorphenylamino)-2-imidazoline hydrochloride, Catapres) in cholinergic mechanisms. Eur. J. Pharmacol. 5:328, 1969.
37. Kobinger, W.: Über den Wirkungsmechanismus einer neuen antihypertensiven Substanz mit Imidazolinstruktur. Naunyn Schmiedebergs Arch. Pharmakol. 258:48, 1967.
38. Schmitt, H., Schmitt, H., Boissier, J. R., and Giudicelli, J. F.: Centrally mediated decrease in sympathetic tone induced by 2-(2,6-dichlorphenylamino)-2-imidazoline (St 155, Catapresan). Eur. J. Pharmacol. 2:147, 1967.
39. Walland, A.: Blutdruck und Herzfrequenz der Ratte nach wiederholter Behandlung mit 2-(2,6-Dichlorphenylamino)-2-Imidazolin. Arzneim. Forsch. 18:833, 1968.
39a. Scriabine, A., Stone, C. A., and Stavorski, J. M.: Studies on the mechanism of St 155 induced cardiac slowing in dogs. Pharmacologist 10:156, 1968.
40. Abreu, B. E.: Mechanism of hypotensive action of therapeutically useful veratrum alkaloids. *In* Moyer, J. H. (Ed.): Hypertension: The First Hahnemann Symposium on Hypertensive Disease. Philadelphia: Saunders, 1959, pp. 327–332.
41. Schmitt, H., Schmitt, H., Boissier, J. R., Giudicelli, J. F., and Fichelle, J.: Cardiovascular effects of 2-(2,6-dichlorphenylamino)-2-imidazoline hydrochloride (St 155). II. Central sympathetic structures. Eur. J. Pharmacol. 2:340, 1968.
42. Hukuhara, T., Jr., Otsuka, Y., Takeda, R., and Sakai, F.: Die zentralen Wirkungen des 2-(2,6-Dichlorphenylamino)-2-Imidazolin-Hydrochlorids. Arzneim. Forsch. 18:1147, 1968.
43. Robson, R. D., Kaplan, H. R., and Laforce, S.: An investigation into the bradycardic effects of ST 155 [2-(2,6-dichlorophenylamino)-2-imidazoline HCl in the anesthetized dog. J. Pharmacol. Exp. Ther. 169:120, 1969.
44. Phelan, E. L., McGregor, D. D., Laverty, R., Taylor, K. M., and Smirk, H.: Properties of Catapresan, a new hypotensive drug, a preliminary report. N. Z. Med. J. 66:864, 1967.
45. Coupar, I. M., and Turner, P.: Relative affinities of some alpha-adrenoceptor blocking drugs in isolated human smooth muscle. Br. J. Pharmacol. 40:155, 1970.
46. Starke, K., and Schümann, H. J.: Zur peripheren sympathikushemmenden Wirkung des Clonidins. Experientia 27:70, 1971.

47. Washizu, Y.: Some effects of clonidine, procaine and tetrodotoxin on crayfish sensory neuron. Eur. J. Pharmacol. 14:384, 1971.

47a. Kobinger, W., and Oda, M.: Effects of sympathetic blocking substances on the diving reflex of ducks. Eur. J. Pharmacol. 7:289, 1969.

48. Li, D. M. P., and Bentley, G. A.: The effects of various antihypertensive drugs on the reflex responses to vasoactive substances. Eur. J. Pharmacol. 12:24, 1970.

48a. Farnebo, L. O., and Hamberger, B.: Drug-induced changes in the release of (^{3}H)-noradrenaline from field-stimulated rat iris. Br. J. Pharmacol. 43:97, 1971.

49. Hoekfelt, B., Dymling, J. F., and Hedeland, H.: The effect of Catapresan on urinary catecholamines, plasma renin and urinary aldosterone in hypertensive patients. *In* Heilmeyer, L., Holtmeier, H. J., and Pfeiffer, E. F. (Eds.): Hochdrucktherapie. Stuttgart: Georg Thieme, 1968, pp. 105–108.

50. Hoekfelt, B., Hedeland, H., and Dymling, J. F.: The influence of Catapres on catecholamines, renin and aldosterone in man. *In* Conolly, M. E. (Ed.): Catapres in Hypertension. London: Butterworth, 1970, pp. 85–98.

51. Hoekfelt, B., Hedeland, H., and Dymling, J. F.: Studies on catecholamines, renin and aldosterone following Catapresan (2-(2,6-dichlorphenylamine)-2-imidazoline hydrochloride) in hypertensive patients. Eur. J. Pharmacol. 10:389, 1970.

52. Iisalo, E., and Laurila, S.: A clinical trial with a new antihypertensive drug, St 155 (Catapresan). Curr. Ther. Res. 9:358, 1967.

53. Andén, N. E., Corrodi, H., Fuxe, K., Hoekfelt, B., Hoekfelt, T., Rydin, C., and Svensson, T.: Part I. Evidence for a central noradrenaline receptor stimulation by clonidine. Life Sci. 9:513, 1970.

54. Sattler, R. W., and Van Zwieten, P. A.: Acute hypotensive action of 2-(2,6-dichlorphenylamino)-2-imidazoline hydrochloride (St 155) after infusion into the cat vertebral artery. Eur. J. Pharmacol. 2:9, 1967.

55. Sherman, G. P., Grega, G. J., Woods, R. J., and Buckley, J. P.: Evidence for a central hypotensive mechanism of 2-(2,6-dichlorphenylamino)-2-imidazoline (Catapresan, St 155). Eur. J. Pharmacol. 2:236, 1968.

56. Li, D. M. F., and Bentley, G. A.: The effect of St 155 on the active reflex vasodilatation induced by adrenaline, noradrenaline and veratrine. Eur. J. Pharmacol. 8:39, 1969.

57. Schmitt, H.: Centrally mediated decrease in sympathetic tone induced by 2-(2,6-dichlorphenylamino)-2-imidazoline (St 155, Catapres). *In* Conolly, M. E. (Ed.): Catapres in Hypertension. London: Butterworth, 1970, pp. 23–41.

58. Maling, H. M., Cho, A. K., Horakova, Z., and Williams, M. A.: The pharmacologic effects of St 155 (Catapres) and related imidazolines in the rat. Pharmacology 2:337, 1969.

58a. Klupp, H., Knappen, F., Otsuka, Y., Streller, I., and Teichmann, H.: Effects of clonidine on central sympathetic tone. Eur. J. Pharmacol. 10:225, 1970.

58b. Shaw, J., Hunyor, S. N., and Korner, P. I.: Sites of central nervous action of clonidine on reflex autonomic function in the unanaesthetized rabbit. Eur. J. Pharmacol. 15:66, 1971.

58c. Folkow, B., Nilsson, N. J., and Yonce, L. R.: Effects of "diving" on cardiac output in ducks. Acta Physiol. Scand. 70:347, 1967.

59. Kobinger, W., and Walland, A.: Evidence for a central activation of a vagal cardiodepressor reflex by clonidine. Eur. J. Pharmacol. 19:203, 1972.

60. Kobinger, W., and Walland, A.: Involvement of adrenergic receptors in central vagus activity. Eur. J. Pharmacol. 16:120, 1971.

61. Rosenblueth, A., and Freeman, N. E.: The reciprocal innervation in reflex changes of heart rate. Am. J. Physiol. 98:430, 1931.

62. Formanek, K., Lindner, A., and Selzer, H.: Die Testung von Antihypertensiva mit protrahierter Wirkung. Wien. Klin. Wochenschr. 80:185, 1968.

63. Laverty, R., and Taylor, K. M.: Behavioural and biochemical effects of 2-(2,6-dichlorphenylamino)-2-imidazoline hydrochloride (St 155) on the central nervous system. Br. J. Pharmacol. 35:253, 1969.

64. Andén, N. E.: Effects of amphetamine and some other drugs on central catecholamine mechanisms. *In* Costa, E., and Garattini, S. (Eds.): International Symposium on Amphetamines and Related Compounds. New York: Raven Press, 1970.

65. Fügner, A., and Hoefke, W.: A sleep-like state in chicks caused by biogenic amines and other compounds; quantitative evaluation. Arzneim. Forsch. 21:1243, 1971.

66. Delbarre, B., and Schmitt, H.: Sedative effects of alpha-sympathomimetic drugs and their antagonism by adrenergic and cholinergic blocking drugs. Eur. J. Pharmacol. 13: 356, 1971.

67. Maskrey, M., Vogt, M., and Bligh, J.: Central effects of clonidine (2-(2,6-dichlorphenyl-

amino)-2-imidazoline hydrochloride, St 155) upon thermoregulation in the sheep and goat. Eur. J. Pharmacol. 12:297, 1970.

68. Kobinger, W., and Walland, A.: Facilitation of vagal reflex bradycardia by an action of clonidine on central alpha-receptors. Eur. J. Pharmacol. 19:210, 1972.

69. Kobinger, W., and Walland, A.: Involvement of adrenergic neurones within the CNS in vagally mediated cardiodepressor reflex. Naunyn Schmiedebergs Arch. Pharmakol. 274(Suppl.):R-67, 1972.

70. Bock, K. D., Merguet, P., Murata, T., and Heimsoth, V.: Klinisch-experimentelle Untersuchungen über die Wirkungen von Dichlorphenylaminoimidazolin. *In* Heilmeyer, L., Holtmeier, H. J., and Pfeiffer, E. F. (Eds.): Hochdrucktherapie. Stuttgart: Georg Thieme, 1968, pp. 28–38.

71. Schmitt, H., Schmitt, H., Mme., and Fenard, S.: Evidence for an alpha-sympathomimetic component in the effects of Catapresan on vasomotor centres: antagonism by piperoxane. Eur. J. Pharmacol. 14:98, 1971.

72. Brodie, D. A., Lotti, V. J., and Bauer, B. G.: Drug effects on gastric secretion and stress gastric hemorrhage in the rat. Am. J. Dig. Dis. 15:111, 1970.

72a. Bolme, P., and Fuxe, K.: Pharmacological studies on the hypotensive effect of clonidine. Eur. J. Pharmacol. 13:168, 1971.

72b. Heller, H.: Über die zentrale Blutdruckwirkung des Adrenalins. Naunyn Schmiedebergs Arch. Exp. Path. Pharmakol. 173:291, 1933.

73. Boissier, J. R., Giudicelli, J. F., Larno, S., and Fichelle, J.: Action de la Clonidine (St 155) sur la sécrétion gastrique et l'ulcère expérimental. J. Pharmacol. 1:109, 1970.

74. Walz, A., and Van Zwieten, P. A.: The influence of 2-(2,6-dichlorphenylamino)-2-imidazoline hydrochloride (clonidine) and some related compounds on gastric secretion in the anaesthetized rat. Eur. J. Pharmacol. 10:369, 1970.

75. Iwata, Y.: Hyperglycemic action of 2-(2,6-dichlorphenylamino)-2-imidazoline hydrochloride in relation to its hypertensive effect. Jap. J. Pharmacol. 19:249, 1969.

76. Rehbinder, D., and Deckers, W.: Stoffwechseleffekte des Catapresan. Naunyn-Schmiedebergs Arch. Pharmakol. Exp. Pathol. 261:162, 1968.

77. Senft, G., Sitt, R., Losert, W., Schultz, G., and Hoffmann, M.: Hemmung der Insulininkretion durch Alpha-Receptoren stimulierende Substanz. Naunyn Schmiedebergs Arch. Pharmakol. 260:309, 1968.

78. Bock, J. U., and Van Zwieten, P. A.: Central hypoglycaemic action of clonidine. Naunyn Schmiedebergs Arch. Pharmakol. 270 (suppl.):R 11, 1971.

79. Kobinger, W.: Die Wirkung von 2-(2,6-Dichlorphenylamino)-2-Imidazolin-Hydrochlorid (St 155, Catapresan) auf die Harnausscheidung von osmotisch freiem Wasser. Naunyn Schmiedebergs Arch. Pharmakol. 260:153, 1968.

80. Laverty, R.: A comparison of the behavioural effects of some hypotensive imidazoline derivatives in rats. Eur. J. Pharmacol. 9:163, 1970.

81. Morpurgo, C.: Aggressive behavior induced by large doses of 2-(2,6-dichlorphenylamino)-2-imidazoline hydrochloride (St 155) in mice. Eur. J. Pharmacol. 3:374, 1968.

82. Kuljyk, S., and Stern, P.: Catapresan-induced tremor and its characteristics. Pharmacol. Res. Commun. 2:17, 1970.

83. Rand, M. J., Rush, M., and Wilson, J.: Some observations on the inhibition of salivation by St 155 (2-(2,6-dichlorphenylamino)-2-imidazoline hydrochloride, Catapres, Catapresan). Eur. J. Pharmacol. 5:168, 1969.

Cardiac and Renal Hemodynamic Effects of Clonidine

By Allan B. Schwartz, M.D., Kwan Eun Kim, M.D., Charles Swartz, M.D., and Gaddo Onesti, M.D.

IN 1966 HOEFKE AND KOBINGER[1] demonstrated that the initial transient hypertensive effect of intravenous clonidine in the anesthetized dog was associated with a decrease in cardiac output, decrease in heart rate, and an increase in total peripheral resistance. The subsequent prolonged fall in blood pressure was associated with a decrease in cardiac output and bradycardia, while the total peripheral resistance returned to control levels.

In 1967 Kobinger and Walland injected clonidine into the cisterna magna[2] and demonstrated that the hypotensive effect was again accompanied by a decrease in cardiac output and a decrease in heart rate. There were no changes in total peripheral resistance. The decrease in cardiac output was secondary to the decrease in heart rate with no change in stroke volume.

Studies in hypertensive patients by Grabner and his co-workers[3] showed that acute administration of intravenous clonidine resulted in a fall in blood pressure associated with a decrease in cardiac output. There were no changes in total peripheral resistance and the stroke volume remained unchanged. Calculated cardiac work was reduced proportionally more than was mean arterial pressure. Schneider and Gattenlöhner[4] also studied the cardiac effect of oral clonidine in hypertensive patients. Four hours after drug administration, there was a fall in blood pressure, a fall in cardiac output, and a modest decrease in total peripheral resistance. The fall in cardiac output was due to a decrease in both heart rate and stroke volume. Circulation time was prolonged. Vorburger, Butikofer, and Reubi[5] investigated the acute effects of intravenously administered clonidine in hypertensive patients. As previously seen in the animal studies,[1,2] intravenously administered clonidine produced a brief hypertensive response in these patients, and a long-lasting decrease in blood pressure followed. During the hypotensive response, there was a decrease in cardiac output while the total peripheral resistance did not change. Heart rate decreased by 5 to 7 percent and stroke volume by 8 to 10 percent. Similarly Michel and co-workers[6] reported a decrease in blood pressure associated with a decrease in cardiac output, stroke volume, and heart rate in hypertensive patients. The calculated total peripheral resistance was actually increased.

From the Division of Nephrology and Hypertension, Hahnemann Medical College and Hospital, Philadelphia, Pennsylvania.

Supported in part by NIH Grant No. T–12–HE–05878.

Cardiac Effects in Essential Hypertension

In the above experiments the patients were studied at rest in the supine position. Studies of the acute cardiac effects of oral clonidine were conducted in our laboratory in patients with essential hypertension,[7] in the supine position and after 45° upright tilt.

To carry out the hemodynamic evaluation, clonidine was administered by mouth in a single dose of 300 to 450 μg to a group of seven patients with essential hypertension. Following oral administration of clonidine, the antihypertensive effect was noted to occur within 30 minutes to 1 hour; and a significant blood pressure reduction was noted within 2 to 4 hours; the duration of action was from 7 to 10 hours (Fig. 1).

The hemodynamic effects of clonidine on the patients in the supine posture are shown in

ROUTE	ONSET OF ACTION	MAXIMUM ACTION	DURATION ACTION
PO	½–1 hour	2–4 hours	7–10 hours

Fig. 1.—Effect of oral clonidine on blood pressure in hypertensive patients.

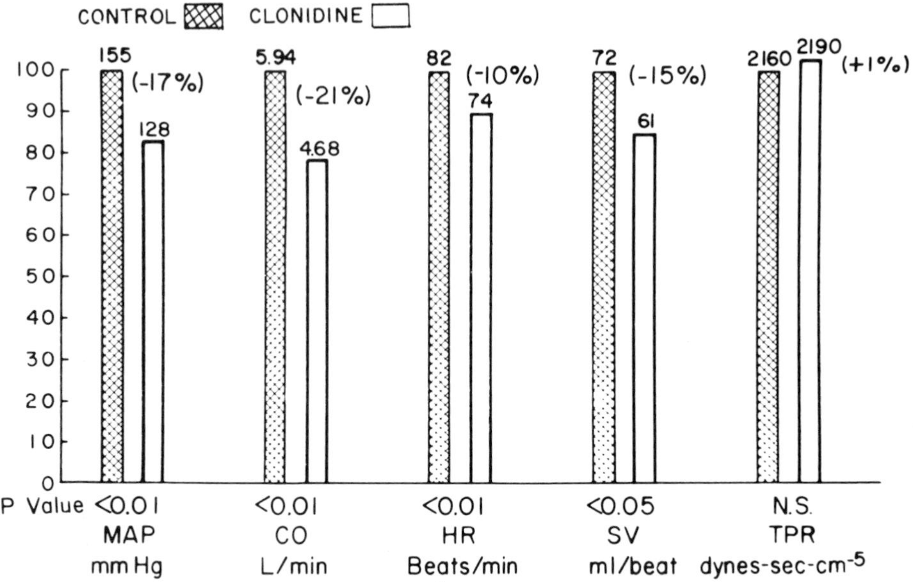

FIG. 2.—Acute effects of clonidine in seven patients with essential hypertension in the supine position. CO, cardiac output; HR, heart rate; MAP, mean arterial pressure; SV, stroke volume; TPR, total peripheral resistance; N.S., not statistically significant. (From Onesti, G., et al.: Anti-hypertensive effect of clonidine. Circ. Res. 28–29 (Suppl. II):53, 1971, by permission of The American Heart Association, Inc.)

Fig. 2. In the supine position, clonidine lowered the mean arterial blood pressure by an average of 27 mm Hg or by 17 percent ($P < 0.01$). Associated with the reduction in blood pressure, there was a decrease in cardiac output of 21 percent ($P < 0.01$). The heart rate decreased by 10 percent and stroke volume decreased by 15 percent. In the supine posture, no significant change in peripheral vascular resistance occurred during the blood pressure-lowering effect.

Figure 3 demonstrates the cardiac effects of clonidine in patients studied in the 45° upright tilt posture. The reduction in mean arterial pressure was greater than in the supine position. In the tilt position, the mean arterial pressure decreased by an average of 50 mm Hg or by 33 percent ($P < 0.05$). This was a lowering of mean arterial blood pressure 16 percent more than occurred in the supine position. Associated with the 33-percent reduction in mean arterial blood pressure, there was a 15-percent reduction of cardiac output. The bradycardic effect of clonidine was again noted as the heart rate decreased by an average of 14 percent ($P < 0.05$). Stroke volume was relatively unchanged. The total peripheral vascular resistance was significantly decreased by 21 percent ($P < 0.02$) in the upright posture, in contrast to the supine evaluation in which no change in peripheral resistance occurred.

PHYSIOLOGIC EFFECTS OF PASSIVE HEAD-UP TILTING IN ESSENTIAL HYPERTENSION

The upper half of Fig. 4 demonstrates the physiologic effects of 45° head-up tilting of this group of seven essential hypertensive patients in a control study before the administration of clonidine. Mean arterial pressure is maintained with passive head-up tilting. Systolic pressure usually decreases slightly and diastolic pressure increases slightly as mean arterial pressure remains relatively unchanged. However, cardiac output usually declines by approximately 25 percent. In this control study of the physiologic changes of passive 45° head-up tilting, the mean arterial pressure was relatively unchanged from 155 mm Hg in the

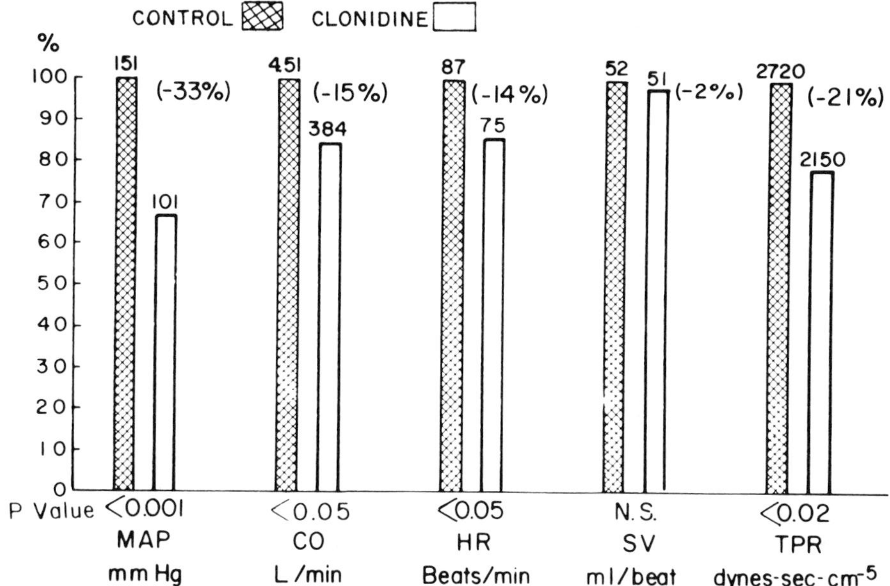

FIG. 3.—Acute effects of clonidine in seven patients with essential hypertension in erect position (45°-tilt). CO, cardiac output; HR, heart rate. (From Onesti, G., et al.: Anti-hypertensive effect of clonidine. Circ. Res. 28–29 (Suppl. II):53, 1971, by permission of the American Heart Association, Inc.)

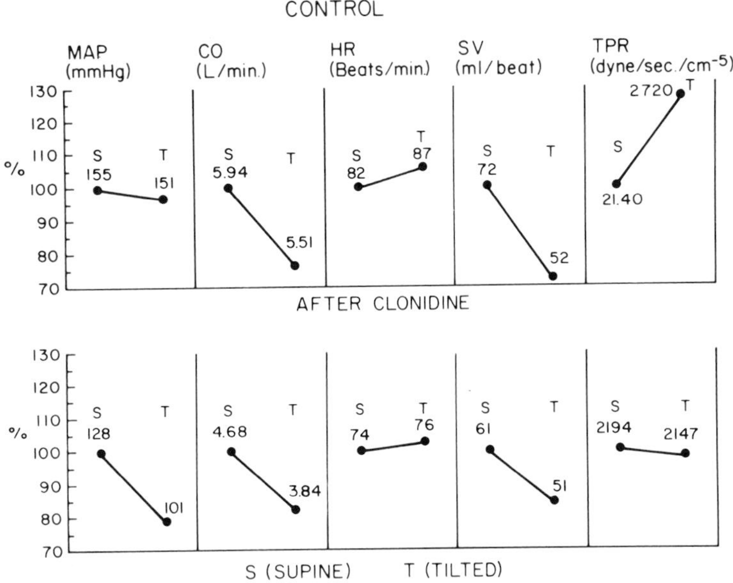

FIG. 4.—Effects of head-up, 45°-tilting before and after administration of clonidine. CO, cardiac output; HR, heart rate. (From Onesti, G., et al.: Anti-hypertensive effect of clonidine. Circ. Res. 28–29 (Suppl. II):53, 1971, by permission of The American Heart Association, Inc.)

supine to 151 mm Hg in the tilt posture. However, cardiac output decreased by 24 percent. Heart rate increased by 6 percent and stroke volume decreased by 28 percent. There was a 27-percent increase in peripheral vascular resistance as the patients were tilted upright. This compensatory increase in peripheral vascular resistance results from an increase in peripheral arteriolar and smooth muscle tone mediated via an increased reflex sympathetic nervous system activity stimulated by the change to the upright posture.

Clonidine Effect on Passive Head-up Tilting in Essential Hypertension

The cardiac hemodynamic effects of tilting during the maximum antihypertensive effect of clonidine are shown in the bottom half of Fig. 4. A 21-percent drop in mean arterial pressure occurred when the patients were tilted upright.

Figure 4 also shows the effect of clonidine on total peripheral vascular resistance. In the upright posture, during the gravity-augmented response to clonidine, the usual compensatory increase of total peripheral resistance of 27 percent did not occur. Instead, peripheral vascular resistance was virtually unchanged.

The failure of total peripheral vascular resistance to rise with upright posture corroborates the impression that clonidine acts to inhibit some portion of the sympathetic reflex mechanism of peripheral arteriolar constriction.

Long-term Hemodynamic Effect and Effect on Exercise

The effects of chronic clonidine therapy (several weeks) on cardiac output were studied by Schneider in 36 hypertensive patients.[8] The decrease in blood pressure was less marked than in acute studies. After an initial antihypertensive response, there was a tendency of the blood pressure to return toward control values. After several weeks of therapy, there was an 11-percent decrease in total peripheral resistance. It is, however, apparent that the overall hemodynamic changes were too small to allow definite conclusions. In the same study, normal subjects performed ergometer exercise before, and 2 hours after, clonidine administration. The exercise heart rate was less after drug administration. Stenberg and co-workers[9] also reported the cardiac effect of bicycle ergometer exercise, before and 1 week after clonidine administration (with the patients in the sitting position): Clonidine did not interfere with the physiologic increase in cardiac output and oxygen consumption induced by exercise.

Renal Effects in Essential Hypertension

The acute renal effects of oral administration of clonidine were studied in our laboratory in seven patients with essential hypertension.[7] Renal blood flow was estimated by the clearance of para-aminohippurate and the hematocrit. The glomerular filtration rate was measured by inulin clearance. Figure 5 shows the acute renal hemodynamic effects of oral clonidine in seven hypertensive patients in the supine position. The blood pressure reduction (17 percent, $P < 0.01$) was not associated with any significant alteration in renal blood flow or glomerular filtration rate. Sodium and chloride excretion decreased markedly.

Figure 6 shows the acute renal hemodynamic effects of oral clonidine with the patients in the erect position (45° tilt). Despite the substantial blood pressure reduction (33 percent, $P < 0.001$) in the erect position, there was no significant change in renal blood flow or the glomerular filtration rate. The renal vascular resistance decreased in every case with an average reduction of 30 percent ($P < 0.01$). During the hypotensive response, excretion of sodium and chloride decreased markedly. Figure 7 depicts the renal hemodynamic effects of tilting before the administration of clonidine (control study). Passive head-up tilting resulted in no changes in renal arterial pressure, a 16-percent reduction in renal blood flow and a 15-percent reduction in the glomerular filtration rate. Renovascular resistance increased with tilting. After clonidine administration (see lower portion of Fig. 7), head-up tilting resulted in a 21-percent orthostatic decrease in blood pressure. Despite the orthostatic blood pressure reduction, the decrease in renal blood flow and the glomerular filtration rate with tilting were the same as those of the control study. In contrast

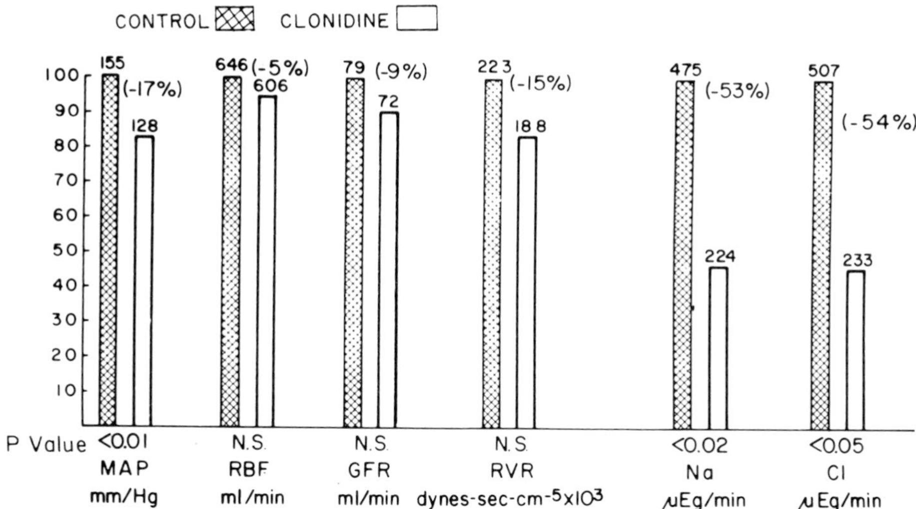

FIG. 5.—Acute renal hemodynamic effects of clonidine in seven patients with essential hypertension in supine position. Cl, urinary chloride excretion; MAP, mean arterial pressure; Na, urinary sodium excretion; RBF, renal blood flow; GFR, glomerular filtration rate; RVR, renovascular resistance; N.S., not statistically significant. (From Onesti, G., et al.: Anti-hypertensive effect of clonidine. Circ. Res. 28–29 (Suppl. II):53, 1971, by permission of The American Heart Association, Inc.)

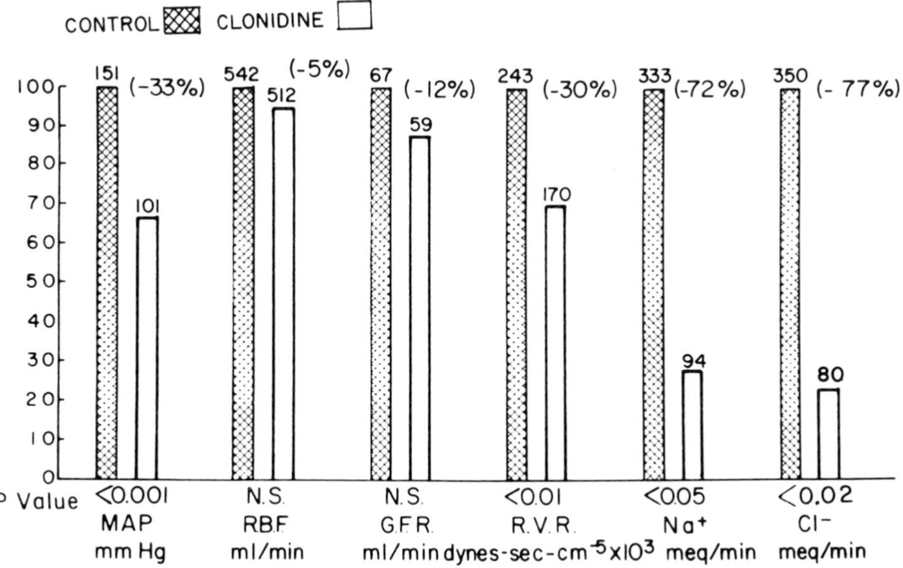

FIG. 6.—Acute renal hemodynamic effects of clonidine in seven patients with essential hypertension in the erect position (45°-tilt). MAP, mean arterial pressure, RBF, renal blood flow; GFR, glomerular filtration rate; RVR, renovascular resistance; N.S., not statistically significant. (From Onesti, G., et al.: Anti-hypertensive effect of clonidine. Circ. Res. 28–29 (Suppl. II):53, 1971, by permission of The American Heart Association, Inc.)

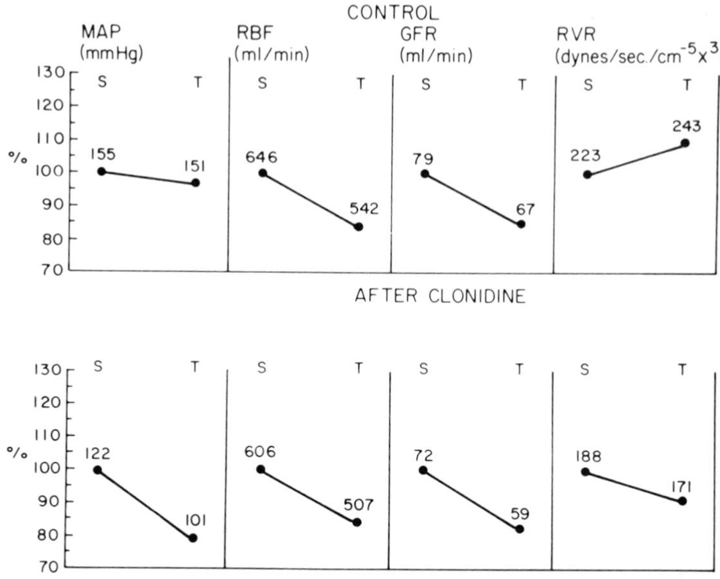

FIG. 7.—Renal hemodynamic effects of passive, head-up 45°-tilting before and after administration of clonidine. MAP, mean arterial pressure; RBF, renal blood flow; GFR, glomerular filtration rate; RVR, renovascular resistance; S, supine; T, tilted. (From Onesti, G., et al.: Anti-hypertensive effect of clonidine. Circ. Res. 28–29 (Suppl. II):53, 1971, by permission of The American Heart Association, Inc.)

with the control period, tilting during clonidine effect resulted in a decrease in renovascular resistance.

The effects of the prolonged administration of clonidine on renal hemodynamics of seven hypertensive patients were studied by Bock and co-workers.[10] Oral administration of clonidine for periods ranging from 11 to 110 days produced no significant change in renal plasma flow or the glomerular filtration rate. The blood pressure was significantly reduced in every case. Ludwig[11] reported that in hypertensive patients, the glomerular filtration rate was slightly decreased after 1 week of clonidine therapy but returned to the control levels after 4 weeks. A modest increase in renal plasma flow occurred while the blood pressure was consistently reduced. This again implies a reduction in renovascular resistance.

Grabner et al.[3] also described minor and inconsistent effects on the clearance of para-aminohippurate and inulin in hypertensive patients administered a single dose of clonidine.

DISCUSSION

Hemodynamic studies in the dog have shown that the decrease in blood pressure is associated with a decrease in cardiac output with no changes in total peripheral resistance.[1,2] The decrease in cardiac output is due primarily to a decrease in heart rate with no change in stroke volume.

Hemodynamic studies with human subjects in the supine position have demonstrated a response similar to that observed in dogs. The decrease in the blood pressure is associated with a decrease in cardiac output with no effect on the total peripheral resistance.[4–7] A fall in the cardiac output is due to a combination of decrease in rate and stroke volume. With the patient in an upright position, however, our human hemodynamic studies have demonstrated, in addition to the fall in cardiac output, a definite decrease in total peripheral resistance. The precise reason for this difference between supine and standing positions is not clear. It may be postulated that clonidine exerts a more potent inhibition of the sympathetic stimuli to the "resistance vessels" during sympathetic overactivity in the upright position. It should also be noted that the peripheral resistance ought to rise in response to drug-induced reduction in cardiac output.[12] This expected compensatory increase in resistance appears to be blocked by clonidine. This last effect together with the obvious effect on peripheral resistance in man in the standing position, the preservation of muscle blood flow during systemic blood pressure reduction,[13] and the consistent decrease in renovascular resistance demonstrates that a major component of the hypotensive effect of clonidine is a decrease in peripheral arteriolar tone.

The clonidine-induced decrease in cardiac output may be theoretically due to either a direct myocardial effect or a decreased venous return to the right side of the heart. Animal studies have failed to demonstrate any change in myocardial contractility.[14,15] In vitro studies on isolated hearts have demonstrated no effect on either rate or force of contraction.[16] The decrease in cardiac output in man is not accompanied by any increase in pulmonary pressure; [9] furthermore, cardiac response to exercise is preserved after clonidine.[8,9] Finally, total capacity of the circulation is increased by clonidine in the heart-lung preparation.[14,15] It is, therefore, logical to conclude that there is no evidence of direct myocardial effect and that the decrease in cardiac output is due to a combination of decrease in heart rate and decrease in venous return, resulting presumably from systemic venous dilatation.[14] These conclusions are based on the experimental data from the acute studies available at this time. Long-term hemodynamic effects await further investigation.

The studies of the cardiac effects of passive head-up tilting in man demonstrate that clonidine administration blocks the compensatory peripheral arteriolar constriction normally occurring in the upright position. Peripheral arteriolar constriction in the upright position is mediated by the sympathetic nervous system. This effect of clonidine is, therefore, in keeping with sympathetic inhibition. Failure of the normal orthostatic reflexes during tilting have been reported with clonidine in the monkey [16] and to a lesser extent in the dog.[16] Failure of compensatory arteriolar constriction results in orthostatic hypotension and has been previously reported with alpha-methyldopa [17] and pargyline hydrochloride.[18]

Acute renal hemodynamic studies in man show that renal blood flow and the glomerular filtration rate are maintained during the hypotensive response to clonidine. Renovascular resistance is decreased. Prolonged administration of oral clonidine results in similar preservation of renal plasma flow and the glomerular filtration rate. This renal effect is similar to the one previously reported with alpha-methyldopa.[17]

The renal hemodynamic effects of tilting appear to be altered by clonidine: The normal increase in renovascular resistance, observed in the upright position in man, is abolished. The decrease in mean arterial pressure, seen with tilting under the effect of clonidine, is associated with an actual decrease in renovascular resistance. It would apear that clonidine preserves the autoregulation of the kidney circulation. The same effect has been reported with alpha-methyldopa. A marked retention of sodium and chloride follows the acute administration of clonidine. The retention occurs with a glomerular filtration rate which is usually unchanged. The most likely mechanism of sodium retention is that the decrease in renal perfusion pressure stimulates enhanced tubular reabsorption of sodium.[19]

References

1. Hoefke, W., and Kobinger, W.: Pharmakologische Wirkungen des 2-(2,6-Dichlorphenylamino)-2-imidazolin-hydrochlorid, einer neuen antihypertensiven Substanz. Arzneim. Forsch. 16:1038, 1966.
2. Kobinger, W., and Walland, A.: Investigations into the mechanism of the hypotensive effect of 2-(2,6-dichlorphenylamino)-2-imidazoline HCl. Eur. J. Pharmacol. 2:155, 1967.
3. Grabner, G., Michalek, P., Pokorny, D., and Vormittag, E.: Klinische und experimentelle Untersuchungen mit der neuen blutdrucksenkenden Substanz 2-(2,6-dichlorphenylamino)-2-imidazolin-hydrochlorid. Arzneim. Forsch. 16:1174, 1966.
4. Schneider, K. W., and Gattenlöhner, W.: Hämodynamische Untersuchungen nach ST 155 2-(2,6-dichlorphenylamino)-2-imidazolin-

hydrochlorid beim Menschen. Dtsch. Med. Wochenschr. 91:1533, 1966.

5. Vorburger, C., Butikofer, E., and Reubi, F.: Die akute Wirkung von St-155 auf die cardiale und renale Haemodynamik. *In:* Heilmeyer, L., Holtmeier, H. J., and Pfeiffer, E. F. (Eds.): Hochdrucktherapie: Symposion über 2-(2,6-dichlorphenylamino)-2-imidazolin-hydrochlorid. Stuttgart: Thieme, 1968, pp. 86–95.
6. Michel, D., Zimmerman, W., Nassehi, A., and Seraphim, P.: Erste Beobachtungen über einen antihypertensiven Effekt von 2-(2,6-dichlorphenylamino)-2-imidazolin-hydrochlorid am Menschen. Dtsch. Med. Wochenschr. 91:1540, 1966.
7. Onesti, G., Schwartz, A. B., Kim, K. E., Swartz, C., and Brest, A. N.: Pharmacodynamic effects of a new antihypertensive drug, Catapres (ST-155). Circulation 39:219, 1969.
8. Schneider, K. W.: Cardiale Hämodynamik im akuten Versuch, nach chronischer Behandlung und im Belastungstest mit St 155. *In* Heilmeyer, L., Holtmeier, H. J., and Pfeiffer, E. F. (Eds.): Hochdrucktherapie: Symposion über 2-(2,6-dichlorphenylamino)-2-imidazolin-hydrochlorid. Stuttgart: Thieme, 1968, pp. 78–83.
9. Stenberg, J., Holmberg, S., Naets, E., and Varnauskas, E.: The hemodynamic effects of Catapresan. Central circulation at rest. Circulation at rest and during exercise. *In* Heilmeyer, L., Holtmeier, H. J., and Pfeiffer, E. F. (Eds.): Hochdrucktherapie: Symposion über 2-(2,6-dichlorphenylamino)-2-imidazolin-hydrochlorid. Stuttgart: Thieme, 1968, pp. 68–75.
10. Bock, K. D., Heimsoth, V., Merguet, P., and Schönermark, J.: Klinische und klinisch-experimentelle Untersuchungen mit einer neuen blutdrucksenkenden Substanz: Dichlorphenylaminoimidazolin. Dtsch. Med. Wochenschr. 91:1761, 1966.
11. Ludwig, H.: Der Einfluss der Langzeitbehandlung mit 2-(2,6-dichlorphenyl-amino)-2-imidazolin-hydrochlorid auf die Nierenhämodynamik beim arteriellen Hockdruck. Arzneim. Forsch. 18:582, 1968.
12. Trapold, J. H.: Role of venous return in the cardiovascular response following injection of ganglion-blocking agents. Circ. Res. 5:444, 1957.
13. Bock, K. D., Merguet, P., Murata, T., and Heimsoth, V.: Klinisch-experimentelle Untersuchungen über die Wirkungen von Dichlorphenylaminoimidazolin. *In* Heilmeyer, L., Holtmeier, H. J., and Pfeiffer, E. F. (Eds.): Hochdrucktherapie: Symposion über 2-(2,6-dichlorphenylamino)-2-imidazolin-hydrochlorid. Stuttgart: Thieme, 1968, p. 28.
14. Nayler, W. G., Price, J. M., Swann, J. B., McInnes, I., Race, D., and Lowe, T. E.: Effect of the hypotensive drug ST-155 (Catapres) on the heart and peripheral circulation. J. Pharmacol. Exp. Ther. 164:45, 1968.
15. Nayler, W. G., Price, J. M., Stone, J., and Lowe, T. E.: Further observations on the cardiovascular effects of ST 155 (Catapres). J. Pharmacol. Exp. Ther. 166:364, 1969.
16. Constantine, J. W., and McShane, W. K.: Analysis of the cardiovascular effects of 2-(2,6-dichlorphenylamino)-2-imidazoline hydrochloride (Catapres). Eur. J. Pharmacol. 4: 109, 1968.
17. Onesti, G., Brest, A. N., Novack, P., Kasparian, H., and Moyer, J. H.: Pharmacodynamic effects of alpha-methyldopa in hypertensive subjects. Am. Heart J. 67:32, 1964.
18. Onesti, G., Novack, P., Ramirez, O., and Brest, A. N.: Hemodynamic effect of pargyline in hypertensive patients. Circulation 30: 830, 1964.
19. Selkurt, E. E.: Effect of pulse pressure and mean arterial pressure on renal hemodynamics and electrolytes and water excretion. Circulation 4:541, 1951.
20. Onesti, G., Schwartz, A. B., Kim, K. E., Paz-Martinez, V., and Swartz, C.: Antihypertensive effect of clonidine. Circ. Res. 28–29 (Suppl. II):53, 1971.

Clinical Efficacy of Clonidine in Hypertension

By Allan B. Schwartz, M.D., Stanley Banach, M.D., I. Sanford Smith, M.D., Kwan Eun Kim, M.D., Gaddo Onesti, M.D., and Charles Swartz, M.D.

OUR EVALUATION OF THE antihypertensive efficacy of clonidine in the treatment of ambulatory patients with essential hypertension has proceeded in three phases. During the first phase (1968) a group of ambulatory patients were treated with clonidine* in doses between 150 and 900 μg per day. Clonidine was used as the sole antihypertensive agent. During the second phase of our investigation (1968) the efficacy of clonidine in combination with the diuretic chlorthalidone was studied. Again the maximum dose of clonidine used was 900 μg per day. Following the reports of Heimsoth and Bock [1] of excellent results with much higher doses, the third phase of our investigation was started in 1969, with doses of clonidine up to 4,000 μg per day, alone and in combination with chlorthalidone.

Low-dose Clinical Study with Clonidine Alone

The first study (1968) included 16 ambulatory patients with resting blood pressures greater than 150/100 mm Hg.[2] They were given placebo medication for at least 4 weeks. The patients returned to the clinic at weekly or biweekly intervals at which time resting cuff blood pressure was recorded with the patients supine and erect. After the control period, administration of clonidine was begun in an initial dosage of 75 μg daily (Fig. 1, Group I). Thereafter, the dosage was increased at biweekly intervals to a maximum of 900 μg per day. Therapy was continued for 12 to 23 weeks.

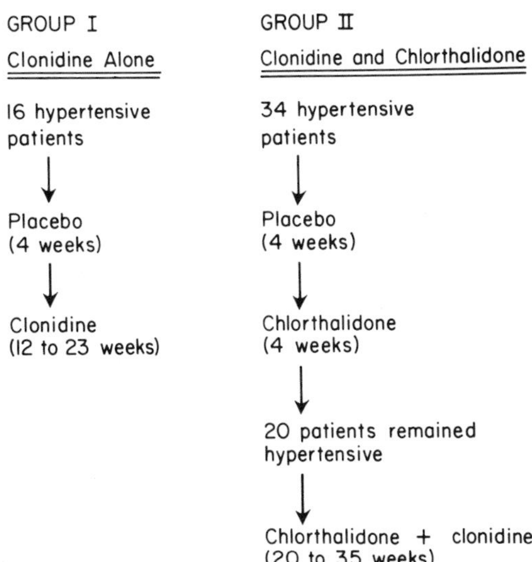

Fig. 1.—Study of the antihypertensive efficacy of clonidine in ambulatory patients with essential hypertension. Group I was treated with placebo, followed by clonidine alone. Group II was treated with chlorthalidone alone, initially. The patients who remained hypertensive after therapy with chlorthalidone alone were then treated with the combination clonidine and chlorthalidone. (From Onesti, G., et al.,[9] with permission.)

The blood pressure response of these 16 patients, treated with clonidine alone, is reported in Table 1. Of the 16 patients treated, three obtained a significant blood pressure reduction in the supine position and one of the 16 became normotensive. When the blood pressure was measured with the patients standing, six patients obtained a significant antihypertensive response. Side effects included: drowsiness (in 11 patients), dryness of the mouth (five patients), and constipation (one patient). The drowsiness improved in three patients and cleared entirely in two others despite continued therapy.

From the Division of Nephrology and Hypertension, Hahnemann Medical College and Hospital, Philadelphia, Pennsylvania.

* Kindly supplied as Catapres by Dr. Paul Kennedy, Geigy Pharmaceuticals, Ardsley, N.Y.

TABLE 1.—*Antihypertensive Effects of Clonidine Alone and in Combination with Chlorthalidone (1968) in a Low-dose Clinical Study*

		Supine				Erect			
		Normotensive *		Responsive †		Normotensive *		Responsive †	
Therapeutic Regimen	*No. of Patients*	*No.*	*%*	*No.*	*%*	*No.*	*%*	*No.*	*%*
Clonidine	16	1	6	3	19	0	0	6	37
Clonidine plus chlorthalidone	20	1	5	16	80	2	10	16	80

* Normotensive = blood pressure reduced to 140/90 mm Hg or less.
† Responsive = mean blood pressure (diastolic plus one-third pulse pressure) reduced 20 mm Hg or more, or normotension.

Low-dose Clinical Study: Clonidine in Combination With Chlorthalidone

The second investigation (1968) included 34 patients with resting blood pressures greater than 150/100 mm Hg who, after at least a 4-week placebo, were given chlorthalidone alone in a single dose of 100 mg per day.[2] After treatment with chlorthalidone, 20 of the 34 patients continued to have blood pressures consistently greater than 150/100 mm Hg. These 20 patients continued to receive chlorthalidone (100 mg per day) and, in addition, clonidine was added to the therapeutic regimen (Fig. 1, Group II). The initial dose ranged from 75 μg to 150 μg per day. Thereafter the dose was increased until significant blood pressure reduction was achieved, side effects became prohibitive, or a maximum daily dose of 900 μg per day was reached. The combination therapy was continued for 20 to 35 weeks.

The blood pressure response of these 20 patients treated with chlorthalidone in combination with clonidine is also reported in Table 1. Of the 20 patients treated, 16 (80%) obtained a significant blood pressure reduction in the supine position and one of the 16 became normotensive. When the blood pressure was measured in the erect position, 16 patients (80%) obtained a significant blood pressure reduction and two of the 16 (10%) became normotensive. Drowsiness, dry mouth, and constipation were the most common side effects encountered.

High-dose Clinical Study: Clonidine Alone and in Combination with Chlorthalidone

The third investigation with higher doses of clonidine started in 1969. After at least 4 weeks of placebo therapy, 41 ambulatory patients with blood pressures greater than 150/100 mm Hg were administered clonidine alone, starting with 600 μg per day. Thereafter, the dose was gradually increased until satisfactory blood pressure reduction was achieved or the side effects became prohibitive. Maximum dosage employed was 5,000 μg per day. Clonidine alone was continued for 4 to 8 weeks. The patients who did not become normotensive or who had severe side effects with clonidine alone were subsequently given the combination of chlorthalidone and clonidine. The doses of chlorthalidone varied from 60 mg per day to 120 mg per day while the doses of clonidine ranged between 400 μg per day and 4,000 μg per day.

At the time of this writing, 41 patients remained on clonidine alone for 2 to 5 months and 37 remained on the clonidine-chlorthalidone combination for 8 to 18 months.

The blood pressure response of the 41 patients treated with clonidine alone is reported in Table 2. Of the 41 patients treated with clonidine alone, 19 (41%) obtained a significant blood pressure reduction and five of the 19 (12%) became normotensive in the supine position. When the blood pressure was measured in the standing position, 18 patients (44%) achieved significant blood pressure re-

TABLE 2.—*Antihypertensive Effects of Clonidine Alone and in Combination with Chlorthalidone (1968–1971) in a High-dose Clinical Study*

		Supine				Erect			
		Normotensive *		Responsive †		Normotensive *		Responsive †	
Therapeutic Regimen	No. of Patients	No.	%	No.	%	No.	%	No.	%
Clonidine	41	5	12	19	41	7	17	18	44
Clonidine plus chlorthalidone	37	13	35	32	86	18	49	35	95

* Normotensive = blood pressure reduced to 140/90 mm Hg or less.
† Responsive = mean blood pressure (diastolic plus one-third pulse pressure) reduced 20 mm Hg or more, or normotension.

duction and seven of the 18 (17%) became normotensive.

The blood pressure response of the 37 patients treated with clonidine-chlorthalidone combination is also reported in Table 2. Of the 37 patients treated with the combination 32 (86%) achieved significant blood pressure reductions in the supine position and 13 of the 32 (35%) became normotensive.

In the erect posture, 35 of the 37 patients treated showed significant blood pressure reduction (95%) and 18 of the 35 became normotensive (49%).

TABLE 3.—*Severity of Blood Pressure in the 41 Patients of the High-dose Study*

Severity	Diastolic Blood Pressure (mm Hg)	No. of Patients
Mild	100–109	9
Moderate	110–129	20
Severe	130 or more	12

An analysis of the results in the patients of this group who exhibited severe hypertension (diastolic pressure 130 mm Hg or more) is of some interest. The sampling of this group treated with high doses with respect to mild, moderate, and severe degrees of diastolic hypertension, is shown in Table 3. Twelve of the 41 patients followed were classified as having severe diastolic hypertension (130 mm Hg or more). The results of clonidine therapy in these patients with severe diastolic hypertension (130 mm Hg or more) are analyzed separately in Table 4. Of these 12 patients nine (75%) showed a significant blood pressure reduction when treated with clonidine alone, both in the supine and in the standing position: none of them became normotensive, however, on clonidine alone. When chlorthalidone was added to clonidine in 10 patients, every patient treated with the combination showed significant blood pressure reduction in the supine and standing position. Furthermore, five (50%) of the

TABLE 4.—*Antihypertensive Effects of Clonidine Alone and in Combination with Chlorthalidone in Twelve Patients with Severe Diastolic Hypertension in a High-dose Clinical Study*

		Supine				Erect			
		Normotensive *		Responsive †		Normotensive *		Responsive †	
Therapeutic Regimen	No. of Patients	No.	%	No.	%	No.	%	No.	%
Clonidine	12	—	—	9	75	—	—	9	75
Clonidine plus chlorthalidone	10	—	—	10	100	5	50	10	100

* Normotensive = blood pressure reduced to 140/90 mm Hg or less.
† Responsive = mean blood pressure (diastolic plus one-third pulse pressure) reduced 20 mm Hg or more, or normotension.

10 patients became normotensive in both body positions.

Drowsiness and dry mouth were each noted in 30 percent of the patients in the high-dose study. In four patients the drowsiness was severe enough to necessitate discontinuance of the drug. In an additional four patients clonidine therapy had to be stopped because of dry mouth. When the drowsiness was mild or moderate and the therapy was continued, an improvement or a disappearance of the symptoms was reported. No orthostatic dizziness nor objective orthostatic hypotension was detected.

Discussion and Appraisal

The largest single clinical experience with clonidine in the treatment of hypertension is by Bock and co-workers and is described in detatil in that section of this book. Following preliminary reports,[3,4] in 1971 Hoobler and Sagastume [5] described an additional large series studied at the University of Michigan Medical Center including 57 hypertensive patients treated with clonidine plus a diuretic. After evaluating their cumulative experience of clonidine in combination with a diuretic these investigators came to the following conclusions: (1) there was no loss of drug effectiveness with the passage of time since the average reduction in blood pressure and dose of drug remained about the same in the sixth and in the final months of treatment; (2) the severity of the original hypertension did not alter the overall success rate (about 66%); (3) of 25 patients with hypertension severe enough to require guanethidine originally, 15 showed improvement on a regimen of clonidine (overall 60% favorable effect); (4) orthostatic hypotension was rarely a problem with clonidine; (5) seven of 12 patients (58%) previously taking alpha-methyldopa (1,000 mg per day or more) were more successfully managed with administration of clonidine.

In addition, Hoobler and Sagastume [5] were able to draw some conclusions on the interrelation of clonidine with other antihypertensive drugs: (1) clonidine showed a slight additive effect with hydralazine and reserpine but not with alpha-methyldopa; (2) clonidine added to guanethidine decreased both the standing and the recumbent blood pressure with a slight increase of the orthostatic gradient; (3) when guanethidine had been progressively totally replaced by clonidine in these patients, the recumbent blood pressure was lower than during the administration of guanethidine with a lesser orthostatic gradient.

Our first study in 1968 [2] demonstrated that clonidine alone, at doses between 400 and 900 μg per day, produced only a modest clinical effect. Our second study in 1968 [2] showed that the combination of clonidine and chlorthalidone is much more effective.

Although evaluation of comparative efficacy of antihypertensive agents is difficult, a fair comparison may be attempted if the study is conducted in the same laboratory and with the same criteria. During the past few years guanethidine,[6] pargyline,[7] and alpha-methyldopa [8] have been evaluated in our clinic in the same hypertensive population and with the same criteria of effectiveness. A comparative impression will, therefore, be attempted (Table 5).

The combination of clonidine and chlorthalidone with doses of clonidine not higher than 900 μg per day gave us significant antihypertensive response in 80 percent of the patients treated, in both the supine and standing position. The results in the supine position compare favorably to what was observed with the combination of guanethidine and hydrochlorothiazide (52%),[6] pargyline and hydrochlorothiazide (36%),[7] and alphamethyldopa and hydrochlorothiazide (63%).[8]

The results obtained with our most recent investigation are interesting because of the higher doses used without greater side effects. It is noteworthy that the combination of clonidine and chlorthalidone is now producing "significant blood pressure reduction" in 95 percent of the patients treated. It is of particular importance that the satisfactory response is obtained in both the supine (89%) and standing (95%) position. Although our acute hemodynamic studies have demonstrated orthostatic hypotension,[2] there is no significant orthostatic effect in the patients on long-term therapy. The results observed with clonidine alone in higher doses (up to 4,000 μg per day) are superior to what was observed with guanethidine,[6] pargyline,[7] and alpha-methyldopa [8]

TABLE 5.—*Comparative Antihypertensive Effects of Guanethidine, Pargyline, Alpha-methyldopa, and Clonidine, Alone and in Combination with Oral Diuretics*

		Supine				Erect			
		Normotensive *		Responsive †		Normotensive *		Responsive †	
Therapeutic Regimen	No. of Patients	No.	%	No.	%	No.	%	No.	%
Guanethidine	30	5	17	12	40	13	43	27	90
Guanethidine plus hydrochlorothiazide	25	6	24	13	52	14	56	22	88
Pargyline	33	5	15	7	21	19	57	27	82
Pargyline plus hydrochlorothiazide	11	1	9	4	36	5	45	9	82
Alpha-methyldopa	38	6	16	13	34	9	24	16	42
Alpha-methyldopa plus hydrochlorothiazide	19	8	42	12	63	10	53	17	89
Clonidine	16	1	6	3	19	0	0	6	37
Clonidine plus chlorthalidone	20	1	5	16	80	2	10	16	80

* Normotensive = blood pressure reduced to 140/90 mm Hg or less.
† Responsive = mean blood pressure (diastolic plus one-third pulse pressure) reduced 20 mm Hg or more or normotension.

used alone. A definite advantage of clonidine is a similar antihypertensive effect in the supine and standing positions.[5]

Of particular interest to us is the efficacy of the clonidine plus chlorthalidone combination in severe hypertension (Table 4).

Drowsiness and dry mouth are serious side effects. After 3 to 4 weeks of therapy, however, drowsiness decreased markedly in 70 percent of our patients. It is therefore very important that the patients are counseled regarding this side effect and its possible transient nature. There has been no evidence of unusual toxicity.[9]

Although in our series, patients with severe diastolic hypertension were included, no experience was gained with patients with hypertension in the malignant phase. Studies of the efficacy of clonidine in the malignant phase are warranted in view of the renin suppression induced by the drug (see chapter entitled "Effect of Clonidine on Renin Release"). It is our impression that clonidine in combination with a diuretic represents a useful addition to our antihypertensive armamentarium.

ACKNOWLEDGMENT

The authors wish to thank Prof. Dr. med. Klaus D. Bock for advice and useful criticism during the years of this investigation, and Dr. Paul Kennedy for his kind cooperation in supplying the drugs that made these studies possible.

REFERENCES

1. Heimsoth, V., and Bock, K. D.: Ergebnisse der Notfall- und Langzeitbehandlung mit 2-(2,6-dichlorphenylamino)-2-imidazolin. *In:* Heilmeyer, L., Holtmeier, H. J., Pfeiffer, E. F. (Eds.): Hochdrucktherapie: Symposion über 2-(2,6-dichlorphenylamino)-2-imidazolin hydrochlorid. Stuttgart: Thieme, 1968, pp. 137-144.
2. Onesti, G., Schwartz, A. B., Kim, K. E., Swartz, C., and Brest, A. N.: Pharmacodynamic effects of a new antihypertensive drug, Catapres (ST-155). Circulation 39:219, 1969.
3. Barnett, A. J., and Cantor, S.: Observations on the hypotensive action of "Catapres" (St-155) in man. Med. J. Aust. 1:87, 1968.
4. Davidov, M., Kakaviatos, N., and Finnerty, F. A., Jr.: The anti-hypertensive effect of an imidazoline compound. Clin. Pharmacol. Ther. 8:810, 1967.
5. Hoobler, S. W., and Sagastume, E.: Clonidine hydrochloride in the treatment of hypertension. Am. J. Cardiol. 28:67, 1971.
6. Brest, A. N., Kodama, R., Naso, F., and Moyer, J. H.: Guanethidine in the treatment of hypertension. Postgrad. Med. 30:260, 1961.
7. Brest, A. N., Onesti, G., Heider, C., and

Moyer, J. H.: Comparative effectiveness of pargyline as an antihypertensive agent. Am. Heart J. 68:621, 1964.

8. Onesti, G., Brest, A. N., Novack, P., and Moyer, J. H.: Pharmacodynamic effects and clinical use of alpha-methyl-dopa in the treatment of essential hypertension. Am. J. Cardiol. 9:863, 1962.

9. Onesti, G., Bock, K. D., Heimsoth, V., Kim, K. E., and Merguet, P.: Clonidine: A new antihypertensive agent. Am. J. Cardiol. 28: 74, 1971.

Effect of Clonidine on Regional Blood Flow and Its Use in the Treatment of Hypertension

By Klaus D. Bock, M.D., Peter Merguet, M.D., and Volker H. Heimsoth, M.D.

THE ANTIHYPERTENSIVE properties of clonidine hydrochloride (2-(2,6-dichlorophenylamino)-2-imidazoline hydrochloride) in both the animal and in man have been described in numerous reports in recent years. The drug was synthesized in 1962 by Stähle, Hauptmann, and Zeile. The first pharmacologic and clinical studies were published in 1966.[1–5] Comprehensive surveys on the experimental and clinical investigation of the drug were given in two international symposia in Ulm (1968) and London (1970).[6,7] Clonidine has been commercially available in numerous countries since 1966. Although more than 365 reports on clonidine have appeared, the mode of its antihypertensive action still is not yet totally clarified. It certainly differs from that of all other antihypertensive agents. Much evidence favors the assumption that the hypotensive effect is mainly due to a centrally mediated adrenergic inhibition.[8–13]

Experimental Studies

The methods used in our experiments have been described in another chapter in this volume and elsewhere.[6,7,14,15] The effects of a single intravenous injection of 0.15 mg of clonidine on arterial pressure, respiration rate, venous pressure, muscle blood flow, and skin blood flow in a hypertensive subject are shown in Figure 1. Immediately after intravenous injection a hypertensive effect of a 1- to 3-minute duration was evident, followed by a slowly developing prolonged reduction in systolic, diastolic, and pulse pressure. This effect lasted 3 to 5 hours. Respiration rate and peripheral venous pressure did not change. In rare instances muscle blood flow showed a slight transient increase, but remained essentially unaltered in most of the experiments in both normotensive and hypertensive subjects. Skin blood flow decreased sharply immediately after intravenous injection, to about 40 to 60 percent of resting blood flow. The extent and the duration of blood-flow reduction in the skin were different in the calf and in the hand. A detailed description of the changes in total, muscle, and skin blood flow in different areas is given in the chapter entitled "Effects of Antihypertensive Agents on Skin and Muscle Blood Flow in Man" (see Figs. 2, 3, and 11). As previously demonstrated, the effects of clonidine on blood pressure and peripheral circulation can be abolished or reversed by tolazoline.[14,15] The preservation of muscle blood flow along with the decrease in systemic arterial pressure reflects a reduction in the regional resistance of skeletal muscle. The sharp initial fall of skin blood flow coincides with the transient initial rise of blood pressure and might be in part responsible for it. Afterward skin blood flow returns slowly to control values whereas the blood pressure decreases. The lack of correlation between blood pressure and skin blood flow indicates that the reduction of skin blood flow is not caused by the fall in blood pressure, but is due to a vasoconstrictor effect of the drug on the skin which might even counteract the pressure decrease.

To investigate the local effect of clonidine on peripheral circulation the drug was injected intra-arterially as well as directly into the skin and into the muscle using the techniques shown in the chapter entitled "Effects of Antihypertensive Agents on Skin and Muscle Blood Flow in Man," (Fig. 4). The results are demonstrated in Fig. 2*A* and *B*. Clonidine given intra-arterially or directly into the muscle did not alter muscle blood flow, indicating the absence of a direct action on the muscle vessels. However, intra-arterial or intracutaneous adminis-

From the Division for Renal and Hypertensive Disease, Medizinische Klinik, Klinikum der Ruhruniversität, Essen, West Germany.

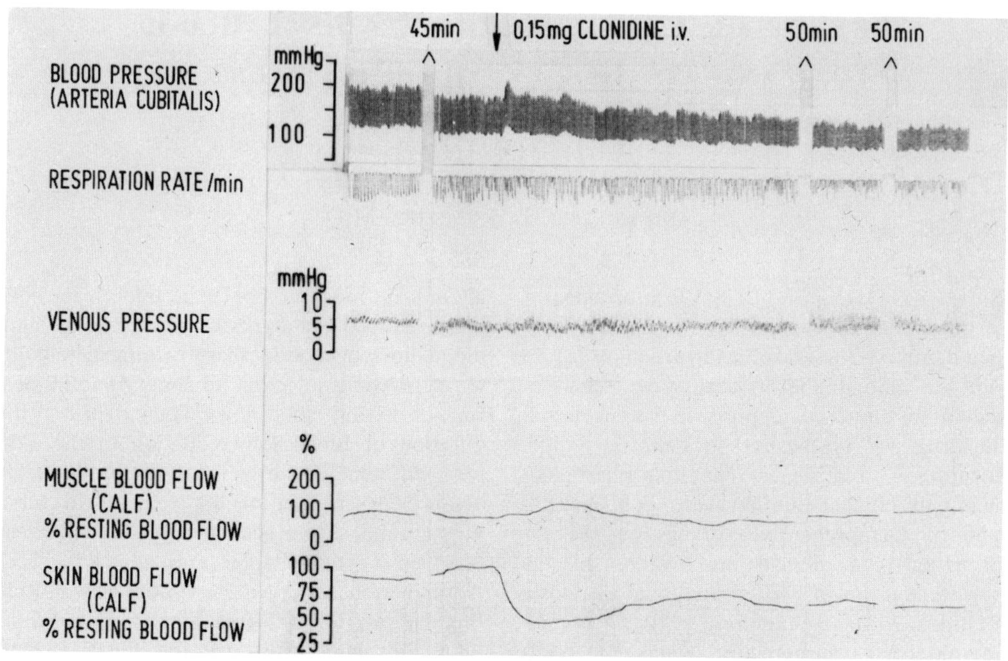

FIG. 1.—Blood pressure, respiration rate, peripheral venous pressure, muscle and skin blood flow in a hypertensive subject before and after intravenous injection of 0.15 mg of clonidine (original record).

tration of clonidine rapidly decreases skin blood flow. Subsequently, locally injected histamine reverses the vasoconstrictor effect of clonidine in the skin into a vasodilatation and also dilates the muscle vessels.

The effects of adrenaline, noradrenaline, and angiotensin on blood pressure, venous pressure, muscle and skin blood flow in normotensive subjects were studied before and after intravenous administration of clonidine. An example of these experiments is given in Fig. 3. The effects of these three agents were not changed qualitatively by pretreatment with clonidine. However, the cutaneous vasoconstriction was less marked because of the reduced flow in the control period after clonidine. Furthermore, a significant prolongation of the depressor effect of adrenaline was demonstrable. Since the fall in blood pressure after adrenaline induces baroreceptor stimulation, the prolonged depressor effect of adrenaline after clonidine might correspond to the inhibition of the carotid occlusion reflex by clonidine which has been observed in animals.[8,12,16]

Our own studies as well as data obtained from the literature [2,4–7,9,14,15,17–32] on the hemodynamic effects of clonidine in man are compiled in Table 1, where the acute and chronic effects are separated.

In acute experiments in the supine position,

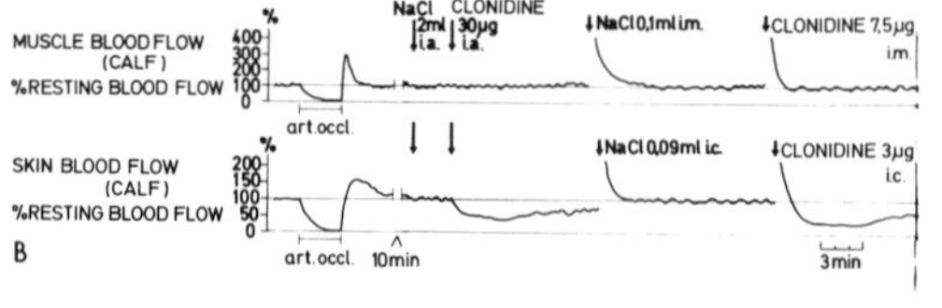

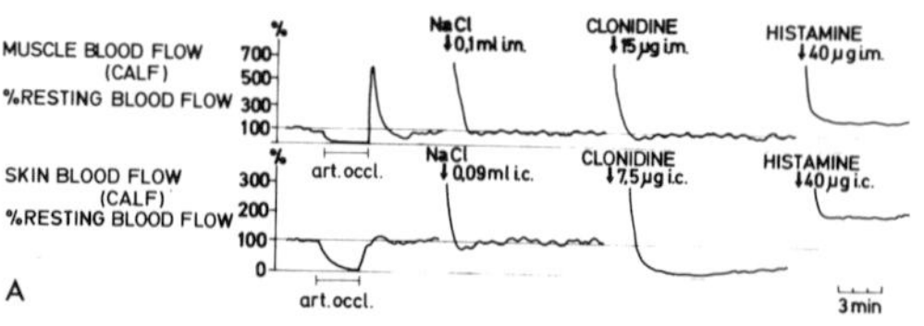

FIG. 2.—*A*, Effects of 0.9% saline and of clonidine on muscle and skin blood flow after intra-arterial and after local injection into the skin and into the muscle. *B*, Local effects of 0.9% saline, clonidine, and histamine on muscle and skin blood flow.

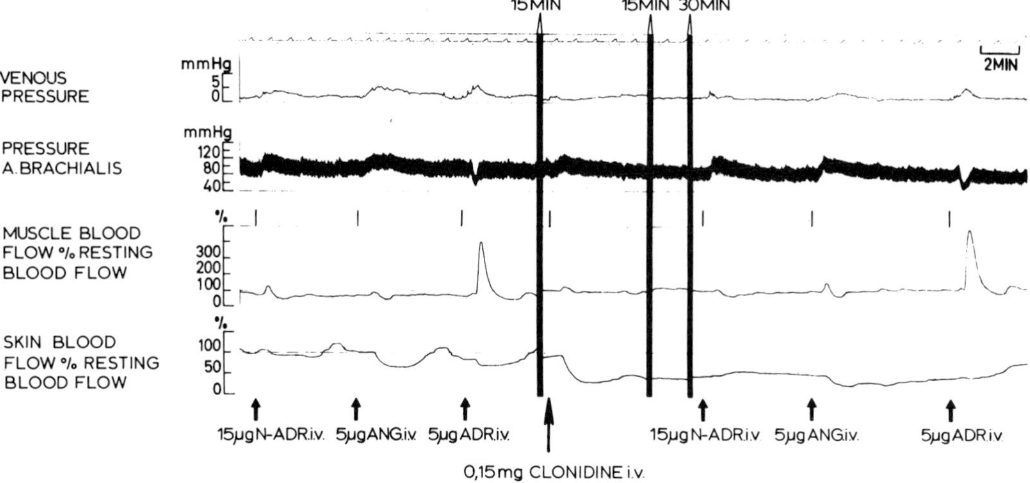

FIG. 3.—Effects of intravenously administered noradrenaline **(N-ADR.)**, angiotensin **(ANG.)**, and adrenaline **(ADR.)** on venous pressure, arterial pressure, muscle blood flow, and skin blood flow (calf) before and after intravenous administration of 0.15 mg of clonidine in a normotensive subject.

blood pressure, cardiac output, stroke volume, and, to a smaller extent, also the heart rate decrease.[17–27] The total peripheral resistance remains essentially unchanged or is slightly reduced.[5,17–22,24–26,28,29] After chronic administration the changes of cardiac output and stroke volume are less pronounced; the total peripheral resistance was often found to be lowered.[7,33] Total blood volume remains unaltered.[14,15] Clinical observations on long-term treated patients show clearly that there is no close correlation between blood pressure reduction and the decrease in heart rate.

TABLE 1.—*Hemodynamic Effects of Clonidine in Man*

		Acute	*Chronic*
Blood pressure		—	—
Heart rate		—	0 —
Stroke volume		0 —	0
Cardiac output		—	0 —
Total peripheral resistance		0 —	0 —
Blood volume			0
Regional blood flow	Brain	0	
	Kidney	—	0
	Muscle	0	
	Skin	—	
	Liver	0	

Symbols used: 0, no change; —, decrease.

Cerebral blood flow was investigated only in acute experiments by two groups of investigators.[31,32] The results were contradictory. In the study of Skinhøj [32] no important change of flow was observed.

In most acute experiments renal blood flow (C_{PAH}) and glomerular filtration rate (C_{In}) were reported to be slightly reduced or unchanged.[15,22,26,29,30] Long-term treatment did not diminish renal blood flow.[2,15] Hepatic blood flow was studied only in acute experiments and was found to be unaltered.[19,20]

CLINICAL OBSERVATIONS

Emergency Treatment

In our hands clonidine has proved to be useful in hypertensive emergencies. We now consider it superior to reserpine and alpha-methyldopa because of its stronger and more rapid effect. We also consider it superior to hydralazine because of less troublesome side effects and lack of tachycardia. For emergency treatment clonidine is given parenterally in single doses of 0.15 to 0.3 mg; according to the response, this dose can be repeated in 1- to 4-hour intervals over the day. Our maximum daily dose was 5 mg. We have never observed a dangerous hypertensive reaction after intravenous injection as has been reported by others.[34,35] To avoid this potential danger, however, the drug may be given intramuscularly. By this route, the onset of effect is nearly as fast as after intravenous injection and, in our experience, no initial blood pressure increase occurs. With clonidine, alone or in combination with furosemide (which is often necessary in emergency situations) we have obtained "good" or "fair" response in about two-thirds of these patients.

In refractory emergency patients or in others with drug-resistant hypertension, we have successfully used a combination of clonidine with diazoxide. The purpose of this combination had been to suppress the tachycardia induced by diazoxide, by the addition of clonidine. To test this, the effects of diazoxide were compared before and after treatment with 0.45 mg per day of clonidine in four hypertensive patients. Figure 4 shows the average blood pressures and heart rates of these patients. In addition, the effects on venous pressure, respiratory rate, and hand blood flow are reported. It is evident that this relatively low dose of clonidine not only reduces the increase in heart rate, but distinctly enhances the hypotensive effect of diazoxide. Clonidine also diminishes the cutaneous vasodilatation induced by diazoxide as is indicated by the record of hand blood flow at the bottom of Fig. 4.

Prolonged Clinical Administration

In our department clonidine has been in clinical use for 6 years. During this time more than 1,000 patients have been treated with the drug. For the evaluation of clinical efficacy and side effects, smaller series of patients were investigated.

One hundred seventy-four hospitalized pa-

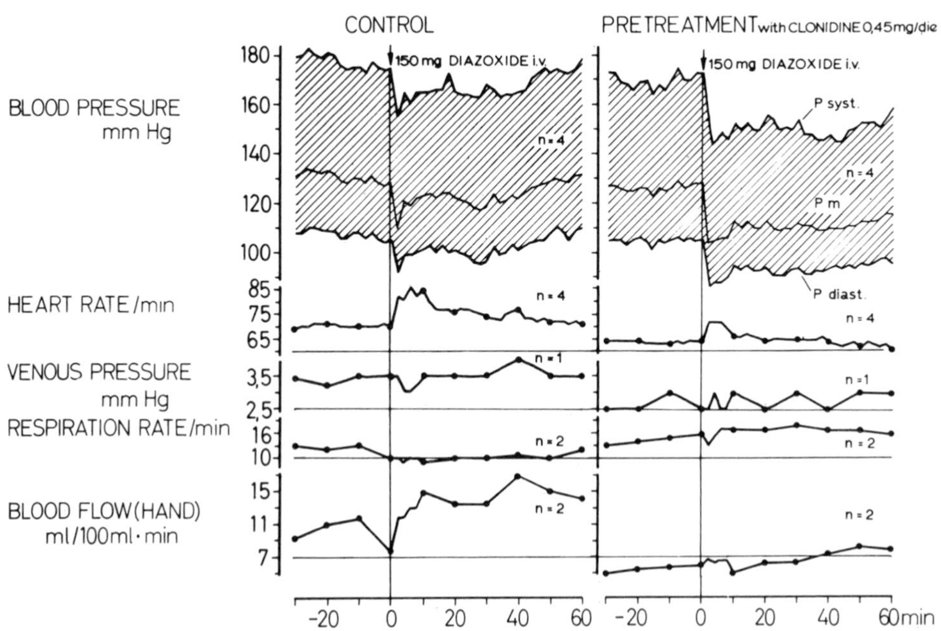

FIG. 4.—Effect of intravenously administered diazoxide on intra-arterial blood pressure, heart rate, and some other parameters before and after pretreatment with clonidine in four hypertensive subjects. Mean values. **n**, number of experiments.

tients (96 men and 78 women, with a mean age of 49 years) received clonidine for 21 days on the average after a control period of 10 to 14 days. One hundred fifteen ambulatory patients (74 men and 41 women, with a mean age of 42 years) were treated with the drug for an average of 344 days, the maximal duration of clonidine therapy in this group being now 1,018 days. Some of the ambulatory patients continued therapy after hospital treatment; others were put on clonidine after an ambulatory control period of at least 3 to 4 weeks' duration. Treatment was started with 0.075 mg of clonidine, given three to four times daily. If there was no satisfying response with clonidine alone in daily doses up to 1.5 mg a diuretic was added. In the hospital the blood pressure was measured two to four times daily with the patient in the supine and erect positions. Among the outpatients, the supine and erect blood pressures were determined at weekly intervals. For the evaluation of drug effect the blood pressures taken at the last 3 days or, in outpatients, at the last three hospital visits of the control and of the treatment period, respectively, i.e., at least 6 values, were averaged and compared. The following criteria were used: "Good" response is defined as systolic and diastolic normotension (140/90 mm Hg or less), "moderate" is defined as systolic *or* diastolic normotension, *or* as a fall in both systolic and diastolic pressure of at least 20 mm Hg. In all other patients the response was defined as "absent."

Table 2 shows the results. The percentage of "good" and "moderate" responses is lower in outpatients than in hospitalized patients and in both groups higher when clonidine is combined with a saluretic. The latter was also shown in a study on 43 hospitalized and 23 ambulatory patients who in addition received a saluretic after a pretreatment period with clonidine alone, because the blood pressure response to clonidine alone was "moderate" or "absent." The improvement of the results is seen in Fig. 5. The reverse, i.e., the additional antihypertensive action of clonidine after unsatisfactory pretreatment with chlorthalidone alone, has been shown by Onesti et al.[15]

Figure 6 demonstrates the results in different forms of hypertension. For this analysis, patients treated with clonidine alone and with the combination clonidine plus a diuretic were put together. There are only slight differences in the responses of patients with primary or with renal hypertension. For the malignant cases (all treated with the combination) in all

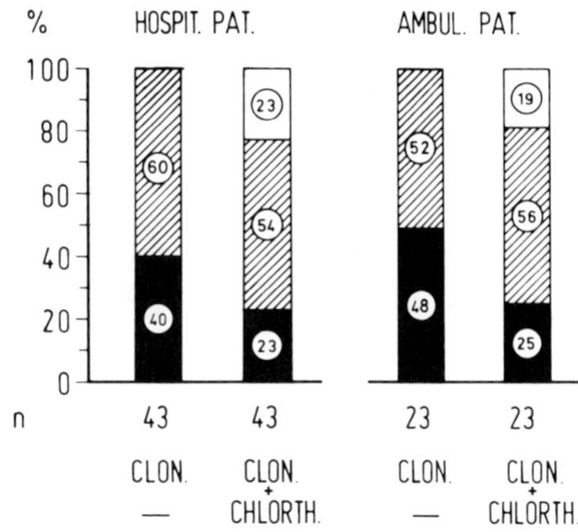

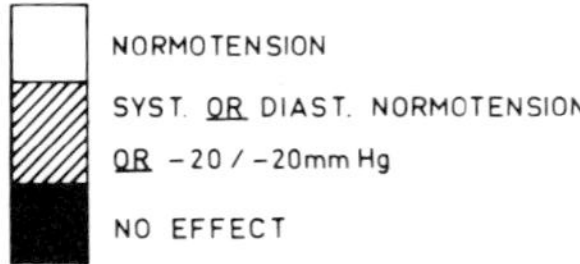

FIG. 5.—Enhancement of the antihypertensive effect of clonidine by adding chlorthalidone in 43 hospitalized (left columns) and 23 ambulatory (right columns) patients.

TABLE 2.—*Antihypertensive Effect of Clonidine in 174 Hospitalized Patients and 115 Ambulatory Patients*

Treatment	*Blood Pressure Response (%)* Good *	Moderate †	Absent ‡
A. 174 Hospitalized Patients			
Clonidine alone	20	41	39
Clonidine and combination of clonidine and diuretic	33	39	28
B. 115 Ambulatory Patients			
Clonidine alone	16	36	48
Clonidine and combination of clonidine and diuretic	29	29	42

* Good: 140/90 mmHg or less.
† Moderate: Systolic 140 *or* diastolic 90 mm Hg or less *or* at least —20/—20 mm Hg.
‡ Absent: All other cases.

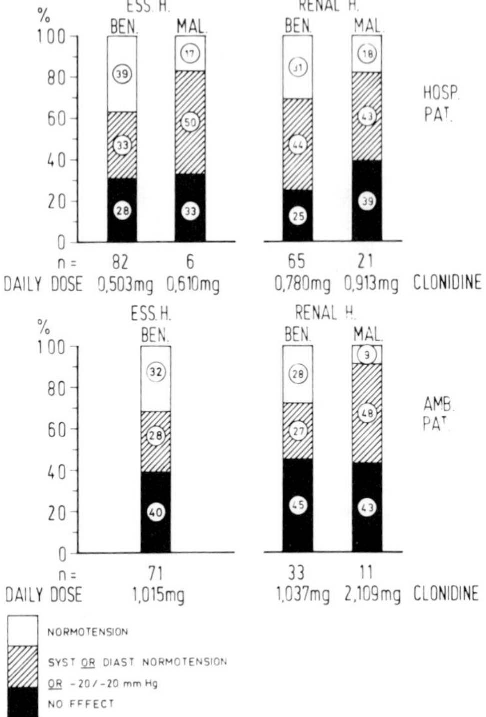

FIG. 6.—Results of treatment with clonidine alone and combined with a saluretic in different forms of hypertension.

groups, "good" responses occurred in 9 to 18 percent and "moderate" responses in 43 to 50 percent. The average daily dose of clonidine was higher in ambulatory than in hospitalized patients, in renal than in essential hypertension, and in malignant than in benign cases, respectively. Patients with azotemia occasionally showed a distinct fall in pressure after very small doses of clonidine, while others needed the same or even higher doses than nonazotemic patients.

Blood urea nitrogen and serum creatinine levels showed minor and inconsistent changes. In 29 patients an oral glucose tolerance test was performed before and during treatment with clonidine; in 15 of them testing occurred 61 to 243 days after starting the drug. No change in the results of the test was observed, regardless of whether the patients previously had a normal response or subclinical diabetes.

Table 3 shows the incidence of side effects of clonidine. The results are based on specific questions asked of 90 patients, in whom the incidence of symptoms had been investigated in the control period. Side effects occurring with similar incidence in the control period and during treatment were regarded as not related to clonidine and omitted from the list. It is apparent that the most prominent side effects are sedation and dryness of mouth. The inhibitory effect of clonidine on the saliva secretion of the parotid gland in man has been previously studied in our laboratory.[36] This effect could also be related to the parotid pain occurring in some patients. Orthostatic hypotension was not a problem. As reported by other authors,[37–39] we also have observed in one patient (not belonging to this series) a Raynaud phenomenon with circumscribed skin necroses at several fingertips which healed after withdrawal of clonidine.

In Table 3, it is shown that some of the side effects disappeared during treatment. This applies especially to sedation and dryness of the mouth. If the patient accepts these symptoms for the first weeks, further therapy is frequently well tolerated. In a few instances the side effects were so troublesome that clonidine had to be discontinued. During the last 6 years the drug has been commercially available in numerous countries. No dangerous or toxic effects have

TABLE 3.—*Side Effects of Clonidine in 90 Subjects*

Side Effect	*Control Period (%)*	*During Administration of Clonidine (%)*		
		Total	*Transitory*	*Persistent*
Sedation	4	64	21	43
Dryness of mouth	4	62	21	41
Vertigo	21	44	10	34
Sleep reversal	—	21	—	21
Shivering	1	17	4	13
Parotid pain	—	10	1	9
Gastrointestinal symptoms	—	7	—	7
Rash	—	4	2	2
Orthostatic symptoms	—	3	—	3
Gynecomastia	—	1	—	1
Impotence *	8	24	2	22

* Evaluated in 59 male subjects only.

been observed by us nor have any been reported to the manufacturer.[40]

Clonidine appears to be a useful, nontoxic antihypertensive agent. We estimate its efficacy as at least similar to that of alpha-methyldopa. Side effects may be sometimes troublesome, but patients who respond to the drug and who tolerate it may be well controlled for many years.

Summary

Experimental studies with the imidazoline derivative, clonidine hydrochloride, in normotensive and hypertensive men showed the following results: Intravenous administration causes an initial transient rise and subsequently a prolonged fall in systolic, diastolic, and pulse pressure. Heart rate decreases slightly; skin blood flow is markedly reduced; muscle blood flow remains unchanged, indicating a decrease of the regional vascular resistance in the muscle. A direct local action on skin vessels, but not on muscle vessels, could be demonstrated. The effects of adrenaline, noradrenaline, and angiotensin on blood pressure and peripheral blood flow were qualitatively not altered. Respiration rate and peripheral venous pressure were not influenced. Tolazoline abolishes or reverses all circulatory effects of clonidine. Parenterally administered clonidine can be successfully used in the treatment of hypertensive emergencies alone or in combination with diazoxide. It enhances the hypotensive action of diazoxide and suppresses its tachycardic effect. Oral administration of clonidine to several groups of patients with hypertension of various degrees and origins revealed a hypotensive efficacy comparable to that of alpha-methyldopa which is enhanced by saluretics. The most frequent side effects are drowsiness and dryness of mouth. During 6 years of clinical experience with clonidine no dangerous or toxic side effects have been reported.

References

1. Hoefke, W., and Kobinger, W.: Pharmakologische Wirkungen des 1-(2,6-Dichlorphenyl-amino)-2-imidazolin-hydrochlorids, einer neuen antihypertensiven Substanz. Arzneim. Forsch. 16:1038, 1966.
2. Bock, K. D., Heimsoth, V., Merguet, P., and Schönermark, J.: Klinische und klinisch-experimentelle Untersuchungen mit einer neuen blutdrucksenkenden Substanz: Dichlorphenylaminoimidazolin. Dtsch. Med. Wochenschr. 91:1761, 1966.
3. Frank, H., and v. Loewenich-Lagois, K.: Therapeutische Prüfung und Untersuchungen zur Nierenfunktion mit einer neuen blutdrucksenkenden Substanz (St 155). Dtsch. Med. Wochenschr. 91:1680, 1966.
4. Michel, D., Zimmermann, W., Nassehi, A., and Seraphim, P.: Erste Beobachtungen über einen antihypertensiven Effekt von 2-(2,6-Dichlorphenylamino)-2-imidazolin-hydrochlorid am Menschen. Dtsch. Med. Wochenschr. 91: 1540, 1966.
5. Schneider, K. W., and Gattenlöhner, W.: Hämodynamische Untersuchungen nach St 155 (2-(2,6-Dichlorphenylamino)-2-imidazolin-hydrochlorid) beim Menschen. Dtsch. Med. Wochenschr. 91:1533, 1966.
6. Heilmeyer, L., Holtmeier, H. J., and Pfeiffer, E. (Ed.): Hochdrucktherapie. Symposion über 2-(2,6-Dichlorphenyl-amino)-2-imidazolin-hydrochlorid in Ulm 20./21.10.1967. Stuttgart: Thieme, 1968.
7. Conolly, M. E. (Ed.): Catapres in Hypertension. A symposium held at the Royal College of Surgeons of England, March 1969. London: Butterworths, 1970.
8. Kobinger, W., and Walland, A.: Kreislaufuntersuchungen mit 2-(2,6-Dichlorphenylamino)-2-imidazolin-hydrochlorid. Arzneim. Forsch. 17:292, 1967.
9. Constantine, J. W., and McShane, W. K.: Analysis of the cardiovascular effects of 2-(2,6-dichlorophenylamino)-2-imidazoline hydrochloride (Catapres). Eur. J. Pharmacol. 4:109, 1968.
10. Nayler, W. G., Price, J. M., Swann, J. B., McInnes, D., Race, D., and Lowe, T. E.: Mechanism of action of "Catapresan". J. Pharmacol. Exp. Ther. 164:45, 1968.
11. Rand, M. J., Rush, M., and Wilson, J.: Inhibition of salivation by "Catapresan". Eur. J. Pharmacol. 5:168, 1969.
12. Sattler, R. W., and van Zwieten, P. A.: Acute hypotensive action of 2-(2,6-dichlorophenylamino)-2-imidazoline hydrochloride (St 155) after infusion into the cat's vertebral artery. Eur. J. Phramacol. 2:9, 1967/68.
13. Schmitt, H., and Schmitt, H.: Mechanism of action of "Catapresan". Eur. J. Pharmacol. 6:8, 1969.
14. Merguet, P., Heimsoth, V., Murata, T., and Bock, K. D.: Experimental study on the

circulatory effects of 2-(2,6-dichlorophenylamino)-2-imidazoline hydrochloride in man. Pharmacol. Clin. 1:30, 1968.

15. Onesti, G., Bock, K. D., Heimsoth, V., Kim, K. E., and Merguet, P.: Clonidine: A new antihypertensive agent. Am. J. Cardiol. 28:74, 1971.
16. Kobinger, W., and Hoefke, W.: Pharmakologische Untersuchungen über Angriffspunkt und Wirkungsmechanismus eines neuen Hochdruckmittels. *In* Heilmeyer, L., Holtmeier, H. J., and Pfeiffer, E. F. (Eds.): Hochdrucktherapie. Symposion über 2-(2,6-Dichlorphenylamino)-2-imidazolin-hydrochlorid in Ulm 20./21.10.1967. Stuttgart: Thieme, 1968, p. 4.
17. Barnett, A. J., and Cantor, S.: Observations on the hypotensive action of "Catapres" (St 155) in man. Med. J. Aust. 55:87, 1968.
18. Brest, A. N., Kim, K. E., Onesti, G., Cangiano, J. L., and Swartz, C. D.: Hemodynamic and clinical effects of a new antihypertensive drug. Circulation 36(Suppl. II):II–76, 1967.
19. Grabner, G., Michalek, P., Pokorny, D., and Vormittag, E.: Klinische und experimentelle Untersuchungen mit der neuen blutdrucksenkenden Substanz 2-(2,6-Dichlorphenylamino)-2-imidazolin-hydrochlorid. Arzneim. Forsch. 16:1774, 1966.
20. Grabner, G., and Michalek, P.: Einige experimentelle Erfahrungen mit Catapresan. *In* Heilmeyer, L., Holtmeier, H. J., and Pfeiffer, E. F. (Eds.): Hochdrucktherapie. Symposion über 2-(2,6-Dichlorphenylamino)-2-imidazolin-hydrochlorid in Ulm 20./21.10.1967. Stuttgart: Thieme, 1968, p. 49.
21. Muir, A. L., and Burton, J. L.: Circulatory effects at rest and exercise of clonidine, an imidazoline derivative with hypotensive properties. Lancet 2:181, 1969.
22. Onesti, G., Schwartz, A. B., Kim, K. E., Swartz, C., and Brest, A. N.: Pharmacodynamic effects of a new antihypertensive drug, Catapres (St-155). Circulation 39:219, 1969.
23. Pozenel, H.: Das Verhalten hämodynamischer Größen von Hypertonikern unter Therapie mit Dichlorphenyl-amino-Imidazolinhydrochlorid. Wien. Klin. Wochenschr. 81:187, 1969.
24. Schneider, K. W.: Cardiale Hämodynamik im akuten Versuch, nach chronischer Behandlung und im Belastungstest mit St 155. *In* Heilmeyer, L., Holtmeier, H. J., and Pfeiffer, E. F. (Eds.): Hochdrucktherapie. Symposion über 2-(2,6-Dichlorphenylamino)-2-imidazolin-hydrochlorid in Ulm 20./21.10. 1967. Stuttgart: Thieme, 1968, p. 78.
25. Stenberg, J., Holmberg, S., Naets, E., and Varnauskas, E.: The hemodynamic effects of Catapresan. Central circulation at rest. Circulation at rest and during exercise. *In* Heilmeyer, L., Holtmeier, H. J., and Pfeiffer, E. F. (Eds.): Hochdrucktherapie. Symposion über 2-(2,6-Dichlorphenylamino)-2-imidazolin-hydrochlorid in Ulm 20./21.10.1967. Stuttgart: Thieme, 1968, p. 68.
26. Vorburger, C., Butikofer, E., and Reubi, F.: Die akute Wirkung von St-155 auf die cardiale und renale Hämodynamik. *In* Heilmeyer, L., Holtmeier, H. J., and Pfeiffer, E. F. (Eds.): Hochdrucktherapie. Symposion über 2-(2,6-Dichlorphenylamino)-2-imidazolin-hydrochlorid in Ulm 21./22.10.1967. Stuttgart: Thieme, 1968, p. 86.
27. Zimmermann, W., Michel, D., and Seraphim, P.-H.: Zur Wirkung von Catapresan auf den kleinen Kreislauf. *In* Heilmeyer, L., Holtmeier, H. J., and Pfeiffer, E. F. (Eds.): Hochdrucktherapie. Symposion über 2-(2,6-Dichlorphenylamino)-2-imidazolin-hydrochlorid in Ulm 21./22.10.1967. Stuttgart: Thieme, 1968, p. 97.
28. Kochsiek, K., and Fritsche, H.: Die Wirkung eines Imidazolin-Derivates auf den arteriellen Blutdruck, die Hämodynamik und die Ventilation. Arzneim. Forsch. 16:1154, 1966.
29. Davidov, M., Kakaviatos, N., and Finnerty, F. A., Jr.: The antihypertensive effects of Catapres. Clin. Pharmacol. Ther. 8:810, 1967.
30. Baum, P.: Experimentelle Untersuchungen zur Nieren-Hämodynamik, und zum Verhalten der Elektrolyte nach einmaliger Verabreichung von 2-(2,6-Dichlorphenyl-amino)-2-imidazolin-hydrochlorid. Arzneim. Forsch. 16:1162, 1966.
31. Deisenhammer, E., and Klausberger, E. M.: Die cerebrale Hämodynamik unter der Einwirkung von 2-(2,6-Dichlorphenylamino)-2-imidazolin-hydrochlorid. Arzneim. Forsch. 16:1161, 1966.
32. Skinhøj, E.: Die zerebrale hämodynamische Wirkung eines Imidazolin-Derivates mit blutdrucksenkender Wirkung. *In* Heilmeyer, L., Holtmeier, H. J., and Pfeiffer, E. F. (Eds.): Hochdrucktherapie. Symposion über 2-(2,6-Dichlorphenylamino)-2-imidazolin-hydrochlorid in Ulm 2.1/22.10.1967. Stuttgart: Thieme, 1968, p. 84.
33. Reubi, F. C., Vorburger, C., and Bütikofer, E.: A comparison of the short-term and long-term haemodynamic effects of antihypertensive drug therapy. *In* Conolly, M. E. (Ed.): Catapres in Hypertension. A symposium held at the Royal College of Surgeons of England,

March, 1969. London: Butterworths, 1970, p. 113.
34. Finnerty, F. A., Jr.: Discussion remark. Circ. Res. 28(Suppl. II):II–69, 1971.
35. Fritsch, H., Bachmann, G. W., and Lenhard, J.: Zur Hypertonietherapie mit 2-(2,6-Dichlorphenylamino)-2-imidazolin-hydrochlorid (Catapresan®). Med. Klin. 64:842, 1969.
36. Bock, K. D., Merguet, P., Brandt, T., and Murata, T.: Experimental studies with clonidine hydrochloride in normotensive and hypertensive subjects. *In* Conolly, M. E. (Ed.): Catapres in Hypertension. A symposium held at the Royal College of Surgeons of England, March, 1969. London: Butterworths, 1970, p. 101.
37. Kellett, R. J., and Hamilton, M.: The treatment of moderate hypertension with Catapres. *In* Conolly, M. E. (Ed.): Catapres in Hypertension. A symposium held at the Royal College of Surgeons of England, March, 1969. London: Butterworths, 1970, p. 197.
38. Vorburger, C.: Discussion remark. *In* Conolly, M. E. (Ed.): Catapres in Hypertension. A symposium held at the Royal College of Surgeons of England, March, 1969. London: Butterworths, 1970, p. 215.
39. Ebringer, A., Doyle, A. E., Dawborn, J. K., Johnston, C. I., and Mashford, M. I.: The use of clonidine ("Catapres") in the treatment of hypertension. Med. J. Aust. 57:524, 1970.
40. C. H. Boehringer Sohn, Ingelheim (manufacturer): Personal communication.

Effect of Clonidine on Renin Release

By Gaddo Onesti, M.D., Virgilio Paz-Martinez, M.D.,
Kwan Eun Kim, M.D., and Charles Swartz, M.D.

The release of renin by the juxtaglomerular apparatus is regulated by several factors, including renal perfusion pressure, sympathetic tone, sodium excretion, and possibly distribution of renal blood flow.[1] Thus, the sympathetic inhibition exerted by clonidine should result in renin suppression, but any decrease in cardiac output, changes in the renal circulation, decrease in renal perfusion pressure, or changes in sodium excretion may modify this effect.

It is the purpose of the present chapter to illustrate the effects of clonidine on renal vein renin activity of the anesthetized dog and on peripheral plasma renin activity in patients with essential hypertension.

Acute Effects on Renal Hemodynamics and Renin Release in Anesthetized Dogs

These studies were carried out in 13 mongrel dogs ranging in weight between 13 and 32 kg under sodium thiopental anesthesia. Intra-arterial pressure and heart rate were continuously monitored. To obtain blood samples from the renal vein a polyethylene catheter was advanced into the left renal vein in the direction of the kidney through cannulation of the ovarian or testicular vein. The following parameters were determined: total renal blood flow (by para-aminohippurate clearance and extraction), glomerular filtration rate (by clearance of exogenous creatinine), sodium excretion and renal vein plasma renin activity (method of Boucher).[2] After control determinations, these measurements were repeated 10, 45, and 85 minutes after clonidine was given intravenously.

Figure 1 shows the effect on renal vein plasma renin activity of 30 μg of clonidine per kilogram of body weight, given intravenously. A dramatic reduction occurred in every dog 10 minutes after clonidine administration with an average decrease of 48 percent ($P < 0.05$). Forty-five and 85 minutes after drug administration renin suppression persisted with an average reduction of 46 percent and 50 percent of control respectively ($P < 0.05$ and $P < 0.01$). In Fig. 2 the effects on renin are reported together with the effects on blood pressure, glomerular filtration rate, total renal blood flow, total renal vascular resistance, and sodium excretion. The mean arterial pressure was essentially unchanged 10 minutes after drug administration. Forty-five minutes after clonidine administration, however, there was a consistent decrease in mean arterial pressure with an average decrease of 26 percent ($P < 0.005$). Eighty-five minutes after drug administration the average decrease in blood pressure was 33 percent ($P < 0.005$). Changes in the glomerular filtration rate were minor. Total renal blood flow showed a 20-percent decrease at 10 minutes, a 19-percent decrease at 45 minutes, and an 11-percent decrease at 85 minutes. These changes, however, were not statistically significant. Total renal vascular resistance increased in every dog 10 minutes after drug administration with an average increase of 16 percent ($P < 0.02$). Forty-five minutes after drug administration renal vascular resistance returned toward the control level and 85 minutes after drug administration the renal vascular resistance was consistently decreased averaging 69 percent of control ($P < 0.005$). Urinary excretion of sodium declined sharply after clonidine was administered. Renal vein plasma renin activity was significantly reduced 10, 45, and 85 minutes after drug administration.

Figure 3 reports the blood pressure, renal hemodynamics, and renin effect of clonidine injected into the cisterna magna of the dog. The small dose of 1 μg per kilogram of body weight did not exert any detectable effect

From the Division of Nephrology and Hypertension, Hahnemann Medical College and Hospital, Philadelphia, Pennsylvania.

Supported in part by NIH Grant No. T–12–HE–05878.

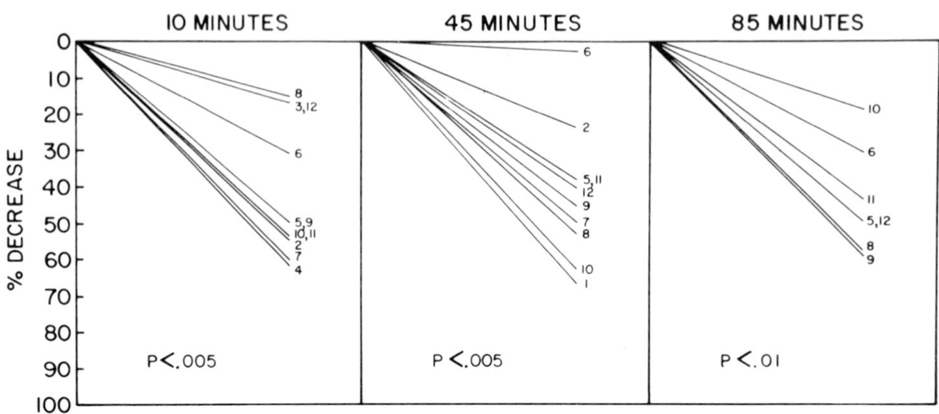

FIG. 1.—Acute effects of intravenous clonidine (30 μg per kilogram of body weight) on renal vein plasma renin activity in 12 anesthetized dogs. Changes in renin activity are expressed as percentage of control. The lines connect determinations for each individual dog. Each dog is identified by the number at the end of the line. Renin determinations were drawn at 10, 45, and 85 minutes after drug administration. (From Onesti, G. et al.: Antihypertensive effect of clonidine. Circ. Res. 28–29 (Suppl. II):53, 1971, with permission of the American Heart Association, Inc.)

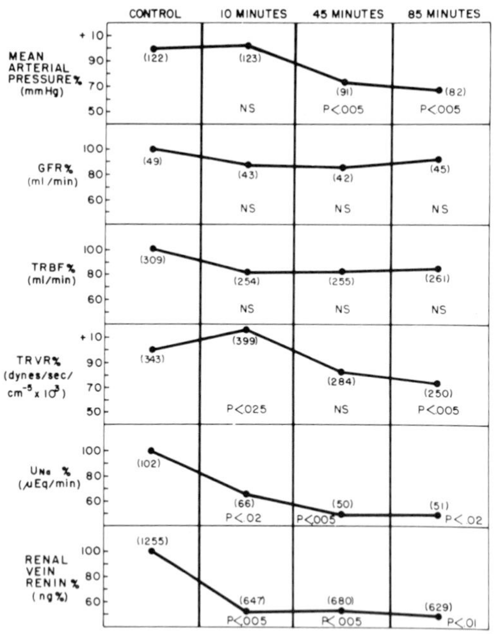

FIG. 2.—Effect of intravenous clonidine (30 μg per kilogram) on mean arterial pressure renal hemodynamics and renal vein plasma renin activity in 12 anesthetized dogs. All changes are expressed in percentage of control. The numbers in parentheses represent the mean values of each parameter. The dimensions for each parameter are listed in parenthesis on the left of the figure. After control, each parameter was determined at 10, 45, and 85 minutes after drug administration. **GFR,** glomerular filtration rate; **TRBF,** total renal blood flow; **TRVR,** total renal vascular resistance; U_{Na}, urinary sodium excretion. (From Onesti, G. et al.: Antihypertensive effect of clonidine. Circ. Res. 28–29 (Suppl. II):53, 1971, with permission of the American Heart Association, Inc.)

when injected intravenously. Intracisternal injection, however, resulted in marked decrease in blood pressure. A moderate decrease in renal blood flow was seen. Renal vein renin activity was markedly suppressed. The timing and the magnitude of renin suppression were similar to those observed with the systemic injection of 30 μg of clonidine per kilogram of body weight.

EFFECTS ON PERIPHERAL PLASMA RENIN IN MAN

Studies on the effects of clonidine on peripheral plasma renin activity were conducted in four patients with essential hypertension in our laboratory. After 4 days on a constant sodium intake (30 mEq per day) peripheral plasma renin activity was first determined by the method of Boucher [2] after 9 hours' rest in the supine position. A second renin determination was done after 30 minutes passive 65° upright tilting. Following this control

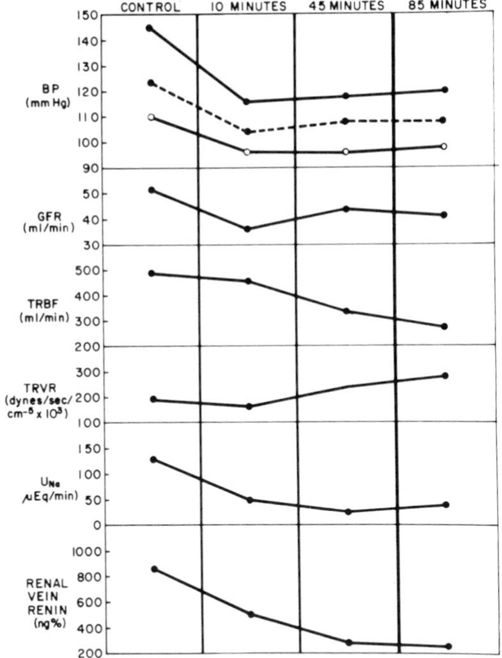

FIG. 3.—Representative experiment illustrating the effect of intracisternal injection of clonidine (1 μg per kilogram of body weight) on the blood pressure (BP), renal hemodynamics (GFR, TRBF, TRVR) and renal vein plasma renin activity. After control, each parameter was determined at 10, 45, and 85 minutes after drug administration. (From Onesti, G. et al.: Antihypertensive effect of clonidine. Circ. Res. 28–29 (Suppl. II):53, 1971, with permission of the American Heart Association, Inc.)

study, 100 μg of clonidine was administered orally four times a day for 4 days. Constant sodium intake was continued. After 4 days of clonidine administration peripheral plasma renin activity was measured again both after 9 hours' rest in the supine position and after 30

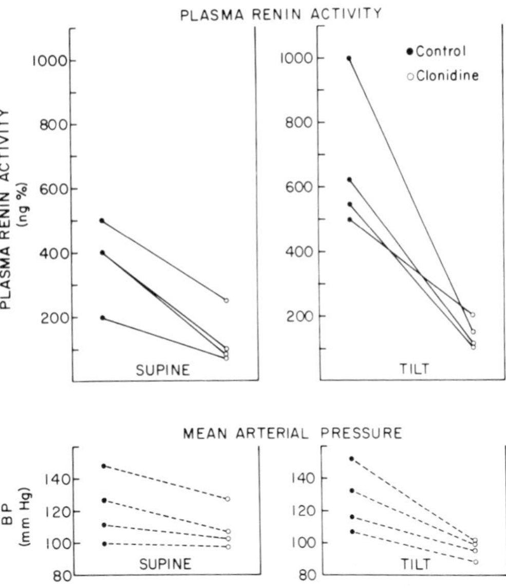

FIG. 4.—Effect of 4 days of orally administered clonidine on peripheral plasma renin activity and mean arterial pressure in four patients with essential hypertension in the supine position and after passive upright tilting. (From Onesti, G. et al.: Antihypertensive effect of clonidine. Circ. Res. 28–29 (Suppl. II):53, 1971, with permission of the American Heart Association, Inc.)

minutes of tilting. The effects of 4 days of clonidine administration are depicted in Fig. 4. Peripheral plasma renin activity was decreased in every case, both in the supine and in the tilted position. The blood pressure was lower after 4 days of drug administration in all patients. In Fig. 5 a representative case is

FIG. 5.—Representative experiment illustrating the effects of 4 days of clonidine administration on peripheral plasma renin activity, blood pressure **(BP)**, urinary sodium excretion **(U_{Na})**, and endogenous creatinine clearance **(C_{cr})** in a patient with essential hypertension. The arrow indicates the increase in plasma renin activity from supine position **(dot)** to upright position **(open circle)** after passive tilt. (From Onesti, G. et al.: Antihypertensive effect of clonidine. Circ. Res. 28–29 (Suppl. II):53, 1971, with permission of the American Heart Association, Inc.)

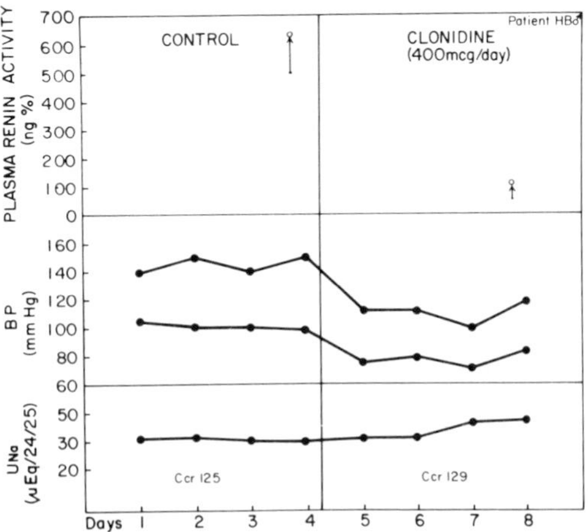

shown. Administration of clonidine (400 μg per kilogram of body weight) resulted in a decrease in blood pressure and peripheral plasma renin activity. Sodium excretion remained constant until the third day of drug administration. On the third and fourth days of drug administration a modest natruresis occurred.

Discussion

The acute renal hemodynamic studies in the anesthetized dog demonstrate an initial increase in renal vascular resistance followed by a progressive return to the control levels and subsequently by an actual decrease. Acute renal hemodynamic studies in man show that renal blood flow and the glomerular filtration rate are maintained during the hypotensive response to clonidine.[3] Renal vascular resistance is decreased. Prolonged oral administration of clonidine results in similar preservation of renal plasma flow and the glomerular filtration rate.[4] This renal effect is similar to the one previously reported with alpha-methyldopa.[5] In the anesthetized dog intravenous administration of clonidine resulted in a consistent decrease in renal vein plasma renin activity. Ten minutes after drug administration the mean arterial pressure had not changed significantly. Forty-five and 85 minutes after drug administration there was a significant decrease in mean arterial pressure. Decrease in renal perfusion pressure is a known stimulus for renin release.[1] Yet in our present study the clonidine-induced fall in perfusion pressure was associated with a significant decrease in renal vein renin. Renal vasodilatation also results in renin stimulation.[6,7] In our present study, however, decrease in renal vascular resistance was associated with a decrease in renal vein renin. Acute sodium retention with less sodium presented to the macula densa may be expected to stimulate renin release.[1] Yet, in the present study the clonidine-induced sodium retention was associated with a consistent decrease in renin release. The most likely explanation of the renin suppression by clonidine is that this is due to sympathetic inhibition.[1] The present study cannot exclude a possible direct effect of clonidine on the juxtoglomerular apparatus. It is important to note that minimal doses of 1 μg of clonidine per kilogram of body weight injected into the cisterna magna results in the same decrease in renin release. This suggests the possibility of interference with a central mechanism of renin regulation. It is of interest to note that sympathetic inhibition by this drug represented the overriding stimulus for renin suppression. Sympathetic inhibition was capable of overcoming the stimuli to increase renin release exerted by decreased perfusion pressure, acute sodium retention, and alteration of renal circulation. The suppressive effect of clonidine on renal vein renin described in the anesthetized dogs was confirmed in patients with essential hypertension to whom the drug was administered for 4 days. These results are similar to the ones reported by Hökfelt, Hedeland, and Dymling.[8] These investigators found a marked decrease in plasma renin activity after clonidine therapy in patients with renovascular hypertension as well as essential hypertension. Concomitantly, with the suppression of plasma renin a decrease in urinary aldosterone excretion was found in their patients.

In contrast with the effect of clonidine, Ayers, Hasris, and Lefer demonstrated that other sympathetic inhibitors (reserpine, trimethaphan) produce increases in plasma renin activity in renal hypertensive dogs.[9] Furthermore, sodium nitroprusside,[10] diazoxide,[6] and hydralazine [7] have each been shown to increase plasma renin activity in normotensive or hypertensive subjects or dogs. The renin-release stimulation by these drugs is presumably due to the reduction in renal perfusion pressure. Only alpha-methyldopa [11] has been reported to decrease plasma renin activity while activating a known stimulus for renin secretion, i.e., a decrease in mean arterial pressure. (See chapters entitled "Effect of Antihypertensive Drugs on Renin Release" and "The Multiple Sites of Action of Methyldopa.")

These observations of the effects of clonidine on renin both in the anesthetized dogs and in hypertensive patients raise the possibility that this effect may also contribute to the antihypertensive efficacy of the drug. In addition, if renin is a factor involved in the pathophysiology of the vascular disease in hypertension, an antihypertensive agent with renin-suppressive abilities may be of significant therapeutic value. (See "Heart Attack and Stroke in Essential Hypertension: The Renin Factor.")

The possible practical therapeutic implication of the effect of clonidine on renin remains speculative at this time.

References

1. Vander, A. J.: Control of renin release. Physiol. Rev. 47:360, 1967.
2. Boucher, R., Veyrat, R., De Champlain, J., and Genest, J.: New procedures for measurement of human plasma angiotensin and renin activity levels. Can. Med. Assoc. J. 30:167, 1964.
3. Onesti, G., Schwartz, A. B., Kim, K. E., Swartz, C., and Brest, A. N.: Pharmacodynamic effects of a new hypertensive drug, Catapres (ST-155). Circulation 39:219, 1969.
4. Grabner, G., Michalek, P., Pokorny, D., and Vormittag, E.: Klinische und experimentelle Untersuchungen mit der neuen Blutdrucksenkenden Substanz 2-(2,6-Dichlorphenylamino)-2-imidazolin-hydrochlorid. Arzneim. Forsch. 16:1174, 1966.
5. Onesti, G., Brest, A. N., Novack, P., Kasparian, H., and Moyer, J. H.: Pharmacodynamic effects of alpha-methyl-dopa in hypertensive subjects. Am. Heart J. 67:32, 1964.
6. Kuchel, O., Fishman, L. M., Liddle, G. W., and Michelakis, A.: Effect of dioxide in plasma renin activity in hypertensive patients. Ann. Intern. Med. 67:791, 1967.
7. Ueda, H., Yagi, S., and Kaneko, Y.: Hydralazine and plasma renin activity. Arch. Intern. Med. 122:387, 1968.
8. Hökfelt, B., Hedeland, H., and Dymling, J. F.: Studies on catecholamines, renin and aldosterone following Catapresan (2-2,6-dichlor-phenylamine)-2-imidazoline hydrochloride in hypertension. Eur. J. Pharmacol. 10: 383, 1970.
9. Ayers, C. R., Harris, R. H., Jr., and Lefer, L. G.: Control of renin release in experimental hypertension. Circ. Res. 24–25 (Suppl. I):103, 1969.
10. Kaneko, Y., Ikada, T., Taxeda, T., and Ueda, H.: Renin release during acute reduction of arterial pressure in normotensive subjects and patients with renovascular hypertension. J. Clin. Invest. 46:705, 1967.
11. Mohammed, S., Fasola, A. F., Privitera, P. J., Lipieky, R. J., Martz, B. L., and Gaffney, T. E.: Effect of methyldopa on plasma renin activity in man. Circ. Res. 25:543, 1969.
12. Onesti, G., Schwartz, A. B., Kim, K. E., Paz-Martinez, V., and Swartz, C.: Antihypertensive effect of clonidine. Circ. Res. 28–29 (Suppl. II):53, 1971.

Effect of Antihypertensive Drugs on Renin Release

By Otto Küchel, M.D., Sc.D., and Jacques Genest, C.C., M.D.

Antihypertensive drugs affect the renin-releasing mechanisms in both directions: they may stimulate the renin release (e.g., hydralazine, diazoxide, diuretics, sodium nitroprusside) or suppress the plasma renin activity (e.g., clonidine, alpha-methyldopa, beta-adrenergic blocking agents). Their effect on the renin release is dependent on their mechanism and site of action; if the action of the antihypertensive drugs is interfering with the physiologic pathways of renin regulation, they usually suppress the renin release in spite of the decrease in the blood pressure which itself is a potent stimulus to renin release. If, however, there is no interference with the physiologic regulation of renin, their hypotensive action (be it a direct blood pressure-lowering effect or a diuretic effect with consequent decrease in the blood pressure) induces a compensatory increase in the renin release and a corresponding activation of angiotensin and aldosterone.

Antihypertensive drugs became in this way an important tool in the study of the mechanisms of renin release. In some cases, the study of their effect on renin release contributed to a better understanding of their hypotensive action and/or of the compensatory reaction to a drug-induced blood pressure decrease. This type of study contributed also to a better understanding of the hypertensive process itself. The gradual decrease in the blood pressure by sodium nitroprusside helped to demonstrate, for example, a higher threshold of responsiveness of the renin-releasing system to blood pressure decrease in renovascular hypertension.[1] A screening of the essential hypertensive population by a diazoxide test for renin stimulation has revealed the existence of the low renin-essential hypertensive group of patients, confirmed later by more elaborate tests.[2]

The great variety of antihypertensive drugs with many different sites of action makes it necessary to deal with every antihypertensive drug individually. The effect of clonidine and alpha-methyldopa on renin release is dealt with in another chapter of this book and only the remaining ones will be discussed here. These are: the hydralazines and sodium nitroprusside, the first ones to be used for these studies; the thiazide diuretics; and diazoxide as a special case of a potent hypotensive agent derived from the thiazides but without diuretic action; finally, adrenergic-blocking agents (guanethidine, phentolamine, and propranolol).

Hydralazine hydrochloride (Apresoline) given intravenously has been reported to cause an increase in plasma renin activity in dogs and in man with renal artery stenosis.[3,4] Further studies have shown that hydralazine given intravenously increases the peripheral plasma renin activity not only in hypertensive subjects (essential or renovascular) but also in normotensives, suggesting a direct renin-releasing effect of the drug from the kidney independent on the blood pressure decrease.[5] Hydralazine, even if increasing the renal blood flow in the long run, induces, following an intravenous injection, an acute reduction in renal perfusion. There is also alteration in the intrarenal hemodynamics, a possible direct effect of the drug on the juxtaglomerular cells and an increased sympathetic discharge following intravenous administration of hydralazine.[6]

Hydralazine was recommended as a tool to dissociate essential and renovascular hypertension, the renin response being higher in the latter group. It may be also useful in differentiating the site of renal artery stenosis by comparing the asymmetric increase in the renal vein renin levels after hydralazine has been intravenously injected, being increased on

From the Clinical Research Institute of Montreal, University of Montreal Medical School, and the Nephrology–Hypertension Service, Hôtel-Dieu Hospital, Montreal, Quebec, Canada.

the side of renal artery stenosis.[4] It has to be considered, however, that such tests are associated with the risk of an intravenous injection of hydralazine. It was shown that the intravenous injection of hydralazine is capable of inducing subjective and objective evidence of coronary insufficiency.[7]

Sodium nitroprusside was studied by Japanese workers in 1966 and 1967 for its renin-stimulating effect in normotensive and hypertensive subjects, using measurements of peripheral and renal venous blood renins.[1,8] The baseline renin activity was significantly higher in the systemic and renal venous blood in hypertensive patients when compared to normotensive controls. Infusion of sodium nitroprusside did not produce an increase in renin unless their blood pressure decreased to pressures below 75 mm Hg. When pressure fell to 60 to 75 mm Hg, there was a significant increase; the increase in renal venous renin activity was detected after 10 to 15 minutes reduction of pressure and recovered after 15 to 30 minutes of normal pressure. The increase in renin activity showed a significant correlation with the decrement of mean arterial pressure.

In patients with renovascular hypertension, nitroprusside infusion caused a significant increase in renin activity from the involved kidneys in all patients and also a significant increase in systemic renin activity with a pressure reduction ranging from 90 to 137 mm Hg, with an average of 103 mm Hg at the end of the infusion (Fig. 1). In contrast, when the uninvolved kidney was sampled, there was no increase in renin release at pressures from 90 to 99 mm Hg. Moreover, for a similar fall of pressure, the renin released in the hypertensive patients was considerably greater than that released in the normotensive patients. This may suggest that the affected kidney was somehow primed against a fall in perfusion pressure.

This work is an important argument in favor of the baroreceptor theory of renin regulation and demonstrates that the threshold of arterial pressure for renin release in renovascular hypertension is shifted to a range much higher than in the normal.[9] Inappropriate release of renin in such patients could be provoked by the fall of blood pressure seen

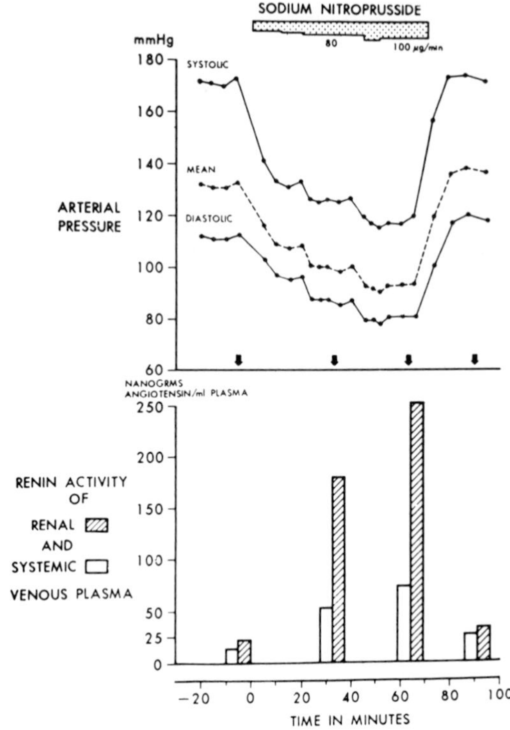

FIG. 1.—Effect of reduction of arterial pressure on renin activity of right renal venous and systemic venous plasma in renovascular hypertension (severe stenosis of the right main renal artery). Marked increase in renin activity occurred at a mean arterial pressure of 100 mm Hg. (From Kaneko, Y., et al.,[1] with permission.)

during sleep, and encourage sodium retention in this period. The increase in renin correlates, however, not only with the fall of blood pressure and its degree but also with the renal blood flow. The renin increase occurred only in patients who present a decrease in the renal blood flow while it is absent if the decrease in renal blood flow is compensated by the renal autoregulation.[10]

This study demonstrates how important it is to apply a dynamic concept of the role of the renin-angiotensin system. The pathogenesis of renovascular hypertension explored by a drug-induced increase in blood pressure is an example of such an approach.

Thiazide diuretics, today the most widely used antihypertensive drugs, have an evident stimulatory effect on renin release in normotensive and hypertensive subjects.[11] This diuretic effect is mainly due to a decrease in the plasma volume secondary to sodium diuresis and is most evident with the use of those diuretics having an acute action such as furosemide and ethacrynic acid.[12,13] The determinant role of the plasma volume was demonstrated by experiments showing that simultaneous intravenous infusion of 20% mannitol or salt-poor concentrated albumin abolished the renin increase in spite of a comparable salt deficit. The furosemide-induced increase in plasma renin activity occurred 10 minutes after the injection of furosemide and remained high thereafter for the whole period of observation, while higher values of free plasma aldosterone occurred only at about 120 minutes.[12] It seems therefore that the rapid activation of renin release secondary to hypovolemia (probably accentuated in hypertensive subjects by a concomitant decrease in blood pressure) leads to an increase in angiotensin and this results in higher plasma aldosterone. Such a chain of events represents a probably typical protective mechanism against drug-induced hypovolemia, in which, in addition to the stretch-receptor stimulation for renin release, an important role could be attributed to the renin stimulation by the sympathetic nervous system.[14] Acutely acting diuretics were shown to increase the excretion of catecholamines and adrenergic-blocking agents to abolish the renin increase in response to these agents.[15,16] Such an example is shown (Fig. 2) in subjects with a plasma renin-activity increase induced by ethacrynic acid.

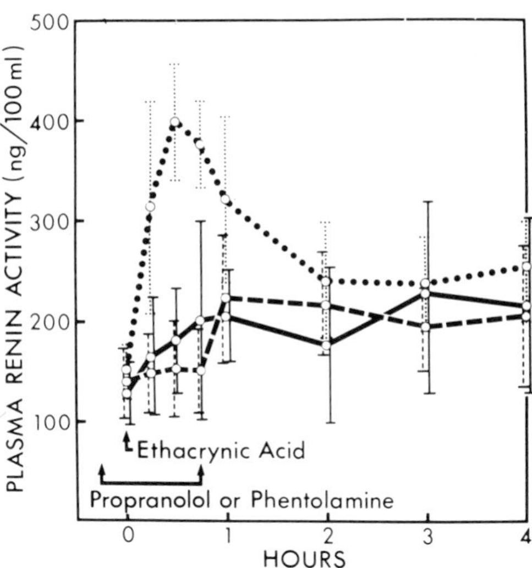

FIG. 2.—Effects of ethacrynic acid and adrenergic blockade on plasma renin activity. The rise in plasma renin activity (mean ± SD) following intravenous ethacrynic acid administration in eight normal subjects **(dotted line)** was prevented by a 1-hour infusion of propranolol in five subjects **(dashed line)** and phentolamine in five subjects **(solid line)** beginning 15 minutes before ethacrynic acid injection. (From Winer, N., et al.,[16] with permission.)

Diazoxide has a special position. It is a benzothiadiazine with sodium-retaining action but possesses a potent and rapid hypotensive action, due to a relaxation of the smooth-muscle cells maintaining the peripheral vascular tone.[17] Its slight sodium-retaining effect is associated with a moderate decrease in renal plasma flow and glomerular filtration rate.[18] Its action in normotensive subjects on blood pressure and renin is weak (Fig. 3). It seems therefore that diazoxide decreases the increased peripheral vascular tone rather than the normal peripheral resistance in normotensive subjects. The decrease of the blood pressure in hypertensive subjects is very rapid with a maximum fall in the blood pressure within 5 to 10 minutes after an intravenous injection. The recovery of the blood pressure is slow and usually after 4 to 8 hours the blood pressure returns to its pretreatment levels. Using diazoxide as a screening test for patients with suppressed plasma renin activity we were able to show that in essential hypertensive patients a subpopulation can be separated (about two-thirds of all patients) presenting a very evident increase in plasma renin activity with a peak usually occurring 2 hours after diazoxide injection.[19] Another group of the patients (about one-third), however, does not respond to diazoxide by an increase in plasma renin activity in spite of having the same order of blood pressure decrease as the patients responding to diazoxide (Fig. 4). Patients unresponsive to diazoxide were also unresponsive to upright posture. Similarly, a low-sodium diet induced an increase in plasma renin activity in diazoxide-responsive patients while patients unresponsive to diazoxide did not increase their plasma renin activity in response to sodium depletion.

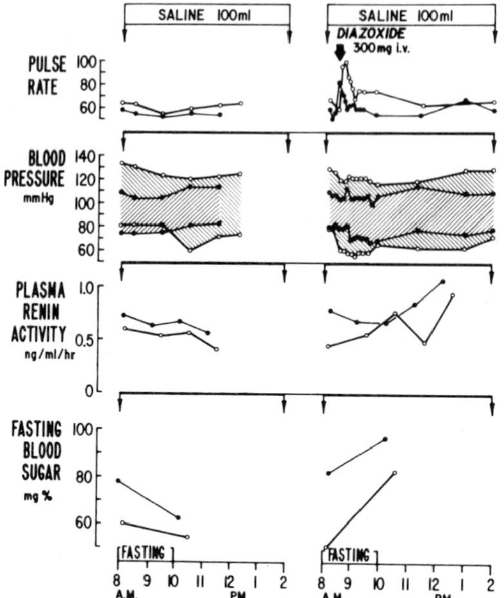

FIG. 3.—The effect of diazoxide (300 mg given intravenously) on pulse rate, blood pressure, plasma renin activity, and fasting blood sugar in two control normotensive, recumbent and 2-hours' fasting subjects on liberal standard sodium diet (100 mEq of sodium). On left are the values recorded on the control day with the subject on a 100-ml saline infusion for 6 hours. On right is the response to diazoxide injected rapidly while the subjects were on the saline infusion as on the previous day. After the diazoxide injection, there is transient tachycardia, but no evident change in the blood pressure, the tendency to plasma renin activity increase is slight, but not significant, the fasting blood sugar increases. The blood pressure-decreasing effect of diazoxide is probably rapidly buffered by a sympathetic discharge of short duration with an evident increase in the pulse rate and slight increase in the plasma renin activity. (From Kuchel, O., Fishman, L. M., and Liddle, G. W.: Unpublished observations.)

If, however, upright posture and diazoxide are combined, the response of the renin-responsive patients is potentiated by this combination while the renin-unresponsive patients do not respond by an additional increase in renin (Fig. 5).

These differences seem to qualify the diazoxide test as a convenient alternative to sodium depletion in screening hypertensive patients for suppression of renin production. This is true in general but in a few patients there may be a dissociated response to diaz-

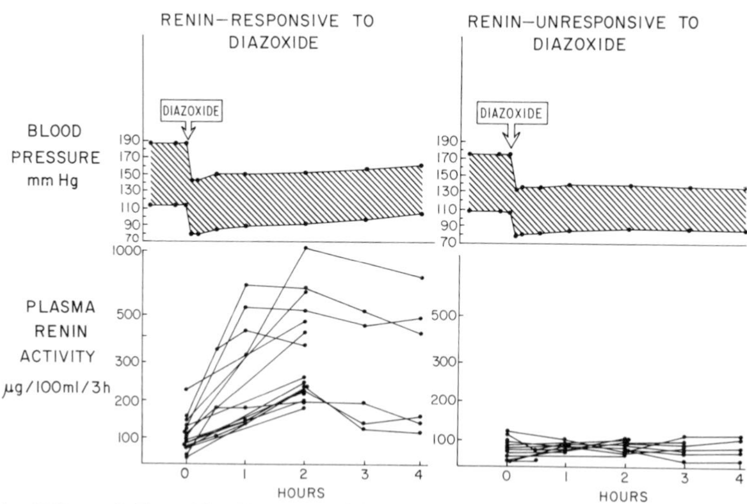

FIG. 4.—Effect of diazoxide (5 mg per kilogram of body weight, given intravenously) on plasma renin activity in 29 patients with essential hypertension on liberal salt diets. The data are subdivided according to the renin response into a group of renin-responsive and renin-unresponsive patients. The blood pressure represents the mean of the pressures of all patients in the respective group of patients. The baseline blood pressures in both groups are not significantly different; the blood pressure response to diazoxide is comparable in both groups, but the recovery from the blood pressure-lowering effect of diazoxide is retarded in the renin-unresponsive group of patients. (See also Fig. 7.)

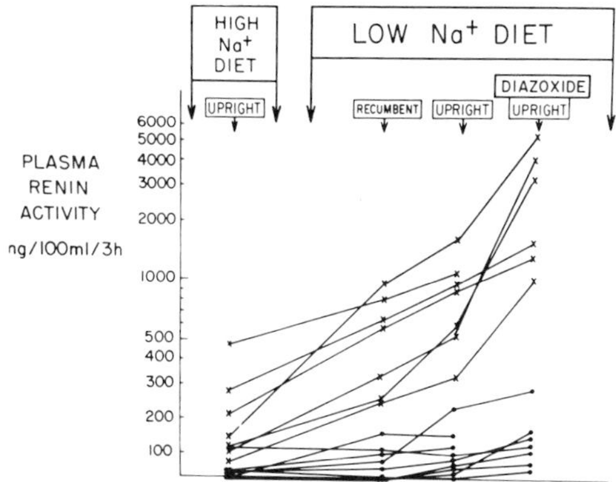

FIG. 5.—Additive effects of low-sodium diet, upright posture, and diazoxide on plasma renin activity of renin-responsive (x) and renin-unresponsive (●) hypertensive patients. (From Kuchel, O., et al.,[19] with permission.)

oxide and sodium depletion.[20] Two types of receptors mediating the renin response to diazoxide and sodium depletion may exist, one being responsive, the other unresponsive in rare cases, but both responding in the same way in the majority of patients.

In response to diazoxide, urinary aldosterone excretion increases within 6 hours following a diazoxide-induced decrease in blood pressure in renin-responsive patients while no increase occurs in a renin-unresponsive patient (Fig. 6). The screening value of this test for detecting primary aldosteronism is diminished by the fact that suppressed plasma renin activity does not signify the presence of an aldosterone-producing adenoma, but a sizable portion (28 percent as a mean of essential hypertensive patients) was shown to have suppressed renin.[21] This portion of patients corresponds very closely to that found by the diazoxide test (32 percent).

Diazoxide is not only a potent hypotensive agent but also a hyperglycemic agent. This is another of its clinical applications.[22] Diazoxide represents therefore a double homeostatic challenge (of the blood pressure and glycemia). Differences in both responses are evident when hypertensive patients who are renin-responsive to diazoxide are compared to those who are renin-unresponsive. As shown in Fig. 7, patients who are renin-unresponsives present a higher rise in blood glucose 2 hours after diazoxide than do the renin-responsives. The renin-unresponsive patients presented, in addition, lower plasma potassium, and in response to diazoxide, less increase in pulse rate; they presented a higher difference between the baseline and the 4 hours after diazoxide blood pressure, pointing to a slower recovery from the diazoxide-induced hypotension of the renin-unresponsive patients than of the renin-responsive patients (see also Fig. 4). The higher hyperglycemic response to diazoxide in renin-unresponsive patients may be related to their lower serum potassium levels since potassium-depleted animals were shown to have an exaggerated hyperglycemic response

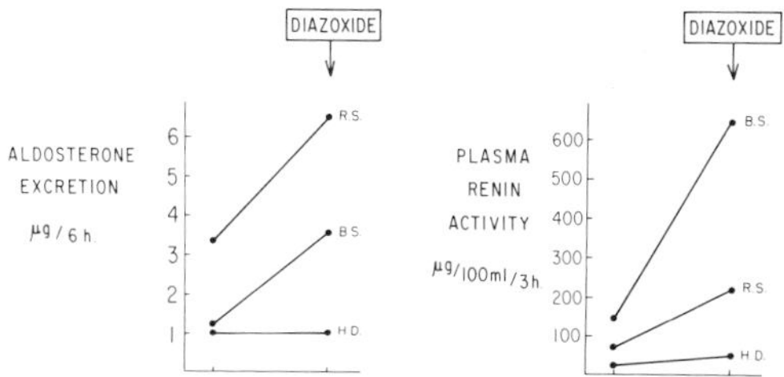

FIG. 6.—Aldosterone excretion (in urine collected 6 hours following injection) and plasma renin activity (2 hours after injection) in response to diazoxide (5 mg per kilogram of body weight given intravenously) in renin-responsive hypertensive patients (R.S., B.S.) and a renin-unresponsive hypertensive patient (H.D.). The absence of renin response coincides with a failure to increase aldosterone excretion in response to diazoxide. (From Kuchel, O., Fishman, L. M., and Liddle, G. W. Unpublished observations.)

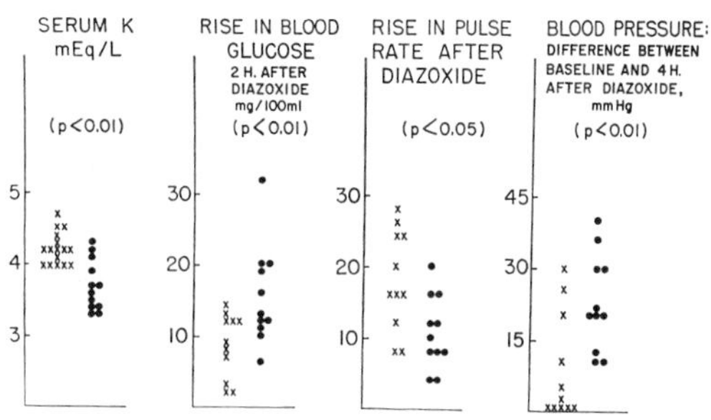

FIG. 7.—Comparison of renin-responsive (x) and renin-unresponsive (●) hypertensive patients with respect to serum potassium levels before diazoxide administration and the changes in blood glucose, pulse rate, and blood pressure after diazoxide administration. (From Kuchel, O., et al.,[19] with permission.)

to diazoxide and some of the patients with hypertension were shown to have lower total body potassium levels.[23,24]

The fact that the renin-unresponsive patients experienced less tachycardia and a more prolonged depression of blood pressure than did the renin-responsive patients speaks in favor of a certain degree of adrenergic insufficiency in the patients with suppressed renin levels. Such a possibility is supported by a very high incidence of orthostatic hypotension in these patients.[25]

The mechanisms by which diazoxide induces a renin increase may be multiple. It was shown recently that the diazoxide-induced renin release in man occurs independently of changes in the extracellular fluid volume.[26] A certain role may be attributed to changes not only in the blood pressure but also in the regional blood flow. We have studied the effect of diazoxide on the regional blood flow in several organs in rats and demonstrated that an evident increase occurs in the heart, thyroid, and less in the adrenals while a decrease occurs in the spleen and to a lesser degree in the kidney (Fig. 8).[27] It may be therefore that a contributing factor at least to the renin-aldosterone stimulation by diazoxide may be a decrease in the renal and increase in the adrenal blood flow.

Probably the most important factor in the renin-stimulating effect of diazoxide is the stimulation of the sympathetic nervous system by the rapid decrease in the blood pressure, a stimulus calling for a compensatory activation of the adrenergic nervous system. Such a mechanism is supported by the finding that adrenergic-blocking agents can prevent completely the diazoxide-induced renin increase (Fig. 9).[16] Since cyclic AMP plays a probably mediating role in the renin increase induced by catecholamines, and diazoxide was shown to be also an inhibitor of the cyclic nucleotide phosphodiesterase, the increase in the intracellular cyclic AMP (due to the adrenergic discharge and also to a lower cyclic-AMP degradation by phosphodiesterase) may represent the final mechanism by which the ad-

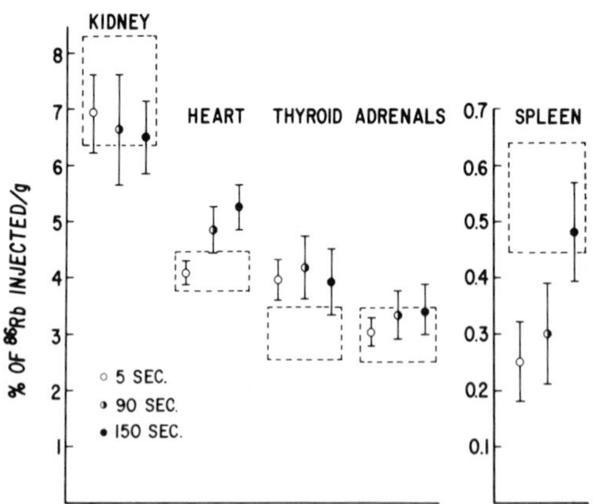

FIG. 8.—Changes in local blood flow in the kidney, heart, thyroid, adrenals, and spleen of rats after intravenous injection of 5 mg of diazoxide. Mean values of the tissue uptake of ^{86}Rb expressed in percentage of injected dose per gram of the tissue at the following time intervals between diazoxide and ^{86}Rb uptake determination: 5 seconds, 90 seconds, 150 seconds. **Verticals:** 95 percent confidence intervals. **Dashed lines:** 95 percent confidence intervals of the control mean values.[27]

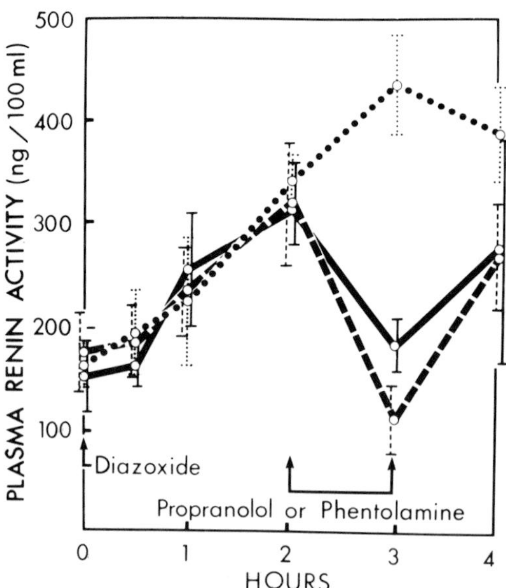

FIG. 9.—Effects of diazoxide and adrenergic blockade on plasma renin activity. The rise in plasma renin activity (mean ± SD) following intravenous diazoxide administration in eight normal subjects **(dotted line)** was suppressed by infusion of propranolol in six subjects **(dashed line)** and phentolamine in five subjects **(solid line)** between the second and third hours. (From Winer, N., et al.,[16] with permission.)

renergic stimulation results in an increased renin secretion and release.[28,29]

The effect of the adrenergic-blocking agents on renin release is, in some cases, rather related to their blood pressure-decreasing effect; sometimes, their renin-decreasing effect may contribute to a better understanding of their long-term beneficial effect on the hypertensive process.

Guanethidine (Ismelin) was used as a part of the stimulating maneuvers in hypertensive patients, to detect patients with suppressed plasma renin activity.[21] Guanethidine given to patients after 4 days of a low-sodium diet led to a further increase in renin. This is probably related to a decrease in the blood pressure (an average decrease of 22 mm Hg in the diastolic blood pressure). In this way responders and nonresponders could be more sharply differentiated on guanethidine than was possible by using a low-sodium diet only. In another type of experiment guanethidine was shown to diminish the upright posture-induced increase in the plasma renin activity while it had no effect on the low sodium diet-stimulated renin increase.[30] This can be interpreted as that the sodium depletion induces renin increase independently of the sympathetic nervous system while the upright posture-induced effect is mediated by the sympathetic nervous system.

Phentolamine was shown to produce a significant rise in plasma renin activity in rats, and pentolinium to produce a very evident increase in the plasma renin activity of sodium-depleted men.[31,32] The stimulatory effects on plasma renin activity are probably due to the blood pressure-decreasing effect of these substances. These data indicate that the blood pressure-decreasing effect is probably in this case a more potent stimulus to renin release than its inhibition resulting from the adrenergic-blocking effect. It may be also explained as an antagonism between the alpha- and beta-blocking agents; the inhibition of one type of receptor may result in an activation of the other.[33] The inhibition of alpha-receptors may result in a stimulation of beta-adrenergic receptors which are believed to be most involved as mediators of the effect of the adrenergic system on renin release.[34]

For this reason, beta-adrenergic-blocking agents, recently used as antihypertensive drugs, are of special interest in relation to renin release. The beta-adrenergic-receptor-mediated renin release can be mimicked by isoproterenol, a beta-adrenergic-stimulating agent known to increase renin release. The probable site of this stimulatory effect of isoproterenol on renin release is the adenylate-cyclase-cyclic AMP system hypertension.[40] Beta-adrenergic receptors are considered to be a part of adenyl cyclase, an enzyme initiating the formation of cyclic AMP in the cells.[35] Cyclic AMP was shown to be a potent stimulus for renin secretion in vivo and in vitro.[28,36]

We have presented recently [37] some evidence that patients with labile hyperkinetic hypertension present renin hyperresponsiveness to upright posture and an excessive and prolonged renin increase in response to beta-adrenergic stimulation by isoproterenol. At the same time, they present an increase in the urinary cyclic AMP excretion with upright posture (while control subjects show a decrease).[38] These data are compatible with an excessive cyclic AMP and renin production in response to beta-adrenergic stimulation by posture or isoproterenol. They correspond well to the description of the condition in those patients as a "beta-adrenergic hyperdynamic state" on the basis of their circulatory behavior.[39]

The treatment by beta-adrenergic-blocking agents was shown to normalize not only the abnormal circulatory responses of these patients (hypertension, tachycardia) but also to decrease renin and its hyperresponsiveness to upright posture as well as the abnormal response in the urinary cyclic AMP excretion. An example of such a patient completely studied is seen in Fig. 10.*

If the described beta-adrenergic-cyclic AMP concept as one of the main factors in renin regulation proves to be correct, it could represent a common mechanism by which several hypotensive drugs with different sites of action

* There is, in addition, recent evidence that the antihypertensive effect of propranolol is closely linked to its renin-inhibiting effect; the higher the baseline levels of plasma renin activity, the greater is the antihypertensive effect of propranolol. Beta-adrenergic blockade may, therefore, become a useful tool in the treatment of renovascular hypertension.

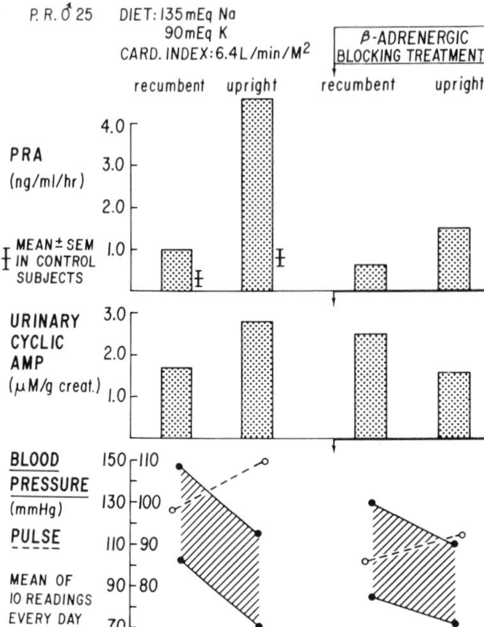

FIG. 10.—The effect of beta-adrenergic-blocking treatment in a patient having labile hyperkinetic hypertension with an elevated cardiac output. In the control period the patient presented an excessive renin response to upright posture when compared to control subjects. Urinary cyclic AMP excretion increased in the upright position, a response typical for labile hypertensive patients with hyperkinetic circulation;[38] he presented an evident tendency to an excessive orthostatic decrease in the blood pressure and baseline tachycardia with a very evident increase in the upright position. With the beta-adrenergic-blocking treatment the blood pressure and pulse rate decreased and their response to the upright position became closer to normal; the plasma renin activity response to upright posture became normal as well as the response of the urinary cyclic AMP excretion in response to upright posture. (From Kuchel, O., Hamet, P., Boucher, R., and Genest, J.: International symposium on the renin-angiotensin-aldosterone-sodium system in hypertension, Sept. 30–Oct. 4, 1971, Mont Gabriel, with permission.)

increase the plasma renin activity. Hydralazine, furosemide, and diazoxide lead to adrenergic activation and renin stimulation. The common link between them may be an increased cellular cyclic AMP concentration in the renin-producing cells. This may be due to a higher cyclic AMP generation because of beta-adrenergic discharge and adenylcyclase activation, or, in another case, to additional inhibition of the phosphodiesterase (in the case of diazoxide), leading to a decreased metabolic degradation of cyclic AMP.

REFERENCES

1. Kaneko, Y., Ikeda, T., Takeda, T., and Ueda, H.: Renin release during acute reduction of arterial pressure in normotensive subjects and patients with renovascular hypertension. J. Clin. Invest. 46:705, 1967.
2. Kuchel, O., Fishman, L. M., Liddle, G. W., and Michelakis, A. M.: Effect of diazoxide on plasma renin activity (PRA) in hypertension. Clin. Res. 14:491, 1966.
3. Yagi, S., Kramsch, D. M., Inoue, G., and Hollander, W.: Stimulation of renin secretion by hydralazine: I. Studies of experimental hypertension of coarctation of the aorta, abstracted. Circulation 32(Suppl. 2):II–222, 1965.
4. Huvos, A., Yagi, S., Mannick, J. A., and Hollander, W.: Stimulation of renin secretion by hydralazine: I. Studies in renovascular hypertension, abstracted. Circulation 32 (Suppl. 2):III–118, 1965.
5. Ueda, H., Yagi, S., and Kaneko, Y.: Hydralazine and plasma renin activity. Arch. Intern. Med. 122:387, 1968.
6. Ablad, B.: A study of the mechanism of the hemodynamic effects of hydralazine in man. Acta Pharmacol. 20(Suppl. 1):1, 1963.
7. Judson, W. E., Hollander, W., and Wilkins, R. W.: Observations on angina pectoris during drug treatment of hypertension. Circulation 13:553, 1956.
8. Ueda, H., Kaneko, Y., and Takeda, T.: Renal pressor system in hypertensive patients. Jap. Circ. J. 30:167, 1966.
9. Skinner, S. L., McCubbin, J. W., and Page, I. H.: Control of renin secretion. Circ. Res. 15:64, 1964.
10. Kaneko, Y., Ikeda, T., Takeda, T., Inoue, G., Tagawa, H., and Ueda, H.: Renin release in patients with benign essential hypertension. Circulation 38:353, 1968.
11. Genest, J.: The renin angiotensin aldosterone system. *In* Brest, A. N., and Moyer, J. H.: Cardiovascular Disorders. Philadelphia: F. A. Davis, 1968, p. 144.
12. Rosenthal, J., Boucher, R., Nowaczynski, W., and Genest, J.: Acute changes in plasma volume, renin activity, and free aldosterone levels in healthy subjects following fursemide ad-

ministration. Canad. J. Physiol. Pharmacol. 46:85, 1968.

13. Meyer, P., Ménard, J., Alexandre, J. M., and Weil, B.: Correlations between plasma renin, hematocrit, and natriuresis. Rev. Canad. Biol. 25:111, 1966.
14. Gordon, R. D., Kuchel, O., Liddle, G. W., and Island, D. P.: Role of the sympathetic nervous system in regulating renin and aldosterone production in man. J. Clin. Invest. 46:599, 1967.
15. Heidland, A., and Hennemann, H.: Aktivierung des sympathicoadrenalen Systems nach Diuretica—Beziehungen zum salidiuretischen Effekt und Glomerulumfiltrat. Klin. Wochenschr. 47:518, 1969.
16. Winer, N., Chokshi, D. S., Yoon, M. S., and Freedman, A. D.: Adrenergic receptor mediation of renin secretion. J. Clin. Endocrinol. Metab. 29:1168, 1969.
17. Rubin, A. A., Taylor, R. M., and Roth, F. E.: A brief review of the development of diazoxide as an antihypertensive agent. Ann. N.Y. Acad. Sci. 150:457, 1968.
18. Ganten, D., Meurer, K. A., and Kaufman, W.: Hämodynamik und Exkretionsfunktion der Niere unter Furosemid und Diazoxid. Med. Welt 22:663, 1971.
19. Kuchel, O., Fishman, L. M., Liddle, G. W., and Michelakis, A.: Effect of diazoxide on plasma renin activity in hypertensive patients. Ann. Intern. Med. 67:791, 1967.
20. Klaus, D., Schmelzle, R., Simsch, A., and Trübestein, G.: Plasma-renin-aktivität nach Orthostase und nach Diazoxid bei primärer und renaler Hypertonie. Klin. Wochenschr. 48:1033, 1970.
21. Jose, A., Crout, J. R., and Kaplan, N. M.: Suppressed plasma renin activity in essential hypertension—Roles of plasma volume, blood pressure, and sympathetic nervous system. Ann. Intern. Med. 72:9, 1970.
22. Graber, A. L., Porte, D., and Williams, R. H.: Clinical use of diazoxide and studies of the mechanism of its hyperglycemic effects in man. Ann. N.Y. Acad. Sci. 150:303, 1968.
23. Kaess, H., Senft, G., Losert, W., Sitt, R., and Schultz, G.: Mechanismus der gesteigerten glykogenolytischen Wirkung des Diazoxids im Kaliummangel. Naunyn Schmiedebergs Arch. Pharmacol. 253:395, 1966.
24. Frankel, H. J., Pierson, R. N., and Hilton, J. G.: Total body potassium (TBK) in hypertension (HT). Clin. Res. 17:241, 1969.
25. Weinberger, M. H., Dowdy, A. J., Nokes, G. W., and Luetscher, J. A.: Plasma renin activity and aldosterone secretion in hypertensive patients during high and low sodium intake and administration of diuretic. J. Clin. Endocrinol. Metab. 28:359, 1968.
26. Baer, L., Goodwin, F. J., and Laragh, J. H.: Diazoxide-induced renin release in man: Dissociation from plasma and extracellular fluid volume changes. J. Clin. Endocrinol. Metab. 29:1107, 1969.
27. Kapitola, J., Kuchel, O., Schreiberova, O., and Jahoda, I.: Influence of diazoxide on regional blood flow in rats. Experientia 24: 242, 1968.
28. Winer, N., Chokshi, D. S., and Walkenhorst, W. G.: Effects of cyclic AMP, sympathomimetic amines, and adrenergic receptor antagonists on renin secretion. Circ. Res. 29: 239, 1971.
29. Moore, P. F.: Effects of diazoxide and benzothiadiazine diuretics upon phosphodiesterase. Ann. N.Y. Acad. Sci. 150:256, 1968.
30. Klaus, D., and Bocskor, A.: Regulation der Reninsekretion beim Natriummangel. Verhandlungen der Deutschen Gesellschaft Für Innere Medizin. Munich: J. F. Bergmann, 1968, pp. 409–413.
31. Peskar, B., Meyer, D. K., Tauchmann, U., and Hertting, G.: Influence of isoproterenol, hydralazine and phentolamine on the renin activity of plasma and renal cortex of rats. Eur. J. Pharmacol. 9:394, 1970.
32. Gordon, R. D., Kuchel, O., and Liddle, G. W.: Unpublished observations.
33. Smith, R. D., and Nash, C. B.: Effects of the beta-adrenergic blocking agents, propranolol, KO592, and MJ-1999 on phenoxybenzamine blockade of norepinephrine. Arch. Int. Pharmacodyn. 181:208, 1969.
34. Assaykeen, T. A., Clayton, P. L., Goldfien, A., and Ganong, W. F.: Effect of alpha- and beta-adrenergic blocking agents on the renin response to hypoglycemia and epinephrine in dogs. Endocrinology 87:1318, 1970.
35. Robison, A., and Sutherland, E. W.: Sympathin E, Sympathin I, and the intracellular level of cyclic AMP. Circulation 26–27 (Suppl. I):1, 1970.
36. Michelakis, A. M., Caudle, J., and Liddle, G. W.: In vitro stimulation of renin production by epinephrine, norepinephrine and cyclic AMP. Proc. Soc. Exp. Biol. Med. 130:748, 1969.
37. Kuchel, O., Cuche, J. L., Hamet, P., Boucher, R., Barbeau, A., and Genest, J.: The relationship between adrenergic nervous system and renin in labile hyperkinetic hypertension.

In Genest, J., and Koiw, E.: Aldosterone Symposium. Heidelberg: Springer, 1972, p. 118.

38. Hamet, P., Kuchel, O., Fraysse, J., and Genest, J.: Effect of posture on cAMP excretion in control subjects and patients with essential hypertension. Clin. Res. 19:760, 1971.
39. Frohlich, E. D., Tarazi, R. C., and Dustan, H. P.: Hyperdynamic β-adrenergic circulatory state. Arch. Intern. Med. 123:1, 1969.
40. Bühler, F. R., Baer, L., Vaughan, E. D., Brunner, H. R., and Laragh, J. H.: Inhibition of renin secretion by propranolol: A specific treatment for renal hypertension? J. Clin. Invest. 51:17a, 1972.

Preliminary Investigation of Levodopa As Adjunctive Therapy for Hypertension

By T. Budya Tjandramaga, M.D., M.Sc., Aaron H. Anton, Ph.D., and Leon I. Goldberg, Ph.D., M.D.

CARDIOVASCULAR AND RENAL actions of levodopa (L-dopa) suggest that the amino acid may be useful for the treatment of hypertension. First, hypotension is a relatively common side effect of levodopa treatment for Parkinson's disease. It has been estimated that approximately 30 percent of treated patients experience this side effect.[1,2] In most cases, the primary reduction in blood pressure occurs in the standing position, but the blood pressure in the supine position is also lowered in some patients. In general, this symptom is well tolerated and becomes less prominent with continuing treatment. In occasional patients reduction of dosage or discontinuation of treatment is necessary. Secondly, oral administration of levodopa in single doses of 1 to 2 gm significantly increases the glomerular filtration rate, renal plasma flow, and sodium and potassium excretion.[3] The natriuretic effect of levodopa persists for more than 150 minutes. Similar increases in renal function have been demonstrated with dopamine, suggesting that these changes are due to generation of dopamine by decarboxylation of levodopa.[4] In support of this interpretation, experiments in the dog have shown that administration of a decarboxylase inhibitor prevents the prolonged increments in renal blood flow produced by intravenous administration of levodopa.[5] The present study was designed to determine the effects of levodopa on blood pressure and renal function of patients with essential hypertension.

From the Department of Medicine (Clinical Pharmacology) of Emory University, Atlanta, Georgia, and the Departments of Anesthesiology and Pharmacology, Case-Western Reserve University, Cleveland, Ohio.

Supported by Grants GM–14270, HE–06491, and FR–39 from the National Institutes of Health, and a grant from Hoffmann-La Roche, Inc.

Methods

Effects of Levodopa on Blood Pressure and Renal Function in Outpatients

Five patients with moderate to severe essential hypertension were selected for this study. All patients required guanethidine and a thiazide diuretic for control of hypertension. Clinical data concerning these patients are shown in Table 1. None had angina, known coronary heart disease, or cardiac arrhythmias. The nature of the study was explained to each participant and written consent was obtained. Four of the patients had decreased renal function (serum creatinine $>$ 1.7 mg per 100 ml; creatinine clearance $<$ 80 ml per minute). The patients were evaluated once weekly in a hypertensive clinic at Grady Memorial Hospital. At each clinic visit, blood pressure and heart rate were recorded with the patient in the supine position and after standing 3 minutes. Serum creatinine, blood urea nitrogen, and uric acid determinations were obtained weekly. Routine urinalysis, complete blood count, liver function tests, serum electrolyte measurements, chest x-ray, electrocardiograms, and funduscopic examinations were performed during the initial evaluation and repeated during the course of levodopa treatment. Guanethidine and thiazide diuretic dosages were adjusted and were maintained at the same level for 3 weeks prior to levodopa administration and throughout the course of the study unless changes were required because of clinical indications. Most patients received placebo tablets resembling levodopa tablets during the control period. After this period, levodopa (Larodopa) was added to the antihypertensive regimen in an initial dose of 250 mg given four times daily. The dose was gradually increased by 0.5-gm increments at intervals depending upon side effects and response. A maximum dose of 3.0 gm per day was attained in most patients.

TABLE 1.—*Effects of Prolonged Levodopa Administration on Renal Function*

Patient	Age	Sex	Levodopa		Other Drugs	mg per day	Blood Urea Nitrogen (mg per 100 ml)		Serum Creatinine (mg per 100 ml)		Serum Uric Acid (mg per 100 ml)	
			Duration (Weeks)	Maximum Dosage (gm per day)			Control	Levodopa	Control	Levodopa	Control	Levodopa
F.W.	49	M	32	3	Guanethidine	75	23	25	1.8	1.8	11.0	10.2
					Trichlormethiazide	4						
L.B.	64	F	31	3	Guanethidine	20	43	49	2.2	2.2	8.1	8.1
					Hydrochlorothiazide	50						
J.F.	59	M	20	2.5	Guanethidine	12.5	40	33	2.9	2.5	10.1	10.0
A.S.	62	M	14	3	Guanethidine	125	35	33	2.2	2.5	10.7	11.2
					Trichlormethiazide	8						
M.H.	47	F	9.5	2	Guanethidine	125	18	17	1.2	1.4	7.8	7.6
					Hydrochlorothiazide	50						
						Average:	31.8 ± 4.9	31.4 ± 5.3	2.06 ± 0.28	2.08 ± 0.21	9.54 ± 0.67	9.42 ± 0.68

Plasma Levels of Dopa and Dopamine

Two serial plasma levels of dopa and dopamine were obtained at different times during levodopa therapy (Table 2) in each of three patients. After an overnight fast, a single oral dose of 1 gm of levodopa was administered at about 9:00 A.M. Heparinized blood samples were obtained before ingestion of the drug and at 15- and 30-minute intervals for the next $3\frac{1}{2}$ hours. Sodium metabisulfite (1 mg per 2 ml blood) was used as preservative. The samples were centrifuged and the supernatant was frozen prior to assays. Plasma levodopa and dopamine levels were determined fluorometrically by the trihydroxyindole method previously described by Anton and Sayre.[6] This method has been shown to be sensitive to a minimum of 100 mμg for levodopa and 50 mμg for dopamine.

Sodium Balance Studies

A 53-year-old man with mild hypertension and a variant of Parkinson's disease was investigated in the Emory University Hospital, Clinical Research Facility. The patient's blood pressure ranged from 180/120 mm Hg to 150/110 mm Hg. Creatinine clearance averaged 100 ml per min; blood urea nitrogen, 18 mg per 100 ml; serum creatinine, 1.0 mg per 100 ml. Increasing amounts of dietary sodium were administered until sodium balance was obtained with an intake of 8 gm (348 mEq) of sodium per day (Fig. 1). Potassium content of the diet was 80 mEq per day. Blood pressure and heart rate were measured three times daily with the patient in the supine position and after standing 3 minutes. Blood pressure readings were averaged to represent the mean readings for the day. Daily measurements of body weight, creatinine clearance, urinary sodium, and potassium excretion were performed. After an initial decrease in blood pressure during the first few days of hospitalization, blood pressure values and sodium balance were essentially stable and 8 days of control values were obtained. Levodopa was then administered in an initial dose of 250 mg every 6 hours. The dose was increased every third day of increments of 0.5 gm until a maximum daily dose of 8 gm was reached. After maintenance of levodopa at this dose

TABLE 2.—*Peak Plasma Levels of Dopa and Dopamine Following Administration of 1 Gm of Levodopa*

Patient	Interval between Study I and Study II (Weeks)	Peak Plasma Levels: Dopa, Study I, Time (hour)	μg per 100 ml	Dopa, Study II, Time (hour)	μg per 100 ml	Dopamine, Study I, Time (hour)	μg per 100 ml	Dopamine, Study II, Time (hour)	μg per 100 ml
F.W.	15 (I–17, II–32)	1	309	2	334	1	21	2	8
L.B.	10 (I–16, II–26)	3	461	3.5	403	2	94	1.5	10
J.F.	11 (I–7, II–18)	3	304	0.5	741	1.5	3.5	1	14.4

for several days, the drug was discontinued and 3 days of post-levodopa values were obtained.

RESULTS

Effects of Prolonged Levodopa Administration on Blood Pressure

Symptomatic orthostatic hypotension, requiring reduction of guanethidine dosage, occurred in two patients during levodopa therapy. The effects of levodopa in Patient F. W. are shown in Fig. 2. Blood pressure in the standing position decreased from levels of approximately 150/115 mm Hg to 70/60 mm Hg after 1 week of levodopa administration in a dose of 1 gm per day. Blood pressure in the supine position was essentially unchanged. Because of severe "dizziness," the dose

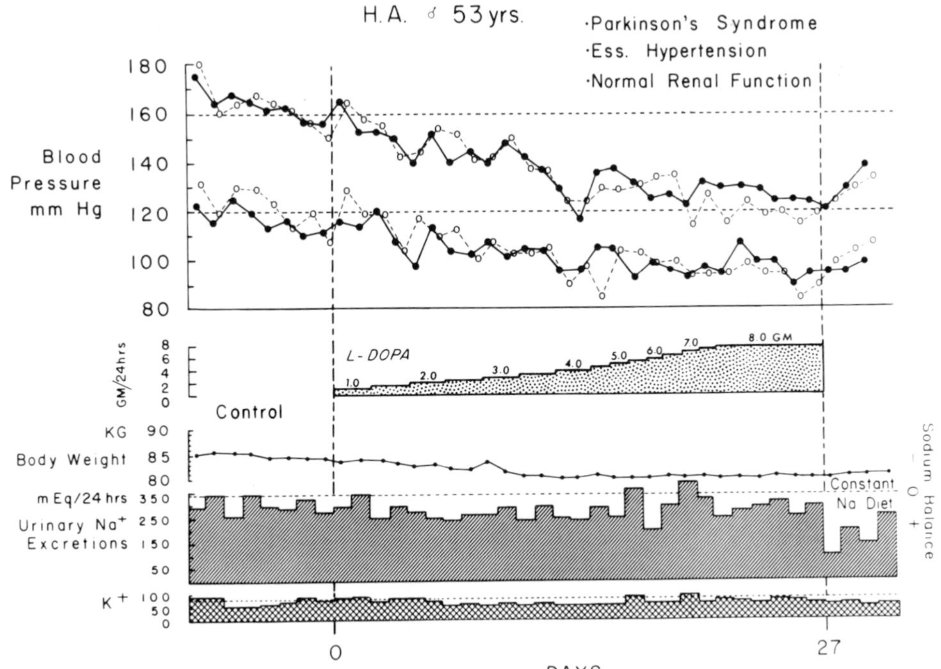

FIG. 1.—Effects of levodopa on blood pressure, body weight, and 24-hour urinary sodium and potassium excretion in Patient H. A.

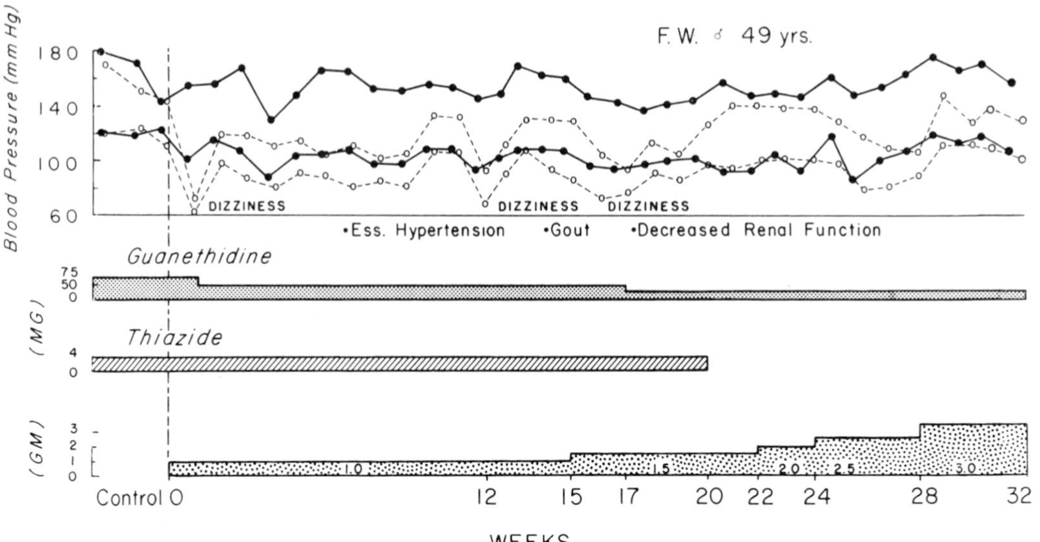

FIG. 2.—Effects of levodopa administration (bottom scale) on blood pressure of Patient F. W. **Closed circles** and **solid lines** refer to blood pressure in the supine position. **Open circles** and **broken lines** denote blood pressure in the erect position. Daily dosages of guanethidine and thiazide diuretic (trichlormethiazide) are also shown.

of guanethidine was decreased from 75 mg per day to 50 mg per day and the standing blood pressure rose to levels of approximately 120/90 mm Hg. The second episode of orthostatic hypotension was recorded during the 12th week, but the blood pressure increased in subsequent weeks despite maintenance of the same dose of guanethidine. After the 15th week, the dose of levodopa was increased to 1.5 gm per day and symptomatic orthostatic hypotension again occurred. Accordingly, the dose of guanethidine was reduced to 37.5 mg per day. Twenty weeks after institution of levodopa therapy, the patient experienced a severe attack of gout, with uric acid levels of 13.1 mg per 100 ml. Trichlormethiazide was discontinued and uric acid levels returned to previous levels of approximately 10 mg per 100 ml. During the subsequent treatment period, the serum uric acid level did not increase again, despite increase of levodopa dosage to 3 gm per day.

Blood pressures of Patient L. B. were approximately 200/120 mm Hg in the supine position and 140/100 mm Hg in the erect position at the time she was receiving guanethidine in a 20-mg dose per day and hydrochlorothiazide in a 50-mg dose per day. After 1 week of levodopa administration in a dose of 1 gm per day, a precipitous reduction in blood pressure occurred to levels of 145/105 mm Hg in the supine position and 90/70 mm Hg in the erect position. Because of symptoms of weakness and dizziness, the dose of guanethidine was reduced to 10 mg per day. Subsequently, blood pressure increased and the dose of guanethidine had to be raised to 15 mg per day on the third week and to 20 mg per day on the sixth week. The dose of levodopa was gradually increased during the subsequent 21 weeks. This patient experienced two additional episodes of reduced pressure. The first occurred in the ninth week after the dose of levodopa was increased to 1.5 gm and the second occurred on the 27th week while she was receiving 3.5 gm of levodopa per day. Both episodes were transient and adjustment of guanethidine dosage was not necessary.

The dose of guanethidine was not altered in the remaining patients. Patient A. S. experienced one episode of orthostatic hypotension 2 weeks after 1 gm of levodopa per day was added to a regimen consisting of 125 mg of guanethidine and 8 mg of trichlormethiazide per day. Despite increase of levodopa dosage of 3 gm per day during the subsequent 14 weeks, no further hypotensive episodes were recorded. Patient M. H. was inadequately treated despite a dose of 125 mg per day of guanethidine and 50 mg per day of hydrochlorothiazide. Before beginning levodopa treatment, blood pressure in the supine position was approximately 190/130 mm Hg, and in the erect position, 190/140 mm Hg. During the subsequent 6 weeks, while receiving 1 gm of levodopa per day, the diastolic pressures in both supine and standing positions were recorded at levels of approximately 110 mm Hg. The systolic pressure in the supine position was not decreased, but there was about a 20-mm Hg decrease in blood pressure recorded in the standing position. Further reduction of blood pressure did not occur despite increase of levodopa dosage to 2 gm per day. This patient complained of frequent episodes of nausea and vomiting and these symptoms became intolerable during administration of 2 gm of levodopa per day. Accordingly, the drug was discontinued after 9½ weeks of therapy. During the subsequent 3 weeks, the blood pressure returned toward levels recorded prior to levodopa treatment. The final patient, J. F., also was inadequately treated with guanethidine, 12.5 mg per day, at the time of initiation of levodopa therapy. The blood pressure of this patient had been more adequately controlled with a thiazide diuretic, but this had to be discontinued because of gout 1 month before levodopa treatment. At the time treatment with levodopa was initiated, blood pressure in the supine position was 210/125 mm Hg, and in the erect position, 190/120 mm Hg. During the initial 5 weeks of treatment with 1 gm levodopa per day, blood pressure in the standing position gradually decreased to levels of approximately 160/110 mm Hg. There was no change of blood pressure in the supine position. Increase of dosage to 2 gm per day did not result in further sustained reduction in blood pressure. When the dose of levodopa was increased to 2.5 gm per day, the blood pressure increased and the patient experienced episodes of flushing and symptoms of "hot flashes." When the dose was reduced to 2 gm per day, the blood pressure was reduced to previous levels and the symptoms were alleviated. Readministration of 2.5 gm per day of levodopa again resulted in elevation of blood pressure and flushing.

Effects of Levodopa on Renal Function

Changes in serum creatinine and blood urea nitrogen were variable and insignificant (Table 1). Serum uric acid levels prior to levodopa administration were abnormally elevated in all patients and were at about the same level at the end of the study. As stated above, thiazide diuretics were discontinued in Patient J. F. before levodopa therapy and had to be stopped in Patient F. W. during levodopa therapy because of an attack of gout.

Plasma Levels of Dopa and Dopamine after a 1-Gm Dose of Levodopa

Peak plasma levels of dopa and dopamine obtained in three patients are summarized in Table 2. In Patient F. W., peak levels of dopa and dopamine during the first and the second studies were reached after 1 and 2 hours respectively. Although the peak plasma level of dopa was higher during the second study, dopamine levels at that time were lower. A similar but more pronounced decrease of dopamine peak levels was found in the second study of Patient L. B. In Patient J. F., the dopa peak level during the first study occurred in 3 hours; peak levels reached during the second study occurred in only 30 minutes. Peak levels of dopa and dopamine were two and a half and four times higher respectively in the second study.

Adverse Effects and Laboratory Values

Nausea or vomiting was experienced by all patients. These side effects were more severe during the initial days of therapy, and were tolerated by all patients except M. H. However, their occurrence dictated a more gradual increment in levodopa dosage. Symptomatic orthostatic hypotension was experienced by patients F. W. and L. B. as described above. No abnormal changes in laboratory values occurred which could be attributed to levodopa therapy.

Effects of Levodopa on Sodium Balance

Results of the study in Patient H. A. are shown in Figure 1. Blood pressure was approximately 160/110 mm Hg in both supine and standing positions during the last 4 days of the control period. During the levodopa treatment period, blood pressure gradually decreased until levels were recorded as low as 130/90 mm Hg in the supine position and 120/85 mm Hg in the standing position. Except for 2 days during administration of 5 and 7 gm of levodopa, the patient remained in positive sodium balance throughout the levodopa treatment period. Thus, the reduction of blood pressure and loss of 2½ kg of body weight could not be related to sodium loss. When levodopa was discontinued after 27 days of continuous administration, blood pressure during the following 3 days rose to levels as high as 140/100 mm Hg in the supine position and 135/110 mm Hg when standing. During this post-levodopa period, the patient retained sodium and his body weight increased by 0.5 kg.

Discussion

This investigation demonstrated that administration of levodopa to hypertensive patients receiving guanethidine and thiazide diuretics can result in further lowering of blood pressure. Unfortunately, the response was extremely variable and not characterized by a dose-response relationship. Renal function as measured by serum creatinine and blood urea nitrogen also did not improve. Accordingly, it is unlikely that levodopa will be a useful addition to the regimens of patients requiring guanethidine and a thiazide diuretic.

Variability of plasma levels of dopa and dopamine may be responsible, in part, for the erratic responses. In two patients, decreased levels of dopamine after prolonged therapy suggested decreased activity of aromatic amino acid decarboxylase, the enzyme responsible for generation of dopamine. Dairman, Christenson, and Udenfriend found a specific reduction of this enzyme in the livers of rats treated with levodopa.[7] Similar findings for the livers of mice were independently reported by Tate et al.[8] Tate and his colleagues also reported that decarboxylase activity in erythrocytes of patients with Parkinson's disease treated with levodopa was significantly lower than that of untreated patients and of normal individuals. Decreased activity of decarboxylase is also suggested by tolerance to the positive inotropic action of levodopa occurring after prolonged levodopa treatment.[9]

Markedly elevated plasma levels of dopa and dopamine during the second study period of the third patient indicated that difference in absorption also occurred. This patient experienced episodes of hypertension and flushing following administration of doses of levodopa which did not produce these effects in the other patients. Previous studies demonstrated that small doses of levodopa and dopamine decrease blood pressure, whereas larger doses increase blood pressure.[5,10–13] However, the finding of a lower dopamine level in Patient J. F. as opposed to Patients L. B. and F. W. during their first studies (Table 2) suggests that considerable variability exists in the sensitivity of the patients to the alpha-adrenergic action of dopamine.

The orthostatic hypotension produced by levodopa suggests decreased function of the sympathetic nervous system. Both central and peripheral mechanisms have been invoked. Watanabe, Chase, and Cardon[14] concluded that a central mechanism was responsible since administration of the peripheral decarboxylase inhibitor, MK-485, did not prevent the hypotensive effects of levodopa in patients with Parkinson's disease. A similar conclusion was reached by Henning and Rubenson[15] after studies in the rat. On the other hand, Farmer,[16] Whitsett, Halushka, and Goldberg[17] and Whitnack et al.[18] demonstrated that administration of levodopa or dopamine to experimental animals attenuated the function of peripheral sympathetic nerves. A similar controversy concerning the mechanism of methyldopa also is unresolved.[19,20]

The present discouraging results do not rule out possible use of levodopa in patients with less severe hypertension. Barbeau[21] reported that levodopa (4.5 gm per day) lowered blood pressure in one patient in both the supine and standing positions. The effect persisted for 3 months, but after that period, rebound hypertension occurred despite continuation of levodopa administration. Reduction of blood pressure in both positions also occurred in our hospitalized patient treated with a maximum of 8 gm of levodopa per day. A persistent natriuretic effect did not occur and thus the reduction of blood pressure could not have been due to sodium loss. Further studies are necessary to confirm these single studies and to determine whether a sustained hypotensive effect can be obtained without orthostasis or nausea and vomiting. Additional measurements of dopa and dopamine plasma levels are needed to confirm the present preliminary observations suggesting that variabilities in absorption and generation of dopamine are responsible for the erratic responses.

Acknowledgment

We wish to thank Dr. Alexander S. McKinney, Miss Marjorie A. Hewett, R.N., and Mrs. Mabel Moorhead, R.N., for their assistance in these studies.

References

1. Yahr, M. D., Duvoisin, R. C., Hoehn, M. D., Schear, J. J., and Barrett, R. C.: L-dopa (1-3,4-dihydroxyphenylalanine): Its clinical effects in parkinsonism. Trans. Am. Neurol. Assoc. 93:56, 1968.
2. Cotzias, G. C., Papavasiliou, P. S., and Gellene, R.: Modification of parkinsonism—chronic treatment with L-dopa. N. Engl. J. Med. 280:337, 1969.
3. Finlay, G. D., Whitsett, T. L., Cucinell, E. A., and Goldberg, L. I.: Augmentation of renal function by levodopa. N. Engl. J. Med. 284: 865, 1971.
4. McDonald, R. H., Jr., Goldberg, L. I., McNay, J. L., and Tuttle, E. P., Jr.: Effect of dopamine in man: Augmentation of sodium excretion, glomerular filtration rate and renal plasma flow. J. Clin. Invest. 43:1116, 1964.
5. Goldberg, L. I., and Whitsett, T. L.: Cardiovascular effects of levodopa. Clin. Pharmacol. Ther. 12:376, 1971.
6. Anton, A. H., and Sayre, D. F.: The distribution of dopamine and dopa in various animals and a method for their determination in diverse biological material. J. Pharmacol. Exp. Ther. 145:326, 1964.
7. Dairman, W., Christenson, J. G., and Udenfriend, S.: Decrease in liver aromatic L-amino-acid decarboxylase produced by chronic administration of L-dopa. Proc. Nat. Acad. Sci. U.S.A. 68:2117, 1971.
8. Tate, S. S., Sweet, R., McDowell, F. H., and Meister, A.: Decrease of the 3,4-dihydroxyphenylalanine (dopa) decarboxylase activities in human erythrocytes and mouse tissues after administration of dopa. Proc. Nat. Acad. Sci. U.S.A. 68:2121, 1971.
9. Whitsett, T. L., and Goldberg, L. I.: Effects of levodopa on systolic pre-ejection period, blood pressure and heart rate during acute and chronic treatment of Parkinson's disease. Circulation 45:97, 1972.
10. McDonald, R. H., Jr., and Goldberg, L. I.: Analysis of the cardiovascular effects of dopamine in the dog. J. Pharmacol. Exp. Ther. 140:60, 1963.
11. McNay, J. L., MacCannell, K. L., Meyer, M. B., and Goldberg, L. I.: Hypotensive effect of dopamine in dogs and hypertensive patients after phenoxybenzamine. J. Clin. Invest. 45: 1045, 1966.
12. McNay, J. L., and Goldberg, L. I.: Hemodynamic effects of dopamine in the dog before and after alpha-adrenergic blockade. Circ. Res. 18:I, 1966.
13. Hunter, K. R., Boakes, A. J., Laurence, D. R., and Stern, G. M.: Monoamine oxidase inhibitors and L-dopa. Br. J. Med. 3:338, 1970.
14. Watanabe, A. M., Chase, T. N., and Cardon, P. V.: Effect of L-dopa alone and in combination with an extracerebral decarboxylase inhibitor on blood pressure and some cardiovascular reflexes. Clin. Pharmacol. Ther. 11: 740, 1970.
15. Henning, M., and Rubenson, A.: Central hypotensive effect of 1-3,4-dihydroxyphenylalanine in the rat. J. Pharm. Pharmacol. 22:553, 1970.
16. Farmer, J. B.: Impairment of sympathetic nerve responses by dopa, dopamine and their alpha-methyl analogues. J. Pharm. Pharmacol. 17:640, 1965.
17. Whitsett, T. L., Halushka, P. V., and Goldberg, L. I.: Attenuation of postganglionic sympathetic nerve activity by L-dopa. Circ. Res. 27:561, 1970.
18. Whitnack, E., Leff, A., Mohammed, S., and Gaffney, T. E.: Effect of L-dopa on chronotropic responses to cardio-accelerator nerve stimulation in dogs. J. Pharmacol. Exp. Ther. 171:409, 1971.
19. Barbeau, A.: L-dopa therapy in Parkinson's disease: A critical review of nine years' experience. Can. Med. Assoc. J. 101:791, 1969.
20. Barger, G., and Dale, H. H.: Chemical structure and sympathomimetic action of amines. J. Physiol. 41:18, 1910.
21. Barbeau, A.: Dopamine and disease. Can. Med. Assoc. J. 103:824, 1970.

Analysis of the Hypotensive Action of Prazosin

Jay W. Constantine, Ph.D., Wilfred K. McShane, B.S., Alexander Scriabine, M.D., and Hans-Jürgen Hess, Ph.D.

PRAZOSIN, 2-[4-(2-furoyl)-piperazine-1-yl]-4-amino-6,7-dimethoxy-quinazoline hydrochloride, was synthesized in our Medicinal Chemistry Laboratories by Dr. Hans-Jürgen Hess. In a preliminary account of the pharmacologic effects of prazosin, Scriabine and coworkers [1] suggested that the hypotensive action of this drug was due, in part, to inhibition of the sympathetic nervous system at some peripheral site and that this action differed in important respects from conventional blockade of alpha-receptors. The purpose of the present study was to further characterize the cardiovascular activity of prazosin and to identify the peripheral site or sites at which it acts.

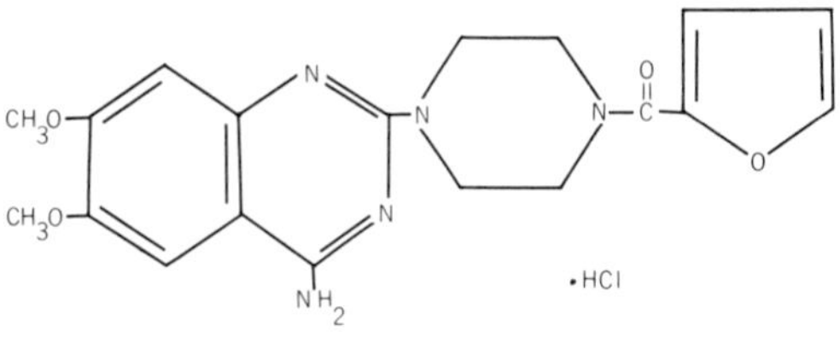

PRAZOSIN

Methods

Renal hypertension was induced in male Charles River rats,[2] with body weights of 400 to 450 gm. Blood pressure in the coccygeal artery was estimated just prior to and at 2 and 24 hours after treatment, using an electrosphygmograph and pneumatic pulse transducer (E & M Instrument Co., Houston, Texas), and recorded with a Sanborn oscillograph. Prazosin was prepared as an aqueous solution and given to rats by gastric gavage; control animals received water only.

Renal hypertension was induced in mongrel dogs [3] of either sex, with body weights of 10 to 18 kg. Blood pressure in the coccygeal artery was estimated [4] just prior to and at intervals ranging from 30 minutes to 48 hours following oral administration of prazosin in capsules. Heart rates were read from electrocardiograms (lead II) recorded simultaneously with blood pressures.

Acute experiments were conducted in anesthetized animals of either sex. Unless otherwise stated dogs were anesthetized with sodium pentobarbital (30 mg per kilogram of body weight) given intravenously and cats with chloralose (75 mg per kilogram of body weight) given intravenously.

Cardiac output was determined in each of six dogs from continuously recorded dilution curves using indocyanine green as indicator. Dye concentrations in femoral arterial blood were detected with a Waters model XP-300 densitometer which was connected to a Sanborn model 130 cardiac output computer.[5] Each dog received prazosin, 0.1 and 0.4 mg per kilogram of body weight, infused intravenously over a 1-minute period, with a 30-minute interval between administration of doses.

The effect of prazosin on electrocardiograms was studied in both conscious and anesthetized normotensive dogs. Silver-faced contact electrodes were employed and lead II tracings were made with a Sanborn polygraph. Conscious dogs were given prazosin orally and their blood pressure was measured indirectly.[4] Anesthetized dogs received prazosin by intravenous infusion (1 mg per kilogram of body weight per minute) and femoral artery blood pressure was measured with a Statham transducer. Heart rates were read from the electrocardiograms.

The effect on the chronotropic response to electrical stimulation of cardiac sympathetic or vagal nerves was studied in a total of 15 mongrel dogs of either sex, intravenously anesthetized with a mixture of urethane (600 mg per kilogram of body weight) and 50 mg of chlo-

From the Department of Pharmacology, Medical Research Laboratories, Pfizer Inc., Groton, Connecticut.

ralose. Blood pressure and heart rate were measured with a Statham transducer and Grass cardiotachograph, respectively, and were recorded with a Grass polygraph (model 5A).

Bilaterally vagotomized dogs were artificially respired with 95 percent oxygen and 5 percent carbon dioxide. The chest was opened on the right side at the fourth intercostal space and a postganglionic cardiac accelerator nerve, originating at the caudal cervical ganglion, was isolated and ligated. Bipolar platinum electrodes were placed on the nerve distal to the ligation and the nerve was stimulated electrically for 15 seconds with square wave impulses of 1-msec duration, at a frequency of 10 per second; voltages were varied from threshold (0.75V) to supramaximal levels (3.5V).

Vagal-stimulation experiments were performed in intact dogs in which both vagi were severed. Bipolar electrodes were placed on the peripheral end of the severed right vagus and the nerve stimulated for a period of 10 seconds with square wave impulses of 1-msec duration, at a frequency of 4 cycles per second, 0.5 to 4.5V.

The effect of intravenously administered prazosin on blood flow in various vascular beds was measured in 15 anesthetized dogs. The left femoral artery was exposed in six dogs. The right renal artery was exposed via a lateral incision in four dogs. In five dogs, the right internal carotid artery was exposed via a lateral incision in the cervical region and, in three of these dogs, the superior mesenteric artery was exposed via a midline incision in the abdomen. Blood flow in the various arteries was measured with an electromagnetic flowmeter (Avionics-Mark 6000) and blood pressure in the right femoral artery was measured with a Statham transducer; each variable was recorded with a Grass polygraph.

Interaction studies were carried out in a total of 25 anesthetized dogs in which femoral artery blood pressure was measured with a Statham pressure transducer and recorded with a Grass or Sanborn polygraph. Antagonists were intravenously given 10 minutes prior to prazosin administration (0.4 mg per kilogram of body weight); they were: atropine (1 mg per kilogram of body weight); propranolol (1 mg per kilogram of body weight); tripelennamine (10 mg per kilogram of body weight); phentolamine (1 mg per kilogram of body weight); sodium nitrite (10 mg per kilogram of body weight); and, as control, 0.9% sodium chloride solution (0.1 ml per kilogram of body weight).

Vasodilator activity was studied in anesthetized dogs in which left femoral arterial blood flow was measured with a Shipley-Wilson flowmeter. Blood pressure in the left femoral artery, proximal and distal to the flowmeter, was measured with Statham transducers. Drugs were injected into the arterial cannula distal to the flowmeter; injection volumes were maintained constant at 0.1 ml. To estimate dependence of the vasodilator effect on interference with sympathetic function, dose responses were obtained both before and after treatment with hexamethonium (2 mg per kilogram of body weight) given intravenously.

The effect of prazosin on segmental vascular resistance was studied in the perfused dog forelimb.[6] The following pressures were measured with Statham transducers and recorded with a Grass polygraph (Model 5A): femoral artery (P_{FA}), brachial artery (P_{BA}), paw artery (P_{PA}), paw vein (P_{PV}), and cephalic vein (P_{CV}). Vascular resistance values, in millimeters of mercury per milliliter per minute, were calculated for the total paw (R_T), arteries (R_A), small vessels (R_{SV}), and veins (R_V).[7] The flow rate (F) in the perfused limb, which varied with each preparation (range, 56 to 108 ml per minute), was maintained constant in each experiment. Drugs were infused into the brachial artery of the perfused limb at the rate of 1 ml per minute for 5 minutes.

The effect of prazosin on the blood pressure response to changes in postural attitude was studied in anesthetized dogs.[8] The animals were tilted prior to, and at 5-minute intervals after administration of drug into a femoral vein.

In seven cat nictitating-membrane preparations, contractions of the membrane were elicited by alternate electrical stimulation of pre- and postganglionic sympathetic nerves,[8] and in three of the animals, with 5 μg epinephrine injected into the lingual artery. Prazosin (0.025 and 0.1 mg per kilogram of body weight) was injected into a femoral vein. In four preparations, *d*-amphetamine (0.5 mg per kilogram of body weight) was given intravenously 30 minutes after prazosin.

Femoral arterial blood pressure in six cats and four dogs was measured with a mercury manometer and recorded on smoked paper. Pressor responses were elicited by bilateral carotid artery occlusion for 30 seconds or with 2 to 4 μg of epinephrine per kilogram of body weight given intravenously. In cats, responses were also obtained with intravenous injections of angiotensin (0.5 μg per kilogram of body weight) and dimethylphenylpiperazinium (DMPP), 5 or 10 μg per kilogram of body weight. Drugs were injected into the right femoral vein.

Seven cats, under ether anesthesia, were pithed by passing a wire through the foramen magnum and down the spinal canal; the wire was left in place for the duration of each experiment. Respiration was maintained with a Starling pump, and the animals were bilaterally vagotomized. Carotid artery blood pressure was measured with a mercury manometer and recorded on smoked paper. In two cats, 2 μg of epinephrine per milliliter was infused into the left femoral vein at the rate of 0.382 ml per minute; three cats received angiotensin, 12.5 μg per milliliter, infused at the same rate. Prazosin was injected into the contralateral vein.

Isolated strips of rabbit aorta were prepared by a previously described [8] modification of the procedure of Furchgott and Bhadrakom.[9] Cumulative concentration-responses were elicited with either norepinephrine or barium alone, and then in the presence of prazosin. For each agonist, two successive concentration-response curves were obtained with a given tissue before addition of prazosin; four different tissues were used for each concentration of prazosin. Isotonic contractions were recorded on smoked paper by means of levers with a 16-fold magnification.

Receptor-protection experiments [10] were conducted with rabbit aorta prepared as described above. After obtaining control contractions to epinephrine (1×10^{-7} gm per milliliter) a high concentration of epinephrine (5×10^{-5} gm per milliliter) was placed in the bath and during the period of maximum contraction, prazosin (5×10^{-5} gm per milliliter) or phenoxybenzamine (2×10^{-8} gm per milliliter) was also added. After 10 minutes, the bath was flushed at 5-minute intervals for 90 minutes at which time epinephrine (1×10^{-7} gm per milliliter) was again added. In control experiments, 0.1 ml of Krebs-Henseleit [11] solution was added in place of the high concentration of epinephrine. Isometric contractions were measured with a Grass force-transducer (model FT-02) and recorded with a Grass polygraph (model 5A).

In additional receptor-protection experiments, two consecutive cumulative concentration-response curves were obtained with norepinephrine. Either prazosin (1×10^{-8} gm per milliliter) or phentolamine (5×10^{-7} gm per milliliter) was added to the bath, followed in 10 minutes by addition of phenoxybenzamine, 1×10^{-7} gm per milliliter. After an additional 20 minutes, cumulative concentration responses to norepinephrine were again obtained. In control experiments, 0.1 ml of Krebs-Henseleit solution was added in place of antagonist. Isotonic contractions were measured with a Phipps and Bird transducer (Model St-2) attached to a Health servorecorder.

Results

Effects on the Blood Pressure in Conscious Animals

In four groups of eight rats each, prazosin (0.08, 0.32, 1.25, or 5 mg per kilogram of body weight) given orally caused dose-dependent decreases in blood pressure within 2 hours after treatment (Fig. 1). The hypotensive effect lasted at least 24 hours, but less than 48 hours in animals given the two higher doses. In rats that received 5 mg per kilogram of body weight, repetition of the treatment caused a hypotensive response similar to that observed on the first treatment day.

Prazosin (0.005 to 1.25 mg per kilogram of body weight) administered orally to 16 conscious, renal hypertensive dogs caused dose-related decreases in blood pressure (Fig. 1). In animals given 0.625 mg per kilogram of body weight or higher doses, the effect lasted at least 24 hours. Heart rate changes were moderate but variable, i.e., either increased or decreased. The pattern of electrocardiograms was not altered and no gross autonomic or behavioral side effects were noted, except for

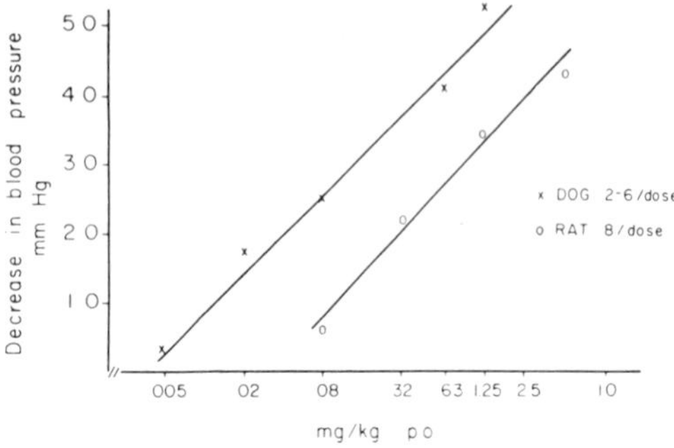

FIG. 1.—Dose-response regression lines for the antihypertensive effect of prazosin in conscious renal hypertensive dogs and rats. Each rat received a single dose of drug, eight rats per dose. Dogs received one or more doses of the drug, 2 to 6 dogs per dose. Slopes of regression lines: $b_x = 19.2$; $b_o = 21.9$.

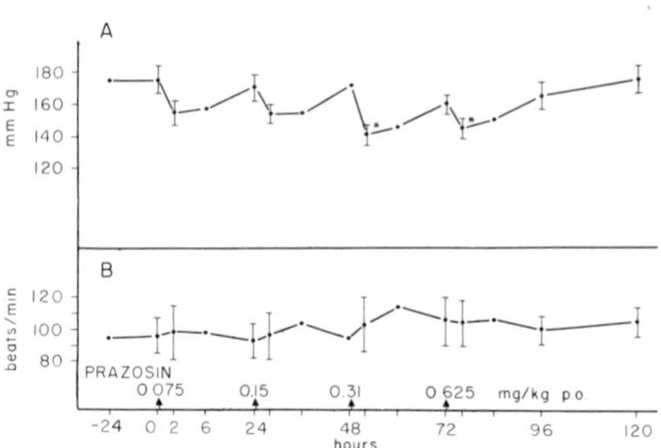

FIG. 2.—Effect of prazosin, administered daily at increasing single oral doses on (*A*) blood pressure and (*B*) heart rate of conscious renal hypertensive dogs. **Graph** indicates the average of values for four dogs, either sex, average weight of 15 kg. **Vertical bars** represent standard error of the mean. **Asterisk (*)** denotes blood pressure is significantly ($P < 0.01$) below control value.

slight relaxation of the nictitating membrane in three dogs given 1.25 mg per kilogram of body weight.

In two groups of four dogs each, prazosin was given orally in increasing daily doses of 1, 10, and 30 mg or 0.075, 0.15, 0.31, and 0.625 mg per kilogram of body weight. In the first group, the hypotensive effect was maximal at 6 hours after treatment with 1 mg per kilogram of body weight and persisted for at least 24 hours. Subsequent administration of 10 and 30 mg per kilogram of body weight caused only slight additional decline in blood pressure and the maximal effect was equivalent to that attained following the 1 mg dose. In the second group, blood pressure falls were dose-related; the maximum hypotensive effect was obtained on the third day after 0.31 mg per kilogram of body weight (Fig. 2). Prazosin had no significant effect on the heart rate in these animals.

In an additional four dogs, prazosin, in a single oral dose of 0.625 mg per kilogram of body weight, caused hypotension which lasted at least 24 hours (Fig. 3). This effect was maximum at 2 to 4 hours; recovery was partial at 24 hours and complete at 48 hours. Heart rate changes were slight, even at the time of maximum hypotension.

The effect of repeated oral administration was studied in two groups of four dogs each given prazosin (0.1 or 0.65 mg per kilogram of body weight) once daily for 10 consecutive days. In dogs given daily doses of 0.1 mg per kilogram of body weight, the maximum hypotensive effect averaged 38 mm Hg within 6 hours after the first treatment, and recovery was complete within 24 hours. Subsequent daily blood pressure falls through the tenth day were equivalent to the response obtained on the first day of the study. In dogs given 0.65 mg per kilogram per day, the maximum hypotensive effect occurred within 6 hours after the first treatment, but recovery was incomplete at 24 hours. The maximum hypotensive effect was maintained throughout the 10

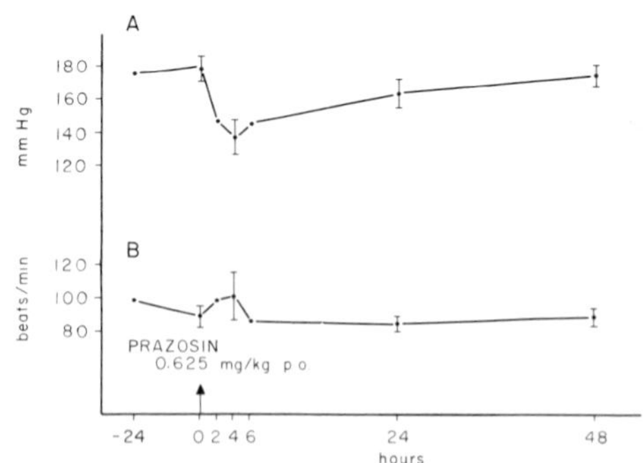

FIG. 3.—Duration of the effect of prazosin on (*A*) blood pressure and (*B*) heart rate of conscious renal hypertensive dogs. Graph indicates the average of values for four male dogs, with an average weight of 17.1 kg. Vertical bars represent standard error of the mean.

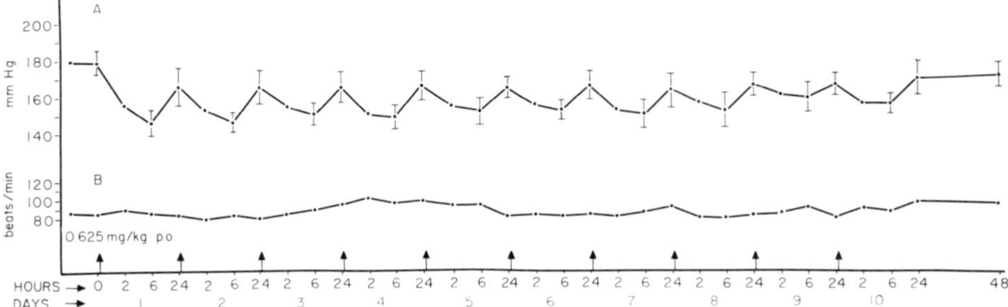

FIG. 4—Effect of repeated oral administration of prazosin (0.625 mg per kilogram of body weight per day) on (*A*) blood pressure and (*B*) heart rate of conscious renal hypertensive dogs. Drug was given (↑) in a single daily dose for 10 days. Graph represents the average of values ± standard error for four male dogs with an average weight of 16.1 kg.

days of treatment (Fig. 4*A*); there was no significant effect on heart rate (Fig. 4*B*).

Effect on Circulatory Factors in Anesthetized Dogs

Six dogs were given prazosin intravenously (0.1 mg per kilogram of body weight) and 30 minutes later, 0.4 mg per kilogram of body weight. Blood pressure was lowered an average of 20 mm Hg following the 0.1-mg dose, and an additional 25 mm Hg following the 0.4-mg dose; it remained at hypotensive levels during the next 60 minutes (Fig. 5*A*). Heart rate increased 20 to 25 beats per minute for 2 to 3 minutes; this effect was associated with the immediate hypotensive response to each dose (Fig. 5*D*). Following the 0.1-mg dose, cardiac output was not significantly affected, but it was increased in each of the six dogs after 0.4 mg per kilogram of body weight (Fig. 5*B*). There was a slight decrease in calculated total peripheral resistance following the lower dose of the drug, and a 40 percent reduction in resistance of at least 60 minutes' duration following the high dose (Fig. 5*C*). In all animals, stroke volume was increased transiently after each dose of the drug (Fig. 5*E*).

Effect on Chronotropic Responses to Electrical Stimulation of Cardiac Nerves

Sympathetic Effect. In five dogs, in which the thorax was open to atmosphere, the cardioaccelerator response to electrical stimulation of postganglionic cardiac sympathetic nerves was not significantly reduced 10 minutes after treatment with prazosin, given intravenously in a 0.1-mg dose per kilogram of body weight.

Vagal Effect. In four anesthetized dogs, cardiac slowing in response to electrical stimulation of the peripheral end of the severed right vagus nerve was not changed by treatment with prazosin, administered in a 0.4-mg dose per kilogram of body weight.

The observation that prazosin increases cardiac output and that it does not alter chronotropic responses to either sympathetic or vagal stimulation is evidence that the drug does not lower blood pressure by decreasing contractile force.

Effect on Regional Blood Flow

When prazosin was given intravenously (0.1 mg per kilogram of body weight) and 30 minutes later (0.4 mg per kilogram of body weight) in each of 15 anesthetized dogs, prolonged hypotension occurred. The effect on blood flow in various vascular beds was as follows:

In six dogs, following intravenous administration of 0.1 mg of prazosin per kilogram of body weight, femoral arterial blood flow was increased transiently by an average of 20 percent. After administration of 0.4 mg per kilogram of body weight, femoral blood flow was increased by 25 percent, but within 4 to 5 minutes flow rate decreased to a level 10 to 12 percent above control values where it remained constant for the next 60 minutes (Fig. 6*A*).

In each of five dogs, 0.1 and 0.4 mg of prazosin per kilogram of body weight given intravenously caused transient increases in right

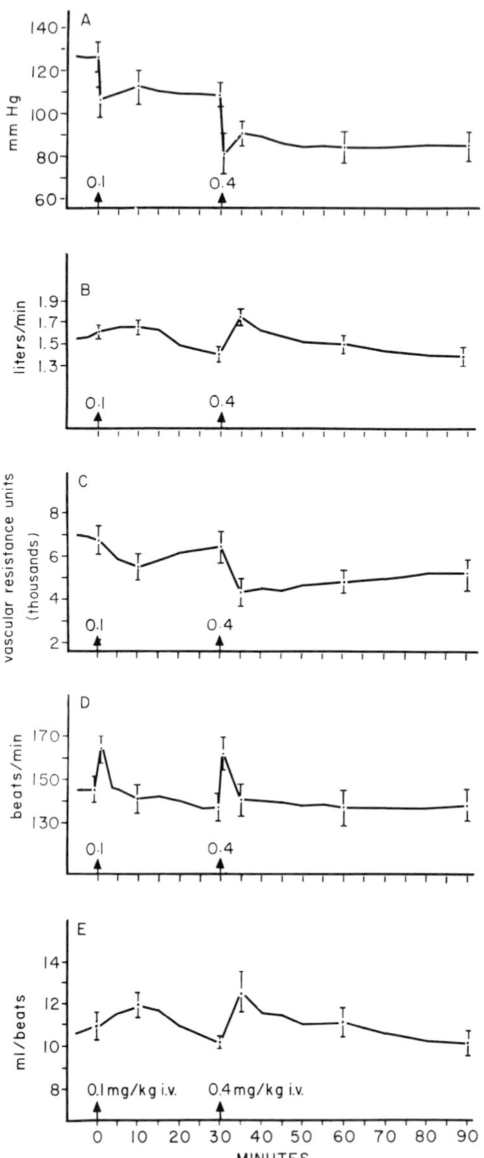

FIG. 5.—Effect of prazosin on (*A*) blood pressure, (*B*) cardiac output, (*C*) total peripheral resistance, (*D*) heart rate, and (*E*) stroke volume of dogs anesthetized with intravenously administered sodium pentobarbital (30 mg per kilogram of body weight). **Graph** represents average of values ± standard error for six dogs, either sex, average weight 14.6 kg. Each dog received prazosin (0.1 mg per kilogram of body weight) given intravenously at 0 time and 30 minutes later in a 0.4 mg dose.

renal artery blood flow (Fig. 6*B*). Calculated renovascular resistance was progressively lowered after each dose of the drug.

In two of five dogs, prazosin, 0.1 mg given intravenously in a 0.1-mg dose per kilogram of body weight, caused a slight transient increase in internal carotid artery blood flow; it was unchanged in the other three dogs. After 0.4 mg of prazosin per kilogram of body weight was given intravenously, changes in flow were minimal (Fig. 6*C*). In each of the three dogs in which superior mesenteric artery blood flow was also measured, prazosin caused transient increases in blood flow (Fig. 6*D*).

Interaction Studies

Four groups of four dogs each were treated with intravenously administered atropine (1 mg per kilogram of body weight); propranolol (1 mg per kilogram of body weight); tripelennamine (10 mg per kilogram of body weight); or by sodium nitrite (10 mg per kilogram of body weight). Ten minutes later, or 1 hour later in the case of sodium nitrite, all animals were intravenously given prazosin (0.4 mg per kilogram of body weight) which caused blood pressure falls averaging 38 to 42 mm Hg. These responses were similar to the average hypotensive response of 42 mm Hg obtained in six animals given prazosin alone.

In an additional four dogs, the combined hypotensive effects caused by intravenously administered phentolamine (1 mg per kilogram of body weight) and 10 minutes later, prazosin (0.4 mg per kilogram of body weight) averaged only 32 mm Hg; this was less than the hypotensive effect of the same dose of prazosin in the absence of phentolamine.

In four dog hindlimb preparations, prazosin (64 μg) given intra-arterially caused transient increases in femoral artery blood flow averaging 22 ml per minute; these responses were unchanged after 1 mg of propranolol per kilogram of body weight was given intravenously.

These observations indicate that the peripheral vasodilator action of prazosin is not mediated by endogenous acetylcholine or histamine, nor is it due to drug interaction with beta-adrenergic receptors.

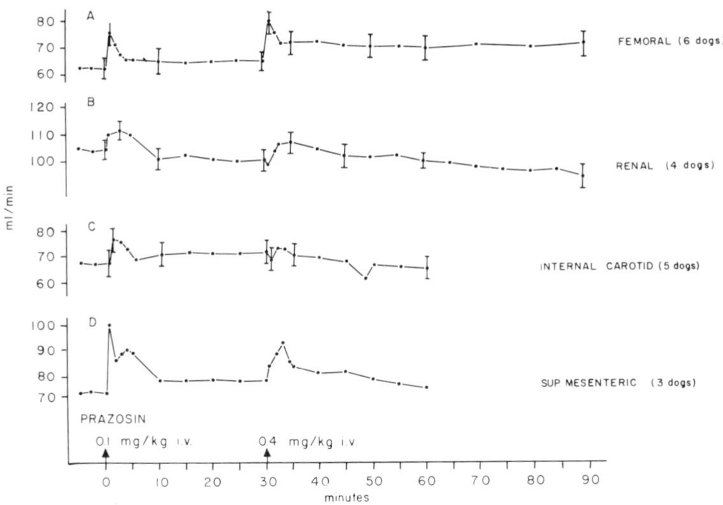

FIG. 6.—Effect of prazosin on femoral (*A*), renal (*B*), internal carotid (*C*), and superior mesenteric (*D*) arterial blood flow in dogs anesthetized with intravenously administered sodium pentobarbital (30 mg per kilogram of body weight). Each dog was given prazosin intravenously (0.1 mg per kilogram of body weight at 0 time and, 30 minutes later, was given 0.4 mg per kilogram of body weight). **Graph** represents the average of values ± standard error for the indicated number of dogs.

Effect of Hexamethonium on the Vasodilator Response

In four dog hindlimb preparations, 1 to 256 μg of prazosin, injected intra-arterially, caused dose-related increases of 5 to 28 ml per minute in femoral artery blood flow. In the same animals, the drug was 17 times less effective in the presence of hexamethonium (2 mg per kilogram of body weight) given intravenously (Fig. 7). The vasodilator effects of the direct smooth-muscle relaxants papaverine and diazoxide were minimally affected by hexamethonium, while the responses to the alpha-receptor-blocking agent, phentolamine, were virtually abolished by hexamethonium.

The decrease in vasodilator activity of a drug following blockade of sympathetic ganglia is considered to represent that portion of drug action due to interference with sympathetic function. The residual response represents that component of drug action due to a direct effect on vascular smooth muscle. Interpreted on this basis, the results indicate that the peripheral vasodilator action of prazosin is due to a combination of these effects, and that the direct relaxant effect is a significant component of action.

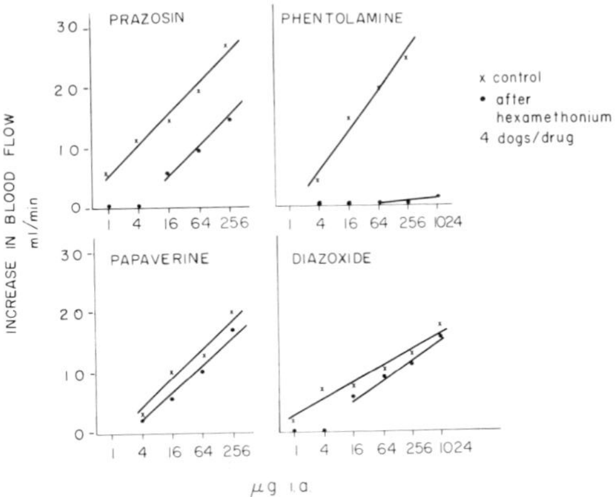

FIG. 7.—Effect of intravenously administered hexamethonium (2 mg per kilogram of body weight) on vasodilator responses in the hindlimb of dogs anesthetized with intravenously administered sodium pentobarbital (30 mg per kilogram of body weight). Each dog received all four or five doses of a drug both before and after hexamethonium; only one of the drugs was given to each dog.

Effect of Segmental Resistances in the Perfused Dog Forelimb

Prazosin, 0.1 mg per milliliter per minute for 5 minutes, infused into the brachial artery of the perfused forelimb, decreased blood pressure in brachial and paw arteries and it increased pressures in paw and cephalic veins. Calculation of the vascular resistance for the various limb segments revealed that 91 percent of the reduction in total paw resistance occurred at the level of the small vessels and only 7 percent in the paw arteries, and that venous resistance was not affected (Fig. 8). Prazosin was similar to diazoxide in this respect. Sodium nitrite and phentolamine exhibited a broader spectrum of vasodilator action, in that decrease in total paw resistance was a consequence of considerable reduction in large- as well as in small-vessel resistance. The distribution of activity in various vascular segments of the perfused forelimb is summarized in Table 1.

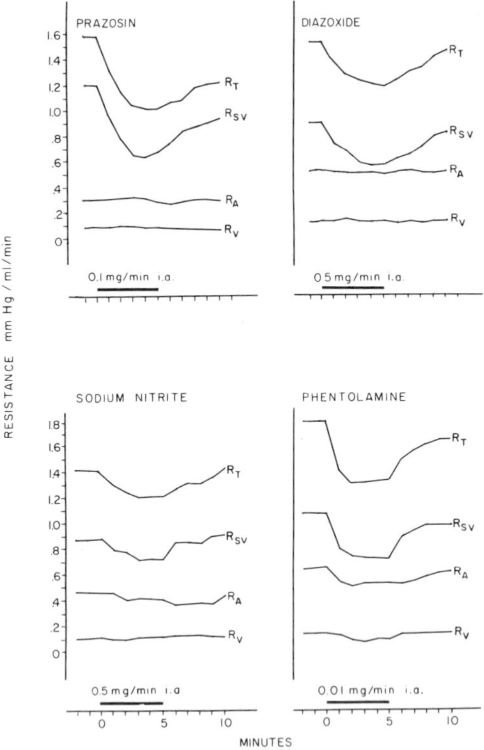

FIG. 8.—Effect of prazosin, diazoxide, sodium nitrite, and phentolamine on vascular resistance in the forepaw of dogs anesthetized with intravenously administered sodium pentobarbital (30 mg per kilogram of body weight). **Horizontal bar** indicates infusion of drug into the perfused brachial artery. **R,** Resistance across: total paw **(T),** arteries **(A),** small vessels **(SV),** and veins **(V).** Each dog received a single infusion, four dogs per drug. Flow rate **(F)** was 72 ml per minute, range of 62 to 97 ml per minute.

Effect on the Blood Pressure of Anesthetized Dogs During Postural Change

In seven of 13 dogs treated with intravenously administered prazosin (0.1 mg per kilogram of body weight), there was a moderate accentuation of the acute depressor response to a vertical tilt; however, prazosin did not interfere with the subsequent compensatory adjustment of the blood pressure (Fig. 9). In the remaining six animals, the compensatory pressor response to tilt was antagonized at 5 to 20 minutes after treatment with prazosin, whereas at 30 minutes, the effect was minimal despite the persistence of systemic hypotension. Diazoxide given intravenously (8 mg per kilogram of body weight) also exaggerated the acute depressor response to tilt; but it had little or no effect on the subsequent compensatory hypertensive response (Fig. 9). Phentolamine (1 mg per kilogram of body weight given intravenously) and sodium nitrite (10 mg per kilogram of body weight given intravenously) each exaggerated the acute depressor response to vertical tilt and markedly inhibited the compensatory reflex adjustment.

Analysis of Effects on Peripheral Sympathetic Function

Nictitating Membrane. Prazosin in 0.025- and 0.1-mg doses per kilogram of body weight, given intravenously, caused equal reduction of nictitating-membrane contractions induced by electrical stimulation of either pre- or postganglionic fibers of the superior cervical ganglion (Fig. 10). This effect was not influenced in each of four cats subsequently treated with *d*-amphetamine, administered intravenously in a 5-mg dose per kilogram of body weight. In three cats, prazosin given intravenously in a 0.1-mg dose per kilogram of body weight also reduced contractions of the nictitating mem-

TABLE 1.—*Distribution of Segmental Vascular Resistance Changes in the Perfused Dog Forelimb*

Compound	*Intra-arterially Administered Dose (mg/ml/min)*	*Resistance Decreases in Indicated Vessels as Percentage of the Total Reduction in Paw Resistance*		
		Small Vessels	*Paw Arteries*	*Paw Veins*
Diazoxide	0.5	93 ± 2	7 ± 0.4	2
Prazosin	0.1	91 ± 8	7 ± 1	2 ± 2
Sodium nitrite	0.5	74 ± 6	24 ± 2	2 ± 0.4
Phentolamine	0.01	68 ± 4	29 ± 3	3 ± 2

Average of values ± standard error for 4 dogs.

brane caused by 5 μg of epinephrine injected into the lingual artery.

Pressor Responses. Prazosin (0.04 mg per kilogram of body weight) given intravenously to three cats caused a slight decrease in the pressor response to epinephrine, but it did not diminish the pressor responses to norepinephrine, angiotensin, or carotid artery occlusion. In six cats intravenously administered 0.5 mg per kilogram of body weight, the drug reversed the pressor response to epinephrine and reduced the pressor response to carotid artery occlusion; the angiotensin response was reduced slightly or not affected (Fig. 11). The pressor response to DMPP was reduced in four cats, and reversed in two cats.

In each of four dogs, prazosin (1 μg per kilogram of body weight) given intravenously decreased the pressor response to epinephrine (Fig. 12). Neither the blood pressure nor the response to bilateral carotid artery occlusion was affected. Following a 50-μg dose per kilogram of body weight, blood pressure was lowered by 20 ± 2 mm Hg. The pressor response to epinephrine was reversed and that to bilateral carotid artery occlusion was diminished.

Spinal-pithed Cats. Prazosin (0.04 mg per kilogram of body weight) given intravenously

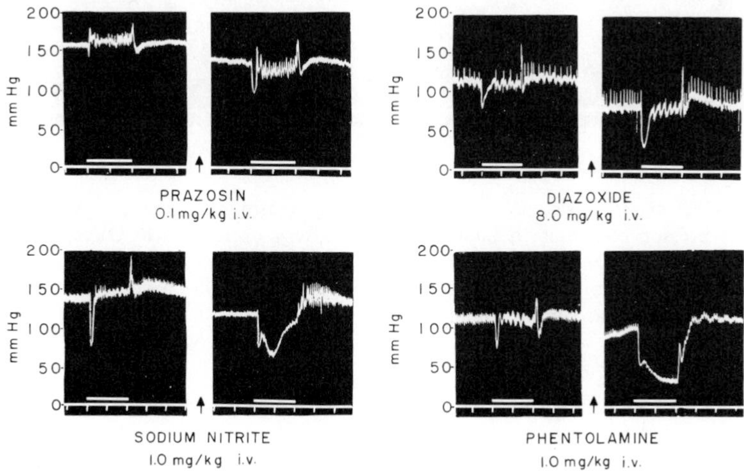

FIG. 9.—Effect of prazosin, diazoxide, sodium nitrite, and phentolamine on the systemic blood pressure response to tilting in dogs anesthetized with intravenously administered sodium pentobarbital (30 mg per kilogram of body weight). **Horizontal bars** indicate a head-up vertical tilt of 2 minutes' duration made 5 minutes before (*left panels*) and 5 minutes after (*right panels*) administration of the indicated drug. Time marks are placed at 1-minute intervals.

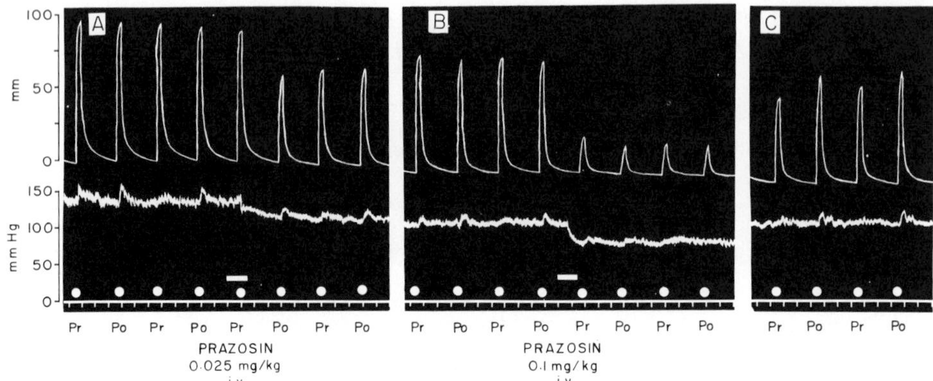

FIG. 10.—Effect of prazosin on the blood pressure (*lower tracing*) and on responses of the nictitating membrane (*upper tracing*) to electrical stimulation of preganglionic **(Pr)** and postganglionic **(Po)** cervical sympathetic nerves of a cat intravenously anesthetized with 75 mg of chloralose per kilogram of body weight. There was a 60-minute interval between panels *A* and *B* and panels *B* and *C*. Time marks are placed at 1-minute intervals.

to two spinal-pithed cats did not affect the blood pressure; it also had no effect in three animals in which the blood pressure was elevated by a continuous infusion of angiotensin. In an additional two cats, 0.04 mg per kilogram of body weight of prazosin, given intravenously, partially antagonized the hypertension caused by infusion of epinephrine.

These results indicate that prazosin does not interfere with nerve-impulse transmission

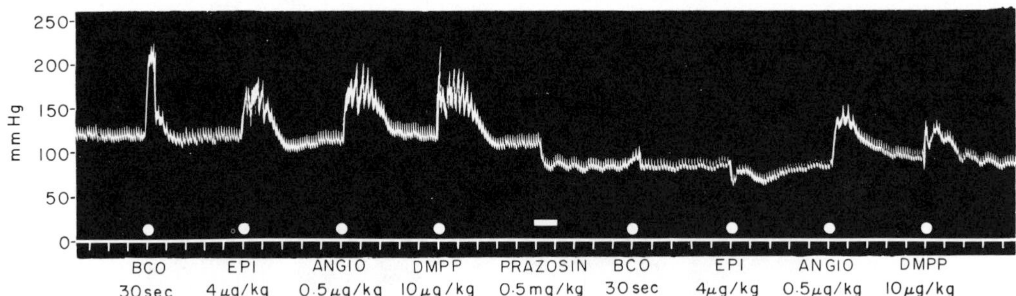

FIG. 11.—Effect of intravenously administered prazosin (0.5 mg per kilogram of body weight) on pressor responses to bilateral carotid artery occlusion **(BCO)**, epinephrine **(EPI)**, angiotensin **(ANGIO)**, and dimethylphenylpiperazinium **(DMPP)** in a cat anesthetized with chloralose, 75 mg per kilogram of body weight. Drugs were administered via a femoral vein. Time marks are placed at 1-minute intervals.

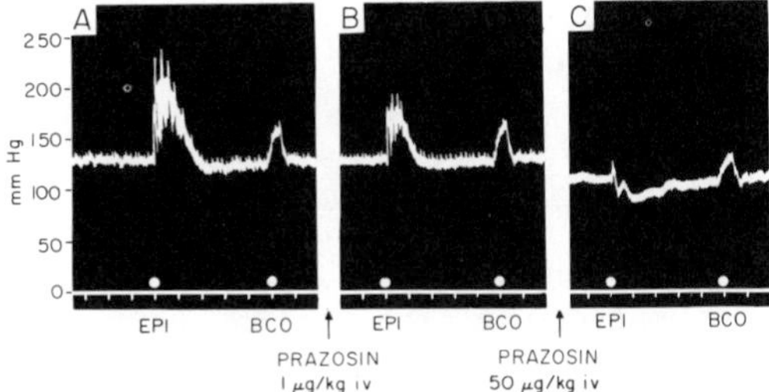

FIG. 12.—Effect of prazosin on pressor responses to intravenously administered epinephrine **(EPI)** in a dose of 2 μg per kilogram of body weight, and to bilateral carotid artery occlusion **(BCO)** for 30 seconds in a dog intravenously anesthetized with sodium pentobarbital (30 mg per kilogram of body weight). There was a 10-minute interval between panels *A* and *B*, and panels *B* and *C*. Time marks are placed at 1-minute intervals.

across sympathetic ganglia since responses of the nictitating membrane to stimulation of either pre- or postganglionic fibers were reduced to an equal extent.

Neuronal adrenergic blockade is eliminated as the site of action of the drug, since there was no effect on cardiac response to electrical stimulation of postganglionic sympathetic nerves. In addition, neuronal adrenergic-blocking agents are characterized by a number of actions, none of which were observed with prazosin, viz., (1) the drug did not cause an initial pressor effect following intravenous administration; (2) it did not potentiate the effects of exogenous catecholamines or of DMPP; and (3) drug-induced inhibition of the nictitating membrane contractions was not reversed by *d*-amphetamine.

Effect on Contractions of Aortic Strips

Antagonism Studies. Prazosin antagonized both norepinephrine- and barium-induced contractions of rabbit aortic strips. Cumulative concentration-response curves for norepinephrine were progressively displaced to the right by increasing concentrations of prazosin, but there was no diminution of the maximum response to norepinephrine (Fig. 13*A*). In contrast, the maximum response to barium was progressively decreased with increasing concentrations of prazosin (Fig. 13*B*).

Receptor Protection Studies. Phenoxybenzamine (2×10^{-8} gm per milliliter) and prazosin (5×10^{-8} gm per milliliter) each inhibited epinephrine-induced contractions of isolated aortic strips. The effect of phenoxybenzamine was irreversible (Fig. 14*A*), while that of prazosin was partially reversible (Fig. 14*C*). Epinephrine (5×10^{-5} gm per milliliter) protected alpha-receptors from phenoxybenzamine blockade (Fig. 14*B*), but it did not afford protection against prazosin (Fig. 14*D*).

In additional experiments, prazosin (1×10^{-8} gm per milliliter) or phentolamine (5×10^{-7} gm per milliliter) caused equivalent displacement to the right of norepinephrine cumulative concentration-response curves, whereas phenoxybenzamine, 1×10^{-7} gm per milliliter, abolished responses to norepinephrine. At the same concentrations, phentolamine and prazosin protected alpha-receptors from irreversible blockade by phenoxybenzamine (Fig. 15). In phentolamine-protected strips, the maximum response to norepinephrine was 55 percent of control value, while in prazosin-protected

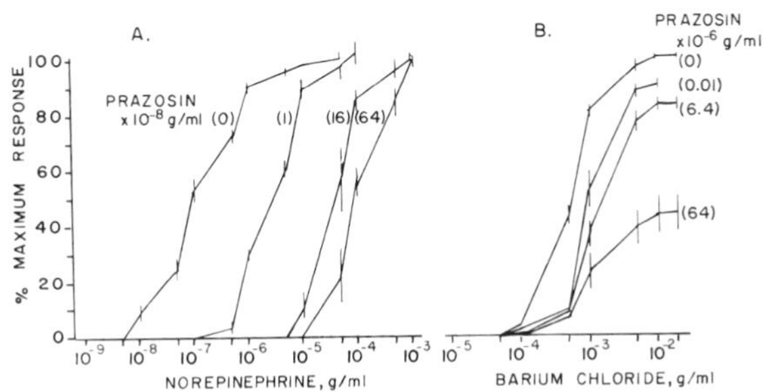

FIG. 13.—Responses of rabbit aorta to norepinephrine (*A*) or to barium (*B*) alone, and in the presence of prazosin. Each **point** on each curve is the mean of responses of at least six tissues; **vertical bars** represent the standard error of the mean. Prazosin concentration is indicated adjacent to each curve.

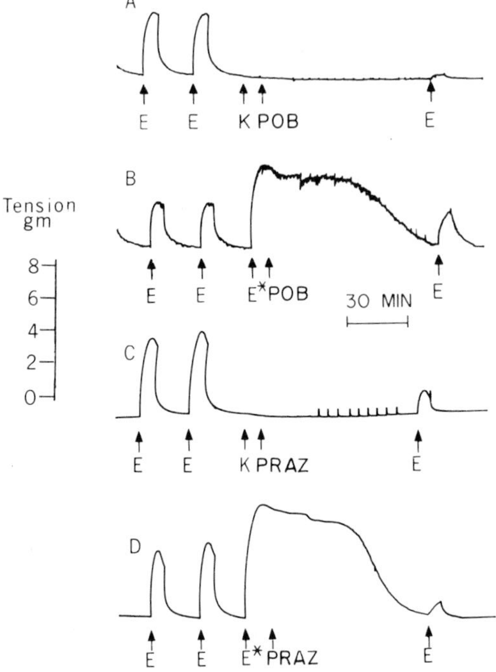

FIG. 14.—Protective effect of high concentrations of epinephrine against phenoxybenzamine, but not prazosin, blockade of alpha-adrenergic receptors in rabbit aorta. **E,** Epinephrine, 1×10^{-7} gm per milliliter; **K,** Krebs-Henseleit solution, 0.1 ml; **POB,** phenoxybenzamine, 2×10^{-8} gm per milliliter; **Praz,** prazosin, 5×10^{-8} gm per milliliter. High concentration of agonist: **E,** Epinephrine, 5×10^{-5} gm per milliliter.

strips, the response was only 20 percent of control value. Thus, the protective effect of prazosin is only half that of phentolamine.

Electrocardiographic Effects

In an anesthetized dog given prazosin (8 mg per kilogram of body weight given intravenously) a normally occurring sinus arrhythmia was abolished and it did not return during the ensuing 4 hours. In an additional three dogs, one received 17.8 mg per kilogram of body weight, and the other two, 20 mg per kilogram of body weight. When doses exceeded 15 mg per kilogram, heart rate increased moderately; T waves were potentiated in two dogs, and a negative T wave became positive and was potentiated in the remaining dog. However, in each animal, heart rate and T waves were normal at 30 to 60 min after completion of the infusion despite persistent hypotension.

Four conscious normotensive dogs were given prazosin orally (20 mg per kilogram of body weight per day) for 3 days, and 1 week later, 80 mg per kilogram in a single oral dose. With the exception of rate changes, the drug did not alter the pattern of electrocardiograms (lead II) taken at 2, 6, and 24 hours after each treatment.

There is no evidence that prazosin causes significant changes in the pattern of electrocardiograms in either conscious or anesthetized

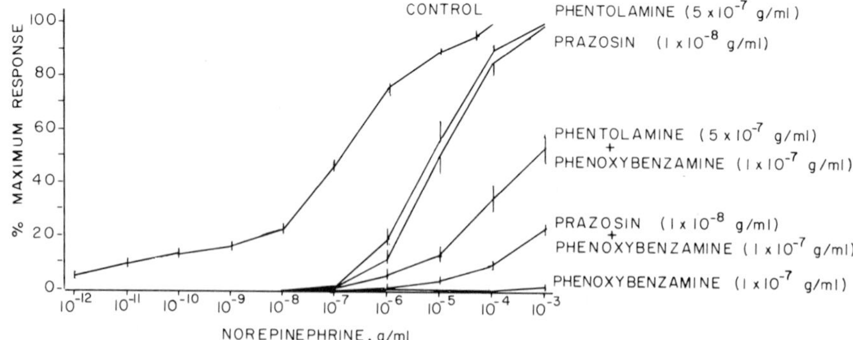

FIG. 15.—Protective effect of prazosin and phentolamine against phenoxybenzamine blockade of alpha-receptors in rabbit aorta. Cumulative concentration-response curves were obtained with norepinephrine alone, in the presence of prazosin, phentolamine, or phenoxybenzamine, and in the presence of prazosin or phentolamine plus phenoxybenzamine. Each **point** on a curve is the mean of responses for at least eight tissues; **vertical bars** represent the standard error of the mean.

dogs. In the latter, elevation of the T wave occurs only after doses of the drug which are in excess of those required to elicit maximal hypotensive effects.

Antidote Studies

In four dogs, prazosin (4 mg per kilogram of body weight) given intravenously caused hypotensive responses averaging 37 mm Hg. At the peak of the hypotensive effect, metaraminol was infused intravenously, initially at 1 μg, and gradually increased to 8 μg per kilogram per minute. Blood pressure was elevated to or near control level and maintained at that level with infusions of 4 to 8 μg per kilogram per minute. When the infusion was discontinued, blood pressure declined to hypotensive levels (Fig. 16).

In an additional three dogs, the hypotension induced by prazosin (4 mg per kilogram of body weight) given intravenously was antagonized with infusions of norepinephrine, 2 to 4 μg per kilogram per minute. Continuous norepinephrine infusions were required to maintain blood pressure at a normotensive level.

DISCUSSION

If a drug is to lower blood pressure by peripheral vasodilatation, it must exert an

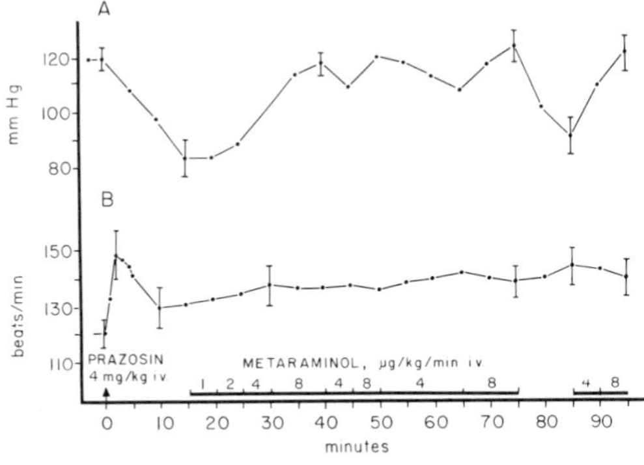

FIG. 16.—Effect of metaraminol on the blood pressure (*A*) and heart rate (*B*) of anesthetized dogs with hypotension induced by prazosin. **Graph** represents the average of values ± standard error for four dogs, either sex, with an average weight of 8.6 kg, who were intravenously anesthetized with sodium pentobarbital (30 mg per kilogram of body weight). Solid bar indicates infusion of metaraminol at indicated doses.

effect, either directly or indirectly, on small vessels (i.e., arterioles), since it is in this segment of the circulation that the greatest resistance to blood flow is encountered.[12] Ideally, the effect would be *confined* to the arterioles; indiscriminate peripheral vasodilatation results in peripheral pooling of blood, decreased venous return to the heart, and a reduction in cardiac output. This sequence of events is especially prominent in the erect position, and causes an exaggerated and prolonged orthostatic hypotension, a limiting side effect of most antihypertensive drugs.

Prazosin is an orally effective hypotensive agent in rats and dogs with a relatively long duration of action, and repeated administration does not provoke tolerance. Its hypotensive effect is a direct result of peripheral vasodilatation. This reduction in tone of vascular smooth muscle is due to two discernible components of drug action: (1) direct smooth-muscle relaxation, and (2) interference with peripheral sympathetic function. Results of the dog hindlimb experiments indicate that the direct relaxant effect may be the dominant component of action because when prazosin is administered to the pharmacologically denervated limb a significant portion of its vasodilator activity is retained. This activity is approximately equivalent to that of diazoxide given under the same conditions.

The results of dog forelimb experiments show that the peripheral vasodilator effect of prazosin is confined mainly to the small vessels. In this respect, prazosin also resembles diazoxide[6] but it contrasts markedly with phentolamine and sodium nitrite, both of which cause diffuse peripheral vasodilation. Since prazosin appears to act mainly at arterioles, it, like diazoxide,[13] should not exaggerate orthostatic hypotension, at least not to the extent that subjective symptoms would limit its usefulness. The fact that neither compound significantly exaggerates orthostatic hypotension in dogs substantially confirms this conclusion. The validity of predictions based on the tilt test is supported by the observation that agents which do cause postural hypotension in man, e.g., phentolamine[14] and sodium nitrite,[15] also depress the tilt response in dogs, and it has recently been reported that prazosin does not exaggerate orthostatic hypotension in humans.[16]

The manner in which prazosin interferes with peripheral sympathetic function is intriguing, and, in fact, analysis of this component of action reveals what may be a unique type of drug action. The studies with cats indicate that the activity of the drug is not due to a blocking action at sympathetic ganglia. Evidence is also presented which makes it unlikely that prazosin interferes with the function of postganglionic adrenergic neurones. Thus eliminated are two sites at which drugs are known to interfere with sympathetic function; there remains only one, the alpha-adrenergic receptor, and the question is thus raised: does prazosin block alpha-receptors?

Among the drugs which interfere with sympathetic function, alpha-adrenergic-blocking agents alone cause reversal of the epinephrine-pressor response. This response is implicitly regarded as proof of alpha-receptor blockade, an interpretation consistent with the prevalent concept which restricts the inactivation of alpha-receptors to an event occurring at the receptor site (i.e., occupancy blockade). But it should be appreciated that the epinephrine-reversal response is an expression of *functional* disruption of alpha-receptors and not, exclusively, of occupancy blockade. Results of the receptor protection experiments indicate that prazosin either does not occupy alpha-receptors or, if it does, the mechanism of such occupancy is different from that of phentolamine. But prazosin does evoke the epinephrine reversal response, hence it must interfere with the function of alpha-receptors. It will be helpful at this point to comment briefly on some recent investigations and current thinking concerning receptor function.

Moran [17] has reiterated the need for a broader conceptual visualization of the events between receptor excitation and response. The assumption that the agonist-receptor interaction is but the first in a sequence of events culminating in a response is symbolized as: $A + R \rightarrow AR \rightarrow a \rightarrow b \rightarrow c \rightarrow n \rightarrow Ef$, where *A* is the agonist, *R* the receptor, *AR* the agonist-receptor complex, and *Ef* the effect. With respect to alpha-adrenergic receptors, phentolamine and phenoxybenzamine are viewed as interfering with the first step: $A + |\alpha - R| \rightarrow$, an example of occupancy blockade. It is clear that drug action further along in the sequence, distal to the receptor, would cause disruption of receptor function without necessarily denying agonists or occupancy blockers access to the receptor site: $A + R \rightarrow AR \rightarrow a \rightarrow |b| \rightarrow$.

Rall and Sutherland [18] proposed that beta-adrenergic responses could be related to increased rate of formation of 3′,5′-AMP caused by stimulation of adenyl cyclase by catecholamines. There is now widespread acceptance of 3′,5′-AMP as a link in the sequence of events between beta-receptor stimulation and response. This may be symbolized as: $A + \beta - R \rightarrow A - \beta - R \rightarrow 3',5'\text{-AMP} \rightarrow b \rightarrow c \rightarrow n \rightarrow Ef$. Sutherland, Øye, and Butcher [19] recently remarked, with reference to events following beta-receptor excitation, ". . . it seems that this sequential messenger system may be of advantage to an organism because it engenders additional opportunities for the amplification or modulation of a given stimulus." To this may be added the advantage to be realized as the result of stimulus modulation by therapeutic agents, an inevitable consequence of investigation now in progress in this area of molecular biology.

On the basis of the available evidence, it is reasonable to consider the possibility that prazosin interferes with peripheral sympathetic function by acting at a site distal to the alpha-receptor. Interference at some point within the sequential process between receptor and response, but close enough to the receptor to modify it, could result in a functional impairment of receptors. Such an effect would account for the epinephrine-reversal response, and for the difference between prazosin and phentolamine in receptor protection experiments. Ariens and Simonis [20] have pointed out that impairment of receptor function in a competitive manner does not necessarily imply "topographical" (i.e., occupancy) blockade by the antagonist. In their view, antagonists can change the properties of receptors without occupying them. Wohl, Hausler, and Roth [21,22] suggest that the vascular smooth-muscle relaxant effect of diazoxide is due to drug action at a site distal to the alpha-receptor because diazoxide competitively inhibits Ba^{++} or Ca^{++}, but not norepinephrine-induced contractions of rat aorta. Prazosin is a noncompetitive antagonist of Ba^{++}, and probably does not act at the same site as diazoxide.

Direct verification of the proposed site of action of prazosin is not now possible. Since the evidence weighs very heavily against drug action at a site proximal to the receptor, the only alternative to the proposal offered is receptor-occupancy blockade. Elimination of this site of action would, therefore, be the strongest evidence in support of the argument. It is recognized that results of receptor-protection experiments require cautious interpretation. For example, it is possible that prazosin does occupy alpha-receptors. The failure of the drug to protect these receptors from phenoxybenzamine to the same extent that phentolamine does might then be due to the ability of phenoxybenzamine to displace prazosin from the receptor; however, the fact that phenoxybenzamine is unable to displace phentolamine from alpha-receptors would indicate that the mechanism of action of prazosin is different from that of phentolamine. The fact that the hypotensive effect of prazosin is not accompanied by postural hypotension in humans [16] is pertinent in this regard, since this undesirable side effect is associated with alpha-receptor occupancy-blockade of the type caused by phentolamine. It appears that this type of blockade constitutes a gross interference with receptor function, with the result that compensatory mechanisms are greatly attenuated. On the other hand, prazosin, acting distal to the receptor or, in a unique way, at the receptor, apparently depresses receptor function in a manner more attuned to normal physiologic function; compensatory stimuli are thus able to provide for homeostatic adjustment.

References

1. Scriabine, A., Constantine, J. W., Hess, H.-J., and McShane, W. K.: Pharmacological studies with some new antihypertensive aminoquinazolines. Experientia 24:1150, 1968.
2. Grollman, A.: A simplified procedure for inducing chronic renal hypertension in the mammal. Proc. Soc. Exp. Biol. Med. 57:102, 1944.
3. Goldblatt, H., Lynch, J., Hanzel, R. F., and Summerville, W. W.: Studies on experimental hypertension: I. The production of persistent elevation of systolic blood pressure by means of renal ischemia. J. Exp. Med. 59:347, 1934.
4. Prioli, N. A., and Winbury, M. M.: Indirect method for blood pressure determination in the dog. J. Appl. Physiol. 15:323, 1960.
5. Benchimol, A., Akre, P. R., and Dimond, E. G.: Clinical experience with the use of computers for calculations of cardiac output. Am. J. Cardiol. 15:213, 1965.
6. Rubin, A. A., Zitowitz, L., and Hausler, L.: Acute circulatory effects of diazoxide and sodium nitrite. J. Pharmacol. Exp. Ther. 140: 46, 1963.
7. Haddy, F. J., Fleishman, M., and Emanuel, D. A.: Effect of epinephrine, norepinephrine and serotonin upon systemic small and large vessel resistance. Circ. Res. 5:247, 1957.
8. Constantine, J. W., and McShane, W. K.: Analysis of the cardiovascular effects of 2-(2, 6-dichlorophenylamino)-2-imidazoline hydrochloride (Catapres). Eur. J. Pharmacol. 4: 109, 1968.
9. Furchgott, R. F., and Bhadrakom, S.: Reactions of strips of rabbit aorta to epinephrine, isopropylarterenol, sodium nitrite and other drugs. J. Pharmacol. Exper. Ther. 108:129, 1953.
10. Furchgott, R. F.: Dibenamine blockade in strips of rabbit aorta and its use in differentiating receptors. J. Pharmacol. Exp. Ther. 111:265, 1954.
11. Krebs, H. A., and Henseleit, K.: Untersuchungen über die harnsstoffbildung in tierkorper. Hoppe Seylers Z. Physiol. Chem. 210: 33, 1932.
12. Haddy, F. J.: Local effects of sodium, calcium and magnesium upon small and large blood vessels of the dog fore limb. Circ. Res. 8:57, 1960.
13. Thomson, A. E., Nickerson, M., and Grahame, G. R.: Clinical observations on an antihypertensive chlorothiazide analog devoid of diuretic activity. Can. Med. Assoc. J. 87: 1306, 1962.
14. Moyer, J. H., and Caplovitz, C.: The clinical results of oral and parenteral administration of 2-(*N'*-*p*-tolyl-*N'*-m-hydroxyphenylamino-methyl)imidazoline hydrochloride (Regitine) in the treatment of hypertension and an evaluation of the cerebral haemodynamic effects. Am. Heart J. 45:602, 1953.
15. Weiss, S., Wilkins, R. W., and Haynes, F. W.: The nature of circulating collapse induced by sodium nitrite. J. Clin. Invest. 16:73, 1937.
16. Cohen, B. M.: Prazosin hydrochloride (CP-12,299-1), an oral antihypertensive agent: Preliminary clinical observations in ambulatory patients. J. Clin. Pharmacol. 10:408, 1970.

17. Moran, N. C.: Pharmacological characterization of adrenergic receptors. Pharmacol. Rev. 18:503, 1966.
18. Rall, T. W., and Sutherland, E. W.: The regulatory role of cyclic 3′,5′-AMP. Symp. Quant. Biol. 26:347, 1961.
19. Sutherland, E. W., Øye, I., and Butcher, R. W.: The action of epinephrine and the role of the adenyl cyclase system in hormone action. Recent Progr. Horm. Res. 21:623, 1965.
20. Ariens, E. J., and Simonis, A. M.: Cholinergic and anticholinergic drugs. Do they act on common receptors? Ann. N.Y. Acad. Sci. 144:842, 1967.
21. Wohl, A. J., Hausler, L. M., and Roth, F. E.: Studies on the mechanism of antihypertensive action of diazoxide: *In vitro* vascular pharmacodynamics. J. Pharmacol. Exp. Ther. 158: 531, 1967.
22. Wohl, A. J., Hausler, L. M., and Roth, F. E.: The role of calcium in the mechanism of the antihypertensive action of diazoxide. Life Sci. 7:381, 1968.

The Use of Diazoxide in Hypertension

By Frank A. Finnerty, Jr., M.D.

During the past several years we have had experience with an agent that chemically resembles chlorothiazide but pharmacologically is quite different (Fig. 1). When administered by mouth, diazoxide reduces arterial pressure only slightly and causes sodium retention and hyperglycemia. When administered by vein, however, it is a very potent vasodilating agent. The average effective dose is 300 mg given rapidly undiluted.[1,2]

Experience has shown that the speed of injection is important in determining both the magnitude of the blood pressure fall and the duration of hypotensive effect.[3] When less than 300 mg of diazoxide is administered or when 300 mg is not administered within a 10- to 15-second period, only a short hypotensive response is noted. In a few hypertensive patients weighing over 150 pounds, 300 mg of diazoxide may produce only a slight reduction in arterial pressure for a short duration, e.g., a duration of 30 to 60 minutes instead of 8 to 9 hours. If a satisfactory fall in arterial pressure does not follow the administration of 300 mg of diazoxide, the dosage should be increased to 5 mg per kilogram of body weight.

Following the rapid intravenous injection of diazoxide a 35-percent average reduction in mean arterial pressure occurs during the first 2 minutes (Fig. 2). During the next 3 to 5 minutes the arterial pressure increases gradually, leveling off at an average 20 percent below control levels. No signs of postural hypotension, cerebral ischemia, or collapse are noted. The average duration of action is 9 to 11 hours.

Mechanism of Action

The fall in arterial pressure with diazoxide is consistently associated with an increase in cardiac output (+40%) and decrease in total

From the Department of Medicine, Georgetown University School of Medicine, and the Department of Medicine and Obstetrics/Gynecology, Georgetown University Medical Division, District of Columbia General Hospital, Washington, D.C.

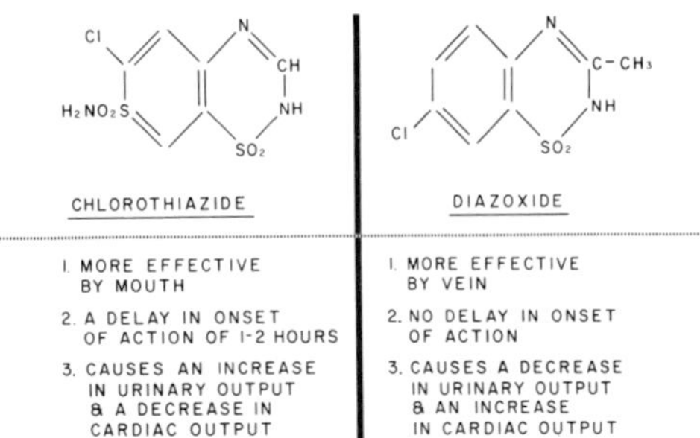

Fig. 1.—Comparison of molecular structures of chlorothiazide and diazoxide.

peripheral resistance (—41%). These changes in cardiac output and total peripheral resistance persist long after the peak action of the drug has been reached. The mechanism of the reduction in total peripheral resistance in man is not clear, but animal data suggest that diazoxide causes reduction in peripheral resistance by a direct action on the arteriolar muscle. From the cardiac hemodynamic standpoint, diazoxide resembles hydralazine, since both agents cause an increase in the cardiac output and heart rate. Determinations of actual cerebral blood flow have not been performed in this laboratory, but the lack of signs of cerebral ischemia accompanying the reduction in arterial pressure and the increase in cardiac output strongly indicate that there is at least maintenance of the cerebral blood flow, even at the point of greatest magnitude of hypotensive action of diazoxide.

Although the fall in arterial pressure with diazoxide is associated with an increase in

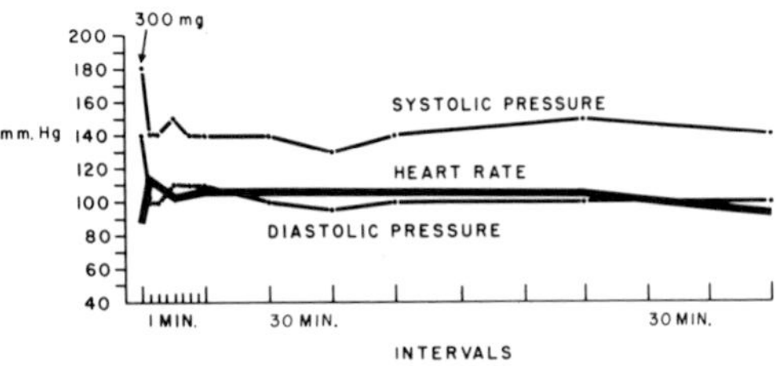

Fig. 2.—Effect of a single 300-mg dose of diazoxide on arterial blood pressure and heart rate.

cardiac output and cerebral blood flow, there is a decrease in renal blood flow, glomerular filtration, urinary output, and urinary sodium excretion. The decrease in urinary output and urinary sodium excretion can be prevented by the concomitant use of thiazide diuretics in hypertensive patients who have normal renal function. Experience in this laboratory has demonstrated, however, that the thiazide diuretics are not sufficiently potent to prevent these diazoxide-induced side effects in patients with impaired renal function.[4]

Increasing the dose of thiazides does not increase their potency, e.g., 2 gm of chlorothiazide administered four times daily does not produce a greater diuresis than does 500 mg administered twice daily. The recent availability of furosemide and the reports of its beneficial effects in high doses, particularly in azotemic patients,[5,6] suggest that combining it with diazoxide might do away with at least some of the detrimental effects of diazoxide in hypertensive azotemic patients. Furosemide by itself has a modest effect on the arterial pressure and a varying effect on the cardiac output and renal blood flow; it produces a marked increase in urinary output and sodium excretion[7] (Fig. 3). Administering these agents together produces a greater decrease in arterial pressure than that from diazoxide alone, increases cardiac output, and increases urinary sodium excretion and urinary output.[4] The combination of diazoxide and furosemide gives the physician a physiologic method for reducing arterial pressure even in patients with impaired renal function.

	DIAZOXIDE	FUROSEMIDE	DIAZOXIDE + FUROSEMIDE
MAP	↓↓	↓	↓↓↓
CO	↑↑	↓↑	↑↑
SODIUM BALANCE	(+)(+)	(−)(−)	(−)
URINARY OUTPUT	↓↓	↑↑	↑

FIG. 3.—Characteristics of 25 hypertensive patients with renal insufficiency.

Aim of Treatment

Whether treating hypertensive encephalopathy, e.g., complicating essential or secondary hypertension, toxemia of pregnancy or malignant hypertension (with or without azotemia), our aim of therapy is to control the diastolic pressure continuously and to insure an adequate urinary output. In adults the diastolic pressure should be maintained under 100 mm Hg; in patients with toxemia, the diastolic pressure should be maintained under 80 mm Hg; and in children with encephalopathy, the diastolic pressure should be maintained under 70 mm Hg. Diazoxide is repeated as often as necessary to keep the diastolic blood pressure below the desired level.

The urinary output should be maintained above 1.5 liters per 24 hours. If the patient has not been receiving diuretics, furosemide is initiated in a dosage of 40 mg. Furosemide is best administered intravenously when treating patients with encephalopathy but may be administered orally to patients with accelerated or malignant hypertension. If the urinary output has not exceeded 100 ml in a 2-hour period, furosemide is repeated and the dose is doubled. This sequential increase in the dosage of furosemide is continued every 2 hours until an adequate diuresis occurs. In our experience, the average effective dosage of furosemide has varied between 80 to 120 mg, administered twice daily in patients with good renal function, and 160 to 200 mg, given twice daily in azotemic patients.

Encephalopathy

In patients with encephalopathy, 24 to 48 hours of intensive therapy usually is all that is necessary to clear the signs of cerebral ischemia. A safe and practical time to discontinue parenteral diazoxide is when 300 mg of diazoxide has kept the diastolic pressure under control for a 24-hour period. Oral antihypertensive therapy can then be started. Furosemide is continued but the dosage is reduced to 80 mg, given twice daily. In our experience, maintenance of a reduced arterial pressure, even for a 24- to 48-hour period, significantly increases sensitivity to oral antihypertensive therapy. To date over 600 patients with various types of hypertensive encephalopathy have been treated with diazoxide. An excellent response (more than 25% fall in mean arterial pressure with complete clearing of the neurologic state and absence of side effects) has occurred in 475 patients (77%).

Except for delivery of the fetus and the obstetric problems attendant upon delivery, we consider severe toxemia (nonconvulsive and convulsive) as another type of encephalopathy; therefore, pregnant patients with toxemia are treated in the same fashion. Induction of labor or cesarean section is advised 12 to 24 hours after cessation of convulsions, control of the arterial pressure, and maintenance of a good urinary output. The details of management of these patients are discussed fully in the chapter entitled "Management of Hypertension in Toxemia of Pregnancy."

Accelerated Hypertension

In patients with accelerated hypertension with or without azotemia, the aim of therapy is again to control and maintain the diastolic pressure under 100 mm Hg and the urinary output above 1.5 liters per day. In these subjects it is usually necessary to extend the duration of intensive therapy to 10 to 14 days. Intensive therapy is again discontinued when a single injection of diazoxide has kept the diastolic pressure under 100 mm Hg for 24 hours or longer. At this point, the dose of furosemide is again reduced and the patient is placed on standard oral antihypertensive therapy. The prolonged (10 to 14 days) control of arterial pressure and maintenance of urinary output usually significantly increase the sensitivity to oral antihypertensive agents, thus allowing use of suboptimal doses.

Several years ago we reported the long-term effects of such intensive therapy in 25 hypertensive azotemic subjects, 20 of whom were in the malignant phase of hypertension.[4] The average mean arterial pressure in these patients was 192 ± 2.9 (Fig. 4). All the patients were placed on full doses of at least five antihypertensive agents in conjunction with a diuretic. One week after intensive therapy (controlled arterial pressure and maintenance of urinary output) the average mean arterial pressure had fallen to 114 mm Hg (Fig. 5). There had been aggravation of renal function, however,

CHARACTERISTICS OF 25 HYPERTENSIVE PATIENTS WITH RENAL INSUFFICIENCY

(DURATION OF HYPERTENSION: 1-10+ years)

BP (mm Hg)	236 ± 42 / 149 ± 29	(Mean: 192 ± 30)
BUN (mg %)	35-103	(Avg: 62 ± 22)
CREATININE (mg %)	3.5-15.2	(Avg: 6.9 ± 2.9)
CARDIOMEGALY (x-ray)	22 PTS	
LVH (ECG)	23 PTS	
CHF	5 PTS	
FUNDI: Grade 4	20 PTS	
Grade 3	3 PTS	
Grade 2	2 PTS	

FIG. 4.—Advantages of diazoxide used in combination with furosemide.

since the creatinine increased from an average of 6.9 to 8.1 mg.

That the aggravation of renal function was temporary was shown by the fact that 3 months later renal function in all patients had returned to control levels and in 6 months a definite improvement was noted. The serial changes in arterial pressure, creatinine, blood urea nitrogen, and renal clearances during the year after intensive therapy in a typical patient are plotted in Fig. 6. The status of the cardiovascular renal disease an average of 26 months after intensive therapy is outlined in Fig. 7. Except for the three patients who died during the period of intensive therapy, none of the subsequent deaths were related to cardiovascular renal disease.

Side Effects

Although the combination of diazoxide and furosemide is extremely valuable for the treatment of all types of hypertensive encephalo-

	CONTROL	ACUTE EFFECT
MAP (mm Hg)	192 ± 30	114 ± 17
BUN (mg %)	62 ± 22	74 ± 32
CREATININE (mg %)	6.9 ± 2.9	8.1 ± 3.7
CARDIOMEGALY	22 PTS	8 PTS
LVH	23 PTS	21 PTS
CHF	5 PTS	0 PTS

DEATHS: 3 PTS

FIG. 5.—Effect of intensive therapy 7 to 14 days after its completion.

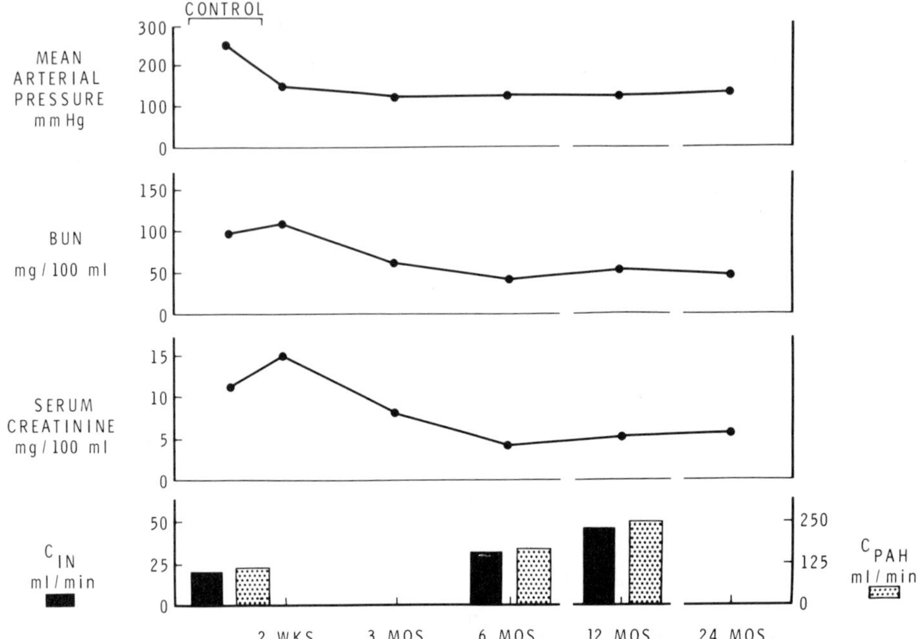

FIG. 6.—The serial changes in mean arterial pressure, BUN, serum creatinine, and renal clearance in one representative patient (Case No. 15).

pathy and accelerated hypertension, certain limitations are present:

1. Transitory hyperglycemia lasting no more than 12 hours occasionally follows intravenous administration of diazoxide. Recent reports of Wolff, Grant, and Wales [8] and studies in our laboratory [9] have demonstrated that pretreatment of patients with tolbutamide will effectively prevent the hyperglycemic effect of diazoxide. Although pretreatment with tolbutamide need not be routine, monitoring of blood sugar in these patients is advised.

	CONTROL	ACUTE EFFECT	LONG TERM EFFECT
MAP (mmHg)	192 ± 30	114 ± 17	120 ± 11
BUN (mg %)	62 ± 22	74 ± 32	26 ± 13
CREATININE (mg %)	6.2 ± 2.9	8.1 ± 3.7	2.2 ± 1.4
CARDIOMEGALY	25 PTS	14 PTS	10 PTS
LVH	23 PTS	21 PTS	11 PTS
CHF	5 PTS	0 PTS	0 PTS
FUNDI			
Grade 4	20 PTS	16 PTS	0 PTS
Grade 3	3 PTS	4 PTS	2 PTS
Grade 2	2 PTS	2 PTS	20 PTS

FIG. 7.—Status of cardiovascular and renal disease 26 ± 7 months after intensive therapy in 22 patients.

2. The alkaline nature of the diazoxide solution makes any extravasation outside the vein painful. Although such extravasation is associated with a severe burning sensation which lasts 1 to 2 hours, no sloughing of tissues has occurred.

3. The fall in arterial pressure following diazoxide given alone is not associated with postural hypotension. The addition of furosemide to diazoxide by decreasing the plasma volume commonly produces postural hypotension.[4] The physician's awareness of the possibility of this complication and the maintenance of the patient in the supine position is all that is necessary to avoid complications.

4. Similar to thiazide diuretics, furosemide may cause significant hypokalemia, hyponatremia, and hyperuricemia. In our experience these electrolyte abnormalities occur only after excessive diuresis and are not particularly common following high doses of furosemide. Monitoring of these electrolytes, however, is mandatory.

Discussion

Experience gained from treating over 600 patients during the past 10 years has convinced us that the combination of diazoxide plus furosemide is the treatment of choice for patients with all types of hypertensive encephalopathy. The standard dosage of diazoxide, e.g., 300 mg (one ampule) bypasses the need for individual titration. The immediate onset of action without aggravating cerebral ischemia or decreasing urinary output gives the physician a simple, immediately effective method for treating the acute situation.

The value of this physiologic method for acutely reducing arterial pressure while maintaining urinary output can also be extended beyond the acute situation. Our experiences would indicate that the combination of diazoxide and furosemide may be life-saving in patients with accelerated hypertension, occurring with or without azotemia. It has been hypothesized that malignant hypertension may be a reversible disease and that survival may be possible if life can be maintained for a reasonable period while healing of the arteriolitis is occurring.[10] It has also been observed that patients with malignant hypertension and renal insufficiency die during the early stages of treatment before the benefits of remission can be realized.[10] The prompt clearing of papilledema and decrease in retinopathy, the significant reduction of blood urea nitrogen and serum creatinine levels 3 months after treatment, and the improvement in renal blood flow and glomerular filtration rate all adequately attest to the reversibility of the malignant phase of hypertension in most of the patients studied here. It would seem that the physiologic reduction of arterial pressure accomplished by diazoxide and furosemide stabilized 22 of the 25 patients until the beneficial effects of a remission could be realized. From this point on, so long as the patients remained on medication, they continued to improve. It seems, therefore, that if the patients could be kept alive during the period of intensive treatment, their chances for survival for at least 1 to 2 years were greatly increased. These findings are in agreement with those of Woods and Blythe.[10] It seems also that aggressive treatment should not be discontinued because of a rise in blood urea nitrogen or serum creatinine for such rises are usually transitory. If further studies verify the reversibility of the malignant phase and the improvement in renal function, it would seem that all patients with severe hypertension, with or without azotemia, would benefit by such aggressive treatment. Such physiologic reduction of arterial pressure seems particularly indicated in those patients with only mild impairment of renal function, for example, in those with low blood urea nitrogen levels, since 1½ years after intensive treatment the levels of blood urea nitrogen and serum creatinine had returned to near normal in all these patients.

Our experience and that of others [11] has convinced us that because of their sodium-retaining properties, potent antihypertensive agents should not be used alone in patients with renal insufficiency. It is not known whether keeping the diastolic pressure at a lower level, the urinary output at a higher level, or prolonging the period of intensive therapy would increase the beneficial effect of intensive therapy. Such studies are currently under way in this laboratory.

It can be concluded from our data that the combination of diazoxide and furosemide is an immediately effective and safe method for reducing arterial pressure; used over a 24- to 48-hour period, this combination is the ideal method for treating patients with all types of encephalopathy; used over a 10- to 14-day period this combination may help reverse the malignant phase of hypertension and actually improve renal function.

References

1. Kakaviatos, N., and Finnerty, F. A., Jr.: Preliminary observations on the value of diazoxide administered intravenously in man. Angiology 13:541, 1962.
2. Finnerty, F. A., Jr., Kakaviatos, N., Tuckman, J., and Magill, J.: Clinical evaluation of diazoxide. Circulation 28:203, 1963.
3. Mroczek, W. J., Leibel, B. A., Davidov, M., and Finnerty, F. A., Jr.: The importance of the rapid administration of diazoxide in accelerated hypertension. N. Engl. J. Med. 285: 603, 1971.
4. Mroczek, W. J., Davidov, M., Gavrilovich, L., and Finnerty, F. A., Jr.: The value of aggressive therapy in the hypertensive patient with azotemia. Circulation 40:893, 1969.

5. Muth, R.: Diuretic properties of furosemide in renal disease. Ann. Intern. Med. 69:249, 1968.
6. Berman, L. B., and Ebrahimi, A.: Experience with furosemide in renal disease. Proc. Soc. Exp. Biol. Med. 118:333, 1965.
7. Finnerty, F. A., Jr., Davidov, M., Mroczek, W. J., and Gavrilovich, L.: Influence of extracellular fluid volume on response to antihypertensive drugs. Circ. Res. 26–27(Suppl. I):71, 1970.
8. Wolff, F. W., Grant, A. M., and Wales, J. K.: Reversal of diazoxide effects by tolbutamide. Lancet 1:1137, 1967.
9. Davidov, M., Kakaviatos, N., and Finnerty, F. A.: Unpublished observations.
10. Woods, J. M., and Blythe, W. B.: Management of malignant hypertension complicated by renal insufficiency. N. Engl. J. Med. 277: 57, 1967.
11. Horowitz, D., and Sjoerdsma, A.: Drug therapy of hypertension. Med. Ann. D.C. 38: 1, 1969.

PART VII. ADRENAL HYPERTENSION

The Regulation of Aldosterone Secretion

By J. R. Stockigt, M.D.

SINCE ITS ISOLATION and characterization in 1954,[1,2] aldosterone has been recognized as a major physiologic factor in the conservation of sodium and the excretion of potassium. Primary hyperaldosteronism is a well-known cause of curable hypertension, and hypoaldosteronism can occur as a distinct entity.[3] In essential hypertension the consensus suggests that aldosterone production is within normal limits [4–6] although markedly elevated levels can occur in malignant hypertension.[7] The suggestion that aldosterone may not be normally suppressible during high-sodium intake in essential hypertension [8] remains to be further evaluated.

A large body of literature demonstrates beyond doubt that the regulation of aldosterone secretion cannot be defined as simply as the relationship between adrenocorticotropic hormone (ACTH) and cortisol. Four major influences on aldosterone production have been identified: (1) the renin-angiotensin system, (2) ACTH, (3) plasma potassium, and (4) plasma sodium, but there are several experimental and naturally occurring variations in aldosterone which cannot be explained in terms of these factors. The possibility that different mechanisms may be involved in the activation and inhibition of secretion adds complexity but may become increasingly important.

Because the circulating level of aldosterone has little direct influence on the adrenal production of aldosterone [9] or on the release of renin from the kidney,[10] feedback results from the effects of aldosterone rather than from the circulating level per se.

The production of aldosterone can be influenced in at least two separate stages of biosynthesis; either early in the pathway probably between cholesterol and pregnenolone,[11] or between corticosterone and aldosterone.[12] Stimulation of aldosterone biosynthesis by angiotensin II has not so far been shown to involve cyclic adenosine monophosphate as a mediator [13] and the available evidence is inconclusive.[14,15]

A complete review of the literature will not be attempted here; this need will be filled by the recent extensive monograph of Gláz and Vecsei,[16] and the reviews of Ganong and Van Brunt,[17] Coghlan et al.,[18,19] Boyd and Peart,[20] and Müller.[21]

Significance of the Renin-Angiotensin System

Despite the well-known association of secondary hyperaldosteronism [7] with elevated plasma renin [22] and angiotensin II [23] in severe or malignant hypertension, the renin-angiotensin system is not the sole regulator of aldosterone secretion because in a number of circumstances fluctuations in aldosterone are inconsistent with the observed changes in renin and angiotensin. In the following lists some close associations of renin-angiotensin with aldosterone are summarized and some major discrepancies outlined.

Evidence *for* the relationship between the renin-angiotensin system and aldosterone is listed below:

1. Administered renin or angiotensin II stimulates aldosterone in most species.
2. Aldosterone responses to hemorrhage and caval constriction involve the kidneys.
3. Passive transfer of antirenin antibodies diminishes the aldosterone response to sodium restriction.
4. There is an elevation of renin, angiotensin II, and aldosterone during the onset of sodium deficiency.

From the Departments of Medicine and Physiology, University of California, San Francisco, California, and Medical Unit, St. Mary's Hospital, London, England.

5. There is an associated elevation of renin, angiotensin, and aldosterone in secondary hyperaldosteronism.

6. Circadian variations and response to upright posture correspond in man.

7. Suppressed renin levels occur in primary hyperaldosteronism.

8. Elevated renin levels occur in adrenal insufficiency.

Evidence *against* a direct relationship between the renin-angiotensin system and aldosterone follows:

1. There is a minimal effect of angiotensin II on aldosterone in the rat.

2. Aldosterone falls *before* renin and angiotensin II when sodium deficit is rapidly corrected in sheep.

3. Aldosterone responses to sodium depletion and repletion persist in sheep despite high doses of infused renin or angiotensin II.

4. Large doses of infused angiotensin II are required in man to simulate the effects of sodium depletion on aldosterone.

5. Aldosterone may remain elevated despite fall in renin during treatment of malignant hypertension.

6. In essential hypertension with subnormal renin, aldosterone is normal.

7. Small changes in posture in man increase aldosterone with a minimal effect on angiotensin II.

8. During adaptation to hypoxia aldosterone falls while renin rises slightly.

9. In natriuresis of fasting aldosterone rises without a renin rise.

10. Aldosterone is present in anephric man.

The suggestion that the kidney could influence the output of aldosterone [24] has been confirmed in many ways. The kidneys are essential for the aldosterone response to hemorrhage in hypophysectomized dogs [25,26] and in the response to inferior vena caval constriction.[27] The aldosterone response to sodium depletion is impaired in nephrectomized dogs [27] and in man,[28] although in the anephric rat aldosterone responds significantly to sodium depletion.[29] In sheep, nephrectomy during sodium depletion is followed by a slow fall in aldosterone but nephrectomy in sodium-replete animals causes no immediate fall in aldosterone.[30] Lee et al.[31] found that passive transfer of antibodies to partially purified renin impaired the aldosterone response to sodium restriction in dogs.

Infused angiotensin II increases aldosterone in man,[32,33] dog,[34] and sheep,[35] but in sheep the effect is not sustained.[36] However, in man the aldosterone response to angiotensin II given at moderate pressor doses was maintained for several days,[37] and in the dog, doses of angiotensin II which caused only minimal elevation of blood pressure sustained the aldosterone response for 4 to 11 days [38] but there is doubt whether the levels of angiotensin during such infusions are within the physiologic range. Boyd et al.[39] showed that infused angiotensin II in man produced a much smaller rise in plasma aldosterone than occurred with comparable levels of naturally secreted angiotensin II during sodium deficiency. This raises the question of whether the aldosterone-producing mechanism becomes more sensitive to angiotensin II during sodium deficiency.

Although it is clear that the sensitivity to the pressor effect of angiotensin II varies widely,[37,40] variations in adrenal sensitivity to its aldosterone-stimulating action are less definite. Ganong, Boryczka, and Shackleford [41] reported some increase in sensitivity in dogs following sodium restriction, but Blair-West et al.[42] found that in sheep both sodium depletion and sodium loading diminished the absolute rise in aldosterone during angiotensin infusion. No clear-cut increase in sensitivity was found in humans.[39]

Aldosterone production in the rat is remarkably resistant to the effects of angiotensin II,[43] although a definite effect is seen with high doses.[44] The facts that nephrectomy does not lower the elevated rate of aldosterone secretion in sodium-depleted rats [29] and that sodium depletion increases aldosterone in anephric rats,[29] suggest that in this species the renin-angiotensin system plays no more than a minor role in the regulation of aldosterone.

In many situations in man there is close correlation between aldosterone and the renin-angiotensin system. Circadian variations during recumbency and the responses to upright posture correspond closely,[45] and both renin and aldosterone rise in response to sodium restriction although the relationship is less clear-cut than with upright posture.[45] In primary hyperaldosteronism where the production of aldosterone is little influenced by changes in sodium balance,[46] renin is markedly suppressed,[47] and in adrenal insufficiency renin levels are elevated.[48] In secondary hyperaldosteronism of various types, renin and aldosterone are often closely correlated. The findings in malignant hypertension,[7,22,23] renin-secreting kidney tumors,[49] sodium-losing renal disease,[50] nephrotic syndrome,[51,52] and Bartter's syndrome [53] suggest a direct relationship between renin and aldosterone. However, McAllister et al.[54] have reported concurrent studies of plasma renin activity and aldosterone secretion rate in 22 patients with malignant hypertension, and have documented serial changes during treatment. While the aldosterone secretion rate was increased in 19 of the 22 patients, plasma renin activity was above normal in only eight patients, and in the course of treatment aldosterone frequently remained above normal for several months after renin had returned to normal. These findings suggest that aldosterone and renin may not be causally related in malignant hypertension, and raise the possibility that a nonrenin-aldosterone-stimulating factor is present, or that excessive stimulation of the adrenal by angiotensin may lead to relatively autonomous aldosterone overproduction.

In several other circumstances there is a dissociation between renin and aldosterone in man. During adaptation to hypoxia at high altitudes aldosterone excretion falls while plasma potassium and renin both tend to rise;[55] although a primary effect of hypoxia on aldosterone secretion has been postulated, this mechanism remains unclear. When total fasting is begun after a period of sodium restriction both renin and aldosterone are elevated at the onset of fasting [56] and the further natriuresis during fasting is associated with a rise in aldosterone which is not accompanied by a rise in renin or potassium.[56] While studies during recumbency and upright posture show close correlation between renin and aldosterone, this relationship may not hold with smaller changes in posture. Tilting of the trunk to 45° after recumbency is associated with a significant rise in plasma aldosterone,[57] but there is only a minimal rise in plasma angiotensin II.[23]

Blair-West et al.[58] have shown several discrepancies between aldosterone and renin-angiotensin in experimental sodium deficiency in the sheep. During sodium loss from a parotid fistula there is a close relationship between aldosterone, renin and angiotensin, and when given access to sodium the animals correct their deficit rapidly and precisely. After correction of the sodium deficit aldosterone falls rapidly within 2 hours, while renin and plasma angiotensin II fall more slowly within 8 to 12 hours.[58] A more rapid fall in the presumed effect than in the postulated cause is strong evidence against such a relationship. The rapid fall in aldosterone does not appear to be the result of the rise in plasma sodium concentration.[59] In further studies either renin or angiotensin II was given as prolonged infusions for several days,[60] during which time sodium depletion and repletion produced a rise and fall in aldosterone despite the constant artificially high levels of renin or angiotensin.

The fact that angiotensin II does not reproduce the biosynthetic effect of sodium depletion is strong evidence against its role as the sole mediator of the aldosterone response to this stimulus. Angiotensin II has been shown to act at an early stage in aldosterone biosynthesis, probably between cholesterol and pregnenolone, and no effect has been demonstrated between corticosterone and aldosterone.[11,14] This is in marked contrast to the effect of sodium depletion which stimulates biosynthesis between corticosterone and aldosterone.[15] In a complex study using ^{3}H-corticosterone infused proximal to the transplanted adrenal in sheep, Blair-West et al.[12] have inferred that the predominant effect in moderate sodium depletion is between corticosterone and aldosterone, but that in very severe sodium depletion an earlier step in biosynthesis is stimulated or an alternative pathway is activated.

The assumption that the renin-angiotensin system is an important regulator of aldosterone synthesis leads to a useful working hypothesis in many situations. However, the statement "It is now clear that angiotensin is the prime regulator of aldosterone secretion" [61] is no longer tenable.

Role of Adrenocorticotropic Hormone (ACTH)

There is abundant evidence that administered ACTH can increase aldosterone production and that maneuvers which suppress or abolish ACTH can diminish aldosterone, but the role of ACTH in the *normal* regulation of aldosterone remains controversial. While exogenous ACTH in doses less than 1.4 international units (IU) daily results in production of normal amounts of glucocorticoid in man,[62] the doses administered to study aldosterone often range between 20 and 80 IU daily. Because the normal output of ACTH is intermittent,[63] the use of large, injected doses may have little relationship to the normal pattern of secretion.

In man the adrenal zona glomerulosa appears normal for up to 9 months after hypophysectomy,[64] but atrophic changes are found after many months in animals.[17] Aldosterone production falls following hypophysectomy in sheep,[35] in dogs,[65] and in rats,[66] and the response to sodium depletion is impaired.[67,68] In man basal aldosterone levels tend to be low in long-standing hypopituitarism with subnormal responses to sodium restriction.[69,70] However, hyponatremia in hypopituitarism does not necessarily indicate mineralocorticoid deficiency because water excretion may be significantly impaired.[71,72]

Spark et al.[73] demonstrated that in man 2 mg of dexamethasone, given daily for 2 days, caused aldosterone to fall by one-third, with impairment in the response to administered angiotensin; and Newton and Laragh [74] showed similar effects with 20 mg of hydrocortisone, given daily for 5 days. However, studies in patients after long-term treatment with pharmacologic doses of glucocorticoids have shown normal aldosterone responses to salt restriction.[75,76] The study of Williams et al.[76] suggests that disease or absence of the pituitary impairs aldosterone production, but that this effect is not reproduced by long-term glucocorticoid treatment. An experimental analogy to this finding exists in dogs,[77] and it has been suggested that a pituitary factor other than ACTH may be involved in aldosterone production.[77]

While administered ACTH can increase aldosterone output, the dose required is much larger than that which gives maximal glucocorticoid output in both dogs [78] and sheep.[36] The threshold for this effect can be markedly lowered by preceding sodium restriction,[78] and both sodium restriction and potassium loading [79] increase the magnitude of the response to ACTH.

When ACTH is administered in man for more than 2 days it fails to sustain high levels of aldosterone, and after cessation of ACTH administration aldosterone commonly falls to below control levels.[80,81] Because this effect is observed both during high-sodium and low-sodium intake [80] and in primary aldosteronism,[46] it seems unlikely to be due to suppression of renin. The possibility that ACTH excess may lead to the accumulation of intra-adrenal steroids which "autoregulate" aldosterone production is supported by the finding that added corticosterone and cortisol can directly inhibit aldosterone production.[82,83]

The levels of aldosterone in Cushing's syndrome have been found to be normal in the majority of cases.[84,85] In the ectopic ACTH syndrome where evidence of mineralocorticoid excess is common, it is an excess of deoxycorticosterone rather than aldosterone which is responsible,[86] and aldosterone has been found to be normal or low.[86] Several patients have been described [87, 88] with unusual forms of hyperaldosteronism which appear to be corrected by glucocorticoid suppression of ACTH, suggesting that in some instances ACTH may be the prime factor responsible for aldosterone excess.

The fact that the aldosterone response to ACTH is augmented by sodium depletion or potassium loading, and that the aldosterone response to exogenous angiotensin II is diminished by dexamethasone, suggests that ACTH may have important interactions with these stimuli. There are few data to indicate whether variations of ACTH within the physiologic range can influence the responses to other stimuli, but the findings of Mulrow and Ganong [89] suggest that when given acutely, ACTH and angiotensin II have independent rather than synergistic effects on 17-hydroxycorticoids and aldosterone. Doses of ACTH sufficient to produce about three-quarters of the maximal 17-hydroxycorticoid response did not augment the aldosterone response to angiotensin in hypophysectomized dogs.

The recent finding [90] that pressor doses of angiotensin II increased immunoreactive ACTH in man suggests a possible interaction between angiotensin II and ACTH. An inhibitory effect of angiotensin on cortisol production is postulated, leading to an increase in ACTH which may augment the aldosterone response. This is consistent with the observation of a diminished aldosterone response to angiotensin during dexamethasone suppression.[73,90]

While the importance of ACTH in aldosterone regulation cannot be defined precisely at present, it may be important to appreciate that neither the known actions of aldosterone nor physiologic variations in the plasma level have been shown to exert direct feedback on ACTH, thus creating a possible "open loop." Since the sensitivity to its aldosterone-stimulating effect can vary greatly, ACTH could contribute to aldosterone overproduction without obvious glucocorticoid excess.

Effect of Potassium

A rise in the level of plasma potassium can stimulate, and a fall in potassium can inhibit, the production of aldosterone. Evidence for these effects is derived from three types of studies: alteration of potassium intake, local alteration of the concentration in adrenal blood supply, and studies with incubated adrenal tissue. In addition to the direct effects of potassium it is important to consider the significance of interactions with other aldosterone-stimulating factors. The important potassium effects are summarized below:

1. Potassium administration increases and depletion diminishes aldosterone output in many species.
2. Potassium balance influences the responses to changes in sodium balance in normal man and in secondary hyperaldosteronism.
3. Potassium status influences the response to ACTH in man.
4. There is a marked effect on aldosterone production in primary aldosteronism.
5. Potassium may be the dominant regulating factor in anephric man.
6. Small changes in plasma potassium influence aldosterone output in sheep.
7. Adrenal potassium accumulation may be common to several factors which stimulate aldosterone secretion.

Potassium has been shown to stimulate aldosterone biosynthesis at an early stage, probably between cholesterol and pregnenolone,[11, 14] but recent studies indicate an influence on the later specific steps in biosynthesis,[15,91] an effect previously thought to occur only in sodium deficiency.[19] In the rat adrenal, potassium appears to stimulate only the zona glomerulosa.[15]

Cannon, Ames, and Laragh [92] demonstrated that potassium loading in man produced a marked increase in aldosterone secretion, with responses of similar magnitude to those produced by angiotensin infusion. The effect appeared to be magnified by sodium depletion, although the rise in plasma potassium was greater during low-sodium intake. Potassium depletion decreased aldosterone secretion and blunted, but did not abolish, the response to sodium depletion.[92,93]

The effect of potassium has also been demonstrated in the rat,[91] in the isolated perfused adrenals of sheep,[36] and in hypophysectomized dogs.[94] Funder et al.[95] found that a rise in local plasma potassium concentration of less than 0.5 mEq per liter significantly increased the output of aldosterone from the transplanted sheep adrenal, but they found no evidence that this effect was augmented during sodium deficiency.

Williams, Dluhy, and Underwood [79] have studied the effect of potassium intake on the aldosterone response to pharmacologic doses of ACTH in man. During high-sodium intake (200 mEq per day) the absolute rise in aldosterone secretion in response to ACTH was increased fourfold by increasing the potassium intake from 40 to 200 mEq per day, but potassium appeared to have a less marked influence on the response to ACTH during low-sodium intake.

In two circumstances potassium appears to be the dominant factor influencing aldosterone secretion. In primary hyperaldosteronism the output of aldosterone is remarkably potassium-dependent while being almost unresponsive to changes in sodium balance.[46] In the presence of severe hypokalemia aldosterone may be reduced into the "normal" range, and aldosterone output can be markedly increased by potassium repletion.[46] In anephric man a rise in plasma aldosterone occurs in association with increasing plasma potassium between dialyses,[28] despite accumulation of sodium and water. Aldosterone fails to rise if the rise in plasma potassium is prevented.[28]

There is strong evidence that the effect of potassium is independent of the renin-angiotensin system. Local infusion of potassium into the adrenal artery influences aldosterone secretion,[95] and potassium is an important stimulus when the renin-angiotensin system is absent[28] or suppressed.[46] Most significantly, hyperkalemia inhibits renin release[96, 97] while stimulating aldosterone.

Baumber et al.[98] have found that in the dog the potassium content of adrenocortical tissue increases in response to angiotensin II, ACTH, sodium depletion, and potassium administration. Although this phenomenon has not yet been directly correlated with aldosterone secretion or shown to be specific to the zona glomerulosa, it does suggest the possibility that local accumulation of potassium in the adrenal cortex may be an important common factor in the regulation of aldosterone secretion.

Effect of Plasma Sodium Concentration

The fact that sodium deficiency stimulates a late stage in aldosterone biosynthesis[12, 15] between corticosterone and aldosterone, while angiotensin does not,[15] is one of several discrepancies between these two stimuli (see above). The possibility that changes in plasma sodium concentration per se might influence aldosterone secretion has been examined using the isolated perfused adrenals of sheep[36] and hypophysectomized, nephrectomized dogs.[94] Local infusions which had a negligible effect on systemic sodium concentration or on total sodium balance produced significant increases in aldosterone secretion when the local sodium concentration was lowered by 20 mEq per liter.[36,94] However, in sheep with increased aldosterone secretion during established sodium deficiency, an elevation in the local sodium concentration produced only a transient 25 percent fall in aldosterone secretion,[99] and the increase in plasma sodium did not account for the very rapid fall in aldosterone secretion which occurred following acute sodium repletion.[58, 59] Lowering the sodium concentration from 148 mEq per liter in the perfusion medium of rat adrenal tissue resulted in only a 40-percent increase in aldosterone secretion (Ref. 21, page 17), suggesting that alteration in local sodium concentration is a weak stimulus to aldosterone secretion. Further, overhydration can lower aldosterone in man in the face of a diminished serum sodium concentration.[100] These results indicate that changes in sodium *concentration* per se do not adequately explain observed variations in aldosterone secretion.

Changes in Aldosterone Clearance

The metabolic clearance rate of aldosterone is approximately equal to liver blood flow,[101] and in several situations changes in the removal of aldosterone can contribute significantly to changes in the peripheral level. Tait et al.[102] showed that the plasma concentration of aldosterone may be raised in subjects with severe cardiac dysfunction in whom the secretion rate of aldosterone is normal. Vecsei et al.[52] found significant diminution of the clearance rate in cirrhosis and congestive cardiac failure, and increased clearance in some cases of severe chronic renal disease and renal hypertension. An increased clearance rate has been reported in hyperthyroidism, with diminished clearance in mxyedema.[103]

The metabolic clearance rate of aldosterone falls during the upright posture,[104] but this has been shown to play a minor role compared with increased secretion in determining the plasma level of aldosterone.[104]

Although evidence for direct physiologic control of aldosterone clearance is lacking, changes in the metabolic clearance rate may significantly influence the plasma concentration.

Other Factors

The assertion that an aldosterone-stimulating factor arises from the region of the pineal[105] has not been confirmed,[17, 106] and it appears that some of the observed effects were mediated by ACTH.

Using the transplanted sheep adrenal, Blair-West et al.[35] showed that direct intra-arterial infusions of lysine vasopressin, acetylcholine, bradykinin, norepinephrine, serotonin, oxytocin, and β-melanocyte-stimulating hormone have no more than minimal direct effects on aldosterone secretion. However, serotonin has been shown to stimulate aldosterone biosynthesis in vitro.[107] Calcium and magnesium appear to have little effect in vivo,[108] but the ammonium ion can augment aldosterone secretion.[108, 109]

Prostaglandin E_1 has recently been shown to have some inhibitory action on aldosterone biosynthesis when infused directly into the blood supply of the transplanted sheep adrenal,[110] but in the dog systemic infusions appear to produce water and electrolyte loss with stimulation of renin release.[111]

Growth hormone has been shown to maintain the aldosterone response to sodium restriction in hypophysectomized rats in the absence of the kidneys,[112] and in both man and dog there is some evidence that a pituitary factor other than ACTH is involved in aldosterone secretion.[76, 77]

CONCLUSION

No attempt has been made in this chapter to oversimplify the current status of aldosterone regulation. Despite the observed discrepancies between aldosterone secretion and its known regulating factors, the hypothesis that the renin-angiotensin system is an important determinant of aldosterone remains useful in most situations.

The salient points may be summarized:

1. While renin and angiotensin often correlate well with aldosterone, there are numerous discrepancies, most notably during the correction of sodium deficiency.
2. Potassium is an important determinant of aldosterone production, both as a primary stimulus and by its interaction with other mechanisms.
3. Physiologic variations in ACTH appear to be of minor importance but some other pituitary factor may be involved.
4. Important aldosterone-regulating mechanisms may so far be unrecognized. The search for such factors may be fruitful in patients with "primary" hyperaldosteronism due to a bilateral adrenal hyperplasia, during the offset of sodium deficiency, or in the rat where the role of the renin-angiotensin system is minimal.

REFERENCES

1. Luetscher, J. A., Johnson, B. B., Dowdy, A., Hanery, J., Lew, W., and Poo, L. J.: Observations on the sodium-retaining corticoid (aldosterone) in the urine of children and adults in relation to sodium balance and edema. J. Clin. Invest. 33:1441, 1954.
2. Simpson, S. A., Tait, J. F., Wettstein, A., Neher, R., Von Euw, J., Schindler, O., and Reichstein, T.: Aldosteron-Isolierung und Eigenschaften über Bestandteile der Nebennierenrinde und verwandte Stoffe. Helv. Chim. Acta 37:1163, 1954.
3. Vagnucci, A. H.: Selective aldosterone deficiency. J. Clin. Endocrinol. 29:279, 1969.
4. Kaplan, N. M.: The steroid content of adrenal adenomas and measurements of aldosterone production in patients with essential hypertension and primary aldosteronism. J. Clin. Invest. 46:728, 1967.
5. Ledingham, J. G. G., Bull, M. G., and Laragh, J. H.: The meaning of aldosteronism in hypertensive disease. Circ. Res. 20–21 (Suppl. II):II–177, 1967.
6. Fishman, L. M., Küchel, O., Liddle, G. W., Michelakis, A. M., Gordon, R. D., and Chick, W. T.: Incidence of primary aldosteronism in "essential" hypertension. JAMA 205:85, 1968.
7. Laragh, J. H., Ulick, S., Januszewicz, V., Deming, Q. B., Kelly, W. G., and Lieberman, S.: Aldosterone secretion in primary and malignant hypertension. J. Clin. Invest. 39:1091, 1960.
8. Collins, R. D., Weinberger, M. H., Dowdy, A. J., Nokes, W., Gonzales, C. M., and Luetscher, J. A.: Abnormally sustained aldosterone secretion during salt loading in patients with various forms of benign hypertension; relation to plasma renin activity. J. Clin. Invest. 49:1415, 1970.
9. Blair-West, J. R., Coghlan, J. P., and Denton, D. A.: Evidence against an aldosterone feedback mechanism within the adrenal gland. Acta Endocrinol. (Kbh) 41:61, 1962.
10. Geelhoed, G. W., and Vander, A. J.: The role of aldosterone in renin secretion. Life Sci. 6:525, 1967.
11. Müller, J.: Aldosterone stimulation in vitro. III. Site of action of different aldosterone-

stimulating substances on steroid biosynthesis. Acta Endocrinol. (Kbh) 52:515, 1966.

12. Blair-West, J. R., Brodie, A., Coghlan, J. P., Denton, D. A., Flood, C., Goding, J. R., Scoggins, B. A., Tait, J. F., Tait, S. A. S., Wintour, E. M., and Wright, R. D.: Studies on the biosynthesis of aldosterone using the sheep adrenal transplant: Effect of sodium depletion on the conversion of corticosterone to aldosterone. J. Endocrinol. 46:453, 1970.
13. Liddle, G. W., and Hardman, J. G.: Cyclic adenosine monophosphate as a mediator of hormone action. N. Engl. J. Med. 285:560, 1971.
14. Kaplan, N. M.: The biosynthesis of adrenal steroids: Effects of angiotensin II, adrenocorticotropin and potassium. J. Clin. Invest. 44:2029, 1965.
15. Müller, J.: Steroidogenic effect of stimulators of aldosterone biosynthesis upon separate zones of the rat adrenal cortex. Eur. J. Clin. Invest. 1:180, 1970.
16. Gláz, E., and Vecsei, P.: Aldosterone. International Series of Monographs in Pure and Applied Biology, vol. 6. Oxford: Pergamon Press, 1971.
17. Ganong, W. F., and Van Brunt, E. E.: Control of aldosterone secretion. *In* Eichler, O., Farah, A., Herken, H., and Welch, A. D. (Eds.): Handbook of Experimental Pharmacology, New Series, vol. XIV/3. Berlin: Springer, 1968, pp. 1–116.
18. Coghlan, J. P., and Blair-West, J. R.: Aldosterone. *In* Gray, C. H., and Bacharach, A. L. (Eds.): Hormones in Blood, vol. 2. New York: Academic Press, 1967, p. 391.
19. Coghlan, J. P., Blair-West, J. R., Denton, D. A., Scoggins, B. A., and Wright, R. D.: Perspectives in aldosterone and renin control. Aust. N. Z. J. Med. 2:178, 1971.
20. Boyd, G. W., and Peart, W. S.: The relationship between angiotensin and aldosterone. *In* Levine, R., and Luft, R. (Eds.): Advances in Metabolic Disorders, vol. 5. New York: Academic Press, 1971, p. 77.
21. Müller, J.: Regulation of Aldosterone Biosynthesis. Monographs on Endocrinology, vol. 5. Berlin: Springer, 1971.
22. Brown, J. J., Davies, D. L., Lever, A. F., and Robertson, J. I. S.: Plasma renin concentration in human hypertension. II. Renin in relation to aetiology. Br. Med. J. II:1215, 1965.
23. Catt, K. J., Cain, M. D., Coghlan, J. P., Zimmet, P. Z., Cran, E., and Best, J. B.: Metabolism and blood levels of angiotensin II in normal subjects, renal disease and essential hypertension. Circ. Res. 27(Suppl. II):II–177, 1970.
24. Gross, F.: Renin and Hypertensin: Physiologische oder pathologische Wirkstoffe. Klin. Wochenschr. 36:693, 1958.
25. Ganong, W. F., and Mulrow, P. J.: Evidence of secretion of an aldosterone-stimulating substance by the kidney. Nature 190: 1115, 1961.
26. Davis, J. O., Carpenter, C. C. J., Ayers, C. R., Holman, J. E., and Bahn, R. C.: Evidence for secretion of an aldosterone-stimulating hormone by the kidney. J. Clin. Invest. 40:684, 1961.
27. Davis, J. O., Ayers, C. R., and Carpenter, C. C. J.: Renal origin of an aldosterone-stimulating hormone in dogs with thoracic caval constriction and in sodium-depleted dogs. J. Clin. Invest. 40:1466, 1961.
28. Bayard, F., Cooke, C. R., Tiller, D. J., Beitins, I. Z., Kowarski, A., Walker, W. G., and Migeon, C. J.: The regulation of aldosterone secretion in anephric man. J. Clin. Invest. 50:1585, 1971.
29. Palmore, W. P., Marieb, N. J., and Mulrow, P. J.: Stimulation of aldosterone secretion by sodium depletion in nephrectomized rats. Endocrinology 84:1342, 1969.
30. Blair-West, J. R., Coghlan, J. P., Denton, D. A., Goding, J. R., Wintour, M., and Wright, R. D.: The effect of nephrectomy on aldosterone secretion in conscious sodium-depleted hypophysectomized sheep. Aust. J. Exp. Biol. Med. Sci. 46:295, 1968.
31. Lee, T. C., Biglieri, E. G., Van Brunt, E. E., and Ganong, W. F.: Inhibition of aldosterone secretion by passive transfer of anti-renin antibodies to dogs on a low sodium diet. Proc. Soc. Exp. Biol. 119:315, 1965.
32. Laragh, J. H., Angers, M., Kelly, W. G., and Lieberman, S.: Hypotensive agents and pressor substances. The effect of norepinephrine, angiotensin II and others on the secretory rate of aldosterone in man. JAMA 174:234, 1960.
33. Biron, P., Koiw, E., Nowaczynski, W., Brouillet, J., and Genest, J.: The effects of intravenous infusions of valine-5 angiotensin II and other pressor agents on urinary electrolytes and corticosteroids, including aldosterone. J. Clin. Invest. 40:338, 1961.
34. Ganong, W. F., Mulrow, P. J., Boryczka, A., and Cera, G.: Evidence for a direct effect of angiotensin II on the adrenal cortex of the dog. Proc. Soc. Exp. Biol. 109:381, 1962.

35. Blair-West, J. R., Coghlan, J. P., Denton, D. A., Goding, J. R., Munro, J. A., Peterson, R. E., and Wintour, M.: Humoral stimulation of adrenal cortical secretion. J. Clin. Invest. 41:1606, 1962.
36. Blair-West, J. R., Coghlan, J. P., Denton, D. A., Goding, J. R., Wintour, E. M., and Wright, R. D.: The control of aldosterone secretion. Recent Progr. Horm. Res. 19:311, 1963.
37. Ames, R. P., Borkowski, A. J., Sicinski, A. M., and Laragh, J. H.: Prolonged infusions of angiotensin II and norepinephrine and blood pressure, electrolyte balance, and aldosterone and cortisol secretion in normal man and in cirrhosis with ascites. J. Clin. Invest. 44:1171, 1965.
38. Urquhart, J., Davis, J. O., and Higgins, J. T.: Effects of prolonged infusions of angiotensin II in normal dogs. Am. J. Physiol. 205:1241, 1963.
39. Boyd, G. W., Adamson, A. R., Arnold, M., James, V. H. T., and Peart, W. S.: The role of angiotensin II in the control of aldosterone in man. Clin. Sci. 42:91, 1972.
40. Kaplan, N. M., and Silah, J. G.: The effect of angiotensin II on the blood pressure in humans with hypertensive disease. J. Clin. Invest. 43:659, 1964.
41. Ganong, W. F., Boryczka, A. T., and Shackleford, R.: Effect of renin on adrenocortical sensitivity to ACTH and angiotensin II in dogs. Endocrinology 80:703, 1967.
42. Blair-West, J. R., Coghlan, J. P., Denton, D. A., Scoggins, B. A., Wintour, M., and Wright, R. D.: Effect of change of sodium balance on the corticosteroid response to angiotensin II. Aust. J. Exp. Biol. Med. Sci. 48:253, 1970.
43. Marieb, N. J., and Murlow, P. J.: Role of the renin-angiotensin system in the regulation of aldosterone in the rat. Endocrinology 76:657, 1965.
44. Dufau, M. L., and Kliman, B.: Pharmacologic effects of angiotensin II amide on aldosterone and corticosterone secretion by the intact anesthetized rat. Endocrinology 82:29, 1968.
45. Michelakis, A. M., and Horton, R.: The relationship between plasma renin and aldosterone in normal man. Circ. Res. 27 (Suppl. I):I–185, 1970.
46. Slaton, P. E., Schambelan, M., and Biglieri, E. G.: Stimulation and suppression of aldosterone secretion in patients with an aldosterone-producing adenoma. J. Clin. Endocr. 29:239, 1969.
47. Conn, J. W., Cohen, E. L., and Rovner, D. R.: Suppression of plasma renin activity in primary aldosteronism: distinguishing primary from secondary aldosteronism in hypertensive disease. JAMA 190:213, 1964.
48. Brown, J. J., Fraser, R., Lever, A. F., Robertson, J. I. S., James, V. H. T., McCusker, J., and Wynn, V.: Renin, angiotensin, corticosteroids and electrolyte balance in Addison's disease. Q. J. Med. 37:97, 1968.
49. Lee, M. R.: Renin-secreting kidney tumours. Lancet II:254, 1971.
50. Fraser, R., James, V. H. T., Brown, J. J., Davies, D. L., Lever, A. F., and Robertson, J. I. S.: Changes in plasma aldosterone, cortisol, corticosterone and renin concentration in a patient with sodium-losing renal disease. J. Endocrinol. 35:311, 1966.
51. Imai, M., and Sokabe, H.: Plasma renin and angiotensinogen levels in pathological states associated with oedema. Arch. Dis. Child. 43:475, 1968.
52. Vecsei, P., Düsterdieck, G., Jahnecke, J., Lommer, D., and Wolff, H. P.: Secretion and turnover of aldosterone in various pathological states. Clin. Sci. 36:241, 1969.
53. Goodman, A. D., Vagnucci, A. H., and Hartroft, P. M.: Pathogenesis of Bartter's syndrome. N. Engl. J. Med. 281:1435, 1969.
54. McAllister, R. G., Van Way, C. W., Dayani, K., Anderson, W. J., Temple, E., Michelakis, A., Coppage, W. S., and Oates, J. A.: Malignant hypertension: Effect of therapy on renin and aldosterone. Circ. Res. 28–29 (Suppl. II):II–160, 1971.
55. Slater, J. D. H., Tuffley, R. E., Williams, E. S., Beresford, C. H., Sönksen, P. H., Edwards, R. H. T., Ekins, R. P., and McLaughlin, M.: Control of aldosterone secretion during acclimatization to hypoxia in man. Clin. Sci. 37:327, 1969.
56. Chinn, R. H., Brown, J. J., Fraser, R., Heron, S. M., Lever, A. F., Murchison, L., and Robertson, J. I. S.: The natriuresis of fasting: Relationships to changes in plasma renin and plasma aldosterone concentration. Clin. Sci. 39:437, 1970.
57. Cain, M. D., Catt, K. J., Coghlan, J. P., Blair-West, J. R., Denton, D. A., Funder, J. W., Scoggins, B. A., Stockigt, J. R., and Wright, R. D.: Further facets of aldosterone regulation. Proceedings of the Third International Congress on Hormonal Ste-

roids, International Congress Series No. 210. Hamburg, 1970. Amsterdam: Excerpta Medica, 1970, p. 42.

58. Blair-West, J. R., Cain, M. D., Catt, K. J., Coghlan, J. P., Denton, D. A., Funder, J. W., Scoggins, B. A., and Wright, R. D.: The dissociation of aldosterone secretion and systemic renin and angiotensin II levels during correction of sodium deficiency. Acta Endocrinol. (Kbh) 66:229, 1971.
59. Blair-West, J. R., Coghlan, J. P., Denton, D. A., Funder, J. W., Scoggins, B. A., and Wright, R. D.: The effect of adrenal arterial infusion of hypertonic $NaHCO_3$ solution on aldosterone secretion in sodium-deficient sheep. Acta Endocrinol. (Kbh) 66:448, 1971.
60. Blair-West, J. R., Cain, M., Catt, K. J., Coghlan, J. P., Denton, D. A., Funder, J. W., Scoggins, B. A., Wintour, M., and Wright, R. D.: The mode of control of aldosterone secretion. *In* Alwall, N., Berglund, F., and Josephson, B. (Eds.): Proceedings of the 4th International Congress of Nephrology, Stockholm. Basel: Karger, 1970.
61. Vander, A. J.: Control of renin release. Physiol. Rev. 47:359, 1967.
62. Nugent, C. A., Eik-Nes, K., Samuels, L. T., and Tyler, F.: Changes in plasma levels of 17-hydroxycorticosteroids during the intravenous administration of adrenocorticotropin. IV. Responses to prolonged infusions of small amounts of ACTH. J. Clin. Endocrinol. 19:334, 1959.
63. Berson, S. A., and Yalow, R. S.: Radioimmunoassoy of ACTH in plasma. J. Clin. Invest. 47:2725, 1968.
64. Jessiman, A. G., Matson, D. D., and Moore, F. D.: Hypophysectomy in the treatment of breast cancer. N. Engl. J. Med. 261:1199, 1959.
65. Davis, J. O., Yankopoulos, N. A., Kliman, B., and Peterson, R. E.: Acute effects of hypophysectomy and diencephalic lesions on aldosterone secretion. Am. J. Physiol. 197: 380, 1959.
66. Palmore, W. P., Anderson, R., and Mulrow, P. J.: Role of the pituitary in controlling aldosterone production in sodium depleted rats. Endocrinology 86:728, 1970.
67. Ganong, W. F., Biglieri, E. G., and Mulrow, P. J.: Mechanisms regulating adrenocortical secretion of aldosterone and glucocorticoids. Recent Progr. Horm. Res. 22:381, 1966.
68. Davis, J. O., Yankopoulos, N. A., Lieberman, F., Holman, J., and Bahn, R. C.: The role of the anterior pituitary in the control of aldosterone secretion in experimental secondary hyperaldosteronism. J. Clin. Invest. 39:765, 1960.
69. Lieberman, A. H., and Luetscher, J. A.: Some effects of abnormalities of pituitary, adrenal and thyroid function on excretion of aldosterone and the response to corticotropin or sodium deprivation. J. Clin. Endocrinol. 20:1004, 1960.
70. Ross, E. J., Van t'Hoff, W., Crabbe, J., and Thorn, G. W.: Aldosterone excretion in hypopituitarism and after hypophysectomy in man. Am. J. Med. 28:229, 1960.
71. Bethune, J. E., and Nelson, D. H.: Hyponatremia in hypopituitarism. N. Engl. J. Med. 272:771, 1965.
72. Agus, Z. S., and Goldberg, M.: Role of antidiuretic hormone in the abnormal water diuresis of anterior hypopituitarism in man. J. Clin. Invest. 50:1478, 1971.
73. Spark, R. F., Gordon, S. J., Dale, S. L., and Melby, J. C.: Aldosterone production after suppression of corticotropic secretory activity. Arch. Intern. Med. 122:394, 1968.
74. Newton, M. A., and Laragh, J. H.: Effects of glucocorticoid administration on aldosterone excretion and plasma renin in normal subjects, in essential hypertension and in primary aldosteronism. J. Clin. Endocrinol. 28:1014, 1968.
75. Thomas, J. P., and El-Shaboury, A. H.: Aldosterone secretion in steroid-treated patients with adrenal suppression. Lancet 1: 623, 1971.
76. Williams, G. H., Rose, L. I., Dluhy, R. G., Dingman, J. F., and Lauler, D. P.: Aldosterone response to sodium restriction and ACTH stimulation in panhypopituitarism. J. Clin. Endocr. 32:27, 1971.
77. Ganong, W. F., Pemberton, D. L., and Van Brunt, E. E.: Adrenocortical responsiveness to ACTH and angiotensin II in hypophysectomized dogs, and dogs treated with large doses of glucocorticoids. Endocrinology 81: 1147, 1967.
78. Ganong, W. F., Boryczka, A., Shackleford, R., Clark, R. N., and Converse, R. P.: Effect of dietary salt restriction on the adrenocortical response to ACTH. Proc. Soc. Exp. Biol. 118:792, 1965.
79. Williams, G. H., Dluhy, R. G., and Underwood, R. H.: The relationship of dietary potassium intake to the aldosterone stimulating properties of ACTH. Clin. Sci. 39: 489, 1970.

80. Newton, M. A., and Laragh, J. H.: Effect of corticotropin on aldosterone excretion and plasma renin in normal subjects, in essential hypertension and in primary aldosteronism. J. Clin. Endocrinol. 28:1006, 1968.
81. Biglieri, E. G., Schambelan, M., and Slaton, P. E.: Effect of adrenocorticotropin on desoxycorticosterone, corticosterone and aldosterone excretion. J. Clin. Endocrinol. 29:1090, 1969.
82. Vecsei, P., Farkas, K., Kemeny, V., and Harangozo, M.: Investigations on the mechanism of reduced aldosterone production caused by the administration of hydrocortisone. Steroids 5:415, 1965.
83. Burrow, G. N., Mulrow, P. J., and Bondy, P. K.: Protein synthesis and aldosterone production. Endocrinology 79:955, 1966.
84. Christy, N. P., and Laragh, J. H.: Pathogenesis of hypokalemic alkalosis in Cushing's syndrome. N. Engl. J. Med. 265:1083, 1961.
85. Biglieri, E. G., Hane, S., Slaton, P. E., and Forsham, P. H.: In vivo and in vitro studies of adrenal secretions in Cushing's syndrome and primary aldosteronism. J. Clin. Invest. 42:516, 1963.
86. Schambelan, M., Slaton, P. E., Jr., and Biglieri, E. G.: Mineralocorticoid production in hyperadrenocorticism: Role in pathogenesis of hypokalemic alkalosis. Am. J. Med. 51: 299, 1971.
87. Sutherland, D. J. A., Rose, J. L., and Laidlaw, J. C.: Hypertension, increased aldosterone secretion and low plasma renin activity relieved by dexamethasone. Can. Med. Assoc. J. 95:1109, 1966.
88. New, M. I., and Peterson, R. E.: A new form of congenital adrenal hyperplasia. J. Clin. Endocrinol. 27:300, 1967.
89. Mulrow, P. J., and Ganong, W. F.: Effect of simultaneous infusions of ACTH and angiotensin II upon aldosterone secretion of hypophysectomized nephrectomized dogs. Proc. Soc. Exp. Biol. 118:195, 1965.
90. Rayyis, S. S., and Horton, R.: Effect of angiotensin II on adrenal and pituitary function in man. J. Clin. Endocrinol. 32:539, 1971.
91. Boyd, J. E., Palmore, W. P., and Mulrow, P. J.: Role of potassium in the control of aldosterone secretion in the rat. Endocrinology 88:556, 1971.
92. Cannon, P. J., Ames, R. P., and Laragh, J. H.: Relation between potassium balance and aldosterone secretion in normal subjects and in patients with hypertensive and renal tubular disease. J. Clin. Invest. 45: 865, 1966.
93. Johnson, B. B., Lieberman, A. H., and Mulrow, P. J.: Aldosterone excretion in normal subjects depleted of sodium and potassium. J. Clin. Invest. 36:757, 1957.
94. Davis, J. O., Urquhart, J., and Higgins, J. T.: The effects of alterations of plasma sodium and potassium concentrations on aldosterone secretion. J. Clin. Invest. 42: 597, 1963.
95. Funder, J. W., Blair-West, J. R., Coghlan, J. P., Denton, D. A., Scoggins, B. A., and Wright, R. D.: Effect of plasma (K) on the secretion of aldosterone. Endocrinology 85: 381, 1969.
96. Vander, A. J.: Direct effects of potassium on renin secretion and renal function. Am. J. Physiol. 219:455, 1970.
97. Sealey, J. E., Clark, I., Bull, M. B., and Laragh, J. H.: Potassium balance and the control of renin secretion. J. Clin. Invest. 49:2119, 1970.
98. Baumber, J. S., Davis, J. O., Johnson, J. A., and Witty, R. T.: Increased adrenocortical potassium in association with increased biosynthesis of aldosterone. Am. J. Physiol. 220:1094, 1971.
99. Blair-West, J. R., Coghlan, J. P., Denton, D. A., Goding, J. R., Wintour, E. M., and Wright, R. D.: The direct effect of increased sodium concentration in adrenal arterial blood on corticosteroid secretion in sodium deficient sheep. Aust. J. Exp. Biol. Med. Sci. 44:455, 1966.
100. Bartter, F. C., Mills, I. H., Biglieri, E. G., and Delea, C.: Studies on the control and physiologic action of aldosterone. Recent Progr. Horm. Res. 15:311, 1959.
101. Tait, J. F., Little, B., Tait, S. A. S., and Flood, C.: The metabolic clearance rate of aldosterone in pregnant and non-pregnant subjects estimated by both single injection and constant-infusion methods. J. Clin. Invest. 41:2093, 1962.
102. Tait, J. F., Bougas, J., Little, B., Tait, S. A. S., and Flood, C.: Splanchnic extraction and clearance of aldosterone in subjects with minimal and marked cardiac dysfunction. J. Clin. Endocrinol. 25:219, 1965.
103. Luetscher, J. A., Cohn, A. P., Camargo, C. A., Dowdy, A. J., and Callaghan, A. M.: Aldosterone secretion and metabolism in hyperthyroidism and myxedema. J. Clin. Endocrinol. 23:873, 1963.

104. Balikian, H. M., Brodie, A. H., Dale, S. L., Melby, J., and Tait, J. F.: Effect of posture on the metabolic clearance rate, plasma concentration and blood production rate of aldosterone in man. J. Clin. Endocrinol. 28: 1630, 1968.
105. Farrell, G.: The physiological factors which influence the secretion of aldosterone. Rec. Progr. Horm. Res. 15:275, 1959.
106. Wurtman, R. J., Altschule, M. D., Greep, R. O., Falk, J. L., and Grave, G.: The pineal gland and aldosterone. Am. J. Physiol. 199: 1109, 1960.
107. Müller, J., and Ziegler, W. H.: Stimulation of aldosterone biosynthesis in vitro by serotonin. Acta Endocrinol. (Kbh) 59:23, 1968.
108. Blair-West, J. R., Coghlan, J. P., Denton, D. A., Goding, J. R., Wintour, M., and Wright, R. D.: The local action of ammonium, calcium and magnesium ions on adrenocortical secretion. Aust. J. Exp. Biol. Med. Sci. 46:371, 1968.
109. Müller, J.: Stimulation of aldosterone production in vitro by ammonium ions. Nature (London) 206:92, 1965.
110. Blair-West, J. R., Coghlan, J. P., Denton, D. A., Funder, J. W., Scoggins, B. A., and Wright, R. D.: Effects of prostaglandin E_1 upon the steroid secretion of the adrenal of the sodium-deficient sheep. Endocrinology 88:367, 1971.
111. Werning, C., Vetter, W., Weidman, P., Schweikert, H. U., Stiel, D., and Siegenthaler, W.: Effect of prostaglandin E_1 on renin in the dog. Am. J. Physiol. 220:852, 1971.
112. Palkovits, M., Strik, J., De Jong, W., and De Wied, D.: Effect of growth hormone on the aldosterone secretory response to sodium restriction in corticotropin-maintained hypophysectomized nephrectomized rats. J. Endocrinol. 51:369, 1971.

Classification of Hypermineralocorticoid Hypertension

By Jacques Genest, C.C., M.D., Otto Küchel, M.D., D.Sc., and Wojciech Nowaczynski, D.Sc.

Hypermineralocorticoid hypertension is defined as hypertension caused by overproduction of mineralocorticoid hormones. These hormones are so called because they exert their major effects on electrolytes by inducing sodium reabsorption at the level of the nephron, sweat, and salivary glands, and by promoting potassium excretion in varying degrees. They are in order of their decreasing potency: aldosterone, deoxycorticosterone (DOC), corticosterone, 11-deoxycortisol and 18-hydroxy-deoxycorticosterone (Fig. 1). In addition, several disturbances in the regulation of these hormones have been described in benign essential, malignant, true renovascular hypertension and in the severe hypertension seen in some patients with terminal renal failure. A classification of hypermineralocorticoid hypertension and of disturbances of mineralocorticoid hormones in other types of hypertension is described below:

I. Hypertension caused by overproduction of mineralocorticoid hormones:
   a. Primary aldosteronism (Conn's syndrome)
   b. 17α-Hydroxylase deficiency (Biglieri's syndrome)
   c. Hypertension form of virilizing adrenal hyperplasia (11β-hydroxylase deficiency)
   d. Cushing's disease or syndrome
   e. Nonendocrine ACTH-producing tumors
   f. Adrenocortical carcinoma
   g. Iatrogenic: anovulatory pills
      licorice
      glucocorticoids and excess salt intake

II. Hypertension apparently not caused by overproduction of mineralocorticoid hormones but with important features of hypermineralocorticoid disturbances:
   a. Malignant hypertension
   b. Hypertension in terminal renal failure
   c. True renovascular hypertension
   d. Benign essential hypertension

Hypertension Caused by Overproduction of Mineralocorticoid Hormones *

These types of hypertension are usually characterized by (1) suppressed plasma renin activity in the great majority of cases, secondary to the retention of sodium and the increase in total exchangeable sodium and in plasma volume and/or extracellular fluid volume; (2) hypokalemia and metabolic alkalosis in many cases; and (3) a high secretion rate of one or more mineralocorticoid hormones.

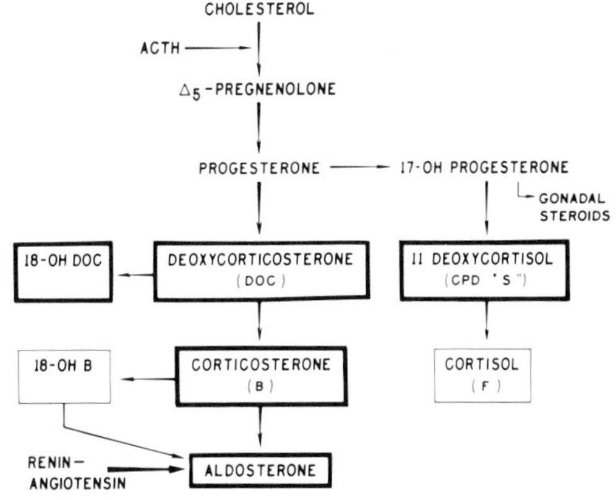

Fig. 1.—Simplified biosynthetic pathways of the mineralocorticoid hormones (in **heavy squares**).

From the Department of Medicine, University of Montreal Medical School, Montreal, Quebec, Canada.

* The reader interested in the detailed biochemical and radiological features of the hypertensive syndromes described is referred to the standard textbooks on endocrinology.

Primary Aldosteronism

This syndrome, described by Conn[1,2] in 1955, is characterized clinically by hypertension usually moderate in degree, persistent headaches, nocturia (despite an adequate renal function), and episodes of weakness of varying intensity. Biochemically it is accompanied by excessive secretion, excretion, and plasma concentration of aldosterone unaffected by administration of deoxycorticosterone[3] or of 9α-fluorohydrocortisone[4] or infusion of isotonic saline,[5–7] hypokalemic alkalosis, high serum sodium, increased plasma volume, decreased ability to concentrate urine, urinary potassium excretion above 30 to 35 mEq per day, and suppressed plasma renin activity unresponsive to the stimuli of upright posture and severe sodium restriction. Hypertensive patients complaining of headaches, fatigability, or asthenia and nocturia in the presence of a normal renal function should be suspected of having primary aldosteronism.

The incidence of hypokalemic primary aldosteronism varies between 0.3 to 0.5 percent of the hypertensive population and that of the normokalemic phase varies between 0.5 to about 3 percent,[8,9] although Conn has lately reported an incidence of 7 percent in his series of patients.[2]

Primary aldosteronism is usually caused by an adenoma of the adrenal cortex in about 80 to 85 percent of the cases. The diagnosis of the localization of the adenoma can be made (1) by adrenal vein catheterization for venography[10] and/or measurement of cortisol and aldosterone in adrenal venous plasma[11]; or (2) by scintillation scanning.[12,13] In the remaining 15 to 20 percent, it is caused by nodular hyperplasia of the adrenal cortex, sometimes restricted only to the zona glomerulosa.[14] Differential diagnosis between cortical nodular hyperplasia and adenoma can be made by the greater suppression of plasma renin concentration as measured by the angiotensin I generation rate and the more marked unresponsiveness of aldosterone to DOC administration in adenoma patients than in those with cortical hyperplasia[15] and even better by the multidimensional computer-assisted analysis developed by the Glasgow group.[16] When primary aldosteronism is associated with cortical nodular hyperplasia, it is responsive in some cases to the administration of glucocorticoids as demonstrated by Salti et al.[17]

In almost all cases, the syndrome can be corrected by the administration of spironolactone at high dosage (200 to 400 mg per day). These patients may also have excessive 18-hydroxycorticosterone secretion and excretion rates.

One of the most intriguing aspects of primary aldosteronism is the persistence of hypertension reported in about 40 percent of patients following surgical removal of an adenoma or more frequently following total or subtotal bilateral adrenalectomy for nodular hyperplasia.[18] The stimulus of the increased aldosterone secretion and of the cortical hyperplasia in the nonadenoma patient is unknown and the mechanism of this persisting hypertension is not understood.

17α-Hydroxylase Deficiency (Biglieri's Syndrome)

This syndrome[19] is seen in hypertensive women with primary amenorrhea, absence of axillary and pubic hair and of secondary sexual characteristics, with hypokalemic alkalosis and low or absent 17-hydroxycorticosteroids and 17-ketosteroids. In its pure form, it is caused by a deficiency in 17α-hydroxylase activity resulting in the almost exclusive production of deoxycorticosterone and corticosterone (Fig. 2). Urinary excretion of aldosterone, cortisol,

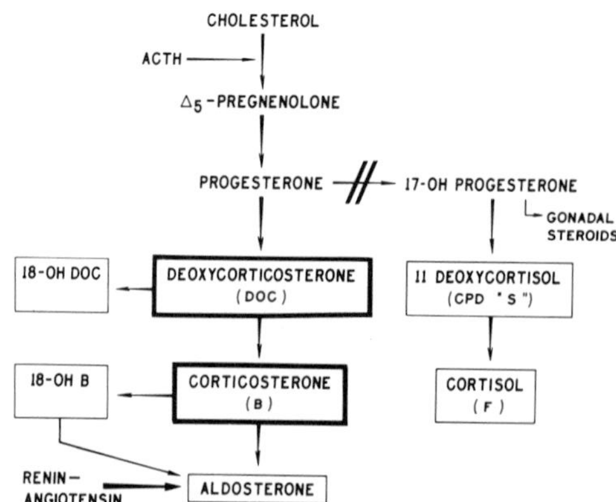

FIG. 2.—A complete deficiency in 17α-hydroxylase leads to almost exclusive overproduction of deoxycorticosterone and corticosterone (in **heavy squares**).

and gonadal steroids is absent or extremely low. Administration of small doses of dexamethasone controls this type of hypertension and corrects the biochemical abnormalities. Varieties of this syndrome with less complete 17α-hydroxylase deficiency have been described in patients with ovarian agenesis [20,20a] and it is believed that patients with Turner's syndrome and hypertension may belong to this broad category.

Hypertensive Form of Virilizing Adrenal Hyperplasia

This is a rare form [21] occurring in young girls with pseudohermaphroditism or in boys with precocious puberty and excessive virilization. It is caused, as first shown by Eberlein and Bongiovanni,[22] by a deficiency in 11β-hydroxylase activity resulting in a decreased production of cortisol and corticosterone (11-hydroxylated steroids) and oversecretion of deoxycorticosterone and 11-deoxycortisol up to 100 times normal (Fig. 3). Aldosterone secretion is low.[23–25] Administration of dexamethasone suppresses ACTH secretion and the overproduction of these two mineralocorticoids and corrects the hypertension and the electrolytes disturbances.

Cushing's Disease

Hypertension is found in about 85 percent of all patients with Cushing's disease, whether of adrenal, pituitary, or hypothalamic origin. It is associated either with an overproduction of deoxycorticosterone, corticosterone,[26] and rarely of aldosterone, or with the excessive intake of salt in the presence of high-cortisol secretion rate.

Nonendocrine ACTH-producing Tumors

The ACTH-like hormone produced by some tumors, mostly of pulmonary origin, provokes an increased secretion of cortisol, deoxycorticosterone, and corticosterone. This ectopic ACTH syndrome is frequently accompanied by many features of the Cushing's syndrome, although the hypokalemia is generally more severe and edema is frequent.[27] The incidence of hypertension in these patients is about the

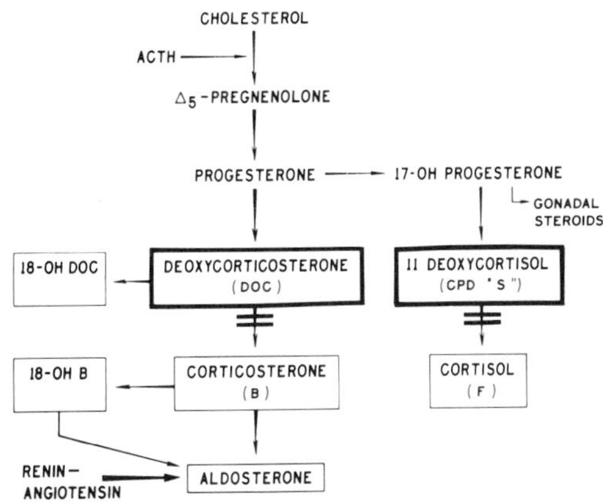

FIG. 3.—11β-Hydroxylase deficiency leads to greatly decreased or absent cortisol production (with resulting oversecretion of ACTH) and overproduction of deoxycorticosterone and 11-deoxycortisol (in **heavy squares**).

same as that seen in those with true Cushing's disease.

Adrenocortical Carcinoma

When hypertension is present in these cases, it is usually associated with the overproduction of one of the main mineralocorticoid hormones, e.g., deoxycorticosterone, corticosterone, and more rarely of aldosterone.[28–30]

Iatrogenic Hypertension

Although this type of hypertension is not secondary to the overproduction of mineralocorticoid hormones, it is usually included in the classification of hypermineralocorticoid hypertension.

It includes hypertension secondary to the administration of moderate to large doses of glucocorticoid hormones, such as prednisone or dexamethasone, to patients with chronic allergic, skin or arthritic disorders, and to those who ingest a disproportionately high amount of sodium in their diet. This hypertension usually responds well to the lowering of dietary sodium intake and/or administration of spironolactone.

Another form is hypertension secondary to the administration of oral contraceptives.[31–37] Depending on the series reported in the literature, this occurs in about 5 to 20 percent of women. It is accompanied by an important increase in plasma renin substrate caused by the estrogenic component, with subsequent increase in plasma renin activity and angiotensin II levels, although the plasma renin concentration itself is decreased. Aldosterone secretion and excretion are frequently increased.

Hypertension also occurs secondary to the chronic and excessive ingestion of licorice rich in ammonium glycyrrhizinate which has a marked mineralocorticoid-like activity. The amounts ingested vary usually from 2 to 5 gm of ammonium glycyrrhizinate equivalent to 20 to 45 gm of licorice extract.[38] Hypertension is accompanied by suppression of plasma renin activity and a decreased aldosterone secretion rate. Hypokalemic alkalosis and severe weakness with occasional paralysis are almost constant features. This syndrome is cured by cessation of licorice ingestion and can be corrected by the administration of spironolactone.[39]

Hypertension from Other Causes but with Important Features of Hypermineralocorticoid Disturbances

This more common form of hypertension is usually associated, except in benign essential hypertension, with a markedly increased activity of the renin-angiotensin system. Serum potassium is usually within the normal range, but can be found below normal levels, especially in patients with malignant hypertension and with true renovascular hypertension with excessive aldosterone secretion, clinically resembling primary aldosteronism.

A very rare form masquerading as hypermineralocorticoid hypertension has been described by Liddle, Bledsoe, and Coppage[40] as a familial renal disorder simulating primary aldosteronism, but with negligible aldosterone-secretion rates. These hypertensive patients present a hypokalemic alkalosis, hyperkaliuria, high salivary sodium:potassium ratio and low 17-hydroxycorticosteroid excretion. The syndrome is unaffected by the administration of spironolactone and stems from a renal defect of sodium conservation and potassium excretion in the virtual absence of aldosterone. It is cured by a low-sodium and high-potassium diet and by the administration of triamterene (Dyrenium).

Malignant Hypertension

It is frequently accompanied by high plasma renin and angiotensin II levels and excessive aldosterone secretion rates.

Hypertension in Terminal Renal Failure

Two forms exist, one that is water- and sodium-dependent and that can be corrected by dietary measures and by ultrafiltration during dialysis, and the second characterized by high plasma renin and angiotensin II levels, which can be corrected by bilateral total nephrectomy.

True Renovascular Hypertension

This type is almost always associated with excessive activity or responsiveness of the renin-angiotensin system[41,42] and is usually accompanied by either excessive aldosterone secretion or high plasma concentration secondary to the decreased metabolic clearance rate of aldosterone.[43]

Benign Essential Hypertension

A review of all the studies of plasma renin activity in patients with essential hypertension indicates that about 28 percent of patients have suppressed plasma renin activity with unresponsiveness to the stimuli of upright posture and severe sodium restriction. Many of these patients show excessive 18-hydroxy-deoxycorticosterone excretion as recently emphasized by Melby, Dale, and Wilson.[44] Other disturbances have also been reported, e.g., higher total exchangeable sodium[45]; increased extracellular fluid volume[46]; decreased salivary sodium:potassium ratio[47]; lack of response of aldosterone secretion or excretion to the stimulus of severe sodium restriction despite the activation of the renin system[48–50]; significant ($p < 0.05$) decrease in mean plasma corticosterone levels.[51]

Several workers believe that the findings of a suppressed plasma renin activity and of its unresponsiveness to the stimuli of upright posture and severe sodium restriction in patients with essential hypertension constitute presumptive evidence of hypermineralocorticoid hypertension.[52,53]

In addition, many important disturbances have also been described in patients with benign essential hypertension, whether their plasma renin activity was normal or suppressed and unresponsive to upright posture and sodium restriction and/or depletion. These disturbances include: a lack of aldosterone stimulation by severe sodium restriction or depletion and by hemorrhage,[50] or a lack of adequate suppression of aldosterone secretion, excretion, or plasma concentration by salt loads to the same degree as observed in normal subjects. In fact, Luetscher and his co-workers have shown that patients with essential hypertension receiving high oral salt loads (over 300 mEq per day) have aldosterone secretion and excretion rates and plasma concentrations about three times those of normal subjects.[54,55] On the other hand, Kem and co-workers found a similar suppression of plasma aldosterone levels in patients with essential hypertension and in normal subjects following the acute intravenous infusion of 290 mEq of sodium (2 liters of isotonic saline) in a 4-hour period [6]; increase in plasma aldosterone levels above the upper range of normal in one-third of patients with benign essential hypertension associated with (1) a significantly decreased metabolic clearance rate of aldosterone,[51,56–58] and (2) an altered ratio of the urinary excretion of aldosterone metabolites (the tetrahydro-aldosterone glucuronide being significantly decreased and the 18-oxo-conjugate increased); [51,58] (3) an increase in plasma progesterone levels above the upper range of normal in 45 percent of patients studied; [58,59] and (4) an increase in 18-hydroxy-deoxycorticosterone secretion rate in 65 percent of patients.[60]

Discussion

The above-mentioned hypermineralocorticoid hypertensive syndromes as well as the significant mineralocorticoid changes in patients with benign essential hypertension are all related to excessive sodium retention. In this respect, one must emphasize caution in the interpretation of measurements of total exchangeable sodium or total body sodium because of the marked variations in individual tissue contents of sodium, even within the arterial system,[61,62] and because of the possibility of significant changes occurring in one tissue without any change in the overall total body sodium content or total exchangeable sodium. The major point that must be resolved in this field is how the excessive sodium retention seen in these hypertensive patients leads to an increased tonicity of the arterial smooth-muscle actomyosin responsible for the increased peripheral resistance and hypertension.

The recent findings of increased plasma progesterone in about 45 percent of patients with benign, uncomplicated essential hypertension is of great interest because it may represent a homeostatic mechanism to protect the patient against the biochemical (mainly hypokalemia) and vascular effects of excessive hypermineralocorticoid secretion. It must be remembered that normal pregnant women do not show any of the biochemical effects of increased aldosterone secretion rate [63] and plasma concentration,[64] and have blood pressure readings within the normal range. It is possible that the rise in plasma progesterone prevents the hypokalemia in patients presenting either increased plasma aldosterone secondary to a reduced metabolic clearance rate or excessive 18-hydroxy-deoxycorticosterone secretion.

References

1. Conn, J. W., Knopf, R. F., and Nesbit, R. M.: Clinical characteristics of primary aldosteronism from an analysis of 145 cases. Am. J. Surg. 107:159, 1964.
2. Conn, J. W.: The evolution of primary aldosteronism 1954–1967. Harvey Lect. 62: 257, 1966–1967.
3. Biglieri, E. G., Slaton, P. E., Kronfield, S. J., and Schambelan, M.: Diagnosis of an aldosterone-producing adenoma in primary aldosteronism: An evaluative maneuver. JAMA 201:510, 1967.
4. Biglieri, E. G., Stockigt, J. R., and Schambelan, M.: A preliminary evaluation for primary aldosteronism. Arch. Intern. Med. 126: 1004, 1970.
5. Espiner, E. A., Tucci, J. R., Jagger, P. I., and Lauler, D. P.: Effect of saline infusions on aldosterone secretion and electrolyte excretion in normal subjects and patients with

primary aldosteronism. N. Engl. J. Med. 277:1, 1967.

6. Kem, D. C., Mayes, D., Weinberger, M., and Nugent, C. A.: Saline suppression of plasma aldosterone and plasma renin activity in hypertension. Ariz. Med. 28:264, 1971.
7. Kem, D. C., Mayes, D., and Nugent, C. A.: Saline suppression of plasma aldosterone and renin in hypertension. Program of the 52nd Meeting of the Endocrine Society, St. Louis, Missouri, June 1970.
8. Peart, W. S., Rovner, D. R., Kaplan, N. M., and Liddle, G. W.: The incidence of aldosteronism and early detection in the population. Panel discussion. Am. J. Clin. Pathol. 54:333, 1970.
9. Fishman, L. M., Kuchel, O., Liddle, G. W., Michelakis, A. M., Gordon, R. D., and Chick, W. T.: Incidence of primary aldosteronism in uncomplicated "essential" hypertension. A prospective study with elevated aldosterone secretion and suppressed plasma renin activity used as diagnostic criteria. JAMA 205: 497, 1968.
10. Conn, J. W., Rovner, D. R., Cohen, E. L., Bookstein, J. J., Cerny, J. C., and Lucas, C. P.: Preoperative diagnosis of primary aldosteronism. Including a comparison of operative findings and preoperative tumor localization by adrenal phlebography. Arch. Intern. Med. 123:113, 1969.
11. Melby, J. C., Spark, R. F., Dale, S. L., Egdahl, R. H., and Kahn, P. C.: Diagnosis and localization of aldosterone-producing adenomas by percutaneous bilateral adrenal vein catheterization. Progr. Clin. Cancer 4:175, 1970.
12. Conn, J. W., Beierwaltes, W. H., Lieberman, L. M., Ansari, A. N., Cohen, E. L., Bookstein, J. J., and Herwig, K. R.: Primary aldosteronism: Preoperative tumor visualization by scintillation scanning. J. Clin. Endocrinol. Metab. 33:713, 1971.
13. Conn, J. W., Morita, R., Cohen, E. L., Beierwaltes, W. H., McDonald, W. J., Ansari, A. N., and Herwig, K. R.: Photoscanning of tumors in primary aldosteronism: Possible distinction from "idiopathic" aldosteronism. *In* Genest, J., and Koiw, E. (Eds.): Hypertension 1972. Berlin: Springer, 1972, pp. 299–312.
14. Genest, J., Koiw, E., Beauregard, P., Nowaczynski, W., Sandor T., Brouillet, J., Bolté, E., Verdy, M., and Marc-Aurèle, J.: Electrolyte and corticosteroid studies in a 15-year-old girl with primary aldosteronism and malignant hypertension. Metabolism 9:624, 1960.
15. Stockigt, J. R., Collins, R. D., Noakes, C. A., and Biglieri, E. G.: Significance of precise determination of basal plasma renin in primary aldosteronism. J. Clin. Invest. 50:89a, 1971.
16. Ferris, J. B., Brown, J. J., Fraser, R., Kay, A. W., Neville, A. M., O'Muircheartaigh, I. G., Robertson, J. F. S., Symington, T., and Levera, A. F.: Hypertension with aldosterone excess and low plasma renin: Preoperative distinction between patients with and without adrenocortical tumor. Lancet 2:995, 1970.
17. Salti, I. S., Stiefel, M., Ruse, J. L., and Laidlaw, J. C.: Nontumorous "primary" aldosteronism: I. Type relieved by glucocorticoid (glucocorticoid-remediable aldosteronism). Can. Med. Assoc. J. 101:1, 1969.
18. Biglieri, E. G., Schambelan, M., Slaton, P. E., and Stockigt, J. R.: The intercurrent hypertension of primary aldosteronism. Circ. Res. 26–27(Suppl. I):I–195, 1970.
19. Biglieri, E. G., Herron, M. A., and Brust, N.: 17-Hydroxylation deficiency in man. J. Clin. Invest. 45:1946, 1966.
20. Hamet, P., Küchel, O., Nowaczynski, W., Rojo-Ortega, J. M., and Genest, J.: A new hypertensive syndrome. Ann. R. Coll. Phys. Surg. Can. 3:31, 1970.
20a. Kuchel, O., Hamet, P., Nowaczynski, W., Cadotte, M., and Genest, J.: Hypertension and hypogenitalism: Two new varieties of this clinical association. Ann. Intern. Med. 72:788, 1970.
21. Eberlein, W. R., and Bongiovanni, A. M.: Congenital adrenal hyperplasia with hypertension: Unusual steroid pattern in blood and urine. J. Clin. Endocrinol. 15:1531, 1955.
22. Eberlein, W. R., and Bongiovanni, A. M.: Plasma and urinary corticosteroids in the hypertensive form of congenital adrenal hyperplasia. J. Biol. Chem. 223:85, 1956.
23. New, M. I., and Seaman, M. P.: Secretion rates of cortisol and aldosterone precursors in various forms of congenital adrenal hyperplasia. J. Clin. Endocrinol. 30:361, 1970.
24. Kowarski, A., Russell, A., and Migeon, C. J.: Aldosterone secretion rate in the hypertensive form of congenital adrenal hyperplasia. J. Clin. Endocrinol. 28:1445, 1968.
25. New, M. I., Miller, B., and Peterson, R. E.: Aldosterone excretion in normal children and

in children with adrenal hyperplasia. J. Clin. Invest. 45:412, 1966.

26. Biglieri, E. G., Slaton, P. E., Schambelan, M., and Kronfield, S. J.: Hypermineralocorticoidism. Am. J. Med. 45:170, 1968.
27. Liddle, G. W:. Cushing's syndrome. *In* Eisenstein, A. B. (Ed.): The Adrenal Cortex. Boston: Little, Brown, 1967, p. 523–551.
28. Crane, M. G., and Harris, J. J.: Desoxycorticosterone secretion rates in hyperadrenocorticism. J. Clin. Endocrinol. 26:1135, 1966.
29. Cost, W. S.: A mineralocorticoid excess syndrome presumably due to excessive secretion of corticosterone. Lancet 1:362, 1963.
30. West, C. D., Kumagai, L. F., Simons, E. L., Dominguez, O. V., and Berliner, D. L.: Adrenocortical carcinoma with feminization and hypertension associated with a defect in 11β-hydroxylation. J. Clin. Endocrinol. 24: 567, 1964.
31. Saruta, J., Saade, G. A., and Kaplan, N. M.: A possible mechanism for hypertension induced by oral contraceptives. Diminished feedback suppression of renin release. Arch. Intern. Med. 126:621, 1970.
32. Laragh, J. H., Sealey, J. E., Ledingham, J. G. G., and Newton, M. A.: Oral contraceptives: Renin, aldosterone and high blood pressure. JAMA 201:918, 1967.
33. Woods, J. W.: Oral contraceptives and hypertension. Lancet 2:653, 1967.
34. Weinberger, M. H., Collins, R. D., Dowdy, A. J., Nokes, G. W., and Luetscher, J. A.: Hypertension induced by oral contraceptives containing estrogen and gestagen: Effects of plasma renin activity and aldosterone excretion. Ann. Intern. Med. 71:891, 1969.
35. Helmer, O. M., and Griffith, R. S.: The effect of the administration of estrogens on the renin-substrate (hypertension) content of rat plasma. Endocrinology 51:421, 1952.
36. Crane, M. G., and Harris, J. J.: Plasma renin activity and aldosterone excretion rate in normal subjects. I. Effect of ethinyl estradiol and medroxyprogesterone acetate. J. Clin. Endocrinol. 29:550, 1969.
37. Cain, M. D., Walters, W. A., and Catt, K. J.: Effects of oral contraceptive therapy on the renin-angiotensin system. J. Clin. Endocrinol. 33:671, 1971.
38. Fournier, A., and Lagrue, G.: Les hypertensions par hyperminéralocorticisme. Sem. Hop. Paris 47:872, 1971.
39. Conn, J. W., Rovner, D. R., and Cohen, E. L.: Licorice-induced pseudoaldosteronism. Hypertension, hypokalemia, aldosteronopenia, and suppressed plasma renin activity. JAMA 205:492, 1968.
40. Liddle, G. W., Bledsoe, T., and Coppage, W. S., Jr.: A familial renal disorder simulating primary aldosteronism but with negligible aldosterone secretion. *In* Bauliey, E. E., and Robel, P. (Eds.): Aldosterone, a Symposium. Oxford: Blackwell, 1964, p. 353.
41. Genest, J., Tremblay, G. Y., Boucher, R., de Champlain, J., Rojo-Ortega, J. M., Lefebure, R., Roy, P., and Cartier, P.: Diagnostic significance of humoral factors in renovascular hypertension. *In* Gross, F. (Ed.): Antihypertensive Therapy (Principles and Practice). Heidelberg: Springer, 1966, pp. 518–540.
42. Genest, J.: The renin-angiotensin-aldosterone system. *In* Brest, A. N., and Moyer, J. H.: Cardiovascular Disorders. Philadelphia: Davis, 1968, pp. 144–160.
43. Kaufmann, W., Steiner, B., Dürr, F., Nieth, H., and Behn, C.: Aldosteronstofewechsel bei Nierenarterienstenose. Klin. Wochenschr. 19:966, 1967.
44. Melby, J. C., Dale, S. L., and Wilson, T. E.: 18-Hydroxy-deoxycorticosterone in human hypertension. Circ. Res. 28–29(Suppl. II):II–143, 1971.
45. Woods, J. W., Liddle, G. W., Stant, E. G., Jr., Michelakis, A. M., and Brill, A. B.: Effect of an adrenal inhibitor in hypertensive patients with suppressed renin. Arch. Intern. Med. 123:366, 1969.
46. Jose, A., and Kaplan, N. M.: Plasma renin activity in the diagnosis of primary aldosteronism. Failure to distinguish primary aldosteronism from essential hypertension. Arch. Intern. Med. 123:141, 1969.
47. Adlin, E. V., Channick, B. J., and Marks, A. D.: Salivary sodium-potassium ratio and plasma renin activity in hypertension. Circulation 39:685, 1969.
48. Helmer, O. M., and Judson, W. E.: Metabolic studies on hypertensive patients with suppressed plasma renin activity not due to hyperaldosteronism. Circulation 38:965, 1968.
49. Streeten, D. H. P., Schletter, F. E., Clift, C. V., Stevenson, C. T., and Dalakos, T. G.: Studies of the renin-angiotensin-aldosterone system in patients with hypertension and in normal subjects. Am. J. Med. 46:844, 1969.
50. Williams, G. H., Rose, L. I., Dluhy, R. G., McCaughn, D., Jagger, P. I., Hickler, R. B., and Lauler, D. P.: Abnormal responsiveness of the renin aldosterone system to acute

stimulation in patients with essential hypertension. Ann. Intern. Med. 72:317, 1970.

51. Nowaczynski, W., Kuchel, O., and Genest, J.: Aldosterone, deoxycorticosterone, and corticosterone metabolism in benign essential hypertension. *In* Genest, J., and Koiw, E. (Eds.): Hypertension 1972. Berlin: Springer, 1972, pp. 244–245.

52. Gunnels, J. C., McGuffin, W. L., Jr., Robinson, R. R., Grim, C. E., Wells, S., Silver, D., and Glenn, J. F.: Hypertension, adrenal abnormalities, and alterations in plasma renin activity. Ann. Intern. Med. 73:901, 1970.

53. Spark, R. F., and Melby, J. C.: Hypertension and low plasma renin activity: Presumptive evidence for mineralocorticoid excess. Ann. Intern. Med. 74:833, 1971.

54. Luetscher, J. A., Weinberger, M. H., Dowdy, A. J., Nokes, G. W., Balikian, H., Brodie, A., and Willoughby, S.: Effects of sodium loading, sodium depletion and posture on plasma aldosterone concentration and renin activity in hypertensive patients. J. Clin. Endocrinol. 29:1310, 1969.

55. Collins, R. D., Weinberger, M. H., Dowdy, A. J., Nokes, G. W., Gonzales, C. M., and Luetscher, J. A.: Abnormally sustained aldosterone secretion during salt loading in patients with various forms of benign hypertension; relation to plasma renin activity. J. Clin. Invest. 49:1415, 1970.

56. Genest, J., and Nowaczynski, W.: Aldosterone and electrolyte balance in human hypertension. J. R. Coll. Physicians Lond. 5: 77, 1970.

57. Nowaczynski, W., Kuchel, O., and Genest, J.: A decreased metabolic clearance rate of aldosterone in benign essential hypertension. J. Clin. Invest. 50:2184, 1971.

58. Genest, J., Nowaczynski, W., and Kuchel, O.: New evidences of disturbances of mineralocorticoid activity in benign, uncomplicated essential hypertension. Am. Clin. Climat. Assoc. 83:134, 1972.

59. Genest, J., Nowaczynski, W., Kuchel, O., and Sasaki, C.: Plasma progesterone levels and 18-hydroxydeoxycorticosterone secretion rate in benign essential hypertension in humans. *In* Genest, J., and Koiw, E. (Eds.): Hypertension 1972. Berlin: Springer, 1972, pp. 293–298.

60. Kuchel, O., Nowaczynski, W., and Genest, J.: Discussion of Melby's paper (see Ref. 44): 18-Hydroxydeoxycorticosterone secretion rates in patients with benign essential hypertension. Circ. Res. 28–29(Suppl. II):II–150, 1971.

61. Hayduk, K., Boucher, R., and Genest, J.: Renin activity content in various tissues of dogs under different physiopathological states. Proc. Soc. Exp. Biol. Med. 134:252, 1970.

62. Hayduk, K., Ganten, D., Boucher, R., and Genest, J.: Arterial and urinary renin activity. *In* Genest, J., and Koiw, E. (Eds.): Hypertension 1972. Berlin: Springer, 1972, pp. 435–443.

63. Watanabe, M., Meeker, C. I., Gray, M. J., Sims, E. A. H., and Solomon, S.: Secretion rate of aldosterone in normal pregnancy. J. Clin. Invest. 42:1619, 1963.

64. Weir, R. J., Paintin, D. B., Brown, J. J., Fraser, R. F., Lever, A. F., Robertson, J. I. S., and Young, I.: A serial study in pregnancy of the plasma concentrations of renin, corticosteroids, electrolytes and proteins: and of hematocrit and plasma volume. J. Obstet. Gynaecol. Br. Commonw. 78:590, 1971.

An Overall View of Primary Aldosteronism

By Jerome W. Conn, M.D.

IN 1954 [1,2] WE DESCRIBED a fascinating new clinical syndrome which we named "primary aldosteronism." The condition is produced by the presence of an aldosterone-secreting adrenocortical adenoma (rarely carcinoma), surgical removal of which results in complete reversal of the entire syndrome. The major clinical features consist of arterial hypertension (average 200/110 mm Hg), and in the most severe cases the hypertension is associated with hypokalemia, hypernatremia, alkalosis, and occasionally hypomagnesemia. Cortisol production is normal but aldosterone secretion and excretion are abnormally elevated. In the severe cases the symptomatology represents merely an expression of the biochemical abnormàlities already mentioned and consists of periodic muscular weakness, episodic tetanic manifestations, nocturnal polyuria, and severe headache. Characteristically edema is absent and hemorrhagic retinopathy *with papilledema* is extremely rare although the milder forms of retinopathy are frequently observed.

From 1954 to 1964 the alerting signal for the possible presence of this syndrome was the coexistence of hypertension and hypokalemia. And on this basis alone thousands of people have been cured of hypertension and the volume of cases detected has increased greatly with each succeding year. Because hypokalemia had become the *sine qua non* of this syndrome, many clinics were screening their hypertensive patients by obtaining values for serum potassium. By 1960 [3] it became apparent that a large number of hypertensive patients had coexisting hypokalemia together with overproduction of aldosterone, but not all of them had primary aldosteronism. Patients with malignant hypertension and with renovascular hypertension were shown to have a newly recognized form of secondary aldosteronism (without edema) associated with hypertension. The demonstration, independently, by both Genest [4] and Laragh,[5] that infusion of angiotensin II in man increased adrenal production of aldosterone, closed the gap in our knowledge. The renin-angiotensin-aldosterone system was thus born and an explanation for secondary aldosteronism in ischemic renal disease became evident. But it also became clear that hypertension, hypokalemia, and overproduction of aldosterone could be produced either by an aldosterone-producing adrenal adenoma or by some forms of renal hypertension.

In 1964 [6] we reported that in primary aldosteronism plasma renin activity is subnormal and that, in the presence of overproduction of aldosterone, this measurement could make the distinction between primary aldosteronism and those forms of secondary aldosteronism produced by renal blood flow abnormalities. In the latter group plasma renin activity is supernormal. These observations have been confirmed repeatedly and the determination of plasma renin activity has become most useful both in the distinction between, and in the diagnosis of, primary aldosteronism and renovascular hypertension. Thus, as we had indicated in 1964, if, in a hypokalemic hypertensive patient with overproduction of aldosterone and normal cortisol production, plasma renin activity can be shown to be subnormal, the diagnosis of primary aldosteronism is established and renal hypertension associated with secondary aldosteronism is ruled out (exceptions are discussed below).

The Detection of Primary Aldosteronism in the Presence of Normal Serum Potassium Levels

In the course of a large experience with primary aldosteronism between 1954 and 1964, it became clear that, even in severely hypokalemic cases, hypertension had preceded hypo-

---

From the Department of Endocrinology and Metablolism and the Metabolism Research Unit, University of Michigan Medical School, Ann Arbor, Michigan.

Supported in part by USPHS Grant AM–10257; USPHS Training Grant AM–05001; 5M01–FR–4204, Division of Research Facilities and Resources.

kalemia by many years. Yet the hypertension and the hypokalemia were corrected by removal of the adrenocortical adenoma. We concluded that a slow-growing adrenal adenoma had been present for many years; that it was the original cause of the hypertension; and that a long period of normokalemic primary aldosteronism had preceded the development of hypokalemia. We had also observed what we called "transitional cases" in which only intermittent hypokalemia occurred. Some of these cases progressed with time to a persistently hypokalemic state. We, therefore, set out deliberately to see if we could detect primary aldosteronism in hypertensive patients before hypokalemia became evident. Our experience with plasma renin activity determinations in the hypokalemic patients indicated that this measurement was subnormal in every proved case. We, thus, had a new exploratory tool in our search for normokalemic primary aldosteronism. If we could find a normokalemic hypertensive patient with overproduction of aldosterone, normal cortisol production, and subnormal plasma renin activity, the chances would be very great that he harbored an aldosterone-producing adrenocortical adenoma. In 1965 we [7] reported the first such case. This patient has now been normotensive for more than 6 years. His left adrenal gland contained two 5-mm aldosterone-producing adenomas and a unilateral adrenalectomy was performed. Preoperatively aldosterone excretion had been four times higher than normal, cortisol production was normal, and no renin activity at all could be detected in his plasma under conditions of sodium restriction followed by 4 hours of upright posture—conditions which, in normal people, result in very high levels of plasma renin activity. After his operation aldosterone production became subnormal and gradually returned to normal over a period of months. This phenomenon of an extremely rapid fall of aldosterone production to subnormal levels in the immediate postoperative period constitutes additional evidence that an aldosterone-producing tumor has been removed,[8] and it occurs in virtually all patients who are eventually cured by the operation. Since then we have been able to prove the existence of normokalemic primary aldosteronism in 28 more patients. Our current figures [9] indicate an incidence of 8 percent for normokalemic primary aldosteronism among hospitalized patients with essential hypertension but a final figure for the prevalence of this disease in essential hypertension is not yet available. The laborious task of screening large numbers of hypertensive patients with aldosterone and renin determinations has limited this research. However, rapid advances have been made during the past 2 years on methods and we now have radioimmunoassay procedures for plasma and urinary aldosterone and for plasma angiotensin I and angiotensin II. Within a relatively short time these tools will become available to practicing physicians so that, on a practical basis, they can screen their hypertensive patients for the possibility of primary aldosteronism.

The Spectrum of Primary Aldosteronism and Its Clinical Classification

From what has already been said, primary aldosteronism can be regarded as a continuum which, at one end of the scale, is indistinguishable from essential hypertension (except by renin and aldosterone measurements), and at the other consists of the classic manifestations as originally described. Between these two extremes are the cases that have various degrees of intermittent hypokalemia. We now classify primary aldosteronism into three main subgroups:

1. Persistently hypokalemic cases. Usually these are the most severe cases.
2. Intermittently hypokalemic cases. These are usually moderately severe.
3. Persistently normokalemic cases. These are usually the mildest cases.

There is, however, some overlapping between these groups. A given patient with intermittent hypokalemia may be periodically normokalemic or hypokalemic. This may have to do with the known variability from time to time of aldosterone secretion by such tumors, as well as to alterations in sodium and potassium intake from time to time.

The following summarizes our experience with 95 surgically explored patients, all of whom exhibited what we believe to be the most crucial diagnostic criteria, namely, overproduction of aldosterone, subnormal plasma renin activity, and normal cortisol production. Of the 95 patients, 82 (86%) proved to have primary aldosteronism (tumor) and 13 (14%) had bilateral hyperplasia which we now classify as "idiopathic" aldosteronism (see section entitled "Pathologic Classification"). At the present time there are no crucial distinguishing characteristics which can separate these cases preoperatively.

In the tumor group (Fig. 1) aldosterone excretion ranged from 17 to 525 μg per day. All patients with aldosterone excretion rates higher than 55 μg per day were persistently hypokalemic. Patients with aldosterone excretion rates between 17 and 55 μg per day fell into three groups: (1) persistently hypokalemic, (2) intermittently hypokalemic, and (3) normokalemic. The 29 normokalemic patients had aldosterone excretion rates between 22 and 55 μg per day. Plasma renin activity was subnormal in all patients, whether they were hypokalemic or not. In the range of aldosterone excretion rates between 22 and 55 μg per day, the degree of suppression of plasma renin activity was similar for hypokalemic and normokalemic patients. When aldosterone excretion exceeded 55 μg per day, suppression of plasma renin activity was more intense.

The development in our laboratory [10] of a very sensitive radioimmunoassay for angiotensin I has allowed us to measure plasma renin activity accurately at very low levels. When this assay is used (Table 1) it is evident that under all conditions studied there is a wide separation between normal people and patients with proved aldosterone-producing tumors. The point of greatest distinction between the two groups is observed when the blood specimen is drawn after 2 hours of ambulation (U) following 3 days of sodium restriction. These are the conditions that we have been employing since 1964.

At the bottom of Table 1 are given plasma renin activity values for four patients who, at operation, disclosed bilateral adrenal hyperplasia without tumor. All had exhibited overproduction of aldosterone, as had the tumor patients. It is of interest that three of the four patients were able to raise their plasma renin activity (10 mEq of sodium and upright pos-

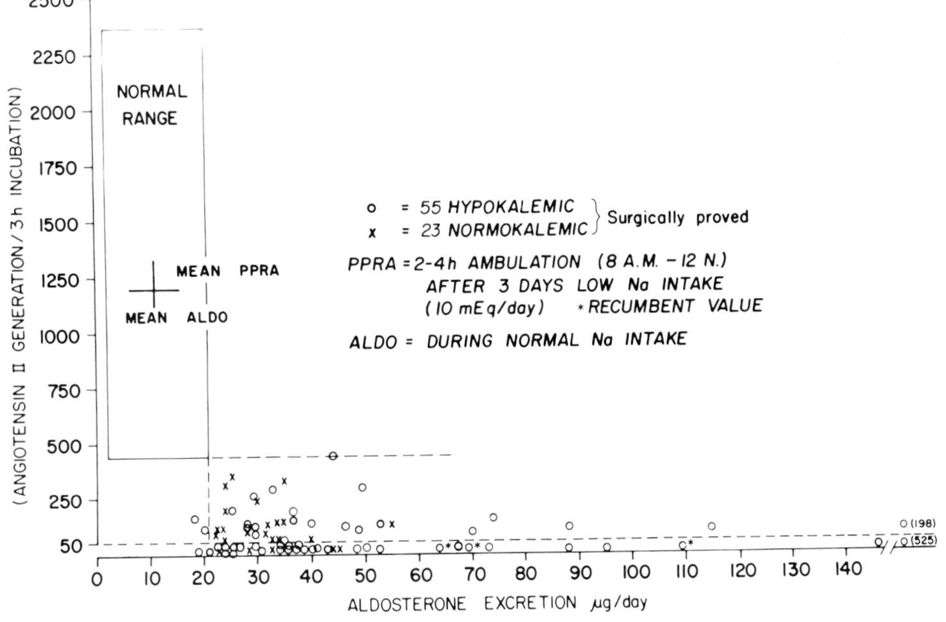

FIG. 1.—Relation between peripheral plasma renin activity **(PPRA)** (bioassay) and aldosterone excretion **(ALDO)** in 78 hypokalemic and normokalemic patients with primary aldosteronism.

TABLE 1.—*Plasma Renin Activity by Radioimmunoassay for Angiotensin I in 18 Patients with Primary Aldosteronism (Tumor) and 4 Patients with "Idiopathic" Aldosteronism (Bilateral Hyperplasia)*

	Normal People				*Primary and "Idiopathic" Aldosteronism*			
Diet	*120 mEq Sodium*		*10 mEq Sodium*		*120 mEq Sodium*		*10 mEq Sodium*	
Posture	*R*	*U*	*R*	*U*	*R*	*U*	*R*	*U*
					Primary (tumor)			
	2.0	17.2	6.6	45.8	.09	1.01		
	1.7	7.6	4.9	13.8	.19	.99	.22	.61
	2.6	10.8	7.2	22.1	.22	.25		.43
	2.2	5.7	6.8	16.6	.30	.34	.18	.46
	1.5	5.7	6.2	9.7	.23	.49		
	3.0	10.9	10.8	24.8	.45	1.10		
		2.7		10.5	.16	.46	.19	.52
		12.2		23.5		.50		
		5.5		19.0		.40		
		3.9		8.2		1.00		1.20
		3.8		9.8		.12		.50
		6.0		37.2		.20		.28
		1.9		6.8		.28		.28
		1.6		6.8		.30		
		15.3		18.8		.15		
		11.3		27.9		1.00		1.40
		4.7		7.0		2.00		
		8.4		11.5		.50		.40
		6.3		16.8				
		10.2		9.7				
Mean ± SEM	2.5 ± .5	7.7 ± 1.0	7.1 ± .8	17.2 ± 2.2	.23 ± .04	.62 ± .11	.20 ± .01	.60 ± .12
					"Idiopathic" (hyperplasia)			
						4.0		5.1
						.20		.60
						1.8		3.2
						1.3		2.3
					Mean ± SEM	1.8 ± .8		2.8 ± .9

Abbreviations used: R, recumbent; U, upright.

ture) higher than any of the tumor patients could, although their values were still subnormal. Thus, although there will be some overlapping, *mild* suppression of plasma renin activity in the presence of overproduction of aldosterone should alert one to the possibility that he may be dealing with "idiopathic" aldosteronism.

The factors which allow some patients to remain normokalemic while others become hypokalemic at similar levels of aldosterone excretion and plasma renin activity (Fig. 1) are not clear. But it is likely that they involve the duration of aldosteronism, the accustomed or acquired level of potassium and sodium intake by the individual patient, and the sex cf the patient.

Mention should be made now of a rare situation [11] in which hypertension and hypokalemia coexist with overproduction of aldosterone, subnormal plasma renin activity, and normal cortisol production. In the two patients described, administration of 1 mg of dexamethasone per day resulted in normalization of all of the abnormalities within 10 days. We have attempted this procedure in many of the patients described above but have not yet encountered one such as Laidlaw's. While the two patients described are well documented (a father and son), we conclude that this must be a very rare situation, indeed. One of these patients was explored surgically and found to have bilateral adrenocortical hyperplasia.

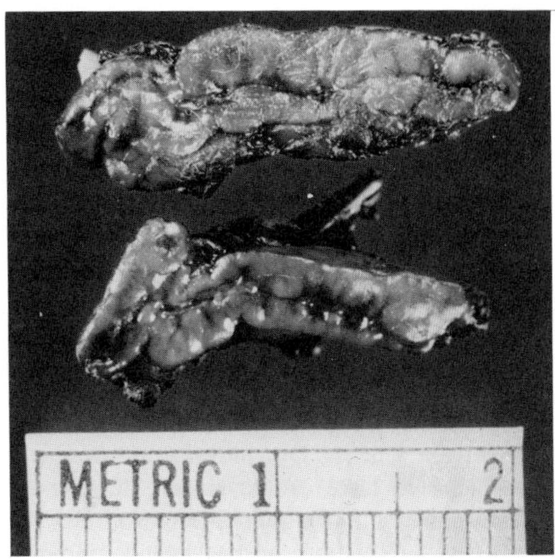

FIG. 3.—Macronodular hyperplasia from a patient with "idiopathic" aldosteronism.

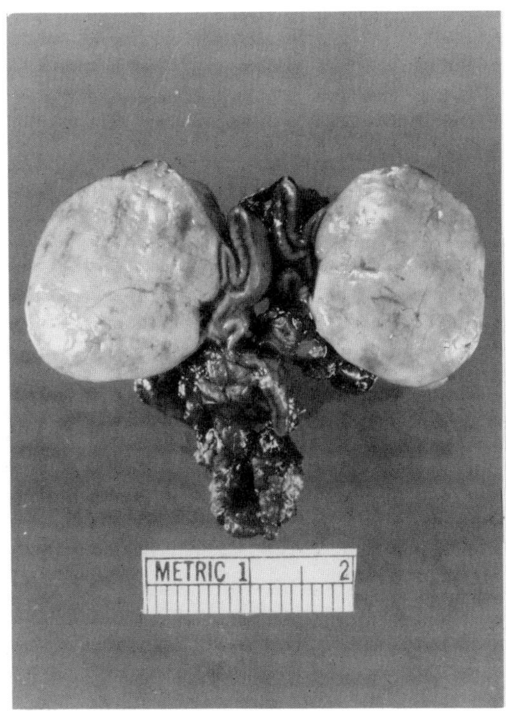

FIG. 2.—Typical aldosterone-producing tumor.

PATHOLOGIC CLASSIFICATION

As stated above, it is not possible to distinguish with precision preoperatively those patients who will be found to have an adenoma at operation from those who will show bilateral adrenocortical hyperplasia, but we have recently reported suggestive progress in this area.[12] Both groups satisfy the preoperative diagnostic criteria that we have stressed above as being diagnostic of primary aldosteronism. Our own experience with 95 patients is as follows: 82 cases (86%) have had tumors (Fig. 2), and 13 (14%) have had micronodular or macronodular hyperplasia (Fig. 3). It is claimed that subtotal or total adrenalectomy in the patients with bilateral adrenal hyperplasia does not result in normalization of blood pressure, as occurs when an adenoma is removed (75 to 80%). Our own experience, however, indicates that this group responds to total or subtotal adrenalectomy just about as well as do patients with primary aldosteronism whose tumors have been removed.

We have reported [13] on successful visualization of small cortical adenomas by selective adrenal venography (Fig. 4) in over 80 percent of patients; Melby et al.[14] have been successful in predicting the site of a tumor by measuring the aldosterone concentration of adrenal venous blood obtained by catheter from each adrenal vein. These techniques help to distinguish tumor from bilateral hyperplasia but they are technically difficult, carry a small risk of adrenal medullary hemorrhage, and are not 100-percent reliable. Our more recent studies [12] in which we have employed an intravenous injection of ^{131}I-19-iodocholesterol, followed by photoscanning of both adrenal glands, indicate that small tumors can be detected by this simple technique (Fig. 5), and suggest that it may be possible to make the preoperative distinction between those patients with bilateral hyperplasia and those with tumor. When this can be accomplished preoperatively with certainty, we will favor surgery for the tumor patient and treatment with spironolactone for the hyperplasia patient, pending clarification of the pathogenesis of this form of hyperplasia.

It is our opinion that, at the present time, the term "primary aldosteronism" should be reserved for those patients subsequently proved to harbor an aldosterone-secreting tumor. The pathophysiology involved in the patients showing bilateral hyperplasia is unclear. If it should eventually be shown that it is the result of a diffuse lesion which is primary in both adrenal glands, one would be justified in classifying it as primary aldosteronism associated with bilateral hyperplasia. If, on the other hand, the bilateral hyperplasia is the result of an, as yet, unknown extra-adrenal stimulus for aldosterone production, the abnormality should be classified as a secondary form of aldosteronism. However, since the nature of the lesion remains unknown, we prefer to classify this form of aldosteronism as "idiopathic" until the situation becomes clarified.

From the above discussion it should be clear that the preoperative diagnosis of the bilateral hyperplasia patients will most likely be primary aldosteronism and that, when no tumor materializes at operation, it will then be classified as idiopathic aldosteronism with bilateral hyperplasia. Once surgery has been embarked upon it would seem wise to carry out a total or subtotal adrenalectomy when bilateral hyperplasia is found. As noted above, when the preoperative diagnosis will be able to be made, we will consider treatment with spironolactone to be preferable pending clarification of the pathophysiology of the condition. Much more information is needed in the area of structure-function relationships in those cases which exhibit diffuse bilateral nodular hyperplasia.

The Pathophysiology of Primary Aldosteronism

Two key points must be realized to properly understand the abnormal physiology involved in primary aldosteronism. First, the patient has had mild to moderate expansion of his extracellular and intravascular volume compartments, usually, for several years. Second, a compensatory adjustment was made early in his disease to prevent further expansion of these spaces. This consisted of a change in renotubular function in which proximal tubular rejection of sodium occurs (decreased proximal tubular reabsorption) and more sodium is shunted to the distal portion of the nephron. In the presence of unsuppressible aldosterone production, this increases the exchange of Na^+ for K^+ at the distal tubular ion exchange site and initiates a period of increased urinary excretion of K^+ which may continue for many years before sufficient body K^+ is lost to produce hypokalemia. However, the major advantage of the mechanism is that it allows for rapid excretion of sudden salt loads which otherwise would so further overload the vascular compartment, including the heart, that acute decompensation and pulmonary edema would occur. Experimentally, this protective phenomenon has been known for many years and has been termed "renal escape" from the sodium-retaining activity of continuously administered mineralocorticoids. This latter adjustment sets up a new steady-state which prevents the formation of edema and restores sodium equilibrium. The mechanism by which the hypertension is induced is not known but it, too, may be a response to chronic mild overexpansion of extracellular and intravascu-

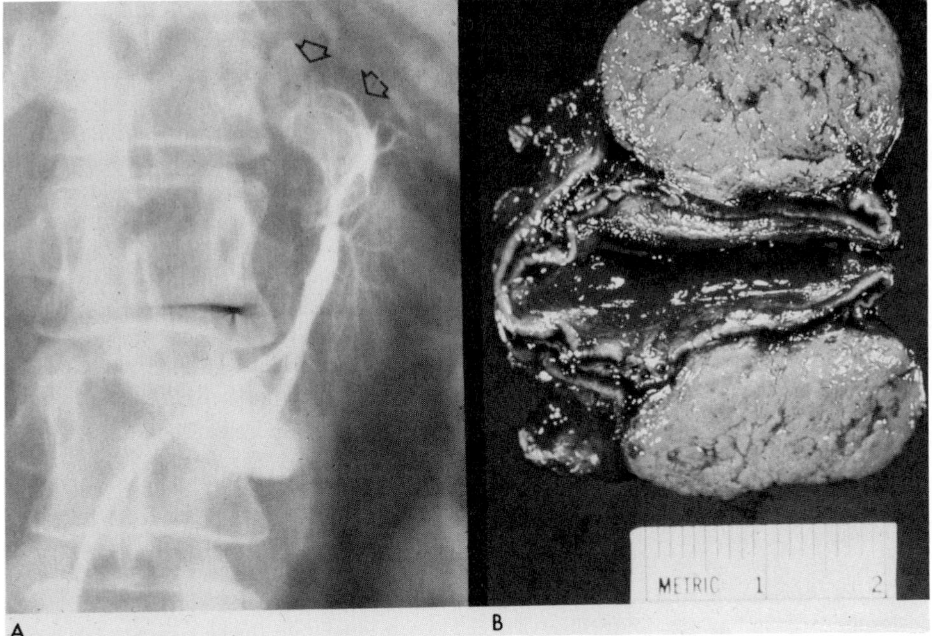

FIG. 4.—*A*, Preoperative visualization of aldosterone-producing tumor **(arrow)** by selective adrenal venography. *B*, Gross appearance of tumor.

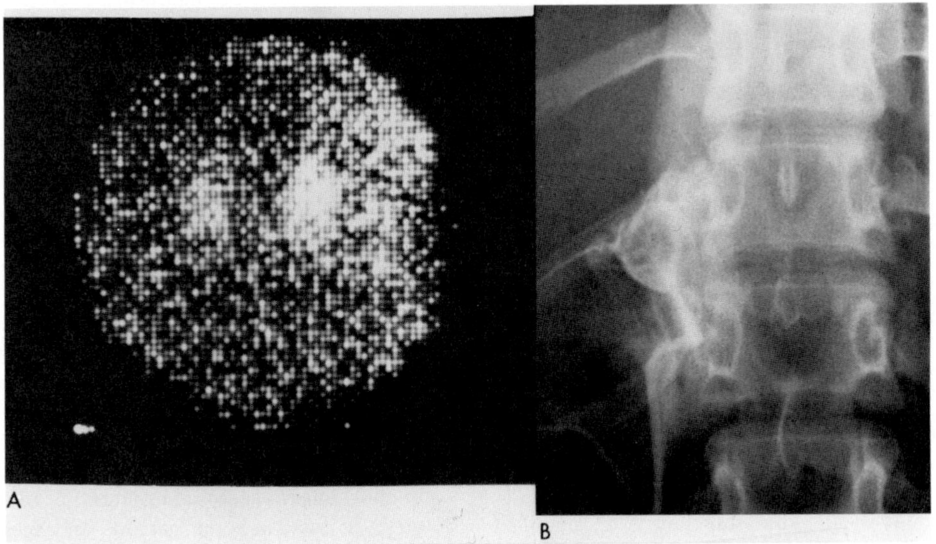

FIG. 5.—Example of visualization of aldosterone-producing tumor after administration of ^{131}I-iodocholesterol. *A*, The scan is a posterior view showing concentration of radioactivity in the right adrenal gland. The radioactivity at the right periphery of the scan is in the liver. *B*, The adrenal venogram is an anterior view showing the right-sided tumor.

lar volumes. It has been well established that mild expansion of intravascular volume diminishes sharply the release of renal renin into the blood stream. It is clear, therefore, that when extracellular fluid volumes are expanded by excessive mineralocorticoid activity in an otherwise normal individual, a series of compensatory reactions occurs which, together with the persistence of mineralocorticoid activity, lead to the clinical and biochemical picture that we recognize as primary aldosteronism.

The simplest experimental approach which would mimic the development of an aldosterone-secreting adrenocortical tumor would be the chronic daily administration of aldosterone, beginning with very tiny amounts and gradually increasing the dosage over a period of years. Such information is not available but short-term experiments of this kind have been carried out in man. Normal people on a fixed sodium intake, given a fixed large daily dose of aldosterone, respond in the following ways. During the first 2 days, urinary sodium falls sharply and total body weight increases 1 to 2 kg. By the third or fourth day urinary sodium has returned to baseline levels and weight has stabilized at the higher value despite continuation of aldosterone injections (renal escape). The latter phenomenon is probably due to liberation, from somewhere in the body, of a salt-losing hormone, sometimes referred to as "third factor." It is presumed that this hormone is responsible for the decreased proximal tubular reabsorption of sodium which occurs under conditions of intravascular volume expansion. Increased amounts of sodium are delivered to the distal tubular ion-exchange site where, under the influence of excessive amounts of aldosterone, a larger than normal exchange of sodium for potassium occurs, leading to increased urinary excretion of potassium. Depending upon the severity of the aldosteronism, this may quickly lead to hypokalemia, or hypokalemia may not manifest itself at all. Negative potassium balance may be minimal so that it would require many years to decrease total-body potassium sufficiently to manifest hypokalemia. We [15] have been able to induce in normal men our diagnostic criteria for primary aldosteronism without the induction of hypokalemia, namely, severe suppression of plasma renin activity, increased aldosterone excretion, and normal cortisol production, after 5 days of administration of aldosterone. Thus, it is the early volume change induced by aldosterone which is responsible for the phenomenon of low plasma renin activity; and this, together with increased aldosterone production, forms the basis for our diagnostic criteria and allows us to make the diagnosis with or without hypokalemia but, particularly, at an early stage in its development. Once chronic hypokalemia appears, the symptoms which ensue are due wholly to potassium depletion and are no different from those of chronic potassium depletion from any other cause. These are muscular weakness or paralysis, tetany, postural hypotension, diminished renal capacity to concentrate and acidify the urine, and polyuria. Chronic potassium depletion also makes the kidneys more vulnerable to infection.

Hypertension, Decreased Plasma Renin Activity, and Normal Aldosterone Production

All investigators who have studied plasma renin activity in hypertensive patients have found a group of them falling into this category. Our figure for this group is 15 percent, but in some studies the figure has been as high as 40 percent (highest in black people with hypertension). We have theorized [16] that endogenously produced, sodium-retaining compounds other than aldosterone, as well as chronic ingestion of unknown compounds having a similar activity, could account for some of these cases. Ingestion of licorice is an example of an exogenous sodium-retainer and desoxycorticosterone-producing tumors and 18-hydroxy-desoxycorticosterone-producing tumors are examples of endogenously produced, nonaldosterone, sodium-retaining compounds. Although no one has found the precise cause of hyporeninemia in this large group of patients with essential hypertension, we believe that the hypertension in all of these situations is via the same mechanism as in aldosterone-producing tumors. In fact, in some patients an excessive end-organ response to normal quantities of aldosterone can, at least, be suggested. Until it is proved otherwise, we shall continue to assume that severely suppressed plasma renin activity in the hypertensive patient is the result of insidious, low-grade, long-term sodium retention; and we will seek to determine the causes which, most likely, are many.

Carbohydrate Tolerance and Insulin-Secretory Capacity in Primary Aldosteronism

In 1965 we reported [17] that over 50 percent of patients with primary aldosteronism exhibited a diabetic type of glucose tolerance test; that in some of them this could be reversed to normal by preoperative potassium loading; and that in many of them glucose tolerance returned to normal in the postoperative period. In studying this phenomenon we found that the plasma insulin response to glucose loading was delayed and subnormal during the first hour after the glucose load. This, too, could be improved by potassium loading and, in many cases, became completely normal in the postoperative period. We suggested that an intracellular potassium deficit within the beta cells of the pancreas might account for this phenomenon, either directly or indirectly. Gorden, Sherman, and Simopoulos,[18] have reported recently that under conditions of potassium deficiency in man the total insulin released into the bloodstream in response to glucose is smaller than normal and is delayed. In addition, it contains a significantly higher proportion of proinsulin than is found in normal people. Proinsulin is physiologically inactive and is the precursor of the smaller molecule that we call insulin. These results confirm our suspicion that intracellular, beta-cell potassium is important with respect to glucose-induced, pancreatic insulin release. These findings may have broad implications in the field of carbohydrate metabolism.

Summary

Primary aldosteronism is much more common among our hypertensive population than has been realized heretofore. A major limiting factor in the recognition of this disorder has been the laborious technical procedures required for the diagnosis, namely, determinations of aldosterone and plasma renin activity. As a result of those difficulties the diagnosis of primary aldosteronism in most parts of the world has been limited to the most severe cases, namely, in those with chronic and persistent hypokalemia. The recent development of radioimmunoassay procedures for both of these determinations will remove part of the limitation.

The pathophysiology of primary aldosteronism has been discussed in relation to the earliest and most crucial diagnostic criteria. It is likely that further study of early cases of primary aldosteronism will lead to a better understanding of the mechanism of hypertension in the large group of patients with essential hypertension who do not exhibit overproduction of aldosterone, but who do have hyporeninemia, a situation currently unexplained.

References

1. Conn, J. W.: Presidential address: I. Painting background. II. Primary aldosteronism, a new clinical syndrome. J. Lab. Clin. Med. 45:3, 1955.
2. Conn, J. W.: Primary aldosteronism. J. Lab. Clin. Med. 45:661, 1955.
3. Laragh, J. H., Ulick, S., Januszewicz, V., Deming, Q. B., Kelly, W. G., and Lieberman, S.: Aldosterone secretion and primary and malignant hypertension. J. Clin. Invest. 39:1091, 1960.
4. Genest, J.: Angiotensin, aldosterone and human arterial hypertension. Canad. Med. Assoc. J. 84:403, 1961.
5. Laragh, J. H.: Interrelationships between angiotensin, norepinephrine, epinephrine, aldosterone secretion, and electrolyte metabolism in man. Circulation 25:203, 1962.
6. Conn, J. W., Cohen, E. L., and Rovner, D. R.: Suppression of plasma renin activity in primary aldosteronism. JAMA 190:213, 1964.
7. Conn, J. W., Cohen, E. L., Rovner, D. R., and Nesbit, R. M.: Normokalemic primary aldosteronism: A detectable cause of curable "essential" hypertension. JAMA 193:200, 1965.
8. Conn, J. W., Rovner, D. R., and Cohen, E. L.: Natural history of recovery of the renin-angiotensin-aldosterone system following long-term suppression of aldosterone-secreting tumors. (Abstract.) Program of the 47th Meeting of the Endocrine Society, New York City, June 1965, Philadelphia: Lippincott, 1965, p. 60.
9. Conn, J. W.: The evolution of primary aldo-

steronism—1954–1967. Harvey Lect. 62:257, 1968.

10. Cohen, E. L., Grim, C. E., Conn, J. W., Blough, W. M., Jr., Guyer, R. B., Kem, D. C., and Lucas, C. P.: Accurate and rapid measurement of plasma renin activity by radioimmunoassay. Results in normal and hypertensive people. J. Lab. Clin. Med. 77:1025, 1971.
11. Sutherland, D. J. A., Ruse, J. L., and Laidlaw, J. C.: Hypertension, increased aldosterone secretion and low plasma renin activity relieved by dexamethasone. Canad. Med. Assoc. J. 95:1109, 1966.
12. Conn, J. W., Morita, R., Cohen, E. L., Beierwaltes, W. H., McDonald, W. J., and Herwig, K. R.: Primary aldosteronism. Photoscanning of tumors after administration of ^{131}I-19-Iodocholesterol. Arch. Intern. Med. 129:417, 1972.
13. Conn, J. W., Rovner, D. R., Cohen, E. L., Bookstein, J. J., Cerny, J. C., and Lucas, C. P.: Preoperative diagnosis of primary aldosteronism. Arch. Intern. Med. 123:113, 1969.
14. Melby, J. C., Spark, R. F., Dale, S. L., Egdahl, R. H., and Kahn, P. C.: Diagnosis and localization of aldosterone-producing adenomas by adrenal-vein catheterization. N. Engl. J. Med. 277:1050, 1967.
15. Conn, J. W., Cohen, E. L., and Rovner, D. R.: Unpublished data.
16. Conn, J. W., Rovner, D. R., and Cohen, E. L.: Licorice-induced pseudoaldosteronism. Hypertension, hypokalemia, aldosteronopenia, and suppressed plasma renin activity. JAMA 205:492, 1968.
17. Conn, J. W., Cohen, E. L., Rovner, D. R., and Nesbit, R. M.: Normokalemic primary aldosteronism: A detectable cause of curable "essential" hypertension. JAMA 193:200, 1965.
18. Gorden, P., Sherman, B. M., and Simopoulos, A. P.: Glucose intolerance with hypokalemia: An increased proportion of circulating proinsulin-like component. J. Clin. Endocrinol. Metab. 34:235, 1972.

Pseudo-Primary Aldosteronism: A Clinical Expression of Low-renin Essential Hypertension?

By Leslie Baer, M.D., Hans R. Brunner, M.D., Fritz R. Bühler, M.D., and John H. Laragh, M.D.

SUPPRESSED PLASMA RENIN activity has become a benchmark in the diagnosis of primary aldosteronism.[1] Plasma renin activity, however, may also be suppressed in at least two other hypertensive disorders. The first, and by far the most common of these, is essential hypertension. Approximately one-quarter to one-third of patients with essential hypertension have been found to have suppressed plasma renin activity.[2–4] In this group, aldosterone secretion is within normal limits, and does not appear to account for the suppression of renin. A second low-renin hypertensive disorder has been described in which hyperaldosteronism is present. We have called this second condition "pseudo-primary aldosteronism" and others have termed it "idiopathic adrenal hyperplasia"[5,6] because these patients differ from those with primary aldosteronism in two respects: First, the adrenal glands are diffusely, usually bilaterally, involved in contrast to the single adenoma that is seen in primary aldosteronism.[5,6] Second, total adrenalectomy and correction of the hyperaldosteronism do not cure the hypertension in pseudo-primary aldosteronism, whereas the majority of patients with primary aldosteronism are cured of their hypertension with removal of the adenoma.[5] These differences between primary aldosteronism and pseudo-primary aldosteronism suggest that these two groups represent biologically different entities. With more appreciation of these differences, the clinical distinction between these two groups has become increasingly important since adrenalectomy is indicated in one group but is not particularly useful in the other.

From the Department of Medicine, Columbia University College of Physicians and Surgeons, New York, New York.

Qualitatively, the biochemical abnormalities are similar in primary aldosteronism and pseudo-primary aldosteronism. But there are a number of quantitative differences. These include differences in the degree of aldosteronism, of hypokalemia, hypernatremia, alkalosis, salivary potassium excretion, and in suppression of plasma renin.[5–10] Although these differences may be useful for separating groups of patients, there is enough overlap to make the absolute differentiation in an individual patient a serious problem.

This chapter further characterizes differences between patients with primary aldosteronism and those with pseudo-primary aldosteronism based on studies made preoperatively and postoperatively which expose differences in renin and aldosterone responses to adrenalectomy. The findings suggest again that the syndrome of hyperaldosteronism, low plasma renin activity, and normal urinary 17-hydroxycorticosteroid and ketosteroid excretion is not a homogeneous entity. Furthermore, these additional observations suggest a remarkable similarity between the group of patients with low-renin "essential" hypertension and patients with pseudo-primary aldosteronism. Thus, it seems possible that pseudo-primary aldosteronism may be a form of low-renin essential hypertension in which aldosterone excretion is increased but in which the adrenal gland is not crucial to the maintenance of the hypertension.

Methodology

Twenty-five patients with hyperaldosteronism who underwent adrenal surgery since 1959 have been studied at the Presbyterian Hospital in New York City. They had no clinical evidence of malignant hypertension, and significant renovascular disease was found in only one patient. Hyporeninemia was documented in 20 of the patients; the other five were evaluated before renin methods were available. The 17-hydroxycorticosteroid and ketosteroid excretion was within normal limits in all patients. Twenty-three of the 25 patients were admitted to the Metabolism Unit and received constant diets of known electrolyte content. All drugs had been discontinued at least 3 weeks before the period of investigation. Preoperative measurements of renin and aldosterone were undertaken only after equilibration for at least 5 days on a given diet. Blood samples for renin determinations were taken at noon when the patients had been ambulant for 4 hours. Aldosterone-secretion or -excretion rates were measured by the double-isotope dilution technique [11] or by a radioimmunoassay of the acid-labile conjugate excreted in the urine.[12] Normal values for aldosterone excretion on a 100-mEq per day sodium diet are below 20 μg per 24 hours in our laboratory. Plasma renin activity was determined by bioassay and by a radioimmunoassay technique,[13,14] and the values are expressed in radioimmunoassay units. A consistent relationship was derived between bioassay and radioimmunoassay units for plasma renin activity. This relationship was used to convert all values into radioimmunoassay units.[14] Submaxillary gland-electrolyte excretion was determined by a method previously described.[7] Mean arterial blood pressures (MABP) were estimated from the following relationship:

$$\text{MABP} = \text{diastolic} + \frac{\text{systolic-diastolic}}{3}$$

Intravenous pyelography was performed in all the patients, and 20 of them also underwent retrograde femoral aortography to rule out renal artery stenosis. Biopsy material was classified without knowledge of the clinical diagnosis of the patient.

The pathologic classification of the adrenal glands may be crucial in the distinction between the two groups described here. The term "nonadenomatous" has been applied to all adrenal glands that did not contain an isolated adenoma, but which were associated with hypersecretion of aldosterone. In the past, these glands have often been termed "multinodular hyperplasia." However, in our experience it has often been difficult, merely by examining the glands microscopically, to be certain that hyperplasia did, in fact, exist.[5] For example, one of the adrenal glands examined in our series appeared normal histologically but this patient was clearly oversecreting aldosterone. Thus, the term "nonadenomatous" need not imply hyperfunction, because many hypertensive and some normotensive patients have multinodular adrenal glands that are not hypersecreting aldosterone.[3,15] The term "nonadenomatous" also need not describe a homogeneous group from a histologic point of view. However, the patients described here with hyperaldosteronism and nonadenomatous adrenal glands appear to represent an entity biologically and clinically distinct from that associated with a single, adrenocortical adenoma typical of primary aldosteronism. We have chosen, therefore, to call this other entity with nonadenomatous adrenal disease pseudo-primary aldosteronism.

Results

The clinical features of the two groups of patients are summarized in Table 1. All 25 patients seen between 1959 and 1971 satisfied the clinical and biochemical criteria of primary aldosteronism and underwent adrenal exploration. Thirteen of the patients were found to have a single adrenocortical adenoma (primary aldosteronism) and the other 12 had the non-adenomatous form of adrenal disease (pseudo-primary aldosteronism).

In the group with primary aldosteronism, the mean age was 40, with 11 Caucasians and two Negroes. Eight were female and five male. Mean duration of hypertension as determined by clinical history was 8 years. Mean arterial blood pressure was 135 mm Hg. All the patients were hypokalemic and alkalotic, with a mean plasma potassium concentration of 2.5 mEq per liter, plasma sodium concentration of 146 mEq per liter, and carbon dioxide content of 32. Submaxillary salivary potassium concentration was 24.6 mEq per liter. Mean aldosterone excretion was 70 μg each 24 hours. Plasma renin activity was low in the 10 patients in whom it was measured.

In the patients with pseudo-primary aldosteronism, the mean age was 41, with six Caucasians and six Negroes. Five were female

TABLE 1.—*Differential Features of Primary Versus Pseudo-Primary Aldosteronism*

	Age	Race	Sex	Duration of Hypertension (yr)	Mean Arterial Blood Pressure (mm Hg)	Plasma (mEq per liter)			Submaxillary K^+ (mEq per liter)	Aldosterone (μg per 24 hr)
						Na^+	K^+	CO_2		
Primary aldosteronism (13) *	40 ± 3	11W 2N	8F 5M	8 ± 1.5	135 ± 3	146 ± 0.9	2.5 ± 0.1	32 ± 0.5	25 ± 0.7	70 ± 7
Pseudo-primary aldosteronism (12) *	41 ± 3	6W 6N	5F 7M	10 ± 2.0	139 ± 5	142 ± 0.9 †	3.5 ± 0.2 †	28 ± 1.3 †	17 ± 1.3 †	46 ± 2 ‡

Values represent the mean ± SEM.
* Number of patients in each group.
† $P < 0.01$.
‡ $P < 0.025$.

and seven male, and mean duration of hypertension was 10 years. Mean arterial blood pressure was 139 mm Hg, and submaxillary salivary potassium concentration was 17.3 mEq per liter. Mean aldosterone excretion was 46 μg each 24 hours. Plasma renin activity was low in all 10 patients in whom it was measured. Three patients had unilateral multinodular glands, while in six a multinodular adrenal cortex was found bilaterally. Two patients appeared to have diffuse hyperplasia and in one patient, the adrenal cortex appeared normal.

Postoperative blood pressures, type of surgery performed, and length of follow-up for the two groups of patients are summarized in Table 2. Four of the 12 patients with pseudo-primary aldosteronism had a total adrenalectomy and five had approximately a 1⅓ subtotal adrenalectomy. The remainder had unilateral adrenalectomy. All 25 patients were normokalemic postoperatively and have remained so. In 10 patients with adenomas and in seven with nonadenomatous adrenal disease, aldosterone excretion, measured from 10 days to 8 years postoperatively, was low or normal. Two additional patients with pseudo-primary aldosteronism redeveloped hyperaldosteronism postoperatively. A striking difference in the postoperative blood pressures is seen in the two groups. Ten of the 13 patients with primary aldosteronism due to a single adenoma were cured of their hypertension. One of the 10 (M.B.) was normotensive for 8 years before redeveloping hypertension with normal renin and aldosterone levels. We consider this patient a surgical cure whose present hypertension appears to be of the essential type. Among the three patients with primary aldosteronism who did not become normotensive after removal of the adenoma, one (G.F.) had renal artery stenosis documented on arteriography. The other two (D.F. and B.K.) had severe and moderately severe degrees of nephrosclerosis on their renal biopsies. Thus, in these patients, renal or renovascular disease may have contributed to the persistent hypertension after adrenalectomy.

Despite a similar length of follow-up in the two groups of patients (37 months), a striking difference was seen in the cure rate of hypertension. In primary aldosteronism, 77 percent of patients were cured of their hypertension

TABLE 2.—*Results of Adrenalectomy in Primary and Pseudo-primary Aldosteronism*

Disease	*Patient*	*Preoperative Blood Pressure (mm Hg)*	*Postoperative Blood Pressure (mm Hg)*	*Length of Follow-up (in months)*	*Type of Surgery*
Adenoma (Primary aldosteronism)					
	GF	176/116	155/100	26	Unilateral Adx
	DF	170/110	160/110	37	Unilateral Adx
	JB	190/110	130/90	29	Unilateral Adx
	AM	170/110	125/78	2	Unilateral Adx
	MR	170/110	110/70	12	Unilateral Adx
	MF	160/110	110/80	34	Unilateral Adx
	HP	160/100	130/88	2	Unilateral Adx
	IW	170/115	110/80	24	Unilateral Adx
	FP	170/120	120/60	48	Total Adx
	LJ	220/126	normal	108	Total Adx
	MB	210/120	135/95 *	96	Unilateral Adx
	DD	160/110	130/80	56	Unilateral Adx
	BK	180/120	170/120	12	Subtotal Adx
				Cure Rate=77%	
Nonadenoma (Pseudo-primary aldosteronism)					
	IJ	170/100	160/100	78	Unilateral Adx
	EW	175/120	160/110	30	Unilateral Adx
	RA	170/120	140/100	18	Total Adx
	JB	180/120	140/110	53	Total Adx
	BW	190/130	170/100	90	Subtotal Adx
	VS	170/110	160/110	48	Total Adx
	LL	216/170	150/110	49	Total Adx
	GM	180/120	160/120	25	Subtotal Adx
	DF	160/110	160/95 *	22	Subtotal Adx
	JJ	170/110	160/96	1	Unilateral Adx
	AK	190/120	160/110	23	Subtotal Adx
	OH	180/120	200/130	17	Subtotal Adx
				Cure Rate=0%	

Abbreviation used: Adx, adrenalectomy.
* On antihypertensive medication.

after removal of the adrenocortical adenoma. In contrast, none of the patients with pseudo-primary aldosteronism became normotensive after surgery. It should be noted in Table 2 that in some instances blood pressures did fall slightly in pseudo-primary aldosteronism patients; however, none of these became normotensive.

In primary aldosteronism the preoperative aldosterone and renin responses to changes in sodium intake are illustrated in Fig. 1. Aldosterone excretion did not change significantly with sodium depletion or sodium loading. Plasma renin activity was low in all the patients. In one patient (B.K.) with primary aldosteronism, in whom renin was measured by the more sensitive radioimmunoassay, renin could be seen to rise during sodium depletion even though it remained subnormal.

In contrast, Fig. 2 illustrates the aldosterone and renin responses in four patients with pseudo-primary aldosteronism. With sodium depletion, aldosterone excretion rose and in three of the four, renin also rose. One patient (L.L.) is of particular interest because she had the highest renin levels in the group of patients with pseudo-primary aldosteronism, and both her renin and aldosterone levels were very responsive to changes in sodium intake. She underwent bilateral adrenalectomy and microscopically the adrenals appeared normal. Four other patients with pseudo-primary aldostero-

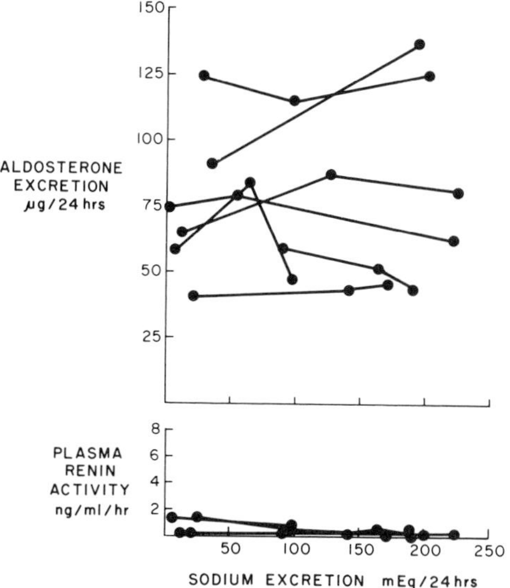

FIG. 1.—Primary aldosteronism. Preoperative response of aldosterone and renin to changes in sodium intake. (From Genest, J., and Koiw, E.,[23] with permission.)

nism whose aldosterone excretion and renin levels were unresponsive to changes in sodium intake are seen in the right half of Fig. 2.

Preoperative and postoperative measurements of aldosterone excretion and plasma renin activity in the two groups of patients are seen in Fig. 3. Patients with pseudo-primary aldosteronism undergoing subtotal adrenalectomy had a lesser fall in aldosterone excretion postoperatively and a lesser rise in renin than did patients with primary aldosteronism. In three patients with pseudo-primary aldosteronism who underwent total adrenalectomy, aldosterone excretion was near zero and renin was variably high.

Postoperative measurements of plasma renin activity and the corresponding 24-hour urinary sodium excretion on the day of the renin measurement are seen in Fig. 4 for the two groups of patients. Hatched lines describe the normal range. In all the patients with primary aldosteronism, renin rose either to normal or to

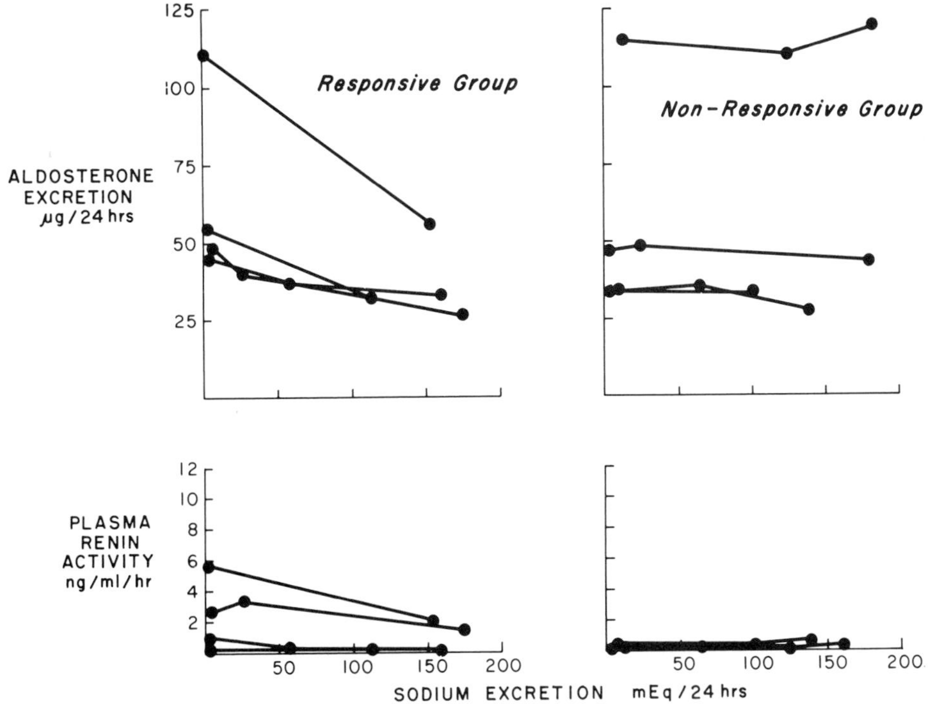

FIG. 2.—Pseudo-primary aldosteronism. Preoperative response of aldosterone and renin to changes in sodium intake. (From Genest, J., and Koiw, E.,[23] with permission.)

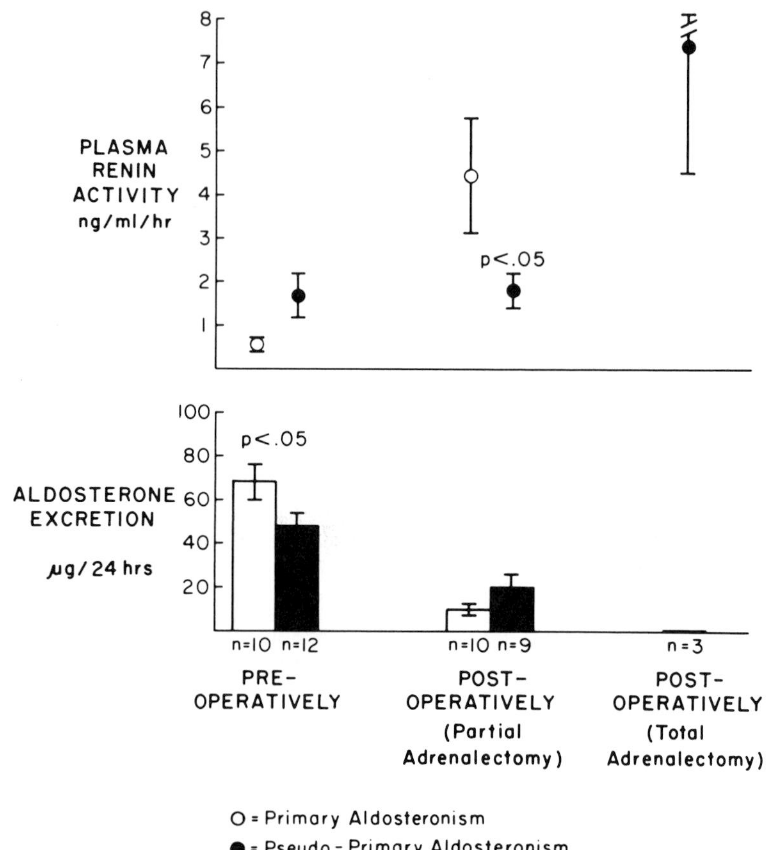

FIG. 3.—Preoperative and postoperative measurements of renin and aldosterone in primary and pseudo-primary aldosteronism. (From Genest, J., and Koiw, E.,[23] with permission.)

supernormal levels within 3 to 5 months after removal of the adenoma. In one patient whose renin level was measured 3 days after removal of the adenoma, renin was clearly still low. In this same patient, however, renin had returned to high normal levels by the third month after adrenalectomy.

In contrast to the consistent rise of renin postoperatively in primary aldosteronism, patients with pseudo-primary aldosteronism often maintained subnormal renin levels for as long as 2½ years after partial adrenalectomy, and despite correction of the hyperaldosteronism. The distribution of renin in pseudo-primary aldosteronism differed from that in primary aldosteronism in both the low and high ranges of renin, although overlap was seen in the two groups in the normal range for plasma renin activity.

Aldosterone and renin responses to changes in sodium intake were studied in seven patients postoperatively and are illustrated in Fig. 5. In the four patients with primary aldosteronism, renin and aldosterone rose normally during sodium depletion. Three patients with primary aldosteronism (Fig. 5) had a unilateral adrenalectomy and the fourth (B.K.) had a subtotal adrenalectomy. Three patients with pseudo-primary aldosteronism had subtotal adrenalectomy. In all of them, an unresponsive or subnormally responsive renin and aldosterone were observed. The absolute aldosterone excretion rate, however, is normal in all three.

Another feature that distinguishes between

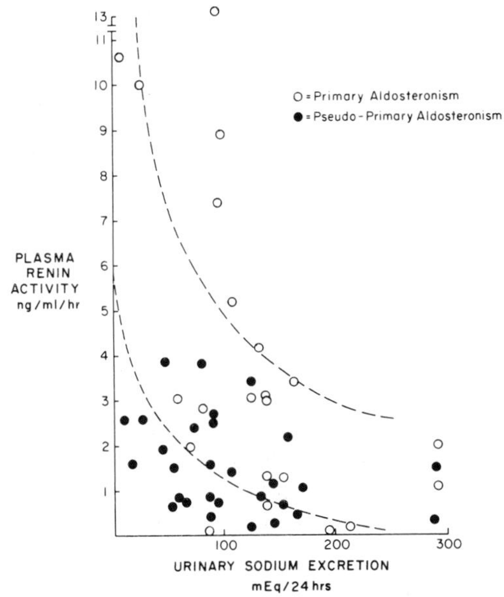

FIG. 4.—Postoperative measurements of plasma renin activity in primary and pseudo-primary aldosteronism. (From Genest, J., and Koiw, E.,[23] with permission.)

the two groups is the fact that aldosterone excretion returned to normal levels in all patients with primary aldosteronism after removal of their adenomas. In contrast, two patients (R.A. and O.H.) with pseudo-primary aldosteronism had a reappearance of hyperaldosteronism 6 months and 8 months respectively after subtotal adrenalectomy. In another patient with pseudo-primary aldosteronism (E.W.) we have observed a progressive rise in aldosterone excretion postoperatively approximately twofold although aldosterone never reached abnormally high levels. Plasma renin activity in this patient also rose slightly for a time, but it never responded normally to sodium depletion. Renin in this patient is still subnormal 2½ years postoperatively.

The relationship of aldosterone excretion to 24-hour urinary sodium excretion is illustrated in Fig. 6 for two groups of patients with low renin hypertension. The first group consists of 59 patients with low-renin essential hypertension who have been studied in our hospital. The second group consists of the patients with pseudo-primary aldosteronism described in this chapter whose aldosterone excretion rates were determined before surgery. The dotted lines indicate the normal range. Considerable overlap of aldosterone excretion is observed in the two groups of patients. Thus, it can be shown that in low-renin essential hypertension, as in pseudo-primary aldosteronism, aldosterone excretion may be inappropriately high, particularly during periods of high-sodium intake.

DISCUSSION

These results illustrate that the syndrome of hypertension associated with low plasma renin activity and hyperaldosteronism comprises at least two different entities that appear to occur with about equal frequency. Forty-eight per-

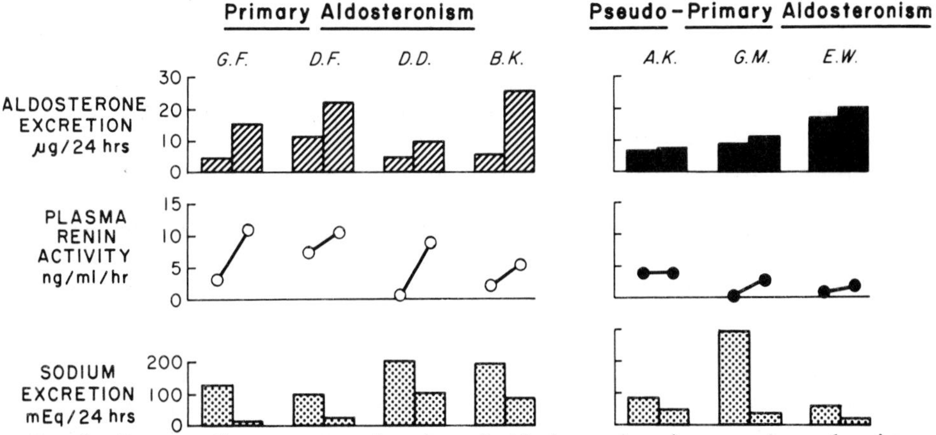

FIG. 5.—Postoperative responses of renin and aldosterone in primary and pseudo-primary aldosteronism. (From Genest, J., and Koiw, E.,[23] with permission.)

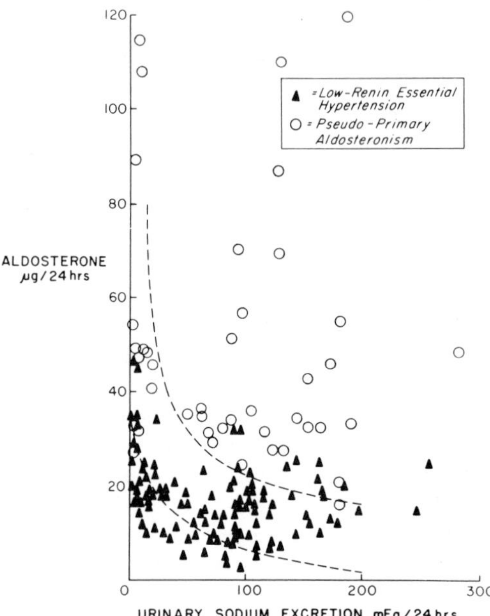

FIG. 6.—The relationship of aldosterone excretion to 24-hour urinary sodium excretion in low-renin essential hypertension and in pseudo-primary aldosteronism. (From Genest, J., and Koiw, E.,[23] with permission.)

cent of the patients in the present series did not prove to have an isolated adrenal cortical adenoma and were classified as having pseudo-primary aldosteronism. In this entity, diffuse nonadenomatous adrenocortical disease was present. In addition, none of these patients were cured of hypertension, even after total adrenalectomy. Our experience with this group of patients is similar to that reported by Biglieri et al.[6] and is quite different from that of Conn, Knopf, and Nesbit.[16]

The consistent failure to cure the hypertension in the nonadenomatous group cannot be attributed to residual hyperaldosteronism, because even total adrenalectomy of five patients failed to remit the hypertension. In contrast to this lack of cure in the first group, 77 percent of patients with primary aldosteronism due to a single adrenocortical adenoma were cured of hypertension after adrenalectomy. This latter experience is similar to that reported by Conn et al.[16] Three patients with primary aldosteronism, however, were not cured of their hypertension. It is possible that renal or renovascular disease may have prevented cure of hypertension of these patients, because two of them had severe and moderately severe degrees of nephrosclerosis on their renal biopsies, and a third was shown on arteriography to have renal artery stenosis. Failure to cure hypertension in the group with pseudo-primary aldosteronism did not appear to be due to renal involvement because, in general, there were no striking differences in these parameters when compared to the group with primary aldosteronism in whom 77 percent were cured.

The similar clinical features of these two disorders pose a delicate problem in differential diagnosis and in management. Certain differences between these two entities (Table 1) may be useful in preoperative classification. Thus, patients with primary aldosteronism are significantly more hypokalemic and alkalotic, more hypernatremic, and tend to have a lower plasma renin activity when compared with patients with pseudo-primary aldosteronism. In fact, one of the more consistent features of pseudo-primary aldosteronism is that the plasma potassium concentration is usually within normal limits when the patients are maintained on a 95- to 100-mEq sodium diet. This is in contrast to patients with primary aldosteronism on the same dietary sodium intake who usually become markedly hypokalemic. The lesser degree of hyperaldosteronism seen in the group with pseudo-primary aldosteronism may explain the less severe electrolyte derangements and lesser renin suppression.[9] It may also explain the consistently higher salivary potassium excretion observed in this group when compared to that in the group with primary aldosteronism.[7]

Other differences in the responses of aldosterone to changes in sodium intake between the two groups may prove helpful in distinguishing these conditions. In pseudo-primary aldosteronism, aldosterone may respond to changes in sodium intake. At every level of sodium intake, however, aldosterone excretion remains too high. In contrast, in patients with primary aldosteronism (and in some patients with pseudo-primary aldosteronism) aldosterone excretion remained high, but fixed, over a wide range of sodium intake. Similar findings have been reported by others in primary aldosteronism.[17] The generally higher plasma renin and potassium concentrations in the group with pseudo-primary aldosteronism may in part explain the response of aldosterone to changes in sodium intake. Whatever the mechanism of this response proves to be, these differences in the two groups may have clinical usefulness because thus far we have not seen a patient with primary aldosteronism who exhibited a significant aldosterone response to either sodium depletion or sodium loading.

Postoperative studies provide further distinctions between primary and pseudo-primary aldosteronism. In primary aldosteronism, there was a greater fall in aldosterone excretion after removal of the adenoma and a significantly greater rise in plasma renin activity, when compared to the group with pseudo-primary aldosteronism who underwent partial adrenalectomy, even though the greatest increases in plasma renin activity were seen in the patients who underwent total adrenalectomy. The relative changes in renin postoperatively, therefore, seem to be directly related to the relative changes in aldosterone. However, the low plasma renin levels observed postoperatively in some patients with pseudo-primary aldosteronism cannot be explained by hyperaldosteronism, because adrenalectomy in this group also returned aldosterone excretion to within normal limits, yet renin remained subnormal. Furthermore, a delayed recovery of renin secretion after prolonged suppression also does not appear to explain this finding, because in primary aldosteronism, the group with a more severe degree of hyperaldosteronism and even more suppressed renins, renin rose to normal or supernormal levels within 3 to 5 months after partial adrenalectomy and removal of the hypersecreting adenoma.

Thus, postoperatively, patients with pseudo-primary aldosteronism exhibit a hormonal profile that has also been observed in certain patients with essential hypertension and low plasma renin activity. Plasma renin activity is similarly suppressed in both disorders, and a number of low-renin essential hypertensive patients also exhibit either fixed or unresponsive renin- and aldosterone-secretory mechanisms.[18–20] This same abnormality has been identified in postoperative studies in patients with pseudo-primary aldosteronism reported herein even when aldosterone excretion is restored to normal. In addition, in both essential hypertension and in pseudo-primary aldosteronism,[21,22] a high incidence of abnormal adrenocortical histology has been described.

Altogether, these similarities suggest a close relationship between patients with low-renin essential hypertension and those with pseudo-primary aldosteronism. Thus, pseudo-primary aldosteronism may be a form of low-renin essential hypertension in which aldosterone secretion, though increased, is not primarily related to the hypertension. Confirmation of this hypothesis must await further study of larger numbers of patients with low-renin essential hypertension and pseudo-primary aldosteronism. However, it is apparent that there are hypertensive patients with hyperaldosteronism who are not cured of hypertension by adrenalectomy even though their metabolic abnormalities are corrected. Thus, the presence of hyperaldosteronism per se cannot be an indication for surgery in these patients.

SUMMARY

The syndrome of hyperaldosteronism, suppressed plasma renin activity, and normal 17-hydroxycorticosteroid and ketosteroid excretion appears to comprise at least two disorders which occur with about equal frequency.

The first condition, primary aldosteronism, is characterized by the presence of a discrete adrenocortical adenoma, removal of which usually corrects the metabolic abnormalities and cures the hypertension. This condition usually presents with marked hyperaldosteronism, hypokalemia and alkalosis, very low plasma renin activity, and high submaxillary potassium excretion.

The second disorder, pseudo-primary aldosteronism, is characterized instead by the presence of diffuse, usually bilateral, adrenocortical disease. In contrast to primary aldosteronism, in pseudo-primary aldosteronism partial or even total adrenalectomy fails to cure the hypertension even though hyperaldosteronism and associated metabolic abnormalities are corrected. This second disorder usually exhibits less aldosteronism, less hypokalemia, less plasma renin suppression, and normal submaxillary potassium excretion.

After partial adrenalectomy and correction of their hyperaldosteronism, patients with pseudo-primary aldosteronism appear to resemble patients with low-renin essential hypertension. Thus, both of these groups exhibit normal aldosterone-excretion rates and low plasma renin levels which may remain fixed or relatively unresponsive to sodium depletion or loading. These similarities suggest that pseudo-primary aldosteronism may be a variant form of low-renin essential hypertension in which aldosterone secretion is increased, but is not primarily related to the hypertension. In this context, it may be possible to understand why partial or total adrenalectomy fails to cure the hypertension. Whatever the explanation, hyperaldosteronism per se is not necessarily an indication for adrenal surgery in pseudo-primary aldosteronism.

References

1. Conn, J. W., Cohen, E. L., and Rovner, D. R.: Suppression of plasma renin activity in primary aldosteronism. JAMA 190:213, 1964.
2. Helmer, O. M.: The renin-angiotensin system and its relation to hypertension. Progr. Cardiovasc. Dis. 8:117, 1965.
3. Ledingham, J. G. G., Bull, M. B., and Laragh, J. H.: The meaning of aldosteronism in hypertensive disease. Circ. Res. 20–21(Suppl. 2):II–177, 1967.
4. Jose, A., Crout, J. R., and Kaplan, N. M.: Suppressed plasma renin activity in essential hypertension. Roles of plasma volume, blood pressure and sympathetic nervous system. Ann. Intern. Med. 72:9, 1970.
5. Baer, L., Sommers, S. C., Krakoff, L. R., Newton, M. A., and Laragh, J. H.: Pseudoprimary aldosteronim. An entity distinct from true primary aldosteronism. Circ. Res. 26–27 (Suppl. 1):I–203, 1970.
6. Biglieri, E. G., Schambelan, M., Slaton, P. E., and Stockigt, J. R.: The intercurrent hypertension of primary aldosteronism. Circ. Res. 26–27(Suppl. 1):I–195, 1970.
7. Wotman, S., Baer, L., Mandel, I. D., and Laragh, J. H.: Submaxillary potassium concentration in true and pseudo-primary aldosteronism. Arch. Intern. Med. 126:248, 1970.
8. Distler, A., Barth, C., Roscher, S., Vecsei, P., Dhom, G., and Wolff, H. P.: Hochdruck und aldosteronismus bei solitaren adenomen und bei nodularer hyperplasie der nebennierenrinde. Klin. Wochenschr. 47:688, 1969.
9. Stockigt, J. R., Collins, R. D., and Biglieri, E. G.: Determination of plasma renin concentration by angiotensin I immunoassay. Diagnostic import of precise measurement of subnormal renin in hyperaldosteronism. Circ. Res. 28–29(Suppl. 2):II–175, 1971.
10. Ferris, J. B., Brown, J. J., Fraser, R., Kay, A. W., Lever, A. F., Neville, A. M., O'Muircheartaigh, I. G., Robertson, J. I. S., and Symington, T.: Hypertension with aldosterone excess and low plasma renin: Preoperative distinction between patients with and without adrenocortical tumor. Lancet 2:995, 1970.
11. Laragh, J. H., Sealey, J. E., and Klein, P. D.: The presence and effect of isotope fractionation in isotope dilution analysis: A factor in the measurement of aldosterone secretory rates in man. *In* Radiochemical Methods of Analysis, vol. 2. Vienna: International Atomic Energy Agency, 1965, p. 353.
12. Sealey, J. E., Buhler, F. R., and Laragh, J. H.: Radioimmunoassay of urinary aldosterone excretion: Correlations with sodium balance. (In preparation.)
13. Newton, M. A., and Laragh, J. H.: Effect of corticotropin on aldosterone excretion and plasma renin in normal subjects, in essential hypertension and in primary aldosteronism. J. Clin. Endocrinol. 28:1006, 1968.
14. Sealey, J. E., Gerten-Banes, J., and Laragh, J. H.: The renin system: Variations in man measured by radioimmunoassay or bioassay. Kidney Int. 1:240, 1972.
15. Kaplan, N. M.: The steroid content of adrenal adenomas and measurement of aldosterone production in patients with essential hypertension and primary aldosteronism. J. Clin. Invest. 46:728, 1967.
16. Conn, J. W., Knopf, R. F., and Nesbit, R. M.: Clinical characteristics of primary aldosteronism from an analysis of 145 cases. Am. J. Surg. 107:159, 1964.
17. Slaton, P. E., Jr., Schambelan, M., and Biglieri, E. G.: Stimulation and suppression of aldosterone secretion in patients with an aldosterone-producing adenoma. J. Clin. Endocrinol. 29:239, 1969.
18. Leutscher, J. A., Weinberger, M. H., Dowdy, A. J., Nokes, G. W., Kalikian, H., Brodie, A., and Willoughby, S.: Effects of sodium loading, sodium depletion and posture on plasma aldosterone concentration and renin activity in hypertensive patients. J. Clin. Endocrinol. 29:1310, 1969.
19. Collins, R. D., Weinberger, M. H., Dowdy, A. J., Nokes, G. W., Gonzales, C. M., and Luetscher, J. A.: Abnormally sustained aldo-

sterone secretion during salt loading in patients with various forms of benign hypertension: relation to plasma renin activity. J. Clin. Invest. 49:1415, 1970.

20. Weinberger, M. H., Dowdy, A. J., Nokes, G. W., and Luetscher, J. A.: Plasma renin activity and aldosterone secretion in hypertensive patients during high and low sodium intake and administration of diuretic. J. Clin. Endocrinol. 28:359, 1968.

21. Shamma, A. H., Goddard, J. W., and Sommers, S. C.: A study of the adrenal status in hypertension. J. Chron. Dis. 8:587, 1958.

22. Gunnells, J. C., McGuffin, W. L., Robinson, R. R., Grim, C. E., Wells, S., Silver, D., and Glenn, J. F.: Hypertension, adrenal abnormalities and alterations in plasma renin activity. Ann. Intern. Med. 73:901, 1970.

23. Genest, J., and Koiw, E. (Eds.): Hypertension. Berlin: Springer, 1972, p. 459.

Management of Primary Aldosteronism

By Edward G. Biglieri, M.D., and Morris Schambelan, M.D.

The importance of the syndrome of primary aldosteronism in correctable hypertension is well established.[1] There are four varieties of this syndrome: (1) primary aldosteronism due to an adrenocortical adenoma (APA); (2) primary aldosteronism due to micro- and macronodular hyperplasia—idiopathic hyperaldosteronism [2,3] (IHA); (3) primary aldosteronism corrected by glucocorticoid hormone treatment [4]; and (4) indeterminate hyperaldosteronism with hypertension, normal to reduced plasma renin activity, and aldosterone levels suppressible by deoxycorticosterone acetate (DOCA).[5]

In considering the management of primary aldosteronism, all efforts should be made to establish clearly the exact diagnosis. This is obviously crucial since treatment and the results of therapy are dependent on the accuracy of the diagnosis.

Diagnosis of Primary Aldosteronism

Adrenocortical Adenoma and Idiopathic Hyperaldosteronism (APA and IHA)

The presence of hypertension with spontaneous hypokalemia or with hypokalemia after sodium loading are strong presumptive signs of hyperaldosteronism. Measurements of increased aldosterone production confirm the diagnosis of primary aldosteronism with a low level of plasma renin activity providing corroborative evidence.

Preoperative distinction between adrenocortical adenoma and idiopathic hyperaldosteronism is not completely established, although there are many suggestive clinical differences. Idiopathic hyperaldosteronism is more prevalent in males.[3] Serum potassium concentrations are lower in patients with an APA who have higher levels of aldosterone excretion; [2–5] however, there is considerable overlap between the ranges in both diseases. Computer quadric analysis of multiple variables [6] shows considerable accuracy in predicting the exact pathology. This laboratory stresses the usefulness of measuring the level of aldosterone after administration of 20 mg of DOCA daily for 3 days (Table 1)[7,8] and the level of basal recumbent plasma renin concentration, which is the least variable of the plasma renin determinations.[8] Patients with APA have significantly lower plasma renin concentrations ($P < 0.01$) than patients with IHA (0.6 vs. 3.0 ng per ml per hour; normal range on a 120-mEq sodium intake is 2.5 to 10.5). Demonstration of persistent hyperaldosteronism is crucial to the diagnosis since low plasma renin concentrations can be observed in up to 30 percent of patients with essential hypertension.[8–11] Comparison of the level of plasma renin

From the Medical Service, San Francisco General Hospital, and the Department of Medicine, University of California, San Francisco, California.

Supported by U.S. Public Health Service Research Grants HL–11046 from the National Heart Institute and AM–06415 from the National Institute of Arthritis and Metabolic Diseases. The studies were carried out in the General Clinical Research Center, RR–83, at San Francisco General Hospital, supported by Division of Research Resources, National Institutes of Health.

Table 1.—*Effect of DOCA on Aldosterone Excretion in Patients with Various Hypertensive Disorders and in Normal Subjects on 120 mEq per day Sodium Intake*

	Mean Urinary Aldosterone (μg per 24 hr)	
Condition	*Control*	*After DOCA* *
APA † (N=40)	33.1	32.2
IHA † (N=12)	25.4	25.3
IndHA (N=12)	21.7	11.9
EHt (N=57)	9.9	6.4
Normal (N=10)	10.2	3.1

Abbreviations used: APA, primary aldosteronism due to adrenocortical adenoma; IHA, idiopathic hyperaldosteronism; IndHA, indeterminate hyperaldosteronism; EHt, essential hypertension.

* On third day after intramuscular administration of 10 mg every 12 hours, for 3 days.

† Subsequently confirmed at surgery.

concentration with the level of aldosterone after DOCA administration, which remains abnormally elevated in both groups of patients, can be used effectively to separate those with idiopathic hyperaldosteronism from those with adrenocortical adenoma. In the 14 patients so studied, the combination of higher levels of aldosterone after DOCA administration with lower levels of plasma renin concentration accurately predicted preoperatively the presence of an adenoma; the less extreme levels indicated the presence of idiopathic hyperaldosteronism.[4]

Indeterminate Hyperaldosteronism

Patients with indeterminate hyperaldosteronism (Table 1) have persistently elevated aldosterone values and normal serum potassium levels with little evidence of potassium wasting. Levels of plasma renin activity are within normal limits or reduced, which is somewhat incongruous in the face of elevated aldosterone production. Two distinctive features separate this group: hypertension is mild and readily controlled and hyperaldosteronism is readily suppressed to normal levels after administration of DOCA (Table 1). Whether these patients represent a distinct clinical entity or forms of early aldosterone-producing adenoma, idiopathic hyperaldosteronism, or a variation of essential hypertension remains to be established.[5]

Glucocorticoid-remediable Hyperaldosteronism

This is an unusual manifestation of the syndrome of primary aldosteronism and is indistinguishable from idiopathic hyperaldosteronism and an adrenocortical adenoma except that glucocorticoid therapy normalizes blood pressure, potassium concentration, and hyperaldosteronism.[4]

Medical Management

Spironolactone Treatment

Short-term Trial (4 to 6 Weeks). Administration of large doses (300 to 400 mg per day) of spironolactone to patients with aldosterone-producing adenoma or idiopathic hyperaldosteronism can reduce blood pressure in many patients and therefore postpone surgery. In 21 of 24 patients with an adenoma, subsequently confirmed at surgery, diastolic blood pressure was reduced to 100 mm Hg or less (Fig. 1); three showed no major changes in blood pressure. Serum potassium concentrations returned to the normal range. In contrast, only two of five patients with IHA had a similar reduction of blood pressure and three showed little change (Fig. 2). Mean aldosterone excretion levels showed a slight fall in patients with an adenoma, but a greater than threefold increase occurred in a single patient with IHA (Fig. 2).

Long-term Therapy (2 to 11 Years). Maintenance therapy with low dosages of spironolactone, ranging from 75 to 300 mg per day, has been employed for up to 11 years in some (N = 6) patients with mild or labile hypertension who have biochemical evidence of aldosterone-producing adenoma or idiopathic hyperaldosteronism (Table 2). Such therapy has maintained normal levels of blood pressure

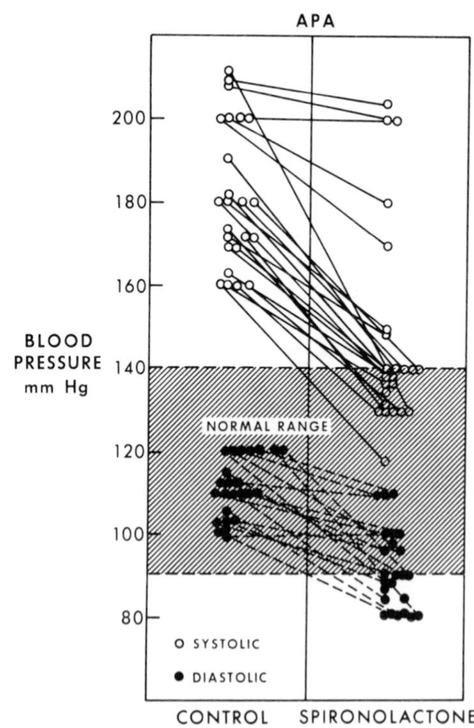

Fig. 1.—Effect of 300 to 400 mg of spironolactone per day on blood pressure in patients with an aldosterone-producing adenoma **(APA).**

TABLE 2.—*Dosages and Duration of Spironolactone Treatment Required to Effect Normalization of Blood Pressure in Patients with Adrenocortical Adenoma or Idiopathic Hyperaldosteronism*

	Spironolactone Therapy	
Patient *	*Dose per Day (mg)*	*No. of Years*
Primary aldosteronism due to adrenocortical adenoma		
1	100	2
2	75–100	11
3	150	8
4	300	2
5	200	3
Idiopathic hyperaldosteronism		
1	500	2

* Diagnosis based on plasma renin concentration compared with urinary aldosterone level after DOCA test.[8]

and serum potassium and prevented renal potassium wasting. Yearly examination of aldosterone production while therapy has been discontinued has shown a remarkable consistency, and no alteration in routine cardiac or renal function has been observed. The use of 100 to 200 mg per day of spironolactone is also effective (4 of 4 patients) in correcting the hypertension in the indeterminate group. Yearly evaluation is crucial in this group since they may represent part of the spectrum of primary aldosteronism due to an adenoma. Even large dosages have been used with good results in patients with an adenoma or idiopathic hyperaldosteronism in whom surgical investigation is contraindicated: two patients with primary aldosteronism have taken 300 to 500 mg per day for 2 years.

The effectiveness of relatively low dosages of spironolactone in managing selected patients with aldosterone-producing adenoma and idiopathic hyperaldosteronism may well be related to the apparently little influence of the drug on the suppressed renin-angiotensin system. Increases in plasma renin activity with short-term treatment with large doses of spironolactone are also minimal and inconsistent[12] (Table 3), but the increases become more consistent with prolonged therapy.[12–14] Aldosterone levels usually remain relatively unchanged (Fig. 3) except when increases in plasma renin concentration occur. In the patient with idiopathic hyperaldosteronism ac-

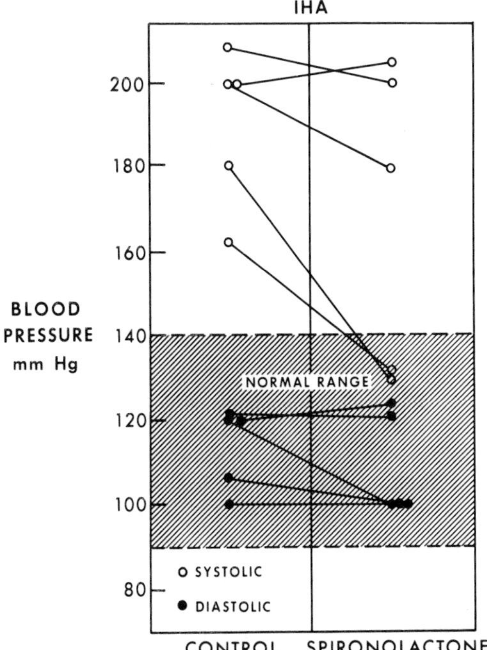

FIG. 2.—Effect of 300 to 400 mg of spironolactone per day on blood pressure in patients with idiopathic hyperaldosteronism (**IHA**).

TABLE 3.—*Effects of Short-term (4 to 6 Weeks) Treatment with Spironolactone on Plasma Renin Concentration in Patients with Adrenocortical Adenoma or Idiopathic Hyperaldosteronism*

	Basal Recumbent Plasma Renin Concentration (ng per ml per hr)	
Patient *	*Control*	*After Spironolactone Therapy* †
Primary aldosteronism due to adrenocortical adenoma		
1	0.13	0.22
2	0.41	0.14
3	0.64	0.69
4	0.15	0.20
5	0.10	1.60
6	0.43	6.60
Idiopathic hyperaldosteronism		
1	1.69	21.10

* Subsequently confirmed at surgery.
† 300 to 400 mg per day.

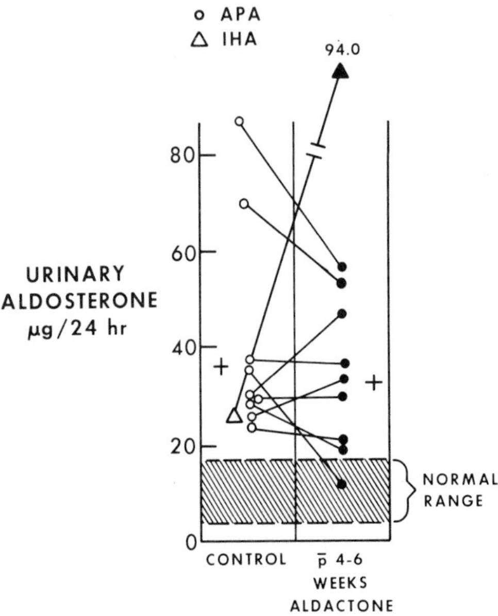

FIG. 3.—Effect of 300 to 400 mg of spironolactone per day on urinary aldosterone levels in patients with aldosterone-producing adenoma **(APA)** or idiopathic hyperaldosteronism **(IHA)**.

companied by a marked increase in aldosterone excretion (Fig. 3), the plasma renin concentrations were also increased 20-fold, reflecting a lesser degree of suppression of the renin-angiotensin system and indicating a potentially useful maneuver in distinguishing IHA from APA. A specific antihypertensive effect of spironolactone appears to occur with small doses in the mildly hypertensive patient where an increase in plasma renin concentration and aldosterone levels might not be expected to occur even with long-term treatment.

SURGICAL MANAGEMENT

Potassium repletion is an essential part of the surgical preparation.[15] Treatment with spironolactone up to the time of surgery has been recommended for both potassium repletion and stimulation of a dormant renin-angiotensin system.[14,15] Short-term treatment with large doses of spironolactone, as shown in Table 2, does not invariably return plasma renin concentration to the normal range, but an increase in plasma renin activity identifies those patients in whom hypoaldosteronism is unlikely to occur postoperatively.[14] In fact, aldosterone levels may actually continue to fall into the normal range after cessation of spironolactone therapy, identifying those patients who most likely will have hypoaldosteronism and hyporeninemia postoperatively. Persistent hypoaldosteronism (4 years postoperatively) is a rare occurrence after removal of a unilateral adenoma (2 of 68 patients) and transient hypoaldosteronism immediately after surgery is also rare (3 of 68 patients) in patients not prepared preoperatively with spironolactone. In six patients treated with large doses of spironolactone for up to 7 days before removal of a unilateral adenoma, transient hypoaldosteronism and hyporeninemia occurred postoperatively in 3, implying a possible direct effect of spironolactone on aldosterone production. The most effective surgical preparation has been sodium restriction with administration of 4 to 6 gm of potassium chloride for 1 to 2 weeks preoperatively.[15]

Patients with APA

Removal of an adenoma by unilateral adrenalectomy has produced beneficial effects in all of our patients so treated. In 77 patients followed for up to 12 years, 65 percent were cured while the remainder required much lower dosages of medication for mild hypertension.[3]

Patients with IHA

Seventeen patients with idiopathic nodular hyperplasia have had adrenal exploration. Our incidence of idiopathic hyperaldosteronism discovered at surgery (17 of 94 patients with primary aldosteronism) is much lower than those in other reported series.[2,3,16] This probably reflects our rigid diagnostic criteria: (1) increased aldosterone production; (2) reduced levels of plasma renin activity; and (3) lack of suppression of aldosterone with DOCA. The number of patients with idiopathic hyperaldosteronism in all of the series is still too small to allow a final evaluation of the results of surgery in this group. However, to date surgery has not corrected or significantly reduced the levels of blood pressure in these patients regardless of whether subtotal (removal of 75% of adrenal tissue) or total adrenalectomy was performed, and the dosage of antihypertensive medication required is similar to that required preoperatively.[3] Only one of our 17 patients has had normalization of blood pressure, which did not occur until 5 years after surgery; the patient died 2 weeks later of a myocardial infarction, suggesting that normalization of blood pressure was a portent of what was imminent.

In the three patients in whom unilateral adrenalectomy was performed who have been followed for up to 4 years, two had reappearance of hyperaldosteronism, hypokalemia, reduced plasma renin activity, lack of suppression of aldosterone levels with DOCA, and persistence of elevated blood pressure.

Comments

While our ability to distinguish aldosterone-producing adenoma from idiopathic hyperaldosteronism has improved considerably, it has not reached a level of predictability that allows denial of surgery in patients with either APA or IHA. In the presence of hypertension that is difficult to control or in cases in which normalization of blood pressure is not continuously achieved, surgery is recommended because of the high cure rate and certainty of improvement in patients with an APA. However, our approach may be revised after we acquire more information on the effects of subtotal or total adrenalectomy in patients with idiopathic hyperaldosteronism. This group will have to be carefully defined. The DOCA test is important in distinguishing IHA and APA from indeterminate hyperaldosteronism. However, at this time the results in significantly reducing the level of blood pressure in patients with idopathic hyperaldosteronism are discouraging.

Summary

The syndrome of primary aldosteronism has a number of variants. Patients with an aldosterone-producing adenoma have marked reduction of blood pressure after short-term treatment with spironolactone and little change in aldosterone levels or plasma-renin concentrations. Surgical removal of a unilateral adenoma results in cure in 65 percent of patients and improvement in the remainder. Patients with idiopathic hyperaldosteronism have had little improvement after administration of large doses of spironolactone. Aldosterone and plasma renin activity levels increased greatly in one patient. Subtotal or total adrenalectomy does not reduce blood pressure, and unilateral adrenalectomy results in reappearance of hyperaldosteronism, hypokalemia, and nonsuppressible levels of aldosterone (2 of 3 patients) after the deoxycorticosterone acetate test. Patients with indeterminate hyperaldosteronism (suppression with deoxycorticosterone acetate) or with labile hypertension and an aldosterone-producing adenoma can be managed effectively for many years with spironolactone therapy.

References

1. Conn, J. W.: The evolution of primary aldosteronism: 1954–1967. Harvey Lect. 62: 257, 1966–1967.
2. Baer, L., Sommers, S. C., Krakoff, L. R., Newton, M. A., and Laragh, J. H.: Pseudo-primary aldosteronism: An entity distinct from true primary aldosteronism. Circ. Res. 26–27(Suppl. I):203, 1970.
3. Biglieri, E. G., Schambelan, M., Slaton, P. E., and Stockigt, J. R.: The intercurrent hypertension of primary aldosteronism. Circ. Res. 26–27(Suppl. I):195, 1970.
4. Sutherland, D. J. A., Ruse, J. L., and Laidlaw, J. C.: Hypertension, increased aldosterone secretion, and low plasma renin activity relieved by dexamethasone. Can. Med. Assoc. J. 95:1109, 1966.
5. Biglieri, E. G., Stockigt, J. R., and Schambelan, M.: Mineralocorticoid hypertension. Third International Congress on Hormonal Steroids. *In* James, W. H. T., and Martini, L. (Eds.): Hormonal Steroids. Amsterdam: Excerpta Medica, 1971, pp. 565–571.
6. Aitchison, J., Brown, J. J., Ferriss, J. B., Fraser, R., Kay, A. W., Lever, A. F., Neville, A. M., Symington, T., and Robertson, J. I. S.: Quadric analysis in the preoperative distinction between patients with and without adrenocortical tumors in hypertension with aldosterone excess and low plasma renin. Am. Heart J. 82:660, 1971.
7. Biglieri, E. G., Slaton, P. E., Kronfield, S. J., and Schambelan, M.: Diagnosis of an aldosterone-producing adenoma in primary aldo-

steronism: An evaluative maneuver. JAMA 201:510, 1967.
8. Stockigt, J. R., Collins, R. D., and Biglieri, E. G.: Determination of plasma renin concentration by angiotensin I immunoassay. Circ. Res. 28–29(Suppl. II):175, 1971.
9. Jose, A., and Kaplan, N. M.: Plasma renin activity in the diagnosis of primary aldosteronism; failure to distinguish primary aldosteronism from essential hypertension. Arch. Intern. Med. 123:141, 1969.
10. Fishman, L. M., Küchel, O., Liddle, G. W., Michelakis, A. M., Gordon, R. D., and Chick, W. T.: Incidence of primary aldosteronism in uncomplicated "essential" hypertension: A prospective study with elevated aldosterone secretion and suppressed plasma renin activity used as diagnostic criteria. JAMA 205:497, 1968.
11. Channick, B. J., Adlin, E. V., and Marks, A. D.: Suppressed plasma renin activity in hypertension. Arch. Intern. Med. 123:131, 1969.
12. Cohen, E. L., Grim, C. E., Conn, J. W., Blough, W. M., Jr., Guyer, R. B., Kem, D. C., and Lucas, C. P.: Accurate and rapid measurement of plasma renin activity by radioimmunoassay: Results in normal and hypertensive people. J. Lab. Clin. Med. 77:1025, 1971.
13. Spark, R. F., and Melby, J. C.: Aldosteronism in hypertension: The spironolactone response test. Ann. Intern. Med. 69:685, 1968.
14. Morimoto, S., Takeda, R., and Murakami, M.: Does prolonged pretreatment with large doses of spironolactone hasten a recovery from juxtaglomerular-adrenal suppression in primary aldosteronism? J. Clin. Endocrinol. Metab. 31:659, 1970.
15. Silen, W., Biglieri, E. G., Slaton, P., and Galante, M.: Management of primary aldosteronism: Evaluation of potassium and sodium balance, technic of adrenalectomy and operative results in 24 cases. Ann. Surg. 164: 600, 1966.
16. George, J. M., Wright, L., Bell, N. H., and Bartter, F. C.: The syndrome of primary aldosteronism. Am. J. Med. 48:343, 1970.

Hypertension in Cushing's Syndrome

By Joseph W. Smiley, M.D.

Cushing's syndrome is the disease state resulting from a chronic excess of cortisol, the main adrenal glucocorticoid. Definitive diagnosis requires the demonstration of an abnormally high concentration of cortisol or its metabolic products in blood and urine.[1] The syndrome is now known to include several well-defined pathologic entities: bilateral adrenal hyperplasia, unilateral adrenal adenoma, adrenocortical carcinoma, nonendocrine ACTH-secreting tumor and steroid administration. Although hypertension has been a well-recognized component of this syndrome since the beginning of the twentieth century, the exact mechanism underlying its pathogenesis has thus far eluded the efforts of investigators in the fields of endocrinology and hypertension.

It is the main purpose of this chapter to review what is presently known concerning the cause of the hypertension. We will briefly mention some of the criteria which diagnose and differentiate the several forms of the syndrome and attempt to formulate a rational plan of therapy, especially for those patients in whom hypertension is a significant problem. Finally, we will suggest some further research which is needed in order for us to understand more clearly the complex role played by hypertension in Cushing's syndrome.

Pathogenesis of Hypertension

Published reviews of the subject of Cushing's syndrome document the fact that hypertension is present in approximately 80 percent of the patients.[2–4] Yet we are able to explain this occurrence with some degree of certainty in only a small minority of cases. It is unlikely that this high frequency of association is coincidental, especially in view of the fact that in those studies in which it was mentioned, blood pressure returned to normal in some 60 percent of the patients in which the syndrome was cured.

Despite the fact that hypertension can be produced in man by the administration of moderate to large doses of glucocorticoid hormones and a high-salt diet,[5] there has been no significant evidence to suggest that cortisol is the most important factor underlying the hypertension in the naturally occurring syndrome. In contrast to its very high incidence in the natural syndrome, hypertension has been found to occur in only 16.6 percent of steroid-treated patients and in 26.6 percent of patients treated with ACTH.[6] This latter observation suggests that there are ACTH-dependent factors other than cortisol that are responsible for hypertension in Cushing's syndrome.

Studies in experimental adrenal hypertension in rats during the 1950s demonstrated the potential importance of mineralocorticoids as a cause of sustained elevations in blood pressure. The phenomena of desoxycorticosterone acetate (DOCA)-induced hypertension[7] and adrenal regeneration hypertension[8] were associated with clinical pictures quite similar to those now seen in humans afflicted with hypertensive disease.

Much of the difficulty in understanding the association of hypertension with Cushing's syndrome stems from three important factors: (1) most published studies have not correlated types of adrenal pathology with incidence of hypertension; (2) the inability during the times most of the experience with Cushing's syndrome was being accumulated to measure accurately the individual chemical compounds produced by the adrenal gland; (3) failure to correlate the occurrence of hypokalemic alkalosis with hypertension. All of these problems now appear to have been at least partially resolved. During the past decade, workers in the field of hypertension have taken an interest in the adrenal cortex and have begun accumulating cases in relatively large numbers. They have been measuring the various secretions of the gland, correlating these measurements with

From the Division of Nephrology and Hypertension, Department of Medicine, Hahnemann Medical College and Hospital, Philadelphia, Pennsylvania.

the clinical aspects of the syndrome and with the various types of adrenal pathology associated with the syndrome.

In recent years, it has become possible to measure the blood levels and secretory rates of the various corticosteroids in patients. In addition to the well-known elevation of plasma cortisol in patients with Cushing's syndrome, the mineralocorticoids, desoxycorticosterone (DOC), and corticosterone (compound B) have been found to be elevated in some patients with Cushing's syndrome due to adrenal hyperplasia, but normal in others. In patients with unilateral adrenal adenoma, DOC and compound B have not been elevated.[9] When hypertension is present in adrenal carcinoma, it is usually associated with the overproduction of DOC, compound B and, occasionally, aldosterone.[9,10] In nonendocrine ACTH-secreting tumors, that form of Cushing's with the highest incidence of hypertension and the highest ACTH levels,[11] there is a markedly increased production of DOC and compound B.[9–12]

Two other examples of ACTH-dependent adrenal hypertension are the 11-hydroxylase deficiency syndrome[13] and the 17-hydroxylase deficiency syndrome.[14] Although they do not fit into the general definition of Cushing's syndrome, these entities are relevant to the discussion in that they are invariably associated with high levels of DOC and, in the case of the 17-hydroxylase defect, also with compound B, in the presence of depressed levels of cortisol, thus demonstrating that the ACTH-dependent mineralocorticoids are capable of causing elevated blood pressure independent of the effect of cortisol. It is noteworthy that the 17-hydroxylase deficiency syndrome and all the forms of Cushing's syndrome with high mineralocorticoid levels, as well as DOC-induced hypertension in rats, are commonly found to show hypokalemic alkalosis and edema.[7,15] This would seem to indicate that when hypokalemic alkalosis occurs in a patient with Cushing's syndrome, one is likely to find elevated levels of mineralocorticoids. Conversely, if it can be shown that there is an even higher incidence of hypertension in these patients, and perhaps, a relationship between the degree of elevation in these mineralocorticoids and the degree of hypertension, then it would certainly seem that the hypertension in these patients could be explained on a mineralocorticoid basis.

Since only about 15 percent of all the reported cases of Cushing's syndrome have demonstrated hypokalemic alkalosis,[2,16] even if 100 percent of these patients turn out to be hypertensive, there remains a large void to be filled in explaining the mechanism of hypertension in the remaining 65 percent of the cases. It appears that a good model to study might be the non-ACTH-dependent, unilateral adrenal adenoma. These tumors have not been shown to secrete excessive levels of the known mineralocorticoids, yet cure of the syndrome and the hypertension by removal of the affected adrenal gland is the rule.

Another problem to be solved is whether there is some unmeasured adrenal hormone that causes hypertension in the absence of hypokalemic alkalosis in cases of adrenal adenoma and in most cases of adrenal hyperplasia. 18-Hydroxy-deoxycorticosterone (18-OH-DOC), which has also been considered as a possible factor in adrenal regeneration hypertension,[17,18] was recently found to be secreted excessively in Cushing's syndrome.[19] This substance is abundantly secreted by the zona fasciculata in response to ACTH. However, implicating 18-OH-DOC as a cause of hypertension in humans is difficult because of its relatively weak mineralocorticoid activity, which is roughly one-half that of DOC and one-fiftieth that of aldosterone.[20] It has recently been postulated that 18-OH-DOC is the precursor of some more potent mineralocorticoid, thus far unrecognized and, therefore, unmeasured. Studies on the structure of the steroid product of 18-OH-DOC are in progress.[20] Concurrently much work is being done in an attempt to relate 18-OH-DOC to hypertensive disease in general. Until the solution of this problem is achieved, its role as a factor in the hypertension of Cushing's syndrome remains at best only a speculation.

The recent report of increased plasma renin substrate in hypertension caused by Cushing's syndrome[21] is of interest since the renin-angiotensin system has not previously been regarded to have etiologic importance in this condition. It is postulated that increased renin substrate may be significant in the patients who are not salt-retainers in that a given level of plasma renin, in the salt-restricted state, can catalyze the formation of larger amounts of angiotensin. Perhaps this is one of the mechanisms by which hypertension is produced in those Cushing's syndrome patients who don't secrete excessive mineralocorticoid.

In discussing the possible hormonal causes of hypertension in Cushing's syndrome, the question arises as to whether the "missing" element is simply cortisol itself, the hallmark of the syndrome. Although "pure" glucocorticoids have been shown to cause hypertension in salt-restricted rats,[7] this has not been shown to occur in humans. Nevertheless, humans taking glucocorticoids chronically for various reasons have been found to become mildly hypertensive or to have an exacerbation of previous hypertension if they overindulge in salt. Therefore, before we dismiss cortisol as a possible important factor in the genesis of hypertension in the syndrome, it is necessary that a large group of patients be studied with regard to their blood pressure levels, sodium balance, and cortisol levels at various grades of salt intake. It could well be that a certain number of patients manifesting mild hypertension could be explained on the basis of a mechanism such as this.

In additional to humoral factors, there may be vascular factors leading to hypertension in these patients, especially in those cases not associated with electrolyte abnormalities. It has been shown in rats that chronic administration of cortisone acetate, a synthetic glucocorticoid, leads to a constant elevation of the serum cholesterol.[7] Abnormal cholesterol metabolism has also been noted in humans with Cushing's syndrome.[22] Another metabolic abnormality predisposing to vascular disease is glucose intolerance, which is one of the hallmarks of the syndrome, occurring in approximately 80 percent of the patients.[16] One study has emphasized the severe vascular changes in these patients and suggested premature development of atherosclerosis as an etiologic factor in their hypertension [22] but no mention is made of a proposed mechanism for the association. There is marked and progressive atherosclerosis in the larger blood vessels in Cushing's syndrome, and the kidneys are commonly noted to show the changes of nephrosclerosis.[2] The incidence of renal arterial stenosis is not known but would be expected to be higher than in the general population less predisposed to atherosclerosis.

Although it is likely that most of the cases of hypertension in Cushing's syndrome will some day be explainable on the basis of hormonal substances produced by the adrenal gland, it is also probable that at least some cases will not correlate well with this theory, and these are the cases in which the hypertension does not respond to bilateral total adrenalectomy. With the early onset of severe atherosclerosis noted in many of these patients, it is likely that some will be found to have renal artery stenosis on this basis, and, for this reason, patients manifesting severe hypertension should be studied arteriographically for this lesion before having adrenal surgery. There will be another group of patients, also small in number, who will have renal parenchymal disease of various etiologies, which is sustaining the hypertension and will cause it to persist after adrenalectomy. Lastly there will be a few patients who have coexisting Cushing's syndrome and hypertension, a not too unlikely possibility in view of the high incidence of essential hypertension in the general population.

DIAGNOSIS [16,23–25]

The presence of three or more of the following symptoms strongly suggests the diagnosis of Cushing's syndrome: extreme weakness with muscle wasting, truncal obesity, red and depressed striae, ecchymosis with normal platelet counts, hypertension, osteoporosis, and glucose intolerance. A recent sudden onset of symptoms suggests adenoma or carcinoma, while a more insidious onset favors bilateral hyperplasia.

Suggestive laboratory findings include neutrophilia, relative lymphocytopenia, decreased direct eosinophil count, elevated fasting blood sugar or abnormal glucose tolerance curve, and hypokalemic, hypochloremic alkalosis.

Diagnostic laboratory studies are those which determine the basal secretory rates of the various hormonal components of the adrenocortical secretory mixture. In Cushing's syndrome, diurnal rhythm is abolished and total secretion of cortisol is increased, with a resulting excess of circulating cortisol reflected in elevated plasma and urinary 17-hydroxycorticoids and 17-ketogenic steroids.[16,23,24]

The overnight dexamethasone suppression test is the first step in screening the patient. One milligram of dexamethasone given just before midnight will suppress ACTH secretion in normal subjects, and cortisol production will stop. In Cushing's syndrome this amount of dexamethasone does not suppress ACTH secretion or excessive autonomous production of cortisol by an adrenocortical tumor. These patients fail to suppress their plasma 17-hydroxycorticoids below 12 μg per 100 ml.

Urinary free cortisol is the measurement of the unbound physiologically active form of cortisol. This will be found to exceed 125 μg per 24 hours in Cushing's syndrome.

Another even more accurate index of adrenal secretory activity is the cortisol secretion rate, in which urine passed after the injection of a tracer dose of ^{3}H-labeled cortisol is collected, and the metabolites of cortisol isolated by thin-layer chromatography. The specific activity of an isolated metabolite is determined and the secretion rate is then calculated.[25]

Since the free cortisol test is not yet generally available to clinicians, one may have to resort to a more readily available test which indirectly reflects cortisol secretion. We are referring, of course, to the 24-hour levels of urinary 17-hydroxycorticoids, 17-ketogenic steroids, and 17-ketosteroids, which are found to be fairly reliable provided one allows for the elevations that are seen with obesity, thyrotoxicosis, acromegaly, emotional disturbances, and surgical stress.

Suppression and stimulation tests are designed to characterize the role of pituitary corticotropin and to differentiate between physiologic overactivity and a truly pathologic state including the presence of tumor.

The metyrapone test is generally available and determines whether there is pituitary secretion of ACTH (as in hyperplasia) or whether it has been suppressed (as in tumor). Metyrapone blocks conversion of the inactive precursor, desoxycortisol, to cortisol. If pituitary ACTH secretion is preserved, it will respond to the falling levels of cortisol with an increased secretion of ACTH and, secondarily, to an increase in urinary 17-hydroxycorticoids. If pituitary ACTH is suppressed, as in an autonomous adrenocortical tumor, there will be no such increase in response to metyrapone. After collecting a baseline 24-hour urine for 17-hydroxycorticoids and 17-ketogenic steroids, on the following day 500 mg of metyrapone is given by mouth at hourly intervals from 7:00 A.M. till 12:00 noon for a total of 3 gm. Throughout this period a second 24-hour urine sample is collected. Patients with adrenal hyperplasia show a doubling of the 17-hydroxycorticoids or the 17-ketogenic steroids, while those with adrenal tumors show little or no change.

Plasma ACTH levels are becoming more generally available and should become a useful diagnostic tool in the near future. In adrenal hyperplasia due to excessive pituitary ACTH, the levels are found to be mildly elevated, while the nonendocrine, ACTH-secreting tumors have been found in association with plasma ACTH levels 50 to 300 times normal. Conversely, when an adrenocortical tumor is responsible for the excess cortisol, ACTH levels are lower than normal.

Another more widely used test for distinguishing between adrenal hyperplasia and tumors is the urinary dexamethasone suppression test. While daily 24-hour urinary steroid collections are performed, 0.5 mg of dexamethasone is given every 6 hours for eight doses. Then 2 mg of dexamethasone is given every 6 hours for another eight doses. Normal or obese subjects show a suppression of 17-hydroxycorticoids of 50 percent or more on the low dose of dexamethasone, but patients with Cushing's syndrome in all its forms do not. Patients with bilateral adrenal hyperplasia do suppress their steroid excretion on the high dose, while those patients with adrenal adenoma or carcinoma fail to suppress.

The differentiation between adrenal adenoma and carcinoma may be determined on the basis of whether the tumor is responsive to ACTH. Twenty-five units of ACTH is given in 500 ml of physiologic saline solution over an 8-hour period. The 17-hydroxycorticoid level will increase three- to fivefold as compared with the control level, and the 17-ketosteroid value increases up to twofold in well over half the cases of adenoma. An increase is rarely found with carcinoma.

Treatment

Recent studies suggest that the diagnosis of Cushing's syndrome now carries a much more favorable prognosis than previously. In the precortisone era, physicians caring for these patients were limited by the need to preserve functioning adrenal tissue in order for their patients to survive. Methods of treatment thus were unsatisfactory, and less than 50 percent of these patients survived 5 years.[2] The present-day philosophy is to do whatever is necessary to cure the patient, including bilateral total adrenalectomy, thus necessitating that the patient remain on glucocorticoid and mineralocorticoid therapy the rest of his life.

The results of surgical treatment of Cushing's syndrome due to adrenal adenoma have been almost uniformly excellent. In reported cases treated by unilateral adrenalectomy and removal of the benign tumor, the cure rate has been close to 100 percent.[26,27] The hypertension has been relieved in about 85 percent of the cases.

The surgical treatment of Cushing's syndrome caused by malignant adrenal tumor has been discouraging. Many patients die before surgery can be performed and most patients operated upon have died within a matter of months postoperatively of previously undiagnosed metastatic disease.[27] In the treatment of patients with inoperable known metastatic adrenal carcinoma, a small degree of success has been achieved with the use of the adrenolytic agent o,p'DDD.[28,29]

Cushing's syndrome due to nonendocrine, ACTH-secreting tumors has been "cured" in those relatively few cases in which the tumors could be successfully resected.[30] Unfortunately the majority of the ectopic ACTH-secreting tumors are malignant and nonresectable. In these cases, it may be possible to correct many of their metabolic complications by using an adrenal inhibitor such as aminoglutethimide or metyrapone,[26] as well as by bilateral adrenalectomy. No large series has yet been published reporting the success rate in amelioration of hypertension in this group of patients, but a good response would be favored by the recent onset of the syndrome in nearly all the patients.

In bilateral adrenal hyperplasia due to excessive pituitary ACTH production, it has become clear that the only dependably curative surgical procedure is total bilateral adrenalectomy. One hundred percent of the patients so treated are cured of the syndrome.[26] In a series reporting cases that were treated during a period of time when subtotal adrenalectomy was considered the treatment of choice, only 59 percent of the surgically treated patients were relieved of their hypertension.[27] Included in these figures are some patients whose condition was not cured by the first operation; the second, more radical procedure cured the syndrome and the hypertension.

Because of the morbidity associated with adrenal surgery and the necessity of life-long steroid-replacement therapy, a recent study advocated the use of pituitary irradiation as the treatment of first choice in patients with adrenal hyperplasia.[26] The authors point out that the complications of this therapy are virtually nil. However, permanent remission of the syndrome is accomplished in only 20 percent of the patients so treated. Total bilateral adrenalectomy is then performed on those patients whose disease is unimproved by irradiation, or as the primary therapeutic procedure in those in whom more rapid correction of hypercortisolism is necessary. This latter group would certainly include those patients with severe intractable hypertension.

In patients whose disease has not yet reached a state of urgency, o,p'DDD has been used experimentally as a possible alternative to pituitary irradiation or bilateral adrenalectomy. This agent has successfully induced remissions in 100 percent of patients with adrenal hyperplasia, in doses much lower than those usually recommended for metastatic adrenal carcinoma.[31] It takes effect slowly over the course of 4 to 6 months, but has the advantage of selectively destroying only the zona fasciculata and zona reticularis, thus making mineralocorticoid-replacement therapy unnecessary. It would be expected that this form of treatment would be applicable to the mildly or moderately severe hypertensive patient who is well controlled on the standard antihypertensive drugs.

References

1. Christy, N. P.: The Human Adrenal Cortex. New York: Harper & Row, 1971, p. 359.
2. Plotz, C., Knowlton, A., and Ragan, C.: The natural history of Cushing's syndrome. Am. J. Med. 13:597, 1952.
3. Soffer, L., Iannaccone, A., and Gabrileve, J.: Cushing's syndrome. Am. J. Med. 30:129, 1961.
4. Ross, E., Marshall-Jones, P., and Friedman, M.: Cushing's syndrome: Diagnostic criteria. Q. J. Med. 35:149, 1966.
5. Genest, J., Kuchel, O., and Nowaczynski, W.: Classification of hypermineralocorticoid hypertension. This volume.
6. Savage, O., Copeman, W. S., Chapman, L., Wells, M. V., and Treadwell, B. L.: Pituitary and adrenal hormones in rheumatoid arthritis. Lancet 1:232, 1962.
7. Knowlten, A. I., Loeb, E. N., Stoerk, H. C., White, J. P., and Heffernan, J. F.: Induction of arterial hypertension in normal and adrenalectomized rats given cortisone acetate. J. Exp. Med. 96:187, 1952.
8. Skelton, F.: Development of hypertension and cardiovascular renal lesions during adrenal regeneration. Proc. Soc. Exp. Biol. Med. 90:342, 1955.
9. Biglieri, E. G., Slaton, P. E., Schambelan, M., and Kronfield, S. J.: Hypermineralocorticoidism. Am. J. Med. 45:170, 1968.
10. Crane, M. G., and Harris, J. J.: Desoxycorticosterone secretion rates in hyperadrenocorticism. J. Clin. Endocrinol. 26:1135, 1966.
11. Lauler, D., Williams, G., and Thorn, G.: Diseases of the adrenal cortex. *In* Harrison's Principles of Internal Medicine, 6th Edition. New York: McGraw-Hill, 1970, p. 495.
12. Cost, W. S.: A mineralocorticoid excess syndrome presumably due to excessive secretions of corticosterone. Lancet 1:362, 1963.
13. Eberlein, W., and Bongiovanni, A.: Plasma and urinary corticosteroids in hypertensive form of congenital adrenal hyperplasia. J. Biol. Chem. 223:85, 1956.
14. Biglieri, E. G., Herron, M. A., and Brust, N.: 17-Hydroxylation deficiency in man. J. Clin. Invest. 45:1946, 1966.
15. Schambelan, M., Slaton, P. E., and Biglieri, E. G.: Mineralocorticoid production in hyperadrenocorticism. Am. J. Med. 51:299, 1971.
16. Williams, R. H.: Textbook of Endocrinology, 4th Edition. Philadelphia: Saunders, 1968, p. 287.
17. Birmingham, M., MacDonald, M., and Rochefert, J.: Adrenal function in normal rats and in rats bearing regenerated adrenal glands. *In* McKerns, K. W. (Ed.): Functions of the Adrenal Cortex, vol. II. New York: Appleton-Century-Crofts, 1968, p. 647.
18. Melby, J. C., Dale, S. L., Grekin, R. J., Gaunt, R., and Wilson, T. E.: 18-Hydroxy-11-deoxycorticosterone (18-OH-DOC) secretion in experimental and human hypertension. This volume.
19. Melby, J. C., Wilson, T. E., and Dale, S. L.: Secretion of 18-hydroxydesoxycorticosterone in human hypertensive disease. (Abstract.) J. Clin. Invest. 49:64a, 1970.
20. Melby, J. C., Dale, S. L., and Wilson, T. E.: 18-Hydroxydesoxycorticosterone in human hypertension. Circ. Res. 48–49 (Suppl. II):143, 1971.
21. Krakoff, L. R., and Amsel, B.: Increased plasma renin substrate in hypertension due to Cushing's syndrome. (Abstract.) Circulation 43–44(Suppl. II):122, 1971.
22. Mannix, H., and Glenn, F.: Hypertension in Cushing's syndrome. JAMA 180:119, 1962.
23. Herrera, M., Cahill, G., and Thorn, G.: Cushing's syndrome—diagnosis and treatment. Am. J. Surg. 107:144, 1964.
24. Smilo, R., and Forsham, P.: Diagnostic approach to hypofunction and hyperfunction of the adrenal cortex. Postgrad. Med. 46:146, 1969.
25. Melby, J. C.: Assessment of adrenocortical function. N. Engl. J. Med. 285:735, 1971.
26. Orth, D., and Liddle, G.: Results of treatment in 108 patients with Cushing's syndrome. N. Engl. J. Med. 285:243, 1971.
27. Raker, J., Cope, O., and Ackerman, I.: Surgical experience with the treatment of hypertension of Cushing's syndrome. Am. J. Surg. 107:153, 1964.
28. Bergenstal, D. M., Lipsett, M. B., Moy, R. H., and Hertz, R.: Regression of adrenal cancer and suppression of adrenal function in man by o,p'DDD. Trans. Assoc. Am. Physicians 72:341, 1959.
29. Bergenstal, D. M., Hertz, R., Lipsett, M. B., and Moy, R. H.: Chemotherapy of adrenocortical cancer with o,p'DDD. Ann. Intern. Med. 53:672, 1960.
30. Liddle, G. W., Nicholson, W. E., Island, D. P., Orth, D. N., Abe, K., and Lowder, S. C.: Clinical and laboratory studies of ectopic humoral syndromes. Recent Progr. Horm. Res. 25:283, 1969.
31. Temple, T. E., Jones, D. J., Liddle, G. W., and Dexter, R. N.: Treatment of Cushing's disease. N. Engl. J. Med. 281:801, 1969.

Adrenal Enzymatic Defects and Hypertension

By Edward G. Biglieri, M.D.

PATIENTS WITH CONGENITAL adrenal hyperplasia, either the 11-β-hydroxylation deficiency syndrome (11-OHDS) or the 17-α-hydroxylation deficiency syndrome (17-OHDS), invariably have hypertension.[1,2] The steroid causing hypertension in both of these disorders is deoxycorticosterone (DOC).[1,2] In the 17-OHDS form, corticosterone (compound B) is increased and aldosterone is decreased.[3–8] Deficiency in the 17-hydroxylating system is also present in the gonads so that virilization is not a feature in the 17-OHDS, but in the 11-OHDS there is no impediment to the formation of excessive androgenic steroids and hypokalemia is not invariably present.[9–11] The 17-OHDS is usually identified during adolescence or early adulthood because of the presence of hypertension and of primary amenorrhea in the female patient and pseudohermaphroditism in the male patient. The characteristics and course of the congenital 17-OHDS and of other clinical hypertensive disorders in which the secretory patterns of the mineralocorticoid hormones suggest an acquired enzymatic hydroxylation inhibitor are examined herein (Table 1).

Materials and Methods

All measurements of blood pressure and electrolyte concentrations were carried out during a sodium intake of 120 mEq per day and a fixed potassium intake of 70 to 80 mEq per day. Steroid measurements[2–5] were made by either gas-liquid chromatography or double-isotope dilution-derivative techniques, as reported previously by this laboratory.[2]

From the Medical Service, San Francisco General Hospital, and the Department of Medicine, University of California, San Francisco, California.

Supported by U.S. Public Health Service Research Grants HL–11046 from the National Heart and Lung Institute and AM–06415 from the National Institute of Arthritis and Metabolic Diseases. The studies were carried out in the General Clinical Research Center, RR–83, at San Francisco General Hospital, supported by Division of Research Grants and Facilities, National Institutes of Health.

Table 1.—*Adrenal Enzymatic Defects and Hypertension*

Congenital adrenal hyperplasia
11-β-Hydroxylation deficiency
17-α-Hydroxylation deficiency
Acquired disorders: effecting altered secretory mixtures
Feminizing adrenocortical carcinoma
Ectopic ACTH-producing syndrome
Cushing's syndrome

Comments

17-OHDS

Salient Clinical Features (*Table 2*). Of the eight reported cases[2–7] (five studied in this laboratory), all were first detected during early adulthood, although hypertension had been observed for a number of years, often dating back to early childhood. The two male patients were first seen because of pseudohermaphroditism. In the female patients, secondary sex characteristics are absent. Blood pressure levels can be slightly to severely elevated. In almost all patients hypokalemia is easily demonstrated and the blood level of bicarbonate is moderately elevated. Plasma renin activity is extremely low or not detectable.

Steroid Patterns (*Table 3; Fig. 1*). Urinary metabolites of the 17-hydroxylated steroids are severely reduced or absent; i.e., pregnanetriol, tetrahydrocortisol, cortisone, and tetrahydro-11-deoxycortisol. The blood levels and secretory rates of cortisol are reduced or absent. Other steroids derived from 17-hydroxyprogesterone and pregnenolone, such as dehydroepiandrosterone and its metabolites, testosterone, and estrogens are also reduced. Ketosteroids are usually reduced since they represent a composite of androgenic steroids

TABLE 2.—*Salient Features in Eight Patients with 17-Hydroxylation Deficiency Syndrome*

Clinical Data	*Reference No.*							
	2	*3*	*4*	*4*	*5*	*6*	*7*	*8*
Age (yr)	36	21	20	19	16	18	24	19
Sex	Female	Female	Female	Female	Female	Female	Male	Male
Duration of hypertension (yr)	20	2	4	4	14	4	?	5
Female secondary sex characteristics	Absent	Absent	Absent	Absent	Absent	Absent	Present	Absent
Blood pressure (mm Hg)	220/140	140/100	150/100	140/100	135–145/90–110	220/120	150/100	160–220/120–150
Serum electrolyte concentration (mEq per liter)								
Sodium	144.0	146.0	145.0	141.0	139.0		133.0	142–150
Potassium	2.7	3.2	2.8	3.1	2.8–3.9	2.1	4.3	2.9–4.0
Chloride	31.0	28.0	28.0	27.0	27–31	40.0		28–33
Carbon dioxide	100.0	105.0	103.0	101.0	100.0			102–106
Plasma renin activity (ng per ml per hr) *	ND	ND	ND	ND	ND		0.1	0–0.18

* Abbreviation used: ND, not detectable.

TABLE 3.—*Steroid Measurements in Eight Patients with 17-Hydroxylation Deficiency Syndrome*

Steroid	*Steroid Assayed* *	*Reference No.* 2	3	4	4	5	6	7	8
17-Hydroxylated steroids									
17-OH-progesterone	Urinary pregnanetriol (mg per 24 hr)	ND	0					1.9	0.43
11-deoxycortisol (compound S)	Tetrahydrodeoxycortisol (μg per 24 hr)	ND	0						
	Secretory rate (mg per 24 hr)							0.051	
Cortisol	Plasma F (μg per 100 ml)	0	7.0			0.4	2.7	5.0	0.4
	THF and THE (mg per 24 hr)	0	1.6	0.7	0.7	2.9		2.7	0.2–2.9
	Secretory rate (mg per 24 hr)	0	3.0	0.5		2.5		2.8	
Steroids derived from 17-hydroxylated steroids									
Ketosteroids (KS)	Urinary KS (mg per 24 hr)	2.0	8.0	1.5	1.1		2.5	5.9	0.8–3.6
Dehydroepiandrosterone (DHEA)	Urinary DHEA (mg per 24 hr)	0.11–0.17							
Testosterone (T)	Plasma T (μg per 100 ml)	0.014	< 0.01					0.04	
Estrogen (E_2)	Urinary E_2 (μg per 24 hr)	< 0.2				1.7		0.11	22
Non-17-hydroxylated steroids									
Progesterone	Plasma (μg per 100 ml)	0.21	2.5				0.8	0.02	4.0
	Pregnanediol (mg per 24 hr)	2–11	21.0					0.29	
DOC	THDOC (μg per 24 hr)	500		107.4	32.1				780
	Secretory rate (μg per 24 hr)	5100	1400	2019		1925		760	
Compound B	Plasma B (μg per 100 ml)	20–30				24.7	14.9		26.8
	THB (μg per 24 hr)			2040	1738	380			
	Secretory rate (mg per 24 hr)	99–124	44.0	29.2		17.9	30.0	34	
18-OHB	TH-18-OHA (μg per 24 hr)	675							
Aldosterone	18-glucuronide (μg per 24 hr)	0–1		0.5	0.5	1.2			0.9–3.2
	TH-aldosterone (μg per 24 hr)	0–5							
	Secretory rate (μg per 24 hr)	10–18	29	36		10.5	12.0	75	

* Abbreviations: THF, tetrahydrocortisol; THE, tetrahydrocortisone; THDOC, tetrahydro-DOC; THB, tetrahydrocorticosterone.

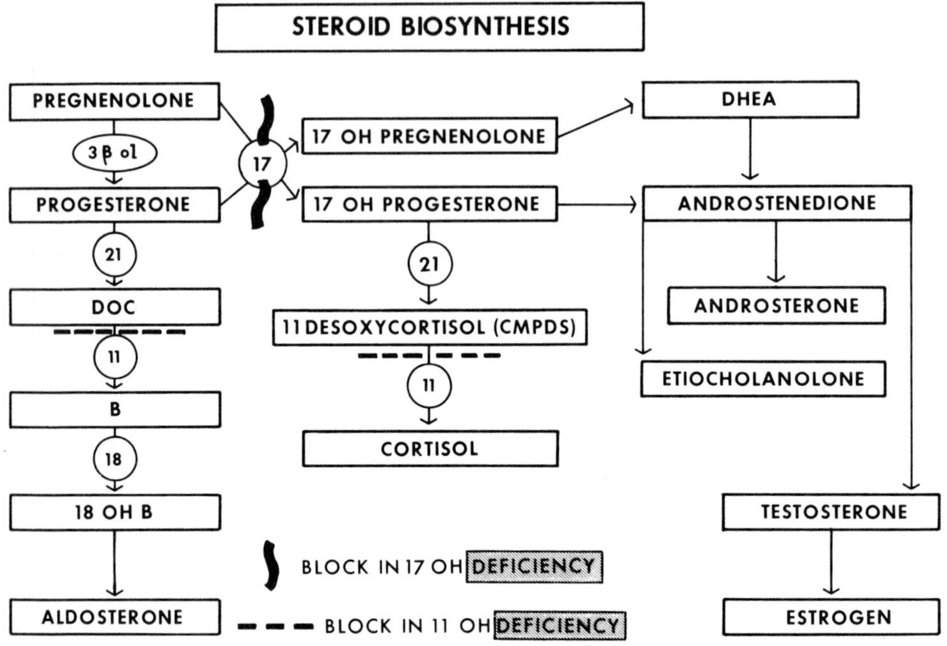

FIG. 1.—Enzymatic blocks in congenital adrenal hyperplasia associated with hypertension.

derived from these precursors. The absence of estrogens and testosterone results in absence of secondary sex characteristics in female patients and pseudohermaphroditism in male patients. These deficiencies are reflected in the elevated levels of follicle-stimulating hormone (FSH).

The adrenal steroids not dependent on 17-hydroxylation are present in elevated amounts. Blood levels, urinary metabolites, and secretory rates of progesterone, DOC, compound B, and 18-hydroxycorticosterone (18-OHB) are invariably elevated. However, aldosterone levels are subnormal or not detectable. Low urinary levels of 17-ketosteroids and 17-hydroxysteroids in a hypokalemic, hypertensive person strongly suggest the 17-OHDS. In addition, the finding of primary amenorrhea makes the diagnosis more likely. The additional observation of a high level of plasma "cortisol" (fluorometric determination) in the presence of reduced urinary 17-hydroxysteroids may also be indicative of this syndrome since the levels of compound B could be measured by this procedure.

Pathophysiology (*Fig. 2*). The reduced ability to synthesize cortisol results in increased ACTH levels [1] that drive the adrenal to produce more of the non-17-hydroxylated steroids DOC and compound B as depicted in Fig. 1. A characteristic of this group of steroids is their limited capacity to reduce the release or formation of ACTH by the pituitary gland. Thus production of progesterone, DOC, compound B, and 18-OHB increases and aldosterone

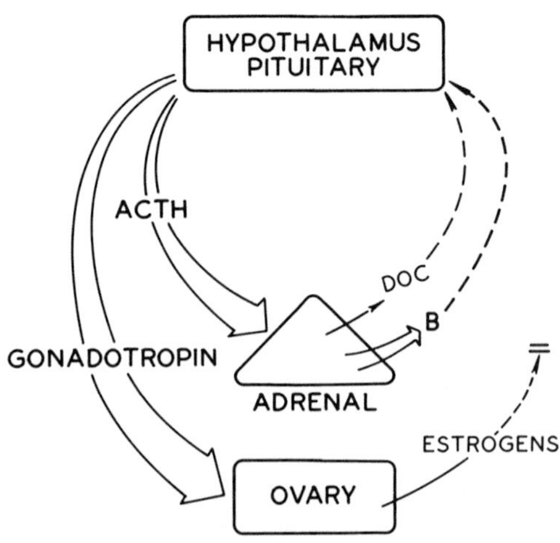

FIG. 2.—Pathophysiology of the 17-hydroxylation deficiency syndrome.

production decreases. The reduction of aldosterone production can result from several factors.[12] Increased amounts of DOC can effect expansion of the extracellular fluid volume and suppression of plasma renin activity, with subsequent reduction of aldosterone production; plasma renin activity levels were low or undetectable in all seven patients studied (Table 2). However, there remains the strong possibility that intra-adrenal modulation of aldosterone production may be affected by substrate inhibition of the major pathways at the final enzymatic formation of aldosterone from 18-OHB. A combination of both of these events may be responsible for the reduced aldosterone production: an initiating event, reduced plasma renin activity, and a sustaining intra-adrenal event. Long-term treatment with large amounts of ACTH in normal subjects and in patients with the "ectopic" ACTH-producing syndrome always results in high secretory levels of compound B and DOC with normal or subnormal levels of aldosterone.[12–15] When ACTH is discontinued, diminution of aldosterone continues to below control levels for up to 7 days.[12] Renin may not be the sole factor in this event because when ACTH is administered to patients with an aldosterone-producing adenoma, in whom plasma renin activity is virtually absent,[16] the usual transient elevation in aldosterone excretion occurs followed by a similar reduction to below control levels after cessation of therapy.

Treatment. Glucocorticoid treatment directed at suppression of ACTH production is definitive. Treatment dosages vary but only replacement doses of 1 mg of dexamethasone or 20 mg of cortisol are required in most patients. Some patients are extremely sensitive to these steroids and treatment should be started with very small doses, especially when cortisol cannot be detected. Initiation of therapy effects a prompt diuresis of sodium, retention of potassium, normalization of blood pressure, return of plasma renin activity, aldosterone, DOC, and compound B to normal values. While aldosterone production increases promptly it may take many months to reach the normal range,[2] and caution must be exercised in the early management to avoid a hyperkalemic crisis. In this context, cortisol with its limited mineralocorticoid action is the treatment of choice.

Implications of 17-OHDS. Subtle alteration in the 17-hydroxylation system may have a significant role in the etiology of hypertension. Partial defects could lead to excessive secretion of such mineralocorticoids as DOC and compound B; however, the steroids are not elevated in patients with essential hypertension.[13,14] Whether other mineralocorticoid hormones are involved is not evident at this time. The role of 18-OH-deoxycorticosterone (18-OH-DOC), which is an ACTH-dependent steroid, is not clear at present, but elevated levels have been found in some patients with essential hypertension and low plasma renin activity levels.[17] There is ample in vitro evidence that the various hydroxylating systems involved in adrenal steroidogenesis can be influenced by various steroids so that the final secretory mixture from the adrenal gland is varied: Interference at positions 11 and 21 by androgens,[18,19] at position 17 by progesterone,[20] and probably at position 11 by estrogens has been demonstrated.[21,22]

Acquired Enzymatic Abnormalities

Feminizing Adrenocortical Carcinoma (Fig. 3). A small number of patients with this disease have hypertension. Greater longevity is associated with the hypertensive patients although the disease is invariably rapid and lethal. In several patients there was strong evidence that a mild degree of 11-β-hydroxylation deficiency was present[22]: the only mineralocorticoid produced in excess was DOC with an associated increase in 11-deoxycortisol excretion (a pattern observed in the congenital 11-OHDS); compound B and cortisol levels were within the normal range and increased promptly after administration of ACTH, and aldosterone levels were low.[22] Could high intra-adrenal levels of estrogens be inhibiting 11-β-hydroxylation?

The "Ectopic" ACTH Syndrome. The pattern of mineralocorticoid hormones secreted in patients with this syndrome is quite similar to that described for patients with the 17-OHDS[14,15]: elevated DOC and compound B secretion and reduced aldosterone production. The levels of DOC and compound B are

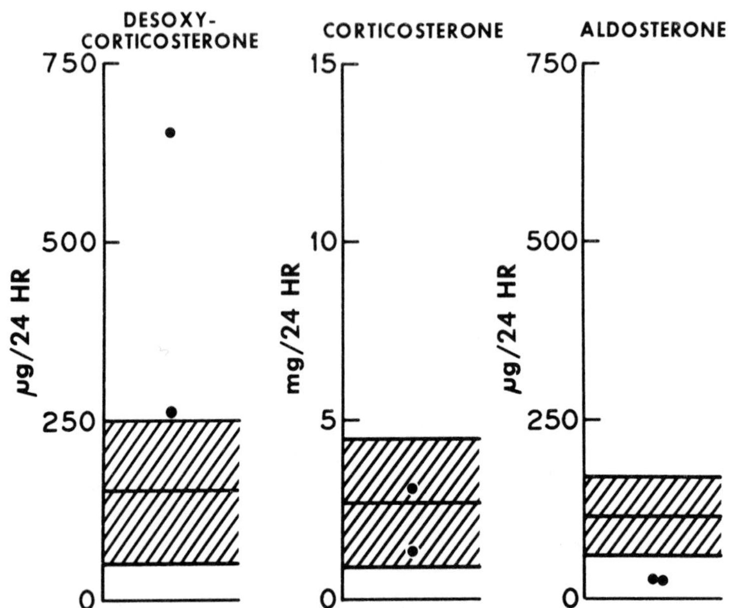

FIG. 3.—Mineralocorticoid secretory rates in the hypertensive form of feminizing adrenocortical carcinoma.

sufficiently elevated that they, by themselves, could account for the frequent occurrence of hypertension and hypokalemia in these patients. The reason for normal or reduced aldosterone production is not clear. The possibility does exist that ACTH might direct steroid precursors to the cortisol pathway rather than to aldosterone; however, the levels of the aldosterone precursors, compound B and DOC, are also increased. Levels of plasma renin activity are usually within normal limits in these patients. The influence of chronic administration of ACTH on plasma renin activity in man is still in dispute.[23,24]

Cushing's Syndrome. In patients with bilateral adrenal hypertension in whom ACTH production is often increased, production of DOC and compound B is occasionally increased.[14] Aldosterone abnormalities have not been observed.[25]

Adrenal Malignancies

While adrenal malignancies do not fall into a category of acquired enzymatic defects, it is important to note that increased production of DOC and compound B are commonly observed. Whether these increased levels represent the production of a particular cell or the modification of the final secretory product of normal cells is not clear.

SUMMARY

The 17-hydroxylation deficiency syndrome in man is identified by hypertension, hypokalemia, primary amenorrhea in the female patient, and pseudohermaphroditism in the male patient. 17-Hydroxylated steroids are not found in the urine of these patients. The principal steroids secreted are DOC and compound B. Levels of ACTH are increased and plasma renin activity levels are reduced. Aldosterone production is subnormal. Treatment with small doses of glucocorticoids suppresses excessive ACTH production and returns DOC and compound B to normal levels. Plasma renin activity and aldosterone are restored to normal levels. Hypertension and hypokalemia are readily corrected. This disorder emphasizes the role of other mineralocorticoids besides aldosterone in the hypertensive process. Partial 17-hydroxylation deficiencies in hypertensive patients could give rise to conditions in which increased production of DOC, compound B, or other still unidentified potent mineralocorticoids could be etiologic factors of hypertension in man. Several disorders may be considered acquired enzymatic defects with patterns similar to those observed in patients with the 17-hydroxylation deficiency syndrome. These are feminizing adrenocortical carcinoma, in which the steroid pattern suggests 11-hydroxylation in appearance, the ectopic ACTH syndrome and, in certain cases, Cushing's syndrome, in which suppression of aldosterone and elevation of DOC and compound B levels follow the same pattern observed in the 17-hydroxylation deficiency syndrome.

References

1. Eberlein, W. R., and Bongiovanni, A. M.: Plasma and urinary corticosteroids in hypertensive form of congenital adrenal hyperplasia. J. Biol. Chem. 223:85, 1956.
2. Biglieri, E. G., Herron, M. A., and Brust, N.: 17-Hydroxylation deficiency in man. J. Clin. Invest. 45:1946, 1966.
3. Goldsmith, O., Solomon, D. H., and Horton, R.: Hypogonadism and mineralocorticoid excess: The 17-hydroxylase deficiency syndrome. N. Engl. J. Med. 277:673, 1967.
4. Malin, S. R.: Congenital adrenal hyperplasia secondary to 17-hydroxylase deficiency; two sisters with amenorrhea, hypokalemia, hypertension, and cystic ovaries. Ann. Intern. Med. 70:69, 1969.
5. Baskin, J. L.: Personal communication.
6. Mills, I. H., Wilson, R. J., Tait, A. D., and Cooper, H. R.: Steroid metabolic studies in a patient with 17-hydroxylase deficiency. J. Endocrinol. 38:19, 1967.
7. New, M. I.: Male pseudohermaphroditism due to 17-alpha-hydroxylase deficiency. J. Clin. Invest. 49:1930, 1970.
8. Mantero, F., Busnardo, B., Riondel, A., Veyrat, R., and Austoni, M.: Hypertension artérielle, alcalose hypokaliémique et pseudohermaphrodisme mâle par déficit en 17-alphahydroxylase. Schweiz. Med. Wochenschr. 101:38, 1971.
9. Gandy, H. M., Keutmann, E. H., and Izzo, A. J.: Characterization of urinary steroids in adrenal hyperplasia: isolation of metabolites of cortisol, compound S, and desoxycorticosterone from normotensive patient with adrenogenital syndrome. J. Clin. Invest. 39:364, 1960.
10. Bergstrand, C. G., Birke, G., and Plantin, L. O.: The corticosteriod excretion pattern in infants and children with the adrenogenital syndrome. Acta Endocrinol. 30:500, 1959.
11. New, M. I., and Seaman, M. P.: Secretion rates of cortisol and aldosterone precursors in various forms of congenital adrenal hyperplasia. J. Clin. Endocrinol. Metab. 30:361, 1970.
12. Biglieri, E. G., Schambelan, M., and Slaton, P. E., Jr.: Effect of adrenocorticotropin on desoxycorticosterone, corticosterone and aldosterone excretion. J. Clin. Endocrinol. Metab. 29:1090, 1969.
13. Biglieri, E. G., Stockigt, J. R., and Schambelan, M.: Mineralocorticoid hypertension. Third International Congress on Hormonal Steroids. *In* James, W. H. T., and Martini, L. (Eds.): Hormonal Steroids. Amsterdam: Excerpta Medica, 1971, pp. 565–571.
14. Biglieri, E. G., Slaton, P. E., Jr., Schambelan, M., and Kronfield, S. J.: Hypomineralocorticoidism. Am. J. Med. 45:170, 1968.
15. Schambelan, M., Slaton, P. E., Jr., and Biglieri, E. G.: Mineralocorticoid production in hyperadrenocorticism: role in pathogenesis of hypokalemic alkalosis. Am. J. Med. 51:299, 1971.
16. Stockigt, J. R., Collins, R. D., and Biglieri, E. G.: Determination of plasma renin concentration by angiotensin I immunoassay. Circ. Res. 28–29(Suppl. II):175, 1971.
17. Melby, J. C., Dale, S. L., and Wilson, T. E.: 18-Hydroxydeoxycorticosterone in human hypertension. Circ. Res. 28–29(Suppl. II):143, 1971.
18. Sharma, D. C., Forchielli, E., and Dorfman, R. I.: Inhibition of enzymatic steroid 11-β-hydroxylation by androgens. J. Biol. Chem. 238:572, 1963.
19. Sharma, D. C., and Dorfman, R. I.: Effect of androgens on steroid C-21 hydroxylation. Biochemistry (Washington) 3:1093, 1964.
20. Mahajan, D. K., and Samuels, L. T.: Inhibition of steroid 17-desmolase by progesterone. Fed. Proc. 21:209, 1962.
21. West, C. D., Kumagai, L. F., Simons, E. L., Dominguez, O. V., and Berliner, D. L.: Adrenocortical carcinoma with feminization and hypertension associated with a defect in 11-β-hydroxylation. J. Clin. Endocrinol. Metab. 24:567, 1964.
22. Soloman, S. S., Swersie, S. P., Paulsen, C. A. and Biglieri, E. G.: Feminizing adrenocortical carcinoma with hypertension. J. Clin. Endocrinol. Metab. 28:608, 1968.
23. Newton, M. A., and Laragh, J. H.: Effect of corticotropin on aldosterone excretion and plasma renin in normal subjects, in essential hypertension, and in primary aldosteronism. J. Clin. Endocrinol. Metab. 28:1006, 1968.

24. Benraad, Th. J., and Kloppenborg, P. W. C.: Plasma renin activity and aldosterone secretory rate in man during chronic ACTH administration. J. Clin. Endocrinol. Metab. 31:581, 1970.

25. Biglieri, E. G., Hane, S., Slaton, P. E., Jr., and Forsham, P. H.: *In vivo* and *in vitro* studies of adrenal secretions in Cushing's syndrome and primary aldosteronism. J. Clin. Invest. 42:516, 1963.

Inheritance of 18-Hydroxydeoxycorticosterone Formation in Genetic Hypertension in Rats

By John P. Rapp, D.V.M., Ph.D., and Lewis K. Dahl, M.D.

In 1962 Dahl et al.[1] reported the selective breeding of rats on the basis of their blood pressure response to a high-salt diet. Two strains were developed; one was highly susceptible (S strain) and the other was highly resistant (R strain) to the hypertensive effect of high-salt intake. Genetic studies have shown that the marked difference in blood pressure response to salt between S- and R-strain rats can be accounted for by a multigenic model consisting of two to four genes.[2] Our present purposes are to: (1) present the genetically controlled differences found in adrenal steroidogenesis between S- and R-strain rats, and (2) show that in genetic experiments differences in steroidogenesis are associated with, and account for, a moderate but significant part of the blood pressure difference between S and R strains. The results will define one of the two to four genes predicted to control blood pressure in this animal model.

Table 1 gives our initial observations on the steroid secretion in adrenal venous blood from S- and R-strain rats. Such secretion rates are obtained under severe surgical stress and probably represent maximal ACTH stimulation. Under these conditions S-strain rats secreted approximately twice as much 18-hydroxydeoxycorticosterone (18-OH-DOC) as R-strain rats, but S-strain rats secreted less corticosterone (compound B) than R-strain animals. There were no differences between strains in deoxycorticosterone (DOC) or aldosterone secretion.

The apparently reciprocal nature of the dif-

From the Penrose Research Laboratory, Philadelphia Zoological Society, and the Department of Pathology, University of Pennsylvania Medical School, Philadelphia, Pennsylvania; and the Brookhaven National Laboratory, Upton, New York.

Dr. Rapp is supported by research grants from the U.S. Public Health Service (USPHS HE–11,293) and The American Heart Association (71–661), and by a Career Development Award (USPHS AM–10,543); Dr. Dahl is supported primarily by the U.S. Atomic Energy Commission with partial support from the USPHS (HE–13,408) and The American Heart Association (70–772) supported by Dutchess County, New York.

Table 1.—*Steroid Secretion in Adrenal Venous Blood of Salt-susceptible (S) and Salt-resistant (R) Female Rats Maintained on Low-salt (0.4% NaCl) Diet.* *

Steroid †	*Resistant*	*Susceptible*	*t-Test Significance*
18-OH-DOC	26.3 ± 4.1	55.7 ± 9.2	0.01–0.025
Compound B	160.5 ± 10.3	116.6 ± 9.0	0.005–0.01
Aldosterone	1.08 ± 0.04	1.06 ± 0.15	NS
DOC	2.33 ± 0.44	2.34 ± 0.33	NS
Body weight (in grams)	235 ± 2	239 ± 6	NS

* The entries in the table are the mean ± standard error of six independent replicates. The significance level is for a t-test comparing R and S strains which was done on logarithmically transformed data, although the untransformed means are given. NS, not significant, i.e., $p > 0.05$. Steroids were measured by gas-liquid chromatography.[3–5]

The data in the table were reported previously by Rapp, J. P., and Dahl, L. K.,[5] and are reproduced by permission.

† Steroid data in μg/rat/hr.

Abbreviations used: 18-OH-DOC, 18-hydroxydeoxycorticosterone; B, corticosterone; DOC, deoxycorticosterone.

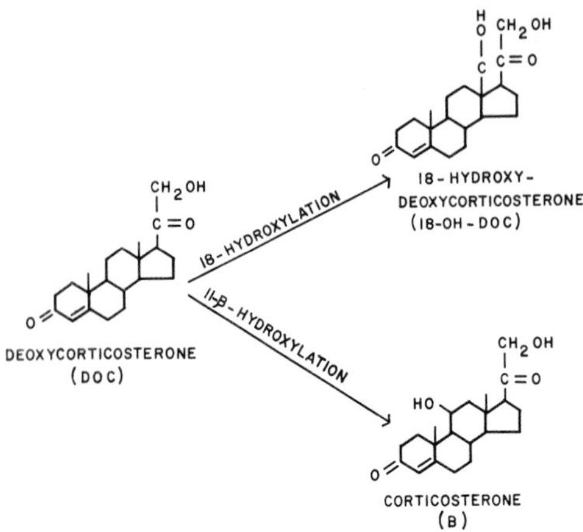

FIG. 1.—Relationship between deoxycorticosterone (DOC), 18-hydroxydeoxycorticosterone (18-OH-DOC) and corticosterone (B) in the steroidogenic pathways of the rat adrenal.

ferences in 18-OH-DOC and compound B in adrenal venous blood of S- and R-strain rats led us to study the in vitro hydroxylation of DOC by S- and R-strain rat adrenals. DOC is the immediate precursor of both 18-OH-DOC and compound B (Fig. 1). Under the appropriate in vitro conditions the amounts of 18-OH-DOC and compound B formed from DOC are a measure, respectively, of 18-hydroxylase and 11-β-hydroxylase activities.

A standard in vitro procedure was developed for characterizing the steroidogenic pattern of an individual rat. The adrenals of a single rat were homogenized (16 mg of adrenal per milliliter) in Krebs-Ringer bicarbonate medium containing 3.81 mM Ca^{+2}. This homogenate was preincubated 15 minutes at 37 C to swell mitochondria, and 0.5 ml of homogenate was incubated with 1.5 ml of Krebs-Ringer bicarbonate medium containing per milliliter: 1.33 mg of TPNH, 33.33 μg of DOC, and 0.133 microcurie DOC-4-^{14}C. The incubation was at 37 C for 10 minutes and was stopped by the addition of 10 ml of cold methylene dichloride. These incubation conditions were carefully selected to provide: (1) a reasonably linear relationship

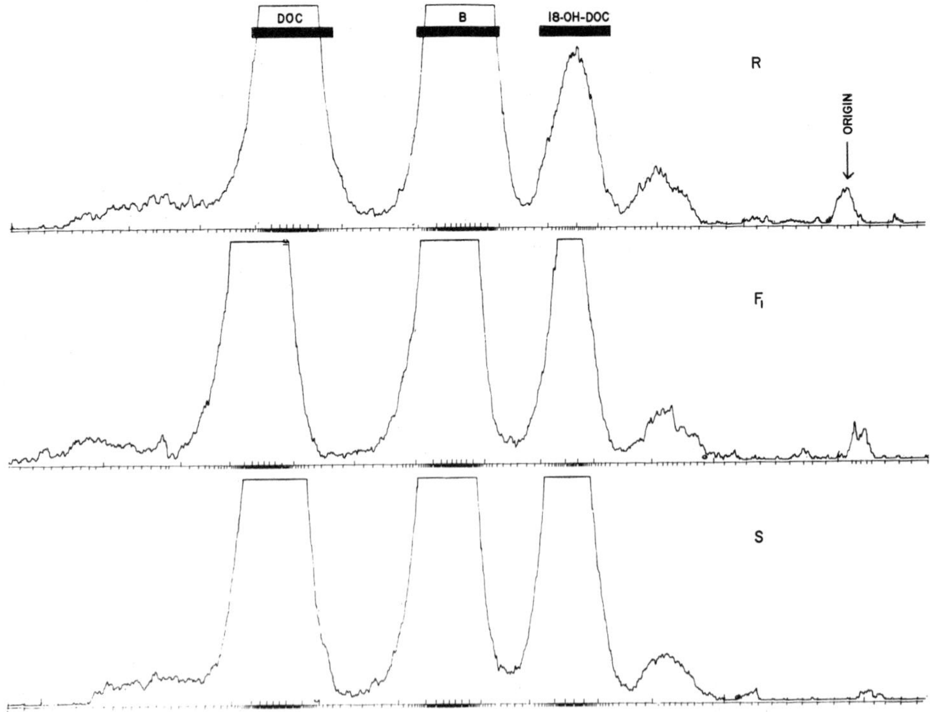

FIG. 2.—Representative radiochromatograms obtained from incubation of DOC-4-^{14}C with adrenal homogenates from individual salt-resistant (R), salt-susceptible (S), or F_1 cross (R×S) rats. The paper chromatographic system was butyl acetate/formamide water. DOC, deoxycorticosterone; B, corticosterone; 18-OH-DOC, 18-hydroxydeoxycorticosterone.

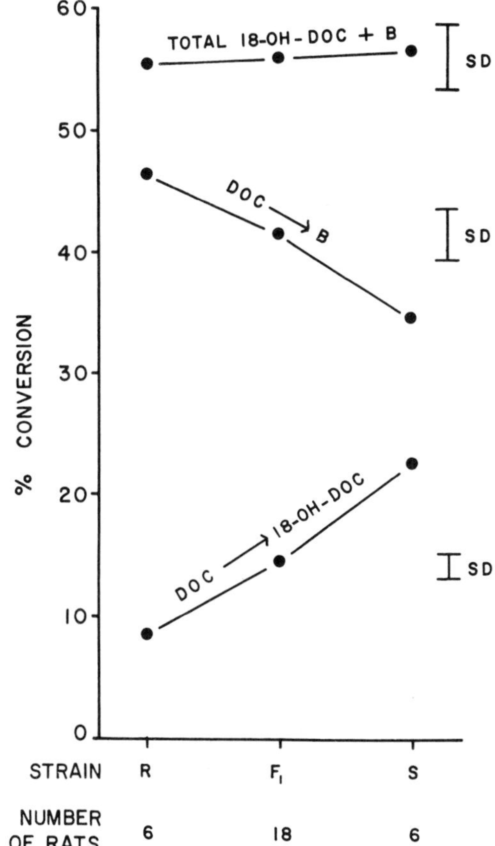

FIG. 3.—Mean percentage conversions of DOC-4-^{14}C in incubations of adrenal homogenates from individual rats of the salt-resistant (R), F_1 cross ($R \times S$), and salt-susceptible (S) strains. The results presented are for female rats; similar results were seen with males. An analysis of variance showed significant strain differences for the percentage conversion DOC → 18-OH-DOC ($p < 0.005$) and the percentage conversion DOC → B ($p < 0.005$), but there were no significant differences between strains in percentage of total DOC converted ($p > 0.05$). The standard deviations (SD) given are from the analysis of variance in which statistical blocking removed day-to-day variation.

between 18- and 11-β-hydroxylation versus time through 10 minutes, (2) a substrate concentration (DOC) high enough to permit approximately zero order kinetics without substrate inhibition, and (3) sufficient ^{14}C conversion to allow accurate radiochromatographic scanning data. Following incubation, methylene dichloride extracts were chromatographed on paper in butyl acetate/formamide water and radioactive steroids were quantitated by radiochromatographic scanning with digital integration. Representative radiochromatographic scans using the above in vitro system are shown in Fig. 2. From such scans the percentage conversion of DOC → 18-OH-DOC, DOC → B, and the percentage of unconverted DOC were readily calculated.

Results with the in vitro system are summarized in Fig. 3, which demonstrates that (1) S-strain rats convert more DOC to 18-OH-DOC (18-hydroxylation) than R-strain rats; (2) S-strain rats convert less DOC to compound B (11-β-hydroxylation) than R-strain rats; (3) total hydroxylation of DOC is constant for S and R strains, as shown by the fact that the sum of 18-OH-DOC plus compound B (18 + 11-β-hydroxylation) was identical for S- and R-strain rats; (4) F_1 rats, produced by $R \times S$ cross, fall halfway between the parental R and S strains for both 18- and 11-β-hydroxylation, and again the total hydroxylation of DOC is constant. The most striking feature of these results is the reciprocal and offsetting nature of the changes in 18- and 11-β-hydroxylase activities.

To study the genetics controlling the differences in steroidogenesis just described one needs some highly reproducible parameter to characterize individual rats. For technical reasons the direct in vitro percentage conversion of, e.g., DOC → 18-OH-DOC, is difficult to use since it is subject to considerable block (day-to-day) variation. This difficulty is overcome by using the ratio of the percentage conversion of DOC → 18-OH-DOC per total percentage conversion of DOC. The total percentage conversion of DOC in the in vitro system is essentially the sum of conversions to 18-OH-DOC and compound B so that the parameter becomes percentage conversion of DOC → 18-OH-DOC per [percentage conversion DOC → 18-OH-DOC + percentage conversion DOC → compound B]. This ratio is hereafter written 18-OH-DOC per (18-OH-DOC plus B) and represents that proportion of the total hydroxylation of DOC that goes along the 18-hydroxylase pathway.[6]

Figure 4 shows the 18-OH-DOC per (18-DOC plus compound B) ratio for R-, S-,

F_1-strain and backcross populations. The R-, F_1-, and S-strain populations are distinct and do not overlap; the F_1 population is intermediate between R and S strains for the 18-OH-DOC per (18-OH-DOC plus compound B) ratio. The backcross to the R strain (R $\times$ F_1) segregates into two distinct groups; one group has an 18-OH-DOC per (18-OH-DOC plus B) ratio similar to R, and the other group has an 18-OH-DOC per (18-OH-DOC plus B) ratio similar to the F_1 or intermediate phenotype. The frequency of individuals in these two groups is approximately 1:1. Similarly, the backcross to the S strain (S $\times$ F_1) segregates 1:1 into two groups which have 18-OH-DOC per (18-OH-DOC plus B) ratios either like the S phenotype or like the intermediate phenotype (Fig. 4).

The 18-OH-DOC per (18-OH-DOC plus B) ratio in F_2 ($F_1 \times F_1$ cross) rats is segregated into a trimodal distribution (Fig. 5). Of the 96 animals studied there were 22 R-type, 55 intermediate-type and 19 S-type individuals. These numbers are not statistically different by a chi-square test ($p > .25$) from a Mendelian ratio of 1:2:1 (expected 24:48:24, observed 22:55:19). We conclude on the basis of a phenotypic ratio of 1:1 in backcross populations, and a phenotypic ratio of 1:2:1 in the F_2 population, that the 18-OH-DOC per (18-OH-DOC plus compound B) parameter is controlled by a single gene inherited by codominance.

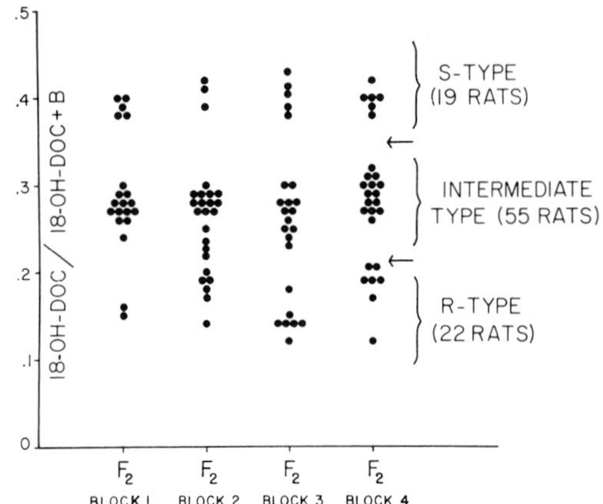

FIG. 5.—Scatter diagram of the ratio of 18-OH-DOC per (18-OH-DOC plus B) determined by in vitro adrenal homogenate incubation with DOC-4-^{14}C for individual rats from an F_2 population. The adrenals were incubated in four approximately equal blocks which are presented separately. The 18-OH-DOC per (18-OH-DOC plus B) ratio is seen to be trimodally distributed and rats were classified by adrenal phenotype as R-type, intermediate-type, or S-type. The horizontal arrows at 18-OH-DOC per (18-OH-DOC plus B) ratios of 0.21 and 0.35 were chosen by inspection of this figure, Fig. 4, and other similar data not presented, and indicate the division points between phenotypes. There was slight block variation in the separation of the R-strain and intermediate phenotypes.

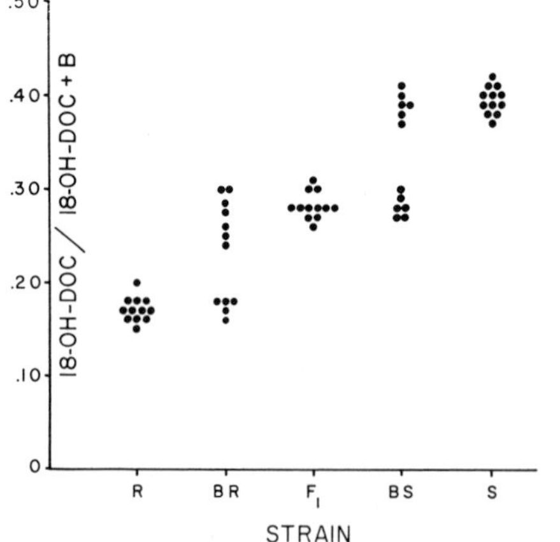

FIG. 4.—Scatter diagram of the ratio of 18-OH-DOC per (18-OH-DOC plus B) determined by in vitro adrenal homogenate incubation with DOC-4-^{14}C for individual rats from R-, F_1-, S-strain and backcross populations. BR and BS are backcrosses of F_1 rats to the R and S strain respectively.

Figure 6 shows that the inverse relationship between 18- and 11-β-hydroxylase activities, which was seen when comparing R, F_1, and S populations, holds also for R-, intermediate-, and S-type adrenals in the (segregating) F_2 population. If 18- and 11-β-hydroxylase activities were controlled by separate, nonlinked genes, they would segregate separately and there would be no relationship between these enzyme activities in F_2 rats. Since 18- and 11-β-hydroxylase activities are related (inversely) in F_2 phenotypes, this implies that both hydroxylase activities are controlled by the same gene. Since 18- and 11-β-hydroxylase activities are both associated with adrenal mitochondria, it is reasonable to speculate that the gene in question actually controls some structural (protein) component of the mito-

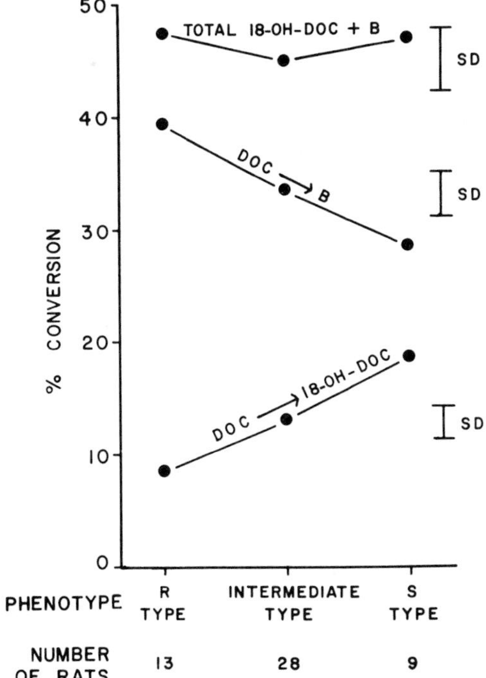

FIG. 6.—Percentage conversions of DOC-4-^{14}C in incubation of adrenal homogenates from individual rats of an F_2 population which had been phenotypically classified as R-type, intermediate-type, or S-type in terms of the 18-OH-DOC per (18-OH-DOC plus B) ratio. The results are presented for female rats; similar results were seen with males. An analysis of variance showed significant differences between phenotypes for percentage conversion DOC → 18-OH-DOC ($p < 0.005$), and the percentage conversion DOC → B ($p < 0.005$), but there were no significant differences between phenotypes in percentage of total DOC converted ($p > 0.05$). The standard deviations (SD) given in the figure are from the analysis of variance.

chondrial membrane which dictates the stoichiometric assembly of 18- and 11-β-hydroxylase units.

What proportion of the blood pressure difference between S- and R-strain rats is accounted for by the gene controlling adrenal steroidogenesis? This question can be answered by comparing the blood pressure responses of adrenal phenotypes in F_2 rats. As noted before, previous genetic experiments have indicated that blood pressure differences between S- and R-strain rats are probably due to from two to four genes. Assuming these genes are nonlinked, then an *individual* F_2 rat that carries a given gene for high blood pressure may also carry by chance all, some, or none of the other genes for high pressure. Consider the comparison of blood pressures between *large numbers* of individuals of the various 18-OH-DOC per (18-OH-DOC plus compound B) phenotypes in F_2 rats. If the genes other than the one for adrenal phenotype segregate at random within each 18-OH-DOC per (18-OH-DOC plus compound B) phenotype, then these other genes cannot cause differences in blood pressure means between the large samples of 18-OH-DOC per (18-OH-DOC plus compound B) phenotypes. The random assortment of other genes can, however, be expected to increase variability of blood pressure within each 18-OH-DOC per (18-OH-DOC plus B) phenotype.

The F_2 rats seen in Fig. 5 had been weaned to a high-salt (8% sodium chloride) diet for the purpose of studying blood pressure response to salt. High-salt diet is the standard test procedure used in studying S- and R-strain rats.[1,2] In addition to the anticipated great variability of blood pressure response in F_2 rats, there was a strong effect of family on blood pressure which accounted for a significant ($p < 0.005$) proportion of the variances in blood pressure between individuals. This family effect was also seen previously in F_1 populations [2] and is probably due to the presence of the heterozygous condition for some (unidentified) hypertensive gene in S-strain rats. It seems likely that such a gene could be lethal in the homozygous condition and that this has prevented genic purification in S-strain animals. The family effect was removed from the data by expressing the blood pressure of each rat as the deviation about its family, sex-specific mean. This also effectively removed the effect of sex on blood pressure. The mean deviations of blood pressure about family, sex-specific means for the three adrenal phenotypes in F_2 rats fall in this order: R-type < intermediate-type < S-type (Table 2). The differences in blood pressure between adrenal phenotypes in F_2 rats are significant by an analysis of variance ($0.01 < p < 0.025$). Thus, increments in blood pressure (Table 2) are associated with increments in adrenal 18-hy-

TABLE 2.—*One-way Analysis of Variance on Deviations of Blood Pressure about the Family, Sex-specific Mean for F_2 Rats Fed High-Salt Diet (8% NaCl) for 10 Weeks from Weaning and Classified by Adrenal Phenotype*

	Adrenal Phenotype			
	R-type	*Intermediate-type*	*S-type*	*Analysis of Variance Significance Level*
Combined ♂ and ♀	−7.48±3.23 *	+0.05±2.26	+8.53±4.45	0.01–0.025
No. of rats	22	55	19	

* mm Hg ± SE.

"Deviations of blood pressure" were defined as $X_i - X_{(sibs,\ sex)}$ where X_i is the average blood pressure of two readings for an individual rat taken at weeks 9 and 10 after weaning to high-salt diet, and $X_{(sibs,\ sex)}$ is the mean of the X_i for all sibs of the same sex in a given family. This transformation removes the effect of sex and family on blood pressure. Blood pressure was measured by the tail microphonic manometer technique.[7]

droxylase activity (or decrements in 11-β-hydroxylase activity; Fig. 6). The difference in 18-hydroxylase (or 11-β-hydroxylase) activity equal to the difference between S-type and R-type adrenals is associated with a blood pressure difference which is best estimated from Table 2 to be the difference between −7.48 and +8.53, or about 16 mm Hg. The difference in blood pressure between the parental R- and S-strains raised on high-salt diet is about 100 mm Hg.[2] The gene controlling the 18-OH-DOC per (18-OH-DOC plus compound B) phenotype accounts, therefore, for about 16/100 or 16 percent of the difference between the two inbred strains. The other 84 percent of this difference is due to the remaining genes predicted to exist by previous genetic experiments.[2]

The above data show that on high-salt intake, genetically controlled increments in 18-hydroxylase activity are associated with increments in blood pressure. What is the mechanism behind such an association? A logical first step is to investigate what effects the described differences in steroidogenesis have on peripheral plasma steroid levels. Peripheral plasma was obtained from nonstressed animals by collection of neck blood following rapid decapitation. The higher adrenal 18-hydroxylation in S- over R-strain rats gives rise to a twofold higher level of peripheral plasma 18-OH-DOC in S- over R-strain animals (Table 3). Interestingly, the peripheral plasma compound B levels are not different between S- and R-strain rats (Table 3) despite the lower 11-β-hydroxylation activity in S-strain rat adrenals. This is not at all surprising when one considers the intact, nonstressed animal. Suppose that S-strain rat adrenals secrete less compound B per unit weight of adrenal than R-strain rat adrenals. It is reasonable to expect that the pituitary (being mainly responsive to peripheral plasma compound B level) will secrete just enough more ACTH in S- than in R-strain animals in order to make the plasma compound B concentrations equal in the two strains. The moderate but significantly higher adrenal weight consistently seen in S- over R-strain rats (Table 3) is due to a larger cortex (unpublished data) and probably results from the anticipated greater ACTH secretion in S- over R-strain rats. This situation is similar to, but quantitatively much less marked than, the congenital adrenocortical hyperplasia seen with various sorts of complete adrenal enzyme blocks.

Table 3 also demonstrates the important point that salt feeding has no effect on 18-OH-DOC or compound B plasma levels. With in vitro studies salt feeding also failed to affect adrenal steroidogenic patterns of 18-OH-DOC and compound B formation.[5]

Given that S-strain rats have higher peripheral plasma 18-OH-DOC levels than R-strain animals, how might this be translated into hypertension? 18-OH-DOC is a weak mineralocorticoid,[8–10] and secretion of excess mineralocorticoid in the presence of high-salt intake is certainly a situation known to favor sodium retention and hypertension. In considering the mineralocorticoid status of an animal one must, however, consider total mineralocorticoid out-

TABLE 3.—*Results of 2×2 Factorial Analysis of Variance on Body and Adrenal Weight, Blood Pressure, and Peripheral Plasma Concentrations of 18-Hydroxydeoxycorticosterone (18-OH-DOC) and Corticosterone (Compound B) for Female Salt-Susceptible (S) and Salt-Resistant (R) Rats Fed High- (8%) or Low- (0.4%) Salt Diets*

	High Salt		*Low Salt*			*Significant Levels*		
	S	*R*	*S*	*R*	*SE*	*Strain*	*Salt Diet*	*Interaction*
Body weight (in grams)	249.3	244.1	246.0	234.3	3.1	0.01–0.025	0.025–0.05	NS
Adrenals weight (in milligrams)	61.9	51.0	60.7	49.1	1.4	< 0.005	NS	NS
	(60.3) *	(50.8)	(60.0)	(51.6)		(< 0.005)	(NS)	(NS)
Blood pressure (mm Hg)	163	117	133	112	3.4	< 0.005	< 0.005	< 0.005
18-OH-DOC (in micrograms per 100 ml plasma)	3.08 ± 0.69 †	1.90 ± 0.41	3.54 ± 0.63	1.20 ± 0.19	—	< 0.005	NS	NS
Compound B (in micrograms per 100 ml of plasma)	12.2 ± 2.2	16.5 ± 3.1	14.4 ± 3.0	11.5 ± 1.9	—	NS	NS	NS

Data reproduced from Rapp, J. P., and Dahl, L. K.,[5] with permission.

There were 24 rats in each group but since the peripheral plasma of three rats was pooled for each steroid sample, there are eight independent replicate determinations in the steroid data. Steroids were measured by gas-liquid chromatography.[4]

Abbreviations used: SE, standard error; NS, not significant, i.e., $p > 0.05$; B, corticosterone.

* Numbers in parentheses are the adjusted means and significance levels from a 2×2 factorial analysis of covariance with body weight as covariate.

† The analysis of variance on plasma steroids was done on logarithmically transformed data to equalize variances between treatments, but the untransformed means and their standard errors are given.

put, which is probably adequately represented for the rat by the sum actions of aldosterone, DOC, 18-OH-DOC, and compound B. Aldosterone is the most potent of the mineralocorticoids and, more importantly, is the only one which is sensitive to salt intake. In order to know that higher 18-OH-DOC secretion in S-strain rats on high-salt intake results in greater *total* mineralocorticoid activity in S- over R-strain rats, it is necessary to evaluate the response of aldosterone to salt in S- and R-strain rats. Table 4 shows preliminary data on the response of aldosterone to salt in S- and R-strain rats. Although further studies are needed on high-salt intakes of longer duration, the results certainly suggest a similar response of aldosterone to salt in both strains.

Theoretical calculations on total mineralocorticoid activity in S- and R-strain rats [11] show that: (1) on low-salt intake the total mineralocorticoid activity in both S- and R-strain rats is approximately equal and is dominated by aldosterone; (2) in both S- and R-strain rats, as salt intake is increased and aldosterone is suppressed, the total mineralocorticoid activity (although decreasing) becomes progressively more dependent on the level of 18-OH-DOC secretion which is constant under variable salt intake; (3) S-strain animals will be at a disadvantage in suppressing total mineralocorticoid activity on high-salt intake. The third possibility certainly favors development of hypertension and may explain the association of blood pressure and 18-OH-DOC observed in these genetic experiments. For a more complete quantitative consideration of these concepts the reader is referred to our original report.[11]

SUMMARY

Adrenal steroidogenesis was studied in two strains of rats which had been selectively bred for susceptibility (S strain) or resistance (R strain) to the hypertensive effects of high-salt intake. In vivo and in vitro data showed that: (1) S-strain rat adrenals had a higher 18-hydroxylase activity than the R-strain; (2) S-strain rat adrenals had a lower 11-β-hydroxylase activity than the R-strain rats; (3) the increment by which 18-hydroxylase was $S > R$ equaled the decrement by which 11-β-hydroxylase was $S < R$. These quantitative differences in steroidogenesis give rise to characteristic patterns of production of 18-OH-DOC and corticosterone (B) which arise respectively from 18-hydroxylation and 11-β-hydroxylation of DOC. Rats were phenotypically classified on the basis of their adrenal steroid production in a standardized in vitro system. It was shown that the reciprocal changes in adrenal 18- and 11-β-hydroxylase activities were controlled by a single Mendelian gene inherited by codominance. In an F_2 population (derived from parental R- and S-strains) rats were classified by adrenal phenotype; their blood pressures fell in this order: R-type adrenals < intermediate-type adrenals < S-type adrenals, with equal increments of blood pressure between types. Thus, in the F_2 population increments in blood pressure were associated with increments in 18-hydroxylase activity. It was shown that

TABLE 4.—*Acute Response of Aldosterone Secretion in Adrenal Venous Blood of Salt-Resistant (R) and Salt-Susceptible (S) Rats to Drinking 1% Saline*

Micrograms per rat per hr ± SE	*Days on 1% Saline*					*Significance Levels*		
	0	*1*	*2*	*4*	*X*	*Strain*	*Saline*	*Interaction*
S	1.074 ±0.106	0.834 ±0.097	0.518 ±0.156	0.357 ±0.117	0.696			
R	1.005 * ±0.019	0.616 ±0.066	0.541 ±0.139	0.537 ±0.156	0.687	NS	< 0.005	NS
X	1.064	0.725	0.530	0.447				

The means ± SE are on three independent replicate samples. Significance levels are from a 2 × 4 factorial analysis of variance done on logarithmically transformed data. NS = not significant, i.e., $p > 0.05$. Aldosterone was measured by gas-liquid chromatography.[3, 5]

* One inordinately high value (probably contaminated with standard aldosterone) was discarded from this mean. Inclusion of this value, however, did not change the conclusions or significance levels presented.

differences in 18-hydroxylase activity could account for about 16 percent of the blood pressure differences between the parental S and R strains. It was suggested that the remaining 84 percent of the blood pressure difference between S and R strains must be due to other unidentified genes known to exist in this multigenic animal model.

It was also shown that S- and R-strain rats secrete equal amounts of aldosterone and that the decrease in aldosterone production in response to acute high-salt intake was equal in S- and R-strain animals. S-strain rats have peripheral plasma levels of 18-OH-DOC which are twofold higher than R-strain rats, and 18-OH-DOC levels are not changed by salt feeding. It was argued that when salt intake is increased and aldosterone is progressively suppressed, the mineralocorticoid activity of 18-OH-DOC will make up a larger and larger part of the total mineralocorticoid activity in both S- and R-strain animals. S-type rats which secrete more 18-OH-DOC than R-type rats will be at a disadvantage in reducing total mineralocorticoid output in the face of high-salt intakes. This situation might account for the positive correlation of 18-OH-DOC production and blood pressure in these genetic experiments.

References

1. Dahl, L. K., Heine, M., and Tassinare, L.: Effects of chronic excess salt ingestion. Evidence that genetic factors play an important role in susceptibility to experimental hypertension. J. Exp. Med. 115:1173, 1962.
2. Knudsen, K. D., Dahl, L. D., Thompson, K., Iwai, J., Heine, M., and Leitl, G.: Effects of chronic excess salt ingestion. Inheritance of hypertension in the rat. J. Exp. Med. 132:976, 1970.
3. Rapp, J. P., and Eik-Nes, K. B.: Determination of deoxycorticosterone and aldosterone in biological samples by gas chromatography with electron capture detection. Anal. Biochem. 15:386, 1966.
4. Rapp, J. P.: Gas chromatographic measurement of peripheral plasma 18-hydroxydeoxycorticosterone in adrenal regeneration hypertension. Endocrinology 86:668, 1970.
5. Rapp, J. P., and Dahl, L. K.: Adrenal steroidogenesis in rats bred for susceptibility and resistance to the hypertensive effect of salt. Endocrinology 88:52, 1971.
6. Rapp, J. P., and Dahl, L. K.: Mendelian inheritance of 18- and 11-β-steroid hydroxylase activities in the adrenals of rats genetically susceptible or resistant to hypertension. Endocrinology 90:1435, 1972.
7. Friedman, M., and Freed, C.: Microphonic manometer for indirect determination of systolic blood pressure in the rat. Proc. Soc. Exp. Biol. Med. 70:670, 1949.
8. Birmingham, M. K., MacDonald, M. L., and Rochefort, J. G.: Adrenal function in normal rats and in rats bearing regenerated adrenal glands. *In* McKerns, K. E. (Ed.): Functions of the Adrenal Cortex, vol. II. New York: Appleton-Century-Crofts, 1968, pp. 647–689.
9. Kagawa, C. M., and Pappo, R.: Renal electrolyte effects of synthetic 18-hydroxylated steroids in adrenalectomized rats. Proc. Soc. Exp. Biol. Med. 109:982, 1962.
10. Porter, G. A., and Kimsey, J.: Assessment of the mineralocorticoid activity of 18-hydroxy-11-deoxycorticosterone (18-OH-DOC) in the isolated toad bladder. Endocrinology 89:353, 1971.
11. Rapp, J. P., and Dahl, L. K.: 18-Hydroxydeoxycorticosterone: Possible role in hypertension. Nature 237:338, 1972.

18-Hydroxy-11-Deoxycorticosterone (18-OH-DOC) Secretion in Experimental and Human Hypertension

By James C. Melby, M.D., Sidney L. Dale, M.S., Roger J. Grekin, M.D., Robert Gaunt, Ph.D., and Thomas E. Wilson, M.S.

In the course of studying patients suspected of having mineralocorticoid hypertension, samples of adrenal venous effluent were obtained by adrenal vein catheterization. From these samples a steroid was isolated which had not been known to be an endogenous secretory product of the human adrenal cortex. This steroid was eventually identified as 18-hydroxy-11-deoxycorticosterone (Fig. 1), which was isolated and identified as a naturally occurring steroid from the medium-bathing, incubated, sectioned rat adrenals by Birmingham and Ward.[2] 18-OH-DOC rivals corticosterone in abundance as a secretory product of the rat adrenal cortex. Because of its predominance it had been anticipated that 18-OH-DOC must have biologic significance for this species, though to the present, no unique role for this steroid has been established. In the rat adrenal cortex, 18-OH-DOC has not been shown to be an important precursor of aldosterone and is regarded as a final product of steroid biosynthesis. 18-OH-DOC appears to be largely derived from the zona fasciculata and to a small extent from the zona glomerulosa as evidenced by measurement of steroid products from decapsulated and capsular adrenal glands. Since the rat adrenal cortex is devoid of 17-α-hydroxylase activity, it is understandable that 18-OH-DOC would be a major secretory product.

In the studies in rats to be described, the procedures for sampling adrenal venous effluent and for steroid analyses were as follows: a left adrenal vein catheter was placed under sodium pentobarbital anesthesia, the animals were heparinized and blood was drawn from the adrenal vein via a pocket in the renal vein for periods of approximately 40 minutes. Steroids were analyzed as described by Melby, Dale, and Wilson.[3]

18-OH-DOC has been implicated in the genesis of two forms of experimental hypertension in rats. Birmingham, MacDonald, and Rochefort[1] found that 18-OH-DOC was the principal steroid secreted by the enucleate adrenal in response to ACTH in the course of the development of adrenal regeneration hypertension. Rapp and Dahl have reported that 18-OH-DOC secretion was uniquely increased in rats genetically susceptible to salt-induced hypertension as compared with rats genetically resistant to the hypertensive effects of salt.

The development of severe hypertensive disease occurs in the rat following unilateral adrenalectomy and nephrectomy and contralateral adrenal enucleation. The mechanism by which the regenerating adrenal initiates the hypertension is not known; however, it seems

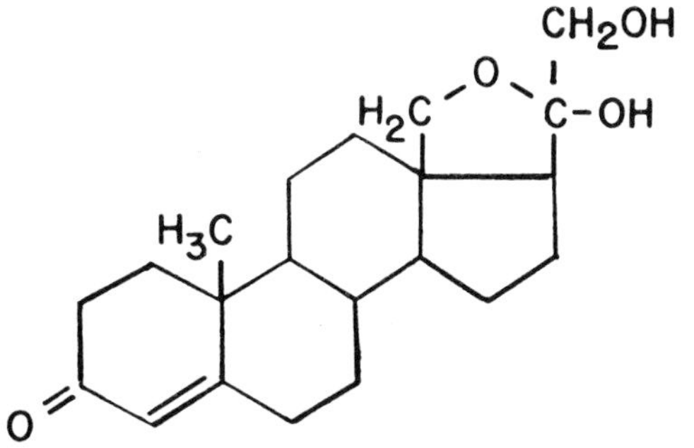

CH$_2$OH
O
H$_2$C
C-OH
H$_3$C
O

Fig. 1.—Structural formula of 18-OH-DOC demonstrates the 18 → 20 hemiketal configuration. The systematic name for 18-OH-DOC is 20,21-dihydroxy-18,20-epoxypregn-4-ene-3-one.

From the Section of Endocrinology and Metabolism, Robert Dawson Evans Department of Clinical Research, Boston University School of Medicine, Boston, Massachusetts.

This work was supported in part by Grants-in-Aid AM–12027–04, TO1–AM–05446–06, and 2–PO2–AM–08657–07 from the National Institutes of Health.

likely that the secretion of one or more adrenocortical steroids is essential to the initiation and perpetuation of the hypertension. Hypophysectomy and suppression of endogenous ACTH secretion by corticosterone administration both block the development of hypertension. Mineralocorticoid antagonists also prevent the hypertensive sequence.

During the first 72 hours following bilateral enucleation of the adrenals, there ensues a marked inability to excrete a sodium load with an attendant antidiuresis. This effect on sodium metabolism diminishes after 72 hours and disappears in 14 days. The phenomenon of acute sodium retention has characteristics in common with the hypertensive sequence occurring later. It is abolished by hypophysectomy and restored by injections of ACTH. Exogenous corticosterone inhibits the sodium retention. Spironolactone also inhibits the sodium retention after adrenal enucleation suggesting that a mineralocorticoid is involved. We have examined the steroid products in the adrenal effluent during the early sodium-retaining phase and also during the development of adrenal regeneration hypertension.

Male rats were used in the "early" or sodium-retaining period (from 24 hours to 2 weeks). The rats underwent bilateral adrenal enucleation, and adrenal vein blood was obtained at 24 and 72 hours after enucleation, corresponding with maximum sodium retention, and also at 1 and 2 weeks after enucleation.

The results of the studies in bilaterally enucleated rats during the early phase of adrenal regeneration hypertension are seen in Fig. 2. 18-OH-DOC, corticosterone, and DOC secretion was negligible at 24 and 72 hours and at 1 week. Aldosterone secretion declined markedly, although there was a detectable increment at 1 week. It is evident from our observations that none of the steroids studied could have induced severe sodium retention. To study the late or hypertensive phase of adrenal regeneration-hypertension female rats were used. Twenty-three intact rats received normal diets and fasted for 18 hours before adrenal vein catheterization. Four groups of six rats each were designated "enucleate." These animals underwent right adrenalectomy and nephrectomy, and the left adrenal was enucleated by slitting the capsule and extruding

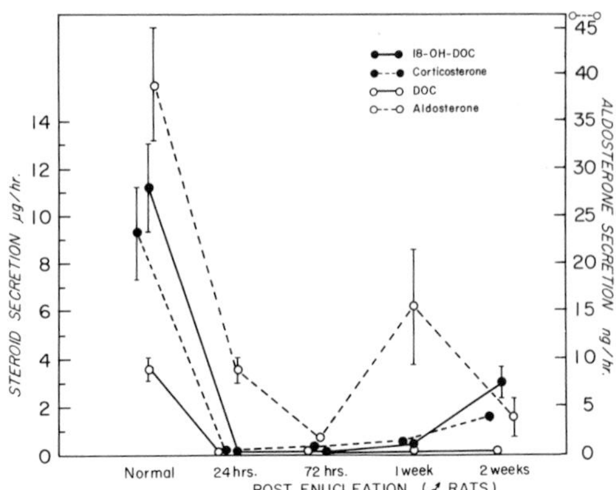

FIG. 2.—Steroid secretion in adrenal venous effluent in male rats following bilateral adrenal enucleation.

the medulla and most of the cortex with gentle forceps pressure. Thereafter they were given 1% sodium chloride solution as drinking water.

Four groups of six rats designated "control" underwent right adrenalectomy and nephrectomy, while the left adrenal remained intact. They also were given 1% sodium chloride solution in place of drinking water. After 24 hours, 1 week, 3 weeks, and 6 weeks, left adrenal vein catheterization was performed.

In adrenal enucleated rats, aldosterone, corticosterone, and 18-OH-DOC secretion fell and was negligible at 24 hours, 1 week, and 3 weeks after enucleation. DOC secretion was restored to the normal range at 3 weeks. In Fig. 3, the secretion of 18-OH-DOC is compared in control and adrenal enucleated rats. Despite high-salt intake, unilateral nephrec-

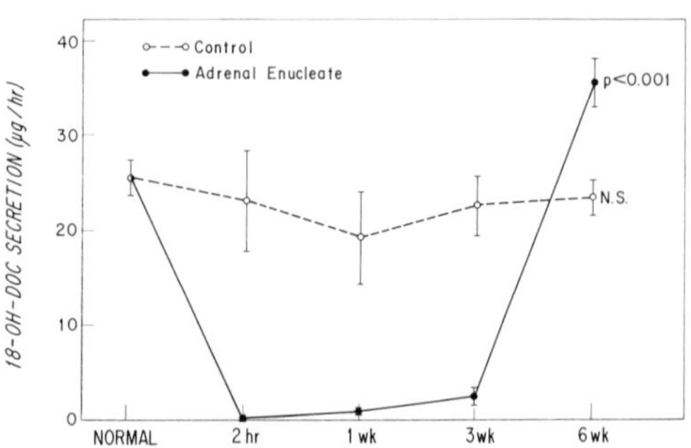

FIG. 3.—18-OH-DOC secretion in adrenal venous effluent of rats during the development of adrenal regeneration hypertension.

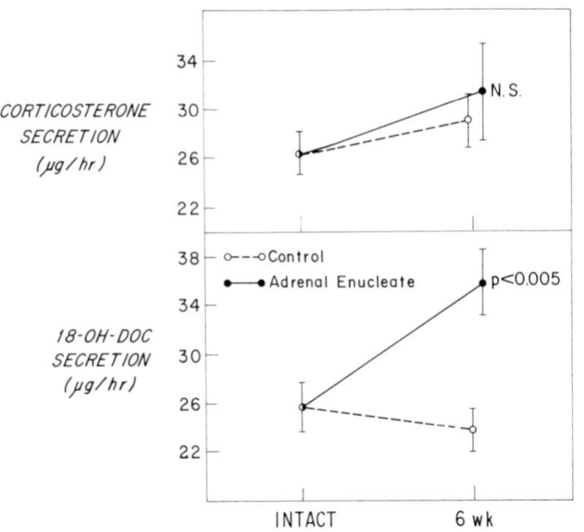

FIG. 4.—18-OH-DOC and corticosterone secretion at 6 weeks after enucleation.

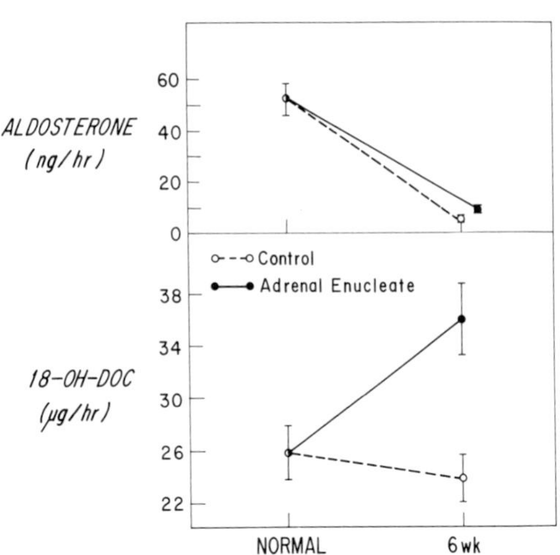

FIG. 6.—18-OH-DOC and aldosterone secretion at 6 weeks after enucleation.

tomy, and adrenalectomy, the secretion of 18-OH-DOC in control rats was not appreciably different from that in intact normal rats. In enucleate animals, 18-OH-DOC secretion was extremely low, at 24 hours, 1 week, and 3 weeks. Six weeks postenucleation, 18-OH-DOC levels were significantly elevated from those of controls. Hypertension started to develop by 3 weeks, but was not fully developed until 6 weeks after enucleation. Elevation in blood pressure occurred before the rise in 18-OH-DOC secretion.

Corticosterone secretion was restored (Fig. 4) within 6 weeks and was not different from controls. 18-OH-DOC secretion is significantly elevated compared to controls. In Fig. 5, DOC levels are restored at 3 weeks earlier than the other steroids. DOC secretion is not elevated at 6 weeks. In Fig. 6, aldosterone secretion in enucleated animals was markedly decreased throughout the 6-week period. Control animals had aldosterone levels as low as those found in enucleated animals. This was no doubt due to the high sodium intake.

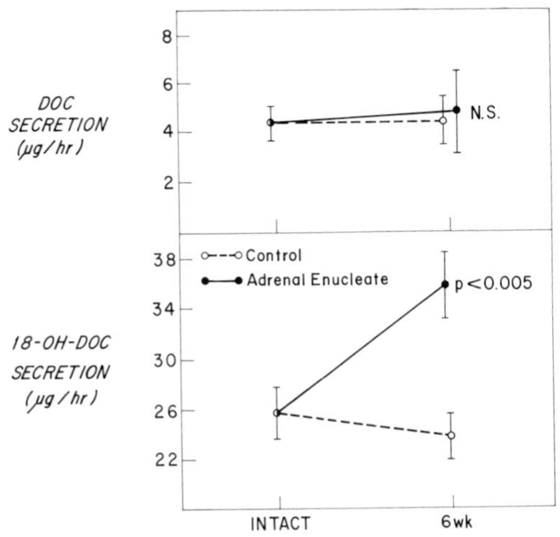

FIG. 5.—18-OH-DOC and DOC secretion at 6 weeks after enucleation.

It is clear that 18-OH-DOC secretion in hypertensive enucleate rats at 6 weeks is significantly increased above comparable controls and normal intact rats. A 40 percent increment in 18-OH-DOC secretion probably has biologic significance if sustained. If 18-OH-DOC possesses 50 percent of the mineralocorticoid activity of DOC, the elevation at 6 weeks is equivalent to a doubling of normal DOC secretion. It is possible that excessive secretion of 18-OH-DOC perpetuates and worsens adrenal regeneration hypertension. We found DOC to be the first steroid measured to return to control levels, and in animals sensitized by uninephrectomy and high-sodium intake it might be a factor in initiating hypertension. The rat adrenal steroid product which behaves as a mineralocorticoid, and is somehow involved in the development of adrenal regeneration hypertension, has not been identified.

18-OH-DOC Secretion in Man

18-OH-DOC was isolated from human adrenal vein blood in concentrations of the same magnitude as was aldosterone, and its structure was proved by a variety of methods including mass spectral analysis. Angiotensin infusions failed to evoke a rise in 18-OH-DOC secretion, whereas ACTH increased 18-OH-DOC secretion up to 20-fold. The secretion rate of 18-OH-DOC, determined by isotope dilution in healthy subjects, was similar to the range of aldosterone secretion. Excretion of the ring A reduced glucuronide metabolite, 18-hydroxy-tetrahydro-deoxycorticosterone (18-OH-TH-DOC), in urine proved to be a valid index of secretion of 18-OH-DOC. (The details of the procedures and methods used appear in an earlier paper.[3])

18-OH-DOC Secretion in Human Hypertension

Since Conn first described the clinical and laboratory manifestations of aldosterone hypersection by an adrenocortical adenoma, a concept of the physiologic consequences of human mineralocorticoid excess has evolved. Hypertension and varying degrees of potassium depletion, accompanied by excessive secretion of DOC, aldosterone, cortisol, and possibly other unknown adrenal steroids are thought to be the principal features of the mineralocorticoid hypertensive syndrome. Another characteristic of this syndrome is that its manifestations may be abolished by the administration of sufficient doses of specific competitive antagonists of mineralocorticoids such as spironolactone.

A most consistent observation in patients with the mineralocorticoid-hypertensive syndrome is that plasma renin activity is usually decreased and it responds not at all or minimally to potent physiologic stimuli such as sodium deprivation or assumption of the erect posture. Hyporesponsiveness or suppression of plasma renin activity is a reliable indicator of mineralocorticoid excess. However, a significant proportion (perhaps 20%) of patients with "essential" hypertension exhibit suppressed plasma renin activity. The majority of these patients have no identifiable cause for the presence of suppressed plasma renin activity.

The possibility that as yet unidentified mineralocorticoids may be responsible for suppressed plasma renin activity in these hypertensive patients is supported by studies of Woods, Liddle, and Stant,[5] in which inhibition of adrenal steroidogenesis by aminoglutethimide restored normal physiologic responsiveness of plasma renin and reduced blood pressure significantly. We have demonstrated a similar restoration of plasma renin responsiveness and reversal of hypertension with large doses of spironolactone in patients with suppressed plasma renin activity and hypertension. Mineralocorticoid antagonism by spironolactone in high dosages did not affect blood pressure in patients with hypertension and normally responsive plasma renin activity.

The isolation and identification of 18-OH-DOC in human adrenal venous effluent coincided with the growing indirect evidence that suppressed plasma renin activity-induced hypertension might be due to a mineralocorticoid, the structure of which was unknown. The possibility that 18-OH-DOC may somehow be involved in suppressed plasma renin activity-induced hypertension has been examined in several patients.

18-OH-DOC Secretion in Patients with Essential Hypertension and Normally Responsive Plasma Renin Activity

Twenty-eight patients with benign essential hypertension were studied. Plasma renin activity was measured after several hours of recumbency and 4 hours after being up and about. Mean upright plasma renin levels averaged 275 ng per 100 ml, with the range from

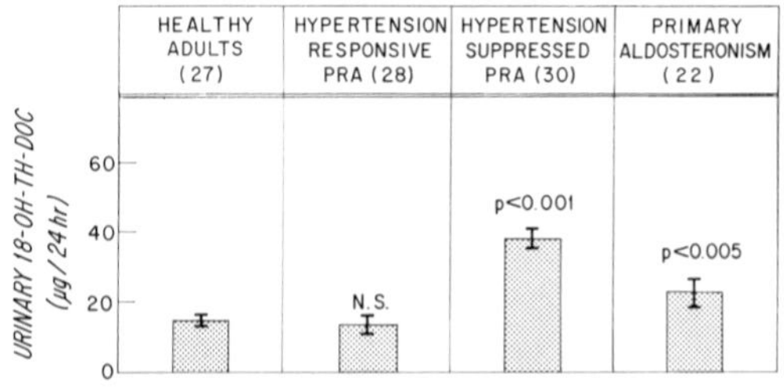

Fig. 7.—Excretion of 18-OH-TH-DOC in urine of patients with hypertensive disorders and in healthy subjects. PRA, plasma renin activity; NS, not significant.

184 to 425 ng per 100 ml. In none of these patients did the aldosterone secretion rate exceed 150 μg per 24-hour period. Urinary 18-OH-TH-DOC excretion in these patients is plotted on the second panel of Fig. 7. The values in the hypertensive population with normally responsive plasma renin activity were not different from those observed in healthy control subjects. Normally responsive plasma renin activity virtually excluded the possibility that there was significant mineralocorticoid excess.

18-OH-DOC Secretion in Hypertensive Patients with Suppressed Plasma Renin Activity

In 30 patients with hypertension, plasma renin activity did not increase significantly from the recumbent to the erect posture. Mean plasma renin levels in the erect posture in these patients was 94 ng per 100 ml. Aldosterone secretion was lower in patients with suppressed plasma renin levels with a mean aldosterone secretion rate of 77 μg per 24-hour period. Urinary 18-OH-TH-DOC excretion in these patients averaged more than twice the mean for hypertensive subjects with normally responsive plasma renin levels. The mean 18-OH-TH-DOC excretion in urine was 38.4 ± 4.3 μg per 24 hours. The difference between the mean excretion of 18-OH-TH-DOC in urine in these patients as compared to both healthy adult controls and patients with normally responsive renin activity is highly significant. Spironolactone was administered in large doses to 22 of the 30 subjects studied. In all of these patients a significant reduction in blood pressure was obtained and in 60 percent, spironolactone reduced the blood pressure consistently into the normal range. Urinary TH-DOC excretion was quantitated in more than 50 percent of these patients and with a single exception, excretion was within normal limits. In Table 1, the essential clinical information and steroid patterns are listed for 10 patients with hypertension, suppressed plasma renin activity, and elevated 18-OH-DOC secretion. Patients 1 through 4 were evaluated in our clinic. In each of these patients an adrenal vein catheterization was performed because of the near certainty that they were producing excessive amounts of a mineralocorticoid. Adrenal venous plasma 18-OH-DOC levels in all four patients were greatly elevated (6.1 to 13.1 μg per 100 ml), whereas in most other patients the 18-OH-DOC levels did not exceed 1 μg per 100 ml. Because venography demonstrated bilateral nodular hyperplasia of the adrenal gland, patient 3 underwent bilateral total adrenalectomy following a short-lived attempt to reduce his blood pressure with dexamethasone in a dosage of 0.75 mg given twice daily. Dexamethasone administration was carried out only for 3 weeks. Blood pressure actually increased during the first week of dexamethasone therapy from 180/120 mm Hg to 202/130 mm Hg. After about 2½ weeks, blood pressure began to fall and at the discontinuation of therapy it was 146/100 mm Hg. After preparation with spironolactone, a bilateral total adrenalectomy was performed and the patient remains normotensive more than 22 months after the operation.

Patient 4, a 37-year-old man with hypertension, hypokalemic alkalosis, suppressed plasma renin levels, and a low aldosterone secretion rate, underwent adrenal venography and the adrenals appeared to be perfectly normal in size. The adrenal venous effluent contained 6.1 μg of 18-OH-DOC per 100 ml of plasma. Urinary 18-OH-TH-DOC was elevated at 115 μg per 24 hours. TH-DOC excretion in urine was 23 μg per 24 hours. After a series of control observations, 0.75 mg of dexamethasone given every 12 hours was begun and continued for a period of 8 weeks. 18-OH-DOC secretion was promptly suppressed with dexamethasone, and within 3 weeks of therapy, blood pressure began to decrease. Therapy was discontinued at the end of the eighth week and the patient became hypertensive 6 weeks after the cessation of therapy. He was again treated with dexamethasone for a prolonged period during which time he remained normotensive. He was then placed on spironolactone for maintenance, to the present.

Patient 5, a hypogonadotropic, hypogonadal man (studied by Dr. C. A. Paulsen of Seattle), has been treated with Depo-testosterone since 1965. He was mildly hypertensive at that time. Hypertension worsened; hypokalemia was induced with a thiazide diuretic and persisted after its discontinuance. He was demonstrated

TABLE 1.—*Clinical Features in Patients Found To Have Increased 18-OH-TH-DOC Excretion and Suppressed Plasma Renin Activity*

Patient	*Sex*	*Age*	*Race*	*Plasma Renin Activity (ng per 100 ml)*	*ASR (μg per 24 hours)*	*Urinary Aldosterone (μg per 24 hours)*	*18-OH-TH-DOC Excretion in Urine (μg per 24 hours)*		*Blood Pressure Response to Dexamethasone*	*Disposition*	*Results of Treatment*
							Control	*Dexamethasone*			
1	F	40	W	< 50 E	50		79			Spironolactone	Normotensive
2	F	54	W	55 E	44		42			Spironolactone	Unknown
3	M	43	W	50 E	38		48		Significant reduction	Bilateral adrenalectomy (nodular hyperplasia)	Normotensive
4	M	37	W	< 50 E	30		115	3	Normotensive	Spironolactone	Normotensive
5	M	54	W	130↓Na^+		12.3	86	9	Normotensive	Spironolactone	Normotensive
6	M	51	N	135↓Na^+		11.9	52			Spironolactone	Normotensive
7	F	8	W			7.3	73		Normotensive	Bilateral adrenalectomy (hyperplasia)	Normotensive
8	F	47	W	87 E		12.7	79			Right adrenalectomy (2 adenomas)	Hypertensive
9	M	60	W	142 E 195↓Na^+		14.2	82, 94			Left adrenalectomy (adenoma)	Hypertensive
10	M	44	W	(1.1 ng angiotensin I per milliliter per hour)		15.2	56		No change	Bilateral adrenalectomy	Normotensive

Abbreviations used: ASR, aldosterone secretion rate; E, erect posture.

to have hyporesponsive renin activity to sodium depletion. Urinary aldosterone secretion was within the normal range, and urinary 18-OH-TH-DOC excretion was significantly elevated. Spironolactone reduced his blood pressure to normal. He then was allowed to become hypertensive and was placed on dexamethasone. During the first 1½-week period, blood pressure increased, but by the third week it was significantly reduced and he eventually became normotensive. No other corticosteroid metabolite was found to be altered in his urine. Urinary TH-DOC excretion was 13 μg per 24 hours.

Patient 7, an 8-year-old girl (studied by Dr. Gerald Kerrigan of Marquette University), had spontaneous hypertensive episodes; and hypertensive paroxysms could be induced by prolonged infusions of ACTH. Spironolactone prevented both the spontaneously occurring and ACTH-induced attacks. Urinary steroid patterns were measured by a number of investigators and no abnormal steroid was demonstrated. Urinary aldosterone excretion was normal; urinary TH-DOC excretion was 20 μg per 24 hours. The patient was studied before the measurement of plasma renin activity became a diagnostic procedure. Glucocorticoids prevented spontaneous hypertensive episodes. Eventually a bilateral total adrenalectomy was performed with the finding of hyperplasia. After adrenalectomy the patient had no further episodes of hypertension. Several years later, frozen specimens of this patient's urine were examined for urinary 18-OH-TH-DOC, which was found to be elevated.

Patient 8 (studied by Dr. Caulie Gunnels, Duke University) underwent bilateral adrenal exploration because of hypertension and suppressed plasma renin activity. The right adrenal gland, which contained two clinically significant adenomas, was removed and the patient remained hypertensive. Increased 18-OH-TH-DOC excretion was found preoperatively. Urinary aldosterone and TH-DOC were in the normal range. The possibility that the remaining adrenal continues to produce a mineralocorticoid must be considered.

Patient 9 (reported by Drs. Rovner, Conn, and Vader), a 60-year-old hypertensive man with hyporesponsive plasma renin activity and normal amounts of urinary aldosterone, underwent adrenal venography, which demonstrated a left adrenal adenoma. A left adrenalectomy was performed and the adenoma was sectioned and incubated and found to convert labeled progesterone to 18-OH-DOC at a rate 10 times as fast as that observed in several other incubated tumors. Urinary 18-OH-TH-DOC excretion measured in this laboratory was elevated. The patient remained hypertensive after the unilateral adrenalectomy.

Patient 10 (studied by Dr. C. Grim), a 44-year-old man with suppressed plasma renin activity, normal aldosterone excretion, and elevated urinary 18-OH-TH-DOC excretion, was given dexamethasone for several weeks without any reduction in blood pressure. Bilateral total adrenalectomy was performed and adrenocortical hyperplasia was demonstrated. The patient is now normotensive.

In nine of these 10 patients exhibiting suppressed plasma renin activity, normal or low aldosterone secretion, and normal TH-DOC excretion, only one steroid abnormality could be found, excessive excretion of 18-OH-TH-DOC in urine. Dexamethasone-suppression of 18-OH-DOC secretion was carried out in five of these patients. Four of the five patients responded; three of these became normotensive.

18-OH-DOC Secretion in Primary Aldosteronism

Twenty-two patients were studied and all were found to have significantly increased aldosterone secretion, suppressed plasma renin activity, spontaneous or easily inducible hypokalemia, and reversal of these manifestations during the administration of large doses of spironolactone. Diagnosis of primary aldosteronism was confirmed by the presence at operation of a solitary adenoma in 16 of the patients and bilateral nodular hyperplasia in six of the patients. Though mean 18-OH-TH-DOC excretion was less than that of patients with suppressed plasma renin-induced hypertension, it was significantly greater than that in healthy subjects ($P < 0.005$).

Of patients with suppressed plasma renin-induced hypertension of unknown etiology, approximately 15 percent excreted markedly abnormal quantities of 18-OH-TH-DOC in urine as the sole alteration from normal steroid pattern. The suppression of ACTH secretion with dexamethasone is associated with a decline in both blood pressure and 18-OH-DOC excretion in urine, in four of five patients studied. Correlation of these events immediately suggests that 18-OH-DOC has some role in the development of hypertension. In limited cases, morphologic abnormalities of the adrenal producing excessive 18-OH-DOC were found to range from hyperplasia to solitary tumor.

The possibility that 18-OH-DOC secretory excess in patients with suppressed plasma renin-induced hypertension is some variant of Biglieri's syndrome of 17-α-hydroxylase deficiency has to be considered. However, the lack of excessive DOC secretion militates against this interpretation. A partial 17-α-hydroxylase deficiency might exist which would increase the secretion of 18-OH-DOC sufficiently to produce hypertension without overloading the 18-OH-steroid dehydrogenase enzyme system of the zona fasciculata, thereby avoiding the build-up of precursor, DOC. The evidence for partial 17-α-hydroxylase deficiency is lacking in this study. A single patient with suppressed plasma renin levels and excessive 18-OH-DOC secretion was also found to have hypogonadism. The possibility that the hypogonadism is related to 17-α-hydroxylase deficiency in the testes is unlikely because gonadotropin secretion was also diminished. Appropriate further studies of these patients might include maximal stimulation with ACTH to make more obvious the presence of 17-α-hydroxylase deficiency.

References

1. Birmingham, M. K., MacDonald, M. L., and Rochefort, J. G.: Adrenal function in normal rats and in rats bearing regenerated adrenal glands. *In* McKerns, K. W. (Ed.): Functions of the Adrenal Cortex, vol. II. New York: Appleton-Century-Crofts, 1968, p. 647.
2. Birmingham, M. K., and Ward, P. J.: Identification of the Porter-Silber chromogen secreted by the rat adrenal. J. Biol. Chem. 236: 1661, 1961.
3. Melby, J. C., Dale, S. L., and Wilson, T. E.: 18-Hydroxy-deoxycorticosterone in human hypertension. Circ. Res. 28–29(Suppl. II):143, 1971.
4. Rapp, J. P., and Dahl, L. K.: Inheritance of 18-hydroxydeoxycorticosterone in genetic hypertension in rats. This volume.
5. Woods, J. W., Liddle, G. W., Stant, E. G., Jr., Michelakis, A. M., and Brill, A. B.: Effect of an adrenal inhibitor in hypertensive patients with suppressed plasma renin. Arch. Intern. Med. 123:366, 1969.

Mechanisms of Hypertension in Spontaneously Hypertensive Rats: The Role of Sodium Balance and the Pituitary-Adrenal Axis

By Leslie Baer, M.D., Abbie I. Knowlton, M.D., J. Dianne Kirshman, and John H. Laragh, M.D.

Congenital forms of hypertension in animals have been useful models for the study of genetic and biochemical determinants in hypertension. At least three strains of congenitally hypertensive rats have been developed.[1-3] These forms bear certain similarities to human forms of hypertension because no drug treatment or surgical procedures are required to raise blood pressure in these animals. Moreover, pathologic changes commonly associated with sustained hypertension in man including cardiomegaly, vascular disease, myocardial infarction, nephrosclerosis, and cerebral hemorrhage have also been observed in the spontaneously hypertensive rats.[4] A number of other histologic abnormalities have been noted including adrenocortical hyperplasia, a finding observed in some human forms of hypertension.[5]

The present studies were designed to further define the role of sodium balance and the adrenal gland in the hypertension of spontaneously hypertensive rats. These two interrelated factors are crucial in a number of animal and human forms of hypertension. In addition, we have carried out a number of studies of the renin-angiotensin system in spontaneously hypertensive rats. Our preliminary impression was that plasma renin concentration was low in spontaneously hypertensive rats. However, subsequent studies from our laboratory using a more sensitive radioimmunoassay technique and from others [6,7] suggest that in fact plasma renin activity in these rats is probably within the normal range. Further studies are needed to characterize the relationship of the renin-angiotensin system to the hypertension of spontaneously hypertensive rats.

From the Department of Medicine, Columbia University College of Physicians and Surgeons, New York, New York.

Methodology

The strain of spontaneously hypertensive rat used in these studies comprised direct descendants of the original strain developed by Okamoto and Aoki. Normotensive Wistar rats matched for sex and weight were used as controls. Blood pressure was measured using the microphonic tail method.[8] For determination of plasma electrolytes, approximately 2 ml of blood was drawn from the jugular vein under ether anesthesia. Plasma and urinary sodium and potassium were measured on a flame photometer (Instrumentation Laboratories, Inc.).

The normal sodium diets consisted of Purina rat chow containing 0.42% sodium. The low-sodium diet consisted of a modified Hartroft low-sodium diet (General Biochemicals). Sodium and potassium balance studies were carried out with these diets with animals housed in individual metabolism cages.

Total adrenalectomy was performed under ether anesthesia through bilateral flank incisions. Following adrenalectomy, the adrenalectomized and nonadrenalectomized control and spontaneously hypertensive rat groups were all placed on a high sodium intake by substituting 0.9% saline for their drinking water and continuing the normal sodium rat chow. In order to assess the adequacy of total adrenalectomy, all the animals were placed on a low-sodium diet at the conclusion of the experiment. The adrenalectomized animals died within 1 week. Those animals that survived the period of sodium depletion after adrenalectomy were considered incompletely adrenalectomized and were excluded from the evaluation.

Results

Figure 1 illustrates sodium and potassium balance in control and spontaneously hypertensive rats during 1-week periods of a normal sodium diet and a low-sodium diet. The data show that there was no significant difference in urinary sodium or potassium excretion in spontaneously hypertensive rats when compared to the normotensive control group.

Plasma potassium and sodium concentrations were measured in three groups of control rats ($n = 26$) and spontaneously hypertensive rats ($n = 26$) while they were maintained on normal sodium diets. Spontaneously hypertensive rats consistently exhibited a lower mean plasma potassium concentration when compared to the control groups ($p < 0.001$). The mean difference between control and spontaneously hypertensive rats in plasma potassium concentration was 0.5 mEq per liter. Thus, this strain when compared to Wistar control rats exhibits a mean depression of plasma potassium concentration of approximately 10 percent. In contrast to these differences in plasma potassium concentration in the two groups of rats, plasma sodium concentration was similar.

Figure 2 illustrates the effect of 4 weeks of sodium depletion on the blood pressure of a group of young control rats and young spontaneously hypertensive rats. The mean blood pressure of the two groups of young spontaneously hypertensive rats, 135 and 137 mm Hg, was already considerably higher than in the control groups, 102 and 104 mm Hg ($p < 0.001$). However, the blood pressure of these young, spontaneously hypertensive rats is still in the prehypertensive range when compared with that of older, spontaneously hypertensive rats. Four weeks of sodium depletion significantly slowed the characteristic rise of blood pressure in the sodium-deprived, spontaneously hypertensive rats (156 ± 3 mm Hg), when compared with the hypertensive group fed a normal sodium diet (174 ± 6): $p<0.02$. In both sodium-deprived, spontaneously hypertensive rats and controls, body weight was significantly lower when compared to the groups fed the normal sodium diet. In contrast to the similar effects of sodium depletion on body weight in both groups, only in sodium-deprived, spontaneously hypertensive rats was the blood pressure significantly altered. However, it should also be noted that the blood

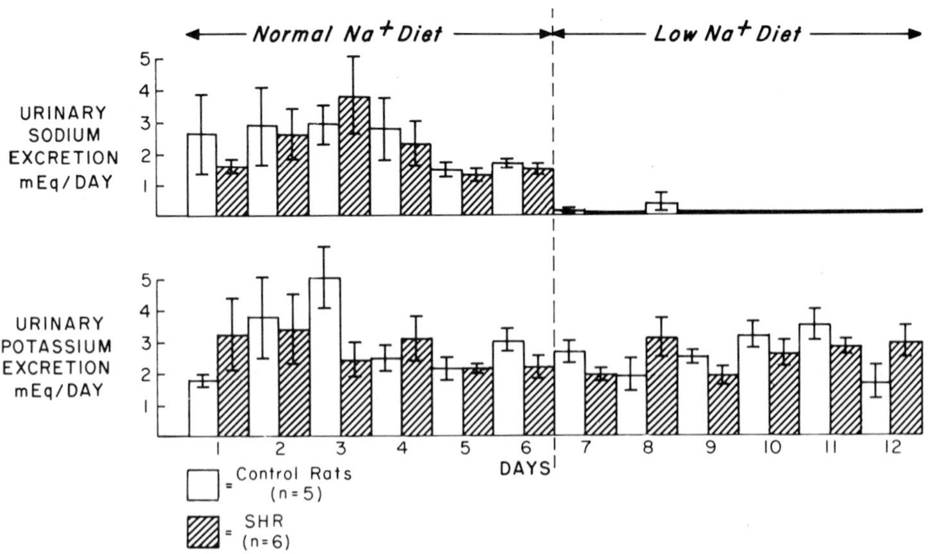

FIG. 1.—Sodium and potassium balance in five control and six spontaneously hypertensive rats (SHR). The **open bars** represent controls and the **hatched bars** represent spontaneously hypertensive rats.

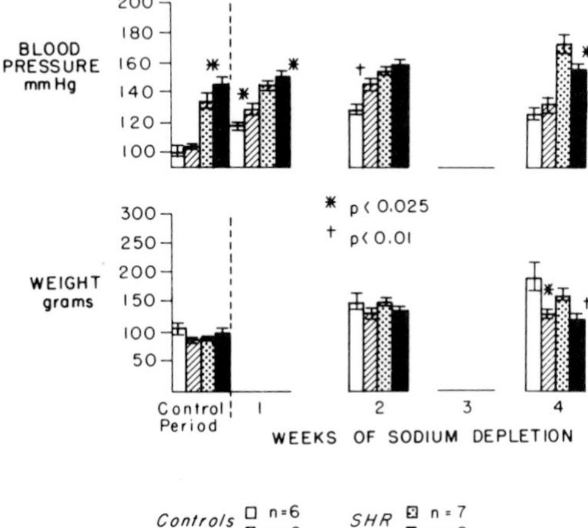

FIG. 2.—Effect of 4 weeks of sodium depletion on the blood pressure of young, normotensive Wistar rats and young, spontaneously hypertensive rats (SHR). The Wistar group (n=6) and the hypertensive group (n=7) maintained on normal sodium diets are indicated by the **open bars** and the **dotted bars** respectively. The sodium-depleted Wistar group (n=9) and the hypertensive group (n=9) are indicated by the **hatched bars** and the **black bars** respectively. The control period refers to measurements while all groups were on a normal sodium diet prior to the start of sodium depletion. (From Okamoto, K. (Ed.): Spontaneous Hypertension—Its Pathogenesis and Complications. Tokyo: Igaku Shoin, 1972, p. 203, with permission.)

pressure of the sodium-deprived, spontaneously hypertensive rats did not fall during the 4-week period of sodium depletion: 147 ± mm Hg versus 156 ± 3 mm Hg, and may even have increased.

Figure 3 illustrates the effect of corticosterone (compound B) administration (1 mg per rat per day) in control rats and spontaneously hypertensive rats. Compound B was administered for 8 weeks to suppress the pituitary-adrenal axis. Compound B had no significant effect on the blood pressure of control rats. In contrast, compound B treatment in spontaneously hypertensive rats slowed the development of hypertension and this effect was maximal at 4 to 5 weeks. At this time the blood pressure of compound B-treated, spontaneously hypertensive rats was consistently 25 to 30 mm Hg lower than in the untreated group. However, with continued compound B treatment blood pressure rose progressively so that by the eighth week, blood pressure was similar in both compound B-treated and untreated spontaneously hypertensive rat groups (186 ± 4 versus 199 ± 6 mm Hg).

Figure 4 illustrates the effect of total adrenalectomy (adx) on young control rats and spontaneously hypertensive rats. The blood pressure of these spontaneously hypertensive rats, while already higher than in age-matched

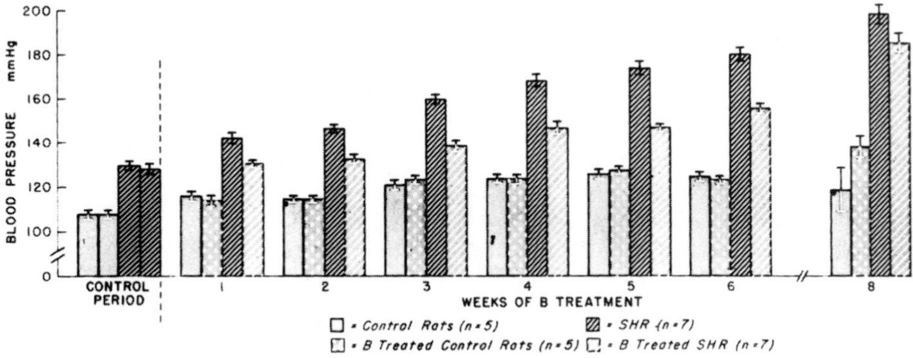

FIG. 3.—Effect of corticosterone (compound B) on the blood pressure of control rats and hypertensive rats. The dose of compound B in these experiments was 1 mg per rat per day. The number of compound B-treated control rats was five and of compound B-treated hypertensive rats was seven. The **black bars** represent untreated control rats and the **black-and-white dotted bars** represent compound B-treated control rats. The **black hatched bars** represent untreated and the **white hatched bars** represent compound B-treated hypertensive rats. (From Okamoto, K. (Ed.): Spontaneous Hypertension—Its Pathogenesis and Complications. Tokyo: Igaku Shoin, 1972, p. 203, with permission.)

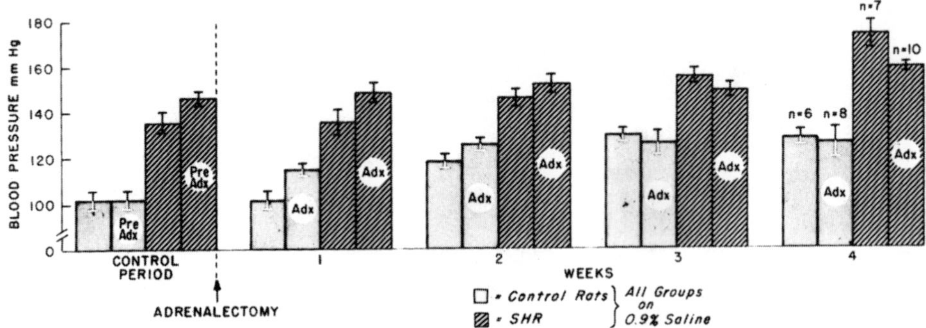

FIG. 4.—Effect of total adrenalectomy **(adx)** on the hypertension of spontaneously hypertensive rats. There were six nonadrenalectomized control and seven nonadrenalectomized hypertensive rats. There were 8 adrenalectomized control rats and 10 adrenalectomized hypertensive rats. The **black bars** represent control rats and the **hatched bars** represent hypertensive rats. Adx, totally adrenalectomized groups. (From Okamoto, K. (Ed.): Spontaneous Hypertension—Its Pathogenesis and Complications. Tokyo: Igaku Shoin, 1972, p. 203, with permission.)

control animals, was considerably lower than that of older, spontaneously hypertensive rats with established hypertension. All groups were given 0.9% saline to drink. Four weeks after total adrenalectomy, the blood pressure of adrenalectomized, spontaneously hypertensive rats rose from 146 ± 3 to 160 ± 2 mm Hg while the blood pressure of the nonadrenalectomized, spontaneously hypertensive rat group rose to higher levels (135 ± 5 to 174 ± 6 mm Hg). Thus, despite adrenalectomy, blood pressure in adrenalectomized, spontaneously hypertensive rats did not fall but rose although the increase in blood pressure in this group was less than in the unoperated, spontaneously hypertensive rat group ($p < 0.02$).

A microscopic study of the kidneys and adrenal glands was performed in five control and in five spontaneously hypertensive rats.* The kidneys were obtained from age-matched males of both groups. The mean weight of the hypertensives prior to nephrectomy was 373 gm, and of the control strain, 369 gm (not significantly different). No striking differences were observed in the kidneys of the two groups with respect to the degree of nephrosclerosis. Juxtaglomerular cell counts were not performed. Bilateral adrenocortical hyperplasia was present in the spontaneously hypertensive group (Fig. 5).

*The renal and adrenal tissue was examined by Sheldon C. Sommers, M.D.

DISCUSSION

A number of considerations led to the study of the effect of sodium balance and the pituitary-adrenal axis on the hypertension of spontaneously hypertensive rats. Sodium is a crucial factor in some forms of congenital hypertension.[2] It also seemed possible that abnormal sodium retention in spontaneously hypertensive rats could be mediated by adrenocortical overactivity. Adrenal hyperplasia was observed in this study and in others[9] and increased aldosterone secretion has been reported in spontaneously hypertensive rats.[10] The lower plasma potassium concentration observed in our studies in the hypertensive rats is compatible with a state of mild mineralocorticoid excess. However, a number of findings in the present study indicate that sodium and the adrenal gland do not play a critical role in the hypertension of spontaneously hypertensive rats.

In the first group of experiments in which sodium balance was measured in spontaneously hypertensive rats, they were not found to differ from controls with respect to sodium excretion during both a normal and a low-sodium diet. In the studies involving chronic sodium depletion, the progressive rise of blood pressure of spontaneously hypertensive rats could not be blocked by a low-sodium diet. Chronic sodium depletion in our experiments delayed the development of the hypertension but it neither

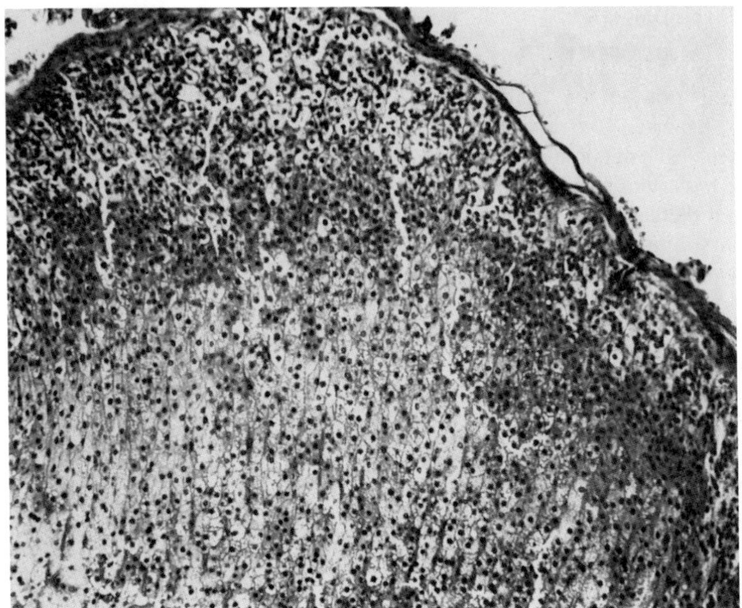

FIG. 5.—Microscopic appearance of the adrenal cortex in spontaneously hypertensive rats. Nodular hyperplasia, primarily of the zona fasciculata, is present.

restored blood pressure to normal levels nor totally blocked the progressive rise of blood pressure in spontaneously hypertensive rats with aging. This finding is similar to that reported by Louis, Tabei, and Spector.[11] Moreover, our results suggest that the effect of sodium depletion on the blood pressure of young, spontaneously hypertensive rats may be related to their failure to grow. Altogether, these findings of the relationship of sodium to the hypertension of spontaneously hypertensive rats indicate that sodium balance is not a crucial factor in the hypertensive process.

The experiments involving corticosterone also seem to rule out the pituitary-adrenal axis as a primary factor in the hypertension of spontaneously hypertensive rats. The administration of corticosterone for 8 weeks slowed the rate of development of hypertension in spontaneously hypertensive rats but it did not cure the hypertension. The delayed development of hypertension in the corticosterone-treated group may support the view that an abnormal pituitary-adrenal axis is present in spontaneously hypertensive rats.[9] However, the failure to normalize blood pressure during corticosterone treatment indicates that the pituitary-adrenal axis is not crucially involved in the hypertension.

A number of the features of spontaneously hypertensive rats described in the present study bear a similarity to another hypertensive disorder that has recently been described in patients and has been termed "pseudo-primary aldosteronism" or "idiopathic adrenal hyperplasia."[12,13] The hypertensive rats and patients with pseudo-primary aldosteronism usually exhibit a normal or mildly depressed plasma potassium concentration and adrenocortical hyperplasia. Total adrenalectomy in these patients cures the hyperaldosteronism but, as in spontaneously hypertensive rats, the hypertension is not fully corrected. Thus, in both spontaneously hypertensive rats and patients with pseudo-primary aldosteronism, the hypertension is not primarily mediated by the adrenal gland, although in both situations adrenal hyperplasia is present. However, before this strain of congenitally hypertensive rat can be used as a model for this and other hypertensive disorders in man, further characterization of adrenal steroid metabolism and the renin-angiotensin system will be necessary.

Summary

The relationship of sodium balance and the pituitary-adrenal axis to the hypertension of spontaneously hypertensive rats was studied. Sodium balance was similar in control rats and spontaneously hypertensive rats during normal and low-sodium diets. Severe sodium depletion for 4 weeks in young, spontaneously hypertensive rats delayed the progression of hypertension but it did not reduce the blood pressure to normotensive levels. The effect of sodium depletion may be nonspecific because severe sodium depletion was also associated with retarded growth of the animals.

Bilateral adrenocortical hyperplasia was observed in spontaneously hypertensive rats. However, suppression of the pituitary-adrenal axis with corticosterone for 8 weeks did not prevent or reverse the hypertensive process although it did delay the development of the hypertension. Total adrenalectomy also did not cũre the hypertension.

These results suggest that sodium and the adrenal gland are not crucially involved in the hypertension of spontaneously hypertensive rats. This animal model resembles at least one form of human hypertension with adrenal hyperplasia (pseudo-primary aldosteronism or idiopathic adrenal hyperplasia) because these patients are similarly not cured by adrenalectomy.

References

1. Smirk, F. H., and Hall, W. H.: Inherited hypertension in rats. Nature (London) 182: 727, 1958.
2. Dahl, L. K., Heine, M., and Tassinari, L.: Effects of chronic excess salt ingestion. Evidence that genetic factors play an important role in susceptibility to experimental hypertension. J. Exp. Med. 115:1173, 1962.
3. Okamoto, K., and Aoki, K.: Development of a strain of spontaneously hypertensive rats. Jap. Circ. J. 27:282, 1963.
4. Okamoto, K., Aoki, K., Nosaka, S., and Fukushima, M.: Cardiovascular diseases in the spontaneously hypertensive rat. Jap. Circ. J. 28:943, 1964.
5. Shamma, A. H., Goddard, J. W., and Sommers, S. C.: A study of the adrenal status in hypertension. J. Chron. Dis. 8:587, 1958.
6. Koletsky, S., Shook, P., and Rivera-Velez, J.: Lack of increased renin-angiotensin activity in rats with spontaneous hypertension. Proc. Soc. Exp. Biol. Med. 134:1187, 1970.
7. De Jong, W., Lovenberg, W., and Sjoerdsma, A.: Increased plasma renin activity in the spontaneously hypertensive rat. Proc. Soc. Exp. Biol. Med. 139:1213, 1972.
8. Friedman, M., and Freed, S. C.: Microphonic manometer for indirect determination of systolic blood pressure in the rat. Proc. Soc. Exp. Biol. Med. 70:670, 1949.
9. Aoki, K., Tankawa, H., Fujinami, T., Miyazaki, A., and Hashimoto, Y.: Pathological studies on the endocrine organs of the spontaneously hypertensive rats. Jap. Heart J. 4:426, 1963.
10. Rapp, J. P., and Dahl, L. K.: Adrenal steroidogenesis in rats bred for susceptibility and resistance to the hypertensive effect of salt. Endocrinology 88:50, 1971.
11. Louis, W. J., Tabei, R., and Spector, S.: Effects of sodium intake on inherited hypertension in the rat. Lancet 2:1283, 1971.
12. Baer, L., Sommers, S. C., Krakoff, L. R., Newton, M. A., and Laragh, J. H.: Pseudo-primary aldosteronism. An entity distinct from true primary aldosteronism. Circ. Res. 26–27(Suppl. 1):I-203, 1970.
13. Biglieri, E. G., Schambelan, M., Slaton, P. E., and Stockigt, J. R.: The intercurrent hypertension of primary aldosteronism. Circ. Res. 26–27(Suppl. 1):I-195, 1970.

Heart Attack and Stroke in Essential Hypertension: The Renin Factor

By Hans R. Brunner, M.D., and John H. Laragh, M.D.

It is now understood that the renin-angiotensin-aldosterone system provides vital regulation of electrolyte and blood pressure homeostasis. Within the past decade, it has been possible to show that a derangement of the system is crucially involved in the pathogenesis of malignant hypertension [1–3] and severe renovascular hypertension,[4] and in the pressor consequences of primary aldosteronism and oral contraceptive use.[5,6] These represent the more dramatic hypertensive disorders and the more easily demonstrated abnormalities of renin and aldosterone. However, altogether they comprise only a small portion of the hypertensive population.

By far the largest group of hypertensives have the less flagrant manifestations that are classified under the term "essential hypertension." That more than one disorder may fall within this classification is suggested by several observations, one of which is that some patients seem to tolerate the condition without apparent deficit, while others incur greatly increased risk of heart attacks and strokes. It occurred to several investigators that the renin- and aldosterone-associated vascular wastage unleashed in the malignant disease might also be at work, but much more slowly, in patients whose more indolent condition ultimately concludes in cardiovascular accident. However, such theories eluded demonstration because of the difficulty of obtaining a clear understanding of renin or aldosterone deviations from normal in these cases. Methods of assay were not adequate for the simultaneous measurements of the hormonal components, nor definitions of normalcy precise enough to expose fine increments of values that could explain the more subtle effects.

Two things led the present investigators to believe that the time was at hand for perceiving the association, if any, between the renin-aldosterone axis and essential hypertension. One was the development of sensitive isotope-dilution and then radioimmunoassay methods permitting consistent, coincident, and reliable quantitative assay of the components of this system; the other was a fresh approach to the concept of normal value that related it to a dynamic of salt balance.

In this chapter, we would like to present to you the findings from a study which has been published in detail elsewhere,[7] in which 219 consecutive hypertensive patients were studied. It turned out that the large majority could readily be fitted into low, normal, or high categories with respect either to renin or aldosterone activity. The implication then emerged that the level of renin activity was related to the incidence of heart attack and stroke, for those patients who had low plasma renin levels suffered no such complications while those with normal or high plasma renin levels had a high frequency of heart attack and stroke. This was so even though the patients in the low-renin category were significantly older on the average and had a comparable duration of arterial hypertension and an equal degree of left ventricular enlargement.

The findings summarized herein and recently reported [7] suggest why certain patients with essential hypertension appear to confound expectations. If, indeed, a low renin level protects while a high renin level predisposes, its value as a diagnostic and prognostic marker may turn out to be surpassed by its importance in therapeutic strategy.

Subjects

Subjects in this study were patients at the Nephritis-Hypertension Clinic or the Doctors' Private Office Facilities of the Columbia-Presbyterian Medical Center. While these institutions accept referrals from the Greater New York area and from more distant points, the

From the Department of Medicine, Columbia University College of Physicians and Surgeons, New York, New York.

principal catchment area consists of upper Manhattan and the Bronx.

There were 219 hypertensive patients. All had diastolic blood pressure elevations greater than 95 mm Hg as determined on three separate occasions. None had been included in any previous studies. Of the patients, 146 were admitted to the metabolic unit of Presbyterian Hospital and the other 73 were studied as outpatients. All antihypertensive and diuretic drugs had been discontinued at least 3 weeks prior to the study, and the patients were put on diets containing normal amounts of sodium. Prior to the study, all were given a complete workup that included intravenous pyelography and occasionally renal arteriography to exclude any known cause of hypertension such as primary aldosteronism, renovascular hypertension, pheochromocytoma, or Cushing's disease. Patients with malignant hypertension, congestive heart failure, or evidence of primary parenchymal kidney disease were also excluded. Thus it was unusual to find among these patients any evidence of impaired renal function.

Study Plan

The renin-angiotensin-aldosterone system in the 146 inpatients was evaluated on the fifth day of a fixed dietary regimen of known electrolyte content. Most were thus studied at two or more different levels of constant sodium intake. Renin activity was measured from plasma samples taken at noon after the patient had been ambulatory at least 4 hours. Matching 24-hour urine samples were saved for the determination of aldosterone and sodium excretion.

Procedures necessarily differed for the 73 outpatients because their dietary regimens could not be standardized. These patients were all instructed not to avoid sodium in their diets, and the state of their salt balance was inferred from 24-hour urinary sodium excretion rate. Among them, the daily rate of sodium excretion ranged from 100 to 250 mEq, and we felt that at such relatively high rates the influence of dietary inconstancy on renin and aldosterone secretion could be expected to be small. On first analyzing the data, the outpatient results were separated from those obtained from inpatients. However, it soon became apparent that the findings among the outpatients, from 24-hour urine specimens for aldosterone determination and midday plasma samples for measurement of renin activity, completely paralleled and reinforced those obtained under more rigidly controlled conditions in the metabolic study unit.

Methodology

Full details of assay methodology are reported elsewhere and need not be provided here. Plasma renin activity was determined by a modified radioimmunoassay of angiotensin I produced during incubation; the method is reproducible to ±12 percent (SD), permits the processing of many samples, and is highly sensitive.[8] The 24-hour aldosterone excretion rate was measured by double-isotope dilution,[9] and more recently by radioimmunoassay.[10] Metabolism unit procedures and analytic methods for measuring plasma and urine electrolytes and blood urea nitrogen have also been reported previously.

Criteria for Normal Values

Normal values were defined by submitting 52 normal volunteers to the same dietary regimens utilized for hypertensive patients and then studying the same parameters. Normal plasma renin activity and rates of aldosterone excretion were related to states of salt balance, as reflected in daily urinary sodium excretion. A close relationship was observed, as seen in Fig. 1. This figure also represents a nomogram of normal expectations at various levels of sodium excretion. This, rather than the more customary use of overlapping bracketed ranges, provided the standard against which the patient group was evaluated.

Results

Renin, Aldosterone and Sodium Balance in Hypertensive Patients

Figure 2 presents a plot of 368 determinations of renin activity and aldosterone excretion, drawn from the 219 hypertensive patients. These, like those for normal volunteers in Fig. 1, are related to the concurrent rate of sodium

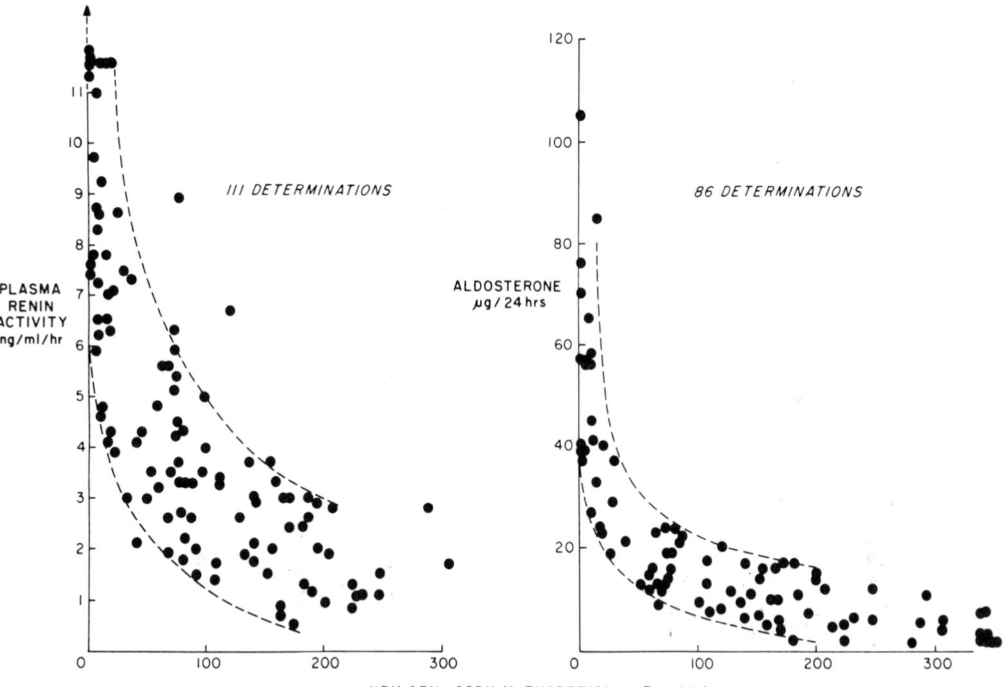

FIG. 1.—Relationship of plasma renin activity measured at noon and of corresponding daily aldosterone excretion to the concurrent rate of sodium excretion in 52 normal subjects. (From Brunner, H. R. et al.,[7] with permission.)

excretion, and normal limits are shown by the dotted lines.

The scatter of both renin and aldosterone values is considerably wider for the hypertensives than for the normal subjects, permitting their classification into high, normal, and low categories.

Thus, 59 patients (27%) showed reduced plasma renin activity, in 36 patients (16%) this parameter was abnormally high, and the

TABLE 1.—*Epidemiologic and Clinical Characteristics in Essential Hypertension*

	No. of Patients	*Mean Diastolic Blood Pressure (mm Hg)*	*Mean Age (years)*	*Known Duration of Hypertension (years)*	*Percentage Black*
Low renin	59 (27%)	104.9 * (±14.2) †	46.5 (±11.3)	8.5 (±6.8)	42
Normal renin	124 (57%)	103.5 (±16.9)	37.5 (±12.0)	7.2 (±6.9)	24
High renin	36 (16%)	124.0 (±19.9)	43.1 (±9.8)	6.8 (±6.2)	11
Total	219 (100%)				27

From Brunner, H. R., et al.,[7] with permission.
* Mean.
† Standard deviation.

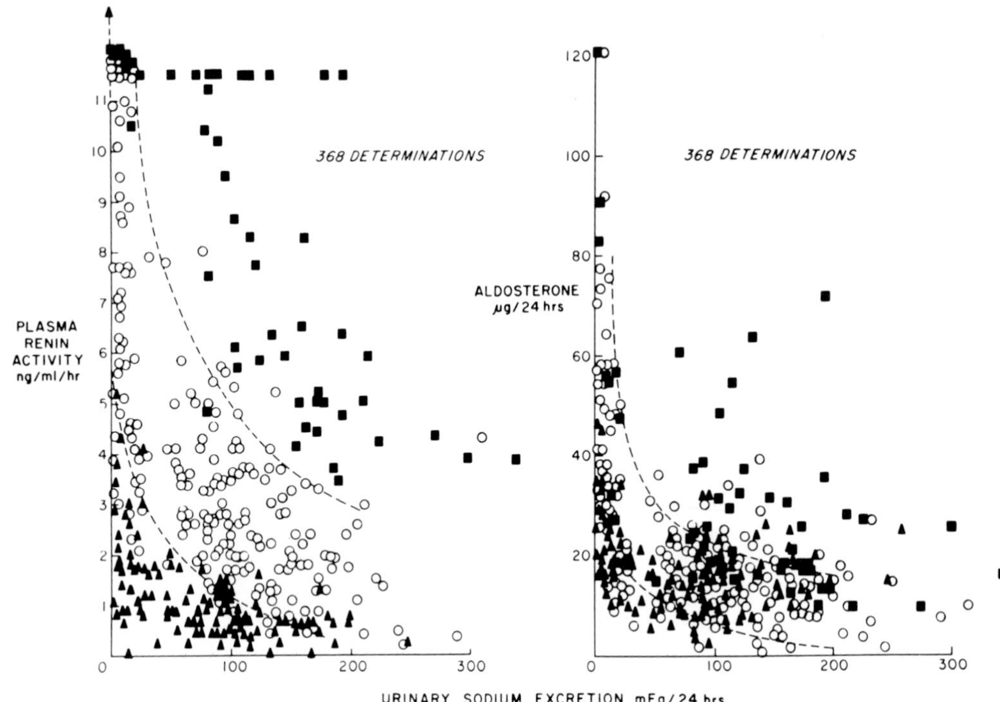

FIG. 2.—Essential hypertension in 219 patients. Relationship of plasma renin activity measured at noon and of corresponding daily aldosterone excretion to the concurrent rate of sodium excretion. ▲, Low renin activity; ○, normal renin activity; ■, high renin activity. (From Brunner, H. R. et al.,[7] with permission.)

remainder of 124 patients (57%) fell within the normal range.

Clinical and Epidemiologic Characteristics of Renin Subgroups

Table 1 presents the clinical and epidemiologic characteristics of the renin subgroups. Of the patients, 71 percent were white, 27 percent black, and 2 percent of Oriental origin. The normal renin group showed about the same racial distribution as the total study population, but the proportion of blacks was considerably increased in the low-renin group (42%) and decreased in the high-renin group (11%). Sex distribution was even among subgroups.

The mean diastolic blood pressure was comparable between low- and normal renin subgroups but it was significantly elevated in the high-renin group. The oldest subgroup was the low-renin category, which averaged 46.5 years; the high-renin group at 43.1 years was slightly younger, while the normal renin group at 37.5 years was significantly younger ($p < 0.01$). All groups were equivalent with regard to the known duration of hypertension. Evaluation of the eye grounds by standard Keith-Wagener criteria revealed a tendency for increased vascular changes in the high-renin group, half of whom showed grade II or grade III changes; no important differences were seen between the low- and normal renin groups.

Clinical Biochemical Characteristics

Table 2 provides clinical biochemical characteristics in the renin subgroups. Mean blood urea nitrogen concentration was normal in the low- and normal-renin groups, but slightly elevated in the high-renin group. The low- and normal renin groups did not differ materially in creatinine clearance or uric acid concentrations, but the high-renin group exhibited more uricemia and a slight tendency to increased albuminuria. Creatinine clearance data were

TABLE 2.—*Clinical Biochemical Data*

	Blood Urea Nitrogen (mg per 100 ml)	*Creatinine Clearance (ml per minute)*	*Uric Acid (mg per 100 ml)*	*Plasma [K⁺] (mEq per liter)*	*Plasma * [Na⁺] (mEq per liter)*	*$U_{Na}V$ * (mEq per liter)*
Low renin	14.8 † (±4.2) ‡	95.1 (±28.8)	6.4 (±1.6)	4.0 (±0.3)	137.9 (±4.0)	16.1 (±10.8)
Normal renin	16.4 (±5.7)	92.8 (±29.1)	6.4 (±1.9)	4.0 (±0.4)	138.0 (±3.9)	12.1 (±6.9)
High renin	24.1 (±15.9)		6.9 (±2.3)	3.6 (±0.6)		

* Fifth day of low-sodium intake.
† Mean.
‡ Standard deviation.
From Brunner, H. R., et al.,[7] with permission.

insufficient for valid analysis in the high-renin group.

As for mean plasma potassium concentration, the low- and normal renin groups did not differ, but the high-renin group was significantly lower. There were no differences between low- and normal-renin groups with regard to mean plasma sodium concentration or urinary sodium excretion, thus providing no evidence of sodium wastage in either group. In the high-renin group, no significant abnormalities of sodium conservation were observed, but these studies were too few in number to be included in the analysis.

Fasting plasma cholesterol levels were obtained on all patients with the routine SMA-12 technique. The mean values of the three groups showed no appreciable difference: 238 ± 68 mg per 100 ml for the low-, 219 ± 49 mg per 100 ml for the normal, and 224 ± 59 mg per 100 ml for the high-renin group.

Classification of Patients

With low, high, or normal values pertaining either in renin or in aldosterone determinations, there are nine theoretically possible classifications. In attempting to classify all patients into these categories, one must consider that their status might vary with time or circumstance. The time factor can tentatively be ruled out, for our preliminary longitudinal studies suggest the unlikelihood that abnormalities of renin activity will change significantly over months or years. As for a change in circumstance, the chief such stimulus would be the level of salt intake, and the only way to deal with this possibility is to measure renin and aldosterone secretion simultaneously at three or more levels of dietary salt. In this study most patients had at least two such measurements, usually at widely separated levels of salt intake. It soon became apparent that some patients could manifest normal values at one level of salt balance but abnormal values at another. Their abnormality could be plotted as a deviation from the curve of the normal nomogram.

This is illustrated in Fig. 3, which details the values obtained for the low-renin group. For this particular group of patients, aldosterone secretion is generally normal or even slightly increased when sodium excretion is greater than 90 mEq per 24 hours, but it becomes subnormal when urinary sodium excretion falls below 40 mEq. Thus, aldosterone secretion is relatively fixed and exhibits a blunted responsiveness in these hypertensive patients.

The distribution of the 219 patients according to the nine possible subgroups is shown in Fig. 4. In each of the boxes can be found two percentages. The smaller number represents the fraction of patients that would fall into this group if "strict" criteria were used, meaning that all the patients so included always exhibited that hormonal pattern without deviation. The higher number represents the percentage obtained with "loose" or less stringent criteria, meaning that it includes all patients who showed that pattern either consistently or inconsistently. Under loose criteria, some patients are included in more than one group.

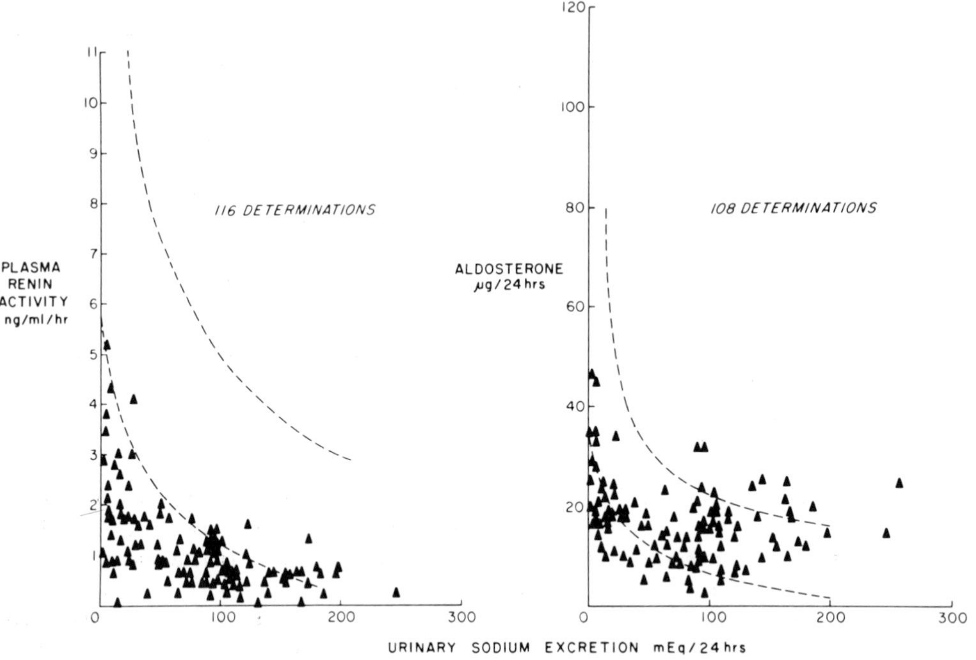

FIG. 3.—Low-renin essential hypertension in 59 patients. Shown here are plasma renin activity measured at noon and the corresponding daily aldosterone excretion in relation to the concurrent daily rate of sodium excretion.

However, study of the figures shows that the percentages of patients distributed into the various categories are not appreciably modified regardless of the criteria, an observation providing some testimony in favor of the validity of the method.

PLASMA RENIN ACTIVITY	ALDOSTERONE EXCRETION: low	normal	high
high	0	8-12 %	6-9 %
normal	2-6 %	36-54 %	3-6 %
low	5-8 %	13-21 %	1-2 %

FIG. 4.—Frequency distribution of hormonal patterns observed in 219 patients with essential hypertension. The first value in each category is derived from application of stringent and the second from less stringent criteria. Whichever criteria are used, the frequency of distribution is not modified appreciably. See text for more complete discussion. (From Brunner, H. R. et al.,[7] with permission.)

The largest fraction of patients was found to have normal renin and aldosterone: 36 percent with strict and 54 percent with loose criteria. Only a small percentage of those with normal renin levels deviated up or down from normal aldosterone values. Especially noteworthy is the high incidence of low-renin essential hypertension, ranging from 19 to 31 percent. These subjects usually showed normal rates of aldosterone secretion, although a small and possibly significant portion showed reduced aldosterone. A rare finding was increased aldosterone in the presence of subnormal renin, possibly suggesting occult primary aldosteronism; however, the few patients with this pattern showed only slightly elevated aldosterone and no hypokalemia. Since we have not found tumors in them and since even total adrenalectomy is not beneficial to their blood pressure, we do not recommend exploratory adrenal surgery in normokalemic patients with excessive aldosterone excretion.[11] High-renin levels appeared in 14 to 21 percent of the group. Among these, aldo-

TABLE 3.—*Incidence of Cardiovascular Complications*

	Left Ventricular Enlargement	*Strokes or Heart Attacks* * *Total*	*Strokes*	*Heart Attacks*
Low renin	12 (20%)	(0%)	(0%)	(0%)
Normal renin	18 (15%)	14 (11%)	8 (6%)	6 (5%)
High renin	8 (22%)	5 (14%)	4 (11%)	2 (6%)
Total	38 (17%)	19 (9%)	12 (5%)	8 (4%)

* One patient in the high-renin group had both a stroke and a heart attack.
From Brunner et al.,[7] with permission.

sterone was either normal or correspondingly elevated. There were no patients with high-renin levels who had reduced aldosterone secretion.

Returning to Figs. 2 and 4, one might draw the conclusion that renin activity is more likely to be abnormal than is aldosterone excretion in patients with essential hypertension. However, we cautiously venture the possibility that some of the seemingly normal values may be inappropriate to the hormonal interaction. What is normal for normals may not be so for hypertensives. One example of this might be the 13 to 21 percent of patients with normal aldosterone excretion but low renin—this might in fact represent an abnormally high aldosterone value for that level of renin activity. A truly "normal" relationship between aldosterone and renin, one in which the adrenocortical response is linearly appropriate to a given renin secretion, is probably the one represented by the three boxes situated on the diagonal from left-lower corner to right-upper corner. In these three groups, from 47 to 71 percent of the hypertensive patients show an appropriate adrenocortical response.

Incidence of Cardiovascular Complications

Thirty-eight patients had left ventricular enlargement by electrocardiogram or routine chest x-ray. Only three were receiving digitalis during the study and none was in a decompensated state of congestive heart failure with fluid retention. Table 3 shows that by these indices left ventricular enlargement was evenly distributed among the patients with low-, high-, or normal renin levels.

Eighteen patients suffered strokes or myocardial infarctions either before or after the study, and one other patient has had both complications: thus, there were 20 instances of stroke or heart attack among 19 patients. The distribution of these complications is markedly and meaningfully uneven: 14 percent of the high-renin group experienced them, 11 percent of the normal renin group, and none of the low-renin group. All of the cardiovascular complications occurred in four subgroups as shown in Fig. 5, those with normal or high-renin levels, or normal or high-aldosterone levels. In none of the four subgroups representing low-renin or low-aldosterone levels has there been a single

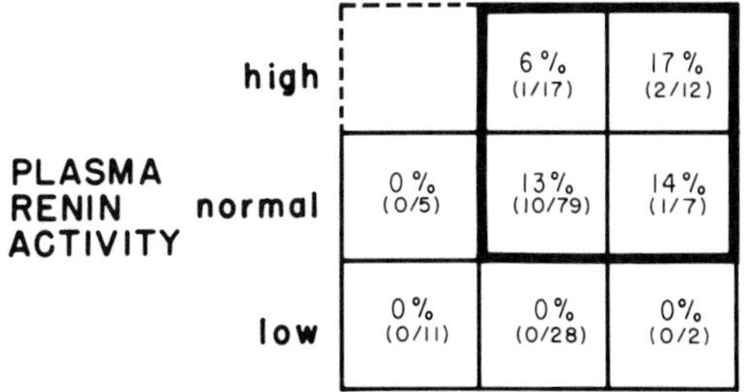

FIG. 5.—Relationship of various hormonal patterns to the incidence of strokes and heart attacks using stringent criteria. See text for more complete discussion. All of the strokes and heart attacks accumulate in four of the categories.

patient to date suffering a myocardial infarction or stroke.

Remarks

This study examines renin and aldosterone levels in patients with essential hypertension to discover whether a classification could be applied with diagnostic or prognostic implications. The hypothesis that improved methodology might reveal such patterns stemmed from the observation of altered renin and aldosterone levels in the more egregious hypertensive disorders.

About a decade ago it was found that marked oversecretion of the sodium-retaining hormone aldosterone almost always occurred in patients with malignant hypertension.[1] The consistent presence of renal damage in this disorder led to studies which demonstrated that aldosterone secretion is activated and controlled by the pressor hormone angiotensin II,[2,3] which is in turn summoned by the action of the renal enzyme renin.

Thus was elucidated the renin-angiotensin-aldosterone system for the normal regulation of sodium balance and, consequently, fluid volume. When perfusion of the kidney is compromised by a fall in arterial blood pressure—induced by such contretemps as hemorrhage or sodium depletion—renin is secreted into the bloodstream. An enzyme, it acts on plasma globulin to release angiotensin II. The most powerful pressor substance known, angiotensin II, also triggers increased aldosterone secretion. The pressor and sodium-retaining effects of this system operate together to restore blood volume and renal perfusion, thus shutting off the initial signal for renal renin release.

A derangement of this system appears to be crucially involved in the more flagrant hypertensive disorders. It has been proposed [3] that the substantial renal damage in malignant hypertension provides false cues for excesses of renin to be released and, in consequence, increased amounts of angiotensin and aldosterone, producing additional excesses of pressor action and fluid volume. The damage in the kidney at the same time renders it unresponsive to the shut-off signal of increased fluid volume. A vicious circle develops in which the damaged kidney calls for more pressor and sodium-retaining action, which further damages the renal vasculature, renders it even less responsive and even more generative of false calls for hormonal action, etc. Some of the accelerated vascular damage may also be attributed to renin, which has been shown in animal experiments to be vasculotoxic.[12–15]

This construction also serves to explain the benign course of the hypertension associated with primary aldosteronism.[1,3,6] Here, oversecretion of aldosterone in the presence of an intact kidney operates to suppress renal renin release, thus preventing the vicious circle described above.

Are the components of this vicious circle insidiously at work in the more indolent forms of hypertension? One can only begin to answer this question by documenting the deviations from normal renin and aldosterone values that occur in hypertensive patients and then determining if any correlation exists between these levels and the incidence of cardiovascular sequelae.

In such a closely interrelated system, the level of any component is dependent on the level of another. Even more significantly, the entire system is closely keyed to the state of sodium balance so that *normal* must be defined in terms of the appropriateness of the hormonal activity in governing this homeostatic function at any given level of salt intake. This interrelationship is dynamic, hyperbolic, and continuous.

Our approach has been to relate these hormonal activities to the 24-hour rate of sodium excretion. Since the kidney is normally the main route by which sodium can be eliminated, the daily rate of urinary sodium excretion obviously reflects the extent to which the kidney is being directed to either retain or release sodium. In this approach, the hormonal activity is thus linked to target organ behavior rather than to changes in the homeostatic function, which probably initiate any changes in the hormonal concatenation, i.e., sodium balance.

Theoretically, one might suspect that it would be most appropriate to relate changes in degrees of hormonal activity to changes in overall sodium balance since this is the homeostatic function which the system seems designed to regulate. In fact, however, not only is this approach more laborious, but, from a practical standpoint, the errors inherent in measurement and calculation of balance also make this parameter an insensitive index as compared with measurement of daily urinary sodium excretion.

It is also more meaningful to relate changes in renin and aldosterone activity to sodium output instead of to the dietary intake since, while sodium intake is held constant, and before equilibrium is achieved, serial daily studies have revealed that changes in renin and aldosterone activity closely parallel changes in sodium excretion rate.[10] From a technical standpoint, too, sodium output from day to day is much more readily monitorable than is dietary intake. In addition, this approach has been applied and validated for use in the study of outpatients.

Therefore, our approach was to plot hormone values from normal subjects over a wide range of sodium balance. The assay of a daily urinary salt excretion proved to be a reliable index of salt balance. From these data a nomographic index could be drawn that clearly showed the continuum of the relationship. Hormone values obtained from patients at a given level of salt excretion could then be related to normal values at the same level. The need for a continuous index of this sort is underlined by the hyperbolic shape of the curve describing the relationship; thus a small change in sodium excretion at a high level of hormonal activity involves a geometrically greater hormonal response than the same quantum of change at other, lower levels. This phenomenon could be completely overlooked in the gaps between bracketed ranges. In this way, it was possible to classify subjects into low-, normal, and high-renin groups over a wide range of salt balance.

The chief finding, that no heart attacks or strokes have yet occurred among the low-renin patients with hypertension, provides intriguing topics for discussion. One is drawn immediately to propose that the low-renin state may be protective against the vascular sequelae of hypertension, a theory apparently supported by the somewhat higher mean age of that hormonally "privileged" group.

Why is plasma renin suppressed in these patients? Some suggest it to be a response to hypervolemia caused by oversecretion of an unidentified mineralocorticoid hormone; [16] others that oversecretion of 18-hydroxydeoxycorticosterone (18-OH-DOC) is involved.[17] Another idea is that low-renin hypertensives are especially susceptible to volume depletion and postural hypertension induced by a low-sodium diet.[18] However, the present study found no abnormalities of sodium conservation in low-renin patients nor did sodium depletion provide any beneficial effect on the arterial hypertension.

As others have found, aldosterone excretion was usually normal among low-renin hypertensives. But, as indicated already, our estimate of normal may not be keeping pace with the dynamics of this system. These apparently normal values could possibly be inappropriately high for low-renin patients. Previous studies indicate that among some patients with essential hypertension the hormone excretion rates are not normally responsive to sodium loading or deprivation.[18–20] The results of this study of low-renin patients seem to bear out these observations.

Of the subjects with normal renin, the largest group, only minor fractions exhibited abnormalities of aldosterone excretion. We do not yet know how to characterize them, except to suggest that they may prove to be a group for whom the term "essential hypertension," though not definitive, may survive. One must also entertain the consideration that the "normal" renin in this group of patients may in fact represent an inappropriately high level; perhaps they should more properly have accommodated to increased arterial blood pressure with suppressed renal renin secretion, as did their more compensatory [7] low-renin associates. More study is needed to define the boundaries of normal for this group; suggested are measurements of other components of the system such as renin substrate and converting-enzyme activity.

The number of subjects with high-renin levels was surprisingly high at 16 percent. Not only did these patients have significantly higher mean diastolic blood pressure, they also had the highest incidence of increased aldosterone secretion, hypokalemia, azotemia, albuminuria, and vascular changes in the optic fundi. The high-renin level seemed to be associated with more severe disease and a greater frequency of cardiovascular complications. All these findings support the possibility that excessive renin secretion is involved in the vascular complications of hypertensive disease.

The association of aldosterone with these vascular complications is less clearly suggested, mostly because the data are too few in those categories with decreased aldosterone excretion. That there is such an association seems likely, if only from the knowledge that the hormone operates within the system to determine sodium balance, which in turn moderates action and secretion of renin. Also, it is known that the vasculotoxic effects of renin are best demonstrated in animals fed salt. In the same way, too, the experimental vascular disease produced by mineralocorticoids requires adequate dietary salt. Thus, physiologic and vasculotoxic effects of renin in patients with essential hypertension may be moderated by aldosterone action. It should be noted that while the numbers are much too small to be meaningful, no vascular complications occurred in any of our low-aldosterone patients, even those with so-called "normal" renin values.

The protected status of the low-renin patients may explain the longevity without complications experienced by certain patients who have had impressive elevations of blood pressure for up to 30 years. A new therapeutic strategy is also suggested. If further study should confirm that low-renin patients have a fundamentally different and more benign disorder, early application of antihypertensive therapy may not be indicated for them. In contrast, such treatment should be instigated earlier and more aggressively in hypertensives with high-renin activity.

One is also led to wonder if the selection of antihypertensive agents with specific action of suppression of renin secretion would correct renin abnormalities to the extent of producing more satisfactory blood pressure responses and reduced incidence of cardiovascular complications. We are presently engaged in studies directed at such questions; we are evaluating blood pressure changes as related to changes in renin levels induced by various antihypertensive drugs prescribed for patients with essential hypertension.

References

1. Laragh, J. H., Ulick, S., Januszewicz, W., Deming, Q. B., Kelly, W. G., and Lieberman, S.: Aldosterone secretion and primary and malignant hypertension. J. Clin. Invest. 39: 1091, 1960 .
2. Laragh, J. H., Angers, M., Kelly, W. G., and Lieberman, S.: Hypotensive agents and pressor substances. The effect of epinephrine, norepinephrine, angiotensin II and others on the secretory rate of aldosterone in man. JAMA 174:234, 1960.
3. Laragh, J. H.: The role of aldosterone in man: Evidence for regulation of electrolyte balance and arterial pressure by renal-adrenal system which may be involved in malignant hypertension. JAMA 174:293, 1960.
4. Dustan, H. P., Tarazi, R. C., and Frohlich, E. D.: Functional correlates of plasma renin activity in hypertensive patients. Circulation 41:555, 1970.
5. Newton, M. A., Sealey, J. E., Ledingham, J. G. G., and Laragh, J. H.: High blood pressure and oral contraceptives. Changes in plasma renin and renin substrate and in aldosterone excretion. Am. J. Obstet. Gynec. 101:1037, 1968.
6. Laragh, J. H., Cannon, P. J., and Ames, R. P.: Aldosterone secretion and various forms of hypertensive vascular disease. Ann. Intern. Med. 59:117, 1963.
7. Brunner, H. R., Laragh, J. H., Baer, L., Newton, M. A., Goodwin, F. T., Krakoff, L. R., Bard, R. H., and Bühler, F. R.: Essential hypertension: Renin and aldosterone, heart attack and stroke. N. Engl. J. Med. 286:441, 1972.
8. Sealey, J. E., Gerten-Banes, J., and Laragh, J. H.: The renin system: Variations in man measured by radioimmunoassay or bioassay. Kidney Int. 1:240, 1972.
9. Laragh, J. H., Sealey, J. E., and Sommers, S. C.: Patterns of adrenal secretion and urinary excretion of aldosterone and plasma renin activity in normal and hypertensive subjects. Circ. Res. 19 (Suppl. I):158, 1966.
10. Sealey, J. E., Bühler, F. R., Laragh, T. H., Manning, E. L., and Brunner, H. R.: Aldosterone excretion: Physiologic variations in man measured by radioimmunoassay or double isotope dilution. Circ. Res. 31:367, 1972.
11. Baer, L., Sommers, S. C., Krakoff, L. R., Newton, M. A., and Laragh, J. H.: Pseudo-primary aldosteronism: An entity distinct from true primary aldosteronism. Circ. Res. 26–27(Suppl. 1):203, 1970.

12. Masson, G. M. C., Mikasa, A., and Yasuda, H.: Experimental vascular disease elicited by aldosterone and renin. Endocrinology 71: 505, 1962.
13. Giese, J.: Acute hypertensive vascular disease. Acta Pathol. Microbiol. Scand. 62:481, 1964.
14. Cuthbert, M. F., and Peart, W. S.: Studies on the identity of a vascular permeability factor of renal origin. Clin. Sci. 38:309, 1970.
15. Gavras, H., Brown, J. J., Lever, A. F., Macadam, R. F., and Robertson, J. I. S.: Acute renal failure, tubular necrosis and myocardial infarction induced in the rabbit by intravenous angiotensin II. Lancet 2:19, 1971.
16. Woods, J. W., Liddle, G. W., Stant, E. G., Jr., Michelakis, A. M., and Brill, A. B.: Effect of an adrenal inhibitor in hypertensive patients with suppressed renin. Arch. Intern. Med. 123:366, 1969.
17. Melby, J. C., Dale, S. L., and Wilson, T. E.: 18-hydroxy-deoxycorticosterone in human hypertension. Circ. Res. 28–29(Suppl. II):143, 1971.
18. Luetscher, J. A., Weinberger, M. H., Dowdy, A. J., Nokes, G. W., Balikian, H., Brodie, A., and Willoughby, S.: Effects of sodium loading, sodium depletion and posture on plasma aldosterone concentration and renin activity in hypertensive patients. J. Clin. Endocrinol. 29:1310, 1969.
19. Williams, G. H., Rose, L. I., Dluhy, R. G., McCaughn, D., Jagger, P. I., Hickler, R. B., and Lauler, D. P.: Abnormal responsiveness of the renin aldosterone system to acute stimulation in patients with essential hypertension. Ann. Intern. Med. 72:317, 1970.
20. Streeten, D. H. P., Schletter, F. E., Clift, G. V., Stevenson, C. T., and Dalakos, T. G.: Studies of the renin-angiotensin-aldosterone system in patients with hypertension and in normal subjects. Am. J. Med. 46:844, 1969.

Adrenal Regeneration Hypertension

By Charles E. Hall, Ph.D., and O. Hall, M.Sc.

Skelton's[1] observation in 1955 that hypertensive vascular disease developed in adrenal-enucleated rats during regeneration of the gland, adrenal regeneration hypertension, was of great theoretic and practical significance. At the time, the only adrenal steroids known to cause a very similar if not identical syndrome in rats were deoxycorticosterone (DOC) and deoxycortisol. Both of these had been isolated from adrenal tissue, but the former then had uncertain status as a circulating hormone, and the latter is secreted by human, but not rat adrenals, raising doubt as to the relevance of biochemical and physiologic changes resulting from treatment with them in rats to like changes accompanying certain forms of spontaneous adrenal hyperactivity in man.

Because there seemed to be a limited number of ways in which function of the enucleate adrenal could be altered, the prospects for early resolution of the etiology of adrenal regeneration hypertension seemed bright. In retrospect, such hopes were illusory, for in 1972 the fundamental processes underlying the disorder still eluded definition. A number of structural and functional changes, that serve to distinguish normal from regenerating adrenal glands, have been described; but their relationship, if any, to the hypertensive state is obscure.

To induce the disorder, it has been customary not only to enucleate the adrenal glands, but also to employ two "sensitizing" procedures, which are the removal of one kidney and the imposition of a high-salt intake. The latter, particularly when combined with unilateral nephrectomy, also causes hypertensive vascular disease, and a high salt intake—often greater in enucleate rats than in controls—has profound effects on adrenal function. It has thus not been easy to differentiate clearly between primary physiologic changes due to adrenal enucleation and secondary changes due to the sensitizing procedures. Then, too, as with hypertension due to a high-salt intake alone,[2] treatment with deoxycorticosterone acetate (DOCA),[3] or constriction of the renal artery,[4] protracted adrenal regeneration hypertension eventually reaches a self-sustaining phase.[5] The mechanism underlying this condition is clearly different from that inductive of the disorder, and hence it is not clear that studies relating to late phases of the disease will prove helpful in unraveling the ultimate causative mechanisms.

Attempts to study factors influencing the course of adrenal regeneration hypertension, either accelerating or delaying onset, modifying severity, etc., are complicated by yet an-

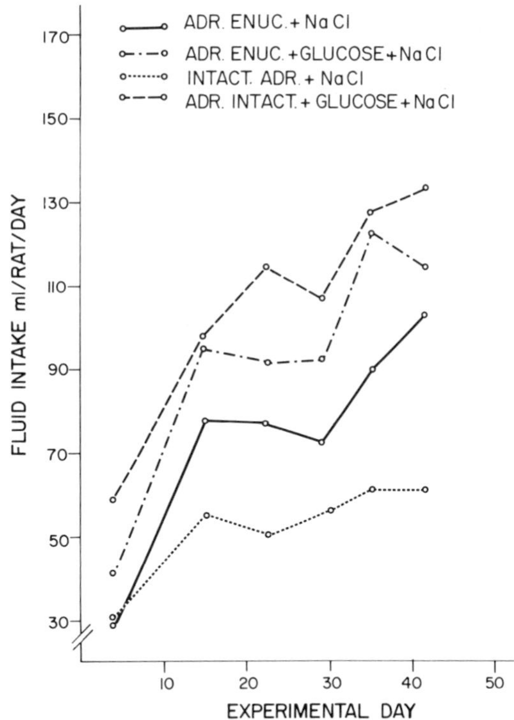

Fig. 1.—Daily fluid consumption in adrenal-enucleated and uninephrectomized control rats drinking 1% sodium chloride and 1% sodium chloride–5% glucose solutions. Note that adrenal-enucleated rats drink more saline than controls, but that both adrenal-enucleated and control rats drink more of the solution with sugar than without.

From the Department of Physiology, University of Texas Medical Branch, Galveston, Texas.

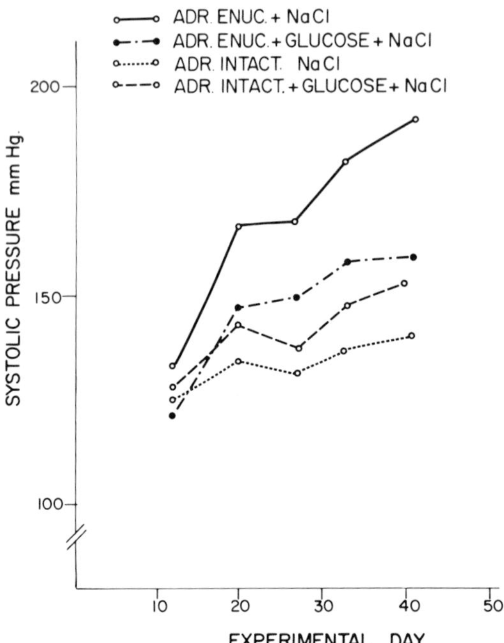

FIG. 2.—Blood pressure response of the groups shown in Fig. 1. Despite their higher level of salt intake, adrenal-enucleated rats drinking glucose saline develop hypertension significantly later and less severely than those that drank saline solution. There is, in fact, an inverse relationship between the level of salt intake and the blood pressure response in adrenal-enucleated rats.

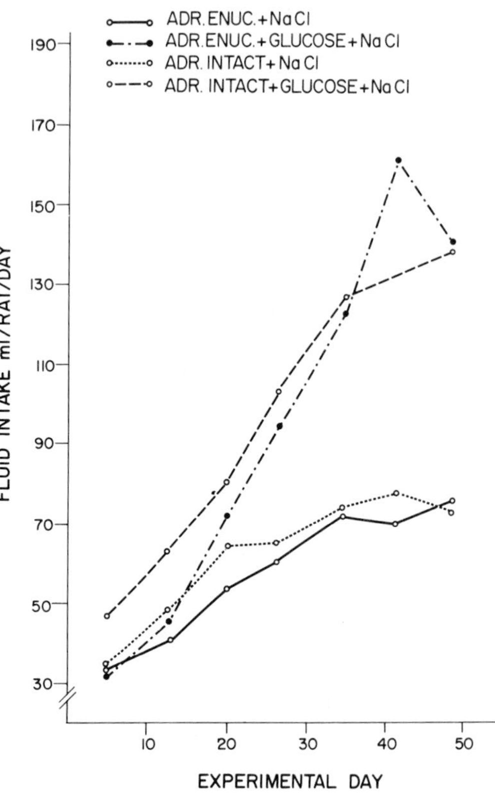

FIG. 3.—Daily fluid consumption of adrenal-enucleated and uninephrectomized control rats drinking 1% sodium chloride and 1% sodium chloride–glucose solutions. Note that adrenal-enucleated rats do not drink more saline than controls, but that both enucleated and control rats have higher consumption of sugar solution than controls. Compare with Fig. 1.

other characteristic of the disorder, namely, the variability in incidence from one experiment to another, first alluded to by Masson and Corcoran.[6] Their contention that this characteristic was unrelated to the surgical skill of the investigator or to any other easily identifiable characteristic is in accord with our experience. A typical example of such variability in response is shown in Figs. 1 through 4. Several obvious factors contribute: genetic differences in susceptibility to the induction of hypertension among the rats themselves, differences in the quantities of salt consumed and variations in the amount of adrenal tissue removed at operation, which affects both the structural repair and the functional secretory capacity of the regenerating gland. Clearly, these variables can interact, complementing or opposing one another in a given instance. Some implications of this characteristic will be presented later, but before doing so it will be necessary to define the requirements of the experimental model, for it is evident from the literature that a number of misconceptions persist.

Sensitizing Procedures and the Induction of Adrenal Regeneration Hypertension

As set forth by Skelton,[7] the experimental induction of adrenal regeneration hypertension had three indispensable requisites: (1) bilateral adrenal enucleation, or unilateral adrenal enucleation and contralateral adrenalectomy; (2) unilateral nephrectomy; and (3) a high-salt intake. The first of these is clearly the primary or inciting cause of the response, whereas the others are sensitizing procedures.

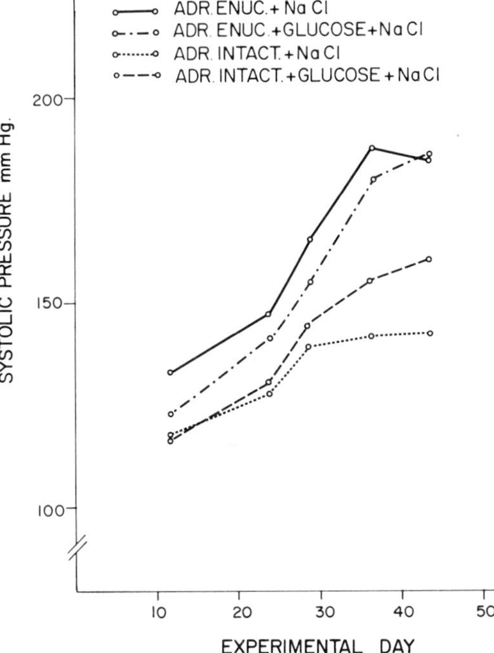

FIG. 4.—Systolic blood pressures of the groups shown in Fig. 2. Here, with a lower level of salt intake, adrenal-enucleated rats on saline developed hypertension at the same rate and with comparable severity as those on glucose–saline solution (see Fig. 3). This is unlike the response shown in Fig. 2.

There can be no doubt as to the indispensability of the first, but such seems not to be the case for the sensitizing procedures, a fact which does not appear to be widely appreciated.

The course and morphologic expression of adrenal regeneration hypertension have been compared with those of DOCA-induced hypertension, it being averred that both require a high-salt intake.[8] The fact is, however, that many forms of experimental hypertension once thought to be dependent upon provision of excess salt are now known not to be. DOCA-induced hypertension in the rat was originally produced with the aid of a high-salt intake,[9] but numerous experiments since have shown it to be dispensable.[10–12] Similarly, methylandrostenediol treatment causes hypertension in rats [13] without imposition of the salt excess, initially believed to be an essential requirement.[14,15] Adrenal regeneration hypertension is no exception. It can be induced without additional dietary salt, although it is greatly accelerated and aggravated thereby. Under conditions where the salt intake is restricted to the content of a commercial ration, adrenal-enucleated rats may take weeks or months to develop hypertension, which usually then follows a relatively benign course causing cardiac hypertrophy but few vascular lesions.[16] Its occurrence, nonetheless, points to the presence of a physiologic disturbance mediated by an abnormal adrenal function. When the diet itself contains relatively large but not unphysiologic quantities of sodium chloride (1.9%), adrenal-enucleated rats given tap water still develop hypertension more rapidly than controls, although it is further exacerbated by increasing salt intake.[17] At very high levels of salt intake, controls develop hypertension so rapidly and severely that adrenal regeneration is incapable of enhancing the process.[18] The fact that adrenal regeneration hypertension can develop without salt excess doubtless has etiologic and pathogenetic significance, but apparently the fact is not yet widely recognized, since a recent article [19] states that "aldosterone production by the regenerating adrenal is less than normal, particularly under the high-sodium intake conditions necessary for development of adrenal regeneration hypertension." Since a high-sodium intake is not essential, it would seem to be preferable to examine the function of enucleated adrenals in situ, under conditions free from the inhibitory influence of sodium chloride excess upon adrenal mineralocorticoid secretion.

What of the alleged requirement of unilateral nephrectomy for the induction of adrenal regeneration hypertension? [7,8,20] It seemed curious that such a requirement should be peculiar to this experimental form of hypertension, since such is certainly not the case for hypertension induced by either salt excess [11,21] or deoxycorticosterone [10–12] treatment, the forms with which adrenal regeneration hypertension seems to be most closely related, even though in both instances hypertension is exacerbated by kidney removal.

Hence, it seemed probable that if the sensitizing sodium load were sufficiently high, higher than is normally afforded by the provision of a 1% saline drinking solution, the greater resistance of rats with intact kidneys to the development of adrenal regeneration hypertension might be overcome. The addition of 5% sucrose to such a saline drinking solution increased consumption two- or threefold in both controls and in adrenal-enucleated rats with intact kidneys. Under these circumstances the latter developed hypertension with greater alacrity and more severely than the former,[22] indicating that regenerating adrenal glands had the effect which is restricted to unilaterally nephrectomized rats at the lesser level of salt consumption prevailing when only 1% saline is given to drink.

The Role of Postoperative Adrenal Insufficiency

Early estimations of the steroid secretory capacity of regenerating adrenal glands, a matter to which we shall return later, indicated subnormal secretion of both aldosterone and corticosterone.[23,24] There being no obvious way of implicating adrenal insufficiency in the hypertensive syndrome which developed in rats bearing such glands, ingenuity was strained in an effort to discern a rational relationship. It could be supposed that although the known hormones were released in lesser quantities, some unidentified and unusual steroid was being elaborated. No evidence for such an occurrence was forthcoming. There was the possibility that the mineralocorticoid:glucocorticoid ratio was elevated, presumably by an increased secretion of mineralocorticoids. Such an alteration might conceivably account for adrenal regeneration hypertension which, like mineralocorticoid but unlike glucocorticoid [25] hypertension, is facilitated by a high-salt intake. A major appeal of implicating an altered ratio of mineralocorticoids to glucocorticoids in the genesis of adrenal regeneration hypertension lay in the fact that during the period of adrenal regeneration there is an overall relative adrenal insufficiency and that such a state in dogs [26] and in patients with Addison's disease [27] sensitizes to the hypertensive effects of DOCA. However, the same is not true of rats. Tobian and Perry [28] found that there was no difference between adrenalectomized and intact rats given an equivalent but very large dose of DOCA insofar as the ultimate incidence and severity of hypertension were concerned. Using graded doses of this hormone, we have shown that the blood pressure response of adrenalectomized rats to both low and high dosages is substantially below that of similarly treated intact rats [29]: they are thus hyporeactive rather than hyperreactive. However, it must be conceded that the absolute adrenal insufficiency of adrenalectomized animals is qualitatively and quantitatively different from the relative insufficiency present during adrenal regeneration and usually in Addison's disease. It is possible that small levels of corticosterone, comparable to those present during the regenerative process, would alter the responsiveness to DOCA, but the presently available data (see below) do not lend attractiveness to the theory that adrenal insufficiency sensitizes adrenal-enucleated rats to the hypertensive effects of their own low hormone levels.

Another suggestion was that during the

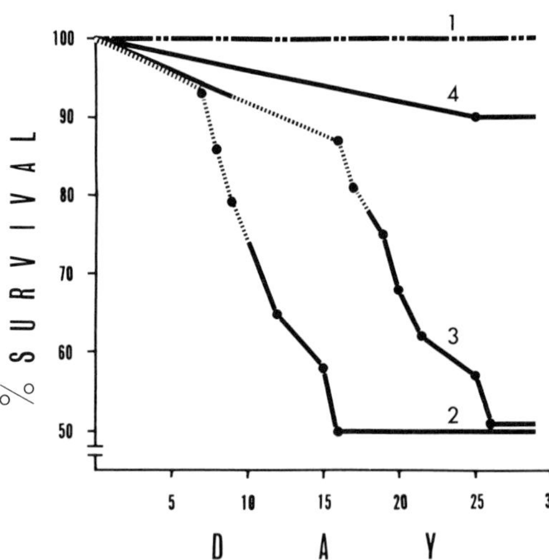

Fig. 5.—Mortality in adrenal-enucleated and control rats: **(1)** 14 untreated adrenal-enucleated rats; **(2)** 16 adrenal-enucleated rats given DOCA and cortisone in declining quantities for the first 10 postoperative days; **(3)** 14 adrenal-enucleated rats given the preceding treatment for 10 days after allowing a week of postoperative adrenal insufficiency; **(4)** 10 controls subjected to right nephroadrenalectomy. The period of hormone treatment is indicated by **cross-hatching** on the respective slopes of groups 2 and 3. Toxicity of the hormone treatment is indicated by the fact that deaths begin to occur in both groups in the first week of treatment and run closely parallel thereafter.

period of adrenal insufficiency the vascular system became "sensitized" to adrenal corticoids; this was first suggested by Grollman [30] and adopted for a time as a working hypothesis by other investigators.[6,8] This seemed to be worthy of examination. A repetition of Grollman's experiment, in which postenucleation adrenal insufficiency was obviated by giving 1 mg per day each of cortisone and deoxycorticosterone on the day of operation, and reducing that dosage by 10 percent each day thereafter, produced a high mortality (Fig. 5) and an aggravated hypertensive response in survivors (Fig. 6) as compared with those in untreated enucleated rats.

A second study was then conducted using the principal adrenal steroid of rat adrenals, corticosterone. Given continuously at a dosage of 1 mg per day, it inhibited adrenal regeneration and prevented adrenal regeneration hypertension; given at a dosage of 1 mg on the day of operation and reduced by 10 percent of that dosage each day for 10 days so as to prevent postoperative adrenal insufficiency, corticosterone did not affect the degree of regeneration and caused a more rapid onset and a severer hypertension than occurred in untreated enucleated rats. Given according to the preceding regimen, but begun on the eighth postoperative day after a period of adrenal insufficiency had occurred, it did not affect the degree of adrenal regeneration nor the manner in which hypertension evolved (Fig. 7). (Further details have been published elsewhere.[31]) It has also been demonstrated that 2 weeks of adrenal insufficiency does not sensitize rats to hypertension caused by corticosterone treatment.[32] Needless to say, these experiments do not support the notion that adrenal insufficiency contributes to the development of adrenal regeneration hypertension.

The Functional Disturbance in Regenerating Rat Adrenals

Because DOCA treatment causes hypertension, because the enucleated adrenal regener-

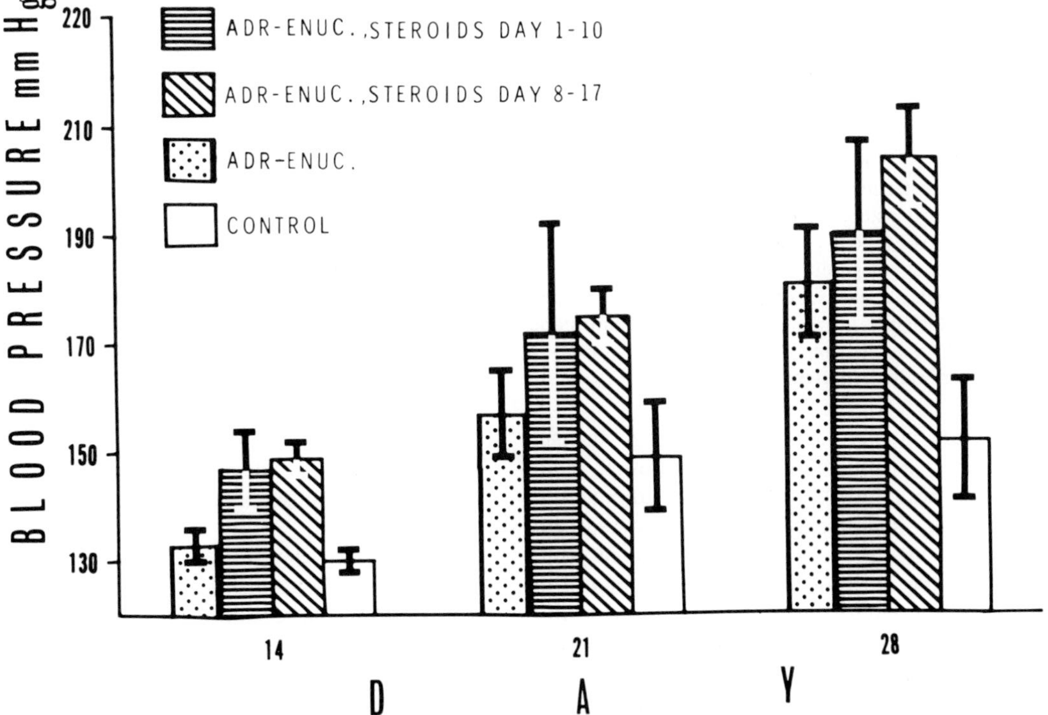

Fig. 6.—Blood pressure response in untreated and hormonally supported adrenal-enucleated rats and their controls. Note that in both groups of hormone-treated rats the blood pressures are somewhat higher than in untreated enucleates and that there is no evidence that hypertension is prevented by such treatment.

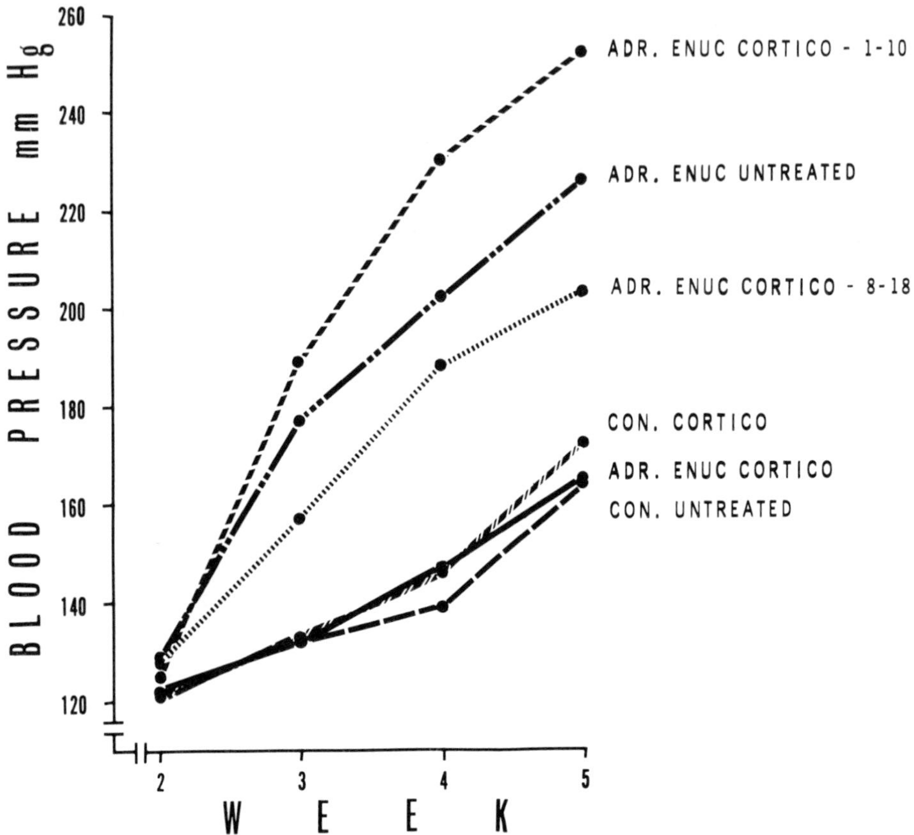

FIG. 7.—Blood pressure response in (1) untreated controls; (2) controls given 1 mg of corticosterone daily; (3) untreated adrenal-enucleated rats; (4) enucleated rats given 1 mg of corticosterone per day; (5) enucleated rats given declining doses of corticosterone for the first 10 postoperative days; (6) enucleated rats given the preceding course of corticosterone treatment beginning on the eighth day after a week of adrenal insufficiency. There are nine animals to each group. Note that the hypertensive response is augmented if acute adrenal insufficiency is prevented but not if hormone treatment is delayed for a week. Continuous corticosterone treatment prevents the early adrenal regeneration hypertension, but not the later "salt" hypertension.

ates from glomerulosa cells, known to be the source of a mineralocorticoid secretion, and because both DOCA-induced and adrenal regeneration hypertension are potentiated by high-salt intake, it was early assumed that regenerating adrenals must secrete something, probably a mineralocorticoid, of crucial importance to the genesis of adrenal regeneration hypertension, despite the overwhelming evidence that the overall secretory activity of enucleate adrenals is depressed, that no unusual steroid is elaborated and that the mineralocorticoid:glucocorticoid ratio is not significantly changed. Nevertheless, there is impressive evidence implicating some type of adrenocortical hyperactivity, although of obscure nature, in the genesis of adrenal regeneration hypertension.

If regenerating glands are removed prior to onset of the self-sustaining phase of adrenal regeneration hypertension, hypertension is "cured."[5] Manipulation of the regenerative process itself has yielded varying results. Adrenal regeneration hypertension is completely prevented although regeneration is incompletely inhibited by thyroparathyroidectomy.[33] Hypophysectomy prevents both occurrences.[34] Interference with adrenal regeneration by injecting steroids has also yielded equivocal results. Cortisol blocks regeneration but not hypertension [35]; however, this steroid can itself cause hypertension,[36] creating interpretive difficulties. Both adrenal regeneration and its hypertension can be prevented when steroids are used which do not themselves cause hypertension [33] or are given in dosages that do not do so.[37] A low dosage of corticosterone typically has that effect, but in this instance ACTH at dosages which fail to repair adrenal atrophy completely restores hypertension.[38] Transplantation of regenerating adrenals to ectopic sites supports adrenal regeneration hypertension to varying degrees depending upon how well the transplants thrive, but transplants to the intestinal mesentery are inadequate, presumably because the hepatic portal drainage of that locus ensures increased inactivation of some essential adrenal hormone by the liver.[39] Pharmacologic agents which depress adrenal function or antagonize aldosterone activity will also inhibit the development of adrenal regeneration hypertension,[40–42] tending to support an important role of aldosterone and related corticoids, despite the fact that the circulating level of these hormones is subnormal in rats with regenerating adrenals. Perhaps aldosterone plays a permissive or supporting role in this form of hypertension, maybe the pharmacologic agents are active not because of their effects on aldosterone but because they have similar effects vis-à-vis another but unidentified hormone that acts like aldosterone, or perchance they have direct antihypertensive effects in addition to their interference with adrenal hormone secretion or action.

Recently it has been reported that a single intravenous injection of 0.3 ml of an antiserum made against the blood of rats with adrenal regeneration hypertension will lower blood pressure of recipient rats with that disorder and cause a concomitant involution of the adrenal zona glomerulosa.[43] Unfortunately, the effect of an antiserum against the blood of normal rats was not tested, and the nature of the antigen is unknown. The results, if confirmed, would be compatible with either an antiadrenal or an antiangiotensin antibody.

Chronic treatment with hydrochlorothiazide will also inhibit the development of adrenal regeneration hypertension or reverse an established hypertension.[8,44] However, there is a tendency for an escape from such suppression despite continued treatment with the natriuretic, leading to a late-onset hypertension.[45] The suppressive effect cannot be attributed solely to natriuresis, since a similar action is exhibited by diazoxide, which causes sodium retention.[46] However, caution is indicated in evaluating the significance of sodium excretion or even serum sodium concentrations: the possibility of occult sodium retention or even an altered sodium distribution in the face of a normal plasma sodium concentration must be recognized. Friedman and Friedman [47,48] have provided persuasive evidence that vascular reactivity is profoundly influenced by the intracellular:extracellular sodium ratio, which might well fluctuate independently of absolute serum levels.

Adrenocortical Enzymatic and Secretory Changes in Regenerating Adrenal Glands

The subnormal level of adrenocortical hormone secretion by enucleate adrenals, alluded to earlier, was subsequently confirmed by both indirect [49] and direct studies.[50–52] Investigators, however, displayed a commendable unwillingness to allow such negative support for the conviction that some form of adrenal hypersecretion caused adrenal regeneration hypertension, to deter them from attempts to determine its nature. For the most part, this has involved studies of enzyme concentrations, substrate dependence, and an analysis of the types and quantities of hormones actually elaborated by adrenal fragments or homogenates studied in vitro. These studies have indicated differences in the secretory profile of regenerating from that of normal adrenal glands. There are discrepancies in the results obtained by different laboratories and differences of opinion as to the significance of various findings in the etiology of adrenal regeneration hypertension.

Brownell et al.[53] found that regenerating adrenal glands were superior to normal adrenal glands in their capacity to synthesize 17-α-hydroxylated steroids from a progesterone substrate, in particular 17-OH-progesterone and 11-desoxy-17-hydroxycorticosterone. The latter has hypertensogenic activity in rats.[54] However, La Plante, Giroud, and Stachenko,[55] using the same substrate, could not detect the formation of either 17-hydroxylated or 11-deoxysteroids, but when 17-α-hydroxyprogesterone was used as a substrate, incubated regenerating adrenals readily synthesized cortisol, cortisone, and 11-deoxycortisol. They suggested that regenerating adrenals had inadequate 17-α-hydroxylase activity. There were certain differences in the models used by the two groups of investigators. The first used the glands from Wistar rats with known adrenal regeneration hypertension, whereas the second used the adrenals from Long-Evans rats in which, although the conditions essential to the development of adrenal regeneration hypertension had been established in some cases, the blood pressures were not measured and the glands were excised 2 weeks postoperatively, which is rather early for the development of this form of hypertension.

Vecsei et al.[56] found an impairment in the ability of regenerating adrenal glands to synthesize 18-hydroxycorticosterone (18-OHB) and aldosterone, but an increased ability to synthesize 18-hydroxy-deoxycorticosterone (18-OH-DOC) and corticosterone. Later Birmingham et al.[57,58] reported that fragments from enucleated adrenals synthesized larger quantities of 18-OH-DOC than normal glands. These studies also indicated that 18-OH-DOC had appreciable sodium-retaining activity without causing potassium excretion, although the small quantities available precluded an evaluation of its hemodynamic properties.[58] Furthermore, both before [59] and after [60] the development of hypertension, regenerating adrenal glands displayed enhanced ability to transform progesterone into 18-OH-DOC, corticosterone, and 11-dehydrocorticosterone, but impaired ability to synthesize aldosterone and 18-OH-OHB.

These studies have led to the presumption that 18-OH-DOC might be the steroid responsible for adrenal regeneration hypertension, but the pertinence of the biochemical findings to the hypertensive state has been rendered somewhat academic, if not null and void, by the recent finding that the systemic blood of rats with that disorder contains less rather than more 18-OH-DOC than blood of normal animals.[61] That investigator has also considered in detail the many factors preventing the adrenal gland from carrying out those functions under in vitro conditions which it does eminently well in vivo. Such differences may well account for the fact that, with regard to 18-OH-DOC at least, the results obtained with the two methods are diametrically opposed.

In fact, even the results obtained with in vitro systems have not been compatible with each other. Brownie and Skelton,[62] using an adrenal homogenate system, found that in contrast to the behavior of normal glands, regenerating adrenals converted progesterone preferentially to DOC at the expense of corticosterone, aldosterone, and 18-OH-DOC, indicating impaired 11-β-hydroxylation, and suggested that increased DOC secretion might account for adrenal regeneration hypertension. Rapp,[63] however, found that, when analyzed by a bioassay depending upon a response in the urinary sodium:potassium ratio, venous effluent blood from regenerating adrenals had less mineralocorticoid activity than that from intact glands, regardless of whether the animals were maintained on saline or water, and could find no evidence for the secretion of an unusual steroid, an abnormal ratio of steroids, or a high mineralocorticoid production relative to sodium intake. In a later study,[64] however, when the actual concentration of DOC in the adrenal venous blood was measured, it was discovered that the concentration in adrenal vein or in peripheral blood was substantially greater in rats with regenerating adrenals than in such blood from intact rats, being increased about fourfold above normal. The results were interpreted as implicating DOC in the genesis of adrenal regeneration hypertension.

Recently another group of investigators has partially confirmed these findings by reporting a several-fold increase above normal in the plasma levels of DOC in rats with regenerating adrenal glands, three weeks postoperatively.[65,66] At that time the hypertension was equally severe but plasma DOC levels were far higher in enucleate rats than in adrenalectomized rats bearing 50-mg DOCA implants, lending credence to DOC as the etiologic agent underlying adrenal regeneration hypertension. Thereafter, the plasma DOC levels fell progressively, reaching normal values at the seventh week, although the blood pressure continued to rise, and at the sixth week plasma 18-OH-DOC levels were greatly increased. The secretory rate of DOC, 18-OH-DOC, aldosterone and corticosterone, as determined in adrenal vein blood, fell precipitously immediately following adrenal enucleation and remained depressed during the period that hypertension was developing.[65,67] These data are in apparent conflict with Rapp's findings regarding the secretory rate of DOC, and it is difficult to reconcile such a diminished rate with a greatly increased plasma concentration, unless one supposes a reduced metabolic turnover.

The known hypertensogenic properties of DOC render the reported augmented level in the plasma of rats with regenerating adrenal glands highly suspect in the causation of adrenal regeneration hypertension. However, there are still a few problems that require resolution before that view can be wholeheartedly adopted.

Rats with DOC-induced hypertension develop hypokalemia, with or sometimes without an associated hypernatremia, whereas a distortion of plasma electrolytes is not typically present in adrenal regeneration hypertension.[63] Rapp [63] has suggested that this particular effect might be characteristic of pharmacologic doses of DOCA. However, it seems reasonable to hold that the fourfold increase of plasma DOC in rats with adrenal regeneration hypertension is a pharmacologic quantity; certainly, it is hypernormal and not to be considered as physiologic if it causes hypertension. It is also difficult to understand why, if both hypertension models are due to DOC excess, it is so easy to cause hypertension in rats having both kidneys by injecting DOCA and giving 1% saline to drink, but impossible to induce adrenal regeneration hypertension under these conditions. Furthermore, DOCA-treated rats given saline to drink invariably exhibit a marked polydipsia, one of the most characteristic and prominent responses of experimental rats under such circumstances, usually involving a two- or threefold increase in volume consumption.[11,12] Such is not the case following adrenal enucleation: in some experiments a saline polydipsia does occur,[18,68] but it is not as great as the increase caused by injected hormone given at a dosage causing hypertension to develop at the same rate and intensity as that which ensues following adrenal enucleation. In other experiments, even by the same groups of investigators, adrenal-enucleated rats have consumed less saline than controls,[1,69,70] though hypertension in them was facilitated nonetheless.

At dosage levels where it fails to cause hypertension, DOCA fails also to cause polydipsia and vice versa.[29] This being so, it is hard to understand why, if adrenal regeneration hypertension is due to DOC hypersecretion, endogenously secreted and exogenously administered hormones do not exert the same effect on salt intake.

We have added sugars such as sucrose or glucose, for which rats exhibit a fondness, to saline drinking solution in order to increase the rate of consumption, thereby hastening the onset of salt hypertension.[71] When this is done with adrenal-enucleated rats, they invariably behave exactly like controls in respect to their pattern of consumption, drinking two to three times as much of this solution as of ordinary saline.[22] Hypertension is accelerated and enhanced in the latter, but not in the former, supporting the inference that the presence of a regenerating adrenal gland so sensitizes rats to the effect of salt that a maximal response occurs at the lower level of intake.[18]

Under the same experimental circumstances DOCA-treated [11] and aldosterone-treated rats [72] behave identically, but quite unlike adrenal-enucleated rats, in that they do not consume more sucrose-saline solution than saline. Apparently the steroids augment saline consumption to about the same degree as does the addition of sucrose to the drinking solution, but the two influences are not additive. The fact that DOCA-treated rats behave quite differently from adrenal-enucleated rats under these experimental circumstances further elides the notion that excess DOCA secretion is responsible for adrenal regeneration hypertension. Finally, it must be recalled not only that the quantities of DOC reported to occur in the plasma of rats with this type of hypertension have not been shown capable of causing hypertension, but also that there is in such rats a concomitant decrease in the circulatory levels of aldosterone which, at certain dosages at least, has an even greater hypertensogenic effect than DOCA.[73] It is of crucial importance that the first of these be answered; the second is of less importance since the same depression of aldosterone secretion occurs when DOCA is administered to normal rats so as to cause hypertension.[52] However, in that circumstance we know that hypertension is caused by DOCA, and the quantities given are usually very large.

At present the evidence supporting a relationship between the hypertension in rats with enucleate adrenals and the level of DOC secretion by the glands is at best exiguous. It is, however, even if flawed, an attractive possibility deserving of every consideration and piercing scrutiny.

Another line of evidence suggesting some form of unusual secretion in enucleated adrenal glands has been provided by Gaunt et al.[74–76] They have reported that between 1 and 4 days following adrenal enucleation the rats are unable to handle a light sodium load normally, retaining more sodium than either control or adrenalectomized rats. The effect of enucleation can be partially reproduced in adrenalectomized rats by small doses of aldosterone, and could be inhibited by corticosterone, spironolactone or hydrochlorothiazide (compare with adrenal regeneration hypertension).[71] It can also be abolished by hypophysectomy and restored by ACTH treatment.[75] The greater retention of a sodium load could not be blocked by aminoglutethimide, metyrapone, or the heparinoid, Ro 1-8307.[75] These studies have been reviewed[77] and the findings have been construed as suggesting that the adrenal gland soon after enucleation acquires the capacity to secrete some physiologically active but perhaps unusual steroid, or combination of steroids. A relationship to the development of adrenal regeneration hypertension has been proposed, although it is difficult, considering the rather short duration of the sodium-retaining effect, to implicate it in the hypertensive response which occurs much later. There is always the possibility that some other irreversible effect occurs during this period, which later causes hypertension. But any attempt to harmonize two events so widely separated in time as the early sodium-retaining aberration and the later hypertension, must necessarily strain somewhat to establish a relationship which intrinsically is obscure.

Conclusions and Speculations

Whole-animal studies have almost uniformly indicated that enucleated adrenals are hypofunctional. Rapp's discovery of a high DOC output constitutes the only major exception, but its significance as regards the etiology of adrenal regeneration hypertension is obscured by the report from the same group that the blood of animals with this form of hypertension does not contain a higher level of mineralocorticoid activity. That would suggest that a high DOC output merely compensates for the reduced level of aldosterone secretion.

Studies of in vitro adrenal systems indicate that the enucleated adrenal functions abnormally prior to development and during the course of adrenal regeneration hypertension. It is always well to have objective evidence, but otherwise such findings merely support what could already be inferred from the fact that adrenal enucleation causes hypertension. The findings in homogenate systems are in accord with the whole-animal experiments, but at variance with the adrenal fragment studies, in suggesting that enucleated adrenals secrete excessive DOC, but, as indicated above, that fact, however attractive from a theoretic point of view, cannot as yet be wholeheartedly adopted as explaining the etiology of adrenal regeneration hypertension.

One of the unsolved mysteries is why the disorder should be restricted to rats. We considered the possibility that only animals having adrenal glands that secrete corticosterone as the principal steroid might develop this form of hypertension. Attempts, however, to induce the disease in mice have been unsuccessful (unpublished observations); and the rabbit, which does not become hypertensive even when treated with DOCA, did not seem to be a suitable test animal.

Thus far, investigators have considered generalized hypersecretion, an abnormal ratio of steroids, the secretion of an unusual steroid, and the possible sensitizing influence of the initial period of postenucleation adrenal insufficiency as being causative of adrenal regeneration hypertension. The first and last are no longer in serious contention and the other two are in dispute. There remains an unexplored alternative which, because of preoccupation with quantitative and qualitative aspects of hormone secretion, does not appear to have been given serious consideration, i.e., that an altered rhythmicity of hormone secretion may be basic to the disorder.

Characteristically, the normal adrenal gland functions cyclically in circadian rhythm. It is questionable whether under such circumstances a concept such as the mean level of hormonal secretion has any real physiologic meaning or significance, but if it does, then it may be said that the body is exposed to higher than "normal" quantities at one time and less than this at other times. Perhaps it would be better to say that in all cases the level of secretion is appropriate to the concurrent physiologic requirements. In any event, the electrolyte shifts and other changes which take place in various tissues and organs under the impact of high levels of circulating hormone are presumably later reversed, or are potentially reversible, when lower amounts are present.

When steroid hormones are administered for the purpose of causing hypertension, they are given as depot material or injected frequently so as to attain a continuous excess level: this is either not rhythmically altered, or oscillates between levels that are higher than normal. This same characteristic also obtains in hypertensive patients with adrenocortical tumors,[73] who also fail to exhibit circadian rhythm. That abnormal temporal relationships of adrenal secretion might be importantly contributory to the development of adrenal regeneration hypertension is suggested by the finding that enucleate adrenals differ from normal glands, at least under in vitro conditions, in their much greater capacity for sustained hormone synthesis under ACTH stimulation.[58] Adrenal enucleation is a procedure certain to stimulate a continuous high level of ACTH output, at least over the period in which hypertension develops, and to disrupt therefore the normal circadian pattern of ACTH and adrenocortical hormone secretion.

The type of hypertensive syndrome in enucleated rats and the experimental studies implicating DOC in its development both suggest a dysfunction of mineralocorticoid secretion. For this reason it would be instructive to learn whether slices from enucleate glands differ from normal glands in their responsiveness to angiotensin stimulation even though DOC secretion seems to be under ACTH control. It would appear that the basal level of aldosterone secretion by regenerating adrenals is lower than normal, but then so is the basal level of corticosterone secretion. If the latter can be secreted for a longer time by enucleated glands in response to ACTH than it can by normal glands, what about the output of mineralocorticoid in response to angiotensin II? It is tempting to speculate that enucleation of the adrenal gland elicits hypersecretion of ACTH in response to the reduced level of corticosterone, and of angiotensin II in response to reduced aldosterone levels, and that at the same time the normal circadian rhythm of the hypothalamico-hypophyseal-adrenal axis is altered. This would cause the adrenal gland to secrete as best it can with the number of cellular units and under the physiologic and biochemical circumstances that prevail. Possibly the abnormal blood supply and other changes so alter the availability of substrates, enzymes, co-factors and the like, that the gland is unable to synthesize corticosterone and aldosterone optimally, with the result that a precursor of both, 11-deoxycorticosterone, is produced in excess, and in a continuous rather than rhythmic fashion.

References

1. Skelton, F. R.: Development of hypertension and cardiovascular renal lesions during adrenal regeneration. Proc. Soc. Exp. Biol. Med. 90:342, 1955.
2. Dahl, L. K.: Effects of chronic excess salt feeding. Induction of self-sustaining hypertension in rats. J. Exp. Med. 114:231, 1961.
3. Friedman, S. M., Friedman, C. L., and Nakashima, M.: II. Sustained hypertension following the administration of desoxycorticosterone acetate. J. Exp. Med. 93:361, 1951.
4. Wilson, C., and Byrom, F. B.: The vicious circle in chronic Bright's disease. Experimental evidence from the hypertensive rat. Q. Med. Rev. 10:65, 1941.
5. Skelton, F. R.: A study of the natural history of adrenal regeneration hypertension. Circ. Res. 7:107, 1959.
6. Masson, G. M. C., and Corcoran, A. C.: Hormonal influence on adrenal regeneration hypertension. Arch. Int. Pharmacodyn. Ther. 114:322, 1958.

7. Skelton, F. R.: Adrenal regeneration and adrenal regeneration hypertension. Physiol. Rev. 39:162, 1959.
8. Gaunt, R., Gross, F., Renzi, A. A., and Chart, J. J.: The adrenal cortex in hypertension (with particular reference to adrenal regeneration hypertension). *In* J. H. Moyer (Ed.): Hypertension. Philadelphia: Saunders, 1959, p. 219.
9. Selye, H., Hall, C. E., and Rowley, E. M.: Malignant hypertension produced with desoxycorticosterone and sodium chloride. Can. Med. Assoc. J. 49:88, 1943.
10. Eades, C. H., Jr., Phillips, G. E., Blaustein, A., Hsu, I. C., and Solberg, V. B.: Coronary atherosclerosis. II. Contrast of DOCA hypertension with renal hypertension in the etiology of coronary atherosclerosis in the adult male Wistar rat. Angiologica 2:61, 1965.
11. Hall, C. E., and Hall, O.: Hypertension and hypersalimentation. II. Deoxycorticosterone hypertension. Lab. Invest. 14:1727, 1965.
12. Hall, C. E., and Hall, O.: Interaction between desoxycorticosterone treatment, fluid intake, sodium consumption, blood pressure, and organ changes in rats drinking water, saline, or sucrose solution. Can. J. Physiol. Pharmacol. 47:81, 1969.
13. Hall, C. E., and Hall, O.: Methylandrostenediol hypertension induced without salt excess, with observations on organ changes and serum composition. Am. J. Pathol. 54:489, 1969.
14. Skelton, F. R.: The production of hypertension, nephrosclerosis and cardiac lesions by methylandrostenediol treatment in the rat. Endocrinology 53:492, 1953.
15. Salgado, E., and Selye, H.: Hormonal factors in the production of experimental renal and cardiovascular disease (synergism between somatotrophic hormone and methylandrostenediol). J. Lab. Clin. Med. 45:237, 1955.
16. Hall, C. E., Holland, O. B., and Hall, O.: Benign and malignant hypertension following adrenal enucleation in the rat. Relationship to salt intake, response to hydrochlorothiazide and similarity to essential hypertension. J. Exp. Med. 126:35, 1967.
17. Rapp, J. R.: Electrolyte and juxtaglomerular changes in adrenal regeneration hypertension. Am. J. Physiol. 206:93, 1964.
18. Oelsner, T., and Skelton, F. R.: Complementary role of adrenal cortex and salt in adrenal-regeneration hypertension. Am. J. Physiol. 200:759, 1961.
19. Skelton, F. R., and Brownie, A. C.: Structure-function studies of the regenerating adrenal. Trans. N.Y. Acad. Sci. Series II, 31: 251, 1969.
20. Skelton, F. R.: Adrenal-regeneration hypertension and factors influencing its development. Arch. Intern. Med. 98:449, 1956.
21. Koletsky, S.: Role of salt and renal mass in experimental hypertension. Arch. Pathol. 68:11, 1959.
22. Hall, C. E., and Hall, O.: Augmented salt ingestion and its effect upon salt hypertension and adrenal-regeneration hypertension. Lab. Invest. 13:1471, 1964.
23. Masson, G. M. C., Koritz, S. B., and Peron, F. G.: Corticosteroid formation in regenerating rat adrenals. Endocrinology 62:229, 1958.
24. Brogi, M. P., and Pellegrino, C.: The secretion of corticosterone and aldosterone by the rat adrenal cortex regenerating after enucleation. J. Physiol. (London) 146:165, 1959.
25. Knowlton, A. I., Loeb, E. N., Stoerck, H. C., White, J. P., and Heffernan, J. F.: Induction of arterial hypertension in normal and adrenalectomized rats given cortisone acetate. J. Exp. Med. 96:187, 1952.
26. Swingle, W. E., Parkins, W. M., and Remington, J. W.: The effect of desoxycorticosterone acetate and of blood serum transfusions upon the circulation of the adrenalectomized dog. Am. J. Physiol. 134:503, 1941.
27. Soffer, L. J.: Diseases of the adrenals. Philadelphia: Lea & Febiger, 1948, p. 163.
28. Tobian, L., and Perry, S.: Effect of adrenal tissue on desoxycorticosterone hypertension. Am. J. Physiol. 134:503, 1941.
29. Hall, C. E., and Ayachi, S.: Dose-effect relationship in desoxycorticosterone hypertension: reduced sensitivity in adrenalectomized rats and its possible significance to the etiology of adrenal-regeneration hypertension. Can. J. Physiol. Pharmacol. 49:139, 1971.
30. Grollman, A.: The pathogenesis of "adrenal-regeneration hypertension." Endocrinology 63:460, 1958.
31. Hall, C. E., Holland, O. B., and Hall, O.: High blood pressure in rats protected against acute post-enucleation adrenal insufficiency and its bearing upon the etiology of adrenal-regeneration hypertension. *In* G. Jasmin (Ed.): Endocrine Aspects of Disease Processes. St. Louis, Mo.: Green, 1968, p. 302.
32. Skelton, F. R.: Increased sensitivity to corticosterone as a possible factor in the develop-

ment of adrenal regeneration hypertension. Circ. Res. 8:772, 1960.

33. Skelton, F. R., Guillebeau, J., and Nichols, J.: Hormonal modification of adrenal regeneration hypertension. Lab. Invest. 10:647, 1961.
34. Skelton, F. R.: Adrenal-regeneration hypertension and factors influencing its development. Arch. Intern. Med. 98:449, 1956.
35. Chart, J. J., Ulsamer, G. M., Quinn, L., Howie, N., Sullivan, B., and Gaunt, R.: Adrenal regeneration hypertension. Endocrinology 61:692, 1957.
36. Friedman, S. M., Friedman, C. L., and Nakashima, M.: The hypertensive effect of Compound F acetate (17-OH-corticosterone-21-acetate) in the rat. Endocrinology 51:401, 1952.
37. Skelton, F. R.: Production and inhibition of hypertensive disease in the rat by corticosterone. Endocrinology 62:365, 1958.
38. Hall, C. E., and Hall, O.: Restoration of adrenal-regeneration hypertension in corticosterone-blocked rats by ACTH. Can. J. Physiol. Pharmacol. 46:837, 1968.
39. Chart, J. J., Ulsamer, G. M., Quinn, L., and Gaunt, R.: Effects of transplantation of regenerating adrenals on adrenal regeneration hypertension. Fed. Proc. 17:25, 1958.
40. Rapp, J. R.: Effect of an aldosterone blocker on electrolyte and juxtaglomerular granularity in adrenal regeneration hypertension. Endocrinology 75:326, 1964.
41. Chappel, C. I., Charest, M. P., Cahill, J., and Grant, G. A.: Reversal of adrenal-regeneration hypertension by amphenone. Endocrinology 60:677, 1957.
42. Sturtevant, F. M.: Prevention of adrenal regeneration hypertension by an aldosterone blocker. Endocrinology 64:299, 1959.
43. Choi, J. H.: The effects of antihypertensive serum in rats with adrenal regeneration hypertension. Can. Med. Assoc. J. 102:283, 1970.
44. Hall, C. E., Holland, O. B., and Hall, O.: Prevention and reversal of adrenal regeneration hypertension with hydrochlorothiazide. Tex. Rep. Biol. Med. 24:73, 1966.
45. Hall, C. E., Holland, O. B., and Hall, O.: Evolution of adrenal-regeneration hypertension in rats with actively regenerating or fully regenerated glands. Lab. Invest. 16:488, 1967.
46. Hall, C. E., Holland, O. B., and Hall, O.: Acute and chronic influence of diazoxide on adrenal-regeneration hypertension. Can. J. Physiol. Pharmacol. 45:491, 1967.
47. Friedman, S. M.: The relation of cations to peripheral vascular resistance. Trans. Roy. Soc. Canad. 56:161, 1962.
48. Friedman, S. M., and Friedman, C. L.: Tonic basis of vascular response to vasoactive substances. Can. Med. Assoc. J. 90:167, 1964.
49. Skelton, F. A., and Hyde, P. M.: Functional response of regenerating adrenal glands to stress. Proc. Soc. Exp. Biol. Med. 106:142, 1961.
50. Fortier, C., and de Groot, J.: Adenohypophysial corticotrophin and plasma free corticosteroids during regeneration of the enucleated rat adrenal gland. Am. J. Physiol. 196:589, 1959.
51. Morimoto, S.: Studies on the pathogenesis of adrenal regeneration in the rat. Folia Endocrinol. Jap. 38:52, 1962.
52. Sheppard, H., Mowles, T. F., Chart, J. J., Renzi, A. A., and Howie, N.: Steroid biosynthesis by rat adrenal during development of adrenal-regeneration and desoxycorticosterone-induced hypertension. Endocrinology 74:762, 1964.
53. Brownell, K. A., Lee, S. L., Beck, R. R., and Besch, P. K.: In vitro 17-α-hydroxylation of steroids by the adrenals of hypertensive rats. Endocrinology 72:167, 1963.
54. Hall, C. E., Hall, O., and McCleskey, O.: A study of the comparative activities of desoxycorticosterone and Reichstein's Compound S. Acta Endocrinol. (Kbh) 9:199, 1952.
55. La Plante, C., Giroud, C. J. P., and Stachenko, J.: Lack of appreciable 17-α-hydroxylase activity in the normal and regenerated rat adrenal cortex. Endocrinology 75:825, 1964.
56. Vecsei, P., Lommer, D., Steinacker, H. G., Vecsei-Görgenyi, A., and Wolff, H. P.: In vitro corticosteroidbiosynthese in proliferierenden Rattennebennieren. Acta Endocrinol. (Kbh) 53:24, 1966.
57. Birmingham, M. K., Rochefort, G., and Traikov, H.: Steroid fractions from incubated normal and regenerated adrenal glands of male and female rats. Endocrinology 76:819, 1965.
58. Birmingham, M. K., MacDonald, M. L., and Rochefort, J. G.: Adrenal function in normal rats and in rats bearing regenerated adrenal glands. *In* K .W. McKerns (Ed.): Functions of the Adrenal Cortex, vol. 2. New York: Appleton-Century-Crofts, 1968, p. 647.
59. de Nicola, A. F., Oliver, J. T., and Birmingham, M. K.: Corticosteroid synthesis in ad-

renal enucleated rats before the onset of hypertension. Endocrinology 85:1205, 1969.

60. de Nicola, A. F., Oliver, J. T., and Birmingham, M. K.: Biotransformation of 1,2-^{3}H-11-deoxycorticosterone and 4-^{14}C-progesterone by rats with adrenal regeneration hypertension. Endocrinology 83:141, 1968.

61. Rapp, J. P.: Gas chromatographic measurement of peripheral plasma 18-hydroxydeoxycorticosterone in adrenal regeneration hypertension. Endocrinology 86:668, 1970.

62. Brownie, A. C., and Skelton, F. R.: The metabolism of progesterone 4-^{14}C by adrenal homogenates from rats with adrenal regeneration hypertension. Steroids 6:47, 1965.

63. Rapp, J. P.: Mineralocorticoid bioassay on adrenal venous plasma from regenerating adrenals. Am. J. Physiol. 208:78, 1969.

64. Rapp, J. R.: Deoxycorticosterone production in adrenal-regeneration hypertension: In vitro vs. in vivo comparison. Endocrinology 84:1409, 1969.

65. Gaunt, R., Melby, J. C., Dale, S. L., Grekin, R. J., and Brown, R. D.: Adrenal regeneration hypertension. *In* Symposium on Mineralocorticoids and Hypertension, Fourth International Congress on Endocrinology, Washington, D.C., 1972 (in press).

66. Brown, R. D., Gaunt, R., Gisoldi, E., and Smith, N.: The role of deoxycorticosterone in adrenal regeneration hypertension. Endocrinology 91:921, 1972.

67. Grekin, R. J., Dale, S. L., Gaunt, R., and Melby, J. C.: Steroid secretion by the enucleated rat adrenal: Measurements during salt retention and the development of hypertension. Endocrinology 91:1166, 1972.

68. Hall, C. E., Holland, O. B., and Hall, O.: Characteristics of adrenal-regeneration and aldosterone hypertension. Proc. Soc. Exp. Biol. Med. 125:1075, 1967.

69. Skelton, F. R., and Guillebeau, J.: Influence of age on the development of adrenal-regeneration hypertension. Endocrinology 59:201, 1956.

70. Bernardis, L. L., and Skelton, R. F.: Effect of crowding on hypertension and growth rate in rats bearing regenerating adrenals. Proc. Soc. Exp. Biol. Med. 113:952, 1963.

71. Hall, C. E., and Hall, O.: Salt hypertension: Facilitated induction in two rat strains. Tex. Rep. Biol. Med. 22:529, 1964.

72. Hall, C. E., and Hall, O.: Hypertension and hypersalimentation. I. Aldosterone hypertension. Lab. Invest. 14:285, 1965.

73. Hall, C. E., and Hall, O.: Comparative hypertensive activities of the acetates of D-aldosterone and desoxycorticosterone. Acta Endocrinol. (Kbh) 54:399, 1967.

74. Gaunt, R., Renzi, A. A., Chart, J. J., and Sheppard, H.: A sodium-retaining influence of enucleate rat adrenals. *In* Sixth Pan-American Congress on Endocrinology, Abstract No. 278. New York: Excerpta Medica, 1965, p. E 125.

75. Gaunt, R., Gisoldi, E., Smith, N., and Giannina, T.: Relation of the pituitary to the sodium retaining effects of adrenal enucleation. Endocrinology 84:1193, 1969.

76. Gaunt, A. A., Gisoldi, E., Herkner, J., Howie, N., and Renzi, A. A.: Sodium retention after adrenal enucleation: Drug and salt appetite studies. Endocrinology 83:927, 1969.

77. Gaunt, R.: The functions of the enucleate adrenal. Trans. N.Y. Acad. Sci. 31:256, 1969.

DOCA- and Aldosterone-Induced Experimental Hypertension

By Charles E. Hall, Ph.D., and O. Hall, M.Sc.

THE HYPERTENSIVE ACTIVITY of desoxycorticosterone acetate (DOCA) has been established both clinically [1,2] and experimentally,[3,4] and human hypertensive disorders associated with adrenal hypersecretion of DOC and a diminished aldosterone secretion have been recognized.[5] This particular secretory pattern is typically found in adrenal 11- or 17-hydroxylase deficiency,[6] these disorders being conspicuously associated with hypertension.

Prior to the discovery of aldosterone, DOC was the most potent naturally occurring mineralocorticoid, causing experimental hypertensive vascular disease at far lower dosages than are necessary when using the less potent, sodium-retaining hormones, 11-desoxycortisol [8] and corticosterone,[9] for the purpose. It was natural to infer from this that should a stronger mineralocorticoid appear, it would prove to be intensely hypertensogenic. Hence, it was not surprising that soon after the discovery of aldosterone the syndrome of aldosteronism, characterized by adrenocortical adenoma, hypersecretion of aldosterone, and hypertension, was identified.[10,11] Quite unexpected, however, was that the early attempts to induce experimental hypertensive disease with aldosterone proved to be singularly disappointing.[12–14] For the most part, treated animals remained normotensive, or when positive results were obtained either a small proportion of the treated animals was affected [15] or hypertensive vascular lesions, so prominent a result of DOCA treatment, were absent.[16] This prompted the observation that aldosterone was virtually incapable of causing hypertension, or was at best weakly active in that respect.[17] Such a conclusion was compatible with the experimental findings, but suspect because it was not in accord with the relationship between sodium-retaining activity and hypertensive potency displayed by the other mineralocorticoids.

From the Department of Physiology, University of Texas Medical Branch, Galveston, Texas.

Later experiments with *d*-aldosterone acetate showed that 0.25 mg per day caused a rapid and severe form of hypertensive vascular disease,[18] more effectively in fact than the same quantity of DOCA.[19] This harmonizes with the known greater sodium-retaining effect of aldosterone, and supports the thesis that the hypertensive effect is dependent on that property. Subsequently Fregly, Kim, and Hood [20] reported that physiologic doses of aldosterone, 10 to 40 μg per day, cause hypertension in rats, supporting the attribution of high intrinsic hypertensogenic activity to the steroid. Besides sharing hypertensive properties, both mineralocorticoids cause sodium retention, potassium diuresis, loss of juxtaglomerular cell granulation, and depletion of renal and plasma renin activity.

Since all four mineralocorticoids cause hypertension and the amount required to induce the disorder appears to be proportionate to the respective sodium-retaining potencies, it would appear that (1) the two properties are dependently related, and (2) whatever mechanism underlies the hypertensive effect, it is evoked by all four.

For these reasons it would appear preferable to use the generic term "mineralocorticoid-excess hypertension," [21] or better, "hypermineralocorticoid hypertension" to designate any hypertensive clinical syndrome due to excess secretion of any one or more of these hormones, and any experimental hypertensive state elicited by them, than to continue the custom of prefixing the word hypertension with the specific name of a hormone.

Mechanism of the Hypertensive Action of Mineralocorticoids

If the mechanism basic to the hypertensive action of the various mineralocorticoids is common to them all, then it should be sufficient to consider the response to DOCA, which has been most intensively studied.

It is generally conceded that DOCA treatment leads to an elevated peripheral resistance. There are a number of ways in which such a condition might be engendered. The retention of sodium might elevate intracellular sodium concentration, thereby inducing mural swelling in the resistance vessels, reducing luminal diameter, and augmenting the mechanical resistance to blood flow.[22] Alternatively, the altered electrolyte composition of the vasculature might either increase its inherent muscle tone, or the degree of constriction evoked by humoral stimuli. Indeed, the vessels of hypertensive animals have been shown to be hyperreactive to pressor stimuli; [23] furthermore, the reactivity of the resistance vessels in the rat tail to norepinephrine is greater in appendages taken from rats treated with DOCA and salt,[24] and there is also evidence that the blood of such animals has increased pressor activity.[25,26] Quite conceivably, these factors might interact, for the demonstrated occurrence of each does not exclude the possible participation of the others.

From time to time there have appeared in the literature concerned with experimental hypertension of various kinds, reports suggesting that the catecholamines play an important role in the condition. Recently, evidence implicating abnormalities in the storage, release, and secretion of norepinephrine from nerve terminals in rats treated with DOCA has appeared,[27–30] and a case has been made for catecholaminergic vascular hyperactivity as the basis of DOCA-induced hypertension. It is difficult to harmonize that view with the reports that DOCA treatment has the usual effects on blood electrolytes and is capable of inducing and maintaining hypertension in rats that have been effectively immunosympathectomized and display a severe sympathetic insufficiency.[31–33] There are a number of pathologic responses induced in tissues and organs by DOCA treatment, but it has not been possible thus far to discriminate between those that are in some way concerned with genesis of the hypertensive response and those that merely coincide with its development.

High-Salt Diets, Salt Intake, and Mineralocorticoid Hypertension

The first experiment in which DOCA was used to induce hypertensive disease involved a high level of salt consumption,[3] it being assumed that the sodium-retaining potency of the steroid was important to its physiologic activity. Since that time the two have almost invariably been used together to produce experimental hypertension, a fact which led to the frequent reference to DOCA-salt-induced hypertension in describing this entity. It was natural therefore that the other mineralocorticoids, 11-deoxycortisol,[7] corticosterone,[8] and aldosterone,[18–20] would be tested for their hypertensive activities under conditions of high sodium chloride intake, but the relationship of salt consumption to mineralocorticoid hypertension is not entirely clear.

A number of investigators have reported DOCA to be ineffective in causing hypertension in the rat excepting under conditions of high-salt intake,[34–36] whereas others have experienced no difficulty in doing so at normal or low levels.[37–40] With 0.9-1% sodium chloride solution as the sole source of fluid, DOCA given in doses capable of causing hypertension invariably increases volume consumption above that of controls. Dosages which do not increase consumption do not cause hypertension, and vice versa.

Corticosterone administration also causes saline polydipsia at a dosage which causes hypertension,[41] but not at dosages which fail to do so.[42] In our hands, aldosterone given in hypertensogenic quantities also increases salt intake,[18,19] and it has been reported that, given acutely in microgram quantities clearly not conducive to the development of hypertension, aldosterone has a marked natroexigenic effect.[43] However, given chronically at these same low dosages, aldosterone causes hypertension, but apparently without a detectable increase in salt consumption.[20] It is also possible to induce hypertension with 11-desoxycortisol without increasing the level of salt consumption above that of controls.[7]

From the foregoing, it seems safe to conclude that the hypertensive property of mineralocorticoids can be manifest at normal levels of salt intake in sensitive animals, but that differences in genetic susceptibility or perhaps other arcane factors may prevent hypertension from developing unless a high-salt diet is afforded. When that is done, then, unless there is a proportionately reduced intake of the medium in which salt is supplied, be it food or water, there will of necessity be an increased level of salt consumption. Usually rats treated with mineralocorticoids will exhibit a higher level of salt intake than controls, thus amplifying the adverse effects of salt, so that the rapid onset of hypertension is understandable. However, the development of mineralocorticoid-induced hypertension in rats that have not been exposed to a high-salt intake suggests that in the presence of hormone excess, normal levels of salt intake can have adverse effects on the cardiovascular system.

It is a part of the conventional wisdom that adrenalectomy sensitizes the cardiovascular system to the hypertensive effects of DOCA. In the rat such is not the case;[44] in fact, these animals are less rather than more sensitive.[45] It is reasonable to suppose that the same would hold for aldosterone.

Recently Park[46] reported that, whereas Sprague-Dawley rats given DOCA and saline developed hypertension, Long-Evans rats developed hypotension. The latter response seemed so unusual and inexplicable that we conducted a study with the two strains.

Materials and Methods

Young female rats of the Sprague-Dawley and Long-Evans strains were unilaterally nephrectomized under ether anesthesia and divided into groups as noted in Table 1. One group of each strain was given 62.5 μg per day of DOCA in sesame oil twice daily, and the other group of each served as uninjected controls. They received Purina Laboratory Chow and a 1% sodium chloride drinking solution and were individually housed. Fluid intake was measured consecutively on 3 days of each week and the average taken as representative of the daily intake for the week. Systolic blood pressures were measured on unanesthetized animals by a tail-microphonic method and values exceeding 150 mm Hg were taken to reflect hypertension. The animals were killed with ether on the 40th experimental day, at which time blood samples were taken by cardiocentesis for biochemical analysis and various tissues removed for weight and histologic examination.

Results

Sprague-Dawley controls consumed substantial and increasing quantities of sodium

TABLE 1.—*Survival, Growth, Organ Weights and Histologic Changes in Control and DOCA-Treated Sprague-Dawley and Long-Evans Rats*

Data		*Sprague-Dawley*		*Long-Evans*	
		DOCA-Treated	*Controls*	*DOCA-Treated*	*Controls*
No Rats	Initial	10	6	10	6
	Final	8	6	10	6
Body wt. g.	Initial	58 ± 1 *	59 ± 1	69 ± 1	68 ± 2
	Final	165 ± 11 †	189 ± 18	194 ± 3	186 ± 6
Organ wt. mg/100g B.W.					
	Kidney	999 ± 45	718 ± 28	664 ± 22	586 ± 12
	Heart	536 ± 30	410 ± 45	334 ± 5	323 ± 16
	Thymus	144 ± 24	200 ± 16	178 ± 8	173 ± 22
	Adrenals	35.1 ± 2.2	36.2 ± 3.6	28.9 ± 0.6	31.7 ± 1.6
Renal Lesions					
	% Incidence	100	50	0	0
	% Severity	2.33 ± 0.16	0.66 ± 0.33	0	0
Cardiac Lesions					
	% Incidence	88.8	0	0	0
	% Severity	1.44 ± 0.29	0	0	0

* Mean ± SEM.
† Underlined figures differ from control values ($P < 0.05$).

chloride solution as the experiment progressed and developed a significant incidence of salt hypertension in the process. Long-Evans controls drank little sodium chloride solution, and none of the rats became hypertensive. DOCA treatment enhanced the fluid intake of Sprague-Dawley rats greatly, and all of them became severely hypertensive. The fluid intake of Long-Evans rats was only slightly increased and the group remained normotensive. Fluid intake is shown in Fig. 1 and the blood pressure response in Fig. 2.

Two of the hormone-treated Sprague-Dawley rats died intercurrently; the others of this group failed to gain weight normally and developed a relatively high blood urea nitrogen, in which respects this group differed from the others.

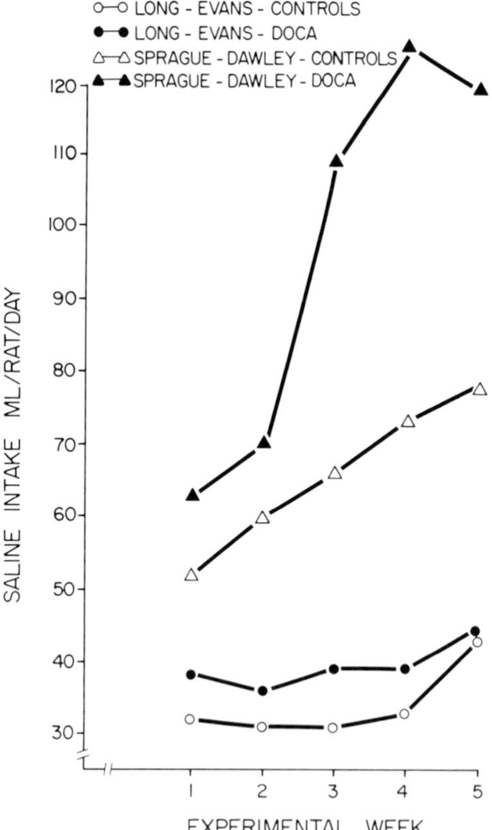

FIG. 1.—Daily saline intake of control and DOCA-treated rats of two strains. Sprague-Dawley controls drink large volumes of saline, which is increased still further by steroid treatment. Neither is true of Long-Evans rats.

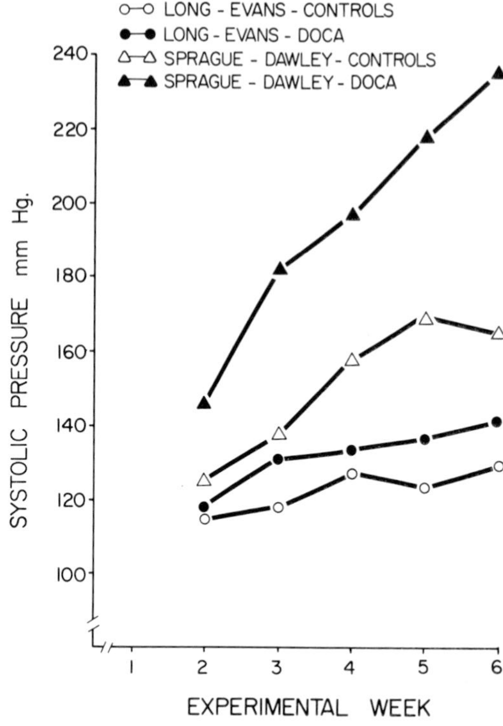

FIG. 2.—Systolic blood pressure response to salt excess (controls) and to DOCA treatment. Sprague-Dawley controls develop salt hypertension, and the hypertensive response is greater when steroid is administered. Neither effect is apparent in Long-Evans rats.

Organ weights revealed that Sprague-Dawley controls had larger hearts and kidneys than Long-Evans rats. Both organs were substantially larger again in the Sprague-Dawley hormone-treated rats, but only the kidneys were enlarged thereby in Long-Evans rats (Table 1).

Histologic examination revealed that hypertensive members of the Sprague-Dawley control group had evidence of nephrosclerosis and that some glomeruli and occasional arterioles showed fibrinoid or hyaline changes. All of the hormone-treated Sprague-Dawley rats had such lesions and they were more widespread and severe; also all but one animal in this group were found to have similar changes in cardiac arterioles and associated cardiac myopathy (Table 1). No such changes were found in any Long-Evans rat, control or hormone-treated.

Conclusions

The quite different response of the two rat strains in respect to saline consumption and the hypertensive effect of DOCA illustrates the danger of alluding to the responsiveness of "the rat" to DOCA, or to the tendency of "rats" given saline as the sole source of fluid to develop a saline polydipsia. Under conditions where it failed to promote saline polydipsia (Long-Evans rats), DOCA also failed to cause hypertension or to induce cardiac hypertrophy or cardiorenal vascular lesions, although the same degree of hypokalemia was exhibited by rats of both groups, indicating that Long-Evans rats did not have a general resistance to hormonal effects.

Regardless of which of the various alternatives purporting to account for DOCA-induced hypertension is actually causative, it is quite evident that Long-Evans rats possess a high degree of resistance to it, at least during the time span of the study. It would be instructive to determine whether or not Long-Evans rats which remain normotensive under DOCA treatment exhibit the same increases in plasma pressor activity and/or the same increased sensitivity to norepinephrine as the hormone has been alleged to cause in strains of rats that develop hypertension under steroid treatment.

Obviously, it will be necessary to compare the responsiveness of control and DOCA-treated rats of the two strains at comparable levels of salt intake, presumably by restricting the voluntary consumption of Sprague-Dawley rats, in order to ascertain whether or not the strains differ in their sensitivity to salt or to DOCA, but with the data in hand it is evident that the hormone fails to cause an increased salt consumption in Long-Evans rats, one of the more dependable actions that have usually been manifest.

References

1. Loeb, R. F., Atchley, D. W., Ferrebee, J. W., and Ragan, C.: Observations on the effect of desoxycorticosterone esters and progesterone in patients with Addison's disease. Trans. Assoc. Am. Physicians 54:285, 1939.
2. Perera, G., Knowlton, A. I., Lowell, A., and Loeb, R. F.: Effect of desoxycorticosterone acetate on the blood pressure of man. JAMA 125:1030, 1944.
3. Selye, H., Hall, C. E., and Rowley, E. M.: Malignant hypertension produced by treatment with desoxycorticosterone acetate and sodium chloride. Can. Med. Assoc. J. 49:88, 1943.
4. Hall, C. E., and Hall, O.: Sensitization to hypertensive action of desoxycorticosterone by unilateral nephrectomy: Relationship to dosage and to interval between surgery and hormone administration. Endocrinology 63: 329, 1958.
5. Biglieri, E. G., Slaton, P. E., Schambelan, M., and Kronfield, S. J.: Hypermineralocorticoidism. Am. J. Med. 45:170, 1968.
6. Forsham, P. H.: The adrenals. *In* Williams, R. H. (Ed.): Textbook of Endocrinology. Philadelphia: Saunders, 1968, p. 369.
7. Hall, C. E., Hall, O., and McClesky, O.: A study of the comparative activities of desoxycorticosterone and Reichstein's Compound S. Acta Endocrinol. (Kbh) 9:199, 1952.
8. Skelton, F. R.: Production and inhibition of hypertensive disease in the rat by corticosterone. Endocrinology 62:365, 1958.
9. Thorn, G. W., Jenkins, D., Laidlaw, J. D., Goetz, F. C., Dingman, J. F., Arons, W. L., Streeten, D. H. P., and McCracken, B. H.: Pharmacologic aspects of adrenocortical steroids and ACTH in man. N. Engl. J. Med. 248:232, 1953.
10. Conn, J. W.: Primary aldosteronism: A new clinical syndrome. J. Lab. Clin. Med. 45:6, 1955.
11. van Buchem, F. S. P., Doorenbos, H., and Elings, H. S.: Conn's syndrome, caused by adrenal hyperplasia; pathogenesis of the signs and symptoms. Acta Endocrinol. (Kbh) 23: 313, 1956.
12. Gaunt, R., Ulsamer, G. F., and Chart, J. J.: Aldosterone and hypertension. Arch. Int. Pharmacodyn. Ther. 110:114, 1957.
13. Fregly, M. J., and Arean, V. M.: Comparison of the effects of aldosterone and desoxycorticosterone acetate on blood pressure of rats. Acta Physiol. Pharmacol. Neerl. 8:162, 1959.
14. Gross, F., Loustalot, P., and Meier, R.: Vergleichende Untersuchungen über die hypertensive Wirkung von Aldosteron und Desoxycorticosteron. Experientia 11:67, 1955.
15. Friedman, S. M., Friedman, C. L., and Nakashima, M.: Effects of aldosterone on blood pressure and electrolyte distribution in the rat. Am. J. Physiol. 195:621, 1958.
16. Gross, F., Loustalot, P., and Meier, R.: Production of experimental hypertension by

aldosterone. Acta Endocrinol. (Kbh) 26:417, 1957.

17. Rondell, P. A.: The role of the adrenal cortex in experimental renal hypertension. Univ. Mich. Med. Cent. J. 27:187, 1961.

18. Hall, C. E., and Hall, O.: Hypertension and hypersalimentation. I. Aldosterone hypertension. Lab. Invest. 14:285, 1965.

19. Hall, C. E., and Hall, O.: The comparative hypertensive potencies of the acetates of *d*-aldosterone and desoxycorticosterone. Acta Endocrinol. (Kbh) 54:399, 1967.

20. Fregley, M., Kim, K. J., and Hood, C. I.: Development of hypertension in rats treated with aldosterone acetate. Toxicol. Appl. Pharmacol. 15:229, 1969.

21. Luetscher, J. A., and Lieberman, A. H.: Aldosterone. Arch. Intern. Med. 102:314, 1958.

22. Folkow, B., Grimby, G., and Thulesius, O.: Adaptive structural changes of the vascular walls in hypertension and their relation to the control of peripheral resistance. Acta Physiol. Scand. 44:255, 1958.

23. Hinke, J. A. M.: In vitro demonstration of vascular hyper-responsiveness in experimental hypertension. Circ. Res. 18:359, 1965.

24. Beilin, L. J., Wade, D. N., Honour, A. J., and Cole, T. J.: Vascular hyper-reactivity with sodium loading and with desoxycorticosterone-induced hypertension in the rat. Clin. Sci. 39:793, 1970.

25. Dahl, L. K., Knudsen, R. D., and Iwai, J.: Humoral transmission of hypertension; evidence from parabiosis. Circ. Res. 24 (Suppl. 1):21, 1969.

26. de Champlain, J., Krakoff, L. R., and Axelrod, J.: A reduction in the accumulation of H^3-norepinephrine in experimental hypertension. Life Sci. 5:2283, 1966.

27. de Champlain, J., Krakoff, L. R., and Axelrod, J.: Catecholamine metabolism in experimental hypertension in the rat. Circ. Res. 20:136, 1967.

28. Krakoff, L. R., de Champlain, J., and Axelrod, J.: Abnormal storage of norepinephrine in experimental hypertension in the rat. Circ. Res. 21:583, 1967.

29. de Champlain, J., Krakoff, L. R., and Axelrod, J.: Relationship between sodium intake and norepinephrine storage during the development of experimental hypertension. Circ. Res. 23:479, 1968.

30. de Champlain, J., Mueller, R. A., and Axelrod, J.: Turnover and synthesis of norepinephrine in experimental hypertension in rats. Circ. Res. 25:285, 1970.

31. Mueller, R. A., and Thoenen, H.: Effect of 6-hydroxydopamine (6HD) and adrenalectomy on the development of desoxycorticosterone trimethyl-acetate (DOC)-NaCl hypertension in rats. Fed. Proc. 29:546, 1970.

32. Varna, D. R.: Antihypertensive effect of methyldopa in metacorticoid immunosympathectomized rats. J. Pharm. Pharmacol. 19:61, 1967.

33. Clarke, D. E., Smookler, H. H., Barry, H., 3rd: Sympathetic nerve function and DOCA-NaCl induced hypertension. Life Sci. 9:1097, 1970.

34. Dahl, L. K.: Effects of chronic salt ingestion. Role of genetic factors in both DOCA-salt and renal hypertension. J. Exp. Med. 118: 605, 1963.

35. Tobian, L., and Redleaf, P. D.: Effect of hypertension on arterial wall electrolytes during desoxycorticosterone administration. Am. J. Physiol. 189:451, 1954.

36. Gross, F., Loustalot, P., and Sulser, F.: Die Bedeutung von Kochsalz für den Cortexon-Hochdruck der Ratte und den Gehalt der Nieren an pressorischen Substanzen. Arch. Exp. Pathol. Pharmakol. 229:381, 1956.

37. Eades, C. H., Jr., Phillips, G. E., Blaustein, A., Hsu, I. C., and Solberg, V. B.: Coronary atherosclerosis. I. Contrast of DOCA hypertension with renal hypertension in the etiology of coronary atherosclerosis in the male Wistar rat. Angiologica 2:61, 1965.

38. Hall, C. E., and Hall, O.: Interaction between desoxycorticosterone treatment, fluid intake, sodium consumption, blood pressure, and organ changes in rats drinking water, saline or sucrose solutions. Can. J. Physiol. Pharmacol. 47:81, 1969.

39. Sturtevant, F. M.: The biology of metacorticoid hypertension. Ann. Intern. Med. 49: 1281, 1958.

40. Bernardis, L. L., and Komura, S.: Blood pressure and dietary sodium as regulators of juxtaglomerular cell function. Fed. Proc. 23: 445, 1964.

41. Skelton, F. R.: Production and inhibition of hypertensive disease in the rat by corticosterone. Endocrinology 62:365, 1958.

42. Hall, C. E., Holland, O. B., and Hall, O.: High blood pressure in rats protected against post-enucleation adrenal insufficiency and its bearing on the etiology of adrenal-regenera-

tion hypertension. *In* Jasmin, G. (Ed.): Endocrine Aspects of Disease Processes. St. Louis, Mo.: Green, 1968, p. 302.

43. Wolf, G., and Handal, P. J.: Aldosterone-induced sodium appetite: Dose-response and specificity. Endocrinology 78:1120, 1966.
44. Tobian, L., and Perry, S.: Effect of adrenal tissue on desoxycorticosterone hypertension. Proc. Soc. Exp. Biol. Med. 108:615, 1961.
45. Hall, C. E., and Ayachi, S.: Dose-effect relationship in desoxycorticosterone hypertension: Reduced sensitivity in adrenalectomized rats and its possible significance to the etiology of adrenal-regeneration hypertension. Can. J. Physiol. Pharmacol. 49:139, 1971.
46. Park, B. E.: The development of a renal hypertensive model. Tex. Rep. Biol. Med. 29:399, 1971.

PHEOCHROMOCYTOMA: INCIDENCE, PATHOPHYSIOLOGY, AND DIAGNOSIS

By ROBERT L. WOLF, M.D.

SINCE THE FIRST antemortem diagnosis of pheochromocytoma was made in 1923 by Masson and Martin,[1] it has been recognized that this tumor produces many variable, interesting clinical problems in diagnosis and treatment in view of the fact that they are associated with a curable variety of hypertension. In the years 1927 and 1929 the first successful surgical removals of pheochromocytomas were demonstrated [2,3]; not until 1949, however, when Grimson et al.[4] introduced phentolamine, was the extraordinarily high surgical mortality associated with the removal of pheochromocytoma reduced. The pharmacologic tests for pheochromocytoma were described in 1945 and greatly enhanced the accuracy of the diagnosis of the illness.[5–8] The discovery of 3-methoxy-4-hydroxymandelic acid (VMA) by Armstrong and McMillan in human urine in 1957 gave further impetus to the accurate antemortem diagnosis of pheochromocytoma.[9] The increased urinary excretion of the catecholamine metabolites has extensively been used since that time in order to establish the diagnosis of pheochromocytoma. It was subsequently shown that metanephrine and normetanephrine are metabolites of epinephrine and norepinephrine. These metabolites may be accurately assayed in the urine of patients with pheochromocytoma, and the increased excretion of these metabolites may be utilized to establish the diagnosis of pheochromocytoma. It is mandatory that the physician test every patient with hypertensive disease for the presence of pheochromocytoma since this tumor is almost always fatal when not surgically treated; the signs and symptoms of pheochromocytoma are frequently identical with those of primary or essential hypertension, the disease of greatest frequency in the United States.

PATHOPHYSIOLOGY

Using the two-dimensional paper chromatographic assay of Armstrong, Shaw, and Vall, the diagnostic value of urinary VMA assays in order to confirm the diagnosis of pheochromocytoma was emphasized by Armstrong.[10] Shortly thereafter, normetanephrine, metanephrine, and 3-methoxy-4-hydroxyphenylglycol were demonstrated to be products of the metabolism of the catecholamines (Fig. 1). The quantities of combined normetanephrine and metanephrine excreted in the urine were at least equal to the amount of VMA excreted; furthermore, smaller amounts of 3-methoxy-4-hydroxyphenylglycol were also present. Not only have the urinary assays for the catecholamine metabolites been utilized to confirm the diagnosis of pheochromocytoma but, also, they have been employed to demonstrate the adequacy of surgical removal of the tumor or tumors.[11–13]

The benign or malignant characteristic of a pheochromocytoma is frequently difficult to establish by historic examination. The malignant nature of pheochromocytoma is inferred by the presence of apparent metastases of the tumor at locations where no neural crest tissue is found and which is distant from the original tumor. Homovanillic acid (HVA) and 3-methoxytyramine may be present in the urine of patients in normal or increased amounts with either benign or malignant pheochromocytoma.[14–16] There is a tendency for pheochromocytoma of adrenal origin to produce disproportionately large amounts of epinephrine.[17]

The metabolic pathways of catecholamine synthesis have been the subject of intensive investigations during the past 20 years. The enzyme tyrosine hydroxylase enhances the conversion of tyrosine to dihydroxyphenylalanine (dopa). This ring hydroxylation of tyrosine to dopa is the rate-limiting step in the

---

From the Department of Medicine, Mount Sinai School of Medicine of the City University of New York, New York.

This work was supported by Grant No. U-1960 from the Health Research Council of the City of New York.

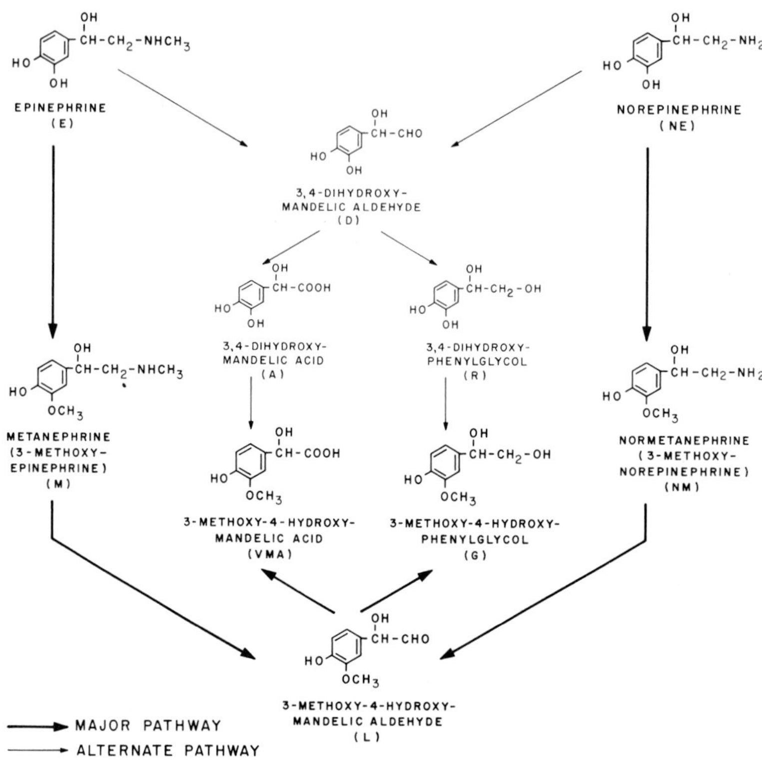

FIG. 1.—Metabolic pathways of norepinephrine and epinephrine degradation.

synthesis of the catecholamines. The conversion of dopa to dihydroxyphenylalanine (dopamine) is catalyzed by the enzyme aromatic-L-amino acid decarboxylase. Aromatic-L-amino acid decarboxylase inhibitors (e.g., methyldopa) are commercially available. Dopamine is converted to norepinephrine by dopamine beta-oxidase; norepinephrine is converted to epinephrine by phenylethanolamine-N-methyltransferase. Aromatic-L-amino acid decarboxylase inhibitors have been employed to inhibit the synthesis of the catecholamines in cases of pheochromocytoma treated by medical methods. Although the quantities of VMA and tyrosine excreted in the urine were occasionally diminished, there was no reproducible beneficial effect on the course of the illness.[18–20] Alpha-methyltyrosine (α-MPT), an inhibitor of tyrosine hydroxylase, has been used to reduce the synthesis of the catecholamines at the rate-limiting step.[18,21] Catecholamine synthesis may be reduced by approximately 50 percent following the administration of α-MPT. The urinary excretions of normetanephrine, metanephrine, and VMA together with the catecholamines were correspondingly reduced. Blood pressure reduction was also associated with these observations. When α-MPT is administered to patients with primary or essential hypertension there is, however, no significant lowering of blood pressure.[18,21,22]

Manifestations and Natural History

A wide variety of manifestations may be associated with pheochromocytoma. These may appear unrelated and have reference to almost any of the organ systems in the human body.[23] Over one thousand cases of pheochromocytoma occur annually in the United States.[24] The presence of pheochromocytoma must be considered in the relatives of all of the patients with this tumor since the familial occurrence has been documented in over 30 kindred.[25,26] Since the description of the familial occurrence of pheochromocytoma in 1947 by Calkins and

Howard, it has been shown that the mode of inheritance is autosomal dominant, with a high degree of penetrance.[27] Familial pheochromocytoma is associated with a higher incidence of sustained hypertension, multiple tumors, bilateral medullary carcinoma of the thyroid with amyloid stroma, a proportionally high incidence of right adrenal gland involvement, and an increased incidence of the neurocutaneous syndromes.[23,28–30] Although pheochromocytomas have been described in all age groups there is an increased incidence in childhood.[31] Pheochromocytomas have been described during pregnancy.[32]

There is no association of pheochromocytoma with the body habitus; it is present with equal frequency in both sexes.[30,33,34] Although an occasional pheochromocytoma is found within the skull or in the neck, 98 percent of all such tumors are located within the abdominal cavity.[35,36] The chest cavity is the location of the remaining pheochromocytomas. These tumors are located in the right adrenal gland with an approximate twofold frequency compared to the left adrenal gland; nine out of 10 intra-abdominal pheochromocytomas occur in the adrenal glands.[31,37] Since multiple pheochromocytomas are frequent, the entire abdominal and pelvic cavity should be thoroughly explored at the time of surgery. There is a wide variation in the size and weight of these tumors although the majority of pheochromocytomas are small in size.

Since pheochromocytoma is inevitably fatal when not recognized and since the clinical manifestations of this disease are variable, all cases of hypertension should be treated for this potentially curable illness. The ensuing paragraphs classify and discuss many of the multifaceted manifestations of this fascinating disease.

Paroxysmal Hypertension

The hypertension associated with pheochromocytoma is characteristically intermittent in slightly more than 50 percent of patients.[23,31] These hypertensive episodes may be associated with palpitations, headache, tachycardia, nausea, perspiration, pallor, chest pain, abdominal pain, anxiety, and weakness. There may be intermittent episodes of trembling, tremor, skin flushing, paresthesias and visual abnormalities. One or a combination of these signs and symptoms may characterize the paroxysmal hypertensive episodes in an individual patient. The rates of onset and defervescence of these symptoms is usually rapid. The duration and frequency of these intermittent hypertensive episodes may vary widely and precipitating factors such as smoking, abdominal pressure, sneezing, sexual intercourse, changes in posture, and eating have been frequently incriminated. The blood pressure may be normal between the intermittent episodes of hypertension; the urinary excretion of the catecholamine metabolites, however, invariably remains elevated.

Sustained Hypertension

Pheochromocytoma frequently presents as primary or essential hypertension and may mimic the clinical course of essential hypertension.[23] The hypertension associated with pheochromocytoma is sustained in almost half of the patients. Signs and symptoms of hypermetabolism characterized by weight loss, excessive perspiration, tremulousness, inability to gain weight, and fever may be associated. Sustained hypertension may develop in patients who initially had intermittent or paroxysmal hypertension; furthermore, paroxysmal hypertensive episodes may develop in patients who have sustained hypertension.

Familial Pheochromocytoma

The familial occurrence of pheochromocytoma is characteristically associated with bilateral involvement, parathyroid adenomas and medullary carcinoma of the thyroid gland.[28,36,37] An association of familial pheochromocytoma with neurofibromatosis or Lindau-von Hippel disease has also been reported.[26,29,38]

Norepinephrine-producing Pheochromocytoma

Pheochromocytomas that predominantly produce norepinephrine may present a triad of symptoms: shock, hypotension, and intermittent episodes. Hypometabolic signs and symptoms are less frequent with such pheochromocytomas.

Other Tumors and Pheochromocytoma

Carcinoma of the thyroid gland may be associated with familial or nonfamilial pheochromocytoma. The thyroid tumor that is associated with the greatest frequency of pheochromocytoma is medullary carcinoma of the thyroid gland with amyloid stroma.[29] When thyroid carcinoma is associated with bilateral pheochromocytomas, then the carcinoma of the thyroid is also bilateral in 75 percent of the cases. The coexistence of pheochromocytoma and parathyroid adenomas is almost always associated with thyroid carcinoma.[25,39]

Childhood and Pheochromocytoma

Childhood pheochromocytomas are characterized by multiple and ectopic tumors and a stormy clinical course. Many of these tumors are bilateral.[40] Pheochromocytomas are more frequently seen in males than in females before puberty; after adolescence there is no apparent sex association related to this tumor. There appears to be an increased incidence of renal artery stenosis, polydipsia, polyuria, and skin manifestations in childhood pheochromocytoma. Signs and symptoms of obstructive uropathy have been reported with increased frequency in pheochromocytoma in childhood.

Pregnancy and Pheochromocytoma

Pheochromocytoma associated with pregnancy is characterized by a high morbidity and mortality.[41] Both the maternal and infant mortality are high. Preeclampsia and toxemia of pregnancy may mimic pheochromocytoma in pregnancy.

Pheochromocytoma of the Urinary Bladder

Unusual manifestations are associated with pheochromocytoma of the urinary bladder wall. Paroxysmal signs and symptoms suggesting the presence of pheochromocytoma of the urinary bladder are frequently associated with the act of urinating. Hematuria is frequently present. Pheochromocytoma of the urinary bladder wall is typically small and located intramurally. Cystoscopy and cystography may be normal.

Pheochromocytoma and the Neurocutaneous Syndromes

Ten to 15 percent of the cases of pheochromocytoma are associated with neurofibromatosis. This association is increased in bilateral pheochromocytoma. Mental retardation, meningiomas, gliomas, congenital vertebral anomalies together with café au lait spots, generalized hyperpigmentation, and axillary freckling are frequently seen with neurofibromatosis. Pheochromocytoma may be associated with Lindau-von Hippel disease with or without neurofibromatosis. Many tumors of the nervous system including astrocytic tumors, hemangioblastomas, paragangliomas, schwannomas, and syringomyelias are not frequently associated with pheochromocytoma.[36,37,42]

DIAGNOSIS

The pharmacologic tests for pheochromocytoma, which were initially described in 1945, measure either the hypertensive response to certain provocative agents or the hypotensive response to adrenergic blocking drugs. Considering the fact that there is an extraordinarily high incidence of serious complications during the pharmacologic testing procedures and that the information obtained from them is less reliable and accurate than that obtained from the urinary assays for the catecholamine metabolites in the diagnosis of pheochromocytoma, these pharmacologic tests are seldom indicated at this time. Only a few of these tests are employed, occasionally, now.[43] Catecholamine and catecholamine metabolite assays in the urine and blood may be simultaneously measured during the course of these provocative tests. Incorrect test results have been recorded in approximately 20 to 25 percent of the histamine-provocative tests; significant mortality and morbidity have also been recorded.[44]

The provocative test for pheochromocytoma employing the pressor responsiveness to tyramine, described by Engelman and Sjoerdsma in 1964, may also be associated with a 20- to 25-percent incidence of false negative responses.[45] It has been asserted that the cold pressor-histamine test may be more sensitive than the tyramine-provocative test.

The phentolamine pharmacologic test for pheochromocytoma, introduced by Emlet et al. in 1951, is still, probably, the safest of these test procedures.[46,47] Occasional deaths, however, have been reported.[48] It is generally agreed that the diagnosis of pheochromocytoma is established with the greatest reliability by urinary assay procedures for the catecholamine metabolites. Many different test procedures have been devised; however, analysis of the urine for the increased excretions of the metanephrines, either combined or separately, is the test procedure associated with the highest degree of accuracy, simplicity, and rapidity of analysis. Emotional stress, hyperglycemia, exogenous dietary catecholamines, nose drops, various drugs, uremia, and high cerebrospinal fluid pressure may be associated with falsely elevated urinary catecholamine metabolite assay results. Pheochromocytomas which are minimally secreting catecholamines may be associated with a urinary catecholamine metabolite test result which is within the normal range. Although several assay techniques for the catecholamines themselves in the plasma and the urine had been described, a new sensitive double-isotope derivative method for total catecholamines in biologic fluids appears to have the important advantages of specificity, reliability, ease of performance, and sensitivity compared to the others.[49] Despite this fact the inherent simplicity and accuracy of the urinary assays for catecholamine metabolites dictate a likelihood that assays for the catecholamines themselves will be used infrequently.

Of all the catecholamine metabolites which are present in the urine, three of them have been utilized with great frequency in order to establish the diagnosis of pheochromocytoma. These metabolites are norepinephrine, metanephrine, and VMA. Shock, drugs, carcinoma, uremia, coronary insufficiency, and dietary factors have been reported to give false positive results with the assay procedures for VMA. Administration of decarboxylase inhibitors and the monoamine oxidase inhibitors may give rise to false low values. Employing any of the tests which are available, which analyze for urinary VMA, the incidence of false positive results is approximately 10 to 15 percent.[50] It is for this reason that almost all hypertensive research laboratories and clinics utilize an assay procedure for the urinary metanephrines in order to establish the diagnosis of pheochromocytoma.[51–53]

Assay of the urine for either the combined or separate metanephrines is the simplest and most suitable assay technique for the diagnosis of pheochromocytoma. These assay techniques employ either periodic oxidation coupled with spectrophotometric measurement or electrophoresis with or without chromatography.[51–62] After the administration of certain pharmacologic agents the concentrations of either the separate or the combined metanephrines may be reduced.[63] Rarely, a patient with pheochromocytoma may have normal or low values for either normetanephrine or metanephrine associated with increased urinary excretion values for the other methylated metabolite. The assay values for the combined urinary metanephrines is, however, always elevated in these cases.[59]

The apparent norepinephrine secretion rate test (ANESR) result is increased in patients with pheochromocytoma.[59,60,62–67] Patients with essential or primary hypertension have a decreased ANESR, patients with renovascular hypertension have a normal ANESR, and patients with pheochromocytoma, as indicated, have an increased ANESR.

Diseases to be considered in the differential diagnosis of pheochromocytoma are of an extraordinarily wide variety and must be carefully distinguished by the attending physician. Neuroblastomas and ganglioneuromas may produce increased amounts of the catecholamines and their metabolites. They may also be associated with hypertension and are not infrequently confused with pheochromocytoma in children. The clinical course of metastatic malignancy characterizes neuroblastoma and the triad of abdominal distention, weight loss, and diarrhea indicates the presence of ganglioneuromas. Pheochromocytoma may mimic patients with Riley-Day syndrome (familial dysautonomia), acrodynia, acute anxiety states, vasodilating headaches, migraine headaches, diencephalic autonomic episodes, coronary insufficiency, hypoglycemia episodes, and even the menopausal syndrome.

Complications

The complications of pheochromocytoma are similar to those of primary or essential hypertension. Coronary artery disease, retinopathy, cerebrovascular accidents, malignant hypertension, diffuse vascular disease, and nephrosclerosis with renal insufficiency have been reported.[23,31,68] A focal myocarditis has been reported in patients with pheochromocytoma.[69] Pulmonary edema and congestive heart failure may complicate myocarditis or pheochromocytoma. Myocardial infarction and cardiac arrhythmias are not infrequent in these patients. Shock and hypotension may dominate the clinical picture, and the presence of ventricular tachycardia and ventricular fibrillation has been emphasized.

There is an increased incidence of cholelithiasis in pheochromocytoma.[36,70] Pheochromocytoma may resemble diabetes mellitus with its initial presentation. The abnormal carbohydrate metabolism associated with pheochromocytoma has been related to inhibition of insulin release and resistance to the hypoglycemic action of insulin.[71,72] Furthermore, pheochromocytoma may coexist with diabetes mellitus in the same patient.

Additional Diagnostic Procedures

Recognizing the fact that over 98 percent of pheochromocytomas are located within the abdominal or pelvic cavity and that approximately 20 percent of adult patients with pheochromocytoma have multiple tumors, together with the recognized relative inaccuracy of tumor location by roentgen procedures, a thorough and complete surgical exploration of the abdomen and pelvis must be performed in all patients with this disease when the tumor is located below the diaphragm. It is recommended, moreover, that additional diagnostic procedures be restricted to a minimum. The possibility of pheochromocytoma of the skull and chest is eliminated by x-rays of these areas. An intravenous pyelogram with laminography of the renal areas is not associated with an excessive morbidity or mortality and provides important information concerning renal function and, occasionally, location of the tumor. Cholelithiasis may be revealed by cholecystography and the diseased gallbladder may be removed electively at the time of abdominal surgery. Other special radiographic techniques have been uniformly associated with significant morbidity and mortality.

Management and Treatment

Surgical removal of the tumor is the treatment of choice for pheochromocytoma. Approximately 90 percent of all patients with pheochromocytoma are valid surgical candidates. Patients who are rejected for surgery include those with metastatic malignant pheochromocytoma and patients who have benign pheochromocytoma but who, for other medical reasons, would not survive the surgical procedure. Patients who are candidates for medical management and treatment include those who are to receive preoperative procedures and medications and those who are not surgical candidates and require chronic medical treatment. Hypertensive patients with pheochromocytoma will usually receive alpha-adrenergic blocking drugs preoperatively. The two alpha-adrenergic blocking agents which are efficacious and currently available are phentolamine and phenoxybenzamine. Phenoxybenzamine may be administered by the oral route and for this reason has distinct advantages over phentolamine which can only be administered parenterally. Phenoxybenzamine has also been used in the chronic treatment of patients with pheochromocytoma.[19,70,74] A tyrosine hydroxylase inhibitor, α-MPT, has been employed in the treatment of patients with pheochromocytoma and it is not unlikely that either this drug or an analog will be used with increased frequency in patients with this disease.

Blood replacement at the time of surgical removal of a pheochromocytoma, or blood volume replacement in excess of the amount of blood estimated to be lost at the time of surgery has been observed to be of importance in the reversal of the hypotension that frequently occurs when the tumor is removed. Patients with pheochromocytoma generally have normal plasma and total blood volume. Rarely, pheochromocytoma may be associated with an increased secretion of an erythropoiesis-stimulating factor and polycythemia. During surgery patients with pheochromocytoma should have continuous and careful monitoring of the arterial blood pressure, electrocardiogram, central venous pressure, and heart rate. Halothane is the anesthetic of choice. The antiarrhythmic drug lidocaine effectively reverses the increased cardiac excitability caused by epinephrine in these patients. The beta-adrenergic blocking drug, propranolol, is effective in the control of catecholamine-induced arrhythmia.

Patients with intra-abdominal pheochromocytoma demand an extensive abdominal exploration since bilateral and multiple tumors are frequent. A transabdominal surgical approach is required in order to expose the entire abdominal cavity. The intra-abdominal areas of chromaffin tissue should be examined with care. These include the adrenal glands, organs of Zuckerkandl at the bifurcation of the aorta, necrotic tissue, and the area adjacent to the pelvic organs. Local tissue invasiveness is the primary criterion for malignancy. If malignancy is established then the local lymph nodes should be removed. Adequacy of tumor removal is documented by the prompt decline of the elevated urinary metanephrine values obtained before surgery and the establishment of normal values within 24 to 48 hours after surgery. Inadequate surgical removal of the tumor or tumors or recurrence of pheochromocytoma is indicated by elevated urinary metanephrine assay results.

There have been distinct and significant advances in the diagnosis and treatment of pheochromocytoma in recent years. These advances have resulted in the designation of pheochromocytoma as a curable form of hypertensive disease.

References

1. Masson, P., and Martin, J.-F.: Paragangliome Surrénal, Étude d'un Cas Humain de Tumeurs Malignes de la Medullo-Surrénale. Bull. Assoc. Franc. Étude Cancer 12:135, 1923.
2. Mayo, C. H.: Paroxysmal hypertension with tumor of retroperitoneal nerve: Report of a case. JAMA 89:1047, 1927.
3. Shipley, A. M.: Paroxysmal hypertension associated with tumor of suprarenal. Ann. Surg. 90:742, 1929.
4. Grimson, K. S., Longino, F. H., Kernodle, C. E., and O'Rear, H. B.: Treatment of patient with pheochromocytoma: Use of adrenolytic drug before and during operation. JAMA 140:1273, 1949.
5. Roth, G. M., and Kvale, W. F.: A tentative test for pheochromocytoma. Am. J. Med. Sci. 210:653, 1945.
6. LaDue, J. S., Murison, P. J., and Pack, G. T.: The use of tetraethylammonium bromide as a diagnostic test for pheochromocytoma. Ann. Intern. Med. 29:914, 1948.
7. Guarneri, V., and Evans, J. A.: Pheochromocytoma. Report of a Case with a New Diagnostic Test. Am J. Med. 4:806, 1948.
8. Goldenberg, M., Snyder, C. H., and Aranow, H., Jr.: New test for hypertension due to circulating epinephrine. JAMA 135:971, 1947.
9. Armstrong, M. D., and McMillan, A.: Identification of major urinary metabolite of norepinephrine. Fed. Proc. 16:146, 1957.
10. Armstrong, M. D., Shaw, K. N. F., and Vall, P. E.: The phenolic acids of human urine. Paper chromatography of phenolic acids. J. Biol. Chem. 218:293, 1956.
11. Sjoerdsma, A., Lepper, L. C., Terry, L. L., and Udenfriend, S.: Studies on biogenesis and metabolism of norepinephrine in patients with pheochromocytoma. J. Clin. Invest. 38: 31, 1959.
12. Armstrong, M. D., Shaw, K. N. F., and Vall, P. E.: The phenolic acids of human urine. Paper chromatography of phenolic acids. J. Biol. Chem. 218:293, 1956.
13. Anton, A. H., Greer, M., Sayre, D. F., and Williams, C. M.: Dihydroxyphenylalanine secretion in a malignant pheochromocytoma. Am. J. Med. 42:469, 1967.
14. Robinson, R., Smith, P., and Wittaker, S. R. F.: Secretion of catecholamines in malignant pheochromocytoma. Br. Med. J. 1:1422, 1964.
15. Weil-Malherbe, H.: Pheochromocytoma catechols in urine and tumor tissue. Lancet 2: 282, 1956.
16. Sato, T. L., and Sjoerdsma, A.: Urinary homovanillic acid in pheochromocytoma. Br. Med. J. 2:1472, 1965.
17. Engelman, K., and Hammond, W. G.: Adrenaline production by an intrathoracic phaeochromocytoma. Lancet 1:609, 1968.
18. Engelman, K., and Sjoerdsma, A.: Chronic medical therapy for pheochromocytoma. A report of four cases. Ann. Intern. Med. 61: 229, 1964.
19. Oates, J. A., Gillespie, L., Udenfriend, S., and Sjoerdsma, A.: Decarboxylase inhibition and blood pressure reduction by α-methyl-3,4-dihydroxy-DL-phenylalanine. Science 131: 1890, 1960.
20. Gillespie, L., Jr., Oates, J. A., Crout, J. R., and Sjoerdsma, A.: Clinical and chemical

studies with α-methyl-dopa in patients with hypertension. Circulation 25:281, 1962.

21. Sjoerdsma, A., Engelman, K., Spector, S., and Udenfriend, S.: Inhibition of catecholamine synthesis in man with alpha-methyltyrosine, an inhibitor of tyrosine hydroxylase. Lancet 2:1092, 1965.
22. Engelman, K., and Sjoerdsma, A.: Inhibition of catecholamine biosynthesis in man. Circ. Res. 18–19:104, 1966.
23. Page, L. B., and Copeland, R. B.: Pheochromocytoma. DM 1, Jan. 1968.
24. Barbeau, A.: Le phéochromocytome. Union Med. Can. 86:1045, 1957.
25. Moorhead, E. L., Jr., Brennan, M. J., Caldwell, J. R., and Averill, W. C.: Pheochromocytoma: A familial tumor, survey of 11 families. Henry Ford Hosp. Med. Bull. 13: 467, 1965.
26. Sarosi, G., and Doe, R. P.: Familial occurrence of parathyroid adenomas, pheochromocytoma, and medullary carcinoma of the thyroid with amyloid stroma (Sipple's syndrome). Ann. Intern. Med. 68:1305, 1968.
27. Calkins, E., and Howard, J. E.: Bilateral familial pheochromocytoma with paroxysmal hypertension: Successful surgical removal of tumors in two cases, with discussion of certain diagnostic procedures and physiological considerations. J. Clin. Endocrinol. 7:475, 1947.
28. Sarosi, G., and Doe, R. P.: Familial occurrence of parathyroid adenomas, pheochromocytoma, and medullary carcinoma of the thyroid with amyloid stroma (Sipple's syndrome). Ann. Intern. Med. 68:1305, 1968.
29. Schimke, R. N., and Hartmann, W. H.: Familial amyloid-producing medullary thyroid carcinoma and pheochromocytoma. Ann. Intern. Med. 63:1027, 1965.
30. Nourok, D. S.: Familial pheochromocytoma and thyroid carcinoma. Ann. Intern. Med. 60:1028, 1964.
31. Moorhead, E. L., Jr., Caldwell, J. R., Kelly, A. R., and Morales, A. R.: The diagnosis of pheochromocytoma. JAMA 196:1107, 1966.
32. Hermann, H., and Mornex, R.: Human Tumours Secreting Catecholamines. New York: Macmillan, 1964.
33. Scott, H. W., Jr., Riddell, D. H., and Brockman, S. K.: Surgical management of pheochromocytoma. Surg. Gynec. Obstet. 120: 707, 1965.
34. Kvale, W. F., Roth, G. M., Manger, W. M., and Priestley, J. T.: Present-day diagnosis and treatment of pheochromocytoma: A review of 51 cases. JAMA 164:854, 1957.
35. Maier, H. C., and Humphreys, G. H.: Intrathoracic pheochromocytoma with hypertension. Ann. Surg. 130:1059, 1949.
36. Green, W. O., and Bassett, F. H.: Intrathoracic Pheochromocytoma: Report of a case. Am. J. Clin. Pathol. 35:142, 1961.
37. Howard, J. E., and Barker, W. H.: Paroxysmal hypertension and other clinical manifestations associated with benign chromaffin cell tumors (pheochromocytoma). Johns Hopkins Med. J. 61:371, 1937.
38. Tisherman, S. E., Gregg, F. J., and Danowski, T. S.: Familial pheochromocytoma. JAMA 182:152, 1962.
39. Sipple, J. H.: The association of pheochromocytoma with carcinoma of the thyroid gland. Am. J. Med. 31:163, 1961.
40. Stackpole, R. H., Meyer, M. M., and Uson, A. C.: Pheochromocytoma in children. J. Pediat. 63:315, 1963.
41. Dean, R. E.: Pheochromocytoma and pregnancy. Obstet. Gynec. 11:35, 1958.
42. Glushein, A. D., Mansuy, M. M., and Littman, D. S.: Pheochromocytoma: Its relationship to the neurocutaneous syndromes. Am. J. Med. 14:318, 1953.
43. Editorial: Diagnosis of pheochromocytoma. N. Engl. J. Med. 227:762, 1967.
44. Chapman, W. P., and Singh, M.: Evaluation of tests used in the diagnosis of pheochromocytoma. Mod. Concepts Cardiovasc. Dis. 23: 221, 1954.
45. Engelman, K., Horwitz, D., Ambrose, I. M., and Sjoerdsma, A.: Further evaluation of the tyramine test for pheochromocytoma. N. Engl. J. Med. 278:705, 1968.
46. Emlet, J. R., Grimson, K. S., Bell, D. M., and Orgain, E. S.: Use of Piperoxan and Regitine as routine tests in patients with hypertension. JAMA 146:1383, 1951.
47. Iseri, L. T., Henderson, H. W., and Derr, J. W.: Use of adrenolytic drug, Regitine, in pheochromocytoma. Am. Heart J. 42:129, 1951.
48. Comens, P., Perry, H. M., Jr., and Schroeder, H. A.: Evaluation of bioassay for urinary catecholamines with strips of rabbit aorta. J. Lab. Clin. Med. 55:748, 1960.
49. Engelman, K., Portnoy, B., and Lovenberg, W.: Sensitive and specific double-isotope derivative method for the determination of catecholamines in biological specimens. Am. J. Med. Sci. 255:259, 1968.

50. Amery, A., and Conway, J.: A critical review of diagnostic tests for pheochromocytoma. Am. Heart J. 73:129, 1967.
51. Wolf, R. L., Mendlowitz, M., Roboz, J., and Gitlow, S. E.: New rapid test for pheochromocytoma: Urinary assay of normetanephrine, metanephrine and 3-methoxy-4-hydroxyphenylglycol. JAMA 188:859, 1964.
52. Wolf, R. L., Mendlowitz, M., and Gitlow, S. E.: Simultaneous urinary assays for the combined metanephrines and 3-methoxy-4-hydroxyphenylglycol in patients with pheochromocytoma and primary hypertension. N. Engl. J. Med. 273:1459, 1965.
53. Wolf, R. L.: A new catecholamine metabolite (CM) test for pheochromocytoma. Heart Bull. 13:96, 1964.
54. Pisano, J. J.: A simple analysis for normetanephrine and metanephrine in urine. Clin. Chim. Acta 5:406, 1960.
55. Wolf, R. L., Mendlowitz, M., Roboz, J., and Gitlow, S. E.: A new rapid test for pheochromocytoma based on the urinary assay of normetanephrine, metanephrine and 3-methoxy-4-hydroxyphenylglycol. Ann. Intern. Med. 60:718, 1964.
56. Wolf, R. L., Mendlowitz, M., and Roboz, J.: A new test for pheochromocytoma based on the assay of 3-methoxy-4-hydroxyphenylglycol, normetanephrine and metanephrine in the urine. *In* Abstracts of VII Inter-American Congress of Cardiology, 1964, p. 210.
57. Wolf, R. L., Mendlowitz, M., Roboz, J., and Gitlow, S. E.: Electrophoretic assay of catecholamine metabolites in human urine. Clin. Res. 13:337, 1965.
58. Wolf, R. L., Mendlowitz, M., Roboz, J., and Gitlow, S. E.: Urinary assays for catecholamine metabolites in essential hypertension and pheochromocytoma. Circulation 32 (Suppl. III): 221, 1965.
59. Wolf, R. L., Mendlowitz, M., Roboz, J., Naftchi, E., and Gitlow, S. E.: Urinary normetanephrine and metanephrine excretion, separately assayed, in normotensive, hypertensive and pheochromocytoma patients. J. Clin. Invest. 45:1088, 1966.
60. Wolf, R. L., Mendlowitz, M., and Roboz, J.: Norepinephrine metabolism in hypertension. Fed. Proc. 27:602, 1968.
61. Wolf, R. L., and Roboz, J.: Urinary normetanephrine and metanephrine excretion, separately assayed, following the oral administration of guanethidine. Fed. Proc. 25:625, 1966.
62. Coward, R. F., and Smith, R.: A new screening test for pheochromocytoma. Clin. Chim. Acta 13:538, 1966.
63. Wolf, R. L., Mendlowitz, M., and Roboz, J.: A new test for primary hypertension: The apparent norepinephrine secretion rate in normotensive and hypertensive man. J. Clin. Invest. 46:1134, 1967.
64. Wolf, R. L., Mendlowitz, M., and Roboz, J.: Distribution kinetics, apparent secretion rate and turnover rate of norepinephrine in man. Circulation 36(Suppl. II):273, 1967.
65. Wolf, R. L., Mendlowitz, M., and Roboz, J.: The metabolism of intravenously injected norepinephrine-H^3 in normotensive and hypertensive subjects. J. Clin. Invest. 47:104a, 1968.
66. Wolf, R. L., Roboz, J., and Mendlowitz, M.: Total body norepinephrine (NE) in hypertensive patients. Circulation 38(Suppl. VI):207, 1968.
67. ———, ———, and Bautz, G.: Norepinephrine metabolism in hypertension. Circulation (In press.)
68. Samellas, W., and Blumberg, N.: Pheochromocytoma. N.Y. State J. Med. 65:2155, 1965.
69. Van Vliet, P. D., Burchell, H. B., and Titus, J. C.: Focal myocarditis associated with pheochromocytoma. N. Engl. J. Med. 274: 1102, 1966.
70. Sjoerdsma, A., Moderator, Combined Clinical Staff Conference at the National Institutes of Health: Pheochromocytoma, current concepts of diagnosis and treatment. Ann. Intern. Med. 65:1302, 1966.
71. Spergel, G., Bleicher, S. J., and Ertel, N. H.: Carbohydrate and fat metabolism in patients with pheochromocytoma. N. Engl. J. Med. 278:803, 1968.
72. Wilber, J. F., Turtle, J. H., and Crane, N. A.: Inhibition of insulin secretion by a pheochromocytoma. Lancet 2:733, 1966.
73. Boijsen, E., Williams, C. M., and Judkins, M. P.: Angiography of pheochromocytoma. Am. J. Roentgenol. Radium Ther. Nucl. Med. 98:225, 1966.
74. Rosenberg, J. C., and Varco, R. L.: Physiologic and pharmacologic considerations in the management of pheochromocytoma. Surg. Clin. N. Am. 47:1453, 1967.

PART VIII. Renal Hypertension

A Survey of Experimental Studies in Renal Hypertension

By Arthur Grollman, Ph.D., M.D.

As an introduction to our considerations of the role of the kidney in hypertension, let us survey the history of these investigations.

Richard Bright's classic publication in 1836,[1] in which he noted that the occurrence of a full pulse, reflecting a high blood pressure, was often present in the face of renal damage, set in motion the inquiry which has been pursued since then concerning the relation of high arterial blood pressure to chronic disease of the kidney. Bright's clinical observation of 100 patients followed to autopsy revealed the coincidence of cardiac and renal disease to be so striking as to convince him that diseases of the heart must be a result of disease of the kidney. He interpreted the cardiac hypertrophy as a compensation for the increased force necessary for propelling the blood through the diseased kidney.

A study of the effects of tissue extracts, which had resulted in the discovery of the pressor action of epinephrine and posterior pituitary extract, led to Tigerstedt and Bergman's[2] discovery of renin in 1898. These investigators injected a crude extract of renal tissue and noted its marked pressor effects. In allusion to its origin they designated the agent responsible for this action as renin. The simplicity of the concept that a pressor agent formed by the kidney would cause the observed elevation in blood pressure has persisted to the present time and has dominated theories of the pathogenesis of hypertension.

From the Laboratory for Experimental Medicine, Department of Pathology, University of Texas Southwestern Medical School, Dallas, Texas.

Previously unpublished studies included in the present paper were supported by a grant (71–1113) from the American Heart Association and the Lilien K. Christy Bequest.

The experimental work of the early decades of the present century was devoted primarily to studies of the effect of nephrectomy and other manipulations of the kidney on the blood pressure. Thus Mosler,[3] in 1912, reported a slight increase in blood pressure of rabbits surviving for 48 hours following nephrectomy. He attributed the rise in pressure to the retention of a pressor agent normally excreted by the kidney. The failure of nephrectomy to result in an elevation in blood pressure led most investigators to conclude that the production of a pressor agent was essential for the manifestation of hypertension.

Pässler and Heinecke,[4] in 1905, showed that partial nephrectomy in the dog resulted in hypertension associated with cardiac hypertrophy. The observed increase in blood pressure varied from 15 to 29 mm Hg. Chanutin and Ferris[5] also noted that partial nephrectomy in rats resulted in an elevation of blood pressure.

A great impetus to the modern study of hypertension was the demonstration by Goldblatt et al.[6] in 1934 that the application of a clamp to a renal artery of a dog with the subsequent removal of the opposite kidney resulted in a chronic elevation in blood pressure. Goldblatt's experiment was based on the assumption that hypertension in man was a result of ischemia of the kidney and that the application of the clamp was comparable to a reduction of the blood flow through the kidney by nephrosclerosis. Although this concept of the pathogenesis of hypertension was refuted by the observations of Bell,[7] Smithwick and Castleman,[8] and others, Goldblatt's procedure for the first time offered a practical method for experimentally inducing a condition analogous to that of essential hypertension, namely, the induction of an elevation in blood pressure without any apparent deficiency in renal excretory function.

Experimental Induction of Hypertension

Numerous procedures are available for inducing an elevation in blood pressure in experimental animals. In some of these, the hypertension is acute in onset and transient; in others, it develops more slowly. The introduction of methods for determining the blood pressure in the rat and operative procedures applicable to this laboratory animal made it possible to carry out experiments that are impracticable with the larger animals. The disease as induced in the rat and in other laboratory animals resembles that occurring spontaneously in the human being in its clinical, hemodynamic, and pathologic features. Despite the reluctance of some to accept results on animals as applicable to the human, the available results indicate that we are dealing with the same disease in the experimental animal and in man.

Most of the experimental procedures used for inducing hypertension involve some manipulation of the kidney or renal artery. Instead of applying a clamp and removing the contralateral kidney, as in the Goldblatt procedure, more consistent results are obtained by applying some form of compression to the kidney, most simply by a figure-of-eight ligature or a clip to the renal artery. A number of other procedures have been used, such as the removal of one kidney and the administration of desoxycorticosterone or other steroids,[9] or enucleation of the adrenals with unilateral nephrectomy.[10]

Other analogues of essential hypertension as it occurs in the human being have also been produced in experimental animals. The species whose manifestations are closest to those in man is the strain of the spontaneously hypertensive rat produced by selective inbreeding.[11,12] Like its human counterpart, the disorder in this case is inherited and genetic in origin and is unaccompanied by obvious renal lesions or evidence of renal excretory deficiency. A similar form of hypertension may be induced by treatment of pregnant rats in various ways.[13] The offspring of such animals are normotensive at birth but their blood pressure gradually rises with age to reach hypertensive levels on attaining adulthood.

Acute Remediable Hypertension

So-called renovascular or "surgically remediable" hypertension is also reproducible in the experimental animal. In fact, restriction of the renal artery or infarction of a kidney, the most commonly used procedures for inducing experimental hypertension, usually results in the production of this form of the disease which, like its human counterpart, is remediable by removal of the restriction or by nephrectomy. This form of hypertension may develop ultimately into chronic hypertension, particularly if the contralateral kidney is removed. During its early stages it has been erroneously used as an experimental model for essential and other forms of chronic hypertension.[14]

Ogden, Collings, and Sapirstein [15] first noted a difference in the mechanism maintaining an elevated pressure during the acute stage following application of a clamp to the renal artery from its subsequent elevation, a difference ignored in many of the preceding as well as the subsequent experimental studies. Another source of confusion has been the development of lesions in the untouched kidney which have been attributed to the effect of the elevated blood pressure but are also attributable in part at least to immune reactions.[16]

The acute hypertension which follows infarction of the kidney or drastic restriction of one renal artery in the rat is accompanied by the appearance of a pressor agent in the renal venous effluent.[14] As in the case of the human being, but unlike the dog, this pressor agent continues to be formed for some weeks. Removal of the kidney during this period results in a decline of the blood pressure to normal with disappearance of the pressor agent from the blood. Ultimately, particularly after removal of the opposite kidney or following bilateral infarction of the kidneys, chronic hypertension ensues in the absence of a circulating pressor agent.

Renoprival Hypertension

Removal of the kidneys in the frog, rat, dog, opossum, and man results in the development of hypertension if the animal survives a sufficiently long time (4 to 6 days) and is maintained in good condition. In animals with mild degrees of hypertension, even unilateral nephrectomy will cause a rise in blood pressure, often to hypertensive levels. The fact that implantation of the ureter into the vena cava, unlike removal of the kidney, does not cause a rise in blood pressure indicates that it is not uremia which is responsible for renoprival hypertension but rather the absence of the kidney.

The hypertensive state induced by restricting the blood flow to the kidney and by nephrectomy appears to be due to a common factor, namely, interference with and removal of that function of the kidney concerned in the maintenance of the normotensive state.

Neurogenic Hypertension

Since the nervous system is concerned with the maintenance of the blood pressure and nervous stimuli induce an elevation in blood pressure, various procedures involving the nervous system have been used to induce hypertension. Trephination of the skull and application of pressure to the dura or brain was shown by Naunyn and Schreiber [17] in 1881 to result in an immediate rise in systolic and diastolic pressures which persists as long as the elevated pressure is maintained. The injection of colloidal kaolin [18] to produce a chronically elevated intracranial pressure has resulted in variable responses, as have ligation of vessels in the neck and stimulation and ablation of the cortical and subcortical areas of the brain.[19] The most successful procedure for inducing neurogenic hypertension has been sectioning of the moderator nerves [20] and subjecting animals to audiogenic or other noxious stimuli.

Although elevations in blood pressure may be induced by the above-mentioned procedures the available evidence indicates that these constitute only hemodynamic alterations and not the reproduction of hypertensive cardiovascular disease.[21] Thus in the case of the elevation in blood pressure induced by section of the moderator nerves in the dog, physical exercise will often reduce the blood pressure to normal, and even when the elevation has persisted for years, the cardiac hypertrophy and arteriolar sclerosis characteristic of hypertensive disease do not appear.

One cannot accept the experimental models of so-called neurogenic hypertension as analogues of hypertensive disease comparable to that induced by the other procedures outlined above. The former are analogous to the hypertension noted in fracture of the skull, encephalitis, and other forms of neurogenic hypertension in the human being which also differ basically from hypertensive cardiovascular disease.[19] Despite many efforts to incriminate the nervous system in the pathogenesis of hypertension the preponderance of evidence supports the view that neither the central nor autonomic nervous systems are concerned in the disorder except as secondary consequences of a generalized disturbance.

Classification of Experimental Hypertension

Much of the confusion and inconsistency noted in the literature on experimental hypertension is a result of considering any elevation of the blood pressure as reflecting the existence of hypertensive disease. Criteria exist for defining essential hypertension and other forms of hypertensive cardiovascular disease in man and the same criteria must be applied in experimental studies before accepting a given preparation as an analogue of the disease as it occurs in the human. As already indicated, for example, experimental neurogenic hypertension, like its clinical analogue, must be looked upon as a hemodynamic variation with an elevation of pressure mediated through stimuli from the nervous system-activating vasomotor function and unrelated to hypertensive cardiovascular disease.

Most laboratory procedures in which hypertension is induced by restricting the renal artery, including the original procedure of Goldblatt, represent analogues of acute, surgically remediable or renovascular, rather than chronic hypertensive, disease, as is usually assumed. Studies carried out on such preparations will give inconsistent results during the period when the elevation in blood pressure is partially due to a circulating pressor agent and in part to chronic hypertensive disease.[22]

Renoprival hypertension manifests all the characteristics of severe chronic hypertension. There is no valid reason for considering it as a specific entity.

PRESSOR AGENTS

Many investigators have been concerned with pressor agents as mediators of the elevated blood pressure observed in hypertension. Braun-Menéndez and his collaborators [23] in Argentina and Page and Helmer [24] in the United States showed that Tigerstedt and Bergman's renin was an enzyme which, acting on its substrate, angiotensinogen, formed a decapeptide, angiotensin I which, in turn, by action of a converting enzyme, formed an octapeptide, angiotensin II.[25] Although it is a potent pressor agent and despite the many attempts to implicate it as the mediator of chronic hypertension, the evidence indicates that this is not the case.[26,27]

Angiotensin, through its action on the adrenal cortex to liberate aldosterone, plays an important role in the maintenance of salt and water homeostasis which indirectly is concerned with the extracellular fluid volume and blood pressure. Accordingly its role in hypertension must be looked upon as a permissive rather than as an etiologic or pathogenetic one.

The source of renin in the kidney is generally accepted as being in the juxtaglomerular zone as first indicated by Goormaghtigh.[28] Changes in the renin content of the kidney, as is to be anticipated, occur with changes in blood pressure since the latter is dependent on the extracellular fluid volume and salt and water metabolism.[29]

Changes in the number of granules present in the juxtaglomerular zone [30,31] and variation in the renin content of the kidneys [32] have been studied widely but, as anticipated from the indirect relation of renin to hypertension, have failed to elucidate the pathogenesis of the hypertensive state. The same has been true of the numerous studies of angiotensin in various conditions associated with hypertension.[27] Of particular interest is the fact that immunization with angiotensin fails to prevent the development of hypertension.[33]

A circulating pressor agent may be demonstrated to be present in the blood during the acute (surgically remediable) stage of hypertension which follows drastic restriction of the renal artery, infarction of the kidney, malignant hypertension, and certain other rare conditions in the human. This pressor agent was originally assumed to be renin and more recently has been claimed to be angiotensin I.[34] Evidence exists to indicate, however, that it is a unique pressor agent of renal origin which has been designated as nephrotensin.[22]

Angiotensin acts as a trophic hormone for aldosterone. Injected in nonpressor doses, it stimulates the secretion of aldosterone without affecting the rate of secretion of hydrocortisone and maintains this action as long as its administration is continued. The pressor action of aldosterone is related to the sodium balance, the crucial determinant of the angiotensin-aldosterone hormonal system.[35]

There is no correlation between the blood renin levels and the height of the blood pressure in either human or experimental hypertension. In sodium-depleted rats, both renal and blood renin levels are elevated [32] but the blood pressure is normal. In adrenalectomized rats the blood pressure is low and the renin level is high; whereas in those given desoxycorticosterone and salt, the blood pressure is high but the renin level is low. Renin and angiotensin, accordingly, play a role in normal homeostasis in the control of renal blood flow and function, aldosterone secretion, and sodium balance, but not in the pathogenesis of renal hypertension. In this way the kidneys maintain a constant blood flow despite changes in arterial perfusion pressure. Plasma renin rises with salt restriction and returns to normal with salt repletion, changes which parallel aldosterone secretion produced by the same maneuver.[36]

Renin is found not only in the kidney but also in the placenta, uterus, arterial wall, salivary glands, and other tissues.[37] It is not a single enzyme; related enzymes, such as the pseudorenin of Skeggs et al.,[38] have been described.

ANTIHYPERTENSIVE RENAL FACTORS

In spite of the preoccupation with renin as the mediator of hypertensive cardiovascular disease, it soon became apparent that it was more likely that the disorder was mediated by some other mechanism, possibly by the production by the kidney of a humoral factor. That extracts of renal tissue were capable of lowering the blood pressure of experimental animals and in several human patients was reported by Grollman, Williams, and Harrison [39] in 1940. The extract used by these investigators was unique in that it was dialyzable, effective when administered orally, and nontoxic, and did not lower the blood pressure in the normotensive. An extract of renal origin prepared by Page and his colleagues [40] was not dialyzable and effective only on parenteral injection. It was pyrogenic and it soon became apparent that like other pyrogens and toxic agents it owed its blood pressure-lowering effects to its noxious actions.

Whole-kidney extracts which reduce the blood pressure in the hypertensive have also been prepared by Milliez et al.[41] Lee et al.[42] and Muirhead et al.[43] have prepared extracts from renomedullary tissue. The acidic lipids present in these extracts have been shown to owe their activity to the presence of prostaglandins E_2 and A_2.[42] Muirhead et al.[43] have also described a neutral lipid which, like that of the previously described extracts of Grollman, Williams, and Harrison,[39] lowers the arterial pressure of the hypertensive rabbit steadily over 24 to 48 hours. After this depressed pressure has remained for a certain period it gradually returns to preinjection levels over another 24- to 48-hour period, the entire response entailing 3 to 4 days. In comparable doses it does not appreciably alter the pressure of normal animals. This antihypertensive, neutral renomedullary lipid is believed to originate from the lipid-laden interstitial cells of the renal medulla, which have characteristics of secretory cells, their lipid content being lowered during the hypertensive state.[44]

A phospholipid has been isolated from kidneys which inhibits renin.[45] It also reduces the blood pressure of rats with acute and chronic renal hypertension but has no effect on the blood pressure of normotensive animals. The significance of this compound and its relation to the other antihypertensive renal agents remains to be established.

The widespread distribution of prostaglandins in the organism and their action on the blood vessels suggest that they function in the local humoral control of the circulation and the permeability of the renotubular epithelium, particularly that of the medulla. It is doubtful, however, that they represent the renohumoral factor concerned in the maintenance of the normotensive state. In the rat, Sokabe and Grollman [46] found that it is the cortex rather than the medulla which is the site of formation of the antihypertensive principle. The fact that medullary extracts afford no protection against arteriolar thickening,[43] a change characteristic of the hypertensive state, and that cystic disease of the medulla is not accompanied by hypertension also speak against the view that it is the medulla which is responsible for the maintenance of the normotensive state.

Hemodynamics of Hypertension

Established hypertension is a state in which hypertonic terminal arteries at one end of the arterial tree and an overactive left ventricle at the other combine to raise blood pressure without markedly altering blood flow. Bright recognized that either of these could be the immediate cause of the elevated blood pressure, but there remains the possibility that the abnormality may involve a more primitive myogenic reaction, i.e., the arterial muscle might become abnormally sensitive to a normal filling tension, or an increase in cardiac output might provoke a secondary vasoconstriction.

Ledingham and Cohen [47] have described a brief period of vasoconstriction followed by a sustained increase in cardiac output during the development of renal hypertension and a transient fall after removal of a Goldblatt clamp. They suggest that an altered relationship between the blood volume and the vascular tone is the cause of experimental hypertension. This conclusion was based on the observation of an increased cardiac output in the early stages of the disease followed later by an increased peripheral resistance. Since these studies were performed shortly after operation, the observed rise in cardiac output may be attributed to the presence of the circulating pressor agent secreted by the kidney that is unrelated to the subsequent development of chronic hypertension.[16] It is of interest in this connection that Olmsted and Page [48] and Grollman et al.[49] failed to note an increased cardiac output in dogs rendered hypertensive by compression of the kidney or nephrectomy, respectively.

Electrolyte Metabolism

That salt intake in the human affects the level of the arterial blood pressure was noted at the beginning of the century and salt restriction was recommended for treatment of the disease over a half-century ago. Experimental studies in animals demonstrated that it was the sodium ion which was responsible for the hypotensive action of salt deprivation and that the effectiveness of the rice and fruit diets was due to their low sodium content.[49]

Dahl and his collaborators [51] have shown that some animals on a high-salt diet develop hypertension while others remain resistant. By selective breeding they developed two statistically separate populations from one unselected strain of rats. One of these was sensitive, the other resistant, to the development of hypertension from a high-salt diet. A similar difference in response was noted after administration of salt and desoxycorticosterone, as well as manipulations of the kidney conducive to hypertension. These results conform with the postulate that the rat like man harbors the genetic defect responsible for hypertension and in many cases manifests a mild degree of this disease as reflected in the wide range of basal blood pressure values generally accepted as normotensive.[51]

Many studies have been directed to establishing the role of sodium in hypertension. Baldwin et al.[53] reported a primary renal defect in sodium reabsorption and concentrating power in the disease. They found afferent and efferent arteriolar vasoconstriction with diversion of blood from some nephrons, a normal para-aminohippuric acid excretion, and an abnormally rapid natriuresis. The latter, however, occurs in any state in which there is an elevation in blood pressure and can be induced by raising the blood pressure with metaraminol. Slight occlusion of the renal artery reduces salt and water excretion, and the presence of unilateral disease results in a similar condition.

Ebihara, Martz, and Grollman [54] have also noted the increased urinary output and the greater reduction in the urinary excretion of sodium in the hypertensive as compared to the normotensive rat on withdrawal of dietary sodium. The hypertensive rat thus retains sodium more efficiently than does the normotensive animal after sodium withdrawal, but this may be secondary to the increased urinary output rather than to the hypertension.

The idea that hypertensive disease is a systemic disorder rather than simply a hemodynamic alteration has been supported by the demonstration of changes in various functions of the organism. Thus changes in the electrolyte and water content of skeletal muscle first demonstrated by Eichelberger [55] have been shown to involve other organs (brain, liver, etc.) with a rise in their sodium and decrease in their potassium content.[56] Similar changes have been observed in blood vessels.[57] The extracellular fluid volume is also expanded in the hypertensive.[58]

Theories of Pathogenesis of Hypertension

Clinical and experimental studies of hypertension have led to a variety of theories regarding its pathogenesis, but none of these has received general acceptance. Some of these theories are in conflict with the available facts, as has already been noted; others are all-embracing and not amenable to experimental test and hence are of no practical value. Any theory of the pathogenesis of hypertension worthy of consideration must be compatible with the available data and offer practical approaches for further study of the disorder. Postulating a multiplicity of factors in the pathogenesis of hypertension would be useful only if the factors could be severally demonstrated and measured.

Malignant Hypertension

The malignant phase of hypertension is also observed in the experimental animal. It may appear spontaneously, as in the human being, or may be induced, for example, by drastic restriction of the renal artery or by other procedures.

Malignant hypertension may be defined as a syndrome in which a systemic arterial pressure well above the normal range coexists with focal, fibrinoid arteriolar necroses, particularly in the kidneys, and with retinal vascular lesions usually accompanied by papilledema. Neither the fibrinoid arteriolar necrosis nor the papilledema is, however, specific for severe hypertension. The former may occur in polyarteritis nodosa without hypertension and at the edges of infarcts or in areas of intense vasoconstriction provoked by vasopressin in the absence of any rise in systemic arterial pressure. The demonstration of the appearance of a circulating pressor agent in malignant hypertension suggests that this agent may also contribute to the inordinate rise in blood pressure and vascular damage induced by this disorder.

References

1. Bright, R.: Causes and observations, illustrative of renal disease accompanied with the secretion of albuminous urine. Guys Hosp. Rep. 1:338, 1836.
2. Tigerstedt, R., and Bergman, P. G.: Niere und Kreislauf. Scand. Arch. Physiol. 8:223, 1898.
3. Mosler, E.: Ueber Blutdrucksteigerung nach doppelseitiger Nierenexstirpation. Zeit. Klin. Med. 74:297, 1912.
4. Pässler, H., and Heinecke, D.: Versuche zur Pathologie des Morbus Brightii. Verh. Dtsch. Pathol. 9:99, 1905.
5. Chanutin, A., and Ferris, E. J., Jr.: Experimental renal insufficiency produced by partial nephrectomy. Arch. Intern. Med. 49:767, 1932.
6. Goldblatt, H., Lynch, J., Hanzal, R. F., and Summerville, W. W.: Studies in experimental hypertension: The production of persistent elevation of systolic blood pressure by means of renal ischemia. J. Exp. Med. 59:347, 1934.
7. Bell, C. T.: The pathological anatomy in primary hypertension. *In* Bell, E. T. (Ed.): Hypertension: A Symposium. Minneapolis: University of Minnesota Press, 1951, pp. 183–185.
8. Smithwick, R. H., and Castleman, B.: Some observations on renal vascular disease in hypertensive patients based on biopsy material obtained at operation. *In* Bell, E. T. (Ed.): Hypertension: A Symposium. Minneapolis: University of Minnesota Press, 1951, pp. 199–201.
9. Grollman, A., Harrison, T. R., and Williams, J. R., Jr.: The effect of various sterol derivatives on the blood pressure of the rat. J. Pharmacol. Exp. Ther. 69:149, 1940.
10. Skelton, F. R.: Development of hypertension and cardiovascular-renal lesions during adrenal regeneration in the rat. Proc. Soc. Exp. Biol. Med. 90:342, 1955.
11. Smirk, F. H., and Hall, W. H.: Inherited hypertension in rats. Nature 182:727, 1958.
12. Okamoto, K., and Kyuzo, A.: Development of a strain of spontaneously hypertensive rats, Jap. Circ. J. 27:282, 1963.
13. Grollman, A., and Grollman, E. F.: The teratogenic induction of hypertension. J. Clin. Invest. 41:710, 1962.
14. Grollman, A.: Pressor activity of circulating blood after focal infarction of the kidney in the rat. Proc. Soc. Exp. Biol. Med. 134:1120, 1970.
15. Ogden, E., Collings, W. D., and Sapirstein, L. A.: A change of mechanism in the course of hypertension of renal origin. N. Y. Acad. Sci. Special Publication, vol. 3, 1946, p. 153.
16. White, F. N., and Grollman, A.: Autoimmune factors associated with infarction of the kidney. Nephron 1:93, 1964.
17. Naunyn, B., and Schreiber, J.: Ueber Gehirndruck. Arch. Exp. Pathol. Pharmak. 14:1, 1881.
18. Griffith, J. Q., Jr., Jeffers, W. A., and Lindauer, M. A.: A study of the mechanisms of hypertension following intracranial kaolin injection of rats; leucocytic reaction and effect on lymphatic absorption. Am. J. Physiol. 113:285, 1935.
19. Tyler, H. R., and Dawson, D.: Hypertension and its relation to the nervous system. Ann. Intern. Med. 55:681, 1961.
20. Heymans, C., Bouchaert, J. J., and Regniers, P.: Le Sinus Carotidien. Paris: Doin et Cie, 1933.
21. Grollman, A.: Experimental studies on the pathogenesis and nature of hypertensive cardiovascular disease. *In* Wolstenholme, G. E. W., and Cameron, M. P. (Eds.): Ciba Foundation Symposium on Hypertension. Boston: Little, Brown, 1954, p. 135.
22. Grollman, A., and Krishnamurty, V. S. R.: A new pressor agent of renal origin: Its differentiation from renin and angiotensin. Am. J. Physiol. 221:1499, 1971.
23. Braun-Menéndez, E., Fasciolo, J. C., Leloir, L. F., Muñoz, J. M., and Taquini, A.: Hypertension arterial nefrogena. Buenos Aires: Libreria y Editorial El Ateneo, 1939.
24. Page, I. H., and Helmer, O. M.: A crystalline pressor substance, angiotonin, resulting from the reaction between renin and renin activator. J. Exp. Med. 71:29, 1940.

25. Helmer, O. M.: Differentiation between two forms of angiotensin by means of spirally cut strips of rabbit aorta. Am. J. Physiol. 188: 571, 1957.
26. Mylon, E., Lund, M., and Heller, J. H.: Limitations of the renin-angiotensin hypothesis. Am. J. Physiol. 152:397, 1948.
27. Kotchen, T. A., Lytton, B., Morrow, L. B., Mulrow, P. J., Shutkin, P. M., and Stansel, H. C.: Angiotensin and aldosterone in renovascular hypertension. Arch. Intern. Med. 125:265, 1970.
28. Goormaghtigh, N.: Existence of an endocrine gland in the media of the renal arterioles. Proc. Soc. Exp. Biol. Med. 42: 688, 1939.
29. Ebihara, A., Martz, B. L., and Grollman, A.: Effect of withdrawal of dietary sodium in hypertensive and normotensive rats, Japanese Heart J. 11:365, 1970.
30. Hartroft, P. M., and Hartroft, W. S.: Renal juxtaglomerular cells. I. Variations produced by sodium chloride and desoxycorticosterone acetate. J. Exp. Med. 94:415, 1953.
31. Tobian, L.: Interrelationship of electrolytes, juxtaglomerular cells and hypertension. Physiol. Rev. 40:280, 1960.
32. Gross, F., Brunner, H., and Ziegler, M.: Renin-angiotensin system, aldosterone and sodium balance. Recent Progr. Hormone Res. 21:119, 1965.
33. Eide, I., and Aars, H.: Renal hypertension in rabbits immunized with angiotensin. Nature 222:571, 1969.
34. Carey, R. M., Schweikert, J. R., and Liddle, G. W.: Radioimmunoassay of renal venous angiotensin I in the diagnosis of renovascular hypertension. Endocrinology 57:A115, 1971.
35. Massani, Z. M., Finkielman, S., Worcel, M., Agrest, A., and Paladini, A. C.: Angiotensin blood levels in hypertensive and non-hypertensive diseases. Clin. Sci. 30:473, 1966.
36. Blair-West, J. R., Coghlan, J. P., Denton, D. A., Orchard, E., Scoggins, B. A., and Wright, R. D.: Renin-angiotensin-aldosterone system and sodium balance in experimental renal hypertension. Endocrinology 83:1199, 1968.
37. Bing, J., and Faarup, P.: Localization and site of formation of extrarenal renin. International Club on Arterial Hypertension. Milliez, P. and Tcherdakoff, P. (Eds.): *In* L'hypertension Artérielle. Paris: L'Expansion Scientifique Francaise, 1966, pp. 75–84.
38. Skeggs, L. T., Lentz, K. E., Kahn, J. R., Dorer, F. E., and Levine, M.: Pseudorenin, a new angiotensin-forming enzyme. Circ. Res. 25:451, 1969.
39. Grollman, A., Williams, J. R., Jr., and Harrison, T. R.: The preparation of renal extracts capable of reducing the blood pressure of animals with experimental renal hypertension. J. Biol. Chem. 134:115, 1940.
40. Page, I. H., Helmer, O. M., Kohlstaedt, K. G., Fouts, P. J., and Kempf, G. F.: Reduction of arterial blood pressure of hypertensive patients and animals with extracts of kidneys. J. Exp. Med. 73:7, 1941.
41. Milliez, P., Meyer, Ph., Lagrue, G., and Boivin, P.: Action hypotensive d'un extrait de rein chez le lapin en hypertension artérielle expérimentale. Pathol. Biol. 9:1887, 1961.
42. Lee, J. B., Covino, B. G., Takman, B. H., and Smith, E. R.: Renomedullary vasodepressor substance, medullin: Isolation, chemical characterization and physiological properties. Circ. Res. 17:57, 1965.
43. Muirhead, E. E., Leach, B. E., Byers, L. W., Brooks, B., Daniels, E. G., and Hinman, J. W.: Antihypertensive neutral renomedullary lipids. *In* Fisher, J. W. (Ed.): Kidney Hormones. New York: Academic Press, 1971, pp. 485–506.
44. Mandal, A. K., Muehrcke, R. C., Epstein, M., and Volini, F. I.: Relationship of the renomedullary interstitial cells to experimental hypertension. J. Lab. Clin. Med. 70:872, 1967.
45. Sen, S., Smeby, R. R., and Bumpus, F. M.: Antihypertensive effect of an isolated phospholipid. Am. J. Physiol. 214:337, 1968.
46. Sokabe, H., and Grollman, A.: Localization of blood pressure regulating and erythropoietic function in rat kidney. Am. J. Physiol. 203:991, 1962.
47. Ledingham, J. M., and Cohen, R. D.: The role of the heart in the pathogenesis of renal hypertension. Lancet 2:979, 1963.
48. Olmsted, F., and Page, I. H.: Hemodynamic changes in trained dogs during experimental renal hypertension. Circ. Res. 16:134, 1965.
49. Grollman, T., Turner, L. B., Levitch, M., and Hill, D.: Hemodynamics of bilaterally nephrectomized dog subjected to intermittent peritoneal lavage. Am. J. Physiol. 165:167, 1951.
50. Grollman, A., Harrison, T., Mason, M., Baxter, J., Crampton, J., and Reichsman, R.: Sodium restriction in the diet for hypertension. JAMA 129:533, 1945.
51. Dahl, L. K., Heine, M., and Tassinari, L.: Effects of chronic excess salt ingestion. Evidence that genetic factors play an important

role in susceptibility to experimental hypertension. J. Exp. Med. 115:1173, 1962.

52. Grollman, A.: The spontaneous hypertensive rat: An experimental analogue of essential hypertension in the human being. *In* Okamoto, K. (Ed.): U.S.–Japanese Symposium on the Spontaneous Hypertensive Rat. Kyoto, 1971, pp. 238–242.
53. Baldwin, D. S., Biggs, A. W., Goldring, W., Hulet, W. H., and Chasis, H.: Exaggerated natriuresis in essential hypertension. Am. J. Med. 24:893, 1958.
54. Ebihara, A., Martz, B. L., and Grollman, A.: Effect of withdrawal of dietary sodium in hypertensive and normotensive rats. Jap. Heart J. 11:365, 1970.
55. Eichelberger, L.: Distribution of water and electrolyte between blood and skeletal muscle in experimental hypertension. J. Exp. Med. 77:205, 1943.
56. Laramore, D. C., and Grollman, A.: Water and electrolyte content of tissue in normal and hypertensive rats. Am. J. Physiol. 161: 278, 1950.
57. Tobian, L., and Binion, J. T.: Tissue cations and water in arterial hypertension. Circulation 5:754, 1952.
58. Grollman, A., and Shapiro, A. P.: The volume of extracellular fluid in experimental and human hypertension. J. Clin. Invest. 32:312, 1953.

Hemodynamics of Experimental Renal Hypertension

By Carlos M. Ferrario, M.D., and James W. McCubbin, M.D.

Renal hypertension is one of the most easily studied forms of experimental hypertension and, especially when compared with essential hypertension in man, it can be investigated with relative ease. Despite this, it is only in recent years that we have begun to understand some of the basic hemodynamic mechanisms that account for rise in arterial pressure of renal origin.

In part, our poor understanding of these mechanisms has been related to lack of adequate methods to measure precisely both flows and pressures in unanesthetized animals before and during the course of the disease. This is why essentially all previous studies have, by necessity, employed anesthetic agents.[1–7] Since we now know that these agents cause profound hemodynamic changes, techniques had to be developed to make chronic measurements in resting animals without inflicting discomfort. Recent refinements in electromagnetic flowmeter technology have provided us with a tool that now makes it possible to make long-term measurements of blood flow in unanesthetized dogs, and thus to follow more precisely the sequence of hemodynamic events that accounts for establishment of renal hypertension.

But lack of adequate methods does not account alone for the seemingly conflicting observations reported throughout the literature. We believe that there are other equally important reasons for this discrepancy. One to be considered is the nature of the stimulus to the kidney that leads to hypertension. It is possible that the stimulus may differ with the method by which renal hypertension is elicited, or that it may vary between animal species. Unilateral stenosis of a renal artery in rats consistently produces hypertension while, in dogs, it is usually necessary to combine clipping with removal of the contralateral normal kidney.[8,9] In addition, the stimulus signaling the kidney to produce hypertension may be of predetermined magnitude, such as renal artery constriction, or may grow progressively stronger, as in hypertension caused by cellophane wrapping.[10] It may even regress, as when collateral circulation develops during the course of renovascular hypertension.

Time is an equally important factor. Different forms of hypertension take different time courses: it appears within days after renal artery constriction but only after weeks or months [10] following wrapping the kidneys in cellophane. While there is general agreement that an increase in total peripheral resistance accounts for the maintenance of elevated blood pressure in the established stage of renal hypertension, it is only recently that evidence has appeared indicating the possibility that other hemodynamic mechanisms are active in the developmental phase of the disease. If arterial hypertension is a disease of regulation, it stands to reason that as the circulatory system maintains equilibrium, one or more hemodynamic mechanisms may predominate at any one time. An example is the upward reset of the carotid baroreceptors which was found by McCubbin [11] to lag behind the gradual rise in blood pressure. It is logical to assume that at this time the baroreceptors oppose, at least in part, the progressive elevation of pressure.

It is only prudent to consider all these influences before a "single mechanism" is assigned as the cause of renal hypertension. With this in mind, we shall examine two of the major outstanding problems in renal hypertension: what is the nature of the intrarenal stimulus that signals the kidney to produce hypertension, and secondly, what hemodynamic changes result in sustained rise in arterial pressure.

From The Cleveland Clinic Foundation, Cleveland, Ohio.

Dr. Ferrario is an Established Investigator of the American Heart Association.

Nature of the Intrarenal Hemodynamic Stimuli Leading to Hypertension

It has been generally held that hypertension associated with renal disease is prompted by a decrease in renal blood flow to the functional components of the kidney.[8–12] The term "renal ischemia" to describe a cause of hypertension has enjoyed common usage by clinicians and researchers alike, though there is, at present, no irrefutable proof that ischemia is a factor concerned with the development of high blood pressure. In fact, studies of Corcoran and Page,[13] Kohlstaedt and Page,[14] and others [15–16] have cast doubt upon the belief that renal ischemia, as proposed by Goldblatt,[12] is a factor signaling the kidney to produce an elevation in systemic blood pressure.

Since precise, serial measurements of renal blood flow have not been made before and after production of hypertension by renal artery constriction, electromagnetic flowmeters were implanted around renal arteries of 15 unanesthetized dogs, and renal blood flow and arterial pressure were measured in each of them daily before, for 15 days after removal of the contralateral untouched kidney and for up to 64 days after narrowing of the renal artery with an externally adjustable clamp.[17] A progressive increase in both pulsatile and mean renal blood flow to the clamped kidney occurred in each of the 15 trained, unanesthetized dogs following removal of the contralateral kidney. These increases stabilized after 8 to 14 days of rising values at 244 ± 20 (SE) ml per minute in mean renal blood flow, an average of 43 percent above control values. This compensatory increase in blood flow to the remaining kidney was not accompanied by significant changes in either mean arterial pressure or cardiac rate.

At this time, the dogs were arbitrarily divided into two groups to study the effect of either a *moderate* or *severe* degree of renal artery constriction on both renal blood flow and development of hypertension. In 10 of the 15 dogs, the clamp placed around the renal artery was tightened sufficiently to cause a 20 ± 2 (SE)-percent decrease in systolic blood flow from the values averaged during the 14 days that preceded adjustment. This mild reduction in the amplitude of the flow pulse was sufficiently small to cause no significant change in mean renal blood flow at the time of adjustment. The course of rise in arterial pressure in these 10 dogs was variable but, in general, a sustained hypertensive plateau developed between the 16th and 23rd days after reducing the lumen of the renal artery. Onset of arterial hypertension was associated initially with a moderate fall in mean renal blood flow (-56 ± 9 ml per minute) lasting for a few days only. As hypertension became established, total mean renal blood flow returned to, or even increased above, the elevated values produced by contralateral nephrectomy (Fig. 1). Despite the absence of a reduction in mean renal blood flow when hypertension became established, the dynamic component of renal flow, i.e., the difference between systolic and diastolic flows, remained strikingly diminished. Narrowing of the flow pulse changed little throughout the period that followed renal artery constriction, despite the fact that the tachycardia observed during the first few days did not endure.

Renal perfusion pressure distal to the clamp was also measured in four of these 10 chronic, benign hypertensive dogs, both immediately before and after constriction of the renal artery, and once again, at 10, 15, and 23 days following adjustment. Measurements were obtained by introducing a fine needle connected to a strain-gauge through a Teflon catheter permanently fastened to a plastic sleeve surrounding the artery. A pressure gradient on the average of 44 ± 4 mm Hg was found between systemic arterial and renal perfusion after moderate constriction of the renal artery. It persisted even after hypertension was established and mean renal blood flow was elevated. At this time, renal perfusion pressure distal to the constriction was above normal (range: 83 to 115 mm Hg) but remained comparatively low with respect to systemic pressure (range: 128 to 153 mm Hg). It is probable that a pressure gradient across the stenotic renal artery persists indefinitely in renovascular hypertension.

These experiments indicate, contrary to current belief, that mean renal blood flow is normal in the chronic, benign form of renovascular hypertension in trained, unanesthetized dogs,[18] and make untenable the suggestion

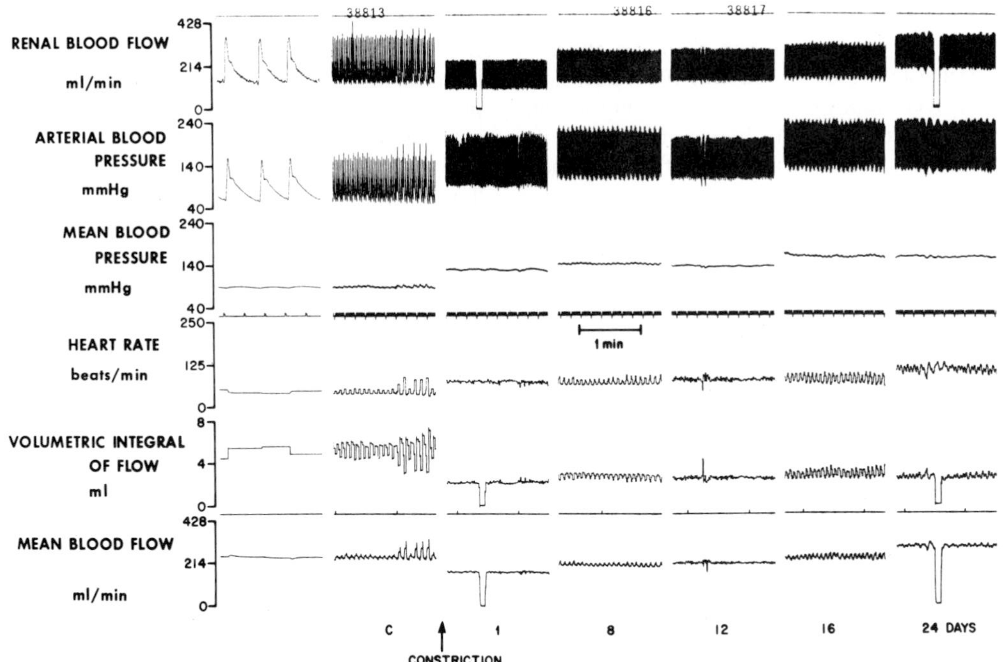

FIG. 1.—Hemodynamic course of arterial hypertension in a trained, unanesthetized dog before and after mild renal artery constriction. Progressive increase in arterial pressure is accompanied by increase in renal blood flow to values above those established after unilateral nephrectomy (*C*). Persistent hypertension is accompanied by moderate cardiac acceleration and a continued decrease in the amplitude of the flow pulse as indicated by the volumetric integral of the flow pulse.

that gross renal ischemia alone is the factor that signals the kidney to produce hypertension.

For reasons that are not now clear, restoration of mean blood flow after development of hypertension was associated with persistent decrease in the amplitude of the flow pulse, which cannot be accounted for by increases in heart rate. Tachycardia usually subsided with time in the hypertensive dogs but the small pulse persisted. Aside from a possible intrarenal redistribution of flow,[19] the majority of the evidence from the experiment makes it more likely that the intrarenal hemodynamic signal accounting for hypertension is reduction in the pulsatile component of renal flow, a fall in renal perfusion pressure with respect to systemic pressure, or a combination of both.

With more severe constriction of the renal artery the situation may be different. In the other five unilaterally nephrectomized dogs, a larger fall in systolic blood flow (average of -46 ± 7 percent) and, hence, pulse flow was produced. This more severe degree of renal artery constriction was accompanied by a fall in mean renal blood flow, and was followed within days by the appearance of accelerated hypertension and marked deterioration of renal function that terminated in death.

IDENTIFICATION OF THE HEMODYNAMIC FACTOR(S) ACCOUNTING FOR RISE IN PERIPHERAL RESISTANCE

The second aspect of our studies is concerned with characterization of the hemodynamic changes that account for renal hypertension. Although, in theory, increases in either cardiac output or peripheral resistance can produce a sustained increase in arterial pressure, it is only recently that the heart has been thought to play some role in the development of high blood pressure. In the nineteenth century, Richard Bright (1836) drew attention to the cardiac hypertrophy that is associated with arterial hypertension and speculated that it may be the cause rather than the effect of hypertension. During the next 100 years, however, hypertrophy was considered only a compensatory response to hypertension. In the early 1950s, interest in the heart as a primary factor in certain forms of hypertension was revived and substantiated by the findings of Widimsky, Fejfarova, and Fejfar; [20] they reported elevation of cardiac output without increase in total peripheral resistance in a substantial group of juvenile hypertensives. In the following years, evidence continued to accumulate suggesting that the heart may play a more important etiologic role than is generally accorded it. In trying to clarify the relation between reduced sodium excretion by the hypertensive kidney of a rat in parabiosis with its pair, and raised blood pressure, Floyer and Richardson [21] produced evidence that suggested an alternative mechanism to the commonly accepted hypothesis of primary arteriolar constriction. By measuring cardiac output with electromagnetic flowmeters in rats, Ledingham and Cohen,[22] and Ledingham and Pelling,[23] demonstrated that in the early phase of hypertension due to renal artery stenosis a transient increase in output accompanied rise in arterial pressure. Olmsted and Page [24] were unable to confirm the results of Ledingham and his co-workers. They implanted electromagnetic flowmeters in dogs and found that both heart rate and cardiac output decreased during the first 4 days after renal artery constriction and contralateral nephrectomy; rise in arterial pressure was due entirely to increased peripheral resistance. Later, output and heart rate returned to normal, but peripheral resistance and pressure remained elevated.

Since it was evident that further work was necessary to clarify these contradictory findings, we reexamined the problem in trained, unanesthetized dogs with chronically implanted flowmeters and produced hypertension by the cellophane perinephritis method.[25] Briefly, this study showed that an increase in cardiac output due solely to a rise in stroke volume preceded for many days any rise in both arterial pressure and total peripheral resistance. Increases in cardiac output occurred as early as

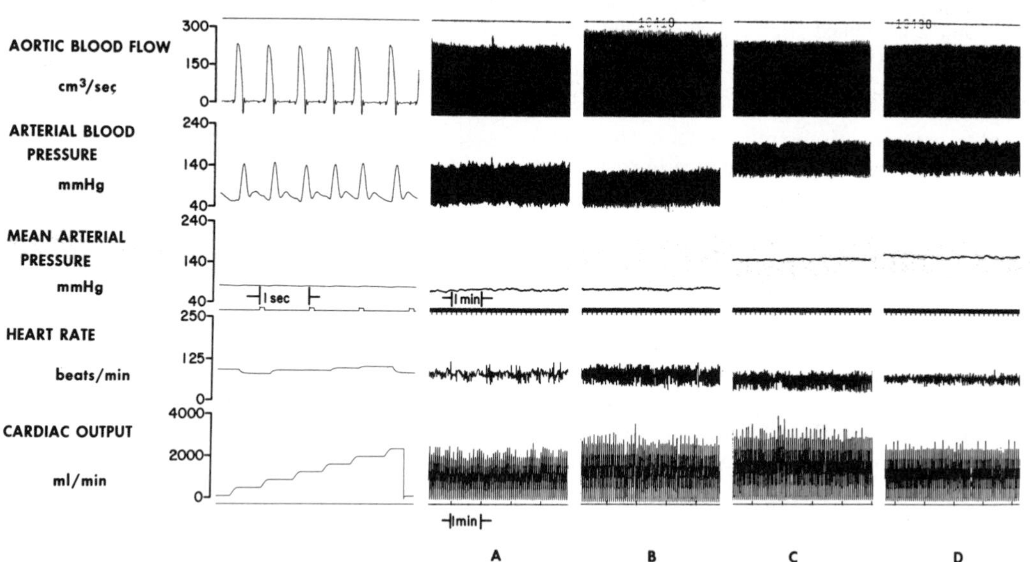

FIG. 2.—Hemodynamic course of arterial hypertension due to perinephritis and nephrectomy as recorded in a trained, unanesthetized dog. *A,* Control. *B,* Moderate increase in cardiac output 12 days after wrapping one kidney in cellophane with the normal kidney still in situ. *C,* Onset of hypertension associated with further increase in cardiac output 16 days after removal of the normal kidney. *D,* Sustained arterial hypertension 41 days after removal of the right kidney with return of cardiac output towards control values. (From Ferrario et al.,[25] by permission of the American Heart Association, Inc.)

8 days after wrapping one kidney in cellophane, with the opposite kidney untouched. Removal of the opposite kidney caused a further increase in cardiac output and, within days thereafter, arterial pressure began to rise. Four weeks after nephrectomy, peripheral resistance became progressively the predominant cause of elevated pressure, while cardiac output returned to control values (Fig. 2).

This sequence of events, particularly the early rise in cardiac output that preceded an increase in arterial pressure, may help provide insight into the mechanism involved in the production of renal hypertension. Several possibilities were considered. Hemodilution was not responsible, since in our experiments,[25] as in those of others,[23] hematocrit was unchanged after production of hypertension.

An increase in myocardial contractility due to enhanced cardiac sympathetic discharge does not account for the increase in output. Dogs with their cardiac sympathetic nerves excised (T1 to T7) also respond to cellophane wrapping with a rise in cardiac output preceding any increase in systemic arterial pressure (Fig. 3).

The remaining possibility, an increase in venous return due to an increased tone of the capacitance vessels without a corresponding change in the volume of their contents, is favored by us as a likely possibility for the increase in cardiac output. This proposal is supported by the findings that mean circulatory pressure increased in the perinephritic dogs prior to a rise in mean arterial pressure and in the absence of changes in plasma and total blood volume.[25] The possibility that venoconstriction is the cause of increased cardiac output in renal hypertension was advanced by Floyer and Richardson,[21] and by Wilson.[26] Richardson, Fermoso and Guyton [7] have reported that mean circulatory pressure, which could have reflected venoconstriction, increased in dogs with hypertension 3 weeks after renal artery constriction and unilateral nephrectomy. Other evidence compatible with participation of capacitance vessels in the genesis of hypertension is the observation that capillary thinning and diminished vascularity of the nail fold and conjunctival vessels occur.[27] There is elevation of the so-called "intrinsic blood pressure," [28,29] which is obtained indirectly and

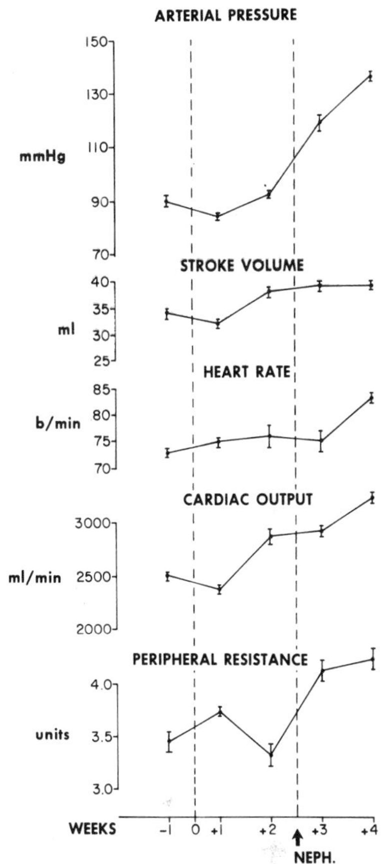

FIG. 3.—Development of arterial hypertension caused by cellophane wrapping of kidney in a trained, unanesthetized dog after sympathetic cardiac denervation. Increase in cardiac output accompanied onset of hypertension despite absence of efferent cardiac sympathetic innervation.

is assumed to reflect size of the capacitance vessels. Hypertensive patients show increased responsiveness to reduction of plasma and extracellular fluid volume, and there is exaggerated natriuresis following small infusions of saline or plasma expanders.[30] On the other hand, Overbeck et al.[31] have disputed the possibility that venoconstriction may play a role in dogs with chronic renal hypertension by assuming that changes in forelimb vein resistance of anesthetized, chronic, renal hypertensive dogs reflect changes in all other venous segments of the circulation. An increase in the tone of postarteriolar resistance (essentially venules and small veins) can occur because of vein geometry without noticeable changes in vein pressure or flow resistance. Folkow and Mellander [32] and Folkow and Neil [33] have very properly stated that: "under ordinary circumstances many veins are in a state of partial collapse with elliptical cross section; marked changes in the volume of the venous reservoir can occur with no change in transmural venous pressure." These characteristics of the venous system make it necessary to interpret with caution the studies of Overbeck et al.[31] Since in their study, only small-vein pressure in skin was low while large-vein brachial pressure was high, it is entirely possible that limb-muscle venous blood flow was increased while that from skin was reduced. This interpretation is consistent with the previous findings of Brod et al.[34] who estimated that total limb resistance is primarily attributable to constriction of skin arterioles.

The possibility that the sequence of hemodynamic events described in perinephritic hypertensive dogs differs from that in hyperten sion produced by constriction of the renal arteries has been recently investigated by us in trained, unanesthetized dogs with chronically implanted flowmeters and catheters. Unilateral nephrectomy was performed in the dogs at least 2 months before commencing the experiment; also, at which time, a clamp, adjustable from the outside,[17] was placed around the remaining renal artery. Preliminary experiments indicate that onset of arterial hypertension due to renal artery constriction is due predominantly to an increase in cardiac output brought about by increases in both stroke volume and heart rate (Fig. 4). Increase in peripheral resistance follows the increase in cardiac output. These results are consistent with those reported by Ledingham and Pelling [23] in rats, and by Bianchi, Tenconi, and Lucca [35] in dogs. Both groups of workers agree, however, that cardiac output is either unchanged or reduced during the first 24 hours that follow renal artery constriction, while there is sharp increment of blood pressure and total peripheral resistance. In the experiments of Bianchi and his co-workers,[35] these initial changes are accompanied by an increase in plasma renin concentration, which, within 3 days, tends to return to control levels. With the reduction in renin concentration, cardiac output increases and hypertension is associated with a partial fall in peripheral resistance. These investigators have suggested that while the early rise in blood pressure might be produced by the increase in plasma renin concentration, both expansion of plasma volume and increase in cardiac output contribute to the maintenance of hypertension. Increase in plasma volume is apparently accompanied by a positive sodium balance [35–36] which has been found by Conway [37] not to be necessary for the emergence of hypertension, but it does appear to play

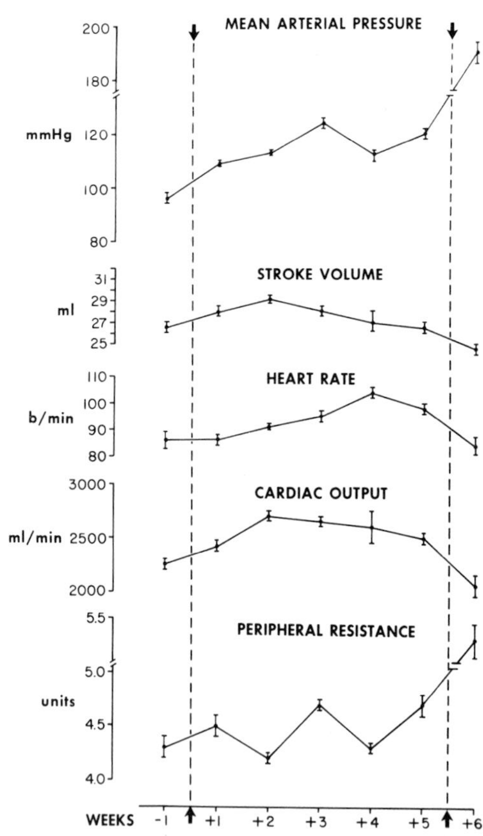

FIG. 4.—Mean hemodynamic changes (± 1 SE) in a trained dog before and after constriction of a renal artery. Onset of arterial hypertension **(first arrow)** is associated with increases in both stroke volume and cardiac output, followed only later by an increase in peripheral resistance. Further constriction of the renal artery **(second arrow)** 5 weeks after onset of hypertension prompted a marked rise in arterial pressure due to increased peripheral resistance. Accelerated hypertension is accompanied by a fall in cardiac output below control levels (+6 weeks).

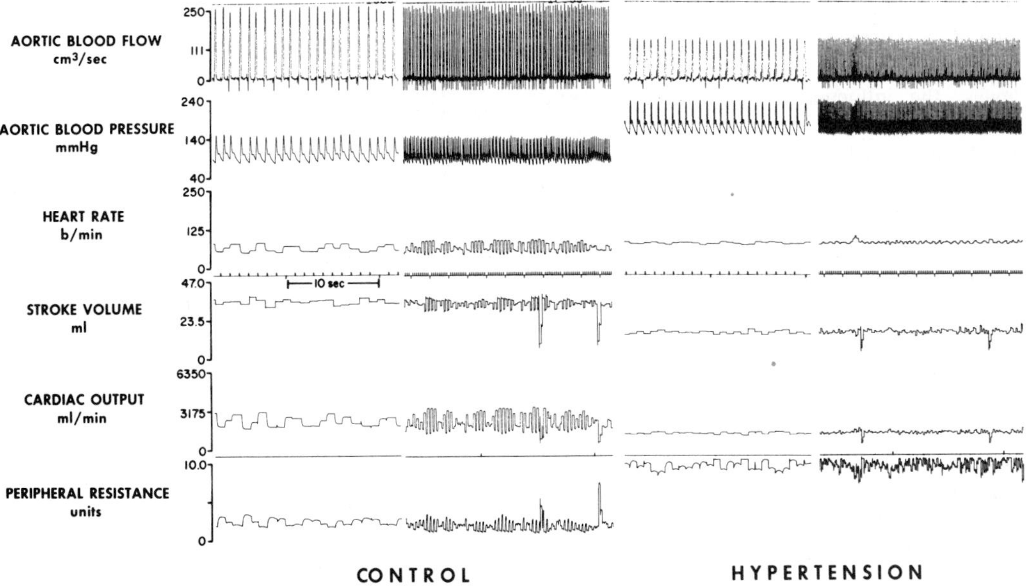

FIG. 5.—Accelerated hypertension following severe constriction of a renal artery and nephrectomy is due to increase in total peripheral resistance alone. Sharp decreases in cardiac output and stroke volume are maintained until death.

some part in determining the magnitude of the rise in pressure.

The basic mechanism of accelerated hypertension, resembling the malignant form of hypertension in man, probably differs from that causing the more benign form of chronic renal hypertension. Accelerated hypertension is associated chiefly with an increase in peripheral resistance and a fall in both stroke volume and cardiac output to below control values (Figs. 4 and 5). This hemodynamic pattern, distinctively different from that occurring in the benign form, may best be explained by assuming an excess amount of circulating vasoconstrictor substances acting directly on the peripheral vessels.[38–41]

It is now reasonably clear that an early increase in cardiac output either precedes [25] or accompanies [23,25,27,35,36] elevation in both arterial pressure and peripheral resistance in most forms of chronic, benign experimental renal hypertension. The increase in cardiac output is probably due either to increased tone of capacitance vessels,[21,25] expansion of plasma and extracellular fluid volumes,[22,23,35,36] or a combination of both. What remains a mystery is the cause of the later increase in resistance which, in the chronic phase of benign renal hypertension, accounts alone for the maintenance of elevated blood pressure.

To explain this puzzle, several investigators have directed their interest to local disturbances in myogenic activity of precapillary resistance vessels as a chief villain.[23,25,35,36,42] If cardiac output were to rise inappropriately to tissue requirements it might be expected that vasoconstriction would take place as a consequence. A form of autoregulation to excess flow was first proposed by Bayliss [43] in 1902, and since then, it has been demonstrated in all vascular territories; [44] recently, it has been demonstrated in the body of both man and animal [45,46] as a whole. In 1956, Ledingham [47] proposed the activation of this autoregulatory mechanism to explain the later increase in peripheral resistance in hypertension of renal origin, a view that in recent years has gained many proponents; [25,27,35,36] Guyton, Granger and Coleman [42] have even applied the technique of system analysis to test the theoretical soundness of the concept.

But as commented recently by Ledingham,[47]

the hypothesis is, as yet, far from being proved. The theory depends upon exclusion of other vasoconstrictor mechanisms acting at tissue levels, the influence of baroreceptor reset,[11] increased sympathetic output to peripheral vessels,[30] increased vascular smooth-muscle responsiveness to vasoactive stimuli,[48] reduction in the wall-to-lumen ratio of resistance vessels due to structural changes,[49,50] and abnormalities in smooth-muscle cell metabolism.[51,52]

Summary

Two major questions were posed at the beginning of this chapter: (1) What is the nature of the intrarenal stimulus that signals the kidney to produce hypertension; and (2) What hemodynamic changes result in the elevated pressure. We hope that the experiments reviewed here provide at least partial answers. From the material presented we conclude the following:

1. It is reasonably clear that production of chronic, benign hypertension by partial occlusion of a renal artery and contralateral nephrectomy is not accompanied by a sustained reduction in renal blood flow. Instead, there is persistent diminution in amplitude of the flow pulse and reduction of renal perfusion pressure in relation to systemic pressure. These latter factors are most likely involved in the etiology of renovascular hypertension. Renal ischemia is present only in the accelerated or "malignant" phase of renal hypertension.
2. Rise in cardiac output precedes rise in arterial pressure and is always present during the development of renovascular hypertension. This rise in output most likely results from increased venous return consequent to contraction of capacitance vessels and/or increase in fluid volumes.
3. The initial increase in cardiac output does not persist but is replaced by an increase in peripheral resistance when hypertension becomes chronic. The increase in resistance may be a response of peripheral resistance vessels to an "inappropriate" increase in cardiac output.

References

1. Holman, D. V., and Page, I. H.: The cardiac output in arterial hypertension. Am. Heart J. 16:321, 1938.
2. Weiss, S., and Ellis, L. B.: The quantitative aspects and dynamics of the circulatory mechanism in arterial hypertension. Am. Heart J. 5:448, 1930.
3. West, W. J., Mercker, H., Wendel, H., and Foltz, E. L.: Effects of renal hypertension on coronary blood flow, cardiac oxygen consumption and related circulatory dynamics of the dog. Circ. Res. 7:476, 1959.
4. Ledingham, J. M., and Cohen, R. D.: Circulatory changes during the reversal of experimental hypertension. Clin. Sci. 22:69, 1962.
5. Page, I. H., Del Greco, F., and Corcoran, A. C.: Effects of pentobarbital anesthesia, high spinal cord section and large doses of ganglioplegic agents on hemodynamic function measured by dye dilution. Am. J. Physiol. 179:601, 1954.
6. Blaquier, P., and Taquini, A. C.: Hemodynamic mechanism by which renal transplants lower the blood pressure of hypertensive animals. Acta Physiol. Lat. Am. 14:138, 1964.
7. Richardson, T. Q., Fermoso, J. D., and Guyton, A. C.: Increase in mean circulatory pressure in Goldblatt hypertension. Am. J. Physiol. 207:751, 1964.
8. Goldblatt, H., Lynch, J., Hanzal, R. F., and Summerville, W. W.: Studies on experimental hypertension. I. The production of persistent elevation of systolic blood pressure by means of renal ischemia. J. Exp. Med. 59:347, 1934.
9. Fasciolo, J. C.: Accion del riñón sano sobre la hipertensión arterial por isquemia renal. Rev. Soc. Argent. Biol. 14:15, 1938.
10. Page, I. H.: The production of persistent arterial hypertension by cellophane perinephritis. JAMA 113:2046, 1939.
11. McCubbin, J. W.: Carotid sinus participation in experimental renal hypertension. Circulation 17:791, 1958.
12. Goldblatt, H.: Renovascular hypertension due to renal ischemia. Circulation 32:1, 1965.
13. Corcoran, A. C., and Page, I. H.: Renal blood flow in experimental hypertension due to constriction of the renal artery. Am. J. Physiol. 133:249, 1941.
14. Kohlstaedt, K. G., and Page, I. H.: Liberation of renin by perfusion of kidneys following reduction of pulse pressure. J. Exp. Med. 72:201, 1940.
15. Hawthorne, E. W., Perry, S. L. C., and Pogue, W.: Development of experimental renal hypertension in the dog following reduction of renal artery pulse pressure without reducing mean pressure. Am. J. Physiol. 174:393, 1953.

16. Bounous, G., and Shumacker, H. B.: Experimental unilateral renal artery stenosis. Surg. Gynec. Obstet. 114:415, 1962.
17. Ferrario, C. M., Blumle, G., Nadzam, G. R., and McCubbin, J. W.: An externally adjustable renal artery clamp. J. Appl. Physiol. 31:635, 1971.
18. Ferrario, C. M., and McCubbin, J. W.: Renal blood flow in renovascular hypertension. Fed. Proc. 30:486, 1971.
19. Ladefoged, J.: Renal cortical blood flow and split function test in patients with hypertension and renal artery stenosis. Acta Med. Scand. 179:641, 1966.
20. Widimsky, J., Fejfarova, M. H., and Fejfar, Z.: Changes of cardiac output in hypertensive disease. Cardiologica 31:381, 1957.
21. Floyer, M. A., and Richardson, P. C.: Mechanism of arterial hypertension. Lancet 1:253, 1961.
22. Ledingham, J. M., and Cohen, R. D.: Role of the heart in the pathogenesis of renal hypertension. Lancet 2:979, 1963.
23. Ledingham, J. M., and Pelling, D.: Cardiac output and peripheral resistance in experimental renal hypertension in rats. Circ. Res. 21(suppl. II):II–187, 1967.
24. Olmsted, F., and Page, I. H.: Hemodynamic changes in trained dogs during experimental renal hypertension. Circ. Res. 16:134, 1965.
25. Ferrario, C. M., Page, I. H., and McCubbin, J. W.: Increased cardiac output as a contributory factor in experimental renal hypertension in dogs. Circ. Res. 27:799, 1970.
26. Wilson, C.: Experimental observations on the role of the kidney in the etiology of hypertension. Am. J. Cardiol. 9:685, 1962.
27. Freis, E. D.: Hemodynamics of hypertension. Physiol. Res. 40:27, 1960.
28. Lanari, A., Bromberger-Barnea, B., and Lambertini, A.: Volume-pressure curves of the human arm. Circ. Res. 5:236, 1957.
29. Anderson, R. M.: Intrinsic blood pressure. Circulation 9:641, 1954.
30. Page, I. H., and McCubbin, J. W. (eds.): Renal Hypertension. Chicago: Year Book, 1968, p. 368.
31. Overbeck, H. W., Swindall, B. T., Cowan, D. F., and Fleck, M. C.: Experimental renal hypertension in dogs. Forelimb hemodynamics. Circ. Res. 29:51, 1971.
32. Folkow, B., and Mellander, S.: Veins and venous tone. Am. Heart J. 68:397, 1964.
33. Folkow, B., and Neil, E.: Circulation. London: Oxford University Press, 1971, pp. 132–145.
34. Brod, J., Fenci, V., Heji, Z., Jirka, J., and Ulrych, M.: General and regional hemodynamic pattern underlying essential hypertension. Clin. Sci. 23:339, 1962.
35. Bianchi, G., Tenconi, L. T., and Lucca, R.: Effect in the conscious dog of constriction of the renal artery to a sole remaining kidney on haemodynamics, sodium balance, body fluid volumes, plasma renin concentration and pressor responsiveness to angiotensin. Clin. Sci. 38:741, 1970.
36. Guyton, A. C., Coleman, T. G., Bower, J. D., and Granger, H. J.: Circulatory control in hypertension. Circ. Res. 26(suppl. II): II–135, 1970.
37. Conway, J.: Changes in sodium balance and hemodynamics during development of experimental renal hypertension in dogs. Circ. Res. 22:763, 1968.
38. Ayers, C. R., Harris, R. H., and Lefer, L. G.: Control of renin release in experimental hypertension. Circ. Res. 24(suppl. I):I–103, 1969.
39. Brown, J. J., Davies, D. L., Lever, A. F., and Robertson, J. I. S.: Plasma renin concentration in human hypertension. I. Relationship between renin, sodium and potassium. Br. Med. J. 2:144, 1965.
40. Bianchi, G., Campolo, L., Vegeto, A., Pietra, V., and Piazza, U.: The value of plasma renin concentration per se, and in relation to plasma and extracellular fluid volume in diagnosis and prognosis of human renovascular hypertension. Clin. Sci. 39:559, 1970.
41. Macdonald, G. J., Louis, W. J., Renzini, V., Boyd, G. W., and Peart, W. S.: Renal-clip hypertension in rabbits immunized against angiotensin II. Circ. Res. 27:197, 1970.
42. Guyton, A. C., Granger, H. J., and Coleman, T. G.: Autoregulation of the total systemic circulation and its relation to control of cardiac output and arterial pressure. Circ. Res. 28(suppl. I):I–93, 1971.
43. Bayliss, W. M.: On the local reactions of the arterial wall to changes of internal pressure. J. Physiol. (London) 28:220, 1902.
44. Ross, G.: The regional circulation. Annu. Rev. Physiol. 33:445, 1971.
45. Granger, H. J., and Guyton, A. C.: Autoregulation of the total systemic circulation following destruction of the central nervous system in the dog. Circ. Res. 25:379, 1969.
46. Coleman, T. G., Bower, J. D., Langford, H. G., and Guyton, A. C.: Regulation of arterial pressure in the anephric state. Circulation 42:509, 1970.

47. Ledingham, J. M.: Mechanisms in renal hypertension. Proc. R. Soc. Med. 64: 409, 1971.
48. Doyle, A. E., and Fraser, J. R. E.: Vascular reactivity in hypertension. Circ. Res. 9:755, 1961.
49. Folkow, B., Grimby, C., and Thulesius, O.: Adaptive structural changes of the vascular walls in hypertension and their relation to the control of the peripheral resistance. Acta Physiol. Scand. 44:255, 1958.
50. Bohr, D. F., Verrier, R. L., and Sabieski, J.: Non-neurogenic tone in isolated perfused resistance vessels. Circ. Res. 28(Suppl. I):I–59, 1971.
51. Olsen, F.: Inflammatory Cellular Reaction in Hypertensive Vascular Disease. Copenhagen: Munksgaard, 1971.
52. Sivertsson, R.: The hemodynamic importance of structural vascular changes in essential hypertension. Acta Physiol. Scand. (Suppl. 343): 1970.

Hemodynamics of the Renal Hypertensions in Man

By Edward D. Frohlich, M.D.

By convention, all hypertension related to renal diseases has been termed "renal." Thus, whether the disease involves the renal arteries (by either atherosclerotic or fibrosing occlusive disease), the renal parenchyma (by inflammatory, cystic, or glomerular diseases), the intrarenal vessels (by nephrosclerosis, necrotizing arteriolitis, or allergic vasculitis), or whether the hypertension is associated with "end-stage" disease (i.e., "renoprival"), the current conception is that they are all "renal hypertension" (Table 1).

Present knowledge of pressor mechanisms in hypertension has developed to such sophistication and complexity that we must consider a myriad of means whereby arterial pressure can be maintained at elevated levels.[1] Thus, hypertension can be produced mechanically, through the renopressor system, by increased participation of catecholamines, by overfunction or increased responsiveness of autonomic nervous factors, by a variety of hormonal mechanisms, or by fluid volume mechanisms (Table 2). Interestingly enough, most of these pressor mechanisms seem to participate to greater or lesser degrees in the variety of hypertensions we term "renal." Perhaps this term "renal" has to no small degree perpetuated our ignorance concerning the pathogenesis and pathophysiologic changes associated with the progression of these renal hypertensions.

Much of our confusion concerning the pathophysiologic alterations associated with the development and progression of the renal hypertensions has come about through those well-controlled experimental laboratory studies which *could* have done much to clear our thinking. Thus, hypertension, whether produced by renal arterial clipping (with or without contralateral nephrectomy),[2] by wrapping the kidney[3] (with cellophane, silk, or Saran), by removal of 70 percent of total functioning renal tissue and then volume overloading with saline,[4] by injecting live organisms,[5] and so forth, all have been termed "renal hypertension" (Table 3).

One purpose of this review is to suggest that at our present state of awareness of pressor mechanisms and with our present availability

From the Departments of Medicine and of Physiology and Biophysics, College of Medicine, The University of Oklahoma Health Sciences Center, Oklahoma City, Oklahoma.

Table 1.—*"Renal Hypertension" in Man*

A. Renal Arterial (Extrarenal)	D. Glomerular Diseases
1. Atherosclerotic	1. Acute glomerulonephritis
2. Nonatherosclerotic	2. Subacute glomerulonephritis
3. Embolic	3. Chronic glomerulonephritis
B. Renal Vascular (Intrarenal)	4. Nodular glomerulosclerosis
1. Nephrosclerosis	E. Cystic Disease
2. Necrotizing arteriolitis	1. Unicystic disease
3. Periarteritis nodosa	2. Polycystic disease
4. Other collagen vascular diseases	3. With associated hepatic cysts
5. Allergic vasculitis	4. Medullary cystic disease
C. Renal Trauma	F. "Renoprival"
1. Perirenal hematoma	1. With kidneys
2. Intrarenal hematoma	2. Anephric (anatomically)
3. Arteriovenous fistula	G. Transplantation Rejection

A deliberate, general, and incomplete classification to emphasize the point that no matter what the cause or mechanism involved, they are all "renal."

TABLE 2.—*Pressor Mechanisms*

1. Mechanical
2. Renopressor—renin, angiotensin I or II, converting enzyme
3. Catecholamines—epinephrine, norepinephrine, dopamine
4. Other pressor and depressor substances
5. Neural factors—transmission, storage, release, re-uptake, response
6. Endocrine factors—adrenal cortical, parathyroid, thyroid, growth hormones
7. Volume—intravascular, extracellular, intracellular

of physiologic, diagnostic, and therapeutic techniques, we ought to revise our consideration of the hypertension associated with renal and extrarenal diseases. Perhaps then we might clarify our understanding of the pathogenesis and pathophysiology of these varieties of renal hypertension. Strong evidence is already available which indicates that these varied types of "renal hypertensive diseases" differ hemodynamically as well as with respect to other pressor mechanisms.[6] The discussion which follows presents current thinking about these "renal hypertensions" in man with respect to their hemodynamic and pressor mechanism characteristics.

TABLE 3.—*"Renal Hypertension" in the Experimental Animal*

1. Renal arterial "clipping," with or without contralateral nephrectomy
2. Perinephritis induced by wrapping the kidney with cellophane, silk, Saran
3. Nephrectomy (70%) plus volume overloading with saline
4. Nephrectomy (unilateral) plus DOCA * plus saline
5. Injection of live organisms with or without massaging the kidneys
6. Total nephrectomy—with various types of diets
7. Experimental glomerulonephritis using anti-kidney serum, foreign proteins, etc.
8. Infusion of subpressor doses of angiotensin intravenously
9. Infusion of pressor doses of angiotensin intravenously
10. Infusion of subpressor doses of angiotensin into the vertebral artery

* DOCA, deoxycorticosterone acetate.

RENAL ARTERIAL DISEASE

Goldblatt placed a clip around the main renal artery [2] because it was impossible to produce an experimental model of the arteriolar constrictor changes produced in man with severe arteriolar nephrosclerosis and hypertension of unknown cause (essential hypertension). By this ingenious maneuver, sustained diastolic hypertension developed in a previously normotensive animal; this was indeed a renal hypertension. Controversy still exists whether the elevated arterial pressure in essential hypertensive man results because of the intrarenal vascular disease or whether the nephrosclerosis is produced by the elevated pressure (i.e., hypertension of undetermined cause). Nevertheless, in the experimental hypertension produced by renal arterial clipping the initial hemodynamic studies suggested that the elevated arterial pressure was a result of increased vascular resistance since cardiac output was found to be normal.[7] Later studies confirmed these findings; [8] however, close inspection of these data indicated that an elevated cardiac output seemed to be present even though vascular resistance was also increased. Other studies in rats, also made hypertensive by placing a clip around the renal artery, showed that early in the development of hypertension there was a phase of increased cardiac output associated with increased vascular resistance; upon removing the clip, reduction of arterial pressure was associated with a fall in cardiac output.[9,10]

Shortly thereafter, we questioned the categorization of all clinical hypertensions into one grouping and suggested that if the variety of hypertensions were subclassified into etiologic types we might understand more about the physiologic characteristics of each. Indeed, this approach allowed further subclassification of clinical types into those patients having similar pressor mechanisms.[11] As a result, we found that when hypertensive patients with fibrosing lesions of renal arteries were compared with patients having essential hypertension who were of the same body habitus, sex, age, and arterial pressure, those with renal arterial disease had significantly higher cardiac output.[12] To be sure, total peripheral resistance was increased in both hypertensive groups; but cardiac output was significantly higher in patients with renal arterial disease and peripheral resistance, and much greater in those with essential hypertension. Later studies, involving patients with atherosclerotic as well as nonatherosclerotic disease, confirmed the finding of a higher cardiac index in patients with renovascular hypertension than in those patients with essential hypertension, or even in normotensive volunteer control subjects.[13] With respect to other hemodynamic indices (than cardiac output), patients with renal arterial disease had a faster heart rate (but normal stroke volume) and a greater left ventricular ejection rate. More recent studies demonstrated an increased overshoot phase of the Valsalva maneuver and an orthostatic hypertensive response during passive upright tilt.[6] Hence, the findings of hyperkinetic circulation and greater reflexive neural activity suggest that adrenergic mechanisms participate actively in renovascular hypertensive patients. That the renopressor system also is an important pressor determinant is shown by the direct relationship between the arterial pressure and plasma renin activity in this type of hypertension.[14] In contrast, intravascular volume is not directly related to the magnitude of arterial pressure; in fact, these two hemodynamic indices are inversely related to each other.[15,16] Thus, patients with renal arterial disease have specific hemodynamic and pressor characteristics which seem to differentiate them from patients with other clinical types of hypertension.

Several patients with renovascular hypertension have had remission of hypertension (either by correction of the arterial lesion or by nephrectomy) and have been studied postoperatively thereby allowing a comparison with their preoperative characteristics. In general, with reduction of arterial pressure to normotensive levels there was a reduction of the increased vascular resistance; changes in cardiac output were not consistent.[16] These findings indicate that the increased cardiac output is not the main hemodynamic factor maintaining the elevated arterial pressure in these patients. Nevertheless, the presence of the hyperkinetic circulatory state serves an important role in indicating the presence of several different pressor mechanisms which actively participate in the maintenance of this pathophysiologic state. Indeed, these clinical hemodynamic findings have permitted certain speculations and hypotheses which have made meaningful other experimental observations relative to renovascular hypertension (i.e., the stimulation of medullary centers by subpressor doses of angiotensin, the hemodynamic characteristics of which are identical with those of renovascular hypertensive man.[17,18]

One final comment concerns the widely accepted term "renovascular hypertension." Since this all-encompassing category might very well include hypertension associated with renal arterial, renal venous, intrarenal arterial and arteriolar, and renal embolic vascular diseases, we have titled this section "Renal Arterial Disease" in keeping with the critique outlined in the introduction. Therefore, we use "renovascular" interchangeably with "renal arterial."

Chronic Pyelonephritis

Patients with renal parenchymal disease also differ hemodynamically from those with essential hypertension or renal arterial disease as well as from normotensive volunteers.[11] Thus, patients with chronic pyelonephritis and hypertension have a normal cardiac output and an increased total peripheral resistance. Later studies confirmed these findings and also related these hemodynamic characteristics and other pressor mechanisms in two types of "renal hypertension": patients having renal arterial disease (nonatherosclerotic) and patients with renal parenchymal (chronic pyelonephritis) disease.[6] Patients were carefully selected so that those with renovascular hypertension did not demonstrate occlusive atherosclerosis involving renal arteries since it might be difficult to know with certainty whether an atherosclerotic lesion had preceded or followed the onset of hypertension. Furthermore, patients with chronic pyelonephritis were selected only if they were nonazotemic, were not anemic, demonstrated repeatedly positive urine cultures indicating a chronic urinary tract infection, and had definite biopsy and radiographic evidence of pyelonephritis. The patients of both groups all had renal arteriography, were matched with respect to age, sex, body-surface area, cardiac size, and hypertensive retinopathy, and their arterial pressures and heart rates were similar. Once more the hemodynamic findings indicated a greater cardiac output and left ventricular ejection rate in the patients with renal arterial disease than in those with chronic pyelonephritis; the reflexive responses of arterial pressure to the Valsalva maneuver and passive upright tilt were greater in the patients with renal arterial disease; and the arterial pressure was inversely related to the intravascular volume in the patients with renal arterial disease but directly with the height of arterial pressure in those patients with chronic pyelonephritis.[6] In addition, other studies indicated that whereas plasma renin activity is an important factor in the maintenance of arterial pressure in normotensive as well as hypertensive individuals, no direct relationship existed between the height of arterial pressure and plasma renin activity in patients with chronic renal parenchymal disease, as it did in patients with renal arterial disease.[14]

Therefore, convincing evidence is available to indicate that whereas renal arterial disease is associated with more active cardiac participation and greater interaction of adrenergic and renopressor mechanisms in the maintenance of hypertension, renal parenchymal disease (at least in nonazotemic patients with chronic pyelonephritis) is related more to those mechanisms which expand intravascular and other body fluid volumes.

Few studies have detailed the regional hemodynamic changes in the various clinical renal hypertensions. Unlike the findings in patients with renal arterial disease or in normotensive subjects receiving an intravenous infusion of angiotensin in which the following regional flows were increased, Brod and his co-workers found that the respective fractions of cardiac output diverted to skeletal muscle, skin and extrarenal tissue were normal in patients with a variety of renal parenchymal diseases. These observations are in contrast to the diminished renal blood flow measured in each of these hypertensive states as well as in patients with essential hypertension.[19]

Glomerulonephritis

Considerable speculation has existed concerning the hemodynamic characteristics associated with acute glomerulonephritis in the oliguric and hypertensive state. The suggestion of Eichna that this altered hemodynamic state is not one of cardiac failure but of a "congested circulation" did much to reorient thinking about this problem.[20,21] At present it is generally held that the oliguric patient in acute renal failure resulting from acute glomerulonephritis has an expanded intravascular (and extravascular) fluid volume; this may or may not be related to the height of resting cardiac output. However, most studies have demonstrated a hyperkinetic circulation and an expanded intravascular volume.[22–26] Since all patients with acute glomerulonephritis are not hypertensive, it has been suggested that other pressor mechanisms, including those involving the adrenergic and renopressor systems, may also participate. Clearly, much additional information is needed to identify with greater confidence the hemodynamics and pathophysiologic characteristics of this renal hypertension. This is particularly necessary in understanding the progression of glomerulonephritis from the acute to the chronic stage—especially before the disease is further complicated by gross impairment of renal excretory function, anemia, pericarditis, and so forth.

Other Renal Parenchymal Diseases

Until now no study has been concerned with the comparison of hemodynamic and other pressor characteristics of the various types of other renal parenchymal diseases. Since these diseases are most complex, involving varying degrees of impairment of renal excretory function and anemia (each being mutually dependent), studies concerned with these questions must be designed and interpreted with great care.

Questions therefore exist whether nonazotemic and nonanemic chronic pyelonephritis and chronic glomerulonephritis (or any other renal parenchymal disease) have similar hemodynamic and pressor mechanism characteristics; whether the hypertension associated with chronic small-vessel disease of the kidney (from nephrosclerosis, necrotizing arteriolitis, periarteritis, and allergic vasculitis) is characterized by similar hemodynamic and other pressor criteria as with occlusive (extrarenal) arterial disease; or whether the hemodynamic and other pressor mechanisms altered by these "renal" diseases may be related to changes in renal excretory function. These and many other problems must be resolved before the hypertensive mechanisms in chronic renal disease can be said to be understood.

Chronic Renal Failure ("Renoprival" Hypertension)

The hemodynamic, metabolic, and other participating pressor mechanisms have become extremely important to the clinician in recent years because of the widespread use of hemodialysis and the strong possibility to restore completely normal function and pressure following renal homotransplantation. Accordingly, it has been of more than academic interest to understand the pathophysiologic changes associated with the normotensive (and hypertensive) patient in chronic renal failure.

In general, it is believed that the hypertensive patient in chronic renal failure is one with a congested circulation and an expanded intravascular (and extravascular) fluid volume.[27–30] The earlier studies have shown that the height of arterial pressure is related directly to the degree of expansion of the intravascular compartment,[28,31] and that careful plasma ultrafiltration during hemodialysis will control arterial pressure.[29] Nevertheless, there are certain patients whose arterial pressure will not be reduced by ultrafiltration (though their numbers are proportionately small); these patients will regain normal arterial pressure following bilateral nephrectomy,[32–34] suggesting that, in some patients with chronic renal failure, a renopressor factor (or absence of a renal depressor factor) may be participating in the maintenance of their elevated arterial pressure over and above the "renoprival" (or volume) factor.

Long-term hemodynamic studies of patients undergoing chronic renal hemodialysis have provided valuable insights into the possible mechanisms associated with this type of "renal" hypertension.[35–40] In general, these studies have indicated that the chronic volume overload in chronic renal failure is associated with an initial increase in cardiac output and arterial pressure. However, these studies also show that overriding the increased cardiac output is a progressive increase in vascular resistance, indicating a process of long-term autoregulation.[38,39] The mechanism for this adaptation of the resistance vessels has not yet been explained, but apparently excluded from consideration is the renopressor system. How persistently aggressive plasma ultrafiltration (with consequent contraction of extravascular water) leads to a reduction of total peripheral vascular resistance is unknown; but perhaps an understanding of this phenomenon may provide insight into the reverse phenomenon which may occur in the development of these and possibly other hypertensions.

The hemodynamic characteristics of these patients with chronic renal failure and hypertension appear to be: chronically expanded intravascular and extravascular fluid volumes, increased cardiac output, and increased total peripheral vascular resistance.[36–40] The mechanisms underlying this type of hypertension are extremely complex with the additional factors of azotemia, anemia, and even possible pericarditis. Moreover, other factors of complicating acute and chronic infections, unknown substances introduced by blood transfusions, varying concentrations of naturally occurring pressor and depressor substances, etc. all compound the problem of evaluating the hemodynamic characteristics involved. In an effort to exclude some of these factors, stable uremic patients without pericarditis, but on maintenance hemodialysis, were studied by Neff and his associates.[40] These patients demonstrated the characteristics described above (increased cardiac output and total peripheral resistance); but some were transfused with packed red blood cells so that their hematocrits were restored to normal levels. Simultaneously, intravascular and extracellular fluid volumes were maintained at normal levels by hemodialysis ultrafiltration, and when these factors had stabilized, cardiac output was reduced to normal levels and arterial pressure and total peripheral resistance increased further. Hence, the elevated cardiac index seen so commonly in uremic patients may be the result of at least two factors: the expanded intravascular and extravascular volumes produced by less-than-aggressive dialysis ultrafiltration and the anemia of renal disease.

In these more recent studies Kim et al.

compared the hemodynamic characteristics of hypertensive and normotensive uremic patients and showed that cardiac output was increased in both groups as a result of the anemia since cardiac output returned to normal levels with correction of anemia.[41] Most important was the finding that the uremic patients with hypertension had significantly higher vascular resistance than the nonhypertensive uremic patients. Moreover, when the hypertensive uremic patients received bilateral nephrectomy (in preparation for renal homotransplantation), there was no change in cardiac output, and hence the fall in their arterial pressure resulted from a fall in vascular resistance.[41] Thus, the elevated arterial pressure in patients with end-stage renal disease (renoprival hypertension) is the result of increased total peripheral resistance. Whether this is the result of a vasopressor substance of renal origin or other factors which promote an adaptation of the resistance vessels remains to be demonstrated.

Dialysis Hypertension and Hypotension

Another type of renal hypertension concerns the sudden unexplained changes in arterial pressure in patients with chronic renal failure *during* hemodialysis. This problem is independent of the presence or absence of hypertension in the intervening period between dialyses and may be found in patients who are hypertensive or normotensive. The mechanism for these explained rises in pressure remains to be defined precisely but recent studies in our laboratory seem to have provided an explanation.[42] In a group of chronic dialysis patients, arterial pressure was raised at will by the rapid intravenous infusion of saline; the pressor rise was associated with a proportional increase in body weight and cardiac output. When these patients lost an equivalent amount of body weight by rapid dialysis ultrafiltration, arterial pressure and cardiac output fell pari passu. Furthermore, we were able to prevent the depressor phenomenon by reducing body weight more slowly to the same level, even though cardiac output was reduced the same extent. These findings were also observed on four occasions when arterial pressure spontaneously changed during dialysis, suggesting that in renoprival man, acute changes in arterial pressure are exquisitely sensitive to changes in intravascular volume during dialysis.

Summary

Evidence is presented to suggest that the term "renal hypertension" is too all-inclusive. Hemodynamic characteristics and participation of the various pressor mechanisms interact in a highly complex fashion in a variety of ways depending upon the type of renal disease. Evidence to support this concept is provided by the difference in hemodynamic and pressor characteristics associated with hypertension in patients with fibrosing lesions of renal arteries and with nonazotemic chronic pyelonephritis. Similar evidence is available in patients with end-stage renal disease with and without hypertension as well as in patients with dialysis hypertension. Yet to be defined are the characteristics in other patients with different types of chronic renal parenchymal disease, the varied types of intrarenal vascular disease, and the relationships of these hemodynamic and pressor mechanism alterations to the changes in renal excretory function.

References

1. Dustan, H. P., Frohlich, E. D., and Tarazi, R. C.: Pressor mechanisms. *In* Frohlich, E. D. (Ed.): Pathophysiology: Altered Regulatory Mechanisms in Disease. Philadelphia: Lippincott, 1972, pp. 41–66.
2. Goldblatt, H., Lynch, J., Hanzal, R. F., and Summerville, W. W.: Studies on experimental hypertension. I. The production of persistent elevation of systolic blood-pressure by means of renal ischemia. J. Exp. Med. 59:347, 1934.
3. Page, I. H.: Production of persistent arterial hypertension by cellophane perinephritis. JAMA 113:2046, 1939.
4. Langston, J. B., Guyton, A. C., Douglas, P. H., and Dorsett, P. E.: Effect of changes in salt intake on arterial pressure and renal function in partially nephrectomized dogs. Circ. Res. 12:508, 1963.
5. Shapiro, A. P., Braude, A. I., and Siemienski, J.: Hematogenous pyelonephritis in rats. II. Production of chronic pyelonephritis by Escherichia coli. Proc. Soc. Exp. Biol. Med. 91:18, 1956.
6. Frohlich, E. D., Tarazi, R. C., and Dustan, H. P.: Hemodynamic and functional mechan-

isms in two renal hypertensions: Arterial and pyelonephritis. Amer. J. Med. Sci. 261:189, 1971.
7. Holman, D. V., and Page, I. H.: The cardiac output in arterial hypertension. II. A study of arterial hypertension produced by constricting the renal arteries in unanesthetized and anesthetized (pentobarbital) dogs. Am. Heart J. 16:321, 1938.
8. Olmsted, F., and Page, I. H.: Hemodynamic changes in trained dogs during experimental renal hypertension. Circ. Res. 16:134, 1965.
9. Ledingham, J. M., and Cohen, R. D.: The role of the heart in the pathogenesis of renal hypertension. Lancet 2:979, 1963.
10. Ledingham, J. M., and Pelling, D.: Cardiac output and peripheral resistance in experimental renal hypertension. Circ. Res. 21 (Suppl. II) 187, 1967.
11. Frohlich, E. D., Tarazi, R. C., and Dustan, H. P.: Re-examination of the hemodynamics of hypertension. Amer. J. Med. Sci. 257:9, 1969.
12. Frohlich, E. D., Ulrych, M., Tarazi, R. C., Dustan, H. P., and Page, I. H.: A hemodynamic comparison of essential and renovascular hypertension. Cardiac output and total peripheral resistance: supine and tilted patients. Circulation 35:289, 1967.
13. Frohlich, E. D., Ulrych, M., Tarazi, R. C., Dustan, H. P., and Page, I. H.: Hemodynamics of renal arterial diseases and hypertension. Amer. J. Med. Sci. 255:29, 1968.
14. Dustan, H. P., Tarazi, R. C., and Frohlich, E. D.: Functional correlates of plasma renin activity in hypertensive patients. Circulation 51:555, 1970.
15. Tarazi, R. C., Dustan, H. P., Frohlich, E. D., Gifford, R. W., Jr., and Hoffman, G. C.: Plasma volume and chronic hypertension. Relationship to arterial pressure levels in different hypertensive diseases. Arch. Intern. Med. 125:835, 1970.
16. Tarazi, R. C., Frohlich, E. D., and Dustan, H. P.: Contribution of cardiac output to renovascular hypertension in man. Circulation 42(Suppl. III):69, 1970.
17. Scroop, G. C., and Whelan, R. F.: A central vasomotor action of angiotensin in man. Clin. Sci. 30:79, 1966.
18. Scroop, G. C., and Lowe, R. D.: Efferent pathways of the cardiovascular response to vertebral artery infusions of angiotensin in the dog. Clin. Sci. 37:605, 1969.
19. Frohlich, E. D., Brod, J., Hoobler, S. W., and Ledingham, J. M.: Hemodynamics. *In* Page, I. H., and McCubbin, J. W. (Eds.): Renal Hypertension. Chicago: Year Book, 1968, pp. 350–370.
20. Eichna, L. W., Farber, S. J., Berger, A. R., Rader, B., Smith, W. W., and Albert, R. E.: Non-cardiac circulatory congestion simulating congestive heart failure. Trans. Assoc. Am. Physicians 67:72, 1954.
21. Eichna, L. W.: Circulatory congestion and heart failure. Circulation 22:864, 1960.
22. DeFazio, V., Christensen, R. C., Regan, T. J., Baer, L. J., Morita, Y., and Hellems, H. K.: Circulatory changes in acute glomerulonephritis. Circulation 20:190, 1959.
23. Glazer, G. A.: Haemodynamic changes in symptomatic renal hypertension. Cor Vasa 6:264, 1964.
24. Fleisher, D. S., Voci, G., Garfunkel, J., Purugganan, H., Kirkpatrick, J., Jr., and Wells, C. R.: Hemodynamic findings in acute glomerulonephritis. J. Pediat. 69:1054, 1966.
25. Agrest, A., and Finkielman, S.: Hemodynamics in acute renal failure. Pathogenesis of hyperkinetic circulation. Am. J. Cardiol. 19: 213, 1967.
26. Birkenhäger, W. H., Schalekamp, M.A.D.H., Schalekamp-Kuyken, M.P.A., Kolsters, C., and Krauss, X. H.: Interrelations between arterial pressure, fluid-volumes, and plasma renin concentration in the course of acute glomerulonephritis. Lancet 1:1086, 1970.
27. Merrill, J. P., Giordana, C., and Heetderks, D. R.: The role of the kidney in human hypertension. Am. J. Med. 31:931, 1961.
28. Merrill, J. P., and Schupak, E.: Mechanisms of hypertension in renoprival man. Canad. Med. Assoc. J. 90:328, 1964.
29. Dustan, H. P., and Page, I. H.: Some factors in renal and renoprival hypertension. J. Lab. Clin. Med. 64:948, 1964.
30. Del Greco, F., Simon, N. M., Roguska, J., and Walker, C.: Hemodynamic studies in chronic uremia. Circulation 40:87, 1969.
31. Klütsch, V. K., Wrede, J. K., Scheitza, E., Grosswendt, J., and Gathof, A. G.: Hämodynamische Veränderungen unter der extrakorporalen Dialyse. Z. Kreislaufforsch. 59:80, 1970.
32. Vertes, V., Cangiano, J. L., Berman, L. B., and Gould, A.: Hypertension in end-stage renal disease. N. Engl. J. Med. 280:978, 1969.
33. Ledingham, J. M.: Blood-pressure regulation in renal failure. J. Roy. Coll. Physicians Lond. 5:103, 1971.
34. Weidman, P., Lupu, A., Massey, S. G., Lewin,

A., Gral, T., and Maxwell, M. H.: Diagnostic value of plasma renin activity in hypertensive terminal renal failure. Circulation 44(Suppl. II):120, 1971.

35. Hampers, C. L., Skillman, J. J., Lyons, J. H., Olsen, J. E., and Merrill, J. P.: A hemodynamic evaluation of bilateral nephrectomy and hemodialysis in hypertensive man. Circulation 35:272, 1967.
36. Coleman, T. G., Bower, J. D., Langford, H. G., and Guyton, A. C.: Regulation of arterial pressure in the anephric state. Circulation 42:509, 1970.
37. Guyton, A. C., Coleman, T. G., Bower, J. D., and Granger, H. J.: Circulatory control in hypertension. Circ. Res. 27(Suppl. II):135, 1970.
38. Guyton, A. C., Granger, H. J., and Coleman, T. G.: Autoregulation of the total systemic circulation and its relation to control of cardiac output and arterial pressure. Circ. Res. 28(Suppl. I):93, 1971.
39. Coleman, T. G., Granger, H. J., and Guyton, A. C.: Whole-body circulatory autoregulation and hypertension. Circ. Res. 28(Suppl. II):76, 1971.
40. Neff, M. S., Kim, K. E., Persoff, M., Onesti, G., and Swartz, C.: Hemodynamics of uremic anemia. Circulation 43:876, 1971.
41. Kim, K. E., Onesti, G., Schwartz, A. B., Chinitz, J. L., and Swartz, C.: Hemodynamics of hypertension in chronic end-stage renal disease. Circulation 46:456, 1972.
42. Frohlich, E. D., Bhatia, S., Matter, B. J., and Pederson, J. A.: Mechanism of acute arterial pressure changes during hemodialysis. J. Lab. Clin. Med. 78:1014, 1971.

Hemodynamic Alterations in Hypertension of Chronic End-stage Renal Disease

By Kwan Eun Kim, M.D., Gaddo Onesti, M.D., Martin S. Neff, M.D., James A. Greco, M.D., Robert F. Slifkin, M.D., and Charles Swartz, M.D.

Although the etiology of essential hypertension remains obscure, extensive studies have revealed a consistent hemodynamic pattern. Early essential hypertension is characterized by a high cardiac output and a normal total peripheral resistance. With advancing age, the patient with essential hypertension will change to a pattern of normal cardiac output and increased total peripheral resistance and, finally, later in the natural course of the disease, into one of low cardiac output and further increase in total peripheral resistance.[1-7]

In contrast with essential hypertension, not only is the etiology of hypertension in chronic renal parenchymal disease and uremia obscure, but also information regarding its basic hemodynamic derangement is limited and conflicting. Elevated cardiac output and normal peripheral resistance have been reported in hypertension of acute glomerulonephritis.[8] This information is of limited importance since most patients with chronic glomerulonephritis never have acute episodes.

In 1961, Brod and co-workers [9] described a cardiac output higher than normal in both chronic glomerulonephritis and polycystic kidney disease. A wide variation of cardiac output was, however, reported.

More recently, Frohlich, Tarazi, and Dustan [6] reported normal cardiac output and increased total peripheral resistance in 11 nonazotemic hypertensive patients with chronic renal parenchymal diseases of varying etiologies.

In hypertension associated with end-stage renal disease and uremia, a higher than normal cardiac output has been described by Goss and associates,[10] and by Mostert and associates.[11] In contrast, Del Greco and co-workers,[12] and Anthonisen and Holst [13] described normal cardiac output in uremic patients.

A knowledge of the hemodynamic alterations in hypertension secondary to chronic renal disease is essential in order to understand the underlying pathophysiologic mechanisms. If the basic hemodynamic change in hypertension of chronic renal parenchymal disease is an increase in cardiac output, then the search for a renal vasoconstrictor material would remain fruitless. Contrariwise, if the hemodynamic change is an increase in total peripheral resistance, then research efforts should be directed toward the causes of peripheral arteriolar constriction. It is possible that both mechanisms operate simultaneously [14] or in chronologic sequence.[15]

During the past 7 years, we have had the opportunity to study the hemodynamic pattern of 75 patients with chronic end-stage renal parenchymal disease and uremia. During the same period, 42 normal volunteers have been studied in the same laboratory.

It is the purpose of the present chapter: (1) to report the hemodynamic changes of chronic end-stage renal disease, and (2) to assess the relative contribution of cardiac output and total peripheral resistance to the hypertension of chronic end-stage renal parenchymal disease.

Hemodynamic Pattern of Chronic End-stage Renal Disease

Seventy-five patients with chronic end-stage renal disease of various etiologies and uremia were studied. There were 39 males and 36 females. Their ages ranged from 16 to 57, with a mean age of 36. Of the 75 patients

From the Division of Nephrology and Hypertension, Department of Medicine, Hahnemann Medical College and Hospital, Philadelphia, Pennsylvania.

Supported by Grants 1-RO-1-HE-09146, HE-06368, and T-12-HE-05878 from the National Institutes of Health.

studied, 23 were normotensive and the remaining 52 were hypertensive. Hypertension was defined as systolic pressure above 150 mm Hg or diastolic blood pressure above 90 mm Hg.

The studies were performed when the patients were clinically at dry weight. There were no differences in the state of hydration between the hypertensive and the normotensive uremic patients. All the uremic patients studied were ambulatory, clinically stable, rehabilitated and free of uremic complications. All antihypertensive medications were discontinued at least 2 weeks prior to the hemodynamic studies. Studies were conducted in the supine position after 1 hour of bed rest. Because of possible acute hemodynamic changes induced by hemodialysis, all the studies were performed at least 48 hours after hemodialysis.

The control group included 42 healthy normal volunteers. Twenty-two were males and 20 were females. Their ages ranged from 22 to 57 with a mean age of 43. The groups of the uremic patients and the normal subjects were of comparable age and sex.

In the uremic patients the hemodynamic studies were performed through an external connector inserted between the arterial and venous ends of the arteriovenous shunt used for hemodialysis. Cardiac output was determined by the dye-dilution technique using a Gilford densitometer with the injection of indocyanine green through the venous side of the external cannula and withdrawal of arterial blood from the arterial side of the external connection. Every cardiac output reported represents the average of at least three determinations. Arterial blood pressure was measured with a Statham strain-gauge transducer from the arterial side of the temporarily occluded external connector. In normal subjects hemodynamic measurements were made through a brachial artery needle with an injection through a venous catheter.

The hemodynamic studies of 75 patients with end-stage renal disease (hypertensives and normotensives) are compared with those of 45 normal subjects in Fig. 1.

The mean value of the hematocrit in normal subjects was 43 percent while the uremic patients were all significantly anemic with a mean hematocrit of 23 percent.

In the 42 normal volunteers, the mean cardiac index was 3.39 ± 0.08 liters per minute per M^2 (mean ± 1 SE). In the 75 patients with end-stage renal disease, the mean cardiac index was 4.44 ± 0.11 liters per minute per M^2. The difference is statistically significant ($p < 0.001$) (Figure 1*A*).

The mean heart rate was 66 ± 1.2 beats per minute in the 42 normal volunteers, and 90 ±

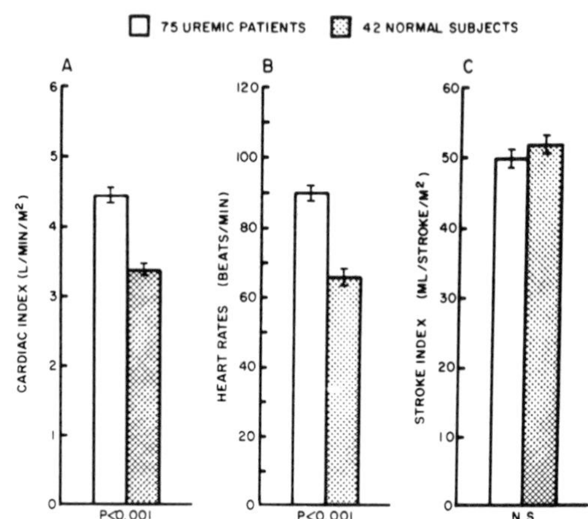

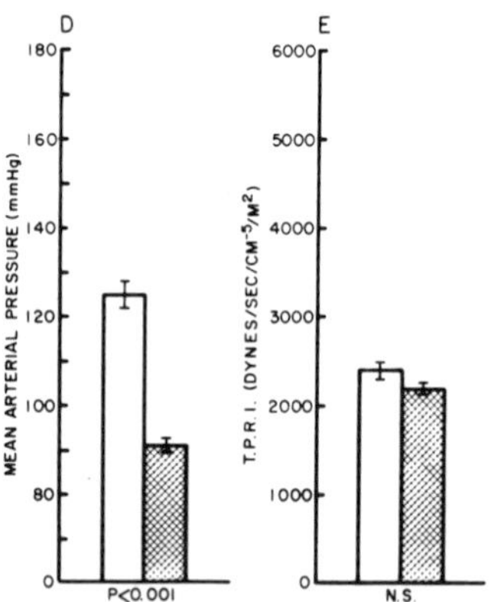

FIG. 1.—Cardiac index (*A*), heart rate (*B*), stroke index (*C*), mean arterial pressure (*D*) and total peripheral resistance index (*E*) of 75 patients with end-stage renal disease (hypertensives and normotensives) compared with those of 45 normal controls. The bars represent the mean ± 1 SE. T.P.R.I., total peripheral resistance index; N.S., not statistically significant. (From Kim, K. E., Onesti, G., Schwartz, A. B., Chinitz, J. L., and Swartz, C.: Hemodynamics of hypertension in chronic end-stage renal disease. Circulation 46: 456, 1972, with the permission of the American Heart Association, Inc.)

1.1 beats per minute in the 75 uremic patients ($p < 0.001$) (Fig. 1*B*). The 42 normal subjects had a mean stroke index of 52 ± 1.4 ml per stroke per M^2; in the 75 uremics, the mean stroke index was 50 ± 1.3 ml per stroke per M^2 (Fig. 1*C*).

The average mean arterial pressure in the 42 normal subjects was 91 ± 1.6 mm Hg, while in the 75 patients with end-stage renal disease, it was 125 ± 3.2 mm Hg. The difference is statistically significant ($p < 0.001$), and reflects the presence of hypertension in 52 of the 75 patients with end-stage renal disease (Fig. 1*D*).

The calculated mean total peripheral vascular resistance index was 2187 ± 59 dynes per sec per cm^{-5} per M^2 in the 42 normal subjects and 2389 ± 103 in the 75 uremic patients. The difference was not statistically significant (Fig. 1*E*).

Hypertensive Uremic Patients Compared with Normotensive Uremic Patients

Within the total group of 75 patients with chronic end-stage renal disease (hypertensive and normotensive), the hemodynamic pattern of the 52 hypertensive patients was compared with that of 23 normotensive patients. The results are shown in Fig. 2.

The mean arterial pressure in the group of hypertensive patients with chronic end-stage renal disease averages 139 ± 2.9 mm Hg while in the group of normotensive patients with chronic end-stage renal disease, the mean arterial pressure was 93 ± 1.8 mm Hg ($p < 0.001$) (Fig. 2*A*).

The mean cardiac index in the hypertensive uremic patients was 4.39 ± 0.14 liter per minute per M^2 and in the normotensive uremic patients, 4.55 ± 0.15 liter per minute per M^2. The difference is not significant (Fig. 2*B*).

The mean heart rate was 91 ± 1.4 beats per minute in the 52 hypertensive patients and 89 ± 2.0 beats per minute in the 23 normotensive patients. The 52 hypertensive patients showed a mean stroke index of 49 ± 1.6 ml per stroke per M^2; mean stroke index in the 23 normotensive patients was 51 ± 1.6 ml per stroke per M^2. Neither of these was significantly different.

Calculated mean total peripheral resistance

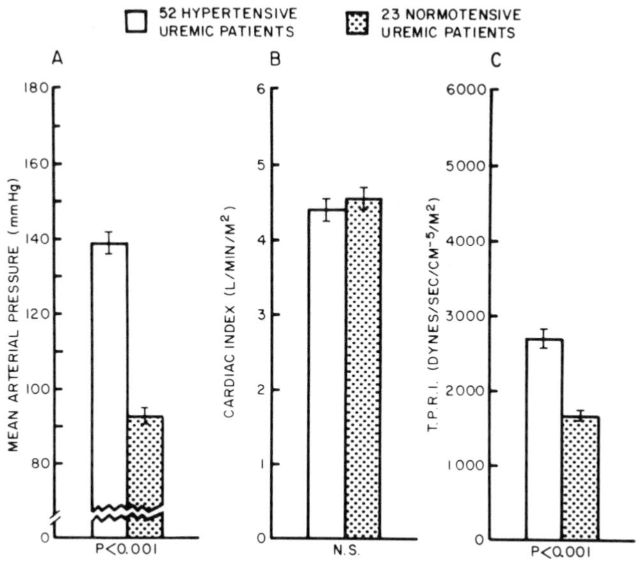

FIG. 2.—Comparison of mean arterial pressure (*A*), cardiac index (*B*), and total peripheral resistance index (*C*) of 52 hypertensive and 23 normotensive patients with end-stage renal disease. **T.P.R.I.,** Total peripheral resistance index. (From Kim, K. E., Onesti, G., Schwartz, A. B., Chinitz, J. L., and Swartz, C.: Hemodynamics of hypertension in chronic end-stage renal disease. Circulation 46:456, 1972, with the permission of the American Heart Association, Inc.)

index was 2703 ± 120 dynes per second per cm^{-5} per M^2 in the hypertensive patients and 1670 ± 61 dynes per second per cm^{-5} per M^2 in the normotensive uremic patients. The difference is highly significant ($p < 0.001$) (Fig. 2*C*).

The mean hematocrit was 23 percent in both the hypertensive and the normotensive uremic patients. In summary, the only significant differences between hypertensive and normotensive uremic patients were an elevated arterial blood pressure and an increased peripheral vascular resistance.

Hemodynamic Effects of Correction of Anemia

Six of the 75 patients with end-stage renal disease had further studies to test the effect of increasing their hematocrit. Hemodynamic studies were performed twice a week prior to hemodialysis at least 48 hours after the patient had received packed red cell transfusions during the previous dialysis. Blood was administered during dialysis as buffy-coat-free, packed red cells. The hematocrit was increased to at least 40 percent in each patient.

Serial transfusion of packed red cells resulted in a linear decrease in cardiac index to a normal level (Fig. 3). Diastolic blood pressure increased as hematocrit increased (Fig. 4). Total peripheral resistance index increased markedly as hematocrit increased (Fig. 5). Neither body weight nor blood volume changed significantly during the study. Figure 6 shows the effect of increase in hematocrit on cardiac index, total peripheral resistance index, and mean arterial pressure in a typical patient. With the increase in hematocrit, there was a progressive decrease in cardiac index. The total peripheral resistance index and mean arterial pressure increased progressively as hematocrit increased.

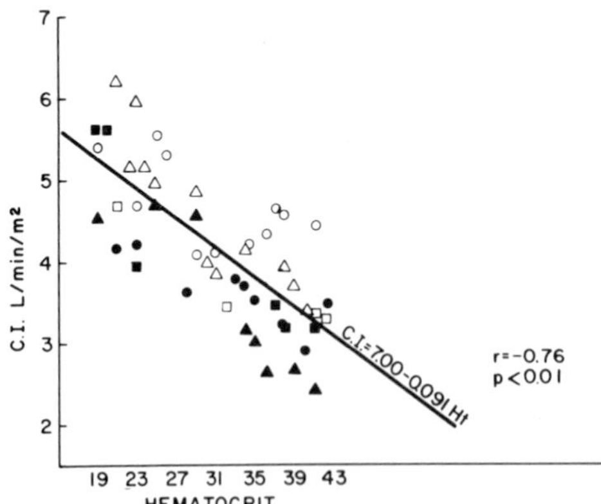

FIG. 3.—The effect of increase in hematocrit on cardiac index in six uremic patients. C.I., cardiac index; r, correlation coefficient. ○, Patient 1; ●, Patient 2; △, Patient 3; ▲, Patient 4; □, Patient 5; ■, Patient 6. (From Neff, M.S. et al.: Hemodynamics of uremic anemia. Circulation 43:876, 1971, with the permission of the American Heart Association, Inc.)

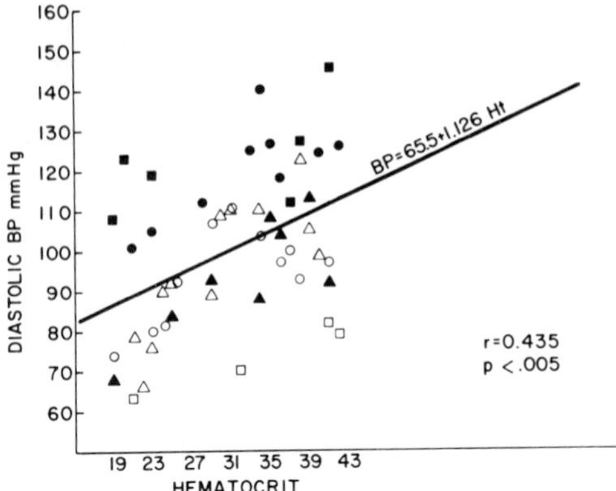

FIG. 4.—The effect of increase in hematocrit on diastolic pressure in six uremic patients. BP, blood pressure; r, correlation coefficient. Symbols are the same as those used in Figure 3. (From Neff, M.S. et al.: Hemodynamics of uremic anemia. Circulation 43:876, 1971, with the permission of the American Heart Association, Inc.)

Discussion

The data obtained in our patients with chronic end-stage renal disease demonstrate that at this phase of the natural history of renal parenchymal disease, the cardiac index is significantly higher than normal. This increase in cardiac index is associated with an increase in heart rate whereas the stroke index is not different from that of controls. The mean cardiac index of 4.44 liters per minute per M^2 in our 75 uremic patients is very close to the value of 4.28 liters per minute per M^2 reported by Goss et al.[10] with the dye-dilution method. Similarly, a mean cardiac index of 4.19 liters per minute per M^2 was reported in 21 uremic patients by Mostert and co-

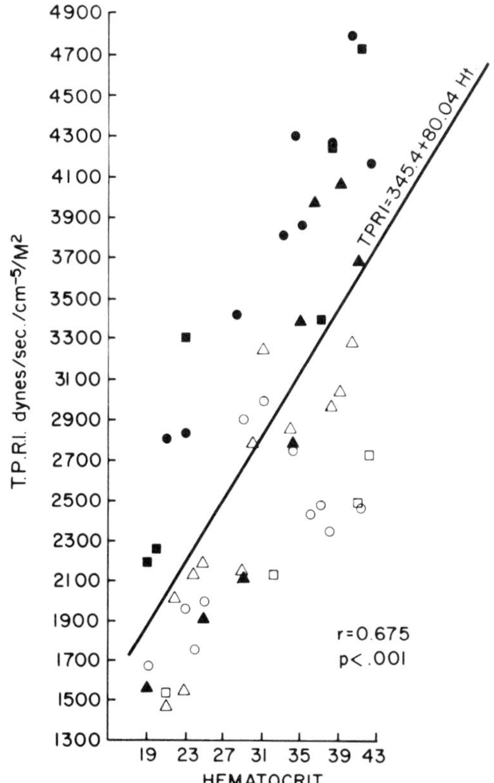

FIG. 5.—The effect of increase in hematocrit on total peripheral resistance index (TPRI) in six uremic patients. r, Correlation coefficient. Symbols are the same as those used in Figure 3. (From Neff, M.S. et al.: Hemodynamics of uremic anemia. Circulation 43:876, 1971, with the permission of the American Heart Association, Inc.)

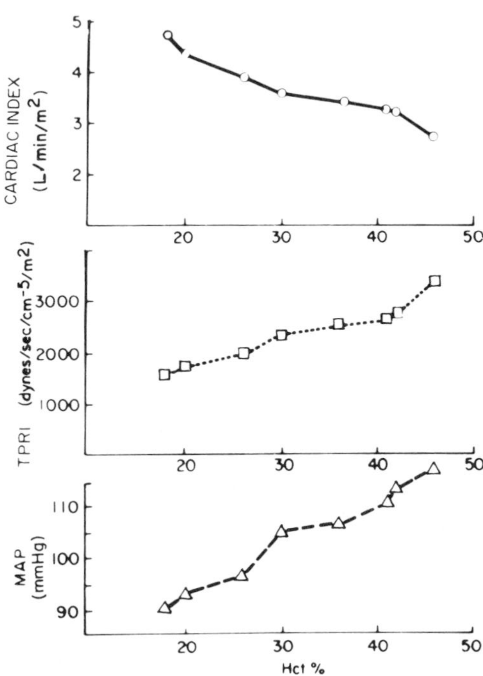

FIG. 6.—The effects of increase in hematocrit on cardiac index (○), total peripheral resistance index (TPRI) (□), and mean arterial pressure (MAP) (△) in one particular patient.

workers.[11] In contrast, Del Greco et al.[12] reported cardiac indices in uremic patients not different from those in their normal controls. The technique for cardiac output used in the Del Greco study, however, was external isotopic counting. This technique gave a cardiac index in normal controls of 4.10 liters per minute per M^2, which is significantly higher than the normal values obtained by the dye-dilution technique in several studies.[1–7] Anthonisen and Holst [13] in 1960 reported that nine patients with chronic uremia had cardiac indices equal to those of their control subjects. However, at the time of their study their uremic patients were not rehabilitated by maintenance hemodialysis and had a uremic syndrome that appeared to be more severe than in the 75 patients reported in the present study.

We conclude that patients with chronic end-stage renal disease and uremia (hypertensive and normotensive) on maintenance dialysis have a higher than normal cardiac output. This increase in cardiac output is associated with an increase in heart rate, whereas the stroke volume remains within the normal limits. Thus, the patients with end-stage renal disease and uremia are characterized by a high cardiac output. Their calculated total peripheral vascular resistance falls within the normal limits. It may, therefore, be suggested that the hypertension, which is present in the majority of these patients, is sustained by such an elevation of the cardiac output. The comparative evaluation of the hemodynamic pattern of the hypertensive uremic patients versus the normotensive uremic patients has now clarified the role of cardiac output in this hypertensive state. Cardiac index, heart rate, and stroke index were entirely similar in these two uremic groups. The 52 hypertensive patients with chronic end-stage renal disease, however, showed a total peripheral resistance index much higher than that of the normotensive patients with chronic end-stage renal disease. Anemia and uremia were equivalent in the two groups. These data support the conclusion that the hypertension of chronic renal parenchymal disease at this stage is sustained by an elevated total peripheral resistance.

Additional information on the role of high cardiac output in this stage of renal hypertension is provided by the studies of the hemodynamic effects of correction of anemia in the six uremic patients. Correction of anemia with serial transfusion of buffy-coat-free, packed red cells decreased cardiac output but raised blood pressure instead of lowering it. Increasing the hematocrit from 20 to 40 percent raised diastolic pressure an average of 20 mm Hg despite a reduction of cardiac index to normal in five of six patients. We maintained a constant body weight, and no significant change in blood volume was noted during the entire study. The most likely explanation for the increasing resistance is related to the fact that severe anemia is associated with inadequate oxygen delivery to the tissues. This produces peripheral vasodilation. Correcting the anemia abolishes hypoxic vasodilation and increases arteriolar resistance and blood pressure. This effect is magnified in previously hypertensive uremic patients. This study indicates that the major factor responsible for high cardiac output in patients with chronic end-stage renal disease is anemia itself. Duke and Abelmann [16] found cardiac index values of 4.73 liters per minute per M^2 and low total peripheral resistance in anemic patients with normal kidney function (a mean hematocrit of 20.3 percent). The hemodynamic pattern of their anemic patients and the degree of their anemia appear to be very similar to those of the normotensive uremic patients discussed in this study. In their study, the correction of anemia in the same patients resulted in a decrease of cardiac index to normal (3.44 liters per minute per M^2) and a significant increase in total peripheral resistance.

The hemodynamic and pathophysiologic conclusions of the present study are limited to the final stage of hypertension of chronic renal disease. No light is shed upon the pathophysiology of the early stages of renal hypertension. In the experimental animal, Bianchi, Tenconi, and Lucca [14] described two phases of experimental hypertension due to renal artery constriction in a single remaining kidney: a first phase, characterized by an increase in resistance and presumably due to the vasopressor effect of angiotensin; and a second phase, in which the hypertension appeared to be secondary to an equal increase in cardiac output and peripheral resistance. Ledingham and Pelling [17] also described sequential changes in cardiac output and resistance in renal hypertensive rats. Ferrario, Page, and McCubbin [18] showed an initial phase of high cardiac output in renal hypertensive dogs followed by a return of cardiac output to normal, while blood pressure and total peripheral resistance were elevated.

The theory of autoregulation in the pathophysiology of hypertension [19–22] minimizes the role of renal vasopressor substances. Demonstration of an initial increase in cardiac output, with return to normal values as arterial pressure and peripheral resistance increase, is an essential aspect of this theoretical relationship between pressure and flow.[22] This has indeed been the case in several types of experimental hypertension,[17,18,23] and in some hypertensive states in man.[4,5,15] If the blood pressure and the peripheral resistance increase without increase in cardiac output, the action of a vasoconstrictor substance must be suggested.[22] This has also been the case in some types and phases of experimental renal hypertension [14,17,18] and, in the present group, of end-stage renal hypertension in man.

The data obtained in the present study leave no doubt that at the end stage of the natural history of hypertension of chronic renal disease in man, the blood pressure elevation is associated with an elevated resistance. Studies of the hemodynamic changes of the early stages of hypertension in chronic renal disease and of their possible evolution appear to be necessary.

Summary

This study was undertaken to define the hemodynamic changes in hypertension of chronic end-stage renal disease. The mean cardiac index in 75 uremic patients was higher ($p < 0.001$) than that of 42 normal volunteers while stroke index was not different from normals. The higher cardiac indices of uremic patients were accounted for by increased heart rates. Despite the significantly higher blood pressure in the uremics, their mean total peripheral resistance index was not different from that of normals.

The total group of 75 uremic patients included 52 hypertensive and 23 normotensive uremics. Cardiac index, heart rate, and stroke index were the same in 52 hypertensive uremics and 23 normotensive uremics while the mean total peripheral resistance index of hypertensive uremics was higher ($p < 0.001$) than that of normotensive uremics. Therefore, the hypertension in end-stage renal disease is sustained by a high total peripheral resistance.

Six patients underwent serial hemodynamic studies over a period of 6 to 12 weeks while being transfused with buffy-coat-free, packed red blood cells to a normal hematocrit. Body weight was maintained constant and blood volume did not change significantly during the study period. Cardiac index decreased during transfusion, reaching a normal level at a hematocrit of 30 percent. Diastolic pressure progressively rose, averaging an increase of 20 mm Hg at a hematocrit of 40 percent. Total peripheral resistance increased by 80 percent at a hematocrit of 40 percent. This study indicates that the major factor responsible for high cardiac output in patients with chronic end-stage renal disease is anemia itself.

These findings imply that a high total peripheral resistance is the major hemodynamic alteration in renal hypertension during the late stage of its natural history.

REFERENCES

1. Finkielman, S., Worcel, M., and Agrest, A.: Hemodynamic pattern in essential hypertension. Circulation 31:356, 1965.
2. Bello, C. T., Sevy, R. W., and Harakal, C.: Varying hemodynamic patterns in essential hypertension. Am. J. Med. Sci. 250:58, 1965.
3. Sannerstedt, R.: Hemodynamic response to exercise in patients with arterial hypertension. Acta Med. Scand. 180(Suppl. 458):1, 1966.
4. Lund-Johansen, P.: Hemodynamics in early essential hypertension. Acta Med. Scand. 181(Suppl. 482):1, 1967.
5. Eich, R. H., Cuddy, R. P., Smulyan, H., and Lyons, R. H.: Hemodynamics in labile hypertension. A follow-up study. Circulation 34:299, 1966.
6. Frohlich, E. D., Tarazi, R. C., Dustan, H. P.: Re-examination of the hemodynamics of hypertension. Am. J. Med. Sci. 257:9, 1969.
7. Julius, S., Pascual, A. V., Sannerstedt, R., Mitchell, C.: Relationship between cardiac output and peripheral resistance in borderline hypertension. Circulation 43:382, 1971.
8. Defazio, V., Christensen, R. C., Regan, T. J., Baer, L. J., Morita, Y., and Hellems, H. K.: Circulatory changes in acute glomerulonephritis. Circulation 20:190, 1959.
9. Brod, J., Hejl, Z., Ulrych, M., Fencl, V., Jirka, J.: Hemodynamic basis of renal hypertension. Cesk. Fysiol. 10:228, 1961.
10. Goss, J. E., Alfrey, A. C., Vogel, J. H. K., and Holmex, J. H.: Hemodynamic changes during hemodialysis. Trans. Am. Soc. Artif. Intern. Organs 13:68, 1967.
11. Mostert, J. W., Evers, J. L., Hobika, G. H., Moore, R. H., Kenny, G. M., and Murphy, G. P.: The haemodynamic response to chronic renal failure as studied in the azotaemic state. Br. J. Anaesth. 42:397, 1970.
12. Del Greco, F., Simon, N. M., Roguska, J., and Walker, C.: Hemodynamic studies in chronic uremia. Circulation 40:87, 1969.
13. Anthonisen, P., and Holst, E.: Determination of cardiac output and other hemodynamic data in uremic patients using dye-dilution technique. Scand. J. Clin. Lab. Invest. 12: 481, 1960.
14. Bianchi, G., Tenconi, L. T., and Lucca, R.: Effect in the conscious dog of constriction of the renal artery to a sole remaining kidney on haemodynamics, sodium balance, body fluid volumes, plasma renin concentration and pressor responsiveness to angiotensin. Clin. Sci. 38:741, 1970.
15. Coleman, T. G., Bower, J. D., Langford, H. G., and Guyton, A. C.: Regulation of arterial pressure in the anephric state. Circulation 42:509, 1970.
16. Duke, M., and Abelmann, W. H.: The hemodynamic response to chronic anemia. Circulation 39:503, 1969.
17. Ledingham, J. M., and Pelling, D.: Cardiac output and peripheral resistance in experimental renal hypertension. Circ. Res. 21 (Suppl. II):187, 1967.
18. Ferrario, C. M., Page, I. H., and McCubbin, J. W.: Increased cardiac output as a contributory factor in experimental renal hypertension in dogs. Circ. Res. 27:799, 1970.

19. Bayliss, W. M.: On the local reactions of the arterial wall to changes of internal pressure. J. Physiol. (London) 28:220, 1902.
20. Folkow, B.: Study of the factors influencing the tone of denervated blood vessel perfused at various pressures. Acta Physiol. Scand. 27:99, 1952.
21. Ledingham, J. M., and Cohen, R. D.: Role of the heart in the pathogenesis of renal hypertension. Lancet 2:279, 1963.
22. Coleman, T. G., Granger, H. J., Guyton, A. C.: Whole-body circulatory autoregulation and hypertension. Circ. Res. 28(Suppl. II): 76, 1971.
23. Coleman, T. G., and Guyton, A. C.: Hypertension caused by salt loading in the dog. III. Onset transients of cardiac output and other circulatory variables. Circ. Res. 25:153, 1969.

The Regulation of Renin Release

By James O. Davis, Ph.D., M.D.

The mechanisms which lead to renin release were first studied in connection with attempts to elucidate the pathogenesis of renal hypertension. With the recognition in 1960 [1–3] of the importance of the renin-angiotensin system in the control of aldosterone secretion, there was renewed interest in the nature of the signal perceived by the kidney. There have been two principal hypotheses for the intrarenal receptors involved in renin secretion,[4,5] namely, (1) the baroreceptor hypothesis, and (2) the macula densa theory. And several factors are now known to influence one or the other of these receptors or to act directly upon the renal juxtaglomerular (JG) cells. These factors include the renal sympathetic nerves and various humoral agents such as epinephrine, norepinephrine, sodium and potassium ions, antidiuretic hormone (ADH) and angiotensin II.[5] This chapter reviews the pertinent observations which form the basis for our present knowledge of the mechanisms of renin release.

Evidence for a Renovascular Receptor for Renin Release

Most of the early evidence supported the view that the JG cells perceive a hemodynamic signal and release renin [4–6] and this explanation was used to account for the renin responses to acute renal artery constriction.[6,7] Also, it is clear from our knowledge of renal autoregulation that the renal arterioles respond to changes in pressure. From the early studies of the isolated kidney in 1940, Kohlstaedt and Page [8] suggested that a decrease in arterial pulse pressure stimulated renin secretion. Against the decreased pulse pressure theory is the finding of Kolff [9] that renin or a renin-like substance was released in response to renal artery constriction irrespective of pulsatile or nonpulsatile blood flow. Also, increased plasma renin activity occurs in dogs with high output failure secondary to a large arteriovenous fistula and with a high arterial pulse pressure.[10]

The present baroreceptor hypothesis was suggested by Tobian, Tomboulian, and Janecek in 1959,[11] in which they proposed that changes in mean renal arterial pressure alter the rate of renin release by the JG cells. Their observations were that a decreased degree of granulation of the JG cells occurred in association with increased mean arterial pressure but it was impossible in their experiments to exclude an influence of an increase in renal blood flow. They proposed that decreased "stretch" of the renal afferent arterioles in the region of the JG cells leads to renin release.

The baroreceptor hypothesis received strong support by Skinner, McCubbin, and Page; [12] with suprarenal aortic constriction they reduced mean renal arterial pressure only slightly without a discernible change in renal blood flow and a renal pressor substance was released. It is noteworthy that under these circumstances the renal arterioles dilated, an autoregulatory response. This association of renal arteriolar dilatation with renin release during aortic constriction and renal autoregulation has been confirmed by Blaine, Davis, and Prewitt,[13,14] and by Eide, Loyning, and Kiil.[15]

The relationship of arteriolar dilatation to renin release was also studied by Ayers, Harris, and Lefer.[16] They found that chronic renal artery constriction produced an initial dilatation followed by gradual constriction of the renal arterioles. The initial decrease in renal arteriolar resistance was associated with increased plasma renin activity, and the later progressive constriction of the arterioles was accompanied by return in plasma renin activity to normal although arterial pressure remained elevated. In this state of chronic renal hypertension with a normal plasma renin activity, vasodilator drugs (dopamine, isoproterenol, nitroprusside, and acetylcholine) increased plasma renin activity but little effect was observed in control experiments on normal dogs. Changes in arterial pressure were not

From the Department of Physiology, University of Missouri School of Medicine, Columbia, Missouri.

correlated with alterations in renin release, nor was renal sodium excretion.

In contrast, the hypersecretion of renin after acute hemorrhage [13,17] or during thoracic caval constriction [18,19] is associated with no change or an increase in renovascular resistance. And mineralocorticoid excess, which leads to decreased plasma renin activity,[20–22] is associated with decreased renovascular resistance.[21,23] Consequently, changes in total renovascular resistance are not necessarily associated with either increased or decreased renin release.

One of the difficulties in attempting to evaluate the response of the so-called "baroreceptor" to various stimuli is that most experimental maneuvers also influence sodium in the renal tubules and could conceivably stimulate the macula densa. For example, the use of diuretics to alter the filtered load of sodium also results in changes in both total renal blood flow and the intrarenal distribution of blood flow. A new approach for evaluation of the baroreceptor hypothesis has been the use of the denervated, nonfiltering kidney model in adrenalectomized dogs.[13,14,17] This model was prepared under sterile conditions by clamping the left renal artery for 2 hours, by removing all visible nervous tissue from the renal vessels and painting them with a 5% phenol solution, by ligating and sectioning the left ureter and, finally, by bilaterally adrenalectomizing the dog; the dogs were maintained on 50 mg of cortisone daily. Three days later the right kidney was removed and on the fourth day the acute response in renin secretion by the denervated, nonfiltering left kidney to hemorrhage or to suprarenal aortic constriction was studied. Renal blood flow was measured in the left kidney with an electromagnetic flowmeter and the venous-arterial renin difference across the kidney determined. Evidence was presented to show that denervation was complete and that the model was nonfiltering.[13,14,17]

The approach was to remove all but one of the possible mechanisms which alter renin secretion and, then, to apply an adequate stimulus. Consequently the renal nerves were abolished, the animals were adrenalectomized to exclude catecholamines, and a nonfiltering kidney was produced to prevent acute changes in sodium load or concentration from occurring in the sodium receptor of the macula densa. Thus, by combining these ablative procedures, it was possible to examine the hypothesis that a receptor mechanism, conceivably a baroreceptor, is located in the renovascular tree.

Dogs prepared in this manner were subjected to acute hemorrhage (20 ml per kilogram of body weight) in an attempt to stimulate renin release; a striking increase in renin secretion occurred (Fig. 1).[13,14] The blood was reinfused in 3 of the dogs and the animals were allowed to recover. The aorta was constricted above the kidney in a stepwise fashion and renin secretion measured at 10-minute intervals. A typical response is shown in Fig. 2. The initial tightening of the aortic ligature reduced renal perfusion pressure approximately 20 mm Hg, but renal blood flow was unchanged; renin secretion increased, as indicated by the increased renal venous-arterial difference in plasma renin activity. These data demonstrate the occurrence of increased renin secretion in association with renal autoregulation and arteriolar dilatation; it should be emphasized that this response occurred in the absence

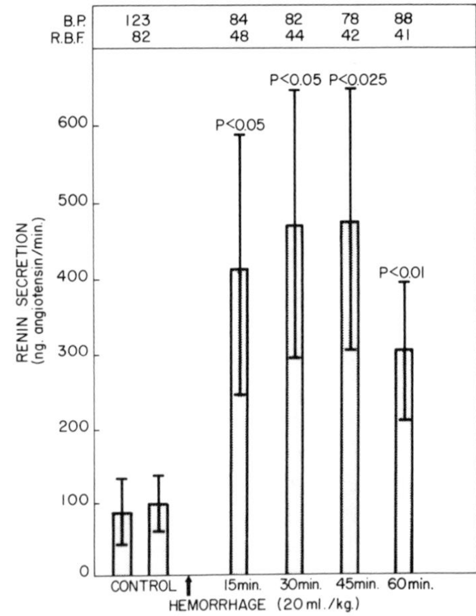

FIG. 1.—Response in renin secretion to hemorrhage in adrenalectomized dogs with denervated nonfiltering kidneys (N=6). B.P., mean blood pressure; R.B.F., mean renal blood flow. (From Blaine, E. H., Davis, J. O., and Prewitt, R. L.,[13] with permission.)

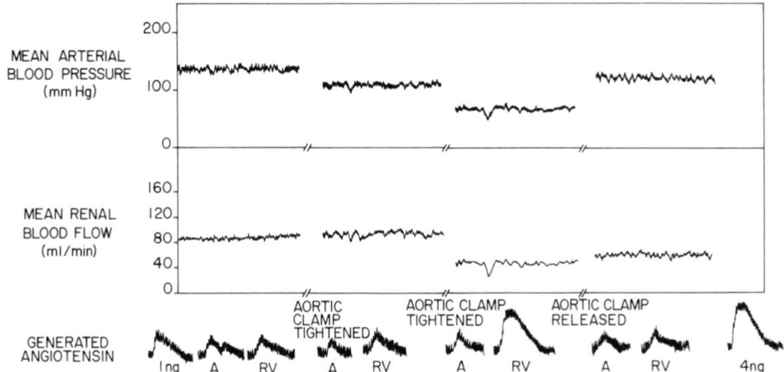

FIG. 2.—Changes in mean arterial pressure, mean renal blood flow, and generated angiotensin, which reflect plasma renin activity in **A** (aortic) and **RV** (renal venous) blood during aortic constriction and release in an adrenalectomized dog with a denervated, nonfiltering kidney. Units of angiotensin (1 ng and 4 ng) were bioassayed as standards. (From Blaine, E. H., and Davis, J. O.: Evidence for a renal vascular mechanism in renin release. New observations with graded stimulation by aortic constriction. Circ. Res.(Suppl. II)28–29:II-118, 1971, by permission of the American Heart Association, Inc.)

of the renal nerves and without a major part of the circulating catecholamines. Further reduction in renal perfusion pressure produced an additional marked increase in renin release. Finally, release of the aortic ligature was accompanied by a reduction in renin secretion to the control level. The findings that the capacity of the nonfiltering kidney to respond to aortic constriction after hemorrhage and after reinfusion of blood, and that renin secretion returned to the control level after release of the aortic ligature, provide convincing evidence of the excellent functional condition of the JG apparatus. Collectively, these observations suggest the presence of an intrarenal vascular receptor which responds to changes in arteriolar hydrostatic pressure and leads to release of renin.

The nature and location of this intrarenal vascular receptor were studied by infusing papaverine into the left renal artery in the denervated nonfiltering model and subjecting the animal to the stimulus of acute hemorrhage.[24] The rationale for this experiment was suggested by the observations of Thurau and Kramer,[25] who gave papaverine intrarenally and completely blocked the renal autoregulatory response. Since renal autoregulation is an afferent arteriolar function, it was reasoned that papaverine might dilate the renal arterioles and block the response of the intrarenal vascular receptor to hemorrhage. As pointed out earlier in this review, either no change or an increase in renovascular resistance occurred in response to acute hemorrhage.[13,17] As a control experiment, the response to acute hemorrhage in the nonfiltering kidney is presented in Fig. 3.[17] Papaverine was infused intrarenally into a denervated nonfiltering kidney at a rate to achieve

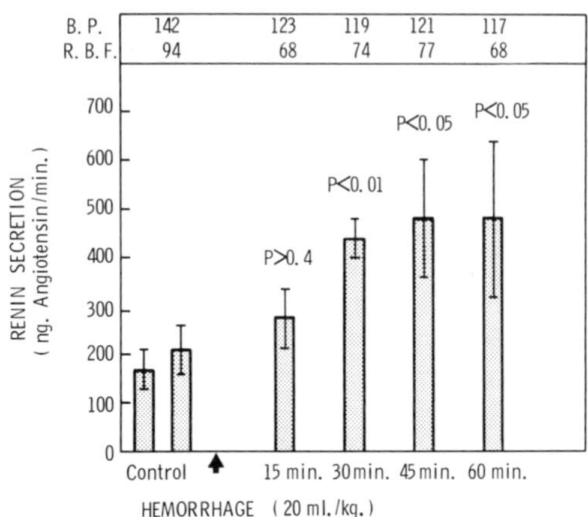

FIG. 3.—Increase in renin secretion following hemorrhage in dogs with a nonfiltering kidney (N=5). B.P., mean arterial pressure; R.B.F., renal blood flow. (From Blaine, E. H., Davis, J. O., and Witty, R. T.: Renin release after hemorrhage and after suprarenal aortic constriction in dogs without sodium delivery to the macula densa. Circ. Res. 27:1081, 1970, by permission of the American Heart Association, Inc.)

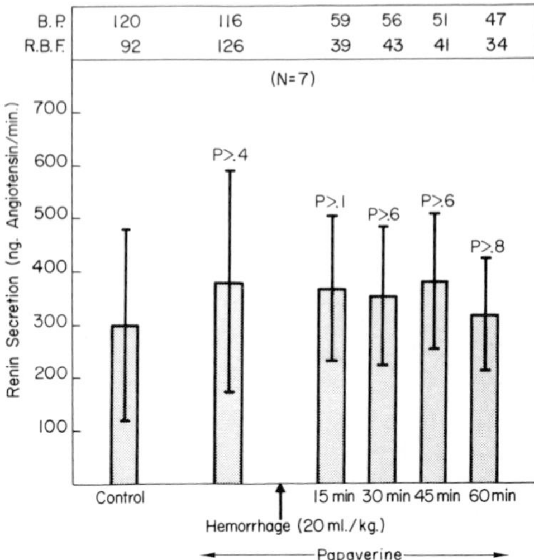

FIG. 4.—Failure of hemorrhage to increase renin secretion in dogs with denervated, nonfiltering kidneys given papaverine intrarenally. (From Witty, R. T., Davis, J. O., Johnson, J. A., and Prewitt, R. L.,[24] with permission.)

maximal arteriolar dilatation with a minimal decrease in arterial pressure. While the kidney was receiving papaverine, the dogs were subjected to hemorrhaging (20 ml per kilogram of body weight). The response in renin secretion was completely blocked (Fig. 4).[24] The data support the original concept of a renovascular receptor for renin release, and they point to an afferent arteriolar locus since papaverine is known to dilate the renal afferent arterioles and to prevent renal autoregulation.

The possible importance of this renovascular receptor in mediating the hypersecretion of renin in low-output heart failure was examined in the experimental model with thoracic caval constriction.[19] A comparative study on renin secretion in dogs with a nonfiltering kidney with or without thoracic caval constriction was performed. In a group of dogs with caval constriction and a nonfiltering left kidney, renin secretion was 1156 ± 188 ng of angiotensin per minute in comparison with 190 ± 50 ng of angiotensin per minute for dogs with the nonfiltering kidney model but otherwise normal ($P < 0.001$). Since the macula densa was nonfunctional in these dogs with nonfiltering kidneys, the data are consistent with the mediation of the high rate of renin secretion during caval constriction by the vascular receptor described earlier. If this interpretation is correct, papaverine given intrarenally should markedly decrease renin secretion in the dog with caval constriction with a nonfiltering kidney and a high renovascular resistance, and this was the response obtained. When this model was given papaverine into the renal artery, renal blood flow increased 50 percent and renin secretion fell from 1156 to 497 ng of angiotensin per minute ($P < 0.005$). Thus, the present data point to an afferent arteriolar receptor for renin release in the dog with thoracic caval constriction since papaverine is known to block renal autoregulation, an afferent arteriolar function. These observations on the effects of papaverine were extended to dogs with thoracic caval constriction with a filtering kidney; again, dilatation of the renal arterioles occurred and a striking fall in renin secretion from 2481 to 697 ng of angiotensin per minute was observed ($P < 0.01$). Thus, the response to papaverine in both the filtering and the nonfiltering kidney of dogs with caval constriction supports the concept of a renovascular receptor for the control of renin release and it seems likely that the receptor is located in the renal afferent arterioles at the level of the JG cells.

Little is known about the nature of the signal perceived by this vascular receptor. According to current theory, a decrease in "stretch" leads to increased renin release, but in considering what is meant by stretch, it seems likely that this receptor responds to changes in wall tension. In this event, the receptor might be influenced by several inputs including (1) changes in the transmural pressure gradient, (2) nervous factors which control arteriolar tone, (3) intrinsic myogenic factors exemplified in renal autoregulation, and (4) alterations in the elastic components of the vessel wall. It is conceivable that alterations in any of these variables produce changes in wall tension and influence the rate of renin release.

THE MACULA DENSA HYPOTHESIS

In 1945, Goormaghtigh[26] suggested a close functional relationship between the macula densa and the JG cells. This hypothesis received its first important support in 1964 when Vander and Miller[27] blocked the increase in renin release induced by aortic constriction by giving diuretics (chlorothiazide, acetazolamide, or osmotic diuretics). They suggested that increased sodium load at the macula densa prevented renin release and, therefore, that the decreased sodium load at the level of the macula densa stimulates renin release. This interpretation seems reasonable if changes in the filtered load of sodium result in similar directional changes of the load of sodium entering the loop of Henle, as suggested by Bunag, Vander, and Kaneko.[28] There is, however, the additional influence of the ascending loop of Henle on renotubular sodium before it reaches the macula densa, and less is known about what happens in this segment than in some other parts of the renal tubules. In contrast to the hypothesis of Vander and Miller, Thurau and associates [29] have proposed that it is increased sodium concentration rather than decreased sodium load to which the macula densa responds and leads to renin release. This view was originally supported with observations from micropuncture experiments [29] in which retrograde injection of isotonic or hypertonic sodium chloride or bromide solutions into the distal tubule near the macula densa produced proximal tubule collapse; in control experiments hypotonic sodium chloride, or hypertonic or isotonic solutions of choline chloride or mannitol injected under the same conditions were without effect on the proximal tubule. They proposed the following sequence of changes: increased renin release, local angiotensin II formation, afferent arteriolar constriction and a decreased glomerular filtration rate with resultant proximal tubule collapse, and they concluded that the sodium ion was necessary for the response. In 1968, Meyer et al.[30] also suggested that increased intratubular sodium concentration at the macula densa leads to renin release; they gave furosemide to rabbits and observed increased plasma renin activity during reinfusion of urine to prevent volume depletion. Since early distal tubule sodium concentration is increased with furosemide, these investigators [30] pointed out the possible association in their experiments of increased sodium concentration at the macula densa and increased renin release. Cooke et al.[31] supported the view that it is increased sodium concentration that the macula densa perceives and leads to renin release. These workers gave ethacrynic acid or chlorothiazide during reinfusion of urine to prevent volume depletion in dogs and noted increased renal venous renin activity only with ethacrynic acid; they cited the evidence [32–34] that ethacrynic acid acts on the ascending limb of Henle whereas chlorothiazide acts more distally. Also, Cooke and co-workers [31] occluded the ureters and observed an increase in renal venous renin activity but ethacrynic acid failed to increase renin secretion until the ureters were released; the increased renin release, therefore, appeared to be associated with increased delivery of sodium to the macula densa from the sodium-rich urine present in the ascending limb of Henle.

In 1968, Nash and associates [35] proposed that renin release is regulated by an intrarenal sodium-sensitive mechanism and possibly by sodium flux across the macula densa cells. Subsequently, Nash [36] referred to this mechanism as a "tubular natriastat" and offered as supportive evidence for it the finding that renal arterial infusion of sodium chloride decreased renin secretion in dogs with acute hypersecretion of renin from ureteral constriction. So the available evidence does indeed point to a sodium-sensitive mechanism in the release of renin but it remains unclear what specifically the macula densa perceives as a signal.

In an attempt to reconcile some of the apparent discrepancies in results as they relate to the sensor, Vander and Carlson [37] suggested that renin release is a function of changes in sodium transport by the macula densa cells. Measurements are needed to determine what does happen to sodium transport in the macula densa cells in association with changes in renin release. With the present available methods, this information has not been forthcoming.

In considering the relationship of the macula densa to the JG cells and the glomerulus, several workers have suggested that an *intrarenal feedback mechanism* is present within each nephron. This intermediate functional connection was proposed by Guyton, Langston, and Navar [38] in a computer model for renal autoregulation. Thurau, Dahlheim, and Granger [39,40] have assembled evidence in favor of such a feedback mechanism; their early evidence [29] from micropuncture experiments has been cited. In a most recent report, Thurau and associates [41] analyzed the vascular pole from single glomeruli in rats for renin activity after retrograde perfusion of the macula densa; a significantly higher level of renin activity was present during perfusion with an isotonic sodium chloride solution compared with an isotonic mannitol infusion. This group of workers has proposed that angiotensin II is formed locally in the JG cells, that increased angiotensin formation leads to afferent arteriolar constriction and decreased glomerular filtration rate, and, finally, that a resultant decrease in sodium concentration at the macula densa decreases renin synthesis in the JG cells to complete the feedback loop. They maintain that all substances available for formation of vasoactive angiotensin are present in the JG apparatus [41] and they point out that myofibrils are present in the JG cells.[40]

This hypothesis has been challenged by Morgan,[42] who perfused the loop of Henle and macula densa in rats and measured glomerular filtration rates for the same nephron. The glomerular filtration rate was found to be remarkably independent of flow and composition of fluid at the macula densa with several experimental sets of conditions and he concluded that an individual nephron feedback system does not exist.

Also, Barajas [43] has reported that in the rat the macula densa is more frequently closely associated with the efferent arteriole and mesangial cells than with the afferent arteriole. He has proposed, as a working hypothesis, that the degree of contact of the macula densa with the afferent arteriole is a function of the sodium load and tubular volume; he suggested that a decreased sodium load and tubular volume leads to decreased contact with the JG cells and increased renin release and vice versa. He pointed out further that this idea might also fit the baroreceptor theory since decreased renal arteriolar volume is frequently an accompaniment of increased renin secretion.

The Role of the Renal Sympathetic Nerves

There is substantial evidence that the renal sympathetic nerves influence renin release. These nerves supply the highly specialized JG cells,[44] other parts of the renal afferent arterioles, and the renal efferent arterioles. Vander [45] reported that application of an electrical stimulus with a loop electrode around the renal artery increased renin release in the dog; this suggested that electrical stimulation of the renal nerves led to renin release. Recently, Johnson, Davis, and Witty [46] stimulated the renal nerves directly by placing electrodes on nerves dissected free from the renal pedicle, and the observations were made before and during intrarenal arterial infusion of papaverine into the nonfiltering kidney model with a nonfunctional macula densa. A striking increase in renin secretion occurred both before and during the infusion of papaverine. Since papaverine appears to block the so-called baroreceptor mechanism in the afferent arterioles and JG cells, these observations indicate that the renin response to direct electrical stimulation of the renal nerves is mediated, at least in part, by a direct effect on the JG cells.

The increase in renin secretion following hemorrhage,[47,48] during sodium depletion,[49] and during chronic thoracic caval constriction [19] appears to be partly mediated by the renal nerves. Bunag, Page, and McCubbin [47] blocked the response to hemorrhage by ganglion blockade and by application of local anesthesia to the renal nerves. Hodge, Lowe, and Vane [48] also blocked the renin response to hemorrhage with a local anesthetic, lignocaine. Vander and Luciano [50] were able to block only partially the release of renin in response to sodium depletion by the combination of surgical denervation, local anesthesia and alpha- and beta-adrenergic blockade. In contrast, Mogil et al.[49] reported failure of plasma renin activity to increase in response to sodium depletion following surgical denervation alone in both normotensive and hypertensive dogs; completeness of denervation was demonstrated by low or absent renocortical norepinephrine. As renocortical norepinephrine returned toward normal with reinnervation, sodium depletion did increase plasma renin activity. In a study by Brubacher and Vander,[51] surgical renal denervation slowed but did not abolish the renin response to sodium deprivation; also no significant changes in arterial pressure, renal hemodynamic function, or plasma electrolytes occurred with sodium depletion. These findings led Brubacher and Vander to postulate the existence of an unidentified hormone to explain the increased renin release in sodium depletion. In dogs with thoracic caval constriction, chronic bilateral renal denervation reduced plasma renin activity from 82 ng per milliliter to 40 ng per milliliter ($P < 0.001$), a value eight times normal ($P < 0.001$), and renal sodium retention with ascites formation continued unabated; [19] renocortical norepinephrine was reduced from a normal value of 0.29 to 0.014 μg per gram of kidney tissue ($P < 0.002$).

The renal nerves also appear to be involved in the renin response to upright posture and physical activity in man [52] and, consequently, contribute to the diurnal rhythm in plasma renin activity in humans.[53] It is well known [54] that assumption of the upright posture and increased physical activity increase renal sympathetic nerve activity and produce renal arteriolar constriction. Gordon et al.[52] found that a patient with severe autonomic insufficiency failed to show an increase in plasma renin activity upon assumption of the upright posture despite a substantial fall in arterial pressure.

The renin response to electrical stimulation of the dorsal region of the medulla oblongata near the obex appears to be mediated by the renal nerves,[55] and it was suggested that beta-adrenergic receptors were involved in the response since it was reduced by propranolol.[56]

Information has only begun to accumulate on the mechanisms whereby the renal nerves increase renin release. They are not essential even for hypersecretion of renin and it has been proposed that the renal nerves modulate the rate of secretion with other more important factors constituting the primary regulatory mechanisms.[5] This interpretation is in agreement with the early suggestion of Tobian [57] that the renal nerves might amplify the signal to the JG cells so that they are more sensitive to small changes in pressure and volume. As previously mentioned, Johnson, Davis, and Witty [46] presented evidence for a direct action of the nerves on the JG cells and Passo et al.[56] have suggested this is mediated by a beta-adrenergic receptor. It should also be pointed out that the renal nerves produce changes in afferent arteriolar constriction which could stimulate the vascular receptor in the JG cells. Also, the renal nerves influence glomerular filtration rate by changing arteriolar tone, and such changes produce alterations in renal tubular sodium which might influence the macula densa to alter renin release. Additional observations are needed to define the precise mechanisms under sympathetic nervous control.

The Role of Humoral Agents in the Control of Renin Secretion

An increasing number of humoral agents is now known to influence the rate of renin secretion. The role of catecholamines has been studied extensively. Wathen and associates [58] demonstrated that intravenous and intrarenal arterial infusion of epinephrine and norepinephrine increased renin release at plasma levels which decreased renal hemodynamic function. Additional information on the mechanism of action of catecholamines was provided by Vander,[45] who induced renin release with an intravenous infusion of epinephrine or norepinephrine during maintenance of a constant arterial pressure by means of an aortic ligature. That catecholamines can act directly on JG cells has been demonstrated from the in vitro studies of Michelakis, Caudle, and Liddle,[59] who reported that "net renin production" was increased with epinephrine, norepinephrine, and cyclic AMP in a dog renal cell suspension. Evidence for a physiologic role of the adrenal medullary hormones in renin release was provided by Otsuka et al.[60] They induced hypoglycemia with insulin, increased arterial plasma epinephrine, and found an increase in plasma renin activity. Infusion of epinephrine at rates which achieved an arterial level comparable to hypoglycemia produced less of an increase in plasma renin activity. Both hypoglycemia and epinephrine infusions decreased the plasma potassium concentration, which may have contributed to the increased plasma renin activity.

Evidence for the mechanism of action of epinephrine and norepinephrine has recently been provided by Johnson, Davis, and Witty [46] from studies in the nonfiltering kidney model. The intra-arterial infusion of either epinephrine or norepinephrine into the kidney increased renin release and this occurred in the absence of a functional macula densa. Simultaneous intrarenal infusion of either epinephrine or norepinephrine with papaverine revealed that papaverine, which blocks the renovascular receptor mechanism, completely abolished the response to epinephrine but failed to influence the action of norepinephrine. It was concluded that norepinephrine acts, at least in part, on the JG cells whereas epinephrine exerts its action on arteriolar smooth muscle, possibly on the renovascular receptor. Further localization of the sites of action of epinephrine and norepinephrine has been provided by studies of adrenergic blocking agents.

The role of adrenergic receptors in renin release was first suggested by Winer et al.[61] They observed an increase in plasma renin activity in normal human subjects following administration of diazoxide, ethacrynic acid, and theophylline, and upon the patient's assumption of an upright posture. They suggested that these stimuli probably act through diverse mechanisms; their influence on sodium excretion was different. With each of these stimuli, the response in plasma renin activity was diminished greatly or blocked when either phentolamine or propranolol was given and adrenergic blockade had little influence on sodium excretion. Subsequently, the mechanism of action of the sympathomimetic amines was investigated by Winer, Chokski, and Walkenhorst [62] in dogs. Cyclic AMP was the only one of several nucleotides tested which increased renin release, and the response was blocked by both phentolamine and propranolol. Winer and his colleagues proposed that cyclic AMP is an intracellular mediator of renin secretion.

Others [63–66] have also suggested a direct action of catecholamines on the JG cells to stimulate renin secretion but they have found renin release is blocked only by beta-adrenergic blockers and not by alpha-antagonists. These observations led Assaykeen et al.[64,65] to suggest that epinephrine stimulates renin secretion via a beta-adrenergic receptor. It has also been found (personal observations) that the beta-blocker propranolol markedly decreases renin secretion in dogs with hypersecretion of renin secondary to thoracic caval constriction with filtering kidneys or in the nonfiltering kidney model; alpha-blockers have not been studied in dogs with caval constriction.

The importance of changes in plasma potassium concentration in the control of renin release was first discovered by Veyrat et al.[66] This relationship has been subsequently investigated by others [67,68] who reported that changes in plasma renin activity occurred independently of associated alterations in either aldosterone secretion [67] or in sodium balance.[68] Recent studies of the effects of intrarenal arterial infusion of potassium in dogs have revealed a striking decrease in renin secretion if the kidney is intact but in the nonfiltering kidney model renin secretion failed to change.[69] These observations suggest that the potassium effect is mediated by the renal tubule system, possibly through the macula densa rather than by a direct action of potassium on either the smooth muscle of the arterioles or on the JG cells.

Attention was called to the possible relation of the sodium ion to renin release when Pitcock and Hartroft [70] noted a significant inverse correlation between the plasma sodium concentration and the degree of granulation of the JG cells. Newsome and Bartter [71] reported that body fluid volume was more important than plasma sodium concentration in the control of renin release since overhydration of normal humans decreased plasma renin activity in spite of a fall in serum sodium concentration. Similar findings and conclusions were reported by Gordon and Pawsey.[72] Nash et al.[35] found a reciprocal relationship between changes in renin secretory activity and renal arterial plasma sodium concentration, filtered sodium load, and urinary sodium excretion in dogs. Conversely, Yamamoto et al.[73] observed an increase in renin secretion by perfused kidneys during a reduction in plasma sodium concentration. In recent studies by Shade et al.[69] in the nonfiltering model, intrarenal infusion of sodium chloride increased renin release only after 45 minutes of infusion while in dogs with filtering kidneys studied similarly a striking decrease in renin secretion was noted during this 45-minute period.

It has been reported that small peptides such as antidiuretic hormone (ADH) and angiotensin II inhibit renin secretion. In the first reports,[74–77] intravenous infusion of pitressin to anesthetized, laparotomized dogs inhibited renin secretion. More recently, Tagawa et al.[78] have found that intravenous pitressin given to conscious, unstressed, sodium-depleted dogs decreased plasma renin activity and this response was reportedly with plasma levels of ADH within the normal range. Infusion of angiotensin II has been found to decrease renin secretion in dog [74,75,77] and man.[79] In a more recent study in sheep,[80] it has been reported that physiologic concentrations of angiotensin II act directly on the kidney to decrease renin secretion and that the response is independent of changes in renal arterial pressure and renal sodium excretion.

Finally, the effects of adrenal steroids and estrogens on plasma renin activity have been studied. Geelhoed and Vander [81] reported that aldosterone had no direct influence on renin secretion but produced its action only by changes in body sodium. Under some conditions, glucocorticoids produced a slight depression of plasma renin activity in humans.[82] In hypophysectomized rats, Goodwin et al.[83] obtained a significant increase in plasma renin concentration while plasma renin substrate fell in response to hypophysectomy. Many years ago, Helmer and Griffith [84] found that a synthetic estrogen, diethylstilbestrol, increased plasma renin substrate but progesterone was without effect. In studies with oral contraceptives, Laragh and associates [85,86] have noted increased plasma renin activity and aldosterone secretion, and occasionally an associated increase in blood pressure occurred; this was confirmed by Weinberger et al.[87] One of the most consistent and impressive abnormalities in these patients was the striking increase in plasma renin substrate. In subsequent and more detailed studies, persistent increases in plasma renin activity occurred in only about half of the patients while plasma renin substrate increased consistently; [86] this led Newton and associates [86] to propose that the true plasma renin concentration was reduced by a negative feedback mechanism.

Summary and Conclusions

Evidence has been presented for the important role of an intrarenal vascular receptor in the renal afferent arterioles in the control of renin release. This receptor probably responds to changes in wall tension but more study is needed to define the inputs which release renin. There is also evidence for a sodium-sensitive mechanism at the macula densa but it is unclear what specifically the macula densa senses as the signal for the control of renin release; it has been proposed that a decreased sodium load or increased sodium concentration at the macula densa provides the signal. In this event, it seems likely that a local humoral mechanism forms a connecting link between the macula densa and the JG cells.[5] It has further been suggested that an intrarenal feedback mechanism is present in each nephron but certain observations have failed to support this hypothesis. A plausible hypothesis is that both intrarenal receptors (vascular receptor and macula densa) are operative and that the extent of dominance varies with the physiologic or pathophysiologic conditions. The observations in the nonfiltering kidney model on the functional autonomy of the renovascular receptor may reflect the fundamental nature of the mechanism. The renal nerves influence renin release but are not essential for hypersecretion of renin; their mechanism of action appears to be, at least in part, by a direct effect on the JG cells, possibly through a beta-adrenergic receptor. The renal nerves influence afferent arteriolar constriction and could, thereby, stimulate the renovascular receptor. Also, arteriolar tone influences the glomerular filtration rate, which is probably an important determinant of tubular sodium load or concentration at the macula densa. Finally, a number of humoral agents are known to influence renin release. These include the catecholamines, sodium and potassium ions, antidiuretic hormone, angiotensin II, adrenal steroids and estrogens; their mechanisms of action have been discussed.

References

1. Davis, J. O.: Evidence for secretion of an aldosterone-stimulating hormone by the kidney. Discussion. *In* Symposium on Aldosterone at the First International Congress of Endocrinology, Copenhagen, 1960.
2. Laragh, J. H.: The role of aldosterone in man. JAMA 174:293, 1960.
3. Genest, J. E., Koiw, E., Nowaczynski, W., and Sandor, T.: Study of urinary adrenocortical hormones in human arterial hypertension. *In* Symposium on Aldosteronism at the First International Congress of Endocrinology, Copenhagen, 1960, p. 173.

4. Vander, A. J.: Control of renin release. Physiol. Rev. 47:355, 1966.
5. Davis, J. O.: What signals the kidney to release renin? Circ. Res. 28:301, 1971.
6. Davis, J. O.: Two important frontiers in renal physiology. Circulation 30:1, 1964.
7. Goldblatt, H.: Experimental renal hypertension. Mechanism of production and maintenance. Circulation 17:642, 1958.
8. Kohlstaedt, K. G., and Page, I. H.: The liberation of renin by perfusion of kidneys following reduction of pulse pressure. J. Exp. Med. 72:201, 1940.
9. Kolff, W. J.: Discussion of reports on renal factors in hypertension. Circulation 17:676, 1958.
10. Davis, J. O., Urquhart, J., Higgins, J. T., Jr., Rubin, E., and Hartroft, P. M.: Hypersecretion of aldosterone in dogs with a chronic aortic-caval fistula and high output heart failure. Circ. Res. 14:471, 1964.
11. Tobian, L., Tomboulian, A., and Janecek, J.: The effect of high perfusion pressures on the granulation of juxtaglomerular cells in an isolated kidney. J. Clin. Invest. 38:605, 1959.
12. Skinner, S. L., McCubbin, J. W., and Page, I. H.: Control of renin secretion. Circ. Res. 15:64, 1964.
13. Blaine, E. H., Davis, J. O., and Prewitt, R. L.: Evidence for a renal vascular receptor in control of renin secretion. Am. J. Physiol. 220:1593, 1971.
14. Blaine, E. H., and Davis, J. O.: Evidence for a renal vascular mechanism in renin release: New observations with graded stimulation by aortic constriction. Circ. Res. (Suppl. II) 28–29:II-118, 1971.
15. Eide, I., Loyning, E. W., and Kiil, F.: Renin release and autoregulation of renal blood flow. Proc. Int. Union Physiol. Sci. 11:564, 1971.
16. Ayers, C. R., Harris, R. H., Jr., and Lefer, L. G.: Control of renin release in experimental hypertension. Circ. Res. 24(Suppl. I): I-103, 1969.
17. Blaine, E. H., Davis, J. O., and Witty, R. T.: Renin release after hemorrhage and after suprarenal aortic constriction in dogs without sodium delivery to the macula densa. Circ. Res. 27:1081, 1970.
18. Davis, J. O., and Howell, D. S.: Mechanisms of fluid and electrolyte retention in experimental preparations in dogs. II. With thoracic inferior vena cava constriction. Circ. Res. 1:171, 1953.
19. Shade, R. E., Davis, J. O., Witty, R. T., Johnson, J. A., and Braverman, B.: Mechanisms regulating renin release in dogs with thoracic caval constriction. Physiologist 14: 228, 1971.
20. Conn, J. W., Cohen, E. L., and Rovner, D. R.: Absence of plasma renin activity in primary aldosteronism. Importance in distinguishing primary from secondary aldosteronism in hypertensive disease. JAMA 190:213, 1964.
21. Robb, C. A., Davis, J. O., Johnston, C. I., and Hartroft, P. M.: Effects of deoxycorticosterone on plasma renin activity in conscious dogs. Am. J. Physiol. 216:884, 1969.
22. Goodwin, F. J., Knowlton, A. I., and Laragh, J. H.: Absence of renin suppression by deoxycorticosterone acetate in rats. Am. J. Physiol. 216:1476, 1969.
23. Davis, J. O., and Howell, D. S.: Comparative effect of ACTH, cortisone and DCA on renal function, electrolyte excretion and water exchange in normal dogs. Endocrinology 52: 245, 1953.
24. Witty, R. T., Davis, J. O., Johnson, J. A., and Prewitt, R. L.: Effects of papaverine and hemorrhage on renin secretion in the non-filtering kidney. Am. J. Physiol. 221: 1666, 1971.
25. Thurau, K., and Kramer, K.: Weitere Untersuchungen zur myogenen Natur der Autoregulation des Nierenkreislaufes. Aufhebung der Autoregulation durch muskulotrope Substanzen und druckpassives Verhalten des Glomerulusfiltrates. Pfluegers Arch. 269:1; 77, 1959.
26. Goormaghtigh, N.: Facts in favour of an endocrine function of the renal arterioles. J. Pathol. 57:393, 1945.
27. Vander, A. J., and Miller, R.: Control of renin secretion in the anesthetized dog. Am. J. Physiol. 207:537, 1964.
28. Bunag, R. D., Vander, A. J., and Kaneko, Y.: Control of renin release. *In* Page, I. H., and McCubbin, J. W. (Eds.): Renal Hypertension. Chicago, Ill.: Year Book, 1968, pp. 100–117.
29. Thurau, K., Schnermann, J., Nagel, W., Horster, M., and Wohl, M.: Composition of tubular fluid in the macula densa segment as a factor regulating the function of the juxtaglomerular apparatus. Circ. Res. 21 (Suppl. II):II-79, 1967.
30. Meyer, P., Menard, J., Papanicolaou, N., Alexandre, J. M., Devaux, C., and Milliez, P.: Mechanism of renin release following

furosemide diuresis in rabbit. Am. J. Physiol. 215:908, 1968.
31. Cooke, C. R., Brown, T. C., Zacherle, B. J., and Walker, W. G.: Effect of altered sodium concentration in the distal nephron segments on renin release. J. Clin. Invest. 49:1630, 1970.
32. Goldberg, M.: Ethacrynic acid: Site and mode of action. Ann. N.Y. Acad. Sci. 139: 443, 1966.
33. Clapp, J. R., and Robinson, R. R.: Distal sites of action of diuretic drugs in the dog nephron. Am. J. Physiol. 215:228, 1968.
34. Laragh, J. H., Cannon, P. J., Stason, W. B., and Heinemann, H. O.: Physiologic and clinical observations on furosemide and ethacrynic acid. Ann. N.Y. Acad. Sci. 139: 453, 1966.
35. Nash, F. D., Rostorfer, H. H., Bailie, M. D., Wathen, R. L., and Schneider, E. G.: Relation to renal sodium load and dissociation from hemodynamic changes. Circ. Res. 22:473, 1968.
36. Nash, F. D.: Renin release: Further evidence for the role of a tubular natriastat. *In* Abstracts of the American Society of Nephrology, 1969, p. 51.
37. Vander, A. J., and Carlson, J.: Mechanism of the effects of furosemide on renin secretion in anesthetized dogs. Circ. Res. 25:145, 1969.
38. Guyton, A. C., Langston, J. B., and Navar, B.: Theory of renal autoregulation by feedback at the juxtaglomerular apparatus. Circ. Res. 15(Suppl. I):I-187, 1964.
39. Thurau, K.: Nature of autoregulation of renal blood flow. *In* Proceedings of the 3rd International Congress of Nephrology, Washington, D.C., 1966, vol. 1. New York: Karger, 1967, p. 162.
40. Thurau, K., Dahlheim, H., and Granger, P.: On the local formation of angiotensin at the site of the juxtaglomerular apparatus. *In* Proceedings of the 4th International Congress of Nephrology, Stockholm, vol. 2. New York: Karger, 1970, p. 24.
41. Thurau, K., Dahlheim, H., Gruner, A., Mason, J., and Granger, P.: The dependence of renin activity in the single juxtaglomerular apparatus of the rat nephron upon NaCl in the fluid of the macula densa segment. Proc. Int. Union Physiol. Sci. 9:564, 1971.
42. Morgan, T.: A microperfusion study of influence of macula densa on glomerular filtration rate. Am. J. Physiol. 220:186, 1971.
43. Barajas, L.: Renin secretion: An anatomical basis for tubular control. Science 172:485, 1971.
44. Wagermark, J., Ungerstedt, U., and Ljungqvist, A.: Sympathetic innervation of the juxtaglomerular cells of the kidney. Circ. Res. 22:149, 1968.
45. Vander, A. J.: Effect of catecholamines and the renal nerves on renin secretion in anesthetized dogs. Am. J. Physiol. 209:659, 1965.
46. Johnson, J. A., Davis, J. O., and Witty, R. T.: Effects of catecholamines and renal nerve stimulation on renin release in the nonfiltering kidney. Circ. Res. 29:646, 1971.
47. Bunag, R. D., Page, I. H., and McCubbin, J. W.: Neural stimulation of release of renin. Circ. Res. 19:851, 1966.
48. Hodge, R. L., Lowe, R. D., and Vane, J. R.: The effects of alteration of blood volume on the concentration of circulating angiotensin in anesthetized dogs. J. Physiol. 185:613, 1966.
49. Mogil, R. A., Itskovitz, H. D., Russell, J. H., and Murphy, J. J.: Renal innervation and renin activity in salt metabolism and hypertension. Am. J. Physiol. 216:693, 1969.
50. Vander, A. J., and Luciano, J. R.: Neural and humoral control of renin release in salt depletion. Circ. Res. (Suppl. II)20–21:II-69, 1967.
51. Brubacher, E. S., and Vander, A. J.: Sodium deprivation and renin secretion in unanesthetized dogs. Am. J. Physiol. 214:15, 1968.
52. Gordon, R. D., Küchel, O., Liddle, G. W., and Island, D. P.: Role of the sympathetic nervous system in regulating renin and aldosterone production in man. Clin. Invest. 46:599, 1967.
53. Gordon, R. D., Wolfe, L. K., Island, D. P., and Liddle, G. W.: A diurnal rhythm in plasma renin activity in man. Clin. Invest. 45:1587, 1966.
54. Pitts, R. F.: Physiology of the Kidney and Body Fluids, 2nd ed. Chicago, Ill.: Year Book, 1968.
55. Passo, S. S., Assaykeen, T. A., Otsuka, K., Wise, B. L., Goldfien, A., and Ganong, W. F.: Effect of stimulation of the medulla oblongata on renin secretion in dogs. Neuroendocrinology 7:1, 1971.
56. Passo, S. S., Assaykeen, T. A., Goldfien, A., and Ganong, W. F.: Effect of α- and β-adrenergic blocking agents on the increase in renin secretion produced by stimulation of the medulla oblongata in dogs. Neuroendocrinology 7:97, 1971.
57. Tobian, L.: Renin release and its role in

renal function and the control of salt balance and arterial pressure. Fed. Proc. 26:48, 1967.

58. Wathen, R. L., Kingsbury, W. S., Stouder, D. A., Schneider, E. G., and Rostorfer, H. H.: Effects of infusion of catecholamines and angiotensin II on renin release in anesthetized dogs. Am. J. Physiol. 209(5):1012, 1965.

59. Michelakis, A. M., Caudle, J., and Liddle, G. W.: *In vitro* stimulation of renin production by epinephrine, norepinephrine, and cyclic AMP. Proc. Soc. Exp. Biol. Med. 130:748, 1969.

60. Otsuka, K., Assaykeen, T. A., Goldfien, A., and Ganong, W. F.: Effect of hypoglycemia on plasma renin activity in dogs. Endocrinology 87:1306, 1970.

61. Winer, N., Chokshi, D. S., Yoon, M. S., and Freedman, A. D.: Adrenergic receptor mediation of renin secretion. J. Clin. Endocrinol. 29:1168, 1969.

62. Winer, N., Chokshi, D. S., and Walkenhorst, W. G.: Effects of cyclic AMP, sympathomimetic amines, and adrenergic receptor antagonists on renin secretion. Circ. Res. 29: 239, 1971.

63. Ueda, H., Yasuda, H., Takabatake, Y., Iizuka, M., Iizuka, T., Ihori, M., and Sakamoto, Y.: Observations on the mechanism of renin release by catecholamines. Circ. Res. (Suppl. II) 26–27:II-195, 1970.

64. Assaykeen, T. A., Clayton, P. L., Goldfien, A., and Ganong, W. F.: Effect of alpha- and beta-adrenergic blocking agents on the renin response to hypoglycemia and epinephrine in dogs. Endocrinology 87:1318, 1970.

65. Assaykeen, T. A., and Ganong, W. F.: The sympathetic nervous system and renin secretion. *In* Ganong, W. F. and Martini, L. (Eds.): Frontiers in Neuroendocrinology. New York: Oxford University Press, 1971.

66. Veyrat, R., Brunner, H. R., Manning, E. L., and Muller, A. F.: Inhibition de l'activité de la renine plasmatique par le potassium. J. Urol. Nephrol. 73:271, 1967.

67. Brunner, H. R., Baer, L., Sealey, J. E., Ledingham, J. G. G., and Laragh, J. H.: Influence of potassium administration and of potassium deprivation on plasma renin in normal and hypertensive subjects. J. Clin. Invest. 49:2128, 1970.

68. Abbrecht, P. H., and Vander, A. J.: Effects of chronic potassium deficiency on plasma renin activity. J. Clin. Invest. 49:1510, 1970.

69. Shade, R. E., Davis, J. O., Johnson, J. A., Witty, R. T., and Braverman, B.: Effects of renal intra-arterial infusion of sodium and potassium on renin secretion in the non-filtering kidney. *In* Abstracts of the Fifth Annual Meeting of the American Society of Nephrology, 1971, p. 71.

70. Pitcock, J. A., and Hartroft, P. M.: The juxtaglomerular cells in man and their relationship to the level of plasma sodium and to the zona glomerulosa of the adrenal cortex. Am. J. Pathol. 34:863, 1958.

71. Newsome, H. H., and Bartter, F. C.: Plasma renin activity in relation to serum sodium concentration and body fluid balance. J. Clin. Endocrinol. Metab. 28:1704, 1968.

72. Gordon, R. D., and Pawsey, C. G. K.: Relative effects of serum sodium concentration and the state of body fluid balance on renin secretion. J. Clin. Endocrinol. Metab. 32:117, 1971.

73. Yamamoto, K., Hasegawa, T., Miyasaki, M., and Ueda, J.: Control of renin secretion in the anesthetized dogs. 2. Relationship between renin secretion, plasma sodium concentration and GFR in the perfused kidney. Jap. Circ. J. 33:593, 1969.

74. Vander, A. J., and Geelhoed, G. W.: Inhibition of renin secretion by angiotensin II. Proc. Soc. Exp. Biol. Med. 120:399, 1965.

75. Bunag, R. D., Page, I. H., and McCubbin, J. W.: Inhibition of renin release by vasopressin and angiotensin. Cardiovasc. Res. 1:67, 1967.

76. Vander, A. J.: Inhibition of renin release in the dog by vasopressin and vasotocin. Circ. Res. 23:605, 1968.

77. Tanaka, K., Omae, T., Hattori, N., and Katsuki, S.: Renin release from ischemic kidneys following angiotensin infusion in dogs. Jap. Circ. J. 33:235, 1969.

78. Tagawa, H., Vander, A. J., Bonjour, J., and Malvin, R. L.: Inhibition of renin secretion by vasopressin in unanesthetized sodium-deprived dogs. Am. J. Physiol. 220:949, 1971.

79. De Champlain, J., Genest, J., Veyrat, R., and Boucher, R.: Factors controlling renin in man. Arch. Intern. Med. 117:355, 1966.

80. Blair-West, J. R., Coghlan, J. P., Denton, D. A., Funder, J. W., Scoggins, B. A., and Wright, R. D.: Inhibition of renin secretion by systemic and intrarenal angiotensin infusion. Am. J. Physiol. 220:1309, 1971.

81. Geelhoed, G. W., and Vander, A. J.: The role of aldosterone in renin secretion. Life Sci. 6:525, 1967.

82. Newton, M. A., and Laragh, J. H.: Effects of glucocorticoid administration on aldoster-

one excretion and plasma renin in normal subjects, in essential hypertension and in primary aldosteronism. J. Clin. Endocrinol. Metab. 28:1014, 1968.

83. Goodwin, F. J., Kirshman, J. D., Sealey, J. E., and Laragh, J. H.: Influence of the pituitary gland on sodium conservation, plasma renin and renin substrate concentrations in the rat. Endocrinology 86:824, 1970.

84. Helmer, O. M., and Griffith, R. S.: The effect of the administration of estrogens on the renin-substrate (hypertensinogen) content of rat plasma. Endocrinology 51:421, 1952.

85. Laragh, J. H., Sealey, J. E., Ledingham, J. G. G., and Newton, M. A.: Oral contraceptives, renin, aldosterone, and high blood pressure. JAMA 201:918, 1967.

86. Newton, M. A., Sealey, J. E., Ledingham, J. G. G., and Laragh, J. H.: High blood pressure and oral contraceptives. Am. J. Obstet. Gynec. 101:1037, 1968.

87. Weinberger, M. H., Collins, D., Dowdy, A. J., Nokes, G. W., and Luetscher, J. A.: Hypertension induced by oral contraceptives containing estrogen and gestagen. Ann. Intern. Med. 71:891, 1969.

Antihypertensive Function of the Renal Medulla

By E. Eric Muirhead, M.D., Byron E. Leach, Ph.D., Lawrence W. Byers, Ph.D., Bennie Brooks, and James A. Pitcock, M.D.

SEVERAL LINES of investigation suggest that the kidney, as a whole, exerts an antihypertensive function.[1,2] Some workers restrict interpretation of this function to control of sodium and volume excess by the kidney through its excretory actions.[3–5] Others [6–8] entertain the possibility of a unique and nonexcretory, antihypertensive renal function, possibly hormonal in type. According to the former view, sodium and volume loads increase the cardiac output, which is followed by some rise in arterial pressure. The rise in arterial pressure, in turn, becomes more pronounced as the periphery adjusts to the elevated flow by what Guyton terms "general autoregulation." By general autoregulation is meant, in part, that the arterial side adjusts flow by constricting, possibly through Bayliss's vascular myogenic reflex, but at the expense of the heightened arterial pressure. The heightened pressure is considered to assist the kidney in regulating the sodium-volume load. Several general reviews of this proposal were published recently.[9–13]

The view that the kidney exerts a nonexcretory, antihypertensive renal function is based primarily on either the prevention or the reversion of the experimental hypertensive state by renal tissue incapable of the external excretion of urine and therefore incapable of the outward control of sodium-volume loads. For this purpose, two renal manipulations were used, namely, the diversion of urine by ureterovenous and ureterointestinal anastomosis [14–19] and the transplantation of fragmented renal tissue.[20–23] A secondary type of support for this thesis was derived by the extraction of antihypertensive renal factors.[24–27]

From the Departments of Pathology, Medicine, and Biochemistry, University of Tennessee Medical Units, and Department of Pathology, Baptist Memorial Hospital, Memphis, Tennessee.

It is the purpose of this chapter to consider the antihypertensive role of the renal medulla. Emphasis will be placed on the renomedullary interstitial cells as potential endocrine-like antihypertensive structures.

The Renal Medulla as an Antihypertensive Organ

The view that the renal medulla exerts an antihypertensive function is based on results with five experimental models.

Model 1

The first model [18,19,28] entailed four manipulations of the dog's kidneys followed by a hypertension-inducing regimen (either a saline-dietary protein intake or a high saline load). The four renal manipulations were: (1) bilateral nephrectomy; (2) ureteral ligation and contralateral nephrectomy; (3) bilateral ureteral ligation; and (4) ureterovenous anastomosis and contralateral nephrectomy. Ureteral ligation, unilateral or bilateral, gave rise to the same level of hypertension as binephrectomy, while ureterovenous anastomosis plus contralateral nephrectomy protected against the hypertensive state in a significant way (Fig. 1). Ureteral ligation, under these circumstances, was associated with extensive damage to the renal medulla and especially the renal papilla,[29] while ureterovenous anastomosis was attended by an intact and hyperplastic medulla. The results of this model suggest that intact renomedullary tissue is implicated in the antihypertensive action of the kidney.

Model 2

In this model [20] (Fig. 2) the left kidney of the dog was removed and either whole kidney, dissected medulla, or dissected cortex was fragmented and injected as an autotransplant.

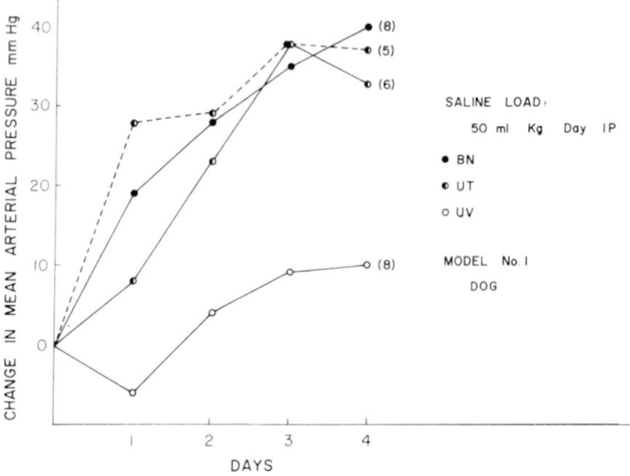

FIG. 1.—Antihypertensive function of the kidney. Results from Model 1 when the hypertension-inducing regimen consisted of the daily intraperitoneal injection of 50 ml of saline per kilogram of body weight. ●, bilateral nephrectomy; ○, ureteral ligation (unilateral plus contralateral nephrectomy is indicated by **solid line,** and bilateral nephrectomy is indicated by **broken line**); ○, ureterovenous anastomosis.

(Splenic and hepatic tissue treated in the same way acted as controls.) Fourteen days later the right kidney was removed, thus creating the renoprival state, and a hypertension-inducing regimen was instituted. Autotransplants of whole kidney and medulla protected against the hypertensive state while autotransplants of renal cortex, spleen, and liver did not. The results of this model demonstrated, in a direct way, the antihypertensive action of

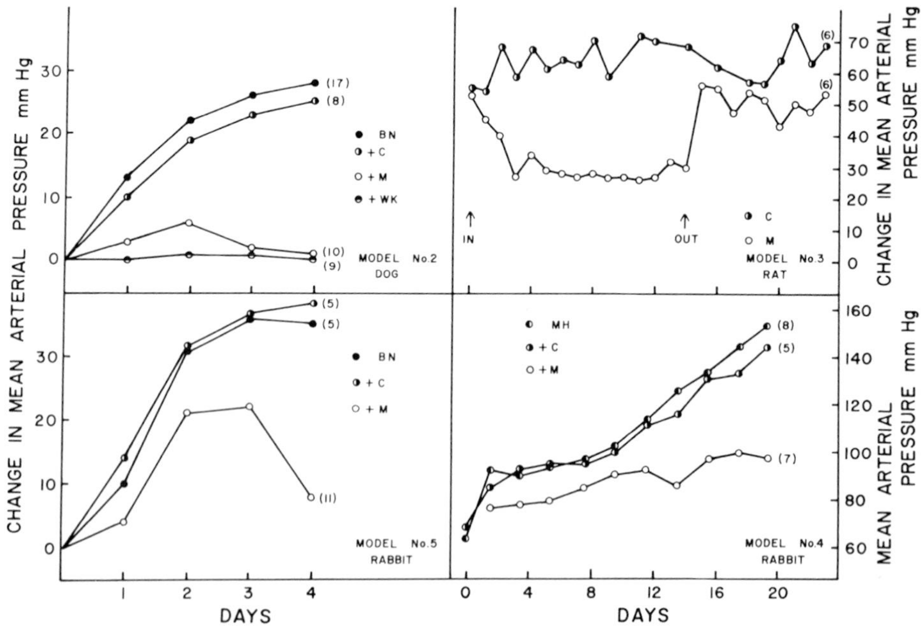

FIG. 2.—Antihypertensive function of the renal medulla. Results with Models 2, 3, 4, and 5. ●, binephrectomy alone; ○, renocortical transplant; ○, renomedullary transplant; ○, whole kidney transplant; ○, malignant hypertension. See text for more complete description.

renomedullary tissue toward renoprival hypertension.

Model 3

The effect of the third model [21,30] was therapeutic rather than preventive.

A Wistar strain of rats capable of accepting each other's renal tissue without rejection was used. After establishing a one-kidney, Goldblatt-type hypertension at a so-called benign level (170 mm Hg), either fragmented renal medulla or fragmented renal cortex was injected subcutaneously as isografts. While medullary tissue was in situ, the arterial pressure dropped significantly (Fig. 2) and remained depressed as long as these transplants were present. The presence of cortical transplants was associated with a continued rise in arterial pressure. The renomedullary effect was dependent on live cells since dead renomedullary transplants did not change the arterial pressure. The results of this model displayed the antihypertensive effectiveness of renomedullary cells in benign renovascular hypertension.

Model 4

The results of this model [22,31] demonstrated the antihypertensive effects of renomedullary tissue toward accelerated (malignant) renovascular hypertension of the rabbit.

The left renal artery was constricted by a rigid, narrow clip [32] having a fixed gap. When the right kidney was removed the arterial pressure rose to lethal levels (140 to 160 mm Hg) within 3 weeks (Fig. 2). Autotransplanted fragmented renal medulla prevented the lethal hypertension while autotransplanted renal cortex did not. Removal of the renomedullary transplants after 3 weeks of protection toward the malignant hypertension was followed by a sharp rise in arterial pressure and death.

Model 5

The purpose of this model [22,23] was to test the ability of renomedullary cells to influence the effect of extreme sodium loading during the renoprival state. Three groups of rabbits were used. Group 1 had binephrectomy alone, group 2 had binephrectomy plus autotransplantation of fragmented renal cortex, and group 3 had binephrectomy plus autotransplantation of renal medulla. The transplantation was performed 10 to 14 days before the second nephrectomy. All three groups received subcutaneously, each day for 4 days, 17 ml of 3% sodium chloride solution per kilogram of body weight. The cumulative sodium load amounted to 35 mEq per kilogram of body weight or about three-fourths of the exchangeable sodium pool. The mean arterial pressure of groups 1 and 2 rose to +35 and +38 mm Hg, respectively, by the fourth day (Fig. 2). The mean arterial pressure of group 3 lagged in elevation for 2 days, leveled off on the third day, and reverted to near baseline levels by the fourth day. The differences in arterial pressure between this group and the first two groups on the third and fourth days were highly significant. The results seem to indicate that renoprival hypertension due to sodium loading is not due entirely to hemodynamic changes, as contended by Ledingham,[9] Guyton et al.,[10] and others. Rather, the hypertension appears to result from hemodynamic and possibly other vascular changes attendant on the sodium excess but made permissible by the absence of renomedullary factors.

Cellular Source of Renomedullary Antihypertensive Function

The cellular source of the renomedullary antihypertensive function, as indicated below, appears to be the renomedullary interstitial cells. These cells are normally situated between Henle's loop, the vasa recta, and the collecting duct (Fig. 3).[34] They are unique in having prominent cytoplasmic processes, many lipid-laden cytoplasmic vesicles, and perinuclear and other cisterns. There appears to be an inverse relationship between the presence of the lipid vesicles and the cistern system. The lipid-laden nature of the interstitial cells was demonstrated by histochemistry.[35–37] The cytoplasmic vesicles contain neutral fats, acidic lipids, including arachidonic acid, phospholipids, and cholesterol. By sucrose-gradient centrifugation the vesicles were shown to contain a vasodepressor lipid, most likely prostaglandin.[36,38] There are indications that these cells are secretory.[39] Their lipid vesicles seem to be extruded into their surroundings.[40,41]

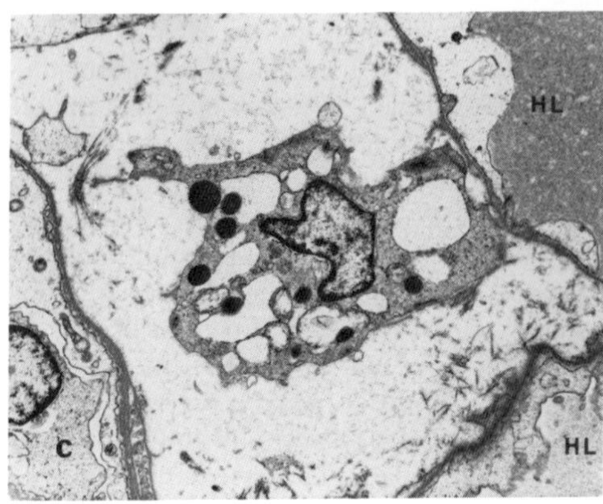

FIG. 3.—Electron microscopic appearance of the renomedullary interstitial cell of the rabbit in its normal habitat. Note prominent osmiophilic vesicles, vacuoles, and cytoplasmic cisterns. **HL**, Henle's loop; **C**, the vasa recta. ×6,860.

Assuming that the interstitial cells are secretory, their secretion most likely would contain lipids.

Muehrcke and associates [42,43] noted a decrease in the lipid vesicles of interstitial cells during DOCA-salt hypertension of the rat and malignant hypertension of man. Muehrcke suggested that these cells were involved in the production of antihypertensive lipids of the type extracted from the normal medulla.[2,44] Tobian and associates [45–47] extended the observations of Muehrcke in a significant way. They noted a decrease in lipid vesicles in salt-sensitive and Goldblatt hypertension of the rat. Tobian also considered the possibility that these cells produce antihypertensive lipid factors.

The observations and suggestions of Muehrcke and Tobian and their associates led us to evaluate the renomedullary interstitial cells within renomedullary transplants which prevent and revert different types of hypertensive states.

Renomedullary Interstitial Cells in the Isografts of Model 3

By light microscopy and the use of hematoxylin and eosin stain, the isografts of Model 3, which reverted benign renovascular hypertension of the rat, appear to consist mostly of nondescript, vascularized connective tissue. A few atrophic and calcified tubules remain; most normal tubular and vascular structures were resorbed. Electron microscopy displays a mixture of collapsed basement membrane, presumably from resorbed tubules, mixed with collagen, many capillaries, and a scattering of renomedullary interstitial cells. Because many of the interstitial cells in these transplants emphasize the cistern pattern, their earlier identification was hindered. Still, the main viable cells within the transplants have the characteristics of the interstitial cells (Fig. 4).

Renomedullary Interstitial Cells in the Renomedullary Transplants of Models 4 and 5

These transplants contain numerous interstitial cells, easily recognized by semi-thin section and electron microscopy (Fig. 4). The cells display typical elongated cytoplasmic processes and contain many osmiophilic vesicles. Histochemistry indicates the presence of neutral fats, phospholipid and cholesterol. The striking arrangement of these cells in clusters suggests proliferation. Moreover, they are often found attached to capillaries. Thus, it seems that the interstitial cells undergo hyperplasia during the time that the transplants exert their antihypertensive action. Since most other cells present (tubules, macrophages, granulocytes, lymphocytes, fibroblasts) are either few in number or in a degenerated state and the endothelial cells of the capillaries present do not appear unique, the indications are that the interstitial cells perform the antihypertensive function.

Interstitial Cells of Renomedullary Transplants Grown in Tissue Culture

The interpretation that renomedullary interstitial cells constitute the main cell type within transplants which prevent the hypertensive state (Models 4 and 5) is supported by the derivation of a monolayer tissue culture of interstitial cells from these transplants.[48] The indications that this monolayer culture consists of renomedullary interstitial cells are morphologic, chromosomal, and functional. The cultured cells maintain the main morphologic features of the renomedullary interstitial cell. The morphologic features include the characteristic lipid vesicles, perinuclear and cytoplasmic cisterns, and the histochemical demonstra-

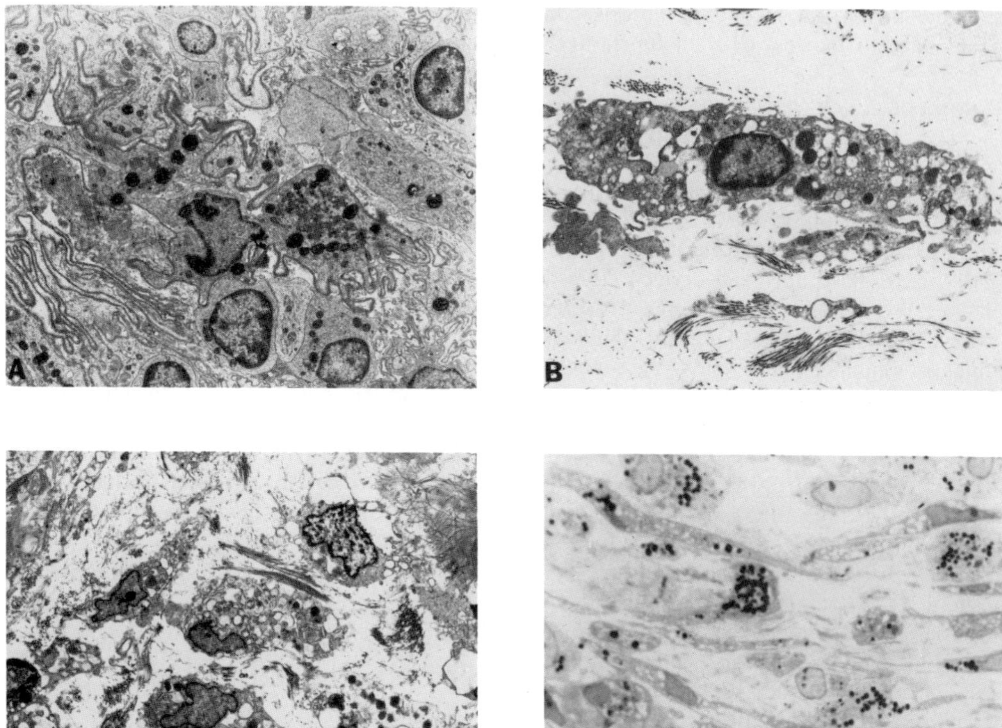

FIG. 4.—*A*, Electron microscopic view of interstitial cells in renomedullary transplant of rat Model 3. ×3,520.

B, An electromicrograph shows an interstitial cell in renomedullary transplant of Model 4. ×7,500.

C, Electron microscopic view shows cells of renomedullary transplant of Model 5. ×2,400.

D, Semi-thin section of a cluster of interstitial cells of Model 4. Toluidine blue. ×450.

tion of neutral lipids, phospholipids, and cholesterol within the vesicles. Even after 25 passages the cell line remained diploid and lapine by chromosome analysis. Moreover, the ability of these cells to synthesize the renomedullary prostaglandins (E_2, A_2, and $F_{2\alpha}$) may be offered additionally in support of their interstitial cell origin.

RENOMEDULLARY FIBROSIS IN HYPERTENSION

In 100 unselected autopsies on human subjects the degree of fibrosis in the inner and outer renal medulla was semi-quantitated.[49] A statistically significant relationship between renomedullary fibrosis in both medullary zones, the hypertensive state of the benign essential type, and arterial and arteriolar sclerosis was detected. The medullary fibrosis could have occurred as a change secondary to the vascular disease. Under the circumstances of the renomedullary fibrosis, the interstitial cells become entrapped in collagen. This represents a change in the habitat of this cell since under normal conditions the cell is surrounded by blood vessels, tubules, and mucopolysaccharide. This finding adds another relationship between the renal medulla and hypertension. Since there is experimental evidence supporting an antihypertensive function exerted by the renal medulla, renal medullary fibrosis could be an index of the loss of such function.

Renomedullary Antihypertensive and Vasodepressor Lipids

The vasodepressor prostaglandins E_2 and A_2,[50–52] and an antihypertensive neutral lipid[2] are extractable from the normal renal medulla. These agents have not been derived from the renal cortex. Despite the passage of several years since the demonstration of these two groups of renomedullary lipids, their possible relationship and, indeed, their relationship to the control of the arterial pressure, remains unresolved.

The recovery of prostaglandin-like substances, most likely PGE_2, from the renal venous effluent during constriction of the renal artery[53,54] and following the infusion of angiotensin II[55] suggests the possible modulation of the arterial pressure, under certain circumstances, by the renomedullary secretion of these compounds. Under such conditions, the renomedullary source of the prostaglandin appears almost certain to be the interstitial cells.

Attempts to demonstrate an antihypertensive action of PGE_2 by its injection into hypertensive rats have yielded inconclusive results. Utilizing high doses, one report[56] indicated a prominent lowering of the arterial pressure of some animals, which was maintained for the duration of the treatment; a prominent lowering of the pressure of other animals followed by escape to prior hypertensive levels during the treatment, and no change in still other animals. Another report[57] indicated a significant lowering of the hypertensive pressure during 1 month of daily injections of PGE_2. Thus far, no published data are available on the effect of PGA_2 on experimental hypertension.

The antihypertensive neutral renomedullary lipid (ANRL) differs from PGE_2 and PGA_2 in that it does not evoke the acute depressor effect in the prepared animal (anesthetized, with the vagi cut, and pentolinium-treated).[58] Rather, this agent acts slowly in reverting the heightened arterial pressure of the hypertensive state. In chronic renal hypertension of the dog[44] and rat[59] ANRL, given daily (with or without the addition of renomedullary prostaglandin), drops the arterial pressure over a period of days. The pressure remains depressed as long as the agent is administered. Upon cessation of this treatment, the pressure returns to its original hypertensive level over a period of days. One or two parenteral doses of ANRL drops the pressure of the hypertensive rabbit[2] over a period of hours (Fig. 5). Return of the pressure to the preinjection level is also slow. The observed temporal difference in response to ANRL between the hypertensive dog, rat, and rabbit may be due to dosage differences but the overall slow effect remains. Thus, ANRL could operate through an indirect system.

The main steps thus far used in the extraction and purification of ANRL include:[2] dehydration of the renomedullary tissue, extrac-

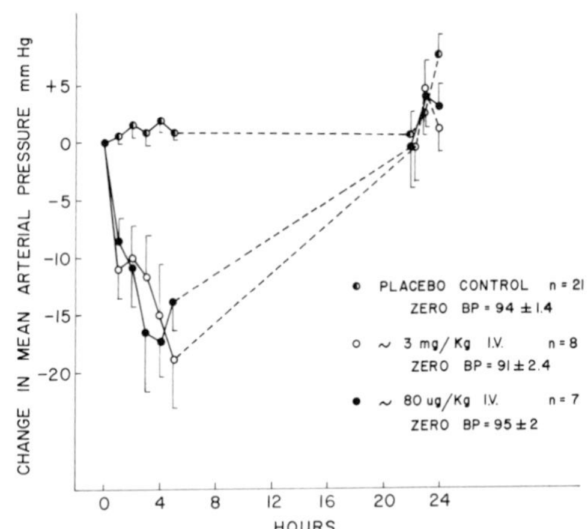

Fig. 5.—Antihypertensive action of ANRL in renoprival hypertension of the rabbit. The kidneys were removed and each day the animal received subcutaneously 25 ml of saline per kilogram of body weight. On the third and fourth days, when the hypertension was sustained (mean blood pressure measured directly from the aorta), the animals were injected intravenously. The blood pressure was recorded for 5 minutes each for 5 hours and 22, 23, and 24 hours after the injection by an automated device while the animals remained quiet in specially designed boxes. ◐, control group receiving the vehicle only (0.05 ml of 95% ethanol); ○, crude ethyl ether extract of normal renal medulla; ●, neutral lipid of the same extract as refined by derivation from a magnesium silicate column (15% ether in hexane eluate). The difference between control and test values at hours 4 and 5 is highly significant ($p < 0.005$).

tion in ethyl ether, removal of the acidic lipids into a buffer, either silicic acid or magnesium silicate column-chromatography and LH-20 Sephadex column-chromatography. Throughout these steps ANRL remains with the neutral lipid fractions. These fractions have a high triglyceride content.

In an additional attempt to purify ANRL, the dry ether extract containing ANRL was passed through a Celite column (dry pack) containing orthophosphoric acid (50%) and then through a Celite column (dry pack) containing a saturated solution of sodium bisulfate, according to the procedure of Parks, Keeney and Schwartz.[60,61] Under these conditions fatty aldehydes liberated in the first column by orthophosphoric acid from alk-1-enyl glyceryl ethers in the ANRL preparation are

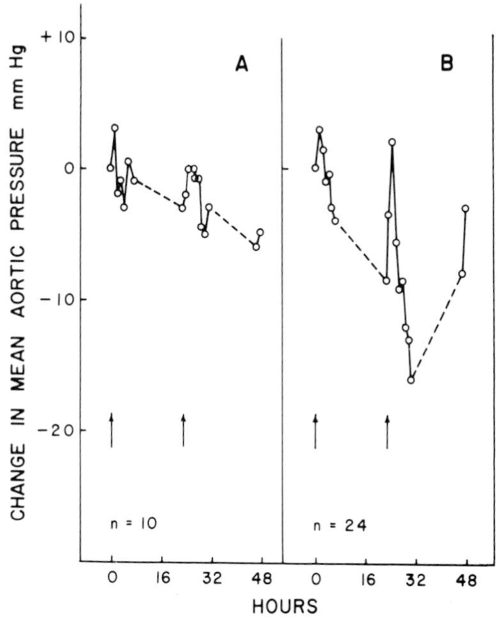

FIG. 6.—Fatty aldehydes derived from ANRL by the Schwartz columns and injected intravenously into rabbits having a one-kidney Goldblatt hypertension. The control versus zero pressure (mean aortic) consisted of the average pressure for 24 hours before the first injection (mean 105 mm Hg ± 2.2 SEM). After each injection the aortic pressure was measured every hour for 5 minutes over 7 hours the first day and 9 hours the second day by the same arrangement as used in Fig. 5. *A*, Vehicle alone (0.05 ml of 95% ethanol); *B*, fatty aldehydes.

trapped as the bisulfite addition product in the second column. Glycerides, alkyl ethers, etc. pass through both columns. The trapped aldehyde can be liberated by stirring the Celite in 20% sodium carbonate. Extraction into hexane and evaporation to dryness yields free fatty aldehydes.

The Schwartz procedure was conducted on the crude ether extract of ANRL, and the "free aldehyde fraction" was taken up into the vehicle (0.05 ml of 95% ethanol) and injected intravenously in two doses 24 hours apart into rabbits having one-kidney Goldblatt hypertension. Since some free aldehydes are very unstable, especially in alkaline solution, the product of the second Schwartz column was immediately taken up in vehicle and injected into the animals. The results (Fig. 6) in 24 unselected and consecutive observations were compared with those of 10 simultaneous control observations (vehicle only injected). The Schwartz-column product caused a gradual decline in arterial pressure over 24 to 32 hours in the same manner as extracts of intact ANRL.[2] (There was, however, a transient pressor effect observed following the second dose.) The differences in results of the treated and control groups were highly significant ($p < 0.001$).

The products yielded by the Schwartz procedure are mixtures. The procedure, as applied, does not eliminate the possibility of preexistent aldehydes within the starting material. The end product did not contain vasodepressor lipids as tested in the prepared rat and presumably was devoid of established prostaglandins. Despite the need for caution, the results of the Schwartz procedure are more consistent with the view that ANRL is an alk-1-enyl-glyceryl ether than other views. This possibility is being pursued.

MEDIATION OF THE ANTIHYPERTENSIVE FUNCTION OF THE RENAL MEDULLA

In terms of modern concepts, two major possibilities may be considered relative to the antihypertensive action of renomedullary cells, namely, (1) the secretion of antihypertensive or depressor substances and (2) the neutralization or suppression of pressor substances. Whichever of these hypotheses pertains, the

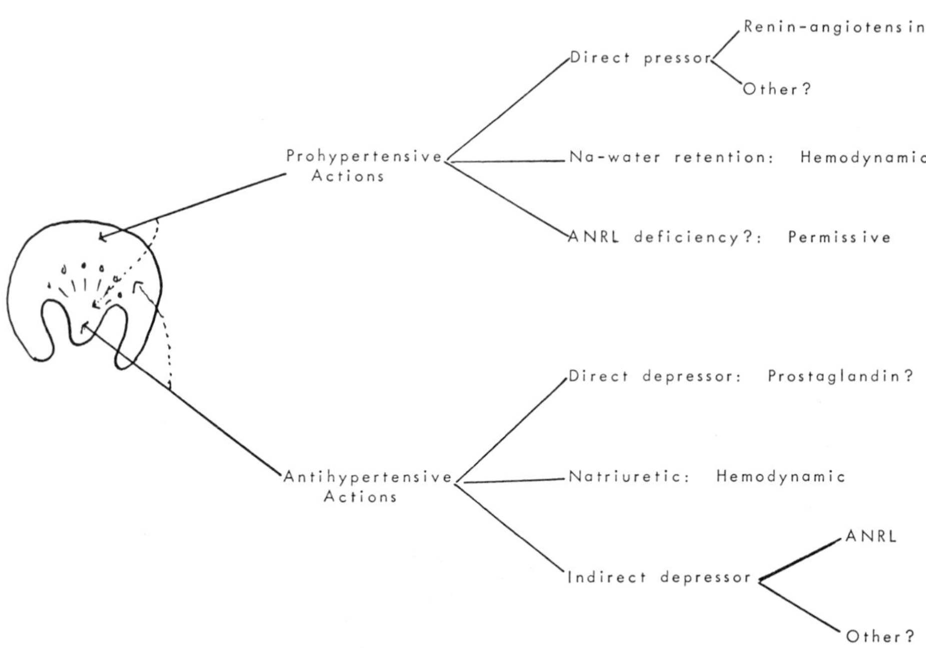

FIG. 7.—Schematic drawing of prohypertensive and antihypertensive actions of the kidney. For further discussion, see section entitled "General Comment."

indications are that the renomedullary interstitial cells are involved in its mediation. Neither the prostaglandins nor ANRL appears to block the pressor effect of angiotensin. The structure of the interstitial cells is such as to indicate their ability to liberate and secrete lipid moieties. There is the distinct possibility that certain of these lipid moieties are depressor and antihypertensive. Taking the presently available information into account, it would seem that the possibility of renomedullary interstitial cells secreting antihypertensive lipids, as suggested by Muehrcke et al., remains the more attractive hypothesis. This hypothesis will not be put to its ultimate critical test until assays for minute quantities of renomedullary prostaglandins are available and the structural formula of ANRL becomes known.

General Comment

It is becoming increasingly evident that the role of the kidney in the pathogenesis of hypertensive states is complex (Fig. 7). Prohypertensive and antihypertensive actions of the kidney have been entertained for some time.[62] As information accrued, it became apparent that these terms relate to multiple factors. For instance, shortly after the Goldblatt experiment the prohypertensive action of the kidney was related to renin,[63] later to renin-angiotensin,[64] and more recently to renin-angiotensin-aldosterone.[65] Doubts concerning the role of these systems in the genesis of hypertension have remained.[66,67] Proposals for new renal pressor systems are being made.[68,69]

In recent times, the ascendance of hemodynamic factors in the instigation and control of hypertensive states has added another dimension to the prohypertensive effects of renal involvement.[11,12,70–73] Thus, sodium-volume loads tend to beget hypertension when the kidney is involved (damaged or missing) and sodium-volume drainage often ameliorates not only renal but other hypertensive states.

Within the framework of these considerations, the crucial question becomes: Is there a unique and specific antihypertensive function of the kidney unrelated to its excretory functions; that is, unrelated to the external sodium-volume control? We support the affirmative position based on the considerations below.

Evidence for a general antihypertensive action of the kidney seems apparent in whole-kidney transplantation and perfusion experiments.[74–79] The rapidity of fall in pressure in certain of these experiments seems to oppose a purely excretory action begetting sodium-volume modulation. The deviation of urine flow by ureteral anastomosis circumvented the external control of sodium loads. It was argued by hemodynamic advocates,[13] however, that the ureterovenous experiment could not be compared to binephrectomy under similar sodium-volume loads because a vascular bed of low resistance (the renal one) was present in one set of observations (ureterovenous) and not in the other (binephrectomy). Thus, hemodynamically speaking, the arterial pressure should have been lower with one kidney in and no outward urine flow, and higher with both kidneys out and no outward urine flow. This analysis overlooked the relationships of Model 1 as herein presented. Ureterovenous anastomosis was not, strictly speaking, compared with binephrectomy. Rather, binephrectomy was used as a standard for hypertension under the impact of sodium or sodium-protein intake and the results of this experiment were compared with those of two other experiments entailing ureteral ligation and ureterovenous anastomosis. Ureteral ligation was attended by the same level of hypertension as binephrectomy but ureterovenous anastomosis significantly blunted the rise in pressure. Moreover, bilateral ureteral ligation did not prevent the hypertensive state under these circumstances. Even if the renal blood flow is halved by the ureteral ligation, as indicated by the data of Blalock and Levy,[80] the hemodynamic argument does not appear secure in view of the results following bilateral ureteral ligation.

The results of Models 2 through 5, as herein reviewed, clearly demonstrate an antihypertensive action of renomedullary cells unrelated to the external control of sodium-water loads. This conclusion pertains not only for different expressions of the hypertensive state (renoprival, benign and malignant renovascular hypertension) but for different species. In addition, the antihypertensive renomedullary action remains in the face of an extreme sodium load.

How and through what target areas renomedullary cells exert their antihypertensive action remains a mystery. Internal volume distribution, as proposed by Green, Lucas, and Floyer [81] for their experiment, and other indirect actions on the cardiovascular system must be kept in mind. As considered above, the most eligible hypothesis at the moment invokes the secretion of antihypertensive lipids by the renomedullary interstitial cells for the mediation of the nonexcretory, antihypertensive function. This hypothesis continues under scrutiny.

Regardless of how and through what target areas renomedullary cells exert their antihypertensive action, certain formulations concerning the pro- and antihypertensive actions of the kidney may not be amiss (Fig. 7). On the prohypertensive side three considerations may be offered: (1) A direct pressor effect, with emphasis on the renin-angiotensin system, despite the continued doubts,[67] must be under continued consideration. (2) Certainly, sodium and water retention, under certain conditions, are contributory and act, according to major indications, via a hemodynamic mechanism. (3) A third possibility may now be considered, namely, the permissive nature of the absence of renomedullary factors. Thus, the absence of renomedullary factors alone does not induce hypertension as indicated by the absence or control of renoprival hypertension by the control of sodium and/or volume loads. The absence of renomedullary factors, on the other hand, appears to allow hypertensive mechanisms to operate. This being the case, the relationship of a deficiency of renomedullary factors to the presence of prohypertensive factors (direct pressor, hemodynamic, etc.) could well be pertinent, especially if this relationship is multiplicatory rather than additive. This thesis would invoke hypertension in the presence of minor and poorly measurable imbalances; i.e., a minor prohypertensive action versus a minor antihypertensive deficiency. On the antihypertensive side, three considerations may also be offered: (1) In view of the seeming presence of renomedullary prostaglandins in renal venous effluent under certain conditions, a direct-depressor action of these agents must also remain under continued consideration. (2) The antihypertensive role of either natriuresis or ultrafiltration, under certain conditions, is undoubted. (3) A third possibility needs consideration also from this viewpoint. ANRL, because of its slow action, appears to operate through a complex or indirect system related to a heightened arterial pressure since, thus far, a preparation of ANRL that depresses the normal arterial pressure has not been derived.

Summary

Consideration has been given to prohypertensive and antihypertensive actions of the kidney. Among the antihypertensive actions of the kidney the renal medulla appears to play a role. This role, according to five experimental models, is nonexcretory and most likely hormone-like. The cells involved in this renomedullary antihypertensive action seem to be the interstitial cells. These cells are lipid-laden and very likely secrete lipid moieties. Since antihypertensive lipid agents can be derived from the renal medulla, it is postulated that the renomedullary antihypertensive function is mediated by lipid agents secreted by the renomedullary interstitial cells. This hypothesis is under continued scrutiny.

References

1. Page, I. H., and McCubbin, J. W.: Renal Hypertension. Chicago: Yearbook, 1968, p. 296.
2. Muirhead, E. E., Leach, B. E., Byers, L. W., Brooks, B., Daniels, E. G., and Hinman, J. W.: Antihypertensive neutral renomedullary lipids (ANRL). *In* Fisher, J. W. (Ed.): Kidney Hormones. London: Academic Press, 1971, pp. 485–506.
3. Ledingham, J. M., and Cohen, R. D.: The role of the heart in the pathogenesis of renal hypertension. Lancet 2:979, 1963.
4. Borst, J. G. G., and Borst de Geus, A.: Hypertension explained by Starling's theory of circulatory homeostasis. Lancet 1:677, 1963.
5. Douglas, B. H., Guyton, A. C., Langston, J. B., and Bishop, V. S.: Hypertension caused by salt loading. II. Fluid volume and tissue pressure changes. Am. J. Physiol. 207:669, 1964.
6. Grollman, A.: A unitary concept of experimental and clinical hypertensive cardiovascular disease. Perspect. Biol. Med. 2:208, 1959.
7. Muirhead, E. E., Hinman, J. W., and Daniels, E. G.: Renoprival hypertension and the antihypertensive function of the kidney. *In* Boorhave Cursus. Leiden: Boorhave Kwattier, 1963, pp. 88–102.
8. Floyer, M. A.: The effect of nephrectomy and adrenalectomy upon the blood pressure in hypertensive and normotensive rats. Clin. Sci. 10:405, 1951.
9. Ledingham, J. M.: Blood pressure regulation in renal failure. J. R. Coll. Physicians Lond. 5:103, 1971.
10. Guyton, A. C., Coleman, T. G., Bower, J. D., and Harris, J. G.: Circulatory control in hypertension. Circ. Res. 27(Supp. 1):135, 1970.
11. Ferrario, C. M., Page, I. H., and McCubbin, J. W.: Increased cardiac output as a contributory factor in experimental renal hypertension in dogs. Circ. Res. 27:799, 1970.
12. Brown, J. J., Dusterdieck, G., Fraser, R., Lever, A. F., Robertson, J. I. S., Tree, M., and Weir, R. J.: Hypertension and chronic renal failure. Br. Med. Bull. 27:128, 1971.
13. Editorial: Renal hypertension. Lancet 1:483, 1971.
14. Katz, L. N., Mendlowitz, M., and Friedman, M.: A study of the factors concerned in renal hypertension. Proc. Soc. Exp. Biol. Med. 37:722, 1938.
15. Grollman, A., Muirhead, E. E., and Vanatta, J.: Role of the kidney in pathogenesis of hypertension as determined by a study of the effects of bilateral nephrectomy and other experimental procedures on the blood pressure of the dog. Am. J. Physiol. 157:21, 1949.
16. Floyer, M. A.: Further studies on the mechanism of experimental hypertension in the rat. Clin. Sci. 14:163, 1955.
17. Kolff, W. J., Page, I. H., and Corcoran, A. C.: Pathogenesis of renoprival cardiovascular disease in dogs. Am. J. Physiol. 178:237, 1954.
18. Muirhead, E. E., Jones, F., and Stirman, J. A.: Hypertensive cardiovascular disease of dog: Relation of sodium and dietary protein to ureterocaval anastomosis and ureteral ligation. Arch. Pathol. 70:108, 1960.
19. Muirhead, E. E.: Protection against sodium overload hypertensive disease by renal tissue and medullorenal extract. Arch. Pathol. 74: 214, 1962.
20. Muirhead, E. E., Stirman, J. A., and Jones, F.: Renal autoexplantation and protection against renoprival hypertensive cardiovascular disease and hemolysis. J. Clin. Invest. 39:266, 1960.

21. Muirhead, E. E., Brown, G. B., Germain, G. S., and Leach, B. E.: The renal medulla as an antihypertensive organ. J. Lab. Clin. Med. 76:641, 1970.
22. Muirhead, E. E., Brooks, B., Pitcock, J. A., and Stephenson, P.: The renomedullary antihypertensive function in accelerated (malignant) hypertension. With observations on the renomedullary interstitial cells. J. Clin. Invest. 51:181, 1972.
23. Muirhead, E. E., Brooks, B., Pitcock, J. A., Stephenson, P. and Brosius, W. L.: Role of the renal medulla in the sodium-sensitive component of renoprival hypertension. Lab. Invest. 27:192, 1972.
24. Hamilton, J. G., and Grollman, A.: The preparation of renal extracts effective in reducing blood pressure in experimental hypertension. J. Biol. Chem. 233:528, 1958.
25. Muirhead, E. E., Jones, F., and Stirman, J. A.: Antihypertensive property in renoprival hypertension of extract from renal medulla. J. Lab. Clin. Med. 56:167, 1960.
26. Milliez, P., Lagrue, G., Meyer, Ph., Devaux, C., and Alexandre, J. M.: Action anti-hypertensive d'un extrait de rein de porc. *In* Milliez, P., and Tcherdakoff, Ph. (Eds.): L'Hypertension Artérielle. Paris: Expansion Scientifique Francaise, 1966, pp. 203–207.
27. Sen, S., Smeby, R. R., and Bumpus, D. M.: Isolation of a phospholipid renin inhibitor from kidney. Biochemistry 6:1572, 1967.
28. Muirhead, E. E., and Stirman, J. A.: Dietary protein and hypertension of dog: Protection by ureterocaval anastomosis with a study of kidneys so treated. (Abstract.) Am. J. Pathol. 34:561, 1958.
29. Muirhead, E. E., Vanatta, J., and Grollman, A.: Papillary necrosis of the kidney, a clinical and experimental correlation. JAMA 142: 627, 1950.
30. Muirhead, E. E., Brown, G. B., Germain, G. S., and Leach, B. E.: The renal medulla as an antihypertensive organ. *In* Alwall, N., Berglund, F., and Josephson, B. (Eds.): Proceedings of the 4th International Congress of Nephrology, vol. 2. Basel: Karger, 1970, pp. 57–64.
31. Muirhead, E. E., and Brooks, B.: Prevention of malignant hypertension of rabbit by renomedullary tissue. Fed. Proc. 29:447, 1970.
32. Brooks, B., and Muirhead, E. E.: Rigid clip for standardized hypertension in the rabbit. J. Appl. Physiol. 31:307, 1971.
33. Muirhead, E. E., and Brooks, B.: Antihypertensive action of renal medulla in salt-loading hypertension. (Abstract.) Fed. Proc. 30:431, 1971.
34. Osvaldo, L., and Latta, H.: Interstitial cells of the renal medulla. J. Ultrastruc. Res. 15: 589, 1966.
35. Nissen, H. M.: On lipid droplets in renal interstitial cells. II. A histological study on the number of droplets in salt depletion and acute salt repletion. Z. Zellforsch. Mikrosk. Anat. 85:483, 1968.
36. Nissen, H. M., and Bojesen, I.: On lipid droplets in renal interstitial cells. IV. Isolation and identification. Z. Zellforsch. Mikrosk. Anat. 97:274, 1969.
37. Nissen, H. M., and Anderson, H.: On the activity of a prostaglandin-dehydrogenase system in the kidney. A histochemical study during hydration/dehydration and salt-repletion/salt depletion. Histochemie 17:241, 1969.
38. Bohman, S. O., and Maunsbach, H. B.: Isolation of lipid droplets from interstitial cells of the renal medulla. J. Ultrastruc. Res. 29: 569, 1969.
39. Osvaldo-Decima, L., and Latta, H.: The renal medulla of diuretic and antidiuretic rats studied by electron microscopy. *In* Alwall, N., Berglund, F., and Josephson, B. (Eds.): Proceedings of the 4th International Congress of Nephrology, vol. 1. Basel: Karger, 1970, pp. 116–123.
40. Simpson, F. O.: Renal vasculature and hypertensive mechanisms. Circ. Res. 27(Suppl. II): 235, 1970.
41. Muirhead, E. E.: Personal observations.
42. Muehrcke, R. C., Mandal, A. K., Epstein, M., and Volini, F. I.: Cytoplasmic granularity of renal medullary interstitial cells in experimental hypertension. J. Lab. Clin. Med. 73: 299, 1969.
43. Muehrcke, R. C., Mandal, A. K., and Volini, F. I.: A pathophysiological review of the renal medullary interstitial cells and their relationship to hypertension. Circ. Res. 27 (Suppl. 1):109, 1970.
44. Muirhead, E. E., Brooks, B., Kosinski, M., Daniels, E. G., and Hinman, J. W.: Renomedullary antihypertensive principle in renal hypertension. J. Lab. Clin. Med. 67:778, 1966.
45. Tobian, L., Ishii, M., and Duke, M.: Relationship of cytoplasmic granules in renal papillary interstitial cells to "post-salt" hypertension. J. Lab. Clin. Med. 73:309, 1969.
46. Ishii, M., and Tobian, L.: Interstitial cell granules in renal papilla and the solute com-

position of renal tissue in rats with Goldblatt hypertension. J. Lab. Clin. Med. 74:1, 1969.

47. Tobian, L., and Azar, S.: Antihypertensive and other functions of the renal papilla. Trans. Assoc. Am. Physicians 84:281, 1971.

48. Muirhead, E. E., Germain, G., Leach, B. E., Pitcock, J. A., Stephenson, P., Brooks, B., Brosius, W. L., Jr., Daniels, E. G., and Hinman, J. W.: Production of renomedullary prostaglandins by renomedullary interstitial cells grown in tissue culture. Circ. Res. Suppl. (In press.)

49. Haggitt, R. C., Pitcock, J. A., and Muirhead, E. E.: Renal medullary fibrosis in hypertension. Human Pathol. 2:587, 1971.

50. Daniels, E. G., Hinman, J. W., Leach, B. E., and Muirhead, E. E.: Identification of prostaglandin E_2 as the principal vasodepressor lipid of rabbit renal medulla. Nature 215:298, 1967.

51. Lee, J. B., Crowshaw, K., Takman, B. H., Attrep, K. A., and Gougoutas, J. Z.: The identification of prostaglandin E_2, $F_{2\alpha}$ and A_2 from rabbit kidney medulla. Biochem. J. 105: 1251, 1967.

52. Crowshaw, K., McGiff, J. C., Strand, J. C., Lonigro, A. J., and Terragno, N. A.: Prostaglandins in dog renal medulla. J. Pharm. Pharmacol. 22:302, 1970.

53. Edwards, W. G., Jr., Strong, C. G., and Hunt, J. C.: A vasodepressor lipid resembling prostaglandin E_2 (PGE_2) in renal venous blood of hypertensive patients. J. Lab. Clin. Med. 74:389, 1969.

54. McGiff, J. C., Crowshaw, K., Terragno, N. A., Lonigro, A. J., Strang, J. C., Williamson, M. A., Lee, J. B., and Ng, K. K. F.: Prostaglandin-like substances appearing in canine renal venous blood during renal ischemia. Circ. Res. 27:765, 1970.

55. McGiff, J. C., Crowshaw, K., Terragno, N. A., and Lonigro, A. J.: Release of a prostaglandin-like substance into renal venous blood in response to angiotensin II. Circ. Res. 27 (Suppl. I):121, 1970.

56. Muirhead, E. E., Leach, B. E., Brooks, B., Brown, G. B., Daniels, E. G., and Hinman, J. W.: Antihypertensive action of prostaglandin E_2. *In* Ramwell, P. W., and Shaw, J. E. (Eds.): Prostaglandin Symposium of the Worcester Foundation for Experimental Biology. New York: Wiley, 1968, pp. 183–200.

57. Somova, L., and Dochev, D.: Changes in the renin activity in rats with experimental hypertension treated with PGE_1 and PGE_2. C.R. Acad. Bulgar. Sci. 23:1581, 1970.

58. Muirhead, E. E., Daniels, E. G., Booth, E., Freyburger, W. A., and Hinman, J. W.: Renomedullary vasodepression and antihypertensive function. Arch. Pathol. 80:43, 1965.

59. Muirhead, E. E., Leach, B. E., Daniels, E. G., and Hinman, J. W.: Lapine renomedullary lipid in murine hypertension. Arch. Pathol. 85:72, 1968.

60. Parks, O. W., Keeney, M., and Schwartz, D. P.: Bound aldehyde in butter oil. J. Dairy Sci. 44:1940, 1961.

61. Parks, O. W., Wong, N. P., Allen, C. A., and Schwartz, D. P.: 6-Trans-Nonenal: An off-flavor component of foam-spray-dried milks. J. Dairy Sci. 52:953, 1969.

62. Braun-Menendez, E.: The prohypertensive and antihypertensive actions of the kidney. Ann. Intern. Med. 49:717, 1958.

63. Goldblatt, H.: The Renal Origin of Hypertension. Springfield, Ill.: Thomas, 1948.

64. Braun-Menendez, E., Fasciolo, J. C., Leloir, L. F., Munoz, J. M., and Taquini, A. C.: Renal Hypertension. Springfield, Ill.: Thomas, 1946, p. 209.

65. Conn, J. W., Rovner, D. R., Cohen, E. L., and Nesbit, R. M.: Normokalemic primary aldosteronism. JAMA 195:111, 1966.

66. Pickering, G. W.: High Blood Pressure. London: Churchill, 1955.

67. Laragh, J. H.: Curable renal hypertension—renin, marker or cause? (Editorial.) JAMA 218:733, 1971.

68. Grollman, A., and Krishnamurty, V. S. R.: Nephrotensin, a newly-described renal pressor agent. (Abstract.) Fed. Proc. 30:432, 1971.

69. Miller, R. P., DeVito, E., Poper, C., Wilson, C., and Shipley, R. E.: Purification and properties of a sustained pressor principle from kidney. (Abstract.) Fed. Proc. 30:432, 1971.

70. Frohlich, E. D., Kozul, V. J., Tarazi, R. C., and Dustan, H. P.: Physiological comparison of labile and essential hypertension. Circ. Res. 27(Suppl. I):55, 1970.

71. Onesti, G., Swartz, C., Ramirez, O., and Brest, A. N.: Bilateral nephrectomy for control of hypertension in uremia. Trans. Am. Soc. Artif. Intern. Organs 14:361, 1968.

72. Ledingham, J. M., and Pelling, D.: Haemodynamic and other studies in the renoprival hypertensive rat. J. Physiol. 210:233, 1970.

73. Dustan, H. P., Bravo, E. L., and Tarazi, R. C.: Volume-dependent essential and steroid hypertensions. (Abstract.) Proc. Cen. Soc. Clin. Res. 44:18, 1971.

74. Merrill, J. P., Giordano, C., and Heetderks, D. R.: The role of the kidney in human hypertension; failure of hypertension to develop in the renoprival subject. Am. J. Med. 31:931, 1961.

75. Muirhead, E. E., Stirman, J. A., Lesch, W., and Jones, F.: The reduction of post nephrectomy hypertension by renal homotransplant. Surg. Gynec. Obstet. 103:673, 1956.

76. Kolff, W. J., and Page, I. H.: Pathogenesis of renoprival cardiovascular disease in dogs. Am. J. Physiol. 178:75, 1954.

77. Kolff, W. J.: Reduction of experimental renal hypertension by kidney perfusion. Circulation 17:702, 1958.

78. Gomez, A. H., Hoobler, S. W., and Blaquier, P.: Effect of addition and removal of kidney transplant in renal and adrenocortical hypertensive rats. Circ. Res. 8:464, 1960.

79. Tobian, L., Schonning, S., and Seefeldt, C.: The influence of arterial pressure on the antihypertensive action of a normal kidney. A biological servomechanism. Ann. Intern. Med. 60:378, 1964.

80. Blalock, A., and Levy, S. E.: Studies on the etiology of renal hypertension. Ann. Surg. 106:826, 1937.

81. Green, J. A., Lucas, J., and Floyer, M. A.: The effect of the kidney in altering the response of the circulation to fluid loading. Clin. Sci. 38:4P, 1970.

Renal Medullary Interstitial Cells and the Antihypertensive Action of Normal and "Hypertensive" Kidneys

By Louis Tobian, M.D.

THERE IS GOOD EVIDENCE to support the idea that the kidney possesses antihypertensive activity. For instance, in the dog, Goldblatt hypertension always becomes more severe when the nonischemic kidney is removed. It is as though removal of this kidney also removes its protective effect, thus allowing hypertension to appear. Moreover, removal of both kidneys in rats and dogs can lead to hypertension, especially when the animal is well hydrated. Muirhead et al.[1] have lowered Goldblatt hypertension by the subcutaneous implantation of cells of the renal medulla. Surgical removal of these implants will cause the blood pressure to bound back up. This provides for an antihypertensive action of the renal medulla. Probably the most striking evidence is the regular way in which successful transplantation of a good kidney can completely abolish the most severe types of hypertension associated with chronic renal failure.

From the Hypertension-Nephrology Division, University of Minnesota Hospitals, Minneapolis, Minnesota.

These observations suggest that the kidney either produces an antihypertensive hormone or has some type of antihypertensive metabolic function. We have found this antihypertensive action to be quite potent during perfusion of an isolated normal kidney when blood pressure levels are high. Conversely, this antihypertensive action is held in abeyance when perfusion

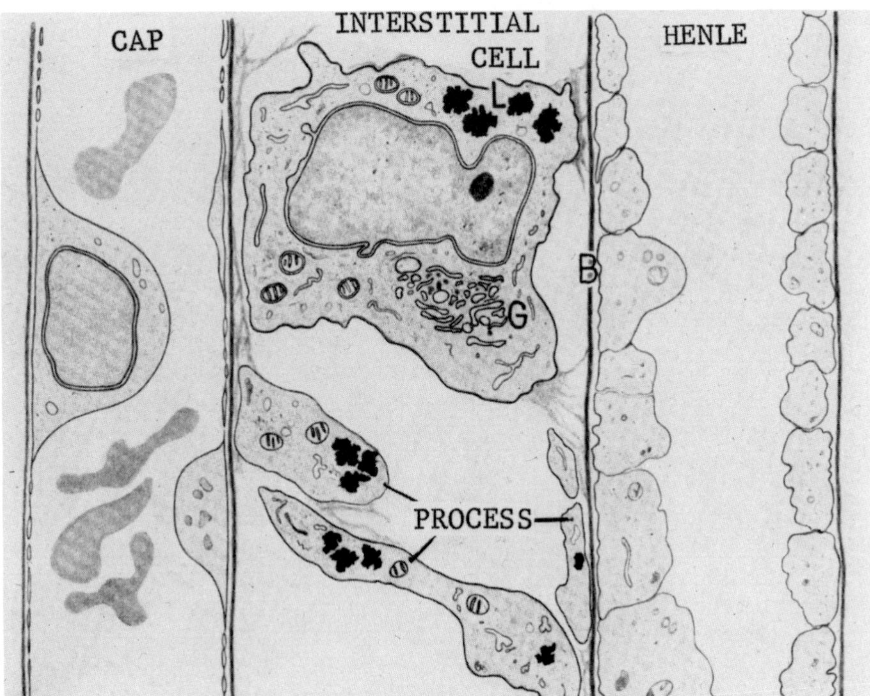

FIG. 1.—Diagrammatic picture of interstitial cells in the renal papilla. (From Gloor, F.: Die interstitiellen Zellen des Nieren markes der Ratte. Z. Zellforsch. Mikrosk. Anat. 68:488, 1965, with permission.)

of the isolated kidney is undertaken when blood pressure levels are in the low normal range.[2] Substances have been extracted from the kidney which can lower blood pressure. We were particularly interested in two such lipid materials that have been extracted from the renal medulla. Lee et al.,[3] Hickler et al.,[4] Strong et al.,[5] and Muirhead et al.[6] have isolated prostaglandin E_2 (PGE_2) from the rabbit renal medulla, and this prostaglandin is capable of lowering blood pressure in both normotensive and hypertensive rats. Moreover, Muirhead et al.[7] have isolated a neutral lipid from the renal medulla, which has clear-cut antihypertensive action when given to rats and rabbits with Goldblatt hypertension. This lipid is not a prostaglandin.

These various findings prompted a study of the lipid granules in the cytoplasm of the interstitial cells of renal papillae from human subjects and rats. These cells have a stellate appearance with many cytoplasmic processes (Fig. 1). They lie horizontally in the interstitial space between the various vertical tubular structures in the renal papilla. In their cytoplasm are large numbers of granules which take up osmic acid and other fat stains and can be dissolved out with fat solvents. The granules definitely contain lipids. Figure 2 is an electronmicrograph of one of these cells. The osmiophilic granules can be easily seen as black cytoplasmic blobs. Dr. Muehrcke[8] of West Suburban Hospital, Oak Park, Illinois, devised a way to stain these granules with a dye mixture of methylene blue and azure II. Figure 3 represents a view under light micros-

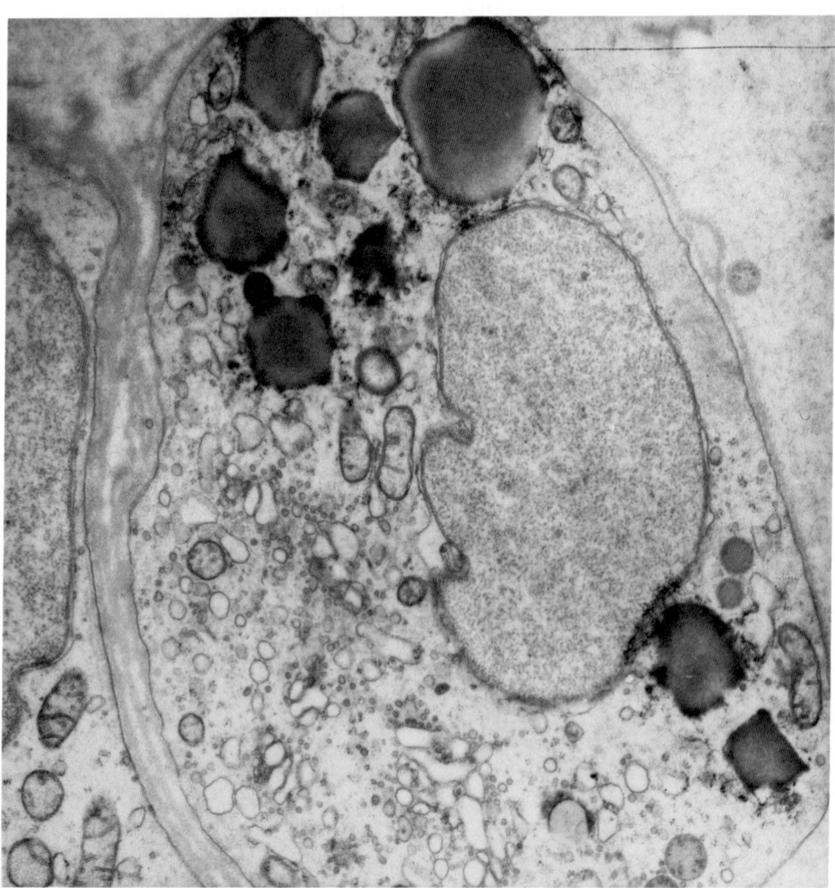

Fig. 2.—Electronmicrograph of a normal interstitial cell in a rat papilla. The black blobs are the lipid granules.

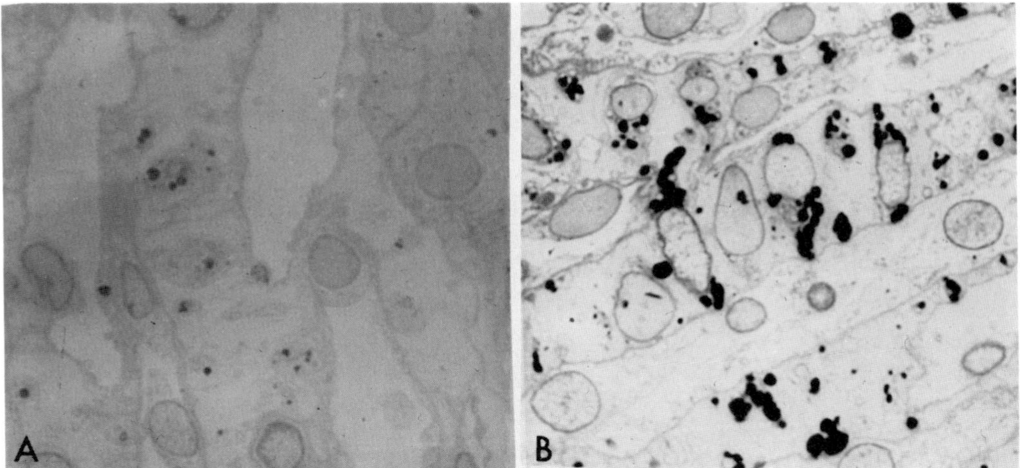

FIG. 3.—Interstitial cell cytoplasmic granules in renal papilla. *A,* Note the numerous prominent dark granules in the papilla of a normotensive control rat. *B,* Relatively few interstitial cell granules are seen in the renal papilla of a rat with post-salt hypertension. Methylene blue—azure II. ×1,100.

copy showing the dark blue granules. By using eyepiece grids, we systematically scan the papilla at 1,100 times magnification and count 1,000 eyepiece squares. The average count per 100 eyepiece squares indicates the abundance of the granules.

With this method we have studied three types of experimental hypertension. First we created a type of "post-salt" hypertension by feeding weanling rats an 8% sodium chloride diet for seven weeks followed by a normal salt diet for 3 months.[9]

As seen in Table 1, the average granule count for the 21 hypertensive rats was 79 per 100 squares, whereas the 10 normotensive control animals had an average count of 136. The difference was significant and indicated a great drop in the number of granules in the hypertensive papillae. Figure 3 shows a papilla from a normotensive control rat and a papilla from a hypertensive rat. The dark blue dots are much fewer and smaller in the hypertensive kidney.

The next type of hypertension was produced in rats by narrowing one renal artery and leaving the contralateral kidney intact.[10] The control group had a sham operation. Four months after the operations both kidneys were obtained for study (Table 2). The papillary granule count in the 38 control kidneys averaged 135 per 100 squares. The granule count in the 38 clipped kidneys averaged 115, significantly lower than control. In the untouched kidneys, which were exposed to the full force of the high blood pressure, the granule count was 99 per 100 squares. Thus the granule count was definitely reduced in both the clipped and untouched kidneys of rats with Goldblatt hypertension.

The third type of hypertension was created by narrowing one renal artery in rats for 9 months, and leaving the opposite kidney intact.[11] At this time the clipped kidney was removed. In 10 of the hypertensive rats blood pressure levels returned to near the normal range after removal of the clipped kidney. In eight other rats hypertension persisted indefinitely (Fig. 4). We can call this "post-Goldblatt" hypertension. Control rats were carried through the whole procedure, with an

TABLE 1.—*Granule Counts in Renal Papilla in Normotensive Rats and in Rats with Post-Salt Hypertension*

Rats	*No.*	*Average Granule Count (per 100 squares)*
Normotensive	10	136
Hypertensive	21	79

$p < 0.001$.

TABLE 2.—*Granule Counts and Sodium Concentration in Renal Papillae of Normotensive Rats and Rats with Goldblatt Hypertension*

Rats	*No.*	*Average Granule Count (per 100 squares)*	*p Value*	*Sodium in Papilla (mEq per kg wet weight)*	*p Value*
Normotensive	38	135	—	136	—
Clipped kidneys	38	115	<0.02	122	<0.07
Untouched kidneys	38	99	<0.001	107	<0.01

initial sham operation and a unilateral nephrectomy 9 months later.

As seen in Table 3, the average granule count in the nine normotensive control rats was 135 per 100 squares. In the rats with "cured" hypertension, the count averaged 112, not significantly different from the controls. However, in the rats with continuing hypertension the average count was 74 per 100 squares, a highly significant reduction. Thus in all three forms of hypertension papillary granules were reduced.

Since the renal papilla also contains very high concentrations of sodium and urea as a result of the countercurrent system, we analyzed the remainder of the papilla as well as a sample of renal cortex for sodium and urea. Figure 5 shows the papilla-to-cortex ratio for sodium concentration in rats with post-salt hypertension. In the normotensive control rats, the concentration of sodium in the papilla

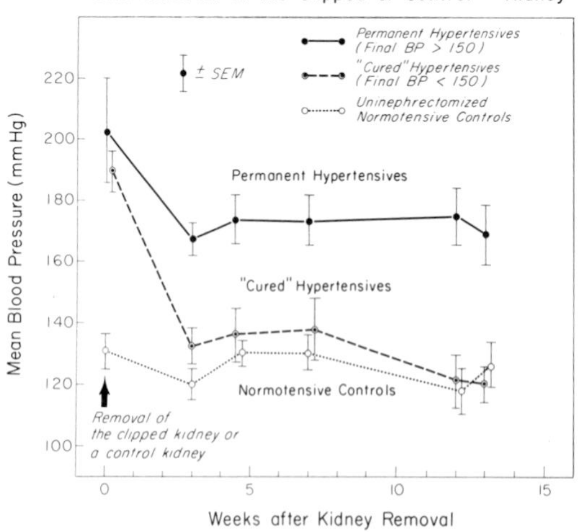

FIG. 4.—Permanent post-Goldblatt hypertension. Average blood pressures are shown for the three experimental groups following nephrectomy.

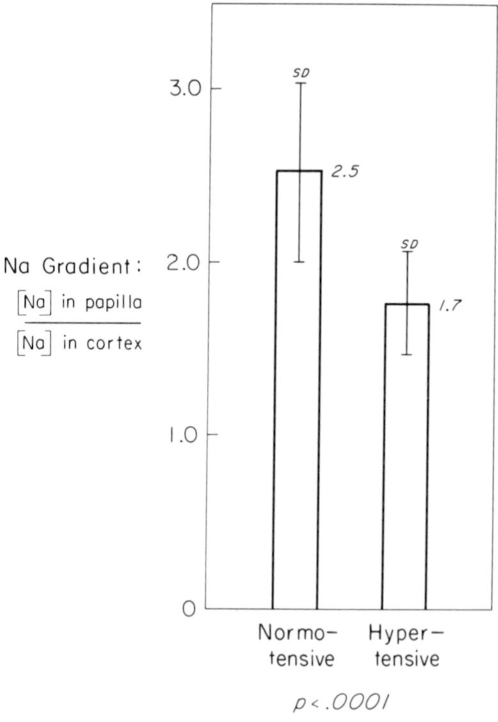

FIG. 5.—Sodium gradients in the renal papilla in relation to post-salt hypertension. (From Tobian, L.: Relationship of cytoplasmic granules in renal papillary interstitial cells to "post-salt" hypertension. J. Lab. Clin. Med., with permission.)

TABLE 3.—*Granule Counts and Sodium Concentration in Renal Papillae of Normotensive Control Rats, Rats with "Cured" Hypertension and Rats with Permanent "Post-Goldblatt" Hypertension*

Rats	*No.*	*Average Granule Count (per 100 squares)*	*p Value*	*Sodium in Papilla (mEq per kg wet weight)*	*p Value*
Normotensive control	9	135	—	153	—
With "cured" hypertension	10	112	>0.1	122	<0.05
With permanent hypertension	8	74	<0.0001	103	<0.001

was 2.5 times greater than that in the cortex. In the rats with post-salt hypertension, the concentration of sodium in the papilla was only 1.7 times that in the cortex. Thus, in these hypertensive rats, the usual steep concentration gradient for sodium in the papilla was not achieved.

In these rats with post-salt hypertension the papilla-to-cortex gradient for sodium is plotted against the papillary granule count in Figure 6. There is a striking correlation. When the granules in a papilla are diminished, the sodium concentration in that same papilla is also lower than normal.

Table 2 shows the sodium concentrations in the papilla in Goldblatt hypertension, 136

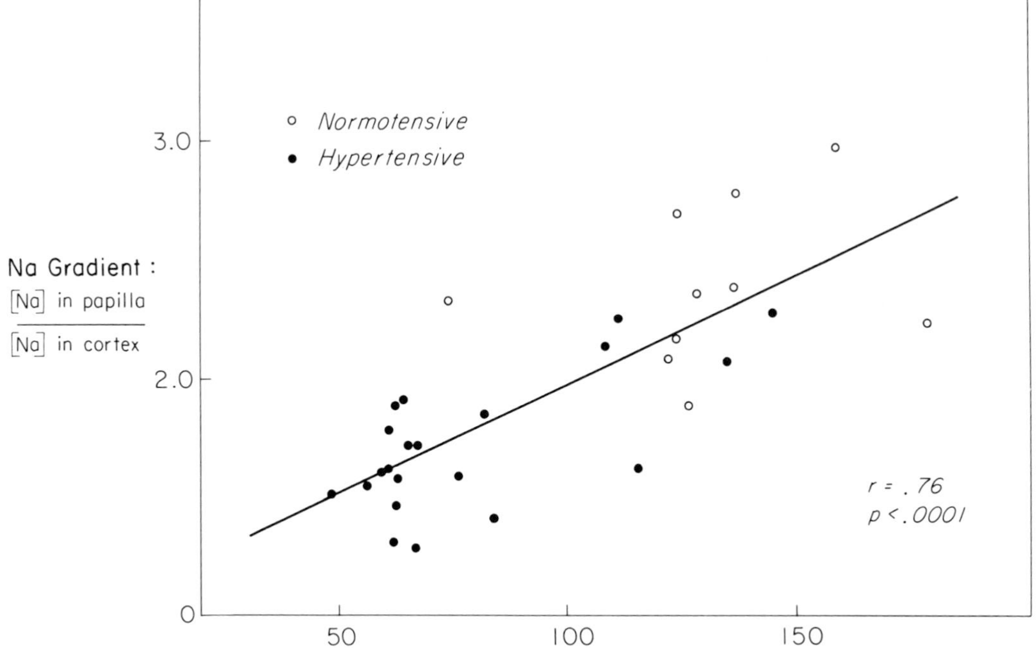

FIG. 6.—Scattergraph relating the sodium (Na) gradient in the kidney to the granule count in papillary interstitial cells. (From Tobian, L.: Relationship of cytoplasmic granules in renal papillary interstitial cells to "post-salt" hypertension. J. Lab. Clin. Med., with permission.)

mEq per kilogram of wet weight in normotensive controls, 122 in the clipped kidney, and 107 in the untouched kidney. Here again the papillae with reduced granules also had a reduced concentration of sodium.

Table 3 shows the concentrations of sodium in the papilla in post-Goldblatt hypertension, 153 mEq per kilogram of wet weight in the normotensive controls, 122 in the cured hypertensive rats, and 103 in the permanent hypertensive rats. Again a reduction in granules is associated with a similar reduction in sodium concentration. In general, the same can be said of the urea concentration in the papilla, i.e., when the granules were reduced, the concentration of urea in the papilla was also reduced.

This relationship was also present in a nonhypertensive setting when rats underwent a massive water diuresis. In such rats, low-sodium and urea levels in the papilla were associated with low levels of papillary granules.[12]

Thus in all these instances, when the granules are few, the sodium in the papilla is also decreased. In the three forms of hypertension, the papillary granules were reduced, as was the papillary concentration of sodium and urea. The papillary granules are also greatly reduced in severe human hypertension. All this would suggest a relationship between a deranged function of the renal papilla and hypertension. We considered the possibility that the low-sodium level in the papilla of the hypertensive rats was due to an increased papillary blood flow, a so-called washout effect. However, when we measured the papillary plasma flow in rats with post-salt hypertension, it was 16 percent lower than that of the normotensive control rats.[13] The low-sodium level in the papilla of hypertensive rats is seemingly not due to a washout.

We also postulated that the decreased num-

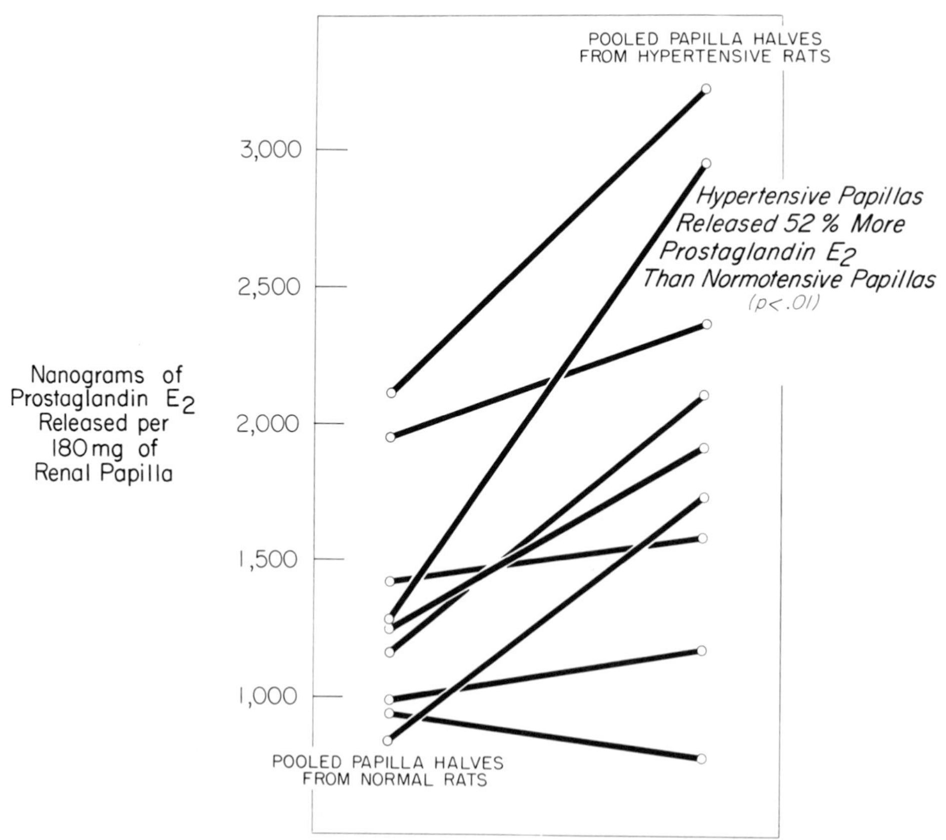

FIG. 7.—Nine comparisons of hypertensive and normotensive renal papillae in regard to their release of PGE_2 into a modified Krebs-Henseleit medium. Each line represents one comparison, with the normal papillae on the left side and the hypertensive papillae on the right side.

ber of interstitial cell granules in the papilla of the hypertensive rats might be a manifestation of sickness or of degeneration of the interstitial cells. Such a situation would be analogous to the atrophic beta cell in the islets of subjects with severe juvenile diabetes. This proposition was tested in two ways. First, it is virtually certain that the interstitial cells secrete PGE_2. The evidence is as follows: The papilla secretes more PGE_2 than any other part of the kidney and contains more interstitial cells. The lipid granules in the interstitial cells contain an unusually high proportion of arachidonic acid in their triglyceride fraction, and arachidonic acid is the sole biochemical precursor of PGE_2. Furthermore, PGE_2 can be extracted from interstitial cells grown in tissue culture. Therefore papillae were obtained from both normotensive control rats and rats with post-salt hypertension. These papillae were halved, pooled, and incubated for 2 hours in a modified Krebs' solution. In eight of nine comparisons the papilla halves from hypertensive rats released more PGE_2 into the medium than did the papillae from normotensive controls. Averaging all nine comparisons, the papillae from hypertensive rats released 52 percent more PGE_2 than the papillae from normotensive rats ($p<0.01$) (Fig. 7).[14]

A second test of the proposition was made by implanting 0.4 gm of fragments of renal papilla under the skin of rats with post-salt hypertension.[14] The effect on the blood pressure of these hypertensive rats was noted 4 days after the implantation (Fig. 8). In 15 hypertensive rats receiving diluent only, the blood pressure fell an average of 8 mm Hg. In 23 hypertensive rats that received implanted fragments of normal "normotensive" renal papilla, the blood pressure fell an average of 23 mm Hg. This drop was significantly greater than that achieved with diluent alone ($p<0.01$). Furthermore, in the eight hypertensive rats that received implanted fragments of "hypertensive" renal papilla (obtained from post-salt hypertensive rats), the blood pressure fell an average of 57 mm Hg. This fall in pressure was significantly greater than that seen with implants of normal papilla ($p<0.01$). Many typical interstitial cells are seen in these medullary fragments. They constitute the chief surviving cell. These studies indicate that the

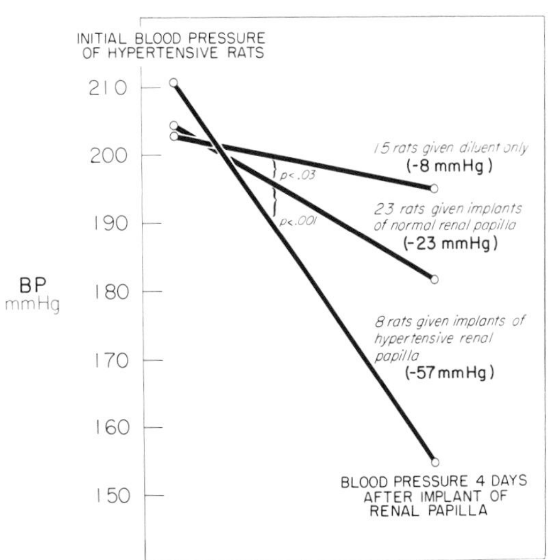

FIG. 8.—The lowering of blood pressure (BP) in hypertensive rats after the subcutaneous implantation of fragments of renal papilla obtained from different sources. See text for more detailed discussion.

interstitial cells of hypertensive papillae are quite capable of secreting antihypertensive agents and prostaglandins and are therefore not comparable to the atrophied pancreatic beta cells in severe juvenile diabetes. Thus, the rat with post-salt hypertension is not hypertensive because of an utter inability of the renal papilla to secrete prostaglandins and other antihypertensive materials. However, it should be realized that the behavior of the hypertensive papilla in a subcutaneous or in an in vitro location may or may not reflect its action in situ as part of an intact kidney. Further experiments are needed to answer these questions.

Another type of experimental hypertension which resembles essential hypertension is that produced by a high-salt intake. Dr. Lewis Dahl has shed much light on this type by breeding one strain of rats that is highly susceptible to salt hypertension and breeding another strain that is highly resistant to salt hypertension. These two strains of rats have been compared in many ways, and it now begins to emerge that the salt-sensitive rats are different partly because the antihypertensive action of their kidneys is deranged.

In an experiment depicted in Figure 9, we

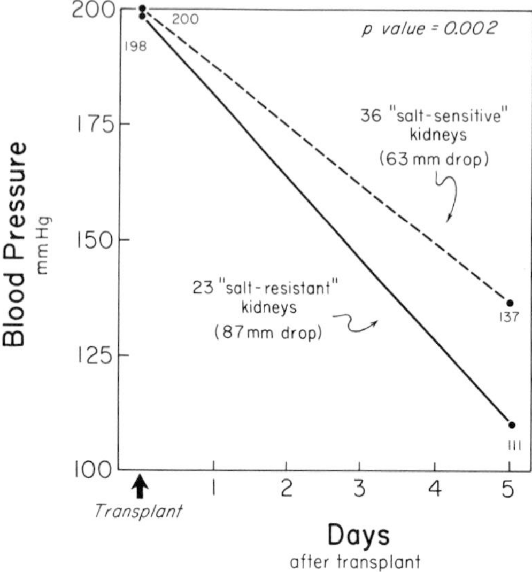

FIG. 9.—The average lowering of blood pressure in Goldblatt-hypertensive rats 5 days after transplantation of a kidney from either a salt-sensitive rat or a salt-resistant rat.

connected kidneys from either salt-sensitive rats or salt-resistant rats into the circulation of rats with Goldblatt hypertension. After the transplanted kidney was connected, we removed the hypertensive rat's own kidney so that the only kidney in the rat was the transplanted one. Over a 5-day period, the transplanted kidneys of the salt-resistant rats reduced the blood pressure markedly, as one can see in the lower line of Figure 9. In this same time, the transplanted kidneys from the salt-sensitive rats did not reduce blood pressure to the same degree, leaving it instead in the range of mild hypertension. Thus, it appeared that the salt-sensitive kidneys had a diminished antihypertensive potency.

Thus, the kidney releases prohypertensive substances and also controls extracellular fluid volume. As indicated above, it may well secrete antihypertensive agents as well. Within this constellation we can find the unique role of the kidney in hypertension.

REFERENCES

1. Muirhead, E. E., Brown, G. B., Germain, G. S., and Leach, B. E.: The renal medulla as an antihypertensive organ. J. Lab. Clin. Med. 76:641, 1970.
2. Tobian, L., Schonning, S., and Seefeldt, C.: The influence of arterial pressure on the antihypertensive action of a normal kidney; a biological servomechanism. Ann. Intern. Med. 60:378, 1964.
3. Lee, J. B., Gougoutos, J. Z., Takman, B. H., Daniel, E. G., Grostic, M. F., Pike, J. E., Hinman, J. W., and Muirhead, E. E.: Vasodepressor and antihypertensive prostaglandins of PGE type with emphasis on the identification of medullin as PGE_2-217. J. Clin. Invest. 45:1036, 1966.
4. Hickler, R. B., Lauler, D. P., Saravis, C. A., and Thorn, G. W.: Characterization of a vasodepressor lipid of the renal medulla. Trans. Assoc. Am. Physicians 77:196, 1964.
5. Strong, C. G., Boucher, R., Nowaczynski, W., and Genest, J.: Renal vasodepressor lipid. Mayo Clin. Proc. 41:433, 1966.
6. Muirhead, E. E., Leach, B. E., Brown, G. B., Daniels, E. G., and Hinman, J. W.: Antihypertensive effect of prostaglandin E_2 (PGE_2) in renovascular hypertension. J. Lab. Clin. Med. 70:986, 1967.
7. Muirhead, E. E., Brooks, B., Kosinski, M., Daniels, E. E., and Hinman, J. W.: Renomedullary antihypertensive principle in renal hypertension. J. Lab. Clin. Med. 67:778, 1966.
8. Muehrcke, R. C., Mandal, A. K., Epstein, M., and Volini, D. I.: Cytoplasmic granularity of the renal medullary interstitial cells in experimental hypertension. J. Lab. Clin. Med. 73:299, 1969.
9. Tobian, L., Ishii, M., and Duke, M.: Relationship of cytoplasmic granules in renal papillary interstitial cells to "post-salt" hypertension. J. Lab. Clin. Med. 73:309, 1969.
10. Ishii, M., and Tobian, L.: Interstitial cell granules in renal papilla and the solute composition of renal tissue in rats with Goldblatt hypertension. J. Lab. Clin. Med. 74:47, 1969.
11. Tobian, L., and Ishii, J.: Interstitial cell granules and solute in renal papilla in post-Goldblatt hypertension. Am. J. Physiol. 217:1699, 1969.
12. Azar, S., Tobian, L., and Ishii, M.: Prolonged water diuresis affecting solutes and interstitial cells of renal papilla. Am. J. Physiol. 221:75, 1971.
13. Ganguli, M., and Tobian, L.: Renal medullary plasma flow in hypertension. Fed. Proc. 31:394, 1972.
14. Tobian, L., and Azar, S.: Antihypertensive and other functions of the renal papilla. Trans. Assoc. Am. Physicians 84:281, 1971.

The Renin-Angiotensin System in Human Renal Hypertension

Jacques Genest, C.C., M.D., and Roger Boucher, Ph.D.

Ever since Goldblatt described in 1934 the production of an "essential-like" type of hypertension in dogs following renal artery constriction,[1] the exact relationship of the renin-angiotensin system to the production of renal experimental hypertension and of human *essential* hypertension has been and is being debated. The following arguments given against the participation of this system are: (1) measurements of plasma renin activity or concentration and of angiotensin II levels are normal in the great majority of animals with chronic renal experimental hypertension and in human benign essential hypertension [2–14]; (2) experimental renal hypertension can be produced in rats or rabbits previously immunized with angiotensin II antibodies. In addition, this type of hypertension when developed is maintained despite administration of angiotensin II antibodies. Blood pressures of both hypertensive immunized as well as nonimmunized rabbits fall to normal levels after removal of the renal clips.[15–17] In contrast, Wakerlin and his group [18,19] and Haas and Goldblatt [20] have demonstrated that administration of renin antibodies from hog renal cortex to renal hypertensive dogs could prevent the appearance of, or decrease blood pressure levels to normal in, experimental renal hypertension in dogs. This effect lasted as long as detectable antirenin titers were present in plasma and could not be obtained by administration of similar homogenates from other tissues such as lungs, liver, or renal medulla. Whatever the arguments for or against these immunization experiments, especially concerning the specificity of the renin antibody preparations, such results serve to emphasize the need for caution and more work on this problem. (3) Cross-transfusions of blood from renal hypertensive animals, whether rats, cats, or dogs, or from hypertensive patients to a normal recipient have no effects on the blood pressure of the latter. (4) Removal of a clipped kidney in hypertensive rats which had the contralateral kidney previously removed has no effect on blood pressure. (5) All parameters of renal function and renal histology are normal in early benign essential hypertension.

From the Clinical Research Institute of Montreal and the Department of Medicine, University of Montreal Medical School, Montreal, Quebec, Canada.

On the other hand, there is definite evidence for the involvement of the renin-angiotensin system in some types of human hypertension. These are described below. In addition, the crucial experiments by Gordon, Drury, and Schapiro [21] of cross-transfusion of blood from a renal hypertensive rabbit to a high-salt-fed rabbit have shown significant increases in blood pressure of the recipient animal persisting for 6 hours after a 1-hour cross-transfusion period. Similar cross-transfusion of blood from a renal hypertensive rabbit to a normally fed rabbit had no effect on blood pressure.[21] These experiments emphasize the importance of the conditioning of the animals by salt to the effect of cross-transfusion of blood from a renal hypertensive animal.

Another reason for keeping an open mind on the relationship of the renin-angiotensin system to benign essential hypertension and to experimental renal hypertension is the recent finding by our group of an isoenzyme of renin in arterial and brain tissues and its persistence at "control" levels despite bilateral nephrectomy in dogs maintained on dialysis for up to 12 days.[22] The role of this arterial and brain-tissue renin must be evaluated in order to define its possible relationship to the hypertensive process and sodium regulation.

The types of human renal hypertension in which the renin-angiotensin system is involved are:

1. Malignant or accelerated hypertension
2. True renovascular hypertension
3. Hypertension in terminal renal failure
4. Renal parenchymatous diseases

Malignant or Accelerated Hypertension

This severe form of hypertension is characterized by the presence of papilledema and retinopathy (exudates and hemorrhages) and frequently of microscopic hematuria secondary to the necrotizing arteriolitis (malignant hypertension) or by the presence of retinopathy with rapid aggravation of the hypertensive condition with increasing diastolic pressures (accelerated hypertension). Plasma renin activity and angiotensin II levels are usually increased in the majority of these patients, presumably because of the necrotizing arteriolitis at the level of the arcuate and interlobular arteries of the kidney, decreasing the renal perfusion pressure to the juxtaglomerular cells with increased liberation of renin. It is not clear whether the malignant hypertension is the cause of the increased renin or its effect, although some experimental evidence would favor the first hypothesis.

True Renovascular Hypertension

We outlined, at the Hypertension Symposium held in Bern in 1965, our experience of over 200 hypertensive patients submitted to surgery because of associated renal artery obstruction.[23] At that time, our failure rate in correcting hypertension was about 50 percent. In reviewing these cases, it appeared clear that measurements of the parameters of systolic pressure gradient beyond the arterial obstruction, plasma renin activity, juxtaglomerular cell count, percentage of granular cells of types II and III, and histological examination of small arteries in the kidneys were most important for the prediction of success or failure of surgery (Table 1).

Thirty-seven of these patients had measurements of at least three of these four parameters. Whatever the arteriographic appearance of the stenosis, nephrectomy or surgical repair of the obstruction resulted in failure if the systolic pressure gradient was greater than 25 to 30 mm Hg.

Recent experimental work in our laboratory has shown that the absence of a gradient or the presence of a systolic gradient of less than 25 to 30 mm Hg in a patient with severe narrowing of a renal artery as seen by angiography is the sign of a markedly increased resistance in the renal parenchyma. In humans, this is most likely due to arteriosclerotic narrowing of the arcuate and interlobular arteries.

In most cases, it was possible to demonstrate a direct correlation between high levels of plasma renin activity in peripheral blood with those in the renal venous blood of the involved kidney, its juxtaglomerular cell count, percentage of granular cells, and the renin content of the renal cortex of the involved kidney.[23,24] But approximately 20 percent of patients had normal plasma renin activity in peripheral blood, and high renal venous blood renin activity and juxtaglomerular cell count and granularity. In those patients with a significant arterial obstruction, as seen on renal arteriograms, who have normal plasma renin

Table 1.—*Hypertension Associated with Renal Artery Obstruction*

Groups	*Systolic Gradient (30 mm Hg)*	*Plasma Renin Activity*	*Juxtaglomerular Granularity*	*Arterial Lesions*	*Percentage Cured or Improved*
I. True renovascular	Greater	High	High	None	86% cured
II. Renovascular plus essential hypertension (?)	Greater	High	High	Present	14% improved * 20% cured
III. Nonfunctional stenosis	Greater	Normal	Normal	Present or not	Rare (2%)
IV. Nonsignificant stenosis	Below	Normal	Normal	—	0

* Patients with long-standing and severe hypertension, and probable contralateral nephrosclerosis.

activity in peripheral blood, it is of utmost importance to repeat those measurements under conditions of stimulation by upright posture and severe sodium restriction.[24,25] Failure to do so is in our opinion the cause of the confusion in the literature concerning the occurrence of normal plasma renin activity in patients cured by surgery. In these reports, no study of the response of renin to the stimuli of upright posture and severe sodium restriction has been made.

Anesthesia is another stimulant of renin liberation and has been known both in animals and in humans to increase its levels two- to threefold in peripheral blood.[26] The case of a 19-year-old male with severe hypertension for the previous 7 years who showed a greatly enhanced response to anesthesia will illustrate this important point. This patient complained only of shortness of breath on exertion and had a blood pressure of 190/130 mm Hg, with marked vasoconstriction of small arteries in both fundi. Renal arteriography showed an almost complete obstruction of the right renal artery with marked collateral circulation to the involved kidney (Fig. 1). Studies of plasma renin activity in peripheral blood repeated on five different days, with the patients in recumbent position and maintained on a dietary intake of 135 mEq of sodium per day, recorded levels of 17, 14, 9, 26, and 20 ng per liter per minute (mean value: 9 with a range of 4 to 24). Although these renin levels were almost all within normal range, the patient was nevertheless submitted to surgery, more, it was thought, for the purpose of saving his right kidney from total atrophy than for the relief of his hypertension. At time of surgery, the systolic gradient was 100 mm Hg, and a vein graft bypass was established with complete correction of this gradient. Blood samples were taken from peripheral blood and left and right renal veins, and biopsies from both kidneys were made. As shown in Fig. 2, the stimulus of anesthesia increased plasma renin activity in peripheral blood more than 20-fold, with the highest level found in blood from the right renal vein. This finding corresponded to a high juxtaglomerular cell count (295 as compared to the average normal of 195 ± S.D. 20) and a very high percentage (20% instead of the average normal of 1 to 3%) of type II and III granular cells in the right kidney. This patient has remained cured of his hypertension since July 1964. The analogy of such patients with cases of pheochromocytoma with normal blood pressure levels between attacks is quite suggestive. Similar observations of greatly increased plasma renin levels during anesthesia for surgery in five patients with renovascular hypertension have been made by Del Greco et al.[11]

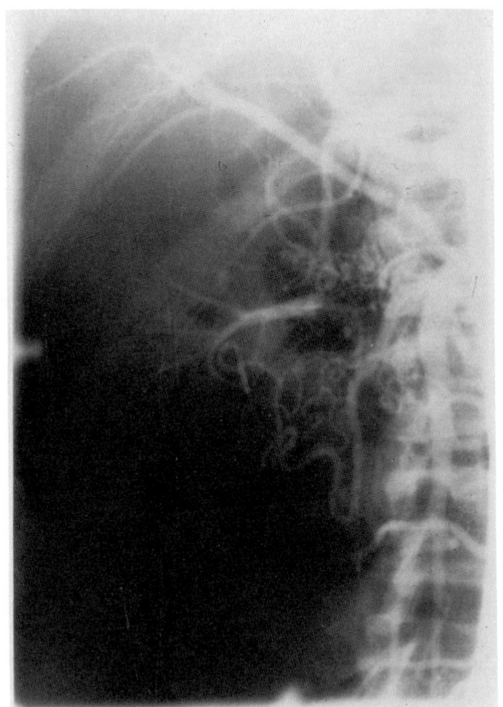

FIG. 1.—Renal arteriogram shows the almost total obstruction of the right renal artery and the marked collateral circulation in a 19-year-old male with severe hypertension of 7 years' duration.

Since renin measurements in renal venous blood necessitate renal vein catheterization with occasional technical difficulties when the effects of upright posture must be studied, and since there is frequent occurrence of more than one renal vein from the same kidney, of branch arterial lesions, of occasionally false positive and negative results, we have adopted the policy of measuring plasma renin activity in peripheral blood under standard conditions of recumbency and fixed sodium intake (135 mEq per day) in hypertensive patients with

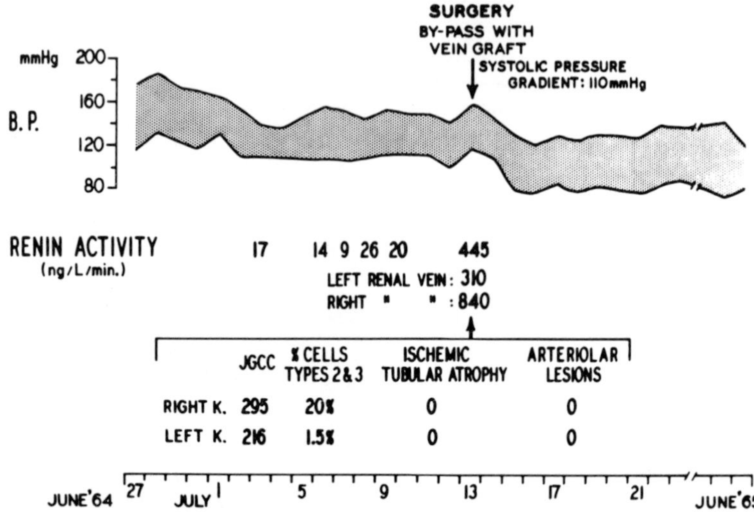

FIG. 2.—This patient was the first one to attract our attention to the importance of stimulatory tests in hypertensive patients with arteriographic evidence of severe renal artery obstruction and normal or paranormal plasma renin activity measurements. Anesthesia in animals and in humans will usually increase plasma renin activity two- to threefold. In this 19-year-old male, laparotomy and anesthesia resulted in a more than 20-fold increase in plasma renin activity, the source being the right kidney with a greatly increased number of juxtaglomerular cells and granular cells of types II and III containing renin. This patient has remained cured of his hypertension for a period of 7 years.

arteriographic evidence of renal artery obstruction. It is important to make sure that these patients have no symptoms or signs of congestive heart failure, are not in a stage of accelerated hypertension and receive no natriuretic or antihypertensive drugs. The protocol which we have been using for the last 6 years with a predictive accuracy in prognosis of 90 to 95 percent of cases is as follows. If peripheral plasma renin levels are high, as they are in 50 to 65 percent of patients, this is sufficient indication for diagnosis of *true* renovascular hypertension. But if the results are borderline or within the normal range, renin measurements should be repeated after stimulation by 4 hours of upright posture and/or 3 days of severe sodium restriction at 10 mEq per day and/or acute sodium depletion by furosemide administration. An excessive response in peripheral renin activity is indicative of renovascular hypertension. But, again, if borderline results are obtained, there are two alternatives: bilateral renal vein catheterization and measurements of renin in renal venous blood from both kidneys under severe sodium restriction and depletion. If renin measurement is greater by a factor of 2 in the blood from the involved side, it may be assumed with a great degree of confidence that this kidney is the cause of hypertension. This protocol gives a prognostic accuracy in 90 to 95 percent of patients. Measurement of peripheral renin activity is easy to accomplish, whereas measurements of renin in renal vein blood necessitate bilateral renal vein catheterization, and have one drawback in cases of branch arterial lesions when the "wrong" vein is catheterized.

It must be pointed out, as shown in Table 1, that a minority of patients belonging to group I (true renovascular hypertension) may remain hypertensive after adequate surgery. In our experience this occurrence was noted in patients with a long-standing hypertension of severe degree who presumably had nephrosclerosis in the contralateral kidney. If this is a correct interpretation, it could well be responsible for the presence of hypertension.

Such a study is illustrated by the case of a

17-year-old girl with severe hypertension of 8 months' duration and a hyperkinetic heart. Blood pressure varied between 180 to 260 and 130 to 160 mm Hg, and the pulse rate often reached 140 to 160 beats per minute during periods of nervousness or when she assumed an upright posture. Intense arteriolar constriction was seen in both fundi. Renal function (phenolsulfonphthalein excretion and creatinine clearance) was normal. Serum sodium and potassium were 137 and 3.7 mEq per liter respectively. An intravenous pyelogram showed a left kidney measuring 13.3 × 6.8 cm and a right kidney measuring 11.5 × 5.5 cm. Renograms were interpreted as normal.

As shown in Fig. 3, renal arteriography revealed a severe stenosis (marked by arrow) of the lower branch of the right renal artery with a post stenotic dilatation. Repeated measurements of plasma renin activity in peripheral blood done either on an *ad libitum* diet or on a carefully controlled sodium-intake diet showed levels (27, 28, and 33 ng per liter per minute) slightly above the upper range of normal (Fig. 4).

There was a markedly enhanced response to upright posture (82 ng per liter per minute) and to severe sodium restriction (104 ng per liter per minute in recumbent position and 500 ng in upright posture). When the patient received a normal sodium diet, a bilateral renal vein catheterization was done and a greater than twofold increase of renin measurement in blood from the right renal vein was observed when compared to the left side.

Normal values of renin activity can be obtained in both peripheral and renal venous blood in patients with true renovascular hypertension and with a high juxtaglomerular cell count and renal cortex renin content. The percentage of such patients is between 15 and 20 percent and it is in this group that the effects of stimulation by upright posture and severe sodium restriction must be studied. In this respect, it is important to emphasize that each laboratory must have its own control values and the range of renin response by normal subjects to these two stimuli. In only one patient did we fail to observe an increase of renin response to these stimuli although the juxtaglomerular cell count was high and the patient was cured by surgery.

In our experience, the value of renin measurements for the diagnosis of true renovascular hypertension and for prognosis of success or failure of surgery surpasses that of rapid sequence intravenous pyelography, renography, and split renal function test. This last test, although most valuable when positive in cases of unilateral main renal artery constriction,

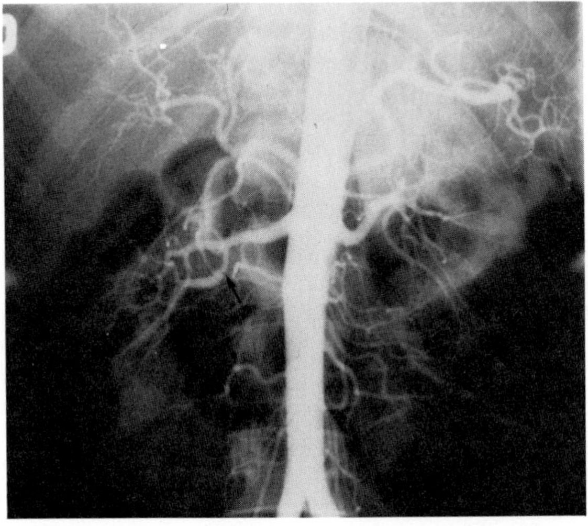

FIG. 3.—Renal arteriography showing **(arrow)** a severe narrowing (arterial dysplasia) of the lower branch of the right renal artery with poststenotic dilatation in a 17-year-old female with severe hypertension of 8 months' duration.

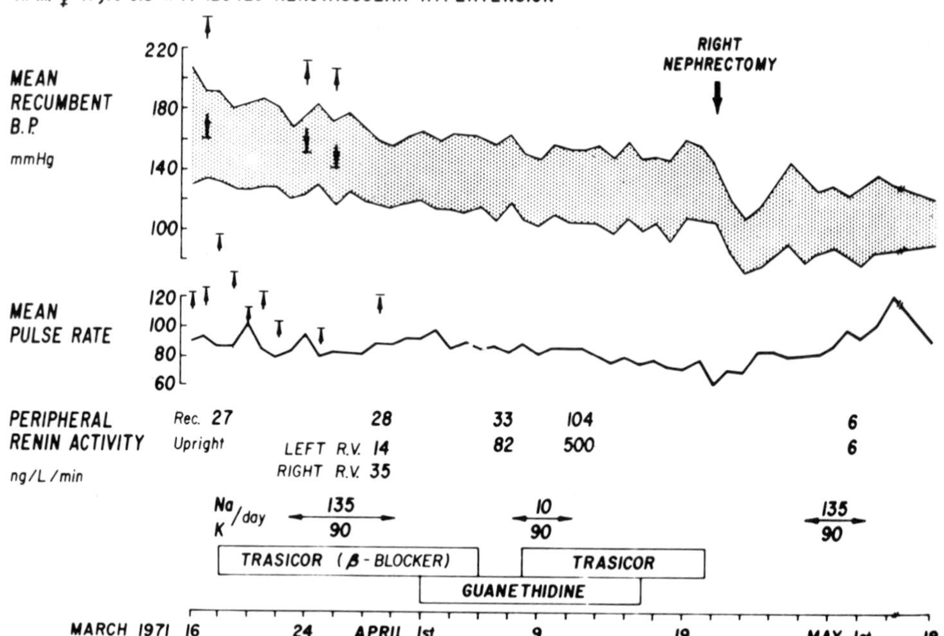

FIG. 4.—Follow-up of the patient seen in Fig. 3 who had true renovascular hypertension. The **arrows** indicate the upper range of blood pressure readings and of pulse rate during slight emotional stresses or in assuming an upright posture. Because of this severe hyperkinetic heart disturbance, the patient was given a beta-adrenergic blocking agent (Trasicor). Plasma renin activity was nevertheless above the upper range of normal. Measurements of plasma renin activity in bilateral renal venous blood were made on a different day from the peripheral measurement (28 ng per liter per minute) and showed a greater than twofold increase on the involved side. These studies illustrated the markedly enhanced response to upright posture and to severe sodium restriction.

has been discarded in most centers because of the discomfort to the patient, the time-consuming aspect of the procedure, and of the many laboratory tests, the risk of infection and obstruction by blood clots, and the not infrequent occurrence of false negative and false positive results.

The physiopathology of true renovascular hypertension, as based on the findings from our laboratory and those of many others, is illustrated in Fig. 5.

Hypertension in Terminal Renal Failure

This type of severe hypertension associated with terminal renal failure depends on two major factors: (1) excessive sodium and water intake and increased plasma volume (such a hypertension is usually controlled by dietary means and by ultrafiltration during dialysis); and (2) excessive renin-angiotensin system activity. In these patients, hypertension is corrected rapidly by bilateral nephrectomy.

Vertes [27,28] and Weidmann [29] and their coworkers have shown that patients with hypertension in terminal renal failure controlled by ultrafiltration had normal plasma renin activity while all patients with uncontrollable hypertension had clearly elevated plasma renin levels. An almost linear correlation between plasma renin activity and mean blood pressure in patients with terminal renal failure has been observed.[27–31]

Renal Parenchymatous Diseases

Following our first findings [32] there have been in the recent literature many reports of measurements of peripheral plasma renin activity in patients with hypertension secondary to such renal parenchymatous diseases

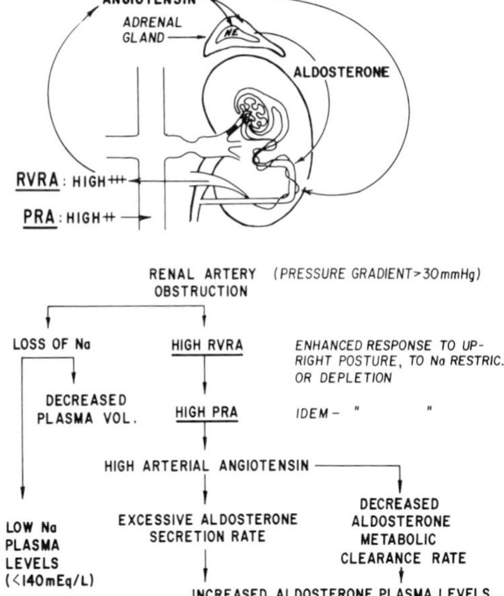

FIG. 5.—Physiopathology of true renovascular hypertension leading in severe cases to a clinical picture similar to that of primary aldosteronism, except for the presence of renal artery obstruction, high renin levels, and lower plasma sodium levels. **RVRA,** renal vein renin activity; **PRA,** peripheral renin activity.

as polycystic kidney disease, acute and chronic glomerulonephritis, pyelonephritis, and hydronephrosis. A wide distribution of values from normal to above normal range has been reported by most workers with about 20 to 25 percent of patients having levels above normal range.

The best documented reports have been those of Warren and Ferris,[33] of Reubi and Hodler,[34] and of Kleinknecht and Maxwell.[35] Warren and Ferris's [33] inpatients with chronic glomerulonephritis showed no change in plasma renin in response to large increases in plasma volume and to upright posture and a lack of suppression by salt loading. Reubi and Hodler [34] studied 70 patients with various parenchymatous nephropathies. Their results show a normal plasma renin activity in acute and in chronic glomerulonephritis without urea retention, whether it was accompanied by hypertension or not. In patients with chronic glomerulonephritis with urea retention and hypertension, the mean plasma renin activity of the group was significantly increased and the plasma renin activity failed to respond to severe sodium restriction. Renin activity in chronic pyelonephritis with urea retention was normal and did not respond to the stimulus of severe sodium restriction. No correlation between plasma renin activity and sodium concentration could be established.

Kleinknecht and Maxwell [35] studied 100 patients with various parenchymatous renal diseases, i.e., chronic glomerulonephritis, nephrotic syndrome, chronic pyelonephritis, polycystic kidney disease, and nephrosclerosis. Although the mean values in each group of patients with these nephropathies are higher than the normal mean, there is a wide scatter of values. Plasma renin activity, measured under conditions of recumbency and after a 5-day period of a normal (100 mEq per day) sodium intake, was increased in 27 out of 43 patients with chronic glomerulonephritis, 7 out of 11 patients with nephrotic syndrome, 6 out of 16 patients with chronic pyelonephritis, and 8 out of 13 patients with polycystic kidney disease. Renin response to severe sodium restriction was similar to that of normal subjects, except for patients with chronic pyelonephritis and polycystic kidney disease in whom no change or even a decrease was noted. On the other hand, patients with nephrosclerosis had an exaggerated response. The effect of upright posture was variable with plasma renin activity increased in some, decreased in others, and unchanged in a few, in contrast to the constant increase in all control subjects studied. These workers found a significant correlation between the logarithm of the plasma renin activity and the diastolic pressure and the logarithm of plasma creatinine concentration. Plasma renin substrate was normal.

REFERENCES

1. Goldblatt, H., Lynch, J., Hanzal, R. F., and Summerville, W. W.: Studies on experimental hypertension. I. The production of persistent elevation of systolic blood pressure by means of renal ischemia. J. Exp. Med. 59:347, 1934.
2. Genest, J., Boucher, R., de Champlain, J., Veyrat, R., Chrétien, M., and Biron, P.: Arterial angiotensin blood levels in hypertensive and edematous diseases. *In* Proceedings of the 2nd International Congress of

Nephrology. Prague: Excerpta Medica, 1963, p. 58.

3. Kahn, J. R., Skeggs, L. T., Shumway, N. P., and Wisenbaugh, P. E.: The assay of hypertensin from the arterial blood of normotensive and hypertensive human beings. J. Exp. Med. 95:523, 1952.
4. Genest, J., Boucher, R., de Champlain, J., Veyrat, R., Chrétien, M., Biron, P., Tremblay, G., Roy, P., and Cartier, P.: Studies on the renin-angiotensin system in hypertensive patients. Can. Med. Assoc. J. 90:263, 1964.
5. Veyrat, R., de Champlain, J., Boucher, R., and Genest, J.: Measurement of human arterial renin activity in some physiological and pathological states. Can. Med. Assoc. J. 90:215, 1964.
6. Boyd, G. W., Adamson, A. R., Fitz, A. E., and Peart, W. S.: Radioimmunoassay determination of plasma renin activity. Lancet 1:213, 1969.
7. Gocke, D. J., Gerten, J., Sherwood, S. M., and Laragh, J. H.: Physiological and pathological variations of plasma angiotensin II in man. Correlation with renin activity and sodium balance. Circ. Res. 24–25(Suppl. I): I–131, 1969.
8. Genest, J., Boucher, R., Nowaczynski, W., Koiw, E., de Champlain, J., Biron, P., Chrétien, M., and Marc-Aurele, J.: Studies on the relationship of aldosterone and angiotensin to human hypertensive disease. *In* Baulieu, E., and Robel, P. (Eds.): Aldosterone, A Symposium. Oxford: Blackwell, 1964, p. 393.
9. Brown, J. J., Davies, D. L., Lever, A. F., and Robertson, J. I. S.: Plasma renin concentration in human hypertension. III. Renin in relation to complications of hypertension. Br. Med. J. 1:505, 1966.
10. Mulrow, P. J., and Goffinet, J. A.: The renin-angiotensin system. *In* Wesseon, L. G., Jr. (Ed.): Physiology of the Human Kidney. New York: Grune & Stratton, 1969, p. 465.
11. Del Greco, F., Simon, N. M., Goodman, S., and Roguska, J.: Plasma renin activity in primary and secondary hypertension. Medicine 46:475, 1967.
12. Yoshinaga, K., Aida, M., Maebashi, M., Sato, T., Abe, K., and Miwa, I.: Assay of renin in peripheral blood. A modification of Helmer's method for the estimation of circulating renin. Tohoku J. Exp. Med. 80:32, 1963.
13. Massani, Z. M., Finkielman, S., Worcel, M., Agrest, A., and Paladini, A. C.: Angiotensin blood levels in hypertensive and nonhypertensive diseases. Clin. Sci. 30:473, 1966.
14. Bourgoignie, J., Kurz, S., Catanzaro, F. J., Scrirat, P., and Perry, H. M.: Renal venous renin in hypertension. Am. J. Med. 48:332, 1970.
15. Eide, I., and Aars, H.: Renal hypertension in rabbits immunized with angiotensin. Nature 222:571, 1969.
16. Eide, I.: Renovascular hypertension in rats immunized with angiotensin. Acta Physiol. Scand. 80:40a, 1970.
17. MacDonald, G. J., Louis, W. J., Renzini, V., Boyd, G. W., and Peart, W. S.: Renal-clip hypertension in rabbits immunized against angiotensin II. Circ. Res. 27:197, 1970.
18. Wakerlin, G. E.: Antibodies to renin as proof of the pathogenesis of sustained renal hypertension. Circulation 17:653, 1958.
19. Wakerlin, G. E., Bird, R. B. Brennan, B. B., Frank, M. H., Kremen, S., Kuperman, I., and Skom, J. H.: Treatment and prophylaxis of experimental renal hypertension with "renin." J. Lab. Clin. Med. 41:708, 1953.
20. Haas, E., and Goldblatt, H.: Effects of ganglionic blocking agents, pressor and depressor drugs on renal hypertension. Am. J. Physiol. 197:1303, 1959.
21. Gordon, D. B., Drury, D. R., and Schapiro, S.: The salt-fed animal as a test object for pressor substances in the blood of hypertensive animals. Am. J. Physiol. 175:123, 1953.
22. Hayduk, K., Ganten, D., Boucher, R., and Genest, J.: Arterial and urinary renin activity. *In* Genest, J., and Koiw, E. (Eds.): Hypertension 72. New York: Springer, 1972, pp. 435–443.
23. Genest, J., Tremblay, G. Y., Boucher, R., de Champlain, J., Rojo-Ortega, J. M., Lefebvre, R., Roy, P., and Cartier, P.: Diagnostic significance of humoral factors in renovascular hypertension. *In* Gross, F. (Ed.): Antihypertensive Therapy (Principles and Practice). Heidelberg: Springer, 1966, p. 518.
24. Genest, J.: The renin-angiotensin-aldosterone system. *In* Brest, A. N., and Moyer, J. H. (Eds.): Cardiovascular Disorders. Philadelphia: Davis, 1968, p. 144–160.
25. Cohen, E. L., Rovner, D. R., and Conn, J. W.: Postural augmentation of plasma renin activity. Importance in diagnosis of renovascular hypertension. JAMA 197:973, 1966.
26. Genest, J., Strong, C. G., and Boucher, R.: Unpublished observations.
27. Vertes, V., Cangiano, J. L., Berman, L. B.,

and Gould, A.: Hypertension in end-stage renal disease. N. Engl. J. Med. 280:978, 1969.

28. Vertes, V., Berman, L. B., and Mitra, S.: Hypertension in end-stage renal failure and anephric man. Circulation 44:120, 1971.
29. Weidmann, P., Maxwell, M. H., Lupu, A. N., Lewin, A. J., and Massey, S. G.: Plasma renin activity and blood pressure in terminal renal failure. N. Engl. J. Med. 285:757, 1971.
30. Wilkinson, R., Scott, D. F., Uldall, P. R., Kerr, D. N. S., and Swinney, J.: Plasma renin and exchangeable sodium in the hypertension of chronic renal failure. The effect of bilateral nephrectomy. Q. J. Med. 39:377, 1970.
31. Stokes, G. S., Goldsmith, R. F., Starr, L. M., Gentle, J. L., Mani, M. K., and Stewart, J. H.: Plasma renin activity in human hypertension. Cir. Res. 26–27(Suppl. II):II–207, 1970.
32. Genest, J., de Champlain, J., Strong, C. G., and Boucher, R.: *In* Milliez, P., and Tcherdakoff, Ph. (Eds.): Le système rénine-angiotensine dans l'hypertension humaine. Club International sur l'Hypertension Artérielle. Paris: Expansion Scientifique Française. 1966, pp. 130–140.
33. Warren, D. J., and Ferris, T. F.: Renin secretion in renal hypertension. Lancet 1:159, 1970.
34. Reubi, F., and Hodler, J.: L'activité rénine au cours des néphropathies parenchymateuses avec ou sans hypertension. Actual. Nephrol. (Paris) 9:221, 1968.
35. Kleinknecht, D., and Maxwell, M. H.: Etude statistique des variations de l'activité rénine plasmatique dans les néphropathies bilatérales. Actual. Nephrol. (Paris) 11:63, 1970.

Experimental Renoprival Hypertension

By Arthur Grollman, Ph.D., M.D.

THE TERM "renoprival hypertension" is used generally in its literal sense to denote the rise in blood pressure that follows bilateral nephrectomy. In this limited sense it is not applicable to hypertension resulting from partial or unilateral nephrectomy; to the hypertension accompanying such obvious morphologic lesions of the kidney as occur in chronic nephritis; or to other forms of hypertension designated as "renal." Nevertheless, all of these forms of hypertension actually involve a loss of renal tissue and function.[1] The use of *renoprival* on the assumption that one is dealing with a specific and unique form of hypertension is accordingly arbitrary, particularly if one accepts the view that most forms of experimental and clinical hypertension are a consequence of the loss of a renal function normally concerned in the maintenance of the normotensive state.[1,2]

The present chapter shall consider the effects of nephrectomy (unilateral and bilateral) on the blood pressure of the normotensive and of the hypertensive experimental animal. Only brief reference will be made to the effects of nephrectomy in man since this is considered elsewhere in this volume.

General Considerations

The earliest work on the effects of nephrectomy on the blood pressure led to the erroneous conclusion that the maintenance of an elevated blood pressure requires the presence of renal tissue. This conclusion was based on the observation that removal of the kidneys resulted in a decline in blood pressure in normal as well as in hypertensive animals. The fact that the elevated blood pressure was not maintained in hypertensive animals following nephrectomy was offered as support for the concept that the observed elevation was maintained by a circulating pressor agent of renal origin. The level of the blood pressure observed in these early studies reflected the premortem state of the animals; and these investigators failed to recognize that in a state of debility, the organism is unable to maintain an elevated blood pressure. This obvious fact was emphasized by Sir Clifford Allbutt[3] in 1915 when he stated, "that the blood pressure does not rise on extirpation of both kidneys . . . may be attributable to the severity of the operation." The same error continued to be made in interpreting observations in many experimental studies as well as in the human beings dying of renal insufficiency. Several days must elapse following bilateral nephrectomy before hypertension develops; failure to note a rise in blood pressure in animals surviving only 3 or 4 days is thus of no significance.[4]

Another source of confusion attending observations on the effect of nephrectomy has been the failure to appreciate the fact that under certain experimental as well as clinical conditions acute hypertension may result from the secretion by the affected kidney of a pressor agent.[2,5] Nephrectomy in such cases will obviously cause a decline in blood pressure rather than the increase which it does in the absence of a circulating pressor agent. The effect of nephrectomy in a given instance will vary, therefore, depending on the mechanism responsible for maintaining the preoperative blood pressure.

In view of the above-described considerations it is not surprising that the available data on the effects of nephrectomy on the blood pressure should be conflicting and confusing. Rather than add to this confusion by recapitulating all of the extant data, therefore, only selected studies which contribute to a better understanding of the pathogenesis of hypertension will be presented here.

From the Laboratory for Experimental Medicine, Department of Pathology, University of Texas Southwestern Medical School, Dallas, Texas.

The previously unpublished experiments reported in this chapter were supported by Grant 71–1113 from the American Heart Association and the Lilien K. Christy Bequest.

Effects of Unilateral Nephrectomy in the Normotensive Animal

Unilateral nephrectomy has been performed frequently in the human and in the experimental animal with no obvious effect on the blood pressure. This is not unexpected since removal of one kidney is followed by compensatory hypertrophy of the remaining organ, which presumably takes over the function of both organs. If the contralateral kidney, however, is unable to maintain this function, or in the presence of already existent hypertension, even of a minimal degree, unilateral nephrectomy, as shown later, results in a further rise in blood pressure.

The incidence of hypertension following unilateral nephrectomy is greater in the rat than in other species. In the dog, for example, chronic hypertension ensues only rarely following removal of one kidney, or other manipulations, if the opposite kidney is left intact.[6] In the rat, on the other hand, approximately 20 percent of the animals in some colonies may develop hypertension following unilateral nephrectomy.[7] This high incidence of hypertension following unilateral nephrectomy is dependent on the status of the contralateral kidney at the time of operation. If lesions are present in the opposite kidney, hypertension develops; if absent, the animals remain normotensive.[8]

The usually encountered colony of laboratory rats manifests a wider variation in blood pressure than one would anticipate to occur as a result simply of normal physiologic variations. Arbitrarily, only those animals with systolic pressures of 150 mm Hg or more are considered hypertensive, but it is more probable that animals with systolic blood pressures over about 100 ± 10 are actually mildly hypertensive. As shown in Fig. 1, unilateral nephrectomy results in the elevation of the blood pressure of the rat to a degree proportional to the preoperative pressure; only in animals with pressures in the lower ranges of normal does unilateral nephrectomy result in no demonstrable elevation in blood pressure. As the basal blood pressure increases, unilateral nephrectomy induces an increasingly greater rise in blood pressure. Removal of one kidney in the spontaneously hypertensive rat, the blood pressure of which is only slightly elevated, also results in the development of hypertension at an accelerated pace, as shown in the uppermost curve of Fig. 1.

The above-described experiments on the effect of unilateral nephrectomy on the normotensive and on the spontaneously hypertensive rat suggest that the laboratory rat has an inheritable congenital tendency to develop hypertensive disease. In most colonies used in the laboratory this congenital defect results in variable moderate rises in blood pressure, but the elevation in blood pressure may be accentuated by age, infection, unilateral nephrectomy, the administration of steroids, high salt intake, the application of a clip to the renal artery, and other procedures having an adverse effect on the renal function concerned in maintaining the normotensive state. This congenital tendency has been taken advantage of by selective breeding to produce strains of animals with spontaneous hypertension.[9,10]

Essential hypertension, like diabetes mellitus and other disorders, affects the organism to a variable degree. Blood pressure levels normally

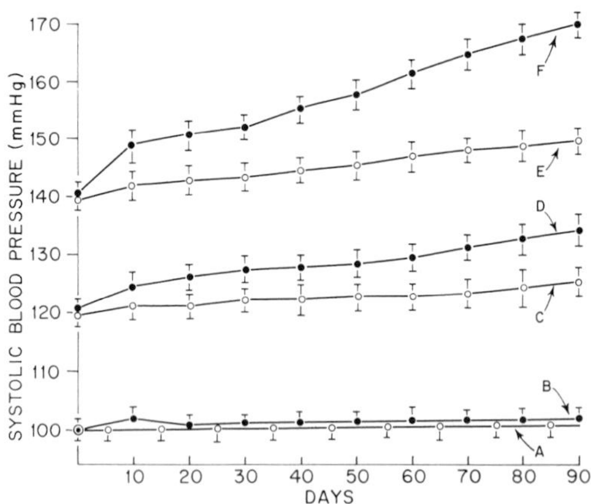

Fig. 1.—The effect of unilateral nephrectomy on the arterial blood pressure of the rat. Curves *B*, *D*, and *F* (●—●) represent the effect of right nephrectomy; curves *A*, *C*, and *E* (○—○), the effect of a sham operation (controls). Operations were performed at day 0. Rats of curves *E* and *F* were from a spontaneously hypertensive colony; those of curves *A*, *B*, *C*, and *D* were from an inbred strain reared in the laboratory. Each point of the curves represents the average of readings on 10 animals ±S.E. (standard error), represented by the **vertical lines.**

considered as being in the upper ranges of normal may accordingly actually constitute a minor degree of hypertension. Unilateral nephrectomy, by reducing an already compromised function, merely intensifies the existent mild degree of hypertension and elevates the blood pressure to a level generally accepted as indicative of the presence of hypertensive cardiovascular disease.[11,12]

Effect of Unilateral Nephrectomy in the Hypertensive Animal

The effect of removing one kidney in the hypertensive animal is dependent upon (1) the level of the blood pressure; (2) whether a renal pressor agent is present in the circulating blood; (3) whether one or both kidneys are present; (4) the condition of the remaining kidney; and (5) whether the kidney which has been manipulated in order to induce the hypertension or the contralateral untouched kidney is removed. Failure to appreciate the influence of these factors has been the cause of the diversity and the confusion in interpreting the observed results.[11]

Effect of Unilateral Nephrectomy in the Presence of Both Kidneys

The original Goldblatt procedure consists of applying a clamp to one renal artery and removing the contralateral kidney.[13] Only occasionally in the dog, but more frequently in the rat, can hypertension be induced by applying a clamp, clip, figure-of-eight ligature, or other constriction unilaterally, leaving the contralateral side untouched. In the rat, removal of a kidney which has been infarcted or the renal artery of which has been restricted, results in a decline of the blood pressure to normal levels.[12,14,15] If removal of the kidney is delayed for some weeks, however, the blood pressure no longer returns to normal. A similar response has been noted in the dog,[16,17] rabbit,[18,19] sheep,[20] and goat,[21] and the same decline in blood pressure follows removal of a restriction on the renal artery as does removal of the ischemic kidney. The observed decline in blood pressure occurs only when acute hypertension is induced by the secretion from the affected kidney of a demonstrable pressor agent. When chronic hypertension in the absence of a circulating pressor agent ensues, removal of the affected kidney no longer results in a decline of the blood pressure.[12,14,19,20]

Although unilateral manipulation of one kidney or its artery does not usually induce hypertension in the dog, it may do so in the rat, with or without a transient stage of acute hypertension.[7,8] This paradoxical effect is a consequence of an immunologic action of the affected kidney on the contralateral one.[22]

Effect of Removing a Single Remaining Kidney

Removal of the remaining kidney of an animal with chronic hypertension induced by constriction of one kidney and removal of the contralateral one does not result in a decline in blood pressure until shortly before death.[6,7] The hypertension in this case is not a result of the liberation of a pressor agent from the kidney as it is in the acutely hypertensive preparation.[2] It is now apparent that under certain conditions in man as well as in the experimental animal, the blood pressure may become elevated as a result of the liberation by the kidney of a pressor agent demonstrable in the renal venous effluent.[2,5] When this is the case, removal of the affected kidney results in a decline in the blood pressure. On the other hand, in chronic hypertension, the rise in blood pressure is not mediated through the presence of a circulating pressor agent, and nephrectomy fails to lower the blood pressure.

The effect of the removal of a single remaining kidney on the blood pressure is complicated by the fact that the ensuing uremic state and moribund condition of the animal may prevent any rise in blood pressure from being manifested unless special measures are taken to assure prolonged survival. In normotensive animals which have undergone prior unilateral nephrectomy, the removal of the remaining kidney results in the development of hypertension similar to that following bilateral nephrectomy as described later. In the case of animals which have been rendered hypertensive by operation on one kidney and removal of the contralateral kidney, the blood pressure, as already indicated, remains elevated following removal of the remaining kidney.[6,7,12,19]

Nephrectomy in Parabiotic Rats

To avoid the complicating effect of uremia on the blood pressure following nephrectomy, rats joined in parabiotic union have been utilized. This preparation permits bilateral nephrectomy of one parabiont with no appreciable loss of renal excretory function. Jeffers et al.[23] first demonstrated that the removal of three kidneys from a pair of rats joined in parabiosis resulted in hypertension in the bilaterally nephrectomized member of the pair. Grollman and Rule [24] found that removal of the kidneys from one member of the pair in parabiosis sufficed to induce hypertension in the nephrectomized animal with only a slight elevation in its intact twin. They interpreted their results as consistent with the view that the kidney elaborated a substance necessary for maintaining the normotensive state.

When rats in which hypertension has been induced by unilateral perinephritis are joined in parabiosis with normotensive animals, the blood pressure falls to normal levels within a few days but returns to hypertensive levels when the parabionts are separated.[25] No change in blood pressure is observed when two hypertensive animals are joined or when a hypertensive rat is joined to a nephrectomized animal.[25] Ledingham [26] also noted that nephrectomy in one member of a parabiotic pair of rats results in hypertension in this member but never in the parabiont with intact kidneys; that adrenalectomy of the nephrectomized member abolished the hypertension; and that arteriolar lesions were limited to the viscera of the nephrectomized rat. Masson, Corcoran, and Page [27] found that animals with DOCA-induced hypertension became normotensive when placed in parabiosis with saline-fed normal rats. The hypertension was restored by removal of the remaining kidney or by separating the parabionts.

The above-described experiments suggest that the removal of normal renal tissue, rather than the release of a pressor agent by abnormal or ischemic tissue, is responsible for the development of hypertension.

Effects of Bilateral Nephrectomy

Early attempts to determine the role of the kidney in the pathogenesis of hypertension were directed to reducing the amount of functioning renal tissue by partial nephrectomy. The most definitive experimental production of hypertension by this means was attained by Chanutin and Ferris,[28] whose procedure in the rat was used by subsequent workers for inducing hypertension in this species. Bilateral nephrectomy of normotensive animals led to equivocal results, with either no rise in blood pressure or a slight rise which could be attributed to the conditions under which the animals were maintained following operation. Moreover, the period of survival of the animals was too brief to permit a rise in blood pressure to manifest itself, as had been predicted by Allbutt.[3]

Braun-Menéndez and von Euler [25] observed a rise in the blood pressure in about a third of bilaterally nephrectomized rats but this rise, as suggested by Braun-Menéndez and Covian,[29] is attributable to expansion of the extracellular fluid volume. Under conditions in which nephrectomized animals are given free access to their usual food and fluids, any observed rise in blood pressure may result from an acute overload of the circulation and tissue edema.[30] When such overloading is avoided, no elevation in blood pressure is observed on the days immediately following nephrectomy, the elevation in blood pressure occurring only in animals surviving for 5 days or more.[8]

Recent workers have often failed also to differentiate between the rise in blood pressure which follows nephrectomy as a result of expansion of the extracellular fluid volume and that occurring after a latent period. Alterations in the extracellular fluid volume induced by allowing the animal free access to salt and water or by failing to replenish the loss of extracellular fluid volume caused by vomiting or dehydration will obviously alter the level of the blood pressure. Only by careful control of the extracellular fluid volume to conform to that obtaining normally in the hypertensive can one draw any conclusions regarding the effects of nephrectomy on the blood pressure.[31,32]

Conclusive results of the effects of bilateral nephrectomy on the blood pressure had to await the elaboration of methods for maintaining the nephrectomized animal alive for prolonged periods. Following the development of the artificial kidney by Kolff, this technique was used to keep the bilaterally nephrectomized dog alive for as long as 16 days during which period the blood pressure rose to hypertensive levels.[33,34] The maintenance of nephrectomized dogs for more prolonged periods was not possible until the introduction of the procedure of intermittent peritoneal lavage by Grollman, Turner, and McLean.[35] This simplified procedure permitted maintenance of bilaterally nephrectomized dogs for periods of 3 to 4 months or more in excellent condition and in a normal state of salt and water balance. Such animals, as shown in Table 1, manifest the hemodynamic features characteristic of hypertension induced by other procedures,[36,37] and at autopsy, display the same anatomic changes, namely, cardiac hypertrophy and proliferative changes in the media of the blood vessels.[38]

The fact that transplantation of the ureter into the vena cava prevents the rise in blood pressure which follows nephrectomy and allows the animal to remain in a normotensive state despite the complete loss of excretory function [33] suggests that either the kidney elaborates a humoral agent necessary for maintaining the normotensive state or otherwise contributes to the metabolism of the organism so as to prevent the development of hypertension.[2,39] Hypertension results after bilateral nephrectomy even when the adrenals are simultaneously removed if the water and electrolyte content of the extracellular fluid is normally maintained by means of intermittent peritoneal lavage. At autopsy such animals reveal the arteriolar and myocardial lesions associated with hypertension induced by nephrectomy alone.[40,41,42]

Most of the studies on the effect of bilateral nephrectomy on the blood pressure have been performed on the dog, but a rise in blood pressure to hypertensive levels has also been noted in rats maintained on a salt- and protein-free diet or by peritoneal lavage in order to prolong their survival.[43] Bilateral nephrectomy in frogs (*Rana pipiens, R. clamita,* and *R. catesbiana*) also results in an elevation in blood pressure, which is most pronounced in animals in which the adrenals are preserved by transplantation into skeletal muscles.[44] In the opossum,[45] bilateral nephrectomy also induces hypertension. Failure of Funder et al.[20] to produce renoprival hypertension in sheep is attributable to the short period of their survival. The similarity in the results obtained in such a variety of species affords further evidence for the basic role of the kidney in the maintenance of the normotensive state.

Effect of Nephrectomy on the Blood Pressure of Normotensive and of Hypertensive Human Beings

Renoprival hypertension in the human being is discussed elsewhere in this volume; it is only necessary to point out here that the same results follow removal of kidney tissue in the human being as in other animals. Unilateral nephrectomy in normotensive individuals results in no appreciable rise in blood pressure, but in patients suffering from renal disease and only a moderate elevation in blood pressure, this operation results in an elevation in pressure as it does in the rat.[46] Bilateral nephrectomy also is accompanied by hypertension as in other animals.[47]

Bilateral nephrectomy in the patient suffer-

TABLE 1.—*Effect of Bilateral Nephrectomy on Hemodynamic Factors in the Dog Maintained by Intermittent Peritoneal Lavage*

Days after Nephrectomy	*Mean Arterial Blood Pressure*	*Venous Pressure*	*Pulse Rate*	*Blood Volume*	*Cardiac Index*
Preoperative	95	−2.0	140	460	3.0
13	145	−2.0	140	440	2.6
20	160	−1.0	120	402	2.6
27	180	−1.0	120	512	2.8
34	150	+1.0	168	498	2.5

Based on data from Grollman, A.[36]

TABLE 2.—*Pressor Activity of Untreated Plasma of the Renal Venous Effluent in Various Clinical Conditions Associated with Hypertension*

Clinical Diagnosis	*Total No. of Patients*	*Positive Pressor Response*	*Negative Pressor Response*
Acute glomerulonephritis	3	1 *	2
Chronic glomerulonephritis	12	0	12
Pyelonephritis	3	2 *	1
Malignant hypertension	10	6 *	4
Occlusion of one renal artery	1	1 †	0
Stenosis of one renal artery	7	2 †	5
Aneurysm of one renal artery	1	1 †	0
Ptosis of right kidney	2	1 †	1 ‡
Essential hypertension	3	0	3
Cyst of kidney	1	0	1 ‡
Gouty kidney	1	0	1
Lipoid nephrosis	1	0	1

* Pressor agent is present in renal venous effluent from both kidneys. In other patients cited, the pressor agent was present only on side of the affected kidney.

† Patients responded to surgery with reduction of blood pressure to essentially normal levels.

‡ Patients failed to respond to surgery or manifested an increase in level of blood pressure following nephrectomy.

ing from malignant hypertension results in an amelioration of the hypertension and has been used therefore as a therapeutic procedure prior to transplanting kidneys in severely ill patients.[48–51] This apparently paradoxical response to nephrectomy is explained by the fact that in malignant hypertension, as shown in Table 2, a circulating pressor agent secreted by the kidney contributes to the inordinate rise in blood pressure observed in this condition.[52] Removal of the kidney therefore causes a decline in blood pressure from this inordinately high level to a lower level consistent with the chronic hypertensive state and the general state of the patient, but not to normal levels unless the patient is in heart failure or a state of debility, or his extracellular fluid volume is reduced.

Renoprival hypertension in man accordingly differs in no way from that noted in the experimental animal.

REFERENCES

1. Grollman, A.: A unitary concept of experimental and clinical hypertensive cardiovascular disease. Perspect. Biol. Med. 2:208, 1959.
2. Grollman, A.: Pathogenesis of hypertension and implications for its therapeutic management. Clin. Pharmacol. Ther. 10:755, 1969.
3. Allbutt, C.: Diseases of the Arteries, Including Angina Pectoris, vol. 1. London: Macmillan, 1915, p. 353.
4. Grollman, A. (Ed.): Alterations in blood pressure with particular reference to hypertension. *In* The Functional Pathology of Disease: The Physiologic Basis of Clinical Medicine, 2nd ed. New York: McGraw-Hill, 1963, pp. 375–376.
5. Grollman, A.: The humoral role of the kidney in hypertension. *In* Milliez, P., and Tcherdakoff, P. (Eds.): International Club on Arterial Hypertension. Paris: Expansion Scientifique Francaise, 1966, pp. 169–176.
6. Grollman, A.: Experimental hypertension in the dog. Am. J. Physiol. 147:647, 1946.
7. Grollman, A., Harrison, T. R., and Williams, J. R., Jr.: The mechanism of experimental renal hypertension in the rat: The relative significance of pressor and anti-pressor factors. Am. J. Physiol. 139:293, 1943.
8. Grollman, A., and Halpert, B.: Renal lesions in chronic hypertension induced by unilateral nephrectomy in the rat. Proc. Soc. Exp. Biol. Med. 71:394, 1949.
9. Smirk, F. H., and Hall, W. H.: Inherited hypertension in rats. Nature 182:727, 1958.
10. Okamoto, K., and Kyuzo, A.: Development of a strain of spontaneously hypertensive rats. Jap. Circ. J. 27:282, 1963.
11. Grollman, A.: The spontaneous hypertensive rat: An experimental analogue of essential hypertension in the human being. *In* Oka-

moto, K. (Ed.): United States-Japanese Cooperative Seminar on the Spontaneous Hypertensive Rat. Tokyo: Igaku Shoin, 1972, pp. 238–242.

12. Floyer, M. A.: The effect of nephrectomy and adrenalectomy upon the blood pressure in hypertensive and normotensive rats. Clin. Sci. 10:405, 1951.
13. Goldblatt, H., Lynch, J., Hanzal, R. F., and Summerville, W. W.: Studies on experimental hypertension. I. The production of persistent elevation of systolic blood-pressure by means of renal ischemia. J. Exp. Med. 59:347, 1934.
14. Ogden, E., Collings, W. D., and Sapirstein, L. A.: A change of mechanism in the course of hypertension of renal origin. Special Publications N. Y. Acad. Sci. 3:153, 1946.
15. Grollman, A.: Pressor activity of circulating blood after focal infarction of the kidney in the rat. Proc. Soc. Exp. Biol. Med. 134:1120, 1970.
16. Blalock, A., and Levy, S. E.: Studies on the etiology of renal hypertension. Ann. Surg. 106:826, 1937.
17. Ebihara, A., and Grollman, A.: Pressor activity of renal venous effluent following constriction of the renal artery in dogs. Am. J. Physiol. 214:1, 1968.
18. Pickering, G. W.: Role of the kidney in acute and chronic hypertension following renal artery constriction in the rabbit. Clin. Sci. 5:229, 1945.
19. Grollman, A.: Experimental chronic hypertension in the rabbit. Am. J. Physiol. 142: 666, 1944.
20. Funder, J. W., Blair-West, J. R., Cain, M. C., Catt, K. J., Coghlan, J. P., Denton, D. A., Nelson, J. F., Scoggins, B. A., and Wright, R. D.: Circulatory and humoral changes in the reversal of renovascular hypertension in sheep by unclipping the renal artery. Circ. Res. 27:249, 1970.
21. Goldblatt, H., Kahn, J. R., and Lewis, H. A.: Studies on experimental hypertension. XIX. The production of persistent hypertension in sheep and goats. J. Exp. Med. 77:297, 1943.
22. White, F. N., and Grollman, A.: Autoimmune factors associated with infarction of the kidney. Nephron 1:93, 1964.
23. Jeffers, W. A., Lindauer, M. A., Twaddle, P. H., and Wolferth, C. C.: Experimental hypertension in nephrectomized parabiotic rats. Am. J. Med. Sci. 199:815, 1940.
24. Grollman, A., and Rule, C.: Experimentally induced hypertension in parabiotic rats. Am. J. Physiol. 138:587, 1943.
25. Braun-Menéndez, E., and von Euler, U. S.: Hypertension after bilateral nephrectomy in the rat. Nature 160:905, 1947.
26. Ledingham, J. M.: The nature of the hypertension occurring in the nephrectomized parabiotic rat. Clin. Sci. 10:423, 1951.
27. Masson, G. M. C., Corcoran, A. C., and Page, I. H.: Rôle du rein dans l'hypertension expérimentale chez le rat. Rev. Canad. Biol. 10:309, 1951.
28. Chanutin, A., and Ferris, E. B.: Experimental renal insufficiency produced by partial nephrectomy. Arch. Intern. Med. 49:767, 1932.
29. Braun-Menéndez, E., and Covian, M. R.: Mecanismo de la hipertension de las ratas totalmente nefrectomizadas. Rev. Soc. Argent. Biol. 24:130, 1948.
30. Grollman, A.: Effect of increasing the extracellular fluid volume on the arterial blood pressure of the normal, hypertensive and nephrectomized dog. Am. J. Physiol. 173: 364, 1953.
31. Grollman, A., Shapiro, A. P., and Gafford, G.: The volume of the extracellular fluid in experimental and human hypertension. J. Clin. Investigation 32:312, 1953.
32. Green, J. A., Lucas, J., and Floyer, M. A.: The effect of the kidney in altering the response of the circulation to fluid loading. Clin. Sci. 38:4P, 1970.
33. Grollman, A., Muirhead, E. E., and Vanatta, J.: Role of the kidney in pathogenesis of hypertension as determined by a study of the effects of bilateral nephrectomy and other experimental procedures on the blood pressure of the dog. Am. J. Physiol. 157:21, 1949.
34. Govaerts, P., Verniory, A., and Lebrun, J.: Recherches sur les relations entre la réactivité à la rénine et l'hypertension rénale expérimentale chez le chien. Bull. Acad. R. Med. Belg. 15:375, 1950.
35. Grollman, A., Turner, L. B., and McLean, J. A.: Intermittent peritoneal lavage in nephrectomized dogs and its application to the human being. Arch. Intern. Med. 87:379, 1951.
36. Grollman, A., Turner, L. B., Levitch, M., and Hill, D.: Hemodynamics of bilaterally nephrectomized dog subjected to intermittent peritoneal lavage. Am. J. Physiol. 165:167, 1951.
37. Pelling, D., and Ledingham, J. M.: Haemodynamics in the renoprival hypertensive rat. Clin. Sci. 38:4P, 1970.
38. Muirhead, E. E., Turner, L. B., and Groll-

man, A.: Hypertensive cardiovascular disease: Vascular lesions of dogs maintained for extended periods following bilateral nephrectomy or ureteral ligation. Arch. Pathol. 51: 575, 1951.
39. Floyer, M. A.: Role of the kidney in experimental hypertension. Br. Med. Bull. 13:29, 1957.
40. Turner, L. B., and Grollman, A.: Role of adrenal cortical activity in experimental hypertension induced by bilateral nephrectomy in the dog. Am. J. Physiol. 166:185, 1951.
41. Ledingham, J. M.: The influence of the adrenal on the water and electrolyte disturbances following nephrectomy and its relation to renoprival hypertension. Clin. Sci. 13:535, 1954.
42. McQueen, E. G.: Vascular reactivity in experimental renal and renoprival hypertension. Clin. Sci. 15:523, 1956.
43. Kolff, W. J., and Page, I. H.: Influence of protein and other factors on postnephrectomy hypertension in rats sustained with an improved method of peritoneal irrigation. Am. J. Physiol. 178:69, 1954.
44. Grollman, E. F., and Grollman, A.: Induction of hypertension in the frog by bilateral nephrectomy. Am. J. Physiol. 199:19, 1960.
45. Grollman, A.: Hypertension in the opossum (*Didelphis virginiana*). Am. J. Physiol. 218: 80, 1970.
46. Mjolnerod, O. K., and Prydz, H.: Prognosen ved nefretomi for ensidig nyrelidelse. Tidsskr. Nor. Laegeforen. 79:826, 1959.
47. Baglin, A., Bedrossian, J., Safar, M., Weil, B., Idatte, J.-M., and Milliez, P.: L'hypertension artérielle des sujets anéphrique. Presse Med. 79:507, 1971.
48. Kolff, W. J., Nakamoto, S., Poutasse, E. F., Straffon, R. A., and Figueroa, J. E.: Effect of bilateral nephrectomy and kidney transplantation on hypertension in man. Circulation 30 (Suppl. II):23, 1964.
49. Onesti, G., Swartz, C., Ramirez, O., and Brest, A. N.: Bilateral nephrectomy for control of hypertension in uremia. Trans. Am. Soc. Artif. Intern. Organs 14:361, 1968.
50. Hampers, C. L., Zollinger, R. M., Skillman, J. J., Gumpert, J. R. W., Bailley, G. L., and Merrill, J. P.: Hemodynamic and body composition changes following bilateral nephrectomy in chronic renal failure. Circulation 40:367, 1969.
51. Toussaint, C., Verniory, A., Vereerstraeten, P., Kinnaert, P., Buchin, R., and Van Geertruyden, J.: Indications de la néphrectomie bilatérale dans l'hypertension du mal de Bright au stade terminal. Actual. Nephrol. (Paris) 1:113, 1970.
52. Grollman, A., and Krishnamurty, V. S. R.: A new pressor agent of renal origin. Am. J. Physiol. 221:1499, 1971.

THE PROSTAGLANDINS

By ROGER B. HICKLER, M.D.

TO DATE THERE IS no definitive evidence of a role for the prostaglandins, and, more specifically, for the renomedullary prostaglandins, in the pathogenesis of hypertension. However, because of their known profound effects on vascular smooth muscle and renal salt and water excretion, as established from numerous pharmacologic studies in recent years, there has been considerable speculation on the subject. On the basis of these speculations, series of ingenious experiments have been devised, the results of which continue to make this line of investigation as promising as any in the field. Any consideration of the fundamental biochemical correlates of primary or secondary hypertension, which, at this time, remain exceedingly elusive, must include a possible role for these ubiquitous, hormone-like polar, cyclized fatty acids.

The time is at hand when we can discuss certain aspects of the prostaglandins without reviewing all of the intriguing historic details of their identification and characterization. A number of excellent monographs are available on the subject. What is intended in this chapter is to present a line of reasoning that may best describe the manner in which these substances could exert an antihypertensive function in the present state of our knowledge. In this summary the reader is urged to distinguish between what is presented as fact and any hypothesis that may be assembled from the accumulated facts.

GENERAL ASPECTS

In a symposium at the New York Academy of Sciences on the prostaglandins in April 1971, Piper and Vane stated: "Mammalian cells seem to disgorge prostaglandins at the slightest provocation. This characteristic can be seen in cells from brain, diaphragm, adrenal and thyroid glands, fat pads, stomach, spleen, skin, liver, intestines, kidney and uterus, and for provocations which can be physiological, pharmacological, or pathological."[1] Fourteen prostaglandins have been identified in mammalian tissue through the pioneering works of Bergström and his associates. These workers demonstrated that all of these 14 related compounds are naturally synthesized from three C_{20} polyunsaturated fatty acid precursors. Dihomo-γ-linolenic acid yields prostaglandin E_1 (PGE_1) and prostaglandin $F_{1\alpha}$ ($PGF_{1\alpha}$). Prostaglandin A_1 (PGA_1) derives from the removal of one water molecule from the cyclopentanone ring of PGE_1, and prostaglandin B_1 (PGB_1) from a rearrangement of the conjugate diene structure of the ring of PGA_1. A substitution of an hydroxyl group on the 19-carbon of PGA_1 and PGB_1 yields 19-hydroxy PGA_1 and B_1 respectively. Similarly, arachidonic acid leads to the derivation of the six prostaglandins of the *2* series: PGE_2, $PGE_{2\alpha}$, PGA_2, PGB_2, 19-hydroxy PGA_2 and 19-hydroxy PGB_2. Finally, eicosa-5,8,11,14,17-pentaenoic acid yields prostaglandin E_3 (PGE_3) and $F_{3\alpha}$($PGE_{3\alpha}$). The subscript number *1, 2,* or *3* refers to the number of double bonds in the noncyclical part of the carbon chain; this is determined by which of the three fatty acids is the precursor of the prostaglandin. The highest concentration of prostaglandin (an admixture of the 14 cited above minus PGF_3) occurs in human seminal plasma at about 300 μg per milliliter.

The profound and diverse actions of the various prostaglandins are generally considered separately for the many systems on which they have pharmacologic effects. A detailed description of these will not be undertaken here, but some major effects may be cited to emphasize the scope of the subject before focusing on the renomedullary prostaglandins and blood pressure homeostasis. Central nervous system effects include sedation, stupor, and an inhibition of norepinephrine release on sympathetic nerve stimulation. In the reproductive system $PGF_{2\alpha}$ increases motility and tone of the pregnant and nonpregnant uterus;

From the Department of Medicine, University of Massachusetts Medical School, and the Medical Division of The Memorial Hospital, Worcester, Massachusetts.

PGE_1 and PGE_2 have a similar effect on the pregnant uterus but inhibit tone and motility of the nonpregnant uterus. The effects of prostaglandins on the gastrointestinal tract are to inhibit gastric secretion and increase intestinal motility. The cardiovascular effects indicate that prostaglandins of the E- and A-series lower blood pressure through a peripheral vasodilatation, associated with an increase in cardiac output; positive inotropy may relate to increased calcium uptake by heart muscle. Conversely, prostaglandins of the F-series raise arterial pressure by increasing peripheral vascular resistance. Renal effects of the prostaglandins include a marked sodium and water diuresis, associated with but not dependent upon an increase in renal blood flow. PGE_1 inhibits and PGE_2 stimulates platelet aggregation. PGE_1 and PGE_2 cause bronchial dilatation; $PGE_{2\alpha}$ produces bronchoconstriction.

A common biochemical denominator to explain these varied activities was proposed some years ago by Bergström, who stated that in those tissues where biosynthesis and release of prostaglandins occur, we may confidently anticipate that they are, in fact, likely to be fulfilling a role in the regulation of hormonal action. Since then an imposing body of information has accumulated to indicate that all but a few cell types containing adenyl cyclase systems are responsive to the prostaglandins, intracellular concentration of cyclic AMP increasing or decreasing on their administration. Thus, PGE_2 increases the cyclic AMP content of the thyroid and corpus luteum, associated with thyroid-stimulating hormone (TSH)- and luteinizing hormone (LH)-like effects, and decreases the cyclic AMP content in the fat cell, associated with an inhibition of hormone-induced lipolysis. According to this concept, the prostaglandins may act as hormone modulators by stimulating or inhibiting the hormonally sensitive adenyl cyclase system of any given tissue. A detailed review of this subject has been presented by Shaw et al.[2]

Renomedullary Prostaglandins

The various contributions toward the identification and characterization of the renomedullary prostaglandins have been admirably described by Daniels.[3] Working with the renal medulla of the rabbit, which has a uniquely high prostaglandin content, Daniels et al.[4] demonstrated conclusively that PGE_2 is the principal vasodepressor lipid substance present; when added to the $PGF_{2\alpha}$ also identified, the prostaglandin concentration totalled 10 to 15 μg per gram, second in concentration only to human and sheep seminal plasma and sheep seminal vesicular tissue. Whether there is also a small amount of PGA_2 present or whether this represents an artifact of the extraction procedure is controversial at the present time. Prostaglandin has also been identified in the renal medulla, but not in the cortex, of the kidney of other species, including man.[3] Figure 1 gives the structure of PGE_2, $PGF_{2\alpha}$, and PGA_2. According to the previous discussion, arachidonic acid is the obligatory unsaturated fatty acid substrate for renomedullary prostaglandin synthetase, yielding prostaglandins of the "two" series.

Figure 2 shows the comparative arterial pressure response in the pentolinium-blocked,

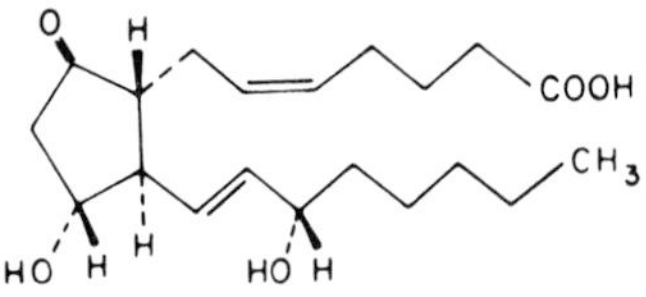

PGE_2

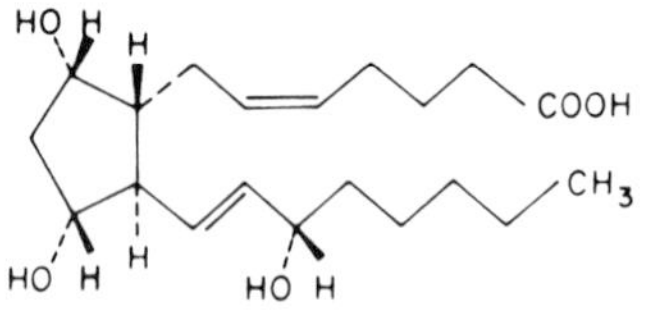

$PGF_{2\alpha}$

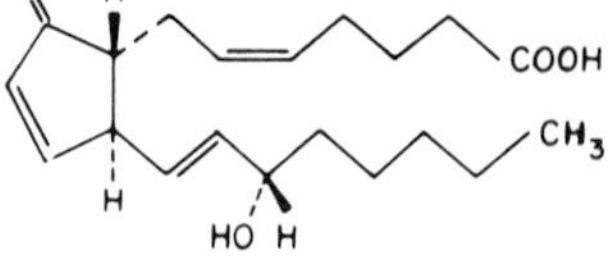

PGA_2

Fig. 1.—The molecular structure of the renomedullary prostaglandins: PGE_2, $PGF_{2\alpha}$, and PGA_2.

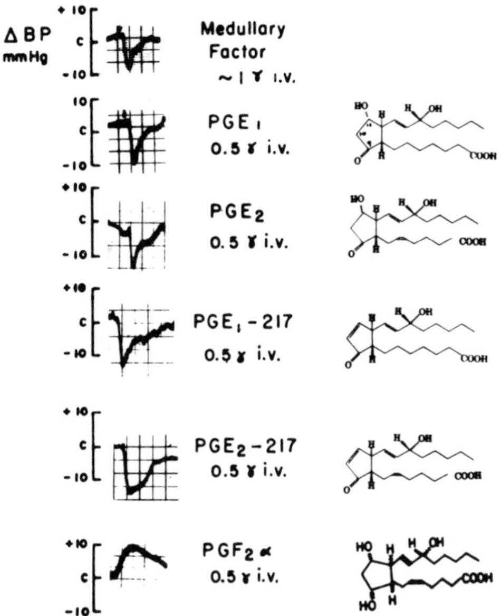

FIG. 2.—Comparative arterial pressure responses to the intravenous injection of medullary lipid and the equivalent dose of several of the prostaglandins in the bioassay rat.

vagotomized, bioassay rat to lapine renomedullary, polar lipid extract and to several synthetic prostaglandins on intravenous administration of comparable doses (0.5 μg). In each instance, the response to PGE_1, PGE_2, PGE_1-217 (PGA_1), and PGE_2-217 (PGA_2) was the same as that to the medullary extract, namely, a transient depression of arterial pressure lasting several minutes. In contrast, the response to 0.5 μg $PGF_{2\alpha}$ indicated a transient *rise* in blood pressure. Since the medullary lipid extract was a vasodepressor, it can be concluded from the previous discussion that the renal medulla contains a relatively high concentration of a vasodepressor lipid in the form of PGE_2 and a low concentration of a vasopressor lipid in the form of $PGF_{2\alpha}$.

The available evidence would indicate two important facts about the prostaglandins. First, the tissue releasing prostaglandin has a relatively low prostaglandin content; thus, the lungs, adrenals, stomach, and spleen have all been shown to release much more prostaglandin than they contain when stimulated, indicating a lively biosynthetic capacity from the effect of prostaglandin synthetase on essential fatty acid precursors.[5] Second, there is much evidence against a peripheral effect through circulation of prostaglandins such that their many actions as described above more likely derive from prostaglandin synthesized in various tissues and released in situ. Samuelsson et al.[6] have reported the rapid biologic inactivation of the prostaglandins through the action of prostaglandin-15 dehydrogenase (and other reductive and oxidative mechanisms), which is widely distributed in mammalian tissue. The highest activity was found in lung, spleen, and kidney. More than 90 percent of PGE_1, administered intravenously in a dose range of 0.1 to 1 μg per kilogram of body weight, is inactivated during a single circulation through the lungs.[7] The normal renal cortex contains about three times more prostaglandin dehydrogenase activity than the medulla. Because of the rapid synthesis and destruction of prostaglandin by various tissues, studies based on the extractable content must be interpreted with great caution. Samuelsson et al.[6] have determined the circulative level of PGE_2 to be less than 1 ng per milliliter. Unlike the other prostaglandins, PGA compounds appear to resist metabolic degradation by the lungs. If the renal medulla does produce and release a small amount of PGA_2, then a peripheral vascular effect for it is conceivable, as proposed by Lee.[8] Whether a circulating level of prostaglandin sufficient to modulate peripheral vascular tone occurs is highly conjectural at this point. From the foregoing it may be more acceptable to base any theoretic antihypertensive function for these substances on an in situ effect of PGE_2 that is synthesized and released within the renal medulla.

Cardiovascular and Renal Effects

Figure 3 shows the cardiovascular effects of the intravenous injection of PGE_1, (above) and $PGF_{2\alpha}$ (below) in anesthetized dogs.[7] PGE_1, PGE_2, and PGE_3 decrease total peripheral resistance through a direct action on vascular smooth muscle. Arterial pressure falls, and heart rate and cardiac output rise significantly. This is associated with an impressive increase in coronary blood flow and myocardial contractile force. These effects are qualitatively similar to those found with PGA_1

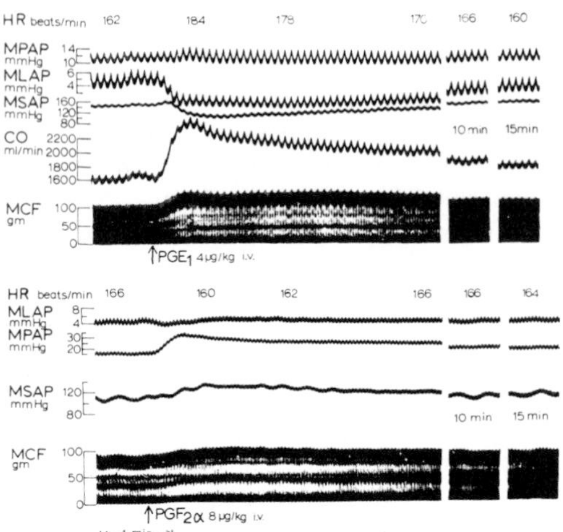

FIG. 3.—Effects of the intravenous injection of PGE_1 (*upper tracing*) and $PGF_{2\alpha}$ (*lower tracing*) on heart rate (HR), mean pulmonary arterial pressure (MPAP), mean left atrial pressure (MLAP), mean systemic arterial pressure (MSAP), cardiac output (CO), and myocardial contractile force (MCF) in dogs. (From Nakano, J.,[7] with permission.)

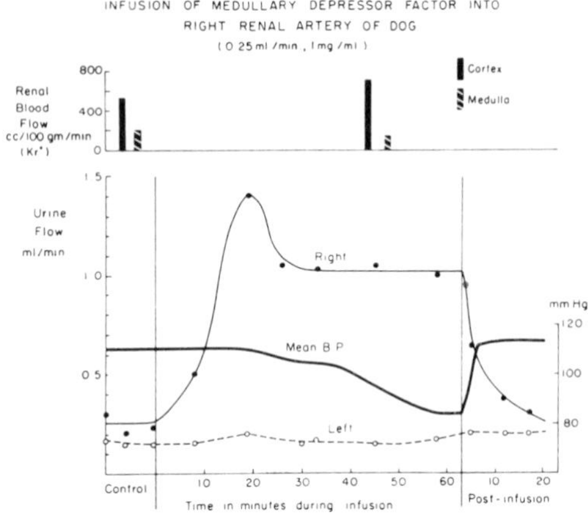

FIG. 4.—Effect of rabbit renomedullary extract, infused directly into the right renal artery of a trained, unanesthetized dog on the distribution of nutrient blood flow to the cortex and medulla by the radio-krypton technique. Total right renal blood flow increased due to large increase in cortical blood flow (medullary blood flow decreased slightly) associated with a large increase in ureteral urine flow, despite an eventual fall in aortic (and renal artery) pressure. (From Hickler, R. B., et al.,[9] with permission.)

and PGA_2. By contrast, $PGF_{2\alpha}$ exerts a mild to moderate hypertensive action, associated with a slight increase in cardiac output and myocardial contractile force, while pulmonary arterial pressure and resistance increase markedly. The major effect is an increase in peripheral and pulmonary vascular resistance through a direct action on vascular smooth muscle. In general, the PGE and PGA compounds are direct vasodilators, and tend to increase regional blood flows, whereas PGF compounds are direct vasoconstrictors and tend to decrease regional blood flows. These effects are not blocked by any of the known blocking agents and are presumed to act independently of any previously described vascular receptor mechanisms.

Figure 4 represents the renal dynamic effects of renomedullary vasodepressor prostaglandin on direct infusion into the renal artery of an unanesthetized, trained laboratory dog.[9] As shown, the initial dose was below that producing any lowering of systemic arterial pressure thereby keeping renal arterial perfusion pressure unchanged from the control period. A marked diuretic effect on the infused kidney is shown, associated with renal vasodilatation as indicated by an increase in total renal blood flow. As measured by the radio-krypton wash-out technique, there was an increase in cortical and decrease in medullary blood flow, the former predominating quantitatively over the latter. Herzog, Johnston, and Lauler subsequently showed that the infusion of prostaglandins of the E-series into the renal artery of the dog, under conditions of blood pressure and glomerular filtration rate unchanged from the control period, caused an increase in renal plasma flow, urine sodium and potassium excretion, urine volume, and free water clearance.[10]

Orloff and Grantham [11] have shown in the toad bladder and isolated rabbit renal-collecting tubule that minute concentrations of PGE_1 can block the permeability response to vasopressin by inhibiting the effect of vasopressin on adenyl cyclase. The resulting block in elaboration of cyclic AMP could account for the increase in free water clearance found in the experiments cited above during prostaglandin infusion.

Several explanations have been proposed

for the natriuretic effect of the prostaglandins under conditions of unchanged ("stable") glomerular filtration rates. One is an increase in sodium excretion due solely to renal vasodilatation, inducing an increased peritubular pressure, mechanically decreasing sodium reabsorptive sites in the loop of Henle. Since, as is shown in Fig. 4, prostaglandin infused into the renal artery produces a redistribution of blood flow away from the medulla to the cortex, this explanation would apply only to those short loops of Henle which fail to reach the medulla. Micropuncture studies by Dirks and Seely [12] failed to show any inhibition of proximal sodium reabsorption by PGE_1. Alternatively, a greater proportion of blood delivered to the relatively short-looped nephron population of the cortex as compared with the juxtamedullary region would of itself afford fewer sodium-reabsorptive sites for filtrate. However, the corresponding lower filtration rate, which has been demonstrated to pertain in the single, shorter-looped nephron, could leave the overall sodium reabsorption and excretion unchanged in the face of a redistribution of an unchanged total glomerular filtrate. Finally, one must consider what is perhaps the most appealing possibility, namely, a direct inhibition of the energy-requiring pumps of the ascending loops by prostaglandin independent of vascular effects.

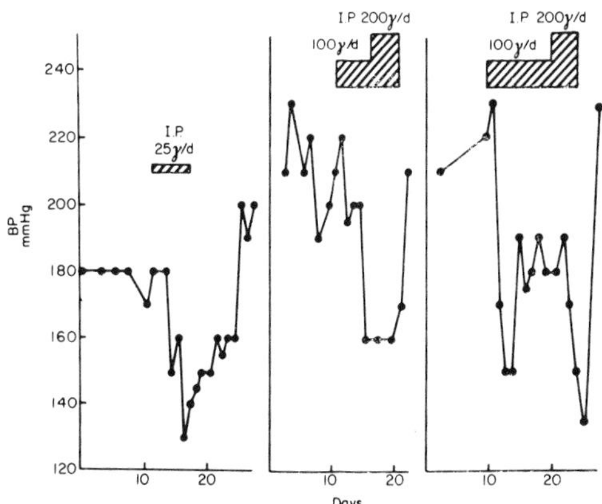

FIG. 5.—Antihypertensive effect of single, daily intraperitoneal injections of PGA_1 (kindly supplied by the Upjohn Co.) in the renovascular hypertensive rat. The three courses of daily injections are shown at the top with the associated reduction in arterial pressure below. On discontinuing each course, the pressure returned to hypertensive levels after a lag period of several days, as shown. (From Alpert, J. S., and Hickler, R. B.,[13] with permission.)

That the prostaglandins do exert a sustained antihypertensive effect is illustrated in Fig. 5.[13] On single, daily intraperitoneal injections of PGA_1 after several days a moderate but *sustained* reduction in arterial pressure was seen in the renovascular hypertensive rat, which disappeared within a few days of discontinuing the injections. This phenomenon should be distinguished sharply from the transient, hypotensive effect described earlier for prostaglandins of the E- and A-series. Muirhead et al.[14] have described the protective effect against the development of canine renoprival hypertension on daily oral administration of PGE_2, PGA_1, and $PGF_{1\alpha}$. It is notable that not only were the vasodilator prostaglandins PGE_2 and PGA_1 protective in this model, but so was the vasoconstrictor prostaglandin $PGF_{1\alpha}$.

An In Situ Locus of Action for Renomedullary Prostaglandins

Van Dorp [15] has investigated the PGE_2 content of various parts of the rabbit renal medulla, both in normal and in essential fatty acid-deficient rats (Fig. 6). The outer medulla contained far less prostaglandins than the inner medulla. Essential fatty acid deficiency was associated with a sharply decreased prostaglandin content. Very little prostaglandin was found if the tissue was homogenized im-

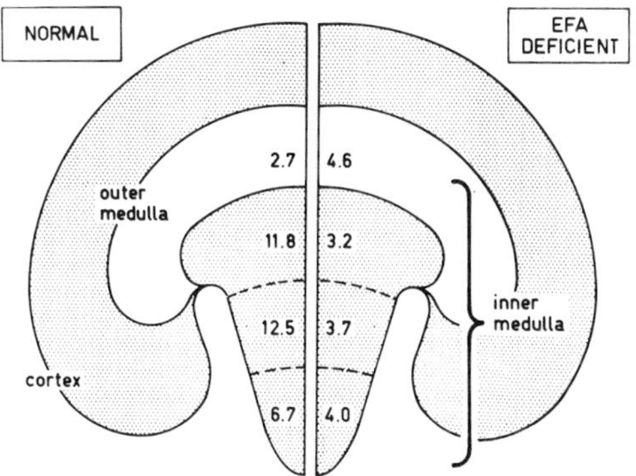

FIG. 6.—PGE_2 content in medulla of rabbit kidney in normal (*left*) and (*right*) essential fatty acid-deficient (EFA) animals measured in micrograms per gram of wet tissue. (From van Dorp, D.,[15] with permission.)

mediately in alcohol, and the figures given are more an indication of biosynthetic activity. The distribution of lipid droplets corresponded to the concentration of lipid droplets in the interstitial cells of the medulla, presumably containing the essential fatty acid precursor. Muirhead et al.[16] showed that tissue culture of lapine renomedullary interstitial cells contained extractable PGE_2, PGA_2, and $PGF_{2\alpha}$. Pulsing the cells with ^{3}H-arachidonic acid indicated synthesis by the cells of prostaglandin, the highest level of radioactivity being in the PGE_2 fraction.[16] The work of Tobian and Azar[17] on the renomedullary interstitial cell and its possible relationship to electrolyte and blood pressure homeostasis is presented elsewhere in this volume and, therefore, will not be included in this short review.

Marumo and Edelman[18] have reported that the adenyl cyclase activity in the kidney of the golden hamster as indicated by the generation of cyclic AMP on vasopressin administration was greatest in the papilla, somewhat lower in the medulla, and lowest in the cortex (Fig. 7).[18] Significant inhibition by PGE_1 of the response of adenyl cyclase to vasopressin was found in the medullary and papillary crude homogenates. The correspondence between the prostaglandin content (Fig. 6) and adenyl cyclase activity in the renal medulla urges the consideration of a primary, in situ, regulatory role of renomedullary PGE_2 on vasopressin function at the tubular level. This consideration for a primary, in situ function for PGE_2 at the tubular level in the renal medulla is enhanced by the observations of Nissen and Andersen,[19] who localized prostaglandin dehydrogenase activity in the kidney by a special cytochemical technique (Fig. 8). The most pronounced activity was observed in the thick ascending limb of the loop of Henle and in the distal tubule, and somewhat lesser activity in the collecting tubules of the medulla. It is tempting to assume that these major tubular sites of inactivation and of salt

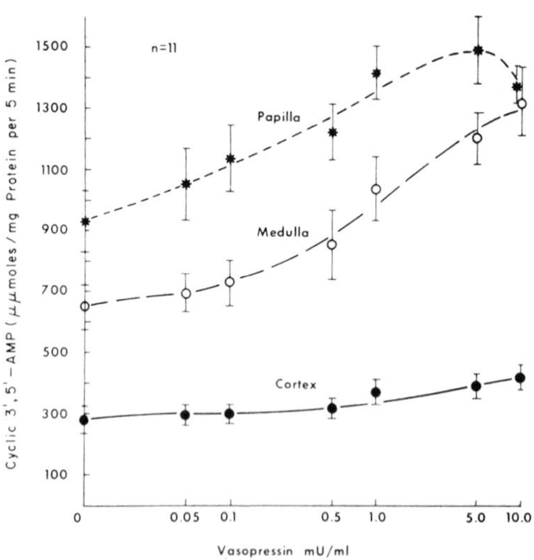

FIG. 7.—Dose response of renal adenyl cyclase activity to vasopressin. Crude homogenates were prepared from cortex (–●–), medulla (–○–) and papilla (–*–) of hydrated hamsters. The concentration of vasopressin is displayed on a log scale. Each point is the mean of 11 determinations. The vertical lines correspond to ±1 SEM. (From Marumo, F., and Edelman, I.,[18] with permission.)

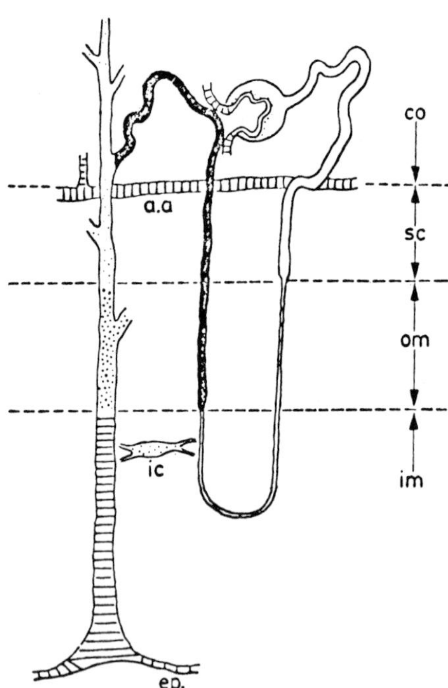

FIG. 8.—The localization in the cortex **(co)**, the subcortical zone **(sc)**, the outer medulla **(om)**, and the inner medulla **(im)** of prostaglandin-dehydrogenase activity. The strength is indicated as faint **(a)**, faint to moderate **(b)**, moderate **(c)**, moderate to strong **(d)**, and strong **(e)**. Arcuate artery **(a.a.)**, epithelial cells at the top of the papilla **(ep)**, and renal interstitial cells **(ic)**. (From Nissen, H. M., and Andersen, H.,[19] with permission.)

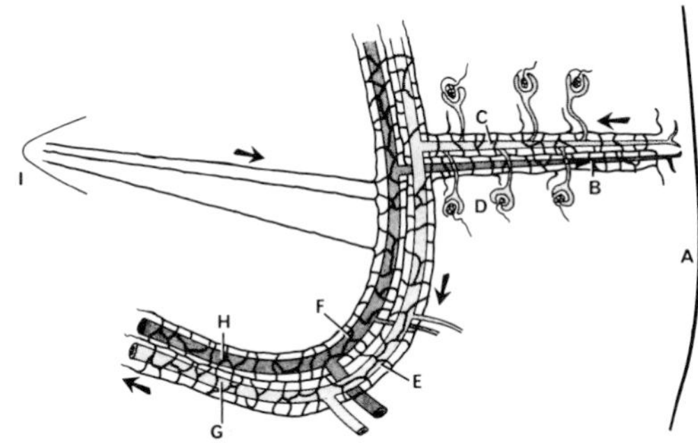

FIG. 9.—Schematic drawing of the lymphatic channels of the human kidney. Two separate systems are demonstrable. One begins in the cortex and accompanies the interlobular vessels toward the corticomedullary junction; the other starts at the papilla and ascends to join the cortical system at the corticomedullary junction. From these long trunks follow the arcuate and interlobular vessels to leave the kidney at the hilus. **Arrows** show the direction of the lymph flow. The structures shown are: **(A)** tunica fibrosa, **(B)** interlobular vein, **(C)** interlobular artery, **(D)** glomerulus, **(E)** arcuate artery, **(F)** arcuate vein, **(G)** interlobular artery, **(H)** interlobular vein and **(I)** papilla. (From Rawson, A. J.,[20] with permission.)

and water transport represent the main potential sites of action of the renomedullary prostaglandins.

The lymphatic drainage of the renal medulla runs from the papilla to the corticomedullary junction and not beyond (Fig. 9).[20] Further, the vasa recta pass down into the papilla and then turn back, entering the venous drainage, and do not penetrate the cortex to any extent. Therefore, it is difficult to conceive how PGE_2 synthesized in the medulla could reach the cortex in significant quantity. This is in contrast to studies where prostaglandin infused directly into the renal artery reaches the cortical circulation immediately from the afferent branches of the interlobular arteries, resulting in a sharp rise in cortical blood flow. It seems reasonable, then, to assume that the primary action of the renal prostaglandins may be limited to the medullary circulation, the loop of Henle of the longer nephrons, and the collecting ducts.

FORMULATION OF A HYPOTHESIS

The evidence that the primary diuretic effect of PGE_2 may be through a blocking of the action of vasopressin on the collecting tubules by an inhibition of medullary adenyl cyclase has been presented. The natriuretic effect may be through a direct blocking of sodium transport along the ascending limb of the loops of Henle that extend into the medulla. Alternatively, renomedullary vasodilatation through the in situ release of prostaglandin would increase deep intrarenal venous pressure. Experimental data indicate that this would produce a rise in peritubular hydrostatic pressure and a fall in peritubular oncotic pressure, reducing sodium and water reabsorption. Loss of sodium would diminish the medullary-concentrating mechanism and facilitate further water loss. In this formulation, a high-sodium intake would stimulate renomedullary prostaglandin synthetase activity, depleting lipid stores of essential fatty acid precursors, releasing prostaglandin in situ, primarily E_2, to promote salt and water diuresis through local medullary tubular and vascular mechanisms. The observations of Lonigro et al.[21] are of interest in this regard. These workers showed that the lowest dose of angiotensin II on infusion into the renal artery of the dog required to release PGE_2 into the renal venous blood was found in dogs which were in the most positive state of sodium balance.[21]

If essential hypertension proves to relate to a constitutional deficiency in the renal antihypertensive function (admittedly highly speculative at this point) and if that deficiency were expressed as a reduction in renomedullary prostaglandin synthetase activity, then the prehypertensive defect should prove to be a difficulty in excreting high sodium loads, according to the preceding formulations. Under these conditions the maintenance of a normal or nonexpanded plasma volume would require an increased filtered sodium load through an increase in cardiac output. As the hypertensive process progressed to the state of increased vascular resistance, which has been related to an autoregulatory, myogenic response of the peripheral arterioles, the elevated cardiac output would become normalized, according to current concepts. Finally, as the disorder progressed to the state of peripheral vascular disease, the higher levels of arterial pressure could lead to a pressure diuresis, leaving the plasma volume reduced, as has been observed by a number of workers. Schrier and de Wardener [22] have commented that "such a predominance of systemic arterial pressure over renal vascular resistance may be involved in the exaggerated response of the hypertensive patient to a saline load." In the final analysis, then, the fixed hypertensive state would be a compensatory mechanism for the failure of a renomedullary mechanism to properly excrete sodium loads. This would be particularly apparent in a society which has acquired a taste for considerably more salt than it requires.

A final word is in order. It is perfectly clear from a great many studies that the kidney, and more specifically, the renal medulla, exerts an antihypertensive "endocrine" function that is independent of its excretory function. Therefore, the hypothesis presented above as to how the renomedullary prostaglandins may function as in situ regulators of salt and water excretion to express a blood pressure-regulating function in no sense precludes the presence of other renal factors. Indeed, we still must postulate a circulatory antihypertensive factor for the renal medulla to account for a number of experimental phenomena, as has been made abundantly clear by the investigations of Muirhead and his associates.[23] It may well prove that there are several renomedullary factors, lipid in nature, that work in concert, both locally and systemically, that express the total antihypertensive function of the normal kidney. Finally, it may develop that renomedullary prostaglandins normally circulate in a quantity sufficient to have a significant effect on peripheral vascular tone, despite the impression held by this author that the available evidence does not seem to favor this concept.

References

1. Piper, P., and Vane, J.: The release of prostaglandins from lung and other tissues. Ann. N. Y. Acad. Sci. 180:363, 1971.
2. Shaw, J., Gibson, W., Jessup, S., and Ramwell, P.: The effect of PGE_1 on cyclic AMP and ion movements in turkey erythrocytes. Ann. N. Y. Acad. Sci. 180:241, 1971.
3. Daniels, E. G.: Extraction of renomedullary prostaglandins. *In* Fisher, J. W. (Ed.): Kidney Hormones. New York: Academic Press, 1971, pp. 507–524.
4. Daniels, E. G., Hinman, J. W., Leach, B. E., and Muirhead, E. E.: Identification of prostaglandin E_2 as the principal vasodepressor lipid of rabbit renal medulla. Nature 215: 1298, 1967.
5. Ramwell, P. W., and Shaw, J. E.: Biological significance of the prostaglandins. Recent Progr. Hormone Res. 26:139, 1970.
6. Samuelsson, B., Granström, E., Green, K., and Hamberg, M.: Metabolism of prostaglandins. Ann. N. Y. Acad. Sci. 180:138, 1971.
7. Nakano, J.: Prostaglandins and the circulation. Mod. Concepts Cardiovasc. Dis. 40:49, 1971.
8. Lee, J. B.: Chemical and physiological properties of renal prostaglandins: The antihypertensive effects of medullin in essential human hypertension. *In* Bergström, S., and Samuelsson, B. (Eds.): Nobel Symposium 2—Prostaglandins. Stockholm: Almqvist and Wiksell, 1967, pp. 197–210.
9. Hickler, R. B., Birbari, A. E., Kamm, D. E., and Thorn, G. W.: Studies on a vasodepressor and antihypertensive lipid of rabbit renal medulla. *In* Milliez, P., and Tscherdakoff, P. (Eds.): L'Hypertension Artérielle. Paris: L'Expansion Scientifique, 1966, pp. 188–202.
10. Herzog, J. P., Johnston, H. H., and Lauler, D. P.: Effects of prostaglandins E_1, E_2, and A_1 on renal hemodynamics, sodium and water excretion in the dog. *In* Ramwell, P. W., and Shaw, J. E. (Eds.): Prostaglandin Symposium of the Worcester Foundation for Experimental Biology. New York: Interscience, 1968, pp. 147–161.
11. Orloff, J., and Grantham, J.: The effect of prostaglandin (PGE_1) on the permeability response of rabbit collecting tubules to vasopressin. *In* Bergström, S., and Samuelsson, B. (Eds.): Stockholm: Almqvist and Wiksell, 1967, pp. 143–146.
12. Dirks, J. H., and Seely, J. F.: Micropuncture studies on the effect of vasodilators on proximal tubule sodium reabsorption in the dog. Clin. Res. 15:478, 1967.
13. Alpert, J. S., and Hickler, R. B.: Cardiovascular and renal effects of renomedullary prostaglandins. *In* Fisher, J. W. (Ed.): Kidney Hormones. New York: Academic Press, 1971, pp. 525–561.
14. Muirhead, E. E., Daniels, E. G., Pike, J. E.,

and Hinman, J. W.: Renomedullary antihypertensive lipids and the prostaglandins. *In* Bergström, S., and Samuelsson, B. (Eds.): Stockholm: Almqvist and Wiksell, 1967, pp. 183–196.

15. van Dorp, D.: Recent developments in the biosynthesis and the analyses of prostaglandins. Ann. N. Y. Acad. Sci. 181:181, 1971.
16. Muirhead, E. E., Germain, G. S., Leach, B. E., Brooks, B., Pitcock, J. A., Stephenson, P., Brosius, W. L., Jr., Hinman, J. W., and Daniels, E. G.: Renomedullary prostaglandins (P.G.) derived from renomedullary interstitial cells (RIC) grown in tissue culture. Clin. Res. 22:69, 1972.
17. Tobian, L., and Azar, S.: Functions of renal papilla. Clin. Res. 19:577, 1971.
18. Marumo, F., and Edelman, I.: Effects of Ca^{++} and prostaglandin on vasopressin activation of renal adenyl cyclase. J. Clin. Invest. 50:1613, 1971.
19. Nissen, H. M., and Andersen, H.: On the localization of a prostaglandin-dehydrogenase activity in the kidney. Histochemie 14:189, 1968.
20. Rawson, A. J.: Distribution of the lymphatics of the human kidney as shown in a case of carcinomatous permeation. Arch. Pathol. 47: 283, 1949.
21. Lonigro, A. J., Terragno, N. A., Malik, K. U., and McGiff, J. C.: Intrarenal release of prostaglandins as determined by the state of sodium balance. J. Clin. Invest. 50:60a, 1971.
22. Schrier, R. W., and de Wardener, H. E.: Tubular reabsorption of sodium ion: influence of factors other than aldosterone and glomerular filtration rate. N. Engl. Med. J. 285: 1231, 1971.
23. Muirhead, E. E., Brooks, B., Pitcock, J. A., and Stephenson, P.: Renomedullary antihypertensive function in accelerated (malignant) hypertension. Observations on renomedullary interstitial cells. J. Clin. Invest. 51: 181, 1972.

Neurogenic Factors in Renal Hypertension

By Paul Kezdi, M.D., J. William Spickler, Ph.D., and R. Karl Kordenat, M.S.

Neurogenic mechanisms in the maintenance of elevated pressure levels in renal hypertension have been suspected for a long time. The first evidence of participation of neurogenic factors in chronic experimental hypertension was provided by Reed and co-workers,[1] who demonstrated that yohimbine and pentobarbital lowered the blood pressure in chronic but not acutely hypertensive rats. The results of these experiments were interpreted as showing that the elevated pressure in renal hypertension is maintained initially by hormonal factors, but later by predominantly neurogenic factors. Considerable evidence has accumulated in the last 20 years to support the concept that neurogenic mechanisms participate in renal hypertension. Blood pressure control by the autonomic nervous system is made up by the afferent, the integrative or central, and the efferent parts of the control system as is shown in a simplified block diagram (Fig. 1). There is an interrelationship between the neurogenic and hormonal regulation of the circulation, and changes in the regulatory function can theoretically occur at any level.

From the Cox Heart Institute, Kettering Medical Center, Kettering, Ohio.

This work was supported by NIH Grant HE-09885, U.S. Public Health Service.

Very little is known about alterations in the integrative centers of the brain and there is no convincing evidence at present that such alterations are causatively involved in the maintenance of chronic renal hypertension. Some evidence has been presented that angiotensin may alter the function of the medullary cardiovascular centers leading to increased central sympathetic outflow. The role of this possible mechanism is not clearly understood.

The efferent sympathetic control of the blood vessels may also be altered by changes in the

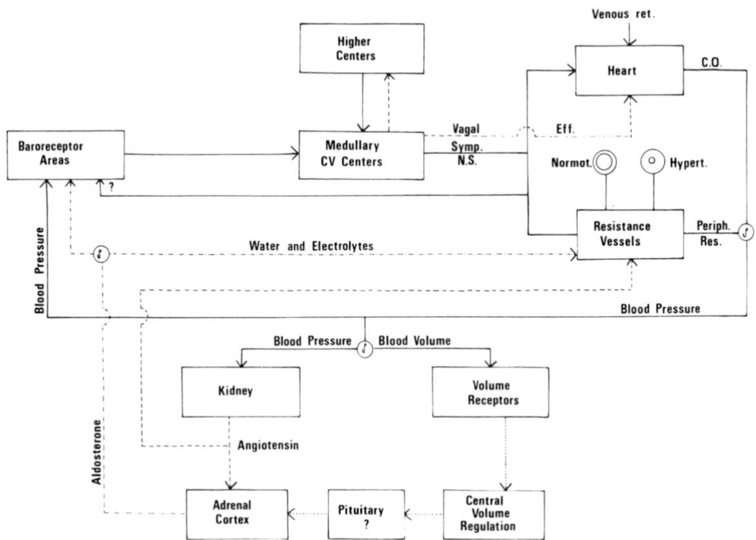

Fig. 1.—Simplified block diagram of the blood pressure control system. In hypertension, vascular resistance is increased due to the decreased cross-sectional area of the resistance vessel. This may be neurogenic or hormonal in origin and also partly the result of anatomic change, namely, thickening of the wall.

sensitivity of the blood vessels to a given sympathetic stimulus. An increase of the norepinephrine pool by blocking the reentry into the receptor by angiotensin was suggested.[2] The role of this mechanism in the maintenance of chronic renal hypertension is also not clear. Circulating angiotensin has to be present, at least in subpressor amounts, to maintain this mechanism. There is no clear-cut evidence that this mechanism is causative in the maintenance of chronic renal hypertension.

The afferent pathways of the autonomic nervous system controlling the circulation are made up by the baroceptors in the carotid sinus and the aortic arterial walls, the carotid sinus and aortic nerves with synapses in the medullary cardiovascular centers.

Since the fundamental works of Hering,[3] Koch,[4] and Heymans et al.,[5] the baroceptors have been suspected to participate in the pathogenesis of systemic arterial hypertension. A complete or partial cessation of carotid sinus and aortic baroceptor function has been considered. However, Goldblatt et al.[6] already concluded that in renal hypertensive dogs the pressor regulator system probably functions normally at a higher level. A change in the threshold of the carotid sinus response in human hypertension was demonstrated by procaine block of the carotid sinus by Lampan et al.[7] and Kezdi.[8] It was theorized that the fundamental change of the baroceptor mechanism in hypertension is an altered response, thus maintaining rather than opposing the elevated pressure. This is not equivalent to a complete cessation of baroceptor function. Subsequently, McCubbin, Green, and Page[9] showed the presence of altered electrical discharge of the carotid sinus nerve in renal hypertensive dogs, while Kezdi and Wennemark[10] documented the altered sympathetic control of the blood pressure.

The mechanism of this resetting then became the subject of investigation. Two facts have been known for some time. First, that the baroceptors respond to the stretch of the arterial wall,[8–11] which acts as a strain on the receptors[12]; and second, that, at least partially, resetting in the experimental animal occurs within a relatively short time.[13,14] Since the strain at the receptors will depend (for a given pressure) on the physical characteristics of the arterial wall, several authors studied the nature of vessel-wall changes in hypertension. Peterson[15] and Jones, Feigel, and Peterson[16] found increased water and sodium in the walls of large arteries including the carotids in renal hypertensive animals and attributed the altered baroceptor function to increased stiffness of the walls. This corresponded with the concept of Volhard,[17] who, based on studies on arterial segments from hypertensive patients, theorized that the fundamental defect is a decreased distensibility of the barosensitive arterial segments. On the other hand, Heymans and van den Heuvel-Heymans[18] suggested a loss of tone and increased distensibility as the fundamental defect. More recently Aars[19] has studied this problem in renal hypertensive rabbits and also came to the conclusion that resetting is probably due to a change in distensibility of the arterial wall.

We have been interested in the resetting process and what role the elevated pressure itself may play in the response of the carotid sinus to stretch and thus to the resetting; and whether resetting can be reversed after prolonged, persistent hypertension by lowering the pressure in the baroceptor area without changing the underlying hypertensive mechanism and thus the total body chemistry at the receptor site.

Methodology

To separate different factors in the resetting mechanism, we have developed an animal model by which, in chronic renal hypertensive animals, the blood pressure in one carotid sinus can be maintained permanently at a low level while in the rest of the animal, and the other carotid sinus, hypertension can develop. We have produced renal hypertension in dogs by cellophane-induced perinephritis and removing the contralateral kidney 1 week to 10 days later. Low pressure in one carotid sinus or permanent protection from hypertensive pressures was produced by the technique outlined below.

One side of the neck, usually the right, was exposed in general anesthesia at about the midportion of the common carotid artery. The carotid sinus area was not exposed. The right jugular vein was isolated and cut between ties. The central segment of the vein was tunneled under the neck muscles to the common carotid artery and, after the common carotid artery was tied centrally, the vein was anastomosed by interrupted vascular sutures to the distal portion of the artery (Fig. 2). The anastomosis immediately lowers the pressure in the sinus and results in a retrograde flow of arterial blood through the sinus area and to the jugular vein and right atrium. The average mean pressure in the carotid sinus following the anastomosis was around 40 mm Hg. The neck was then closed and the animal permitted to recover. In one group of animals (Group I) hypertension was produced 2 to 3 weeks after the neck operation. After 6 to 8 months of persistent hypertension, acute studies were performed to compare the function of the right and left carotid sinus in the same animal. In another group of animals (Group II) hypertension was produced first; 6 to 8 months later anastomosis of the right common carotid artery was performed. The same lowering of the pressure in the sinus occurred. Four weeks were allowed before the function of the two carotid sinuses in the same animal was compared in an acute experiment.

The reflex function of the carotid sinus was studied in the following way. The animals were anesthetized with chloral-urethane, were intubated, and artificially respirated, after which repeated small doses of succinylcholine were given. The neck was exposed by a median incision and both carotid sinuses were isolated. Extreme care was taken not to damage the carotid sinus nerves. Arterial branches of the sinus were isolated and suture slings were placed around the internal, external, common carotid, and lingual arteries. The rest of the vessels were tied under a dissecting microscope. A polyethylene catheter was placed into the lingual artery for pressure measurement. The external carotid artery was cannulated for perfusion of the sinus by a pump producing sine wave pressures at different levels using oxygenated Ringer's solution (Fig. 3). The blood circulation to the sinuses was not interrupted until the tests were performed. When pressure in the sinus was controlled by the pump the internal and common carotid arteries were clamped by bulldog clamps. One sinus was tested first while the pressure in the opposite sinus was decreased to zero by clamping its inflow and outflow, and by opening the lingual catheter to air in order to eliminate modifying effect of the reflex response by the opposite sinus. Prior to this, the aortic nerves running in the vagus were isolated on both sides, electroneurographically identified, and cut to eliminate their modifying effect on the

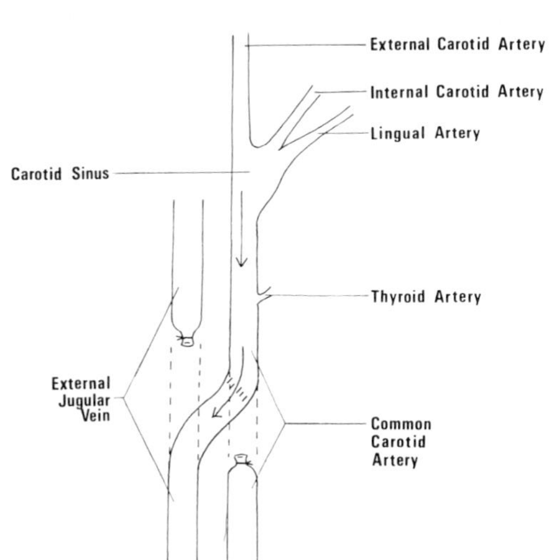

FIG. 2.—Schematic diagram of the technique of anastomosing the carotid sinus to the jugular vein.

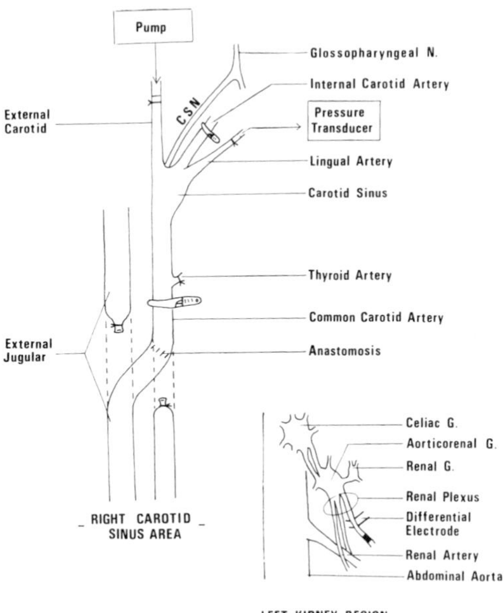

FIG. 3.—Schematic diagram for the study of reflex function of the isolated carotid sinus.

reflex function of the tested sinus. The vagus trunks were left intact.

The reflex function of the sinus was tested by its reflex inhibition of renal sympathetic discharge, heart rate, and systemic pressure. For this purpose the left kidney was retroperitoneally isolated and the renal sympathetic nerve placed on platinum-iridium bipolar electrodes for nerve recording. The peripheral end of the nerve was crushed by clamp to eliminate afferent activity. Femoral arterial pressure was measured by placing a catheter in the artery and the heart rate was obtained from the pressure tracing. The pressure in the sinus was gradually raised from 50 mm Hg to 225 mm Hg in 25-mm increments, using a sine wave with a pulse pressure 25 mm ± and a frequency of 100 beats per minute. Following the test of one side, blood flow was reestablished in the sinuses for several minutes before the other side was tested. After a set of satisfactory recordings was obtained the carotid sinus nerves were isolated under mineral oil and the sheath was removed. The nerve to be tested was placed on platinum-iridium electrodes and the electrical activity of the sinus nerves to changing intrasinus pressures was recorded. This way, not only the reflex function of the two sinuses but also their electrical activity could be obtained and the results compared.

For recording of the nerve activity, a Tektronics 122 low-level preamplifier was connected to an Astrodata direct current amplifier. Recordings were made on a Honeywell 1507 visicorder. The nerve activity was rectified and integrated, and phasic and mean nerve activity was obtained on the same paper. Pressures were recorded by Statham P-23 DB gauges and Astrodata amplifiers. The nerves were submerged in mineral oil, but they were not moved from their original position, and the gains were kept the same for the entire time of the experiment. The quantitate nerve activity the distance of the mean activity from zero activity was measured. For comparison the measured sympathetic nerve activities were normalized, carotid sinus nerve activities were expressed in microvolts, and both were plotted as a function of the intrasinus pressure. Heart rate and blood pressure responses were also plotted as a function of the intrasinus pressure. The response to forcing the pressure in the right and left sinuses was compared by calculating the mean responses and the standard errors of the means for both groups.

Since it has been assumed that baroceptor resetting might be in part the result of a change in arterial wall distensibility at the receptor location, changing the stress-strain relationship and receptor stimulation, and since these changes in the wall might relate to changes in water and sodium content, we have studied the water and sodium content of hypertensive, normotensive, and protected and nonprotected carotid sinuses. For this purpose, segments of the carotid artery, including the sinus, were removed at the end of the experiment. All excess connective tissue was carefully removed by sharp scissors; the artery was rapidly weighed and then dried in an oven at 110°C for 20 hours to remove all water. The tissues were then weighed again. Components of tissue were extracted with 1.0 ml of 0.75N nitric acid for 40 hours. Sodium and potassium content was determined on a 1:100 dilution of the extract by flame photometry. The data were expressed in milliequivalents of 100 gm of tissue.[20]

In another series of experiments, the static stress-strain characteristics of isolated vascular rings cut from the carotid sinus were determined for hypertensive and normotensive animals, and also for protected and nonprotected sinuses of hypertensive animals. In this discussion, stress is defined as the force per unit area tending to deform or stretch the vessel ring. Strain is the resulting deformation. The experimental procedure was first to determine the response of the baroceptors to intraluminal pressures by recording from the carotid sinus nerve as described above, and then to determine the static stress-strain characteristics as follows: a 1-mm long section of the carotid sinus was cut just distal to the root of the internal carotid artery and was immediately placed in a warm Ringer's solution bath. Photomicrographs were taken of the section under unstressed conditions in order to accurately determine the mean length and thickness of the section. The ring was then mounted on an isometric stress-strain apparatus and the force in grams was determined as a function of the circumference. Since the changes in circumference were small compared to the unstressed circumference, the unstressed cross-sectional dimensions of the ring were used to convert the measured force to an equivalent intravascular pressure.

Results

Reflex Responses to Forcing in the Protected and Nonprotected Sinuses

In eight dogs of Group I, where the sinus was anastomosed prior to hypertension, the average systemic pressure rose following cellophane wrapping of the kidney from mean baseline pressure of 117 ± 18 to a mean pressure of 170 ± 21 mm Hg. At the time of the acute test under anesthesia the average systemic pressure was 155 ± 20 mm Hg while the pressure in the protected sinus was 45 ± 12 mm Hg. Occlusion of the anastomosis by a bulldog clamp always led to increase of the pressure in the protected sinus but this never reached the hypertensive level of the other side. This occlusion of the anastomosis caused a marked increase in the ipsilateral carotid sinus nerve activity, which usually changed from a previous phasic to continuous discharge (Fig. 4). On the other hand, the hypertensive side always showed phasic activity at the hypertensive level, as described previously.[21]

When the reflex response to forcing pressures in the protected and nonprotected sinuses was compared a significant difference in response was found. The protected sinus inhibited heart rate, blood pressure, and sympathetic activity more markedly for a given intrasinus pressure than the nonprotected sinus (Fig. 5). The degree of inhibition in the protected sinus corresponded to that found in normotensive animals. The inhibition on the nonprotected side, on the other hand, corresponded to the hypertensive resetting previously seen in hypertensive animals (Fig. 6). After testing the reflex response to intrasinus pressure changes in the same animals, the carotid sinus nerve activity was analyzed. The typical shift in the response curve downward could be seen in the nonprotected sinus while the response of the protected side was similar to the normotensive response curve.

In Group II (five dogs) both sinuses were exposed to hypertension for a prolonged time (6 months) and the pressure was afterward lowered in one sinus by the anastomosis. Testing of the carotid sinus was performed 4 weeks after the anastomosis was prepared, leading to permanent lowering of the pressure on this side while the other sinus was continuously exposed to the hypertensive pressures. The pressure in the protected sinus was 45 ± 20 mm Hg at the time of testing while the average systemic pressure was 175 ± 30 mm Hg (control, 115). Only in one dog was the reflex inhibition by the now-protected sinus greater than by the nonprotected. This difference, however, appeared to be less than the average difference seen when the sinus was protected prior to hypertension.

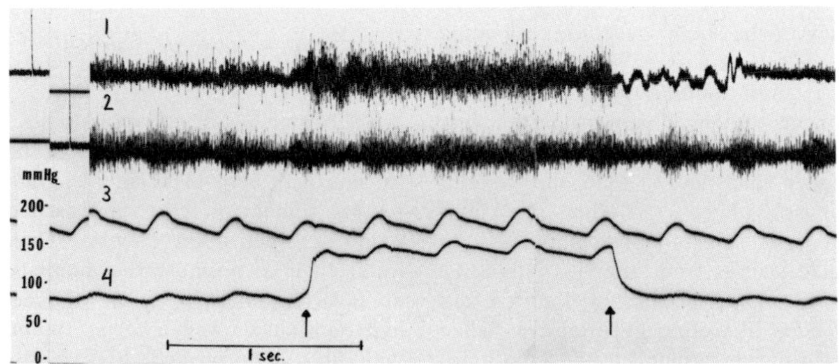

FIG. 4.—Simultaneous recording of carotid nerve activity and blood pressure in a hypertensive dog. (*1*) Nerve activity from the protected and (*2*) the nonprotected sinus; (*3*) blood pressure in the nonprotected and (*4*) the protected sinus. Between **arrows,** jugular anastomosis was clamped. Note increase of pressure (*4*) and nerve activity (*1*) during clamping.

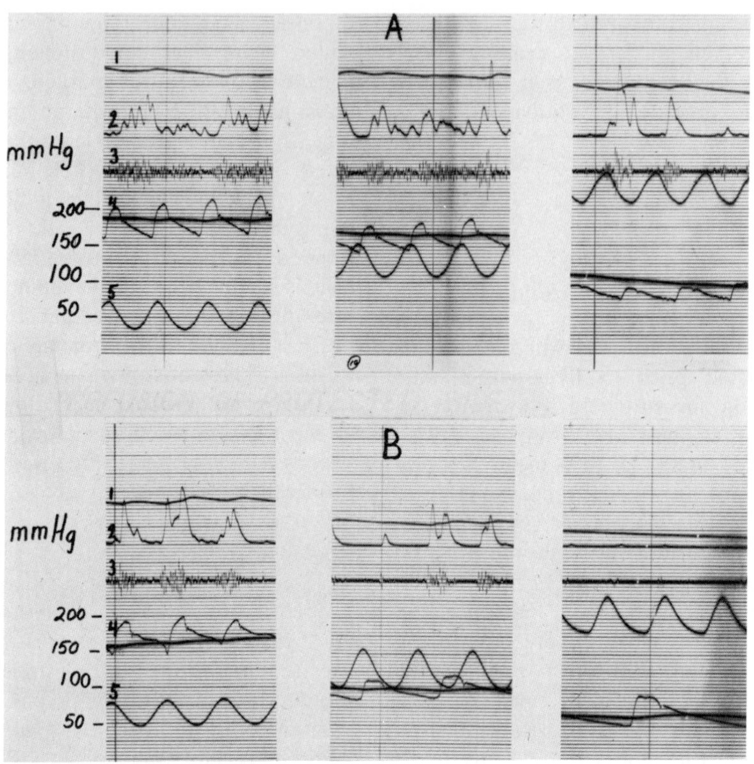

FIG. 5.—Actual recording from a chronic renal hypertensive dog. *A,* Nonprotected sinus. *B,* Protected sinus. **1,** average sympathetic nerve activity; **2,** phasic sympathetic nerve activity; **3,** actual nerve activity recording; **4,** systemic blood pressure (**solid line** is electrical mean); **5,** sine wave perfusion pressure in the isolated carotid sinus. Only three levels of carotid sinus perfusion pressure are shown. Note the markedly greater response of the protected sinus.

In the other four dogs only a little difference between the two sides was seen (Fig. 7).

Distensibility of the Carotid Sinus

The study of the stretch response to loading of the isolated carotid sinus segments showed that, for a given load, hypertensive carotid artery segments responded with proportionately greater stretch at all load levels, particularly at the higher load levels, than did normotensive sinuses (Fig. 8). When the nonprotected carotid sinuses were compared with the protected sinuses from animals with anastomosis prior to hypertension, the nonprotected sides responded like other hypertensives while the protected sinuses responded like the normotensive carotid sinus segments. All carotid sinus arteries and rings from the hypertensive or nonprotected sinuses were larger and more distended when compared in situ before removal in the same animals with the protected sinuses. The nerve activity curves showed downward displacement of the hypertensive side (Fig. 9).

Water and Electrolyte Content of the Carotid Sinus

The water and electrolyte studies of hypertensive and normotensive carotid sinuses have shown that there is a significantly increased sodium content of the hypertensive wall. The water and potassium content, however, was lower than in normotensive animals. The sinuses protected prior to development of the hypertension showed a lower sodium content than the nonprotected hypertensive sinuses (Table 1). Water and potassium content was similar. The differences in the latter were not significant. However, results of only few experiments were available at this writing. Four

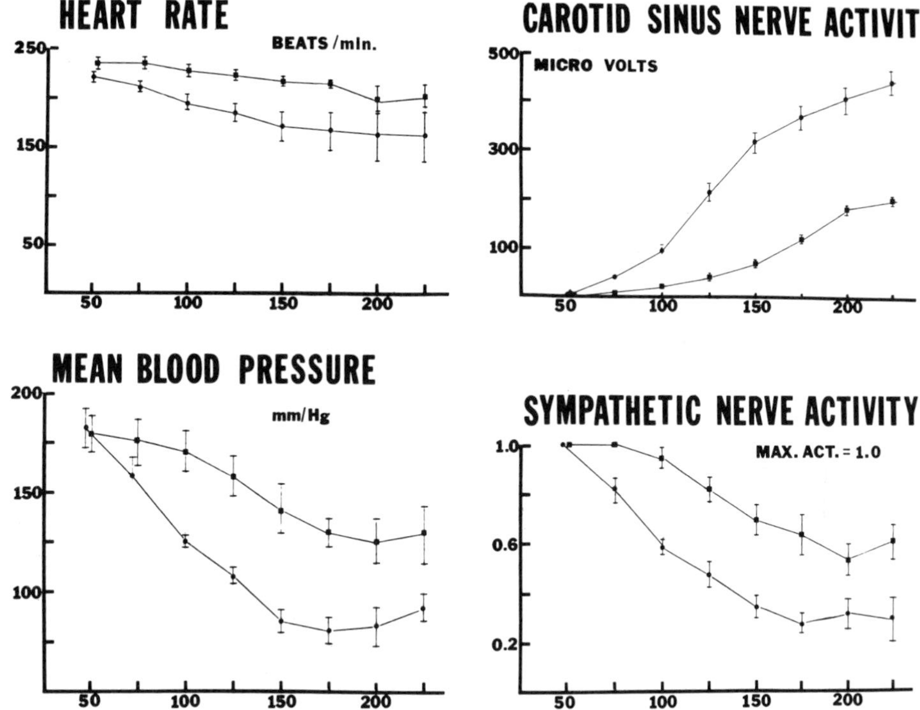

FIG. 6.—Heart rate, mean blood pressure, and carotid sinus and sympathetic nerve activity plotted as a function of intrasinus pressure in the protected (–●–) and nonprotected (–■–) sinuses of hypertensive dogs. **Vertical bars** show the standard error of the mean.

of the post-hypertension-protected carotid sinuses showed similarly increased sodium and decreased potassium and water, as did the opposite hypertensive sinuses.

DISCUSSION

The experiments described confirmed previous results that the carotid sinus is reset in experimental renal hypertension at the hypertensive blood pressure level. The resetting appears to be predominantly located in the baroceptor areas themselves since the reflex responses in hypertension, measured by the heart rate, blood pressure, and sympathetic nerve activity (like the measure of the efferent response of the baroceptor reflex arch), showed quanti-

TABLE 1.—*Water, Sodium, and Potassium Content of Carotid Sinus Arterial Wall*

Type of Carotid Sinuses Analyzed	*Water (%)*		*Sodium (mEq per gm)*		*Potassium (mEq per 100 gm)*	
Normotensive (9)	70.1 ± 3.9		39.7 ± 1.8		9.4 ± 1.5	
		*		*		*
Hypertensive (6)	60.8 ± 5.9		44.3 ± 3.8		6.9 ± 2.9	
						*
Protected sinus (prior to hypertension) (4)	61.3 ± 6.5		39.7 ± 2.7		6.0 ± 1.7	
Protected sinus (after hypertension) (4)	64.0 ± 6.0		43.0 ± 4.5		6.0 ± 4.0	
Nonprotected sinus (8)	60.3 ± 10.6		43.2 ± 3.6		6.9 ± 3.4	

* Difference significant at the 2-percent level.
Numbers in parentheses in the first column represent the number of carotid sinuses analyzed.

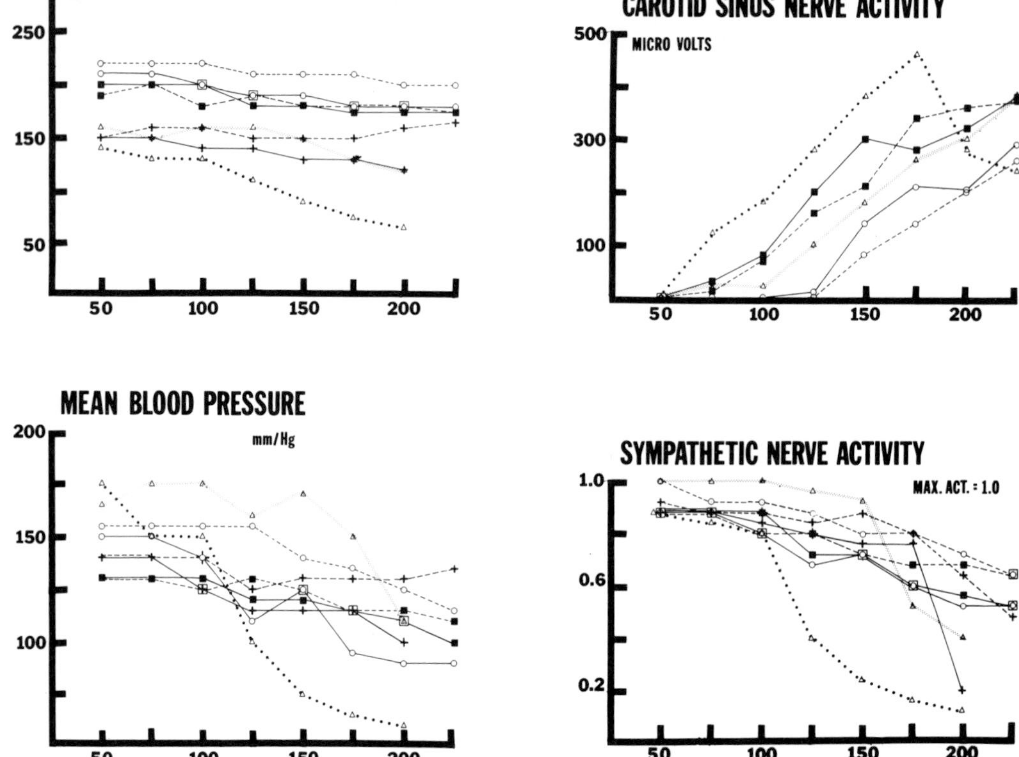

FIG. 7.—Reflex response of heart rate, mean blood pressure, carotid sinus nerve activity, and sympathetic nerve activity during perfusion of the protected and nonprotected sinuses in four renal hypertensive dogs. Each symbol represents the response in an individual dog. Protected sinus is shown by **solid line,** nonprotected by **interrupted line.** Protection by anastomosis was achieved after 6 months' exposure to hypertension. Test was performed 4 weeks after anastomosis. Only in one dog (△) is significant separation of the two curves seen as sign of reversed resetting (note greater response of △ . . . . △).

tatively about the same degree of displacement in the opposite direction as the baroceptor nerve activity. If resetting would have a significant central or efferent peripheral component, a discrepancy between the degree of resetting at the carotid sinus and the reflex response for a given strain at the sinus could be expected. The set point, i.e., the point at which the pressure in the isolated sinus is the same as the systemic pressure, for the hypertensive side was around 150 mm Hg mean pressure while for the protected side it was around 110 mm Hg. The ratio between the two sides at the set point for blood pressure-inhibition or inhibition of the sympathetic activity and displacement of carotid sinus activity in the opposite direction was about the same (1:1.37). The relatively high set point for the protected sinus, when compared to the measured pressure in that sinus during anesthesia at the time of the acute experiment, indicates probably that the pressure during the awake state was higher in that artery than at the time of the measurement when also the systemic pressure and the pressure in the other carotid sinus were lower because of the anesthetic effect. Nevertheless, there probably was a significant difference between the pressures in the two sinuses during the entire course of hypertension. Since all the conditions regarding biochemistry and nervous innervation were the same on both sides during the development of hypertension and only the

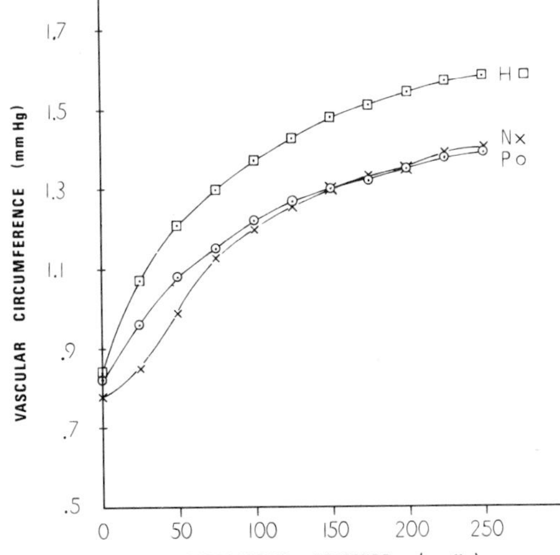

FIG. 8.—The circumference of rings excised from the carotid sinus plotted as a function of the equivalent intracarotid pressure for six normotensive dogs **(N)**, five hypertensive carotid sinuses **(H)** and four protected carotid sinuses **(P)**. There is no significant difference between **P** and **N** at all pressures but a significant difference ($p < 0.1$) exists for all pressures above 75 mm Hg for the **H** curve.

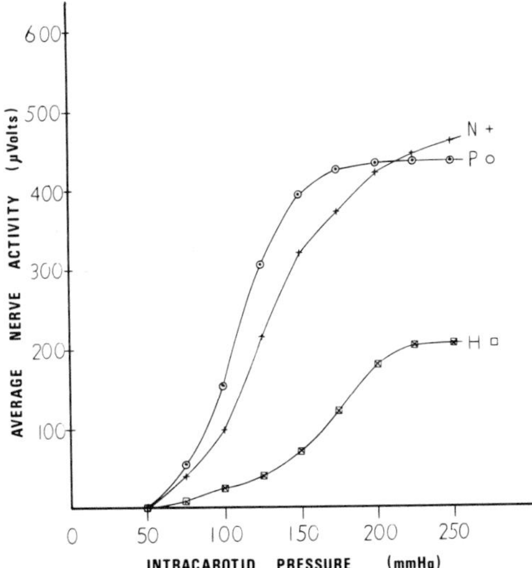

FIG. 9.—Nerve activity plotted as a function of intracarotid pressure for six normotensive dogs **(N)**, five hypertensive carotid sinuses **(H)** and four protected carotid sinuses **(P)**. There is no significant difference between **P** and **N** at all pressures with a significant difference ($p < 0.1$) at all pressures above 75 mm Hg for the **H** curve.

exposure to the level of intra-arterial pressure was different, it can be concluded that the hydrostatic pressure itself either directly or indirectly is responsible for the resetting phenomenon occurring in the unprotected sinus and in hypertension in general.

Our findings of the water and sodium content of the carotid sinus arterial wall only partially confirmed the findings of Peterson et al.[15] We found, as did Tobian and Redleaf,[20] that in experimental renal hypertension there is an increased sodium and decreased potassium content of the vascular walls. The curious fact is that while increased sodium content could be found on the nonprotected side of the sinus there was not a statistically significant increase on the protected side in the same animal. This is not greatly surprising since it appears that the elevated pressure itself is partially responsible for the increased sodium. Hollander et al.[22] found no increase of sodium below the experimentally constricted segment of the aorta when the aorta was constricted below the diaphragm, where the pressure was normal or below normal, but they did find increased sodium content in the upper segment of the aorta where hypertension existed. They concluded that the pressure itself was a driving force for sodium to enter the interstitial tissues of the arterial wall while the hormonal influences played only a secondary role.

In our experiments, the findings may not be surprising that segments of hypertensive carotid sinuses had less resistance to forces of stretch or were more distensible than normotensive sinuses or sinuses from the protected side of the hypertensive animals. At first sight one might think that this is contradictory since it may be assumed that increased sodium and water lead to increased stiffness and greater resistance to stretch. However, we have shown only increased sodium but not water. One must take into consideration that from a purely physical standpoint there must be a difference between the effect of increased sodium and water whether it occurs in the small or resistance vessels, in the large arteries with thick media or thin media as in the carotid sinus. Since resistance relates to the power of the radius of the arteriole, it can easily be seen that increased sodium and water as well as hypertrophy of the smooth muscles will affect the wall-lumen ratio in the direction that it will result in increased resistance. However, the increased sodium in the large arteries, specifically in the carotid sinus with thin media, few smooth muscles, and predominant elastic fibers, may not affect the resistance to stretch or distensibility since there was no increased water and the sodium is probably intracellular.

We have noticed for some time that the carotid arteries, specifically the carotid sinuses, are usually markedly distended and bulging in hypertensive animals and that in the same animal the nonprotected sinus was distended sometimes to twice the size when compared in situ with the protected sinus. Apparently the forces of constantly elevated pressure will lead to overextension of the elastic fibers and eventually to stretching of the collagen of the connective tissue which provides the support and the limit to which elastic fiber can be stretched. When a carotid sinus segment is removed and is not under pressure load, its elastic fibers will reduce the ring to a certain size. When successive loads are applied the hypertensive ring will stretch more easily because the collagen support of its wall has been previously stretched by the hypertension. Now, if the receptors are so located that the stress-relaxed collagen also transmits the stretch of the vessel to the receptor, then the receptors will not be deformed as much for the same vessel-wall deformation and therefore, the response of the receptors will be less.

Another possible hypothesis is that the overextension of the vessel wall damages the baroceptor nerve endings and thereby reduces the total number of active fibers in the nerve bundle.

There is, of course, a third alternative, and that is that the receptors merely adapt to the elevated pressure of hypertension. This may be due to their increased sodium content affecting their depolarization. Short-term adaptation of receptors to steady pressures has not been observed; however, the time scale of such experiments has not been long enough to indicate what happens after a period of days or weeks of exposure to elevated pressure.

It is possible to make an educated guess about the *primary* mechanism involved with resetting, understanding of course that the receptor properties of the vessel cannot be isolated from each other and, in fact, the resetting probably involves a number of mechanisms. If the resetting mechanism were purely a neural adaptation, then it would be expected that the nerve activity would respond in the same general way to pressures, but a higher pressure level would be required to elicit the same nerve response. Such a situation is depicted by the curves shown in Fig. 10, which indicate that an increased pressure and circumference are required for the same nerve activity, whereas the pressure-circumference characteristics, i.e., the elastic properties of the vessel, remain unchanged.

An alternative hypothesis is that, as has been proposed in the past, the vessel wall becomes stiffer so that there is less vessel strain for the same change in pressure. This hypothesis is

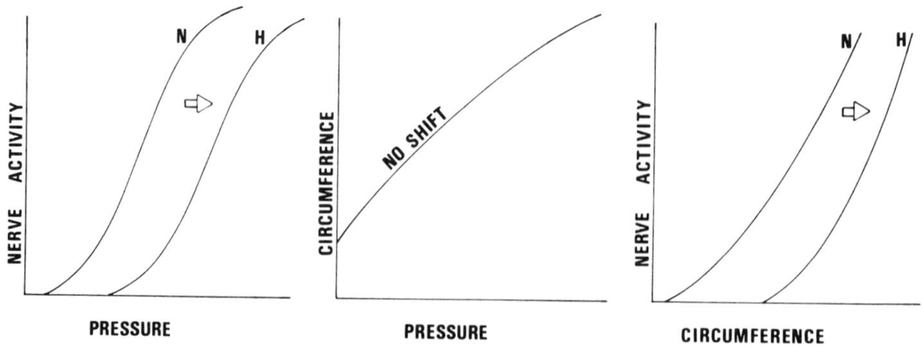

FIG. 10.—Neural adaptation. A greater pressure and an increased circumference are required to stimulate the same nerve activity. There is no change in the pressure circumference relationship. **N,** normotensive; **H,** hypertensive; **arrows** indicate principal direction of shift of the curves.

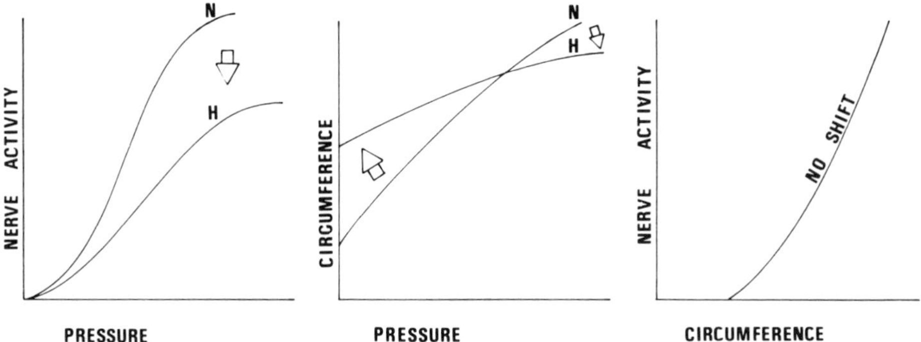

FIG. 11.—Increased wall stiffness. A greater change of pressure is required for the same change in circumference and nerve activity. The circumference versus nerve activity characteristic is unchanged. **N,** normotensive; **H,** hypertensive; **arrows** indicate principal direction of shift of the curves.

depicted by the curves of Fig. 11. This pressure-nerve activity characteristic better agrees with the experimental result in that the nerve activity saturates at a lower pressure and never reaches the maximum level of the normal case at any pressure. The elastic characteristic however, is not what we have observed in these experiments. In fact, what we have observed perhaps can best be explained by the hypothesis previously described in which there are structural changes in the vessel wall such that the wall becomes more distended and more distensible, but this distention does not stimulate the receptors either because they have been damaged or their mechanical attachment within the vessel wall has been changed. This hypothesis is represented by the curves shown in Fig. 12, which agree with the experimental results obtained. Now, if our additional future experiments will confirm our preliminary studies that the receptors are not able to recover when they are protected by an arteriovenous anastomosis after chronic hypertension has been established, then we can conclude that the primary mechanism may be an actual change of threshold or destruction of the receptors so that there are fewer active fibers in hypertension for a given intrasinus pressure. If, on the other hand, the receptors do recover, then the primary mechanism may be a modification in the structural relationships of the receptors and the vessel wall. Surely the two mechanisms could simultaneously be present and reversal of resetting toward normal pres-

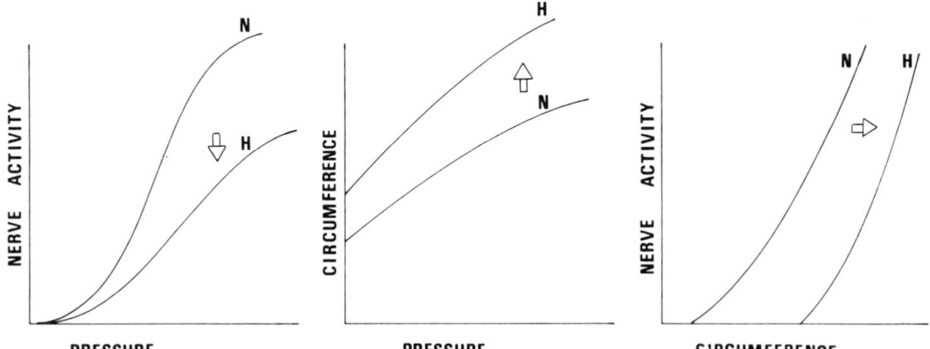

FIG. 12.—Vessel-wall structural changes. For the same pressure level the vessel maintains a greater circumference but a reduced neural activity because the relationship between the receptors organs and the gross structure of the vessel has changed. **N,** normotensive; **H,** hypertensive; **arrows** indicate principal direction of shift of the curves.

sure would then depend on which mechanism is dominant. Whatever the mechanism of resetting, it appears that it plays a role in the maintenance of the elevated vascular resistance, jointly either with structural changes of the resistance vessels or a pressor mechanism, in chronic renal hypertension. Since we know that resetting can occur within a few days but that it lags behind the gradual increase of pressure there must be a delay of structural changes in the arterial wall or change in receptor threshold, and only if the pressure is consistently and for a prolonged time elevated will these changes become established. The question of reversibility of these changes in renal hypertension is obviously important.

REFERENCES

1. Reed, R. K., Sapirstein, L. A., Southard, F. D., Jr., and Ogden, E.: The effects of nembutal and yohimbine on chronic renal hypertension in the rat. Am. J. Physiol. 141: 707, 1944.
2. McCubbin, J. W., and Page, I. H.: Renal pressor system and neurogenic control of arterial pressure. Circ. Res. 12:553, 1963.
3. Hering, H. E.: Die Karotissinusreflexe auf Herz und Gefasse. Dresden-Leipzig: Steinkopf, 1927.
4. Koch, E.: Die reflektorische Selbststeuerung des Kreislaufes. Dresden-Leipzig: Steinkopf, 1931.
5. Heymans, C., Bouckaert, J. J., and Regniers, P.: Le Sinus Carotidien et la Zone Homologue Cardioaortique. Paris: Coin et Fils, 1933.
6. Goldblatt, H., Kahn, J. R., Bayless, P., and Simon, M. A.: Studies on experimental hypertension. XI. The effect of excision of the carotid sinuses on experimental hypertension produced by renal ischemia. J. Exp. Med. 71:175, 1940.
7. Lampan, H., Kezdi, P., Koppermann, E., and Kaufmann, L.: Experimenteller Entzugelungschochdruck bei arteriellen Hypertonie. Arch. Int. Pharmacodyn. Ther. 38:19, 1949.
8. Kezdi, P.: Sinaortic regulatory system: Role in pathogenesis of essential and malignant hypertension. Arch. Intern. Med. 91:26, 1958.
9. McCubbin, J. W., Green, J. H., and Page, I. H.: Baroceptor function in chronic renal hypertension. Circ. Res. 4:205, 1956.
10. Kezdi, P., and Wennemark, J. R.: Baroceptor and sympathetic activity in experimental renal hypertension in the dog. Circulation 17: 785, 1958.
11. Hauss, W. H., Kreuziger, H., and Asteroth, H.: Uber die Reizung der Pressor-rezeptoren in sinus carotis beim Hund. Z. Kreislaufforsch. 38:28, 1949.
12. Peterson, L. H.: Systems behavior, feedback loops, and high blood pressure research. Circ. Res. 12:585, 1968.
13. McCubbin, J. W.: Carotid sinus participation in experimental renal hypertension. Circulation 17:791, 1958.
14. Krieger, E. M.: Time course of baroreceptor resetting in acute hypertension. Am. J. Physiol. 218:486, 1970.
15. Peterson, L. H.: Some studies of the regulation of cardiovascular functions. Arch. Int. Pharmacodyn. 140:281, 1962.
16. Jones, A. W., Feigel, E. O., and Peterson, L. H.: Water and electrolyte content of normal and hypertensive arteries in dogs. Circ. Res. 15:386, 1964.
17. Volhard, F.: Uber die Pathogenese des roten (essentiellen) arteriellen Hochdrucks und der malignen Sklerose. Schweiz. Med. Wochenschr. 78:1189, 1948.
18. Heymans, C., and van den Heuvel-Heymans, G.: New aspects of blood pressure regulation. Circulation 6:581, 1951.
19. Aars, H.: Relationship between aortic diameter and aortic baroreceptor activity in normal and hypertensive rabbits. Acta Physiol. Scand. 75:406, 1969.
20. Tobian, L., and Redleaf, P. D.: Ionic composition of the aorta in renal and adrenal hypertension. Am. J. Physiol. 192:325, 1958.
21. Kezdi, P.: Resetting of the carotid sinus in experimental hypertension. *In* Proceedings Baroreceptors and Hypertension International Symposium, Dayton, Ohio, November 17, 1965. New York: Pergamon Press, 1967, pp. 301–306.
22. Hollander, W., Madoff, I. M., Kramusch, D., and Yagi, S.: Arterial wall metabolism in experimental hypertension of coarctation of the aorta. Hypertension 8:191, 1964.

Experimental Pyelonephritis and Hypertension

By Robert H. Heptinstall, M.D.

NUMEROUS EXPERIMENTS have been performed to explain the association of hypertension and chronic pyelonephritis encountered in man. Briefly these experiments are designed to determine whether chronic pyelonephritis produces hypertension, or whether a hypertensive kidney is unduly susceptible to the development of pyelonephritis.

Before the experimental findings are discussed some of the observations in man should be considered. When patients with chronic pyelonephritis are analyzed, a high incidence of hypertension is noted,[1–4] amounting to over 66 percent in all of these series. Similarly, if groups of patients with clinical malignant hypertension are studied to determine the underlying cause of the hypertension, an appreciable incidence of chronic pyelonephritis is encountered, invariably over 15 percent.[2,5–7] In two of these series a unilateral lesion was encountered in a proportion of patients.[3,5] This is of interest in that such cases provide evidence for the pyelonephritis producing hypertension, because removal of a unilateral pyelonephritic kidney may cause an alleviation of the hypertension.[8] Further reasons for considering the chronic infective process to be the cause of the hypertension are as follows. First, the relationship between chronic pyelonephritis and hypertension is most convincing in childhood. Here, because of the rarity of essential hypertension and renovascular hypertension, the chances of a hypertensive kidney becoming infected, the alternative idea, are remote. Secondly, recurrent attacks of acute pyelonephritis cause an increase in blood pressure in patients who were initially normotensive. Thirdly, the calyceal deformities and anomalies such as bifid pelvis or ureter are more consistent with the idea of infection being the first event.

A further complicating factor emerges from the study of Bengtsson, Högdahl, and Hood [9] who have shown, in a group of patients 20 to 40 years of age with chronic nonobstructive pyelonephritis and hypertension, that there is a high incidence of a positive family history of hypertension. The incidence was twice that seen in a group of patients with chronic pyelonephritis and normal blood pressure. The possibility is therefore raised that chronic infection might cause essential hypertension to appear earlier than usual. This possibility is lessened, although not excluded, by the observation that the incidence of a positive family history is much higher in patients with essential hypertension than in the hypertensive patients in the chronic pyelonephritic series.

The first experiments to be considered are those performed to determine whether chronic pyelonephritis can produce hypertension in the laboratory animal. In the rabbit it has proved possible to produce hypertension only when one kidney is infected and the other removed.[10] Unilateral pyelonephritis with an intact opposite kidney produces no such elevation of pressure. In the rat, Spitznagel and Schroeder [11] produced hypertension by infecting one kidney following intravenous injection of *Escherichia coli* and tying off the ureter. It should be noted that in this experiment the ureter of the infected kidney was permanently occluded. Vivaldi et al.[12] caused hypertension in over half the rats in their experiment following introduction of *Proteus vulgaris* into the bladder. This resulted in a bilateral renal infection. We were able to produce hypertension in the rat by infecting one kidney with *E. coli* with the other removed, and less consistently when both were infected.[13] Little success was achieved when one kidney was infected with the opposite kidney intact. Shapiro, Braude, and Siemienski,[14] and Shapiro and Kobernick [15] were unable to

From the Department of Pathology, The Johns Hopkins University School of Medicine and Hospital, Baltimore, Maryland.

This work was supported by Grant HE-07835 from the U.S. Public Health Service.

produce hypertension in the rat either by bilateral infection or by unilateral infection with one kidney removed. They produced infection by massage of the kidney coupled with intravenous injection of *E. coli, Proteus morganii,* or *Streptococcus faecalis* separately, or all three together. Similarly Guze [16] was unable to produce any elevation of blood pressure in rats with chronic infection induced by intravenous injection of *S. faecalis.* The evidence is rather conflicting, but on balance it can be concluded that a large amount of renal parenchyma must be compromised before hypertension is produced.

The other experiments are those carried out to see whether the kidney is more susceptible to infection in an animal with hypertension than in one with a normal blood pressure. The evidence again is conflicting. On the one hand both Woods [17] and Shapiro [18] were able to show an increased susceptibility of the kidney to infection by *E. coli* when rats were made hypertensive by injection of deoxycorticosteroid. Heptinstall and Stryker [19] were unable to show an increased susceptibility of the kidney to infection by *E. coli* when hypertension was produced by the application of a silver clip to one renal artery in the rat. The discrepancies are likely to be accounted for by the differences in the "virulence" of the organism used to produce the infection. This is almost certainly the case when our experience is compared with that of Woods,[17] who used a strain of *E. coli* which from time to time was capable of causing infection in the untouched kidneys of control animals. The organism used in our experiment is one that will not cause a lesion in an untouched kidney.

There are two ways in which hypertension could bring about increased susceptibility, through parenchymal damage, or through changed hemodynamics. There is good evidence to show that damage to the parenchyma of the kidney makes it easier for organisms to localize and proliferate there.[20,21] We were not impressed with parenchymal damage in the hypertensive kidneys in our study; apparently this was also true in the experiments where organisms localized with increased facility. Jones and Shapiro [22] tested the hemodynamic aspects by injecting 10 μg of angiotensin into rats, a procedure which caused an elevation of blood pressure which was sustained for 5 minutes. When *E. coli* was injected simultaneously a high proportion of the rats developed pyelonephritis. Several of the rats in our experiments achieved blood pressures of a comparable magnitude which were sustained for longer periods. However, they did not show increased localization of organisms in the kidney. The explanation for the discrepancy is not apparent.

The results from the various experiments, well reviewed by Shapiro,[23] are therefore conflicting and not altogether satisfactory to answer the various questions posed from studies in man. Certainly it is difficult to understand why the alleged incidence of hypertension in chronic pyelonephritis in man is so high. Although this is not the place to attempt it, a reassessment of the blood pressure findings in pyelonephritis is needed. Over the past few years I have become increasingly unhappy over the entity of chronic pyelonephritis of the nonobstructive variety in adults. We have recently surveyed the incidence of this entity, using strict criteria, in the autopsy service of the Johns Hopkins Hospital.[24] We found only eight cases among 2,970 adult autopsies, an incidence of less than 0.3 percent. In pediatric practice it still remains an important condition as a cause of chronic renal failure and hypertension.

The reason for the overdiagnosis is a failure to realize that the parenchymal changes are entirely nonspecific. These changes may be brought about in several different ways and by many different agents.[25] The diagnosis can only be made with certainty when calyceal deformities are present. A dilated calyx with an overlying scarred parenchyma must be seen before chronic pyelonephritis can be diagnosed. Intravenous pyelography reveals these abnormalities. The explanation is that pyelonephritis begins in the forniceal region, organisms having been transmitted up the ureters from an infected bladder by vesicoureteric reflux. Eventually the papilla is destroyed, thereby increasing the calyceal size and giving rise to the club-shaped defect seen on pyelography. Papillary necrosis is the only other condition that can give rise to a similar radiologic and pathologic picture.

Assuming this overdiagnosis, we must question the figures quoted for the association of hypertension and chronic pyelonephritis. Many of the kidneys so frequently diagnosed as chronic pyelonephritis are kidneys with arteriosclerosis, and it would therefore not be surprising to find hypertension in this group.

References

1. Longcope, W. T.: Chronic bilateral pyelonephritis: Its origin and its association with hypertension. Ann. Intern. Med. 11:149, 1937.
2. Weiss, S., and Parker, F., Jr.: Pyelonephritis: Its relation to vascular lesions and to arterial hypertension. Medicine 18:221, 1939.
3. Kincaid-Smith, P.: Vascular obstruction in chronic pyelonephritic kidneys and its relation to hypertension. Lancet 2:1263, 1955.
4. Brod, J.: Chronic pyelonephritis. Lancet 1: 973, 1956.
5. Heptinstall, R. H.: Malignant hypertension: A study of 51 cases. J. Pathol. Bacteriol. 65: 423, 1953.
6. Kincaid-Smith, P., McMichael, J., and Murphy, E. A.: The clinical course and pathology of hypertension with papilloedema (malignant hypertension). Q. J. Med. 27:117, 1958.
7. Kimmelstiel, P., Kim, O. J., Beres, J. A., and Wellmann, K.: Chronic pyelonephritis. Am. J. Med. 30:589, 1961.
8. Pickering, G. W., and Heptinstall, R. H.: Nephrectomy and other treatment for hypertension in pyelonephritis. Q. J. Med. 22:1, 1953.
9. Bengtsson, U., Högdahl, A.-M., and Hood, B.: Chronic nonobstructive pyelonephritis and hypertension: A long-term study. Q. J. Med. 37:361, 1968.
10. Heptinstall, R. H., and Gorrill, R. H.: Experimental pyelonephritis and its effect on the blood pressure. J. Pathol. Bacteriol. 69:191, 1955.
11. Spitznagel, J. K., and Schroeder, H. A.: Experimental pyelonephritis and hypertension in rats. Proc. Soc. Exp. Biol. Med. 77:762, 1951.
12. Vivaldi, E., Zangwill, D. P., Cotral, R., and Kass, E. H.: Experimental pyelonephritis consequent to induction of bacteriuria. *In* Quinn, E. L., and Kass, E. H. (Eds.): Henry Ford Hospital International Symposium on Biology of Pyelonephritis. Boston: Little, Brown, 1960, p. 27.
13. Heptinstall, R. H.: Experimental pyelonephritis: the effect of chronic infection on the blood pressure in the rat. Br. J. Exp. Pathol. 43:333, 1962.
14. Shapiro, A. P., Braude, A. I., and Siemienski, J.: Hematogenous pyelonephritis in rats. IV. Relationship of bacterial species to the pathogenesis and sequelae of chronic pyelonephritis. J. Clin. Invest. 38:1228, 1959.
15. Shapiro, A. P., and Kobernick, J. L.: Effects of unilateral nephrectomy and mixed infection on blood pressure of rats with experimental chronic pyelonephritis. Circ. Res. 7:936, 1959.
16. Guze, L. B.: Experimental pyelonephritis: Observations on the course of enterococcal infection in the kidney of the rat. *In* Quinn, E. L., and Kass, E. H. (Eds.): Henry Ford Hospital International Symposium on Biology of Pyelonephritis. Boston: Little, Brown, 1960, p. 11.
17. Woods, J. W.: Susceptibility of rats with hormonal hypertension to experimental pyelonephritis. J. Clin. Invest. 37:1686, 1958.
18. Shapiro, A. P.: Susceptibility of rats with DCA hypertension to experimental pyelonephritis and aggravation of DCA hypertension by renal infection. J. Lab. Clin. Med. 55:715, 1960.
19. Heptinstall, R. H., and Stryker, M.: Experimental pyelonephritis: A study of the susceptibility of the hypertensive kidney to infection in the rat. Bull. Hopkins Hosp. 111:292, 1962.
20. De Navasquez, S.: Further studies in experimental pyelonephritis produced by various bacteria, with special reference to renal scarring as a factor in pathogenesis. J. Pathol. Bacteriol. 71:27, 1956.
21. Beeson, P. B., Rocha, H., and Guze, L. B.: Experimental pyelonephritis: Influence of localized injury in different parts of the kidney on susceptibility to hematogenous infection. Trans. Assoc. Am. Physicians 70:120, 1957.
22. Jones, R. K., and Shapiro, A. P.: Increased susceptibility to pyelonephritis during acute hypertension by angiotensin II and norepinephrine. J. Clin. Invest. 42:179, 1963.
23. Shapiro, A. P.: Experimental pyelonephritis and hypertension: implications for the clinical problem. Ann. Intern. Med. 59:37, 1963.
24. Farmer, E. R., and Heptinstall, R. H.: Chronic non-obstructive pyelonephritis—a reappraisal. *In* Kincaid-Smith, P., and Fairley, K. F. (Eds.): Renal Infection and Renal Scarring. Melbourne, Australia: Mercedes, 1970, p. 233.
25. Heptinstall, R. H.: The enigma of chronic pyelonephritis. J. Infect. Dis. 120:104, 1969.

Pyelonephritis as a Cause of Hypertension in Man

By Priscilla Kincaid-Smith, M.D., K. F. Fairley, M.D., and W. F. Heale, M.B.

THE MAJOR DIFFICULTY in obtaining precise information about pyelonephritis as a cause of hypertension in man lies in defining pyelonephritis in a manner which is uniformly acceptable to microbiologists, radiologists, pathologists, and clinicians.

If we adopt a simple definition of pyelonephritis, namely, "renal damage due to bacterial infection" we immediately face the difficulty of determining which urinary tract infections arise in the kidney and how to estimate the damage which they produce.

Over the past few years we have evolved methods which allow us to determine the site of urinary tract infection in all patients presenting to us and have correlated this with other findings such as the blood pressure, functional damage, and radiologic damage.

Some of these findings will be presented in this chapter and discussed in relation to other views about pyelonephritis as a cause of hypertension in man.

Historical Review

At the last Hahnemann Symposium on hypertension 10 years ago Smythe [1] outlined and reviewed the contradictory theories which have accumulated since Weiss and Parker's [2] classic paper was published in 1939. Goldring and Chasis [3] and Bell [4] believed that the apparent association between pyelonephritis and hypertension represented a fortuitous coincidental occurrence of two common conditions. Since then most authors have agreed that renal damage due to recurrent infection either directly causes hypertension or that it stimulates an underlying hereditary predisposition to hypertension.[1,5–15] The latter suggestion arises from the observation that patients with chronic pyelonephritis have a significant family history of hypertension.[7,14,16] The opposite view has been expressed by Shapiro and his coworkers,[17,18] who believe that hypertension is the primary disorder which predisposes to urinary tract infection and pyelonephritis.

Bacteriuria has been found in 3 to 6 percent of adult women [12,13,19–22] and may recur in 80 percent of patients within 18 months of treatment.[23–25] If bacteriuria were a manifestation of underlying renal damage or pyelonephritis one would expect a significant morbidity and possibly even mortality due to pyelonephritis in adult women.

Evidence is, however, accumulating to show that one-third to one-half of urinary tract infections are confined to the bladder [26–32] and that even when they arise in the kidney a sensitive test of function such as ability to concentrate the urine is impaired in only 30 to 40 percent of patients.[27,32] Other evidence of the benign course of bacteriuria was apparent from following a large series of adult women with recurrent urinary tract infection—no impairment of function or development of hypertension was noted over 7 years.[33]

The situation is quite different in children and more and more evidence is accumulating to show that almost all pyelonephritic scarring and radiologic damage which we recognize as pyelonephritis represents damage which occurred in childhood. Not only do scars develop more frequently in childhood but children provide the most convincing evidence of an association between hypertension and pyelonephritis. The rarity of hypertension in childhood makes the common association of pyelonephritis and hypertension in children [34] of far greater significance. Even in adults under the age of 40 the frequency of hypertension in patients with pyelonephritis makes it very unlikely that this is a chance association.[16] The radiologic lesion which we recognize as pyelonephritis has been clearly shown to develop in

From the University Department of Medicine at the Royal Melbourne Hospital, Melbourne, Victoria, Australia.

Supported by grants from the National Health and Medical Research Council, The Wellcome Trust, the Victor Hurley Research Fund, and the Royal Australasian College of Physicians.

association with vesicoureteric reflux in childhood.[35,36] It is now generally accepted that reflux and bacterial infection are the two factors which produce nonobstructive pyelonephritic scarring.[37] Scarring rarely develops in adults, perhaps because adults rarely show reflux.[38] We have, however, recently observed progressive scar formation in two adults who continued to show gross reflux (unpublished data). Bilateral atrophic pyelonephritis proved by nephrectomy accounted for one-third of 120 patients presenting to our dialysis and transplantation program (unpublished data). Hypertension played a part in rapid progression to renal failure in the latter part of the course of most of these patients. Therefore, we must recognize the association of pyelonephritis and hypertension as an important cause of morbidity and mortality.

One of the aims of our careful studies of the site of urinary tract infection has been to understand the apparently benign character of recurrent bacteriuria in most women in the face of undoubted cases of renal failure due to pyelonephritis and hypertension which we see in older children and young adults.

In this chapter we have attempted to eliminate some of the problems in this area and to define clinically recognizable forms of pyelonephritis and to relate these to the blood pressure.

What Is Pyelonephritis?

When reviewing the association between hypertension and pyelonephritis some years ago, we encountered major difficulties in defining pyelonephritis on precise clinical, bacteriologic, radiologic, or pathologic grounds.

Since that time our group has been able to overcome some of these difficulties by careful studies of the site of infection in relation to clinical features, urinary findings, natural history, and radiologic and pathologic findings in a large number of patients.[27–33,39] We have also been able to define more accurately the radiology,[40] pathology,[41] and clinical features [42] of the quite distinct condition, analgesic nephropathy, which has often been confused with pyelonephritis. The whole subject of the relationship between bacteriuria, pyuria, pyelonephritis, vesicoureteric reflux, and analgesic nephropathy was the subject of a recent symposium in this department.[36]

We now have more clearly defined views about what constitutes pyelonephritis, and in order to consider the relationship between pyelonephritis and hypertension, we shall attempt in the following pages to define pyelonephritis.

Acute Pyelonephritis

Acute attacks of loin pain, loin tenderness, rigors, and pyrexia occur relatively frequently in patients presenting to their general practitioners.[39] Clinical attacks of acute pyelonephritis are particularly liable to occur during pregnancy when asymptomatic bladder bacteriuria has been shown to ascend the ureter and cause symptomatic acute pyelonephritis.[32]

Clinical attacks of acute pyelonephritis are also more liable to occur in association with some underlying lesion such as a stone, vesicoureteric reflux, or renal papillary necrosis.

Although hypertension may occur as an acute manifestation in acute pyelonephritis, we have not been able to find reports of a follow-up of such patients except in relation to pregnancy bacteriuria. Following pregnancy bacteriuria and pyelonephritis, hypertension has not developed as a complication in our own series.[33]

Chronic Pyelonephritis

It has been usual to consider as having chronic pyelonephritis those patients with evidence of radiographic scars of the type which develop in childhood in association with vesicoureteric reflux.[35,36] These scars when advanced correspond in their appearance to the pathologic descriptions of the irregular atrophic pyelonephritic kidney.[2,7,35,36,38,43] Because we have little information about the time course of the development of scars and because failure to grow, rather than progressive scar formation, may be an important factor in the natural history of pyelonephritis, the term "chronic" is perhaps not warranted as it implies evidence of bacterial infection over a long time. The term "pyelonephritis" implies that the scarring results from bacterial infection and, whereas it is very likely that this is so, either obstruction or vesicoureteric reflux is almost invariably present at the time at which a scar develops. It has even been implied [36] that vesicoureteric reflux and not bacterial infection may cause the scar formation.

For these reasons we shall not use the term "chronic" in the remaining discussions but will refer to pyelonephritis and to focal or generalized pyelonephritic scarring.

Bacteriuria, Pyuria, and Pyelonephritis

If pyelonephritis implies bacterial infection within the kidney, it becomes important to define the relationship between recurrent symptomatic urinary tract infections, asymptomatic bacteriuria, and pyelonephritis. Stamey's group have shown that both in men [44] and in women [45,46] recurrent urinary tract infections usually arise from reinfection with organisms persisting in the urethra, prostate, and vulval area. Once organisms reach the bladder it is assumed that some are able to overcome the normal valve mechanism of the vesicoureteric junction and ascend the ureter. We have observed this in pregnancy [32] but assume that it also occurs in other infections. Even in acute urinary tract infections about half are renal.[31]

In assessing the presence of urinary tract infection in the individual patient one cannot adhere strictly to Kass's [11] definition of bacteriuria, namely, over 100,000 organisms per milliliter. This definition is of use in epidemiologic studies, but in the individual patient, because bladder urine is normally sterile, any organisms in the bladder urine may represent an infection provided contamination can be excluded. In carefully collected midstream specimens 10,000 organisms per milliliter usually represent infection [47]; where doubt arises needle aspiration of the bladder will prove or exclude the presence of infected bladder urine even when counts are below 1,000 organisms per milliliter.[26,47]

When bladder urine is known to be infected, either the method described by Stamey, Govan, and Palmer,[26] or the simpler method which we use [30] will provide a diagnosis of renal or bladder infection. We have applied such methods routinely to patients presenting with urinary tract infection over the past 5 years.[32] In a group of patients currently attending our clinic we shall consider the blood pressure in relation to the presence of renal bacteriuria and to the presence of radiologic scars.

We have come to recognize that pyuria, particularly when it persists after disappearance of bacteria from the urine, may have serious significance. Pyuria correlates well with the presence of underlying lesions both in pregnancy bacteriuria [33] and in other conditions.[39] Pyuria may indicate persistence of occult bacterial infection and may be the only manifestation of persistent infection in patients during progression to renal failure.[39]

Pyelonephritis and Damage to the Renal Parenchyma

Apart from impairment of concentrating ability which develops during an infection but improves again when the infection is cured, radiology provides us with the best evidence that bacterial infection may damage the kidney. Characteristic pyelonephritic scars [35] have been shown to develop in children in association with vesicoureteric reflux and recurrent infection. These correspond in their pathologic features [35] to scars which pathologists accept as pyelonephritic.[43,48]

Although radiologic shrinkage may occur in analgesic nephropathy [40,49] this condition has quite separate and well-recognized clinical and pathologic features.[36,41,42] We have, however, deliberately excluded from this study patients with a history of a high intake of analgesics.

Renal infection and renal atrophy may also develop in the presence of obstruction and the appearances may be indistinguishable from the generalized clubbing seen in association with marked vesicoureteric reflux. The present chapter deals only with nonobstructive pyelonephritis.

If we exclude obstruction and renal papillary necrosis there remain a fairly well-defined group of patients in whom pyelonephritic scarring probably developed in childhood in association with urinary tract infection and vesicoureteric reflux. These scars rarely progress after the second decade. This sequence of events, well described by Hodson and Wilson,[35] has been assumed to be due to infection in the presence of vesicoureteric reflux. Vesicoureteric reflux usually disappears in childhood most commonly between the ages of 6 and 16 and is therefore relatively rare in adults.

In a follow-up of Hodson and Wilson's patients, Smellie and Normand [50] have claimed that progressive scar formation can be prevented by long-term sulfonamide administration. Hodson [51] suggests that the scars form because of introduction of organisms into the renal parenchyma during intrarenal reflux.

Certain studies [52,53] raise the possibility that the scarring may develop even in the absence of infection. However, since in these studies, infection was excluded only on the basis of the absence of overt bacteriuria and because occult infection associated with sterile pyuria may be important in patients with deteriorating function,[39] it is possible that occult infection was missed in these patients.

Recurrent urinary tract infection is often such a benign condition that it is important to recognize the features which may imply a worse prognosis. A history of childhood infection increases the likelihood of vesicoureteric reflux and scarring. When marked pyelonephritic scarring is present, sterile pyuria or microscopic hematuria persisting after treatment suggests active progressive disease.[39]

The finding of persistent microscopic hematuria in some patients suggested that glomerular lesions may play a part in progression of chronic pyelonephritis. Renal biopsies in such patients may reveal proliferative glomerular lesions at a stage before either renal failure or hypertension is present and perhaps these glomerular lesions play a part in progressive renal failure and hypertension in this disease.

Bacteriuria, Pyelonephritis, and Hypertension

One hundred and nine adult women who presented with urinary tract infection to the Renal Unit at the Royal Melbourne Hospital are included in this study. Although otherwise unselected, most patients had been referred because of a long history of recurrent urinary tract infection. To exclude bias all patients known to be hypertensive before they presented to us have been excluded. We also excluded all with a history of excessive intake of analgesics or in whom calculi or any other obstructive lesion had been present at any time.

Fifty-eight patients had abnormalities judged to represent pyelonephritic scarring of the type described by Hodson and Wilson.[35] Fifty-one patients had normal intravenous pyelograms. The mean ages in the two groups were 36.0 (range: 16 to 64) and 31.6 years (range: 18 to 65) respectively.

Site of Infection

This had been determined recently by the bladder washout technique in most patients with normal renal radiography but in only a third of those with pyelonephritic scarring. In the latter group infection is much more likely to be renal.[32] The results are shown in Table 1 and show a marked preponderance of renal infection in the group with scars compared with the group without scars.

Prevalence of Hypertension

The blood pressures were recorded by one observer using the London School of Hygiene and Tropical Medicine sphygmomanometer, which eliminates observer bias. Two casual blood pressure recordings were made at consecutive outpatient visits. These visits were usually 4 weeks apart. The readings were made on the left arm with the patient in a sitting position. The study was conducted over a 3-month period and patients were only included if their urine remained free of infection during this period. The systolic blood pressure was recorded at the appearance of sounds and the diastolic blood pressure at the disappearance of sounds. Hypertension was defined as a mean of four readings greater than 140 mm Hg systolic and 90 mm Hg diastolic. Table 2 shows that there is no apparent correlation between hypertension and the site of infection. The findings listed in Table 2 show that bladder infection is rare in patients with scars and that

TABLE 1.—*Site of Urinary Tract Infection in Patients with or without Radiologic Evidence of Pyelonephritic Scars*

Radiologic Findings (No. of Patients)	*Kidney*	*Bladder*
No scars (47)	19	18
With scars (23)	19	4

TABLE 2.—*Site of Urinary Tract Infection in Relation to Hypertension in Patients with Pyelonephritic Scars*

Clinical and Radiologic Status	*Kidney Infection (No. of patients)*	*Bladder Infection (No. of patients)*
Hypertension		
Pyelonephritic scars (10 patients)	9	1
No hypertension		
Pyelonephritic scars (13 patients)	10	3
Hypertension		
No pyelonephritic scars (3 patients)	2	1
No hypertension		
No pyelonephritic scars (44 patients)	27	17

hypertension is rare in patients without scars. The most significant group are those with renal bacteriuria but no scars, only two of whom had a raised blood pressure.

At the time of examination 26 patients were receiving hypotensive drugs for hypertension, which had been diagnosed previously although this had not been their initial complaint. All these patients had shown persistent diastolic blood pressures above 100 mm Hg before the start of treatment and thus the diagnosis of hypertension was clearly established. Twenty-five had radiographic findings consistent with a diagnosis of pyelonephritic scarring and one patient had a normal intravenous pyelogram.

During the present blind study six more patients with hypertension were detected. Four of these patients had radiographic evidence of pyelonephritic scarring.

Hypertension was thus present in 50 percent of patients with radiographic abnormalities of pyelonephritis and in only 5.9 percent of patients with radiologically normal kidneys (Table 3). One of the three patients with hypertension but normal kidneys on a renal radiograph was 44 years old and had had repeated urinary tract infections for 21 years. She had also had toxemia of pregnancy and had a family history of renal disease. The only other two patients with blood pressures above 140 mm Hg systolic and 90 mm Hg diastolic were well above the average age (56 and 45 respectively).

TABLE 3.—*Prevalence of Hypertension in Patients with or without Pyelonephritic Scars*

Scarring	*No. of Patients*	*No. with blood pressure of 140/90 mm Hg or higher*
Without scars	51	3 (5.9%)
With scars	58	29 (50%)

The age at which hypertension was diagnosed in patients with radiographic evidence of pyelonephritis is shown in Table 4. Nearly half the patients developed hypertension before the age of 30 and 65.5 percent developed hypertension before the age of 40.

DISCUSSION

Although there have been many previous reports of the prevalence of hypertension in pyelonephritis, as far as we are aware this is the only study in which the blood pressure measurement has been related to the site of urinary tract infection.

It is apparent from the results that hypertension correlates with the presence of renal damage in the form of scars which are large enough to be seen on an intravenous pyelogram.

Women with recurrent infection and renal bacteriuria but no scars showed raised blood pressures in only 5.9 percent of those examined. These three patients were aged 44, 45, and 56. This contrasts with the early age of onset of hypertension in the group of patients with pyelonephritic scars and with the fact that 50 percent of patients with pyelonephritic scars were hypertensive. This correlates well with other studies in "chronic" pyelonephritis (Table 5).

It is probably correct to use the term "pyelo-

TABLE 4.—*Age at Which Hypertension Was First Detected in Patients with Pyelonephritic Scars*

Age range (in years)				
10–19	*20–29*	*30–39*	*40–49*	*50–59*
4	10	5	4	6

Mean age at time of detection was 33.8 years.

TABLE 5.—*The Prevalence of Hypertension in Other Studies of Patients with Pyelonephritic Scars*

Study	*Percentage with Hypertension*
Longcope (1937)[5]	55
Weiss and Parker (1939)[2]	75
Platt and Davson (1950)[8]	58
Kincaid-Smith (1955)[37]	67
Brod (1956)[6]	60
Grieble and Jackson (1960)[9]	25–38 (clinical; cf. autopsy series)
Kleeman, Hewitt, and Guze (1960)[10]	44–70 (clinical; cf autopsy series)
Bengtsson (1962)[14]	47
Hodson and Wilson (1965)[35]	36
Heale (1971)[15]	47
Present series (1971)	50

nephritis" to describe patients who may have tens or even hundreds of millions of organisms in every milliliter of ureteric urine.[29,39] There is, however, little evidence to show that even heavy infection accompanied by heavy pyuria produces demonstrable scarring or loss of renal parenchyma in man in the absence of vesicoureteric reflux or some obstructive lesion. Even in experimental pyelonephritis it has usually been necessary to produce reflux or to damage the kidney or ureter in some way to produce lesions of pyelonephritis in the renal parenchyma.

It is difficult to imagine what factors are necessary to permit the discharge of countless millions of organisms down the ureters in the absence of any detectable parenchymal lesion. Renal-concentrating ability may be impaired during renal infection but returns to normal following treatment. We have considered the possibility that the lesion is pyelitis not pyelonephritis[28,32] but an increase in urine flow does not necessarily decrease the rate of excretion of bacteria as one would expect in pyelitis. The accompanying pyuria implies inflammation, and further work is in progress in an attempt to determine whether parenchymal infection is present in such patients. At the present state of our knowledge patients with infected ureteric urine should probably be regarded as having pyelonephritis without demonstrable parenchymal scarring.

It is clearly apparent from this study that in adult women hypertension correlates not with pyelonephritis in the sense of renal bacteriuria but with the presence of pyelonephritic scars, the markers of previous vesicoureteric reflux.

In man the best evidence that hypertension can be caused by pyelonephritic scars still rests on the cure of hypertension by removal of a unilateral atrophic pyelonephritic kidney.[54] Of the factors in the scarred renal parenchyma which may cause hypertension ischemia still remains the most likely possibility.[55] The relationship between vessel lesions, ischemia, and hypertension is, however, not as simple as it appeared to be 16 years ago.[54]

Although there is some evidence that hypertension is more frequently associated with pyelonephritis in patients with impaired renal function,[5,6,14] the suggestion that hypertension may be renoprival is clearly untenable for the group cured by unilateral nephrectomy. Renoprival factors may operate in end-stage renal failure in pyelonephritis as well as other forms of end-stage renal disease; however, bilateral nephrectomy undoubtedly further assists in control of the blood pressure in such patients.

The common occurrence of hypertension in children with pyelonephritis,[34] together with the early age of onset in the present series of patients with pyelonephritic scars, supports the thesis that pyelonephritic scarring causes hypertension.

Although population studies have shown an association between hypertension and bacteriuria,[12,13,21,22] our patients with proved renal bacteriuria without scars showed a far lower prevalence of hypertension than our patients with renal parenchymal scars. Population studies would automatically include patients with scars; our own study in pregnant women[20] and Asscher and Waters's study in nonpregnant women[19] both showed a high incidence of pyelonephritic scars and other radiographic abnormalities in patients with bacteriuria detected by screening techniques. We also found that women with bacteriuria were more prone to develop hypertension and preeclamptic toxemia,[20] and this has been confirmed in other studies.[21] Hypertension associated with pregnancy bacteriuria may well reflect the fact that some patients within the group have underlying pyelonephritic scarring.

It is interesting to consider the possible relationship between the glomerular lesions which we have found in some of our pyelonephritic patients and hypertension. Although glomerular lesions were observed many years ago very little has been written about them. Both Kimmelstiel and Wilson's [56] original description and Heptinstall's [57] book suggest that they are confined to scarred areas and mainly present in association with renal failure and hypertension. In biopsies we have found that glomerular lesions may precede both hypertension and renal failure, and have not found them only in scarred areas. The fact that microscopic hematuria is a relatively bad prognostic sign in pyelonephritis both in our view [31,32] and in that of others [58] may indicate that glomerular lesions play some part in the development of both hypertension and progressive parenchymal damage in pyelonephritis.

It is possible that the glomerular lesions represent a form of antibody-complex glomerulonephritis related either to autoantibody formation following renal tissue necrosis or possibly to bacterial antigen. We have so far been unable to substantiate this using immunofluorescent staining techniques. Only one patient in whom the primary disease was clearly pyelonephritis had positive IgG and IgM staining in glomeruli and she could conceivably have had coincident glomerulonephritis. None have shown positive staining with antibody against the common *Escherichia coli* antigen.

The fact that 100 percent of our patients with pyelonephritis coming to dialysis and transplantation show glomerular lesions suggests that these may play some part in progression to renal failure.

References

1. Smythe, C. M.: Renal infection and hypertension—cause or effect. *In* Brest, A. N., and Moyer, J. H. (Eds.): Hypertension—Recent Advances. Philadelphia: Lea & Febiger, 1961, p. 143.
2. Weiss, S., and Parker, F., Jr.: Pyelonephritis: Its relationship to vascular lesions and arterial hypertension. Medicine 18:221, 1939.
3. Goldring, W., and Chasis, H.: Hypertension and Hypertensive Disease. New York: Commonwealth Fund, 1944.
4. Bell, E. T.: Renal Diseases. Philadelphia: Lea & Febiger, 1946.
5. Longcope, W. T.: Chronic bilateral pyelonephritis and its association with hypertension. Ann. Intern. Med. 11:149, 1937.
6. Brod, J.: Chronic pyelonephritis. Lancet 1: 973, 1956.
7. Kincaid-Smith, P., McMichael, J., and Murphy, E. A.: The clinical course and pathology of hypertension with papilloedema (malignant hypertension). Q. J. Med. 27:117, 1958.
8. Platt, R., and Davson, J.: A clinical and pathological study of renal disease. Part II. Diseases other than nephritis. Q. J. Med. 19: 33, 1950.
9. Grieble, H. G., and Jackson, G. G.: Bacteriuria, pyelonephritis, and hypertension. *In* Quinn, E. L., and Kass, E. H. (Eds.): Biology of Pyelonephritis. London: Churchill, 1960, p. 485.
10. Kleeman, C. R., Hewitt, W. L., and Guze, L. B.: Pyelonephritis. Medicine 39:3, 1960.
11. Kass, E. H.: Asymptomatic infection of the urinary tract. Trans. Assoc. Am. Physicians 69:56, 1956.
12. Kass, E. H., Miall, W. E., and Stuart, K. L.: Relationship of bacteriuria to hypertension. An epidemiological study. J. Clin. Invest. 40: 1053, 1961.
13. Miall, W. E., Kass, E. H., Ling, J., and Stuart, K. L.: Factors influencing arterial pressure in the population in Jamaica. Br. Med. J. 2:497, 1962.
14. Bengtsson, U., Högdahl, A. M., and Hood, B.: Chronic nonobstructive pyelonephritis and hypertension. Q. J. Med. 37:361, 1968.
15. Heale, W. F.: Chronic pyelonephritis in the adult. Aust. N.Z. J. Med. 1:283, 1971.
16. Breckenridge, A., Preger, L., Dollery, C. T., and Laws, J. W.: Hypertension in the young. Q. J. Med. 144:549, 1967.
17. Shapiro, A. P., Moutsos, S. E., Krifcher, E., and Sapira, J. D.: Hypertension, pyelonephritis and renal failure. Am. J. Cardiol. 17: 638, 1966.
18. Shapiro, A. P., Sapira, J. D., and Scheib, E. T.: Development of bacteriuria in a hypertensive population. Ann. Intern. Med. 74: 861, 1971.
19. Asscher, A. W., and Waters, W. E.: Significant bacteriuria in non-pregnant women. *In* Kincaid-Smith, P., and Fairley, K. F. (Eds.): Renal Infection and Renal Scarring. Mel-

bourne, Australia: Mercedes Press, 1971, p. 25.
20. Kincaid-Smith, P., and Bullen, M.: Bacteriuria in pregnancy. Lancet 1:396, 1965.
21. Stuart, K. L., Cummings, G. T. M., and Chin, W. A.: Bacteriuria prematurity and the hypertensive disorders of pregnancy. Br. Med. J. 1:554, 1965.
22. Kunin, C. M., and McCormack, R. C.: An epidemiological study of bacteriuria and blood pressure among nuns and working women. N. Engl. J. Med. 278:635, 1968.
23. Kunin, C. M.: Epidemiology of bacteriuria and its relation to pyelonephritis. J. Chronic Dis. 120:1, 1969.
24. Kunin, C. M.: The natural history of recurrent bacteriuria in schoolgirls. *In* Kincaid-Smith, P., and Fairley, K. F. (Eds.): Renal Infection and Renal Scarring. Melbourne, Australia: Mercedes Press, 1971, p. 3.
25. Little, P. J., and de Wardener, H. E.: Acute pyelonephritis: Incidence of recurrence in 100 patients. Lancet 2:1277, 1966.
26. Stamey, T. A., Govan, D. E., and Palmer, J. M.: The localization and treatment of urinary tract infection. The role of bactericidal urine levels as opposed to serum levels. Medicine 44:1, 1965.
27. Seng, O. B., and Kincaid-Smith, P.: Urine concentration after Pitressin administration in upper and lower urinary tract infection. Med. J. Aust. 1:982, 1969.
28. Bremner, D. A., Fairley, K. F., and Kincaid-Smith, P. The serum antibody response in renal and bladder infection. Med. J. Aust. 1:1069, 1969.
29. Fairley, K. F., Bond, A. G., and Adey, F. D.: The site of infection in pregnancy bacteriuria. Lancet 1:539, 1966.
30. Fairley, K. F., Bond, A. G., Brown, R. B., and Habersberger, P.: Simple test to determine the site of urinary tract infection. Lancet 2:427, 1967.
31. Fairley, K. F., Carson, N. E., Gutch, R. C., Leighton, P., O'Keefe, C. M., Grounds, A. D., Laird, E. C., McCallum, P. H. G., and Sleeman, M. B.: Site of infection in acute urinary tract infection in general practice. Lancet 2: 615, 1971.
32. Fairley, K. F.: The routine determination of the site of infection in the investigation of patients with urinary tract infection. *In* Kincaid-Smith, P., and Fairley, K. F. (Eds.): Renal Infection and Renal Scarring. Melbourne, Australia: Mercedes Press, 1971, p. 107.
33. Bullen, M., and Kincaid-Smith, P.: Asymptomatic pregnancy bacteriuria. A follow-up 4–7 years after delivery. *In* Kincaid-Smith, P., and Fairley, K. F. (Eds.): Renal Infection and Renal Scarring. Melbourne, Australia: Mercedes Press, 1971, p. 33.
34. Still, J. L., and Cottam, D.: Severe hypertension in children. Arch. Dis. Child. 42:34, 1967.
35. Hodson, C. J., and Wilson, S.: The natural history of pyelonephritic scarring. Br. Med. J. 2:191, 1965.
36. Kincaid-Smith, P., and Fairley, K. F. (Eds.): Renal Infection and Renal Scarring. Melbourne, Australia: Mercedes Press, 1971.
37. Kincaid-Smith, P.: Vascular obstruction in chronic pyelonephritic kidneys and its relation to hypertension. Lancet 2:1263, 1955.
38. Kincaid-Smith, P.: (Discussion) *In* Kass, E. H. (Ed.): Progress in Pyelonephritis. Philadelphia: Davis, 1965, p. 683.
39. Fairley, K. F., and Butler, H. M.: Sterile pyuria as a manifestation of occult bacterial pyelonephritis. *In* Kincaid-Smith, P., and Fairley, K. F. (Eds.): Renal Infection and Renal Scarring. Melbourne, Australia: Mercedes Press, 1971, p. 51.
40. Dawborn, J. K., Fairley, K. F., Kincaid-Smith, P., and King, W. E.: The association of peptic ulceration, chronic renal disease and analgesic abuse. Q. J. Med. 35:69, 1966.
41. Kincaid-Smith, P.: Pathogenesis of the renal lesion associated with abuse of analgesics. Lancet 1:859, 1967.
42. Kincaid-Smith, P.: Analgesic nephropathy: A common form of renal disease in Australia. Med. J. Aust. 2:1131, 1969.
43. Heptinstall, R. H.: The limitations of the pathological diagnosis of chronic pyelonephritis. *In* Black, D. A. K. (Ed.): Renal Disease. Oxford: Blackwell, 1967, p. 350.
44. Stamey, T. A.: Workshop summary and comment. *In* Stamey, T. A., and Hinman, F. (Eds.): Urinary Infections in the Male. Washington D.C., National Research Council, National Academy of Sciences, 1967.
45. Fair, W. R.: Observations on the origin of urinary tract infections. *In* Kincaid-Smith, P., and Fairley, K. F. (Eds.): Renal Infection and Renal Scarring. Melbourne, Australia: Mercedes Press, 1971, p. 89.
46. Stamey, T. A., Timothy, M., Millar, M., and Mihara, G.: Recurrent urinary infections in adult women—the role of introital enterobacteria. Calif. Med. 115:1, 1971.
47. Kincaid-Smith, P., and Fairley, K. F.: The

diagnosis of urinary tract infection. Hosp. Med. 1:993, 1967.

48. Farmer, E. R., and Heptinstall, R. H.: Chronic non-obstructive pyelonephritis—A reappraisal. *In* Kincaid-Smith, P., and Fairley, K. F. (Eds.): Renal Infection and Renal Scarring. Melbourne, Australia: Mercedes Press, 1971, p. 233.
49. Hare, W. S. C.: The radiology of analgesic nephropathy. *In* Kincaid-Smith, P., and Fairley, K. F. (Eds.): Renal Infection and Renal Scarring. Melbourne, Australia: Mercedes Press, 1971, p. 233.
50. Smellie, J. M., and Normand, I. C. S.: Experience of follow-up of children with urinary tract infection. *In* O'Grady, F., and Brumfitt, W. (Eds.): Urinary Tract Infection. London: Oxford University Press, 1968, p. 123.
51. Hodson, C. J.: The mechanism of scar formation in chronic pyelonephritis. *In* Kincaid-Smith, P., and Fairley, K. F. (Eds.): Renal Infection and Renal Scarring. Melbourne, Australia: Mercedes Press, 1971, p. 327.
52. Shannon, F. T.: The significance and management of vesicoureteric reflux in infancy: Clinical aspects. *In* Kincaid-Smith, P., and Fairley, K. F. (Eds.): Renal Infection and Renal Scarring. Melbourne, Australia: Mercedes Press, 1971, p. 241.
53. Rolleston, G. L.: The significance and management of vesicoureteric reflux in infancy: Radiological aspects. *In* Kincaid-Smith, P., and Fairley, K. F. (Eds.): Renal Infection and Renal Scarring. Melbourne, Australia: Mercedes Press, 1971, p. 246.
54. Kincaid-Smith, P.: Renal ischemia and hypertension: A review of the results of surgery. Australas. Ann. Med. 10:166, 1961.
55. Heptinstall, R. H.: *In* Heptinstall, R. H.: Pathology of the Kidney. Boston: Little, Brown, 1966, p. 448.
56. Kimmelstiel, P., and Wilson, C.: Inflammatory lesions in glomeruli in pyelonephritis in relation to hypertension and renal insufficiency. Am. J. Pathol. 12:99, 1936.
57. Heptinstall, R. H.: *In* Heptinstall, R. H.: Pathology of the Kidney. Boston: Little, Brown, 1966, p. 430.
58. Zinsser, H. H., and Dryfus, J.: Prospective pyelonephritis study. Abstracts, American Society of Nephrology, 1970, p. 89.

Morphologic Abnormalities of the Renal Artery Associated with Hypertension

By Lawrence J. McCormack, M.D., M.S. Path.

Fifteen years ago my colleagues and I pointed out that other pathologic processes besides atherosclerosis and thrombosis could obstruct the main renal artery and/or its major branches, thereby initiating hypertension.[1] Unfortunately, one of the terms used, "fibromuscular hyperplasia," was more euphonious than the rest and was seized upon by many as an overall generic term for the fibrotic lesions encountered. Recently, Dr. E. G. Harrison and I have been able to agree on a classification that has totally eradicated the classification "fibromuscular hyperplasia."[2] Unfortunately, no etiologic factor has been elucidated for any of the fibrous dysplasias other than sex. As a consequence the classification we have recommended is based primarily on the location of the alteration (or dysplasia). The classification is as follows:

Dysplasias of the Renal Artery

- I. Intimal—Intimal fibroplasia
  - a. Primary
  - b. Secondary
- II. Medial
  - a. Medial dissection
  - b. Medial hyperplasia
  - c. Medial fibroplasia with aneurysms
  - d. Perimedial fibroplasia
    - 1. Isolated
    - 2. With intimal fibroplasia
- III. Periadventitial fibroplasia

Primary Intimal Fibroplasia. Although among the rarest of the fibrotic lesions of the renal artery, primary intimal fibroplasia is one of the most intriguing. The lesion basically consists of a circumferential occluding mass of primitive collagen that occupies varying amounts of the arterial lumen (Fig. 1). It involves the main renal artery for varying distances and can be seen to extend into the main branches of the vessel. There appears to be a difference between lesions demonstrated in childhood and those in adult life. In childhood, it appears that there is a major disorganization of arterial formation since not only is the intima involved but there are important changes within the internal elastic membrane, i.e., it may be reduplicated, fragmented, or partially absent (Fig. 2). Although not invariably so, the childhood variety unfortunately may involve other systemic arteries, and evidence of occlusive vascular disease in the extremities or in the gastrointestinal tract may also be present.

The changes found in older people are not nearly so severe since the lesions appear limited to the intima alone (Fig. 3). Once again, however, this is not a lesion solely characteristic of the renal artery; we have seen evidences of it in other arteries of the body including the brachial and intestinal. Other investigators also have noted a widespread distribution of the disorder. Some of the lesions reported from

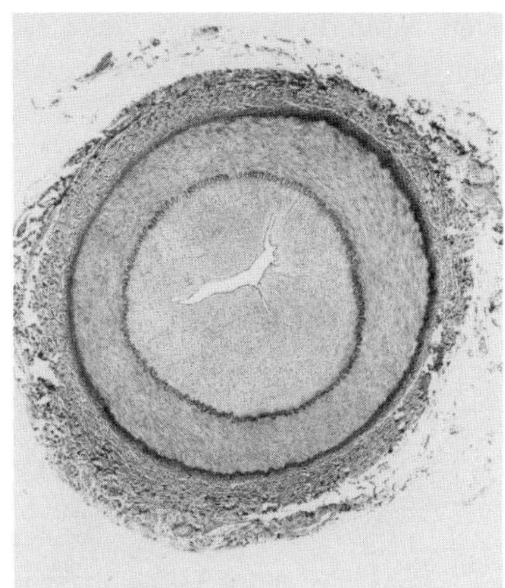

Fig. 1.—Photomicrograph of intimal fibroplasia in adult shows an enormous increase of collagen superficial to the internal elastic lamella that stains black (inner line). Verhoeff elastic-van Gieson. ×15.

From The Cleveland Clinic Foundation and The Cleveland Clinic Educational Foundation, Cleveland, Ohio.

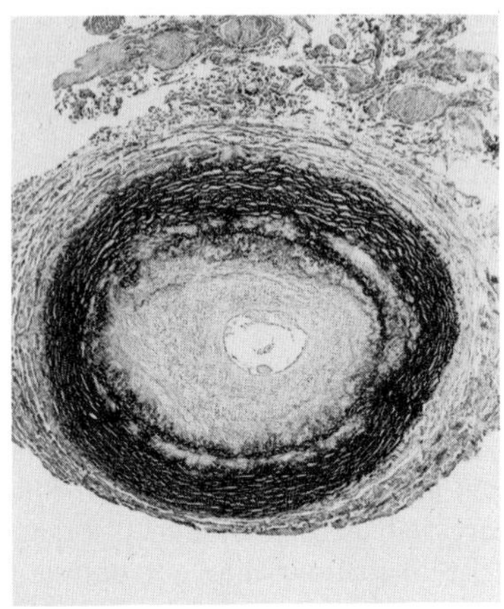

FIG. 2.—Intimal fibroplasia close to aorta in a child. Verhoeff elastic-van Gieson. ×55.

other countries of the world, where there supposedly is a low incidence of atherosclerosis, demonstrate that this arterial lesion can occur even in coronary arteries of young Korean soldiers. It must be emphasized that these lesions show no evidence of being part of atherogenesis. Special stains for lipids demonstrate none of this material to be present. These disorders occur predominantly in young people and if only the renal artery is involved, long-term cures can be anticipated as a result of carefully planned therapy.

Secondary Intimal Fibroplasia. The perplexing part of the primary lesion is its possible relationship to what we have classified as "secondary intimal fibroplasia." This disorder occurs under a wide variety of circumstances. It apparently may be a part of aging so far as the branches of the uterine artery are concerned. It can be also introduced by an inflammatory reaction since such thickening is a prominent feature of pyelonephritis. Actually it can be seen in inflammatory scars of any organ; the margins of old tuberculous foci in the lung will show such a marked intimal proliferation. In these circumstances I believe the cause to be an acute arteritis of the vessel itself. Recent studies of kidneys removed from individuals on long-term dialysis demonstrate a large accumulation of immature collagen within the arterial intimae; the production of intimal collagen seems to be a basic body mechanism designed to exclude a structure that is no longer useful. The purpose of such accumulation could be an attempt on the part of the body to conserve its blood supply for other uses. Another factor in production of intimal collagen may be that it is caused initially by platelet deposition as a result of marked slowing of blood flow through an organ system. Some time ago Beland, Schneckloth, and I called attention to the fact that this lesion is prominent in certain patients with treated malignant hypertension.[3] There the extreme hypertension recurs after a period of time, accompanied by renal failure; but the kidneys appear atrophic, showing only intimal fibroplasia of the larger arteries but no other evidence of the acute reactions seen in the untreated group. Finally, so far as secondary intimal hyperplasia is concerned, Harrison and I decided to exclude from the group of primary intimal fibroplasias those that had medial dissection plus intimal fibroplasia and place them in a separate category. I originally had included them in the intimal fibroplasia group, since I believed that the dissection occurred secondary to the damage of the renal artery indirectly produced by the intimal fibroplasia, postulating that some type of a "jet lesion" destroyed the intima and caused damage to the internal elastica distal to the stenosis.

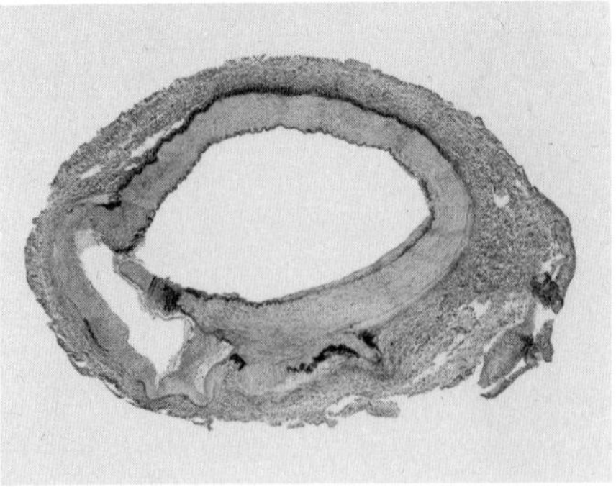

FIG. 3.—Medial dissection; this shows defect in internal elastic membrane as the probable mechanism for blood entering the media. Verhoeff elastic-van Gieson. ×15.

As experience was accumulated I found that the origin of the dissecting hematoma could occur proximal to the area of intimal fibroplasia. I now believe that the intimal fibroplasia must occur as a result of a secondary accumulation of fibrous tissue, due to hemodynamic changes in the area of narrowing caused by the dissection, similar to those that apparently occur in coarctation of the aorta. Coarctation in very young individuals has a different morphologic appearance from that in young adults. In older individuals large amounts of intimal collagen apparently accumulate, further narrowing the lumen of the coarctation.

Medial Dissection. This is most protean in its morphologic characteristics. The lesion may occur in either sex and in any age group. We have carefully excluded these lesions from those dissections that are associated with a lipid-containing atheroma. The remaining lesions probably have a pathogenesis related to a defect in the internal elastica of the renal artery that allows blood to escape into the muscular media (Fig. 3). The hematoma may extend for varying distances along the renal artery but does not dissect proximally into the aorta. Failure to do so is probably related to the peculiar morphology of the relationship between the aortic elastic tissue and the muscular media of the renal artery. Remember that the elastica of the aorta blends obliquely with the muscular media in such a manner that a channel in the media would not be able to penetrate the aortic elastic tissue because of sidetracking. The hematoma itself usually contains clot. Depending upon the age of the process, the clot may or may not be organized. Organization of the clot produces a mass of fibrous tissue that contains many vascular channels; some might be tempted to use the descriptive term "angiomatoid transformation of the intima" (Fig. 4). The clot also can stimulate a major and productive reaction in the media with the formation of much immature collagen; it therefore requires very careful study to demonstrate the exact nature of the lesion (Fig. 5). As was mentioned earlier, an intimal proliferative reaction can occur that may be located either proximally or distally to the point of dissection. Complete occlusion of the original arterial lumen by an old thrombus can also be found in association with the dissection. It therefore appears that the intimal reaction is entirely dependent upon the blood attempting to flow past the point of compression. These dissections can involve main branches as well as the renal artery itself. Surgical problems occur when dissections extend into several branches of the renal artery and under such circumstances it may be impossible to save the kidney.

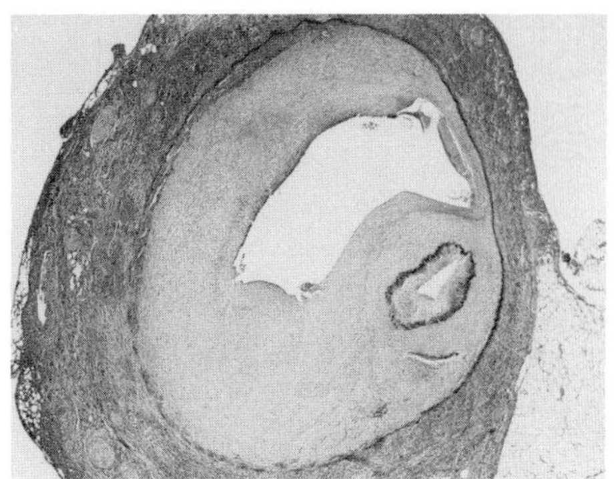

FIG. 5.—Photomicrograph of dissecting hematoma with intimal fibroplasia in a branch artery. Verhoeff elastic-van Gieson. ×20.

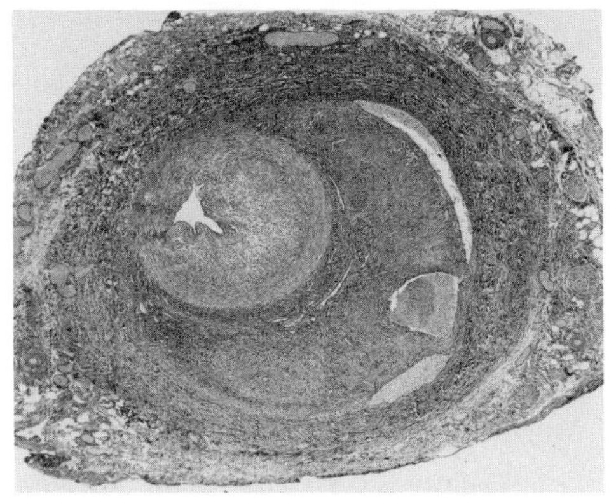

FIG. 4.—Medial dissection; this shows organization and angiomatous transformation, with associated intimal fibroplasia. Masson trichrome. ×22.

Fibrotic lesions of the media are totally perplexing so far as pathogenesis is concerned. On the one hand, a lesion like perimedial fibroplasia would seem to be acquired. On the other hand, lesions like muscular hyperplasia and fibrous dysplasia with microaneurysms certainly appear to be related to a defect in the internal elastica or in the formation of the muscular media.

Medial Hyperplasia. This entity was originally represented by some of us [4] under the term "fibromuscular hyperplasia" (Fig. 6). Our initial encounter with it was in a case of

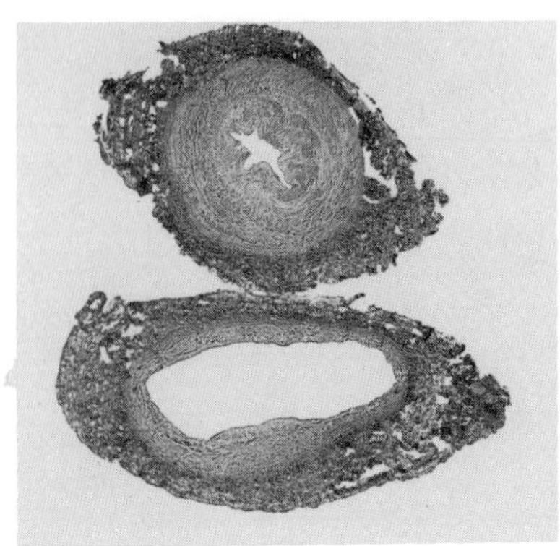

FIG. 6.—Medial hyperplasia and the somewhat dilated segment of artery found distal to the hyperplasia. Mallory-Heidenhain. ×15.

a young boy with bilateral renal arterial lesions. In both arteries, the media had localized accumulations of both muscle and collagen, with varying losses of internal elastica. The bilateral stenosis was extreme and was accompanied by poststenotic dilatation. However, overall, the lesion appears to be much more muscular in the majority of the patients, occurring primarily in young women. The mass of muscle may be variable as to both degree of concentricity and degree of longitudinal involvement, although most characteristically, the segment of involvement is short. There may be some defects of the internal elastica associated with it, and small areas of lesion may resemble medial dysplasia with aneurysms.

Medial Fibroplasia with Aneurysms. This classification remained an enigma to me for a considerable period of time. For some reason, while I was accumulating cases of perimedial fibroplasia, Dr. Harrison was accumulating an equal number of cases of medial fibroplasia with microaneurysms but few cases of perimedial fibroplasia. This led to some confusion between us since neither could quite understand the other's findings. It now seems reasonable to accept medial fibroplasia with microaneurysms as a disorder mostly but not exclusively of women, usually young, which commonly occurs bilaterally. Again, this lesion may not be limited exclusively to the renal artery, although this is usually the vessel involved. Arteriograms from other areas than the main renal artery and its major branches have been interpreted as meaning that such vessels as the carotid may be involved. Being a morphologist, I am unconvinced when no tissue is available as I have seen beautifully beaded angiograms of the renal artery, with nothing demonstrable at autopsy so far as the vessel is concerned. Spasm in a large artery can mimic the changes caused by a morphologic lesion.

I was further confused by the fact that I have found renal arteries extremely difficult to examine. No matter what method one follows, there are many instances when one wishes he had used another. All of these arteries can be studied by either transverse or longitudinal sections. The transverse or cross sections many times appear entirely different from the longitudinal ones and it is only when one has studied several by both methods that the true morphologic pattern emerges (Fig. 7). The most prominent feature of medial dysplasia is the discontinuity and loss of the internal elastica. In focal areas it appears completely intact and in others lost. In the areas where it is intact, the surrounding media contains large quantities of collagen as well as smooth muscle. There is no doubt that these large fibrocollagenous masses do constrict and serve as barriers to arterial blood flow. In the areas where the internal elastica is lost, there is marked thinning to complete loss of the media, and the outer wall of the segmental dilatation of the lumen may be

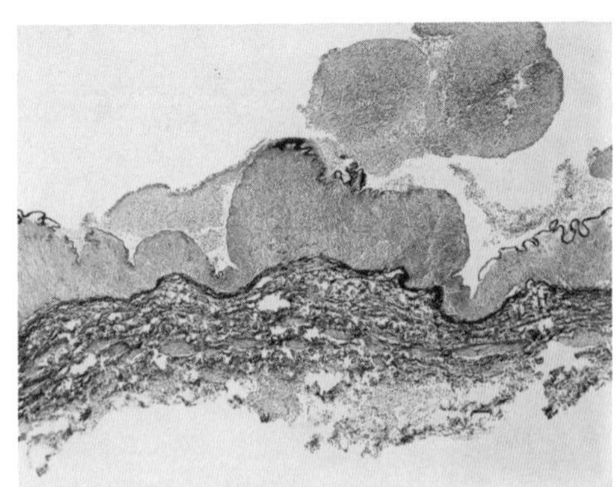

FIG. 7.—Medial fibroplasia with aneurysms; this shows the extreme variability in thickness of the media and the thinned areas that form the aneurysmal outpouchings or "breading." Verhoeff elastic-van Gieson. ×20.

formed entirely by the adventitia and the elastica externa. It is these losses of media that are responsible for the "beads," larger than the diameter of the lumen of the vessels, that appear on the roentgenogram. Although this lesion can extend into branches of the renal artery, often it is not seen involving the first portion of the renal artery. It is therefore possible to use this area for comparison. Why such lesions occur dominantly on the right side and at times are bilateral is totally obscure. I have seen only one instance of a large aneurysm associated with the small ones. Other intriguing facts are the total lack of thrombosis within these lesions and the total lack of evidences of any proximal or distal dissection, a phenomenon one might expect. I believe the explanation for the lack of this dissection rests in the large amount of collagen present within the remaining media that serves as a tether for that particular segment of musculature and does not allow blood to dissect within the media. Here also there can occur some intimal accumulation of collagen. I suspect once again it is secondary and related to platelet deposition and subsequent organization due to turbulence in blood flow.

Perimedial Fibroplasia. This is a most fascinating lesion.[5] My original descriptions were a bit confusing since I first classified the lesion merely as a medial scar. At that particular time I was studying the vessels only by longitudinal section and had a great deal of difficulty in understanding their appearance. Later, with cross sections, I determined that the lesion consisted of a thick layer of mature collagen that completely surrounded the media, partially to completely replacing it and sometimes replacing a portion of the external elastic layers as well (Fig. 8). However, extensive remnants of this particular structure, the external elastica, can be demonstrated. It also can be demonstrated that this collagenous zone is of variable thickness and will thereby produce varying degrees of constriction of the arterial lumen (Fig. 9). Whereas the beads seen in medial dysplasia with aneurysm are larger than the diameter of the proximal normal vessel, the beads of perimedial fibroplasia are smaller than the diameter of the proximal arterial segment. This lesion also occurs mostly in young women; but again, not exclusively, so that it cannot be stated that it is related to pregnancy. The lesion may be bilateral, but if it is unilateral, it occurs most commonly on the right. The reason for this peculiar distribution is totally inexplicable. However, I have on rare occasions encountered what I believe to be the earliest change wherein irregular masses of collagen can be seen lying just internally to the external elastic membranes.

At times one can also encounter a thickening of the intima by collagen, but in such irregular quantity that, once again, I believe it to be a secondary phenomenon as a result of variable blood flow related to old fibrin and platelet deposition. Only once in more than 40 cases

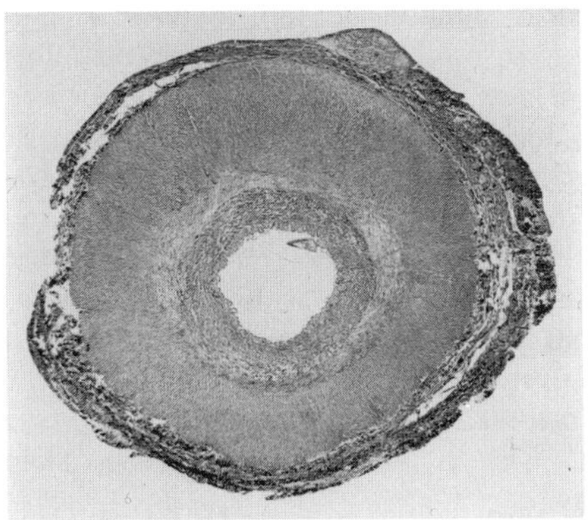

FIG. 8.—Photomicrograph shows cross section of perimedial fibroplasia with a dense collar of collagen that occurs just outside the media. Masson trichrome. ×20.

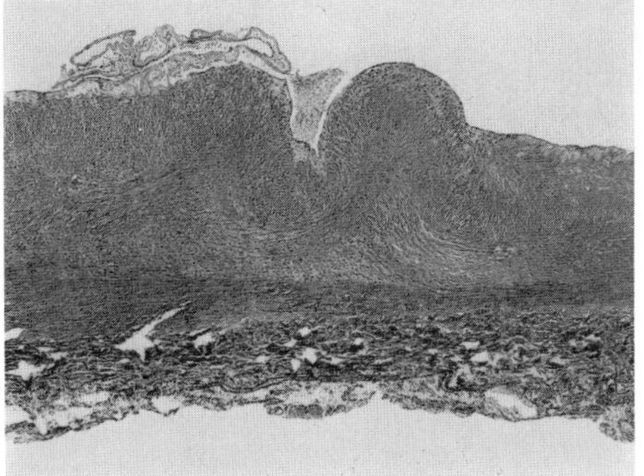

FIG. 9.—Perimedial fibroplasia in longitudinal section shows the variability in thickness of the collagenous collar. Mallory-Heidenhain. ×50.

have I encountered what I believe to be a secondary phenomenon, i.e., an associated complete thrombotic occlusion of the renal artery. Certainly, dissection is not a feature of this particular renal arterial lesion.

Periadventitial Fibroplasia. This is an extremely rare lesion and the only instances I have seen are those that Dr. Harrison demonstrated to me. I suspect that this disorder is related to the problem of sclerosing retroperitonitis and is some type of inflammatory reaction within the adventitia of the renal artery.

I would be remiss if I did not briefly mention the most common cause of renal artery obstruction, *atherosclerosis* (Fig. 10). The lesions can occur as either eccentric (Fig. 11) or concentric plaques, and dominantly occur in the first part of the renal artery, especially at the orifice. However, atherosclerosis is not limited to this distribution and may even be encountered as obstructing lesions of branches of the renal artery. The morphologic pattern is no different from that found anywhere else; all stages of lipid deposition can be found, varying from many lipophages to the accumulation of a "pool of putty." Further complications can occur in the form of either thrombosis or dissection. I suspect that these last two may be at times responsible for the sudden appearance of extreme hypertension. It is known that an individual can have atheromatous involvement of his renal arteries and yet be completely normotensive.

The occurrence of a renal artery totally occluded by thrombus only is also associated with hypertension. The distinction as to whether the occlusion is an embolus or a thrombus is usually beyond the morphologist's skill. These lesions seem to occur in both a primary form without prior incident and, rarely, secondarily, apparently in association with some inflammatory reaction in the medial and the adventitial areas although it may be difficult to prove that the arteritis was not the primary cause. Secondary lesions can also occur as a result of trauma. Dr. Gifford, our associates, and I have recently reported our experiences with the relationships of renal trauma and hypertension, and have included several of these occlusions within the group.[6]

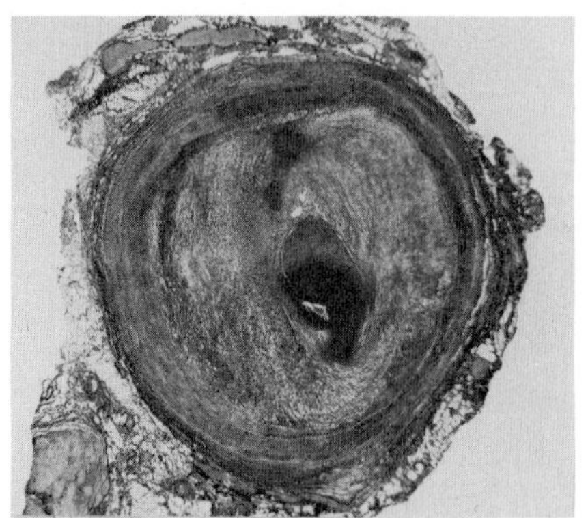

FIG. 10.—Severe concentric atherosclerosis with recent thrombus. Mallory-Heidenhain. ×10.

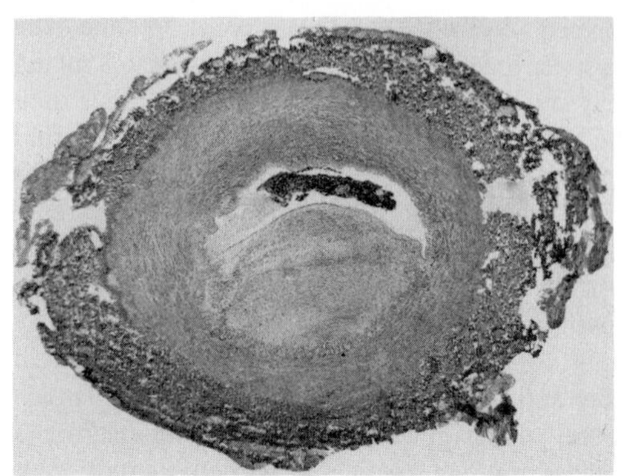

FIG. 11.—Eccentric atherosclerotic plaque. Masson. ×20.

In summary, the renal artery is beset by a large variety of lesions attempting to interfere with its blood flow. Atherosclerosis is by far the most common, but individuals in a younger age group suffer a wide variety of fibrotic lesions that may be classified on the basis of their location within the renal artery. It is unfortunate that we cannot at this time classify them on an etiologic basis. I therefore recognize intimal fibroplasia, medial hyperplasia, intimal fibroplasia with microaneurysms, medial dissection, perimedial fibroplasia and periadventitial fibroplasia. Each of these is a separate and distinct morphologic entity and each has a singularly different biologic behavior.

REFERENCES

1. McCormack, L. J., Hazard, J. B., and Poutasse, E. F.: Obstructive lesions of the

renal artery associated with remediable hypertension. Am. J. Pathol. 34:582, 1958.

2. Harrison, E. G., and McCormack, L. J.: Pathologic classification of renal arterial disease in renovascular hypertension. Mayo Clin. Proc. 46:161, 1971.
3. McCormack, L. J., Beland, J. E., and Schneckloth, R. E.: Morphologic changes in malignant nephrosclerosis after treatment with potent antihypertensive drugs. Am. J. Pathol. 33:622, 1957. (Abstract)
4. Poutasse, E. F., Humphries, A. W., McCormack, L. J., and Corcoran, A. C.: Bilateral stenosis of renal arteries and hypertension; treatment by arterial homografts. JAMA 161:419, 1956.
5. McCormack, L. J., Noto, T. J., Meaney, T. F., Poutasse, E. F., and Dustan, H. P.: Subadventitial fibroplasia of the renal artery, a disease of young women. Am. Heart J. 73: 602, 1967.
6. Grant, R. P., Gifford, R. W., Jr., Pudvan, W. R., Meaney, T. F., Straffon, R. A., and McCormack, L. J.: Renal trauma and hypertension. Am. J. Cardiol. 27:173, 1971.

Renovascular Hypertension as a Clinical Syndrome

By Harriet P. Dustan, M.D., Morton H. Maxwell, M.D., Norman M. Simon, M.D., and Joseph J. Bookstein, M.D.

IN THE 20 YEARS since translumbar aortography was recommended for diagnosis of stenosing lesions of arteries arising from the abdominal aorta,[1] renal arterial disease has become recognized as an important cause of hypertension. This technique made possible the antemortem diagnosis of a type of hypertension that had been suggested by the earlier demonstration of experimental hypertension produced by partial renal artery clamping,[2] by the first descriptions of the renal pressor system,[3,4] and two reports in children of obstructed renal arteries associated with hypertension.[5,6]

Although these occlusive lesions are a numerically significant cause of hypertension, they do not occur very frequently. Further, definitive diagnosis is neither simple nor inexpensive since it is based on renal arteriography, which is expensive and unpleasant, and requires hospitalization. Thus, there is need for easy clues that will indicate those patients who have renovascular hypertension. With the early descriptive studies of this type of hypertension, the possibility of such clues seemed very real. These studies were clearly influenced by two reports of unilateral renal disease causing hypertension that were published before the era of aortography [7,8] and also by the types of patients in whom the diagnosis was first made; these, for the most part, were unusual patients who had either symptoms or signs suggesting a type of hypertension not usually seen. Subsequently it became clear that renovascular hypertensives cannot be surely separated from other patients on clinical grounds alone; in retrospect, considering what was known about the broad spectrum of hypertension, it seems naïve to have thought that they might be.

Before renal arteriography had become available, Sensenbach,[7] as well as Perera and Haelig,[8] had suggested that surgically remediable renal hypertension has distinctive clinical features. Both reports stressed hypertension of short duration and severe vascular disease occurring in young people (<25 years) and in older people (>50 years), at ages when hypertension does not usually begin. Howard et al.[9] were likewise impressed by these findings. When arteriography first became available it was not widely used because of concern over its safety and consequently was usually reserved for study of patients with unusual symptoms or gross urographic abnormalities. Thus it is not surprising that suggestions of distinctive clinical characteristics continued to be reported. Some of these included no family history of hypertension [10]; flank pain preceding either onset of hypertension or acceleration of vascular disease in patients known to be hypertensive [10]; an "overwhelming inner tension and restlessness" [11]; hypokalemia because of secondary aldosteronism [12]; relative orthostatic hypotension [13]; and an upper abdominal bruit.[14]

With increasing use of arteriography, based primarily on the presence of urographic abnormalities, enough experience was gained to begin assessing the scope of renovascular hypertension and its clinical characteristics.[15,16] In 1963, Wilson et al.[15] compared findings in 139 patients with renal arterial stenosis with 127 patients with essential hypertension. One of the unusual features of the report, for that time, was that all the essential hypertensives had had renal arteriography. The report stressed the absence of distinctive clinical characteristics and the frequency of urographic ab-

From the Research Division, The Cleveland Clinic Foundation and The Cleveland Clinic Educational Foundation, Cleveland, Ohio; Cedars-Sinai Medical Center, Los Angeles, Calif.; Passavant Memorial Hospital, Chicago, Ill.; and University of Michigan Medical Center, Ann Arbor, Mich.

This study was supported in part by Grant HE-6835 from the National Heart and Lung Institute, National Institutes of Health, and USPHS Grants HE-10356 and HE-06652.

normalities but suggested that certain clinical features could indicate patients more likely to have renovascular than essential hypertension. With the exception of upper abdominal bruits, these features related to inappropriate hypertension or vascular disease.[17] The term "inappropriate hypertension" was used to describe the onset of hypertension at an unusual age—either early (less than 35 years) or later (after 50 years)—and symptoms of atherosclerosis preceding the onset of hypertension because atherosclerosis caused by hypertension occurs after years of elevated arterial pressure. "Inappropriate vascular disease" described malignant hypertension of abrupt onset in a recently normotensive person, and the sudden acceleration of vascular disease.

In 1966, Maxwell, Kaufman, and Bleifer[16] reported on 180 patients with essential and renovascular hypertension, the latter being divided into those with atherosclerotic and nonatherosclerotic stenoses. They found that hypertensive heart disease and renal damage were more frequent in patients with atherosclerotic lesions than those with essential hypertension, without differences in the degree of hypertension. They also found that hypokalemia, taken to indicate secondary aldosteronism as Laidlaw, Yendt, and Gornall had suggested,[12] was related to the severity, rather than the cause, of hypertension.

These reports served to emphasize that hypertension caused by renal arterial stenosis presents the same broad spectrum of signs and symptoms found in other types, whether associated with renal parenchymal disease, pheochromocytoma or primary aldosteronism, or of unknown cause, essential hypertension. Further, they suggested that no matter how carefully a history is taken or a physical examination done, the best that information available from such sources can provide is varying degrees of probability that the hypertension is caused by occlusive renal arterial disease.

The Cooperative Study of Renovascular Hypertension

Early in the 1960s a national Cooperative Study of Renovascular Hypertension was begun, supported by Public Health Service research grants. Fifteen institutions participated and among them they studied a total of 2,442 hypertensive patients, of whom 880 had renal arterial disease. Reports on various aspects of renovascular hypertension and its comparison with essential hypertension are just now appearing. Since this constitutes the largest series of patients studied similarly—which was not the case for any of the other series—and is a definitive study of renovascular hypertension, the report concerning clinical characteristics is here summarized.[18]

The finding of renal arterial stenosis in a hypertensive patient does not constitute a diagnosis of renovascular hypertension. At the present time there is no way to make this diagnosis other than retrospectively as judged by cure of hypertension by nephrectomy or successful renal revascularization. Thus, in order for the Cooperative Study to assess the clinical characteristics of renovascular hypertension it was necessary to analyze those patients cured of hypertension by operation. There were 175 patients; 91 had atherosclerotic lesions and 84, fibrous or fibromuscular dysplasia. These patients were compared with 339 essential hypertensives chosen from the large pool of 1,128 patients because of their unequivocally normal intravenous urograms and renal arteriograms, similarity of function of the two kidneys as shown by "split function" tests, and absence of any evidence suggesting other known causes of hypertension. The results of this comparison (Table 1) clearly show that there are no distinctive clinical characteristics but that there are a number of features the presence of which strongly increases the likelihood of renovascular hypertension. In many ways this study strengthens the conclusions of previous studies.

In regard to sex distribution, the group of patients with fibrous dysplasia contained more women (81%) than the other two groups, a finding stressed by earlier studies. Also, as previously noted, there were significantly fewer blacks among the renal hypertensives than among essential hypertensives.

Several differences in regard to age appeared. The mean age of the patients with essential hypertension was 41 years and this was significantly older than that of patients with fibrous dysplasia (35 years). Known duration of hypertension was shorter in both renal hy-

TABLE 1.—*Clinical Characteristics of Essential and Renovascular Hypertension*

History and Physical Examination	Essential Hypertension	Renovascular Hypertension: Atherosclerosis	Renovascular Hypertension: Fibrous Dysplasia
History			
Age–years	41	50 *	35 *
History of hypertension			
Age at onset (years)	35	46 *	33
Duration (in years)	3.1	1.9 *	2.0 *
Sex (females) (%) †	40	34	81 *
Race (black) (%)	29	7 *	10 *
Acceleration of hypertension (%)	13	23 *	14 *
Family history			
Hypertension (%)	67	58	41 *
No vascular disease (%)	19	30	46 *
Atherosclerotic symptoms or signs (%)	10	20 *	6
Physical Examination			
Systolic blood pressure (mm Hg)	169	181 *	174
Fundi–Groups 3 and 4 (%)	12	26 *	10
Abdominal bruit (%)	7	41 *	57 *

Adapted from Simon, N. M., et al.[18]
* Indicates significant difference ($p < 0.05$ or $p < 0.01$) from essential hypertension.
† Percentage of patients in each group.

pertensive groups than in essential hypertensives and as a corollary there were significantly more essential hypertensives who had been hypertensive for longer than 10 years.

As suggested by earlier reports, the onset of hypertension after age 50 was more frequent in patients with atherosclerotic stenosis than in those with essential hypertension. Surprisingly, there was no difference between essential hypertensives and those with fibrous dysplasia in numbers of patients whose hypertension had developed prior to age 20.

It will be remembered that at one time lack of a family history of hypertension was thought a characteristic of renovascular hypertension. Although it did not emerge from this study as distinctive a feature as previously thought, there was a significantly lesser family history of hypertension as well as strokes, coronary artery disease, diabetes, and renal disease in patients with fibrous dysplasia than in the other two groups. Also, as would have been expected, those with atherosclerotic renal arterial disease, who were also older and had higher serum cholesterol levels, had previously had significantly more episodes of myocardial infarction, strokes, and symptoms of peripheral arterial occlusive disease.

For the three groups—essential hypertension, atherosclerotic stenoses, and fibrous stenoses—average arterial pressures were 169/109, 181/108, and 174/108 mm Hg, respectively. Only systolic pressure for the atherosclerotic renovascular hypertensives was significantly different. Even though average diastolic pressures were similar among the three groups, those with atherosclerotic stenoses had significantly more exudative and hemorrhagic retinopathy with or without papilledema (Keith-Wagener-Barker classification: Groups 3 and 4).

Abdominal bruits warrant special emphasis because of their potential usefulness in indicating those patients with renal arterial disease. Either upper abdominal or flank bruits were found in 41 percent of patients with atherosclerosis and in 57 percent of those with fibrous dysplasia, in contrast to only a 7-percent occurrence in patients with essential hypertension. This report of the Cooperative Study stresses that since essential hypertension is many times more frequent than renovascular hypertension and since such patients occasionally have bruits, the finding of an upper abdominal bruit, of itself, signifies nothing diagnostically. However, the report does not calculate the possibility of a bruit having greater diagnostic significance in women less than 35 years of age or in children. Surely, such a calculation would increase the significance because essential hypertensives with bruits are more apt to be older patients who have abdominal atherosclerosis.

Urographic Abnormalities As Part of the Clinical Syndrome

Although urographic findings in renovascular hypertension cannot be taken strictly as clinical characteristics, urography is so readily available and so widely used that it becomes an extension of the clinical examination of a hypertensive patient. Howard et al.[9] drew attention to the presence of urographic abnormalities in patients with renal arterial disease and this point has been stressed in all subsequent reports.[19] The matter of importance with this test is, of course, the frequency of urographic abnormalities in such patients and thus the value of urography as a screening procedure.

Reports from the Cooperative Study should settle the question concerning the frequency of abnormalities because they will analyze results from the largest number of patients ever studied. Although the entire experience is not available for review, a study of urography in unilateral renal arterial disease has been completed [20] and will be summarized here (Table 2).

Urograms done with rapid-sequence filming were available for review in 771 essential hypertensives and 398 patients with renal arterial disease. Films were considered acceptable for review if their quality was such as to allow an accurate measurement of renal lengths, assessment of disparity in calyceal appearance time of contrast material, and estimation of differences in concentration of contrast material on late films. Not only were the features compared between the essential and renal hypertensive groups but in the latter, they were also related to the degree of stenosis as judged from the renal arteriogram to be: less than 50 percent, 50 to 80 percent, 80 to 99 percent, or complete.

Disparities in renal length, in calyceal appearance time on early films, and in concentration of the contrast medium on late films were found to be the most important urographic features of renal arterial disease. Other features that may be present in a few patients were considered ancillary; these include ureteral notching by collateral vessels, decreased volume of a collecting system or narrow calyces and infundibulae, segmental parenchymal atrophy and degree of renal ptosis on films taken in the upright position.

Because the left kidney is normally longer than the right, disparity in length was considered significant if the left kidney was 2 cm or longer than the right, or the right 1.5 cm

Table 2.—*Frequency of Urographic Abnormalities in Patients with Essential Hypertension and Renal Arterial Stenosis*

		Abnormalities (% of patients)		
	Abnormal Urograms (%)	*Calyceal Appearance Time*	*Medium Concentration (Late)*	*Renal Length*
Essential Hypertension	11.4	2.0	4.3	5.6
Renal Arterial Stenosis				
< 50% *	22.3	5.6	7.2	5.6
50–80%	64.0	47.7	24.9	26.6
80–99%	82.8	60.5	49.0	36.0
100%	95.7	80.8	67.8	74.3

Adapted from Bookstein, J. J., et al.[20]
* Degree of stenosis as judged from arteriogram.

or longer than the left. Disparity in calyceal appearance time was considered significant if there was at least a 1-minute difference between the two sides.

Among the 771 patients with essential hypertension, 11.4 percent had abnormal urograms; in 5.6 percent there was disparity in length, and in 2.0 percent a disparity in appearance time; 4.3 percent showed hyperconcentration on late films. Practically none had more than one of the three major abnormalities.

Among the renal hypertensive group, for those with less than 50 percent stenosis, urograms were abnormal in 22.3 percent, but for greater degrees of stenosis (> 50-100%), the occurrence of abnormal urograms rose to 78.2 percent and often more than one abnormality was found. Considering each feature separately in this subgroup, 38.6 percent had a disparity in length, 59.0 percent in appearance time, and 42.4 percent had hyperconcentration. It was not surprising to find that with increasing degrees of stenosis the frequency of abnormalities, singly or in combination, increased. When stenosis was less than 50 percent, there was a slightly increased frequency in disparity of appearance time (5.6%) and in hyperconcentration (7.2%) over that found in essential hypertensives, but only one of these patients had more than one urographic sign. In contrast, when stenoses had produced 80 to 99 percent luminal narrowing, 83 percent of patients had abnormalities. Delayed appearance time, either alone or in combination, was the most frequently encountered abnormality and 65 percent of patients had two or more abnormalities.

Several other points emerged from this study. For instance, for any degree of stenosis, the urogram was never invariably abnormal. Even among the 47 patients who had complete occlusion of the main renal artery, there were two with normal urograms; presumably this was because of good collateral blood flow which was apparent from the arteriogram. The ancillary urographic features, although sometimes present, did not improve the urogram as a screening test. And finally, as could have been predicted, neither major nor minor urographic abnormalities had any value in discriminating between hypertension with renal arterial disease and renovascular hypertension curable by an operative procedure.

This report deals only with urographic features of main renal arterial disease, so it does not discuss the value of urography in indicating those patients who have bilateral main renal arterial lesions or stenosis of one or more primary arterial branches. In regard to unilateral lesions, the study is invaluable because for the first time the urographic features of large groups of similarly studied patients with essential and renovascular hypertension are compared.

Summary

Study of patients with occlusive renal arterial disease during the past 20 years has shown that renovascular hypertension causes no exclusively distinctive, clinical characteristics that permit diagnosis without arteriography. There are, however, several clinical features which, when present, increase the probability of finding arterial lesions.

Patients with fibrous dysplasias, when compared with essential hypertensives, are younger, are more often women, are less often black, have hypertension of shorter duration, a lesser family history of hypertension, atherosclerotic complications, diabetes, renal disease, and a markedly increased frequency of upper abdominal bruits.

Patients with atherosclerotic stenoses, when compared with essential hypertensives, are older, are less often black, may have onset of hypertension after the age of 50 years, have shorter duration of hypertension, are more likely to have exudative and hemorrhagic retinopathy with or without papilledema, have more symptoms of extrarenal atherosclerosis, and have a higher frequency of upper abdominal bruits.

The available information emphasizes the importance of rapid-sequence intravenous urography as a screening test for unilateral renal arterial occlusive disease. The important urographic features, in order of their numerical significance, are: delay in calyceal appearance time of contrast material, hyperconcentration of contrast material on late films, and disparity of renal length. In patients with essential hypertension, urographic abnormalities were found in 11.4 percent. In renovascular hypertensives, with less than 50 percent stenosis, only 22.3 percent had abnormalities; with increasing degrees of stenosis the frequency of abnormalities rose progressively, so that for the group with complete occlusion it reached 95.7 percent.

References

1. Smith, P. G., Rush, T. W., and Evans, A. T.: The technique of translumbar arteriography. JAMA 198:255, 1951.
2. Goldblatt, H., Lynch, J., Hanzal, R. F., and Summerville, W. W.: Studies on experimental hypertension. I. The production of persistent elevation of systolic blood pressure by means of renal ischemia. J. Exp. Med. 59:347, 1934.
3. Page, I. H., and Helmer, O. M.: A crystalline pressor substance, angiotonin, resulting from the reaction between renin and renin activator. Proc. Soc. Clin. Invest. 12:17, 1939.
4. Braun-Menendez, E., Fasciolo, J. C., Leloir, L. F., and Munoz, J. M.: The substance causing renal hypertension. J. Physiol. 98: 283, 1940.
5. Butler, A. M.: Chronic pyelonephritis and arterial hypertension. J. Clin. Invest. 16:889, 1937.
6. Leadbetter, W. F., and Burkland, C. E.: Hypertension in unilateral renal disease. J. Urol. 39:611, 1938.
7. Sensenbach, W.: Effects of unilateral nephrectomy in treatment of hypertension. Arch. Intern. Med. 73:123, 1944.
8. Perera, G. N., and Haelig, A. W.: Clinical characteristics of hypertension associated with unilateral renal disease. Circulation 6:349, 1952.
9. Howard, J. E., Berthrong, M., Gould, B. M., and Yendt, E. R.: Hypertension resulting from unilateral vascular disease and its relief by nephrectomy. Bull. Johns Hopkins Hosp. 94:51, 1954.
10. Poutasse, E. F., and Dustan, H. P.: Arteriosclerosis and renal hypertension. JAMA 165: 1521, 1957.
11. Birchall, R., Batson, H. M., Jr., and Moore, C. B.: Hypertension due to unilateral renal arterial obstruction: Preliminary observations on the contribution of differential renal clearance studies. Am. Heart J. 56:616, 1958.
12. Laidlaw, J. C., Yendt, E. R., and Gornall, A. G.: Hypertension caused by renal artery occlusion simulating primary aldosteronism. Metabolism 9:612, 1960.
13. Smithwick, R. H.: Surgery in treatment of hypertension of adrenal and renal origin. *In* Moyer, J. H. (Ed.): Hypertension. Philadelphia: Saunders, 1959, pp. 633–640.
14. Moser, R. J., Jr., and Caldwell, J. R., Jr.: Abdominal murmurs, an aid in the diagnosis of renal artery disease in hypertension. Ann. Intern. Med. 56:471, 1962.
15. Wilson, L. L., Dustan, H. P., Page, I. H., and Poutasse, E. F.: Diagnosis of renal arterial lesions. Arch. Intern. Med. 112:270, 1963.
16. Maxwell, M. H., Kaufman, J. J., and Bleifer, K. H.: Stenosing lesions of the renal arteries. Postgrad. Med. 40:247, 1966.
17. Dustan, H. P., and Page, I. H.: Renal hypertensive suspect: Clinical characteristics. Am. J. Surg. 107:35, 1964.
18. Simon, N. M., Franklin, S., Bleifer, K. H., and Maxwell, M. H.: Clinical characteristics of renovascular hypertension. JAMA 220: 1209, 1972.
19. Dustan, H. P. (Chap. Ed.): Renal arterial stenosis and parenchymal diseases. *In* Page, I. H. and McCubbin, J. W. (Eds.): Renal Hypertension. Chicago: Year Book, 1968, pp. 306–349.
20. Bookstein, J. J., Abrams, H. L., Buenger, R. E., Lecky, J., Franklin, S. S., Reiss, M. D., Bleifer, K. H., Klatte, E. C., Varady, P. D., and Maxwell, M. H.: Cooperative study of renovascular hypertension. Radiologic aspects of renovascular hypertension. Part II. Unilateral renovascular disease: the role of urography. JAMA 220:1225, 1972.

Renal Histologic Observations in Occlusive Disease of the Renal Artery

By Lawrence J. McCormack, M.D., M.S. Path.

Unfortunate disputes have marred the accumulation of knowledge concerning renal reaction to injury. At times it seems as though the remarks by prominent disputants have blocked further independent study of phases of the problem. The careful student of renovascular disease is acquainted with these errors of history and the difficulties engendered. I shall do my best to dwell upon what are known to be current areas of debate. No doubt there will be exceptions taken to my opinions as much as the exceptions I take to those of others. The facts are real; the interpretations may be transient. I only hope that I can select those that have stood well the test of time.

One must agree that the morphologic changes of renal reaction to injury involve the nephron and its surrounding investitures, the renal vasculature, and the problem of an inflammatory infiltrate. The relationships among these changes have been causes of considerable debate. This chapter will be limited to the changes in relationship to renovascular disease.

Most investigators agree that hypertension plays a major role in destroying renal vasculature. No segment of the renal arterial tree appears immune, be it large artery, small artery, or arteriole. However, pyelonephritis can have, in its acute phase, an associated violent arteritis or arteriolitis resulting in permanent changes in the renal vasculature. The inflammatory infiltrate of pyelonephritis can in part be mimicked by that seen in renal arterial disease. It is such overlappings of events with influences upon all segments of the kidney that have created so much difference of opinion.

I hope also that there is agreement that the closer the area of damage of the vascular tree is to the nephron, the more violent is the reaction of the nephron to this interference with its blood supply. Dislocation of an arteriole or an intralobular artery usually produces a zone of infarction and subsequent fibrosis and depressed scar. Involvement of the interlobular, arcuate, and large hilar arteries can also result in infarction but if the process is chronic such involvement seems to result in parenchymal atrophy with glomerular sparing. It is apparently this latter reaction of atrophy that occurs when the main renal artery is slowly occluded. Hopefully there is agreement (1) that primary involvement or obstruction of the main renal artery, under both experimental and natural conditions, can be responsible for the hypertension; and (2) that such blockade also exerts a protective influence upon the vasculature of the kidney distal to the blockade if infarction does not occur. This lack of renal necrosis may be related to some of the peculiarities of collateral circulation to the kidney wherein the capsular vessels seem to penetrate deep within renal parenchyma

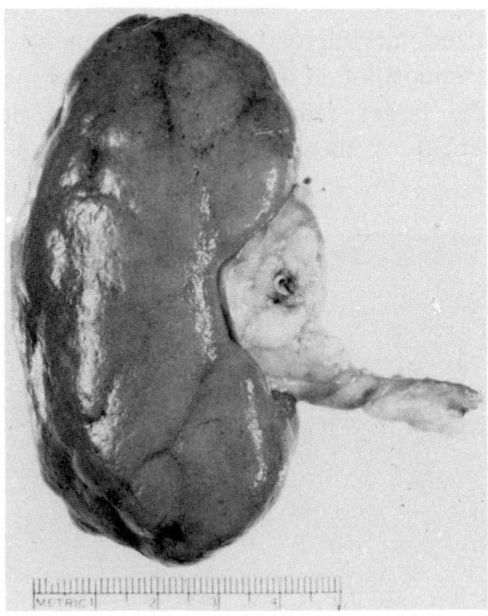

Fig. 1.—The small, smooth kidney of parenchymal atrophy, secondary to general ischemia caused by renal artery stenosis.

From The Cleveland Clinic Foundation and The Cleveland Clinic Educational Foundation, Cleveland, Ohio.

before making anastomoses with the main arterial channels.

The end-point of chronic major occlusion of the renal artery of a previously undiseased kidney is a small kidney with marked parenchymal atrophy (Fig. 1). Such a kidney is smooth and shows none of the granularities or focality of scarring seen in other renovascular or inflammatory diseases. Microscopic study demonstrates closely crowded, normal-appearing glomeruli without any evidences of arteriolar damage (Fig. 2). Various components of the renotubular system can no longer be positively identified. The tubules appear to be lined by a single layer of low cuboidal, undifferentiated cells. The individual nephrons appear separated by an increased amount of collagen. Whether this increase is real or merely a phanerosis is unknown to me. The larger renal arteries also show no evidences of morphologic damage. Scattered within the renal parenchyma may be found aggregates of "chronic inflammatory cells." Close examination reveals these cells to be lymphocytes, with occasionally a few progenitors. However, plasma cells and granulocytes are not a feature. It is our interpretation that such aggregates do not indicate pyelonephritic activity.

If, however, the kidney has previously been the site of chronic vascular disease in the form of arteriolar sclerosis and atherosclerosis, the superimposition of a major blockade at the level of the larger renal artery does not destroy evidences of the previous renovascular damage. The occurrence of a fresh atheroma at a renal arterial orifice or the superimposition of a thrombus upon a chronic atheroma at a renal orifice does not obliterate evidences of previously existing vascular disease. It is entirely possible that an individual can have extensive renal parenchymal vascular disease and remain normotensive. However, some type of internal balance may be disturbed by the further addition of either more atheromata or thrombosis and as a result hypertension ensues. It is entirely possible then to have an individual with major renal arterial occlusion as the genesis of his hypertensions and with parenchymal vascular disease. It therefore follows that biopsy of such a kidney and the recognition of these vascular changes really play no role in determining whether the vascular disease seen should influence the type of therapy.

There is ample evidence to suggest that a period of hypertension may ensue before any evidence of renal arterial damage is present. However, in the experimental animal, necrotizing arteriopathy can occur in as short a period as a week. It seems, however, that sooner or later damage to the entire arterial side of the renal vasculature does occur. For purposes of definition we shall call these changes those found in the unprotected kidney. In cases of essential hypertension, both kidneys are unprotected. If only a branch lesion is responsi-

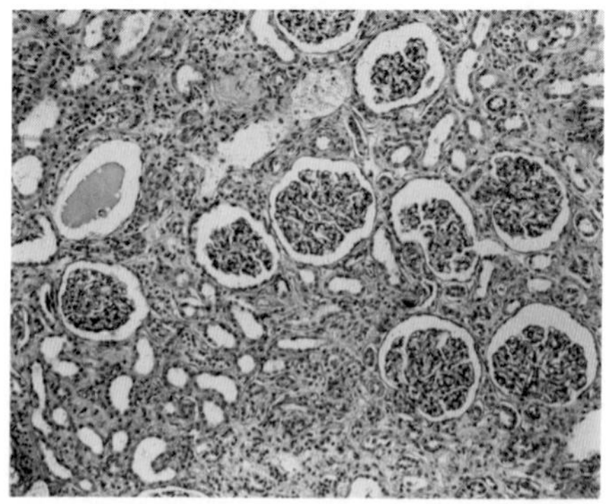

FIG. 2.—Photomicrograph shows crowded glomeruli and atrophic tubules due to secondary ischemic atrophy. Hematoxylin-eosin. ×100.

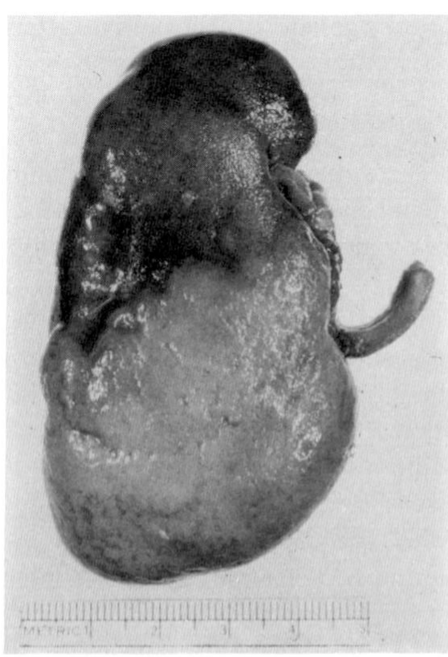

FIG. 3.—Secondary polar atrophy due to blockade of renal hilar artery.

ble for the disorder (Figs. 3 and 4), one kidney plus a segment of the other may be considered as unprotected and it is in those areas that varying degrees of arterial and arteriolar disease can be found. The variability can be graded.

In our institution we have recently had an opportunity to review the case histories of 33 patients with unilateral renal arterial stenosis who had bilateral renal biopsies performed at the time of surgery. As can be imagined, the specimens of the renal parenchyma at times were rather small. Many surgeons do not like to invade what they believe to be the kidney of the future so far as the patient is concerned and this is especially true if they find it necessary to sacrifice the ischemic kidney. As is commonly the fate of the morphologist, I was forced to review these biopsies without knowing anything other than that the specimens were removed from kidneys. I used certain criteria and developed five grades of vascular nomenclature. Grade 0 was normal. Grade I was minimal, when I believed that muscular thickening only or muscular hyperplasia was present; Grade II, mild, in which the arteriolar lumen was narrowed by less than one-third with hyaline material (Fig. 5). Grade III, moderate, where in my estimation one-third to two-thirds of the arterial lumen was narrowed (Fig. 6). Grade IV severe, in which the narrowing was greater than two-thirds, necrosis, or thrombonecrosis of the arteriole (Fig. 7). I was unable to grade accurately the ischemic changes at the same time since the size of the biopsy precluded such

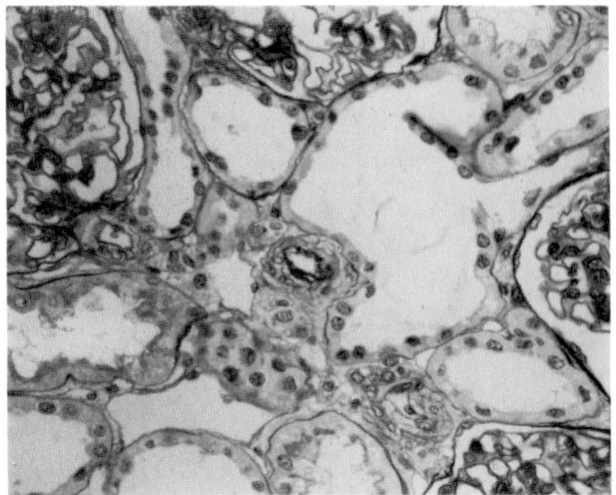

Fig. 5.—Photomicrographs of Grade II arteriolar sclerosis found in renal biopsy. Periodic acid-Schiff. ×400.

an evaluation. Later we reviewed the sections from the renal artery lesions and were able to separate the group into atherosclerotic and fibrotic diseases. The fibrotic lesions were further subdivided into the subgroups of intimal fibroplasia, medial fibroplasia with aneurysm, muscular hyperplasia, or perimedial fibroplasia. Bilateral renal vein assays were obtained in 10 of these patients. All patients were followed for at least 12 months after surgery with two exceptions. One patient died of hypertension and bronchopneumonia and one died of unknown causes; both had responded poorly to surgery. Of the 33 patients, 17 had atherosclerotic lesions and 16 had fibrous disease in the main renal artery. The average age of the patients with atherosclerotic

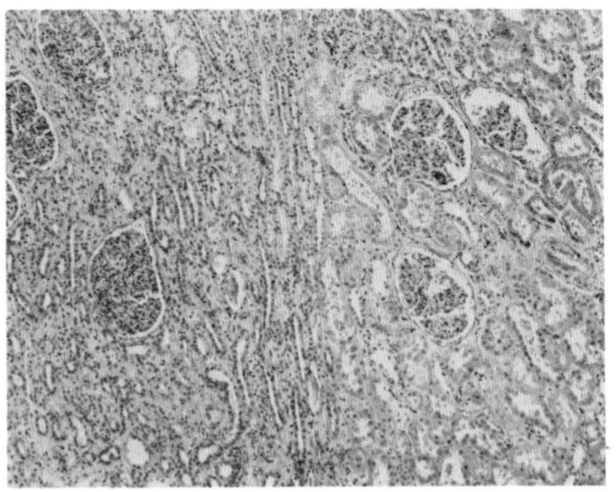

Fig. 4.—Photomicrograph shows boundary between ischemic and normal kidney found in branch blockade. Hematoxylin-eosin. ×100.

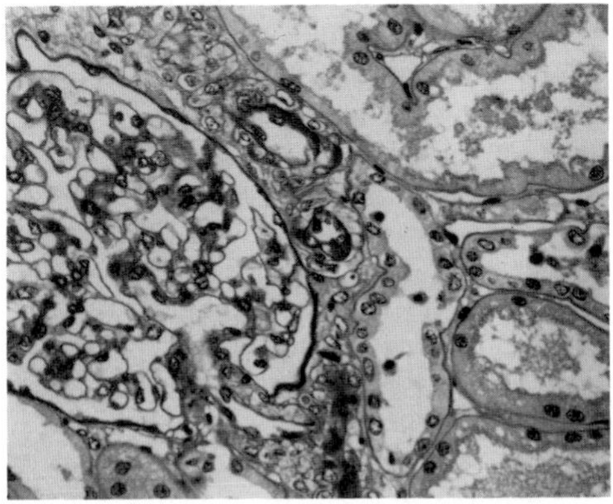

Fig. 6.—Photomicrograph of Grade III arteriolar sclerosis in renal biopsy. Periodic acid-Schiff. ×400.

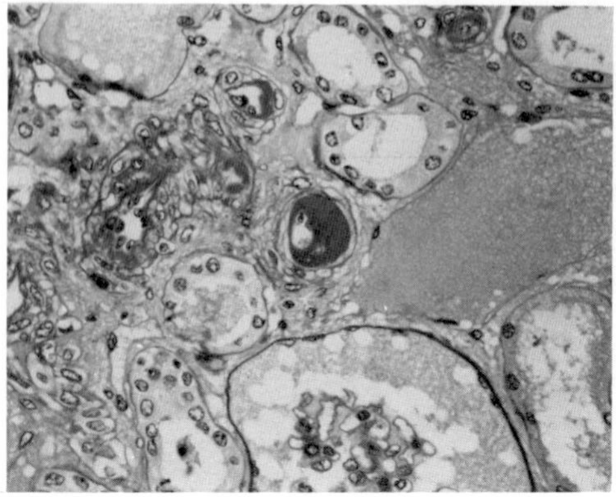

FIG. 7.—Photomicrograph of Grade IV, arteriolar sclerosis in renal biopsy. Periodic acid-Schiff. ×400.

lesions was 49.3 years, and the average age of the 16 patients with fibrous disease was 29.3 years. Of the 17 atherosclerotic patients, nine were women and eight were men; of the 16 patients with fibrous disease, 14 were women. Twelve of the patients with fibrous disease had complete relief from diastolic hypertension, representing an excellent to good response to surgery, with four of the patients considered fair to poor. Eight with atherosclerotic lesions had complete relief of diastolic hypertension while nine had fair or poor responses. For purposes of discussion we shall consider a fair to poor response as no relief. An excellent or good response means diastolic pressures below 100 in the older groups and below 90 in the younger; a good response with a systolic pressure somewhat higher than the limits of 130 to 160 mm Hg; and fair with a diastolic blood pressure at least 20 mm Hg less than preoperative levels without medication but not within normal limits, or a decrease in therapeutic demands. A poor response is no response.

Arteriolar sclerosis was noted in the contralateral kidney in 18 patients. Nine of the 20 had relief from diastolic hypertension and nine of 13 failed to respond to corrective surgery. Arteriolar sclerosis was moderate to severe in four of the former group and in three of the latter group. The ipsilateral kidney showed minimal to moderate changes of arteriolar sclerosis in only five patients and none had severe involvement. Most of those with vascular changes in the ipsilateral kidney had atherosclerosis as the underlying renal arterial lesion. So far as changes in the contralateral kidney were concerned, no distinction could be made between atherosclerosis or fibrotic lesions as to the severity of intrarenal arteriolar sclerosis.

Ischemic tubular atrophy without infarction was found in the ipsilateral kidney of 10 of 20 patients who had relief of their diastolic hypertension. All these changes were present in the contralateral kidney of only one patient. Ischemic changes without infarction were noted in the ipsilateral kidney of 9 of 13 patients who did not benefit from surgery. These changes were present in the contralateral kidneys of three patients in this group. As stated previously, we did not grade these changes for severity. The renal vein determinations that were available on the 10 patients showed that five of the seven patients who had complete relief from diastolic hypertension had a renal vein renin activity ratio of 1.5 or greater when the ipsilateral kidney was compared to the contralateral activity. Three who had a poor result had renal vein values less than this.

Although others have demonstrated to their satisfaction a statistical correlation between numbers of cells in juxtaglomerular apparatus and hypertension, I must admit to a total failure so far as study of this system is concerned. First of all, I have never been able to find a sufficiency of such bodies in biopsy material to allow adequate study. Originally, in the totally nephrectomized individuals I thought that I could recognize a group when careful study of the microscopic section revealed juxtaglomerular apparatuses that appeared to be of greatly increased cellularity. This alteration was on a gross recognition basis and therefore I do believe that they were truly of an increased cellularity. However, I was unable to correlate this group with anything of prognostic significance. From that experience I formed the opinion that although it did not correlate with anything, some individuals had larger juxtaglomerular apparatuses or at least more prominent ones in the ischemic kidney. I further made the unsupported judgment that these were of such an increase in size as to alter a statistical study markedly and give a high level of confidence in the final result. In addition, I have never been able to determine when one should count the cells in the apparatus. I am always torn by the process of selection. No matter how hard I try, the moment I see an ischemic kidney, I look for the biggest juxtaglomerular apparatus to count that I can find. As a result, my counts are spectacular, but I still don't have anything for comparison.

I therefore find myself adhering to the concept that a protective function can be exerted on the ipsilateral kidney by renal arterial blockade, but I can make no correlations between the vascular changes in the ipsilateral and contralateral kidney so far as prognosis is concerned. Therefore, I believe that needle biopsies or other biopsies prior to attempts at surgical correction are of no value whatsoever, and may expose the patients to an unnecessary hazard. I would certainly be most saddened by the loss of a contralateral kidney at the time when the ipsilateral kidney was rather markedly atrophic. I also find little solace in enumerations of juxtaglomerular cellularity.

There is one final facet that I have not as yet mentioned; I hesitate to do so, and will only briefly. My own rather incomplete studies from removed atrophic kidneys suggest that there is an intermediate phase wherein the renal parenchyma superficially looks rather normal. However, alkaline phosphatase stains demonstrate that this activity has been lost so far as the renotubules are concerned, and I hope that future studies may demonstrate that this tool can be of value in determining early renal ischemia.

Renal Hypertension: Does It Relate to Essential Hypertension?

By W. Stanley Peart, M.D.

IT IS OBVIOUS that the title of this chapter requires explanation since essential hypertension is that form for which no cause can be found and is therefore defined by exclusion, while renal hypertension can only be accepted as such when an operation on the kidney either to improve it or remove it has cured the hypertension. This latter situation must be contrasted with those cases of hypertension associated with renal disease in which this ultimate proof is lacking. There is a long history of controversy in which the sound of axes being ground has drowned the still, small voices of those asking for the hard facts. There are a number of questions which require answers:

1. How can renal hypertension be recognized?
2. What are the functional effects of renal hypertension in respect of (a) kidney; (b) hemodynamic effects including cardiac output, peripheral resistance, plasma and extracellular fluid volume; and (c) endocrinologic effects, including renin, angiotensin and aldosterone?
3. How does hypertension itself affect the kidney and the other parameters mentioned in (2), and does hypertension of unknown origin lead ultimately to renal hypertension?
4. Are there differences in the epidemiologic and familial aspects of renal and essential hypertension?

Renal hypertension, as stated at the outset, can only be accepted as such by cure following surgery, since the absolute cause of hypertension is still unknown despite all the efforts that have been made since the experimental model was established in 1934.[1] As I have elaborated elsewhere,[2] I believe that ischemia of the kidney is the most important aspect, whatever the nature of the underlying renal disease. For this reason it is best to concentrate on renal artery stenosis in man since this type of kidney always shows signs of ischemia, whether compared functionally with its normal partner, or in its histology.[3] This has been disputed by reference to data from experimental clipping of the renal artery,[4] but the situation seems so clear-cut in man, where I think there is the best data, that I could say that with renal artery stenosis there is a negligible chance of curing the hypertension by reparative surgery or nephrectomy unless the functional changes and the evidence of pressure drop across the stenosis leave no room for doubt.[5] This does not exclude the fact, however, that there are certain types of uni-

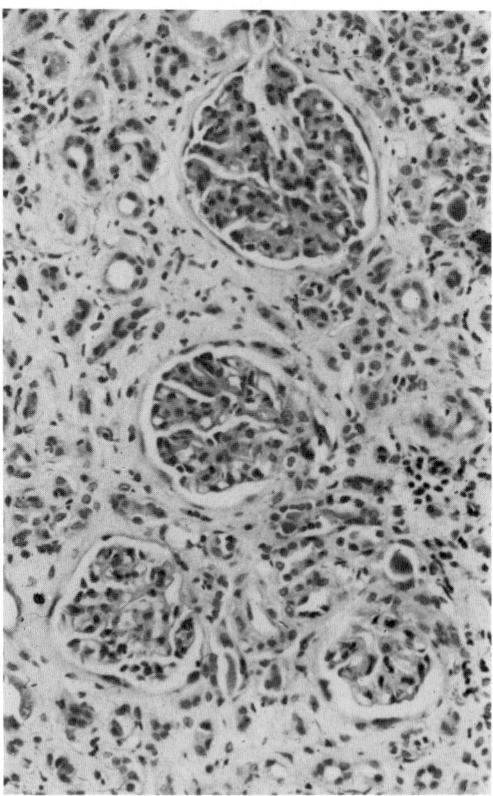

Fig. 1.—Renal biopsy from a patient with renal artery stenosis showing the crowding of the glomeruli and the tubular atrophy.

From the Medical Unit, St. Mary's Hospital, London, England.

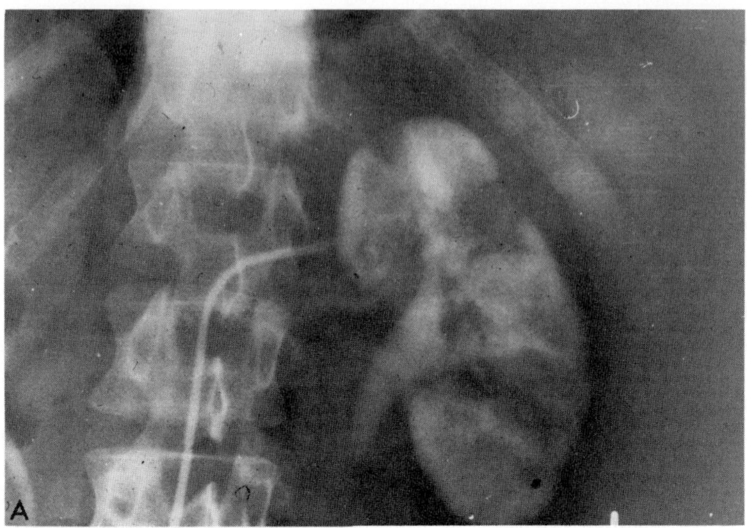

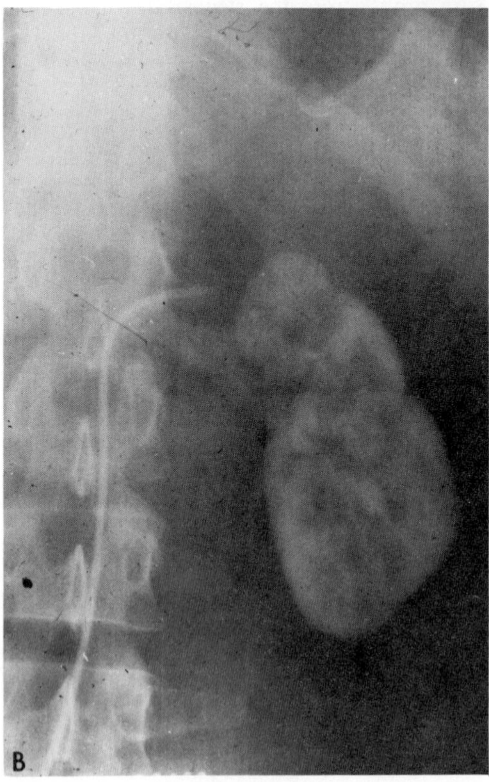

FIG. 2.—This patient presented with a pain in the left loin and was subsequently found to develop hypertension. *A,* A selective renal arteriogram at this stage showed a slight indentation in the upper outer cortical border. The blood pressure was controlled by means of drugs but over the next 12 months these were gradually diminished and he became normotensive without treatment. *B,* A repeat arteriogram showed again, in the nephrographic phase, shrinkage of the upper pole, which was presumably the site of an infarct thought to have caused his hypertension, and then by continued atrophy to have undergone spontaneous cure. (From Benraad, H. B., et al.,[59] with permission.)

lateral renal disease with hypertension such as pyelonephritis in which the same functional evidence of ischemia cannot be obtained. However, examination of the kidney still shows in most cases viable glomeruli, whatever may have happened to the tubules in between. Therefore, there must be a poor blood supply to certain definite elements of the kidney, and damage or loss of tubules is characteristic (Fig. 1).[6,7] An important aspect of this is that while it is not quite certain how small an amount of ischemic renal tissue will cause hypertension, it may be very small (see Figs. 2–4) despite the presence of large amounts of normal functioning kidney. For this reason the occasional success of polar nephrectomy in curing hypertension is of particular interest.[8] It also makes it possible to miss small scattered lesions in the kidney, small enough to escape the single biopsy and too small to affect overall renal function even if occurring on one side only.[9–12] This, of course, makes the difficulty of excluding such renal disease on histologic, functional, and even arteriographic grounds very difficult. At the moment we probably have to look for further improvements in renal arteriography to better define such lesions. The points made are all illustrated in Figs. 2–4: The first, self-curing hypertension following a small infarct in the upper pole of the kidney[13] (Fig. 2*A* and *B*); the second, shrinkage of the lower pole of the kidney following an attack of pyelonephritis (Fig. 3*A* and *B*); and the third, a localized area of renal ischemia due to a branch stenosis on the basis of fibromuscular disease (Fig. 4*A* and *B*). Therefore, we might be left with the conclusion that it is almost impossible to exclude a renal cause for hypertension. It is perhaps only if the degree of proteinuria is excessive in relation to the prevailing blood pressure that this possibility comes readily to mind. This is why quantitative measurement of proteinuria over a 24-hour period is important. Unsuspected glomerulonephritis is by no means rare and renal biopsy is the only way in which this can be proved in many cases (Fig. 5). With more severe grades of hypertension, the difficulty can be quite great without renal biopsy since proteinuria may increase quite markedly at the higher levels of blood pressure, especially when the malignant phase is present. Finally, hypertension itself causes severe vascular damage in the kidneys[14,14a] (Fig. 6) and has been held

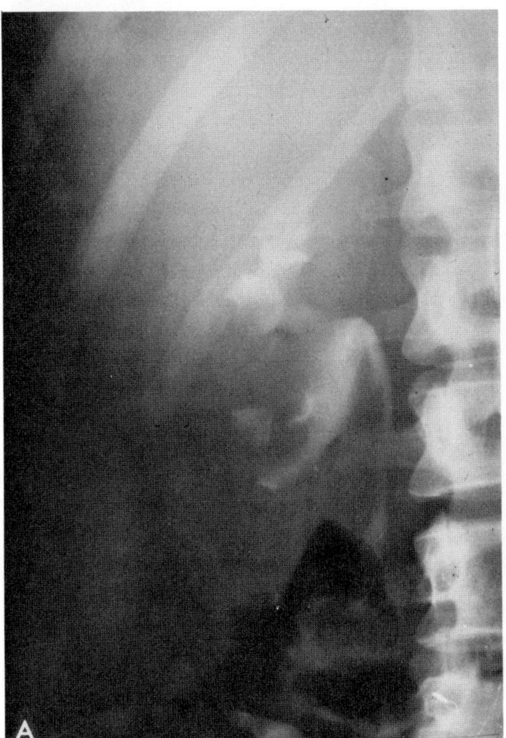

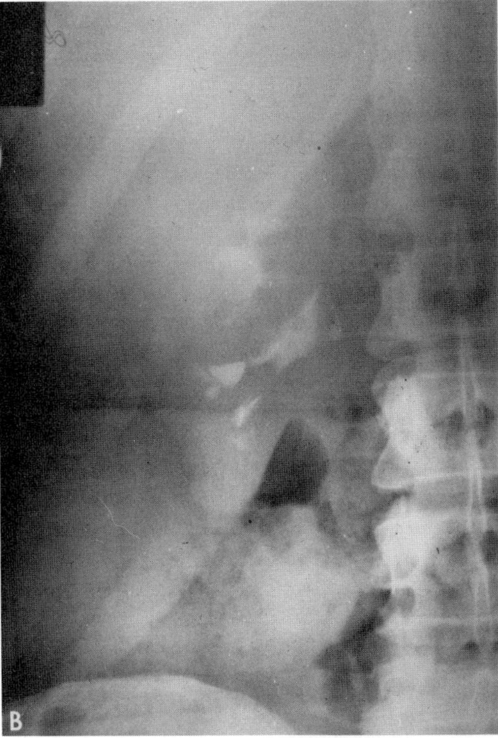

FIG. 3.—This young woman presented with pain in the loin and a fever and infection in the urine. *A*, The initial intravenous pyelogram showed involvement of the lower calyces. She was subsequently found to become hypertensive and a repeat pyelogram 9 months later (*B*) showed shrinkage of the lower pole and evidence of necrosis of the tip of the papilla in the lower calyces.

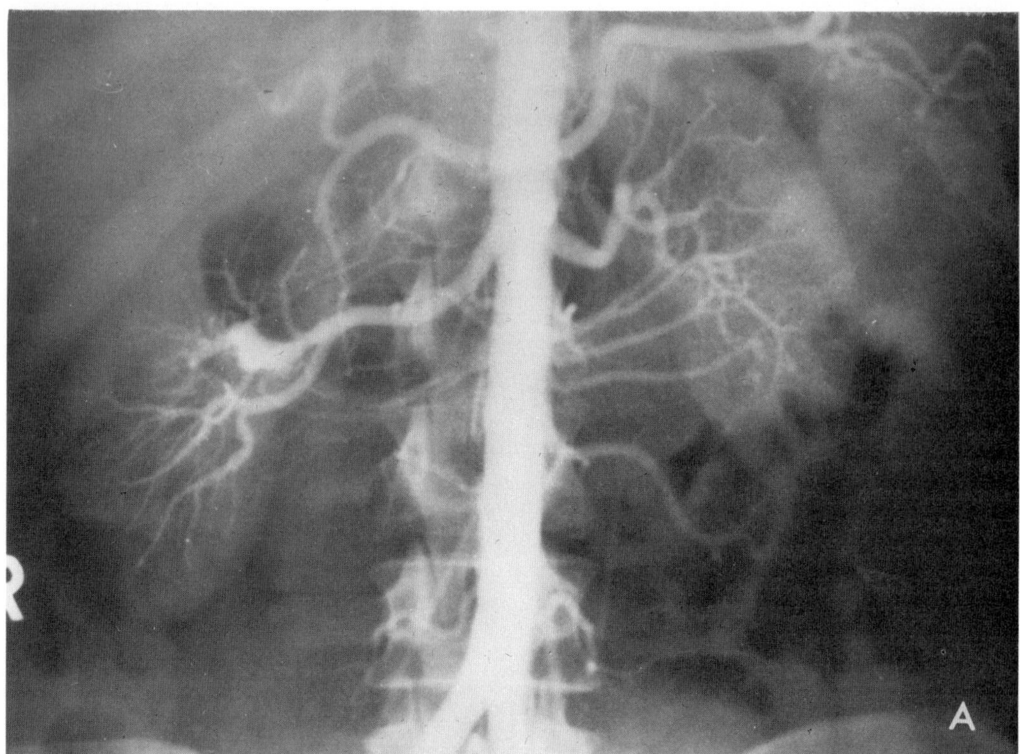

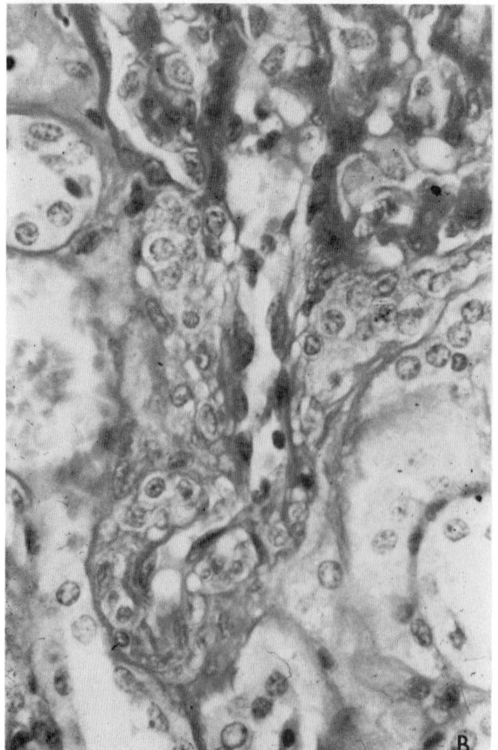

FIG. 4.—*A*, Aortogram of a young woman with hypertension showing aneurysmal dilatation of the artery to the upper third of the right kidney. *B*, Histologic appearance of the upper third of the right kidney shows gross hyperplasia of the juxtaglomerular cells in the afferent arteriole. The histology in the remainder of the kidney is normal and nephrectomy was followed by cure of the hypertension.

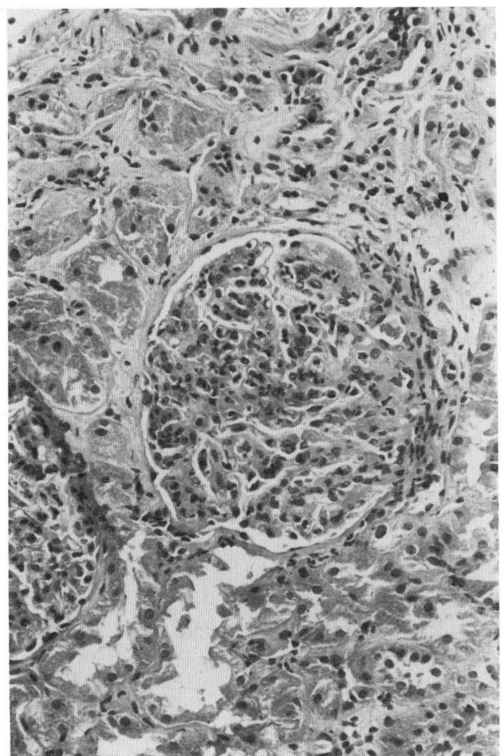

FIG. 5.—Renal biopsy from a patient who presented with severe hypertension (180/120 mm Hg), pulmonary edema and papilledema. Initially there was no proteinuria and his passage of urine was good. Proteinuria developed over the course of the next few days and the renal biopsy taken 2 weeks later showed hypercellular glomeruli.

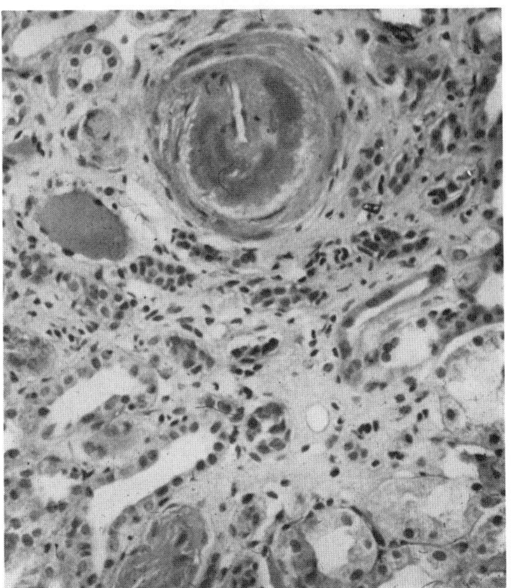

FIG. 6.—Severe hypertensive vascular changes shown in a medium-sized artery within the kidney. The lumen is reduced to a slit and there is fibrinoid necrosis within the media.

responsible for the persistence of hypertension following adequate surgery on stenosed renal arteries or even removal of pheochromocytoma.[15]

The functional effects of renal hypertension are best discussed first in relation to unilateral renal disease, and especially the effects of renal artery stenosis where the typical reduction of perfusion pressure leads to increased water reabsorption, increased concentration of filtered substances such as creatinine, inulin, and para-aminohippuric acid (PAH), and increased sodium reabsorption which exceeds that of water leading to a lowering of its concentration (Table 1). Following the work of Baldwin and his colleagues,[16] who claimed that there was often a functional difference between the two kidneys under certain circumstances in patients who would otherwise be regarded as having essential hypertension, it becomes necessary to see whether this could be used as

TABLE 1.—*Period of Time in Which Urine Was Collected from the Right and Left Ureters Without Bladder Leak*

	Right Ureter	*Left Ureter*
Urine volume (ml per minute)	1.0	3.1
Sodium (mEq per liter)	101.0	119.0
Chloride (mEq per liter)	90.0	119.0
Urine PAH concentration (mg per 100 ml)	392.0	158.0
Urine inulin concentration (mg per 100 ml)	1982	915
PAH clearance (ml per minute)	165.0	210.0
Inulin clearance (ml per minute)	58.0	85.0

It can be seen that the urine flow was less on the right with increased sodium and chloride reabsorption and increased water reabsorption leading to higher concentrations of PAH and inulin but with lower clearances on the affected side. Usually endogenous creatinine is used instead of inulin as a measure of filtration rate.

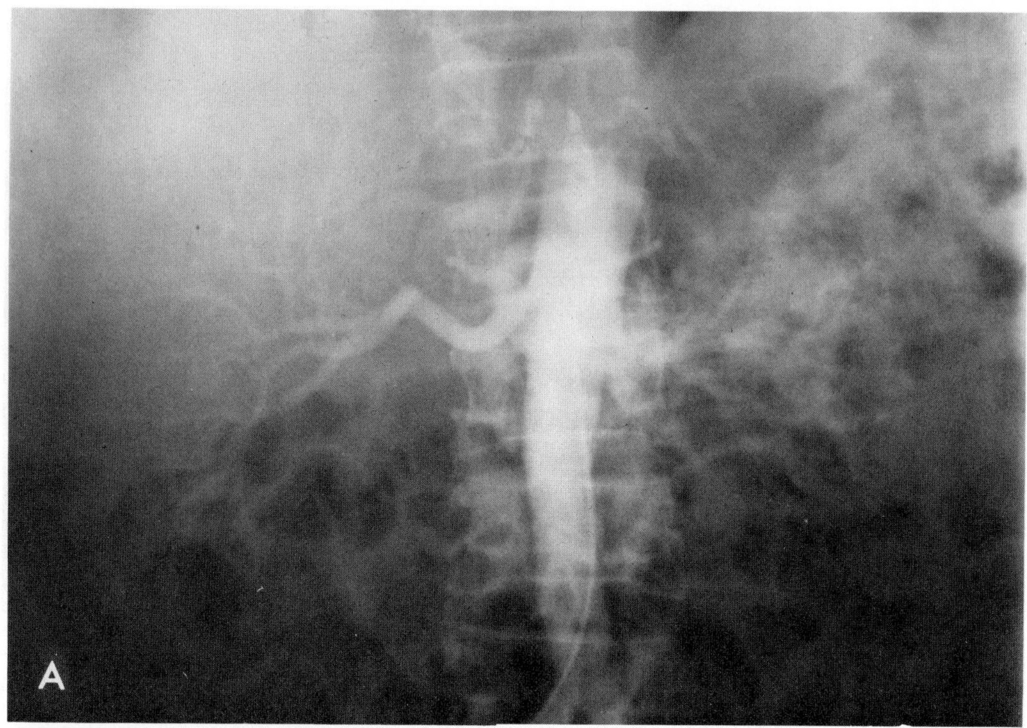

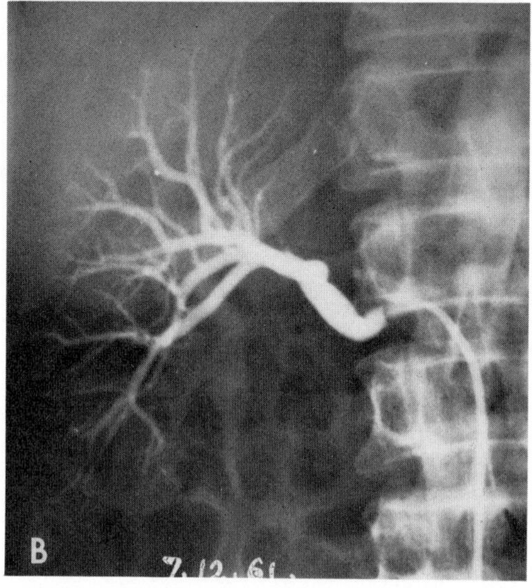

Fig. 7.—Male patient aged 50 years with severe hypertension (240/140 mm Hg) who developed a pain in the left loin. *A,* He was shown at aortography to have a thrombosed left renal artery but the right renal artery seemed normal. Nephrectomy was followed by cure of his hypertension for 2 years. *B,* He then became hypertensive again and a repeat, selective renal arteriogram showed a stenosis had developed at the origin of the right renal artery.

evidence that renal disease was causing the hypertension observed in their patients. It is certain that in their patients the pattern of renal function was not like that observed in curable renal artery stenosis and where the changes have to be clearly recognizable if successful surgery is to be achieved.[17,18,18a] From what has been said about functional changes in pyelonephritis, it equally follows that external urinary function will not be the best guide. Since, in the patients reported by Baldwin and his colleagues,[16] the ultimate proof of renal hypertension is lacking, namely correction or removal of the renal abnormality, then it cannot be certain that the change observed is not caused by the hypertension itself. Vascular disease in the kidneys may not always be uniform in its effects on function because of the varying damage in the smaller blood vessels within each kidney.[10,19] It is often difficult, for example, to decide whether atheromatous, renal artery stenosis is secondary to previously existing hypertension of other cause,[20] and certainly atheromatous plaques at the entrance to the renal arteries are common at autopsy in hypertensive subjects. Force is lent to this argument by the observation of such stenoses occurring subsequently in the opposite renal artery when correction has been applied to the other (Fig. 7*A* and *B*).

Turning to hemodynamic effects, the "pattern of the circulation" or the relation between cardiac output and peripheral resistance in different segments of the circulation has been studied in various forms of hypertension. One of the problems in man is, of course, the simultaneous measurement of cardiac output and blood flow in different parts of the body, but various approaches to the problem have been made.[21,21a,21b] In essential hypertension a fairly well-distributed increase in peripheral resistance was noted in most organs, except in voluntary muscle.[22] It has been suggested, however, that there are differences in cardiac output, plasma volume, and peripheral resistance between groups of patients with essential and renal hypertension,[23,24] and this has been related to changes in the pattern of activity of the renin-angiotensin system.[25] There is no doubt that in most of the forms of established hypertension, the peripheral resistance is more commonly raised than not, but careful studies on the hemodynamic state at rest and on exercise indicate that there are some hypertensive patients where the rise in pressure seems more dependent on increase in cardiac output.[26–28,28a] This, of course, is important in relation to the concept initially stressed by Borst and Borst-de Geus [29] and supported by Ledingham [30] that the initiating step, even in renal hypertension, was rise of cardiac output followed in some way by increase of peripheral resistance and later by return of the cardiac output to normal levels. Using a computer-assisted model of the circulation, Colman, Granger, and Guyton [31] strongly favor this view, but the piece of physiologic knowledge which is lacking at the present time is the way in which a rise in cardiac output could lead to a rise in peripheral resistance, and the hypothesis will not be convincing until this important piece of information is provided. One of the factors which might make all forms of well-established hypertension have a similar circulatory pattern lies in the observations of Folkow,[32] who showed in various human and animal studies that certain forms of hypertension were associated with a structural change in the arteriolar wall, which represented the anatomic basis for some part of the increased peripheral resistance. Therefore, the concept that all hypertension might be self-perpetuating by the fixed organic changes produced in the main vessels of peripheral resistance is attractive and there is evidence for support. Nevertheless, the relief of quite long-standing, severe hypertension as in renal artery stenosis suggests that this may only be a minor part of the overall peripheral resistance. The experimental observations of Bianchi, Tilde Tenconi, and Lucca,[33] in dogs made hypertensive by renal artery clipping, where changes in plasma and extracellular fluid volume during the development of hypertension were believed to be of some importance, lead to the need to consider control of the plasma volume and extracellular fluid volume, which are intimately concerned, not only with excretory function of the kidney, but with the renin-angiotensin system and the adrenal.

Since electrolyte and aldosterone metabolism was the first of these groups of variables to be seriously studied, it may be helpful to comment on the different views that have been taken from time to time on their role in hypertension. The importance of the role of sodium in hypertension is still unsettled. That excess sodium will exacerbate established hypertension, especially in the presence of severe renal disease, has been brought out by studies on man in renal failure.[33a] Its primary role, which receives support from the work of Dahl,[34] is less certain. If there are true differences of plasma and extracellular fluid volume between patients with renal and essential hypertension, then there will be differences in total-body sodium, but whether secondary to hypertension or a primary event is the important question. From the first suggestion of Gross [35] that renal hypertension was intimately connected with the adrenal, to the description by Conn [36] of the syndrome which bears his name, the discussion has ranged over the question of aldosterone excess as a prime cause of hypertension,[37,38] or as a consequence of hypertension.[39,40] With some difficulty, the small group of patients with Conn's syndrome due to a tumor in one suprarenal, removal of which leads to cure, have been separated out in a still imperfect manner.[41] There is no doubt also that patients with severe malignant hypertension usually have an excess production of aldosterone and even more so if they fall into the group with hyponatremia.[42] Many of these patients have hypertension of acute onset due to sudden diminution of blood supply to the kidney. Lowering the blood pressure by any means, including drugs, will return the excess aldosterone production to normal.[43] It should be stressed that this picture can certainly occur in malignant hypertension of quite unknown and subsequently unproved origin. Soon after the suggestion that the kidney and adrenal were functionally related, Genest and his colleagues,[39] and Laragh and his colleagues [44] showed the effect of angiotensin in stimulating aldosterone production and it is impossible to look at groups of hypertensive patients without considering both together. Originally Genest and his colleagues [39,45] believed that excess aldosterone production was quite common in essential hypertension but gradually this claim received less and less support elsewhere as more studies were made using different techniques.[45a] Now it seems that only in those patients with severe or malignant hypertension, Conn's tumor and hyperplastic adrenals are excess aldosterone production and plasma level observed.[46] Obviously in some of these patients aldosterone is extremely important in maintaining hypertension, as in Conn's tumor; in others it seems to be a secondary phenomenon since removing hyperplastic adrenals has not been followed by cure of the hypertension. This latter group has assumed greater importance with studies on renin activity which have a double relationship with aldosterone in the sense that those conditions which stimulate the kidney to produce large amounts of renin and thus of angiotensin, such as renal artery stenosis, are usually associated with high aldosterone production and plasma level, while those in which an adenoma exists in the suprarenal as a supposed primary event are associated with barely detectable renin and angiotensin levels. Close to this range, however, lies the group with hyperplastic suprarenals without one definite large adenoma, where the

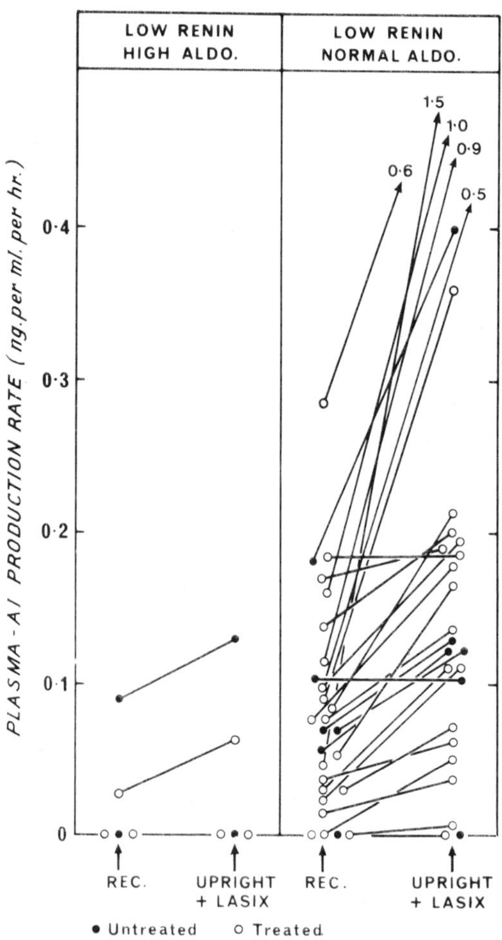

FIG. 8.—Studies on patients with low plasma renin and high plasma aldosterone levels shown in the left-hand column. The three subjects, whose values remain at zero despite stimulation by upright posture and Lasix, have Conn's tumors, whereas the other two with rather higher but still subnormal values of plasma renin are thought to have hyperplastic suprarenals. The large number of subjects with subnormal plasma renin levels (below 0.1 ng per milliliter per hour on the ordinate) who have normal plasma aldosterone levels is clearly shown in the right-hand column with the varying effects of upright posture and Lasix.

plasma renin activity may be very low although not usually as low as occurs in Conn's tumor,[46] and where the plasma aldosterone is often as high. In the group of patients with essential hypertension, there are many patients of this type, and furthermore, there are many patients with a low plasma renin activity who have a normal plasma aldosterone level (Figs. 8 and 9). The percentage of patients with hypertension of unknown origin with a low plasma renin activity rises in black populations.[47] The reason for this is uncertain, but it is not due to hyperaldosteronism. In contrast, it is uncommon in patients with renal disease and hypertension, even if it can only be described as renal disease associated with hypertension rather than renal hypertension itself, to find low renin levels. More commonly the levels are high, so much so that it is worth investigating patients with supposed essential hypertension if the plasma renin activity is high in case some underlying renal disease is present. The reason for this not being such a good index is that hypertension itself, presumably due to a secondary stimulus or damage to the kidney, leads to elevation of plasma renin activity, and treatment of the hypertension by drugs reduces the plasma renin activity and also the aldosterone levels to normal.[43] Again, if subjects with normal blood pressures are examined, there are examples of low plasma renin activity present.[48] The quite large numbers of patients with hypertension of unknown origin who have lower than normal plasma renin activity might point to a common inhibitory factor. This certainly does not seem to be aldosterone and its effects, and efforts to incriminate another mineralocorticoid, such as 18-hydroxy-desoxycorticosterone, have not been too rewarding.[49] It still is true, however, that usually the presence of renal disease elevates plasma renin activity but the scatter of figures is such that the use of either aldosterone or renin levels to define essential or renal hypertension is not very certain (Fig. 10). Attempts have therefore been made to see whether any other variables are related and it has been suggested that differences in the plasma and extracellular fluid volume may be the key.[25] Frohlich and his colleagues [24] have suggested that unlike previous findings, there is a difference between larger groups of patients in respect of cardiac output and plasma volume so that patients with renal disease and hypertension have higher cardiac outputs and lower blood volumes than those with essential hypertension. One problem here, of course, is the definition of cardiac failure but Bianchi and his colleagues [25] found that where there was normal or low plasma renin activity in patients with renovascular hypertension, the plasma and extracellular fluid volumes were increased compared with those with a raised plasma renin activity (Fig. 11). The differentiation, therefore, between many patients with renal hypertension and normal plasma renin activity from those with essen-

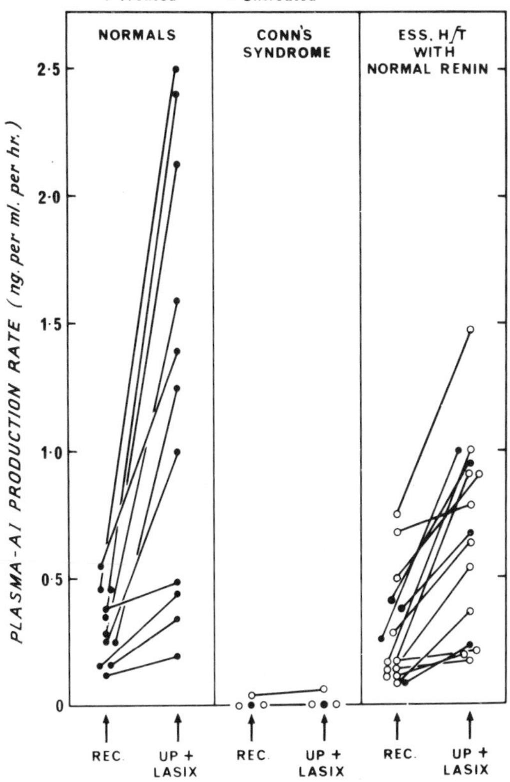

FIG. 9.—The presence of low plasma renin activity, slightly affected in some cases by upright posture and Lasix, in patients with essential hypertension, is shown in the right-hand column, and compared with patients having Conn's tumors in the central column, and the normal population in the left-hand column. Note that some normal subjects have low levels which do not respond a great deal to posture and intravenous administration of Lasix.

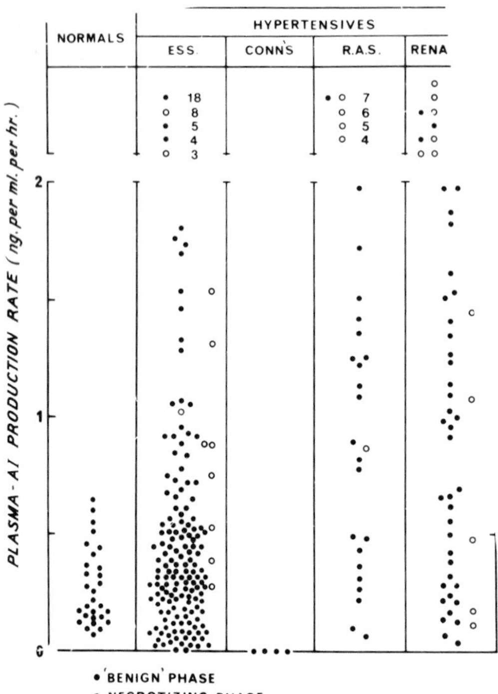

FIG. 10.—Plasma renin activity in a variety of subjects with different types of hypertension compared with normal levels. The overlap and scatter of values are self-evident.

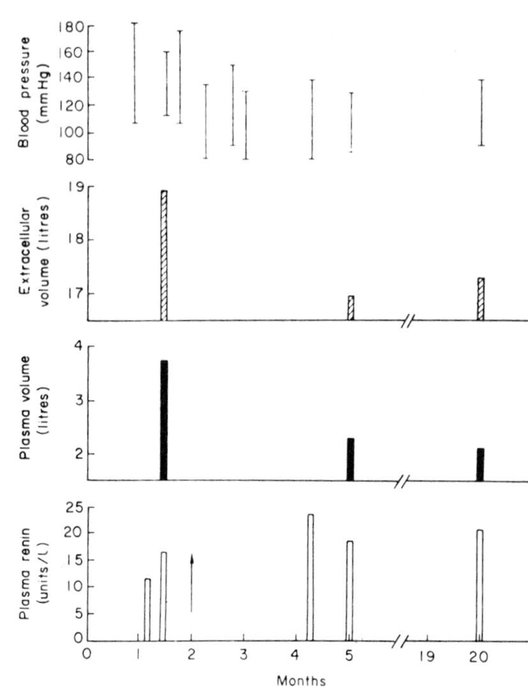

FIG. 11.—Following surgery (2), there was a fall in extracellular fluid volume and plasma volume, while the plasma renin rose slowly from the middle to the top end of the normal range (normal range 5 to 20 units per liter). (From Bianchi G. et al.,[25] with permission.)

tial hypertension, turns back on the differentiation of renal disease by other means. Looked at another way, as with cases of scattered renal disease of small degree, it becomes very difficult to say with confidence that the kidney could not be playing a causal role in the hypertension. The lack of demonstration of differences in histology, excretory function, aldosterone production, and plasma renin and angiotensin activity, would still allow of a renal cause for hypertension in many patients now classified as essential. However, these patients cannot be differentiated from normal subjects without hypertension so there is not much to be gained along these lines. The wheel has turned full circle, and an adequate definition of renal hypertension from knowledge of cause is still required.

Epidemiologic and family studies do not help too much in this differentiation of renal from essential hypertension. The truly inherited, familial renal causes are usually of a type which produces easily recognizable changes, such as polycystic disease, and Alport's syndrome with glomerulonephritis and deafness. These groups are obviously rare and have little bearing on the great mass of patients with hypertension. Inheritance of hypertension in the great majority of cases of unknown origin is, however, well established and of a multifactoral nature.[50] Some families, of course, have an easily determined line of severe hypertension running through several generations where underlying causes are never found, and in fact, apart from the examples given, the existence of a strong family history would be a point against finding an obvious renal cause. However, there are some interesting and unexplained correlations. This was best brought out by the studies of Hamilton and his colleagues [51] who showed that what they called pyelonephritis in the patients they studied was associated with a higher incidence of hypertension within their families.

Either hypertension itself leads to a higher incidence of pyelonephritis, or alternatively there might be some underlying inherited tendency to pyelonephritis associated with hypertension. The diagnosis of pyelonephritis, however, requires consideration and this is a very difficult area of definition in the adult, and perhaps too much should not be made of this supposed association at the present time. There is another important familial relation to hypertension and that is the effect of pregnancy on blood pressure. It has been clearly shown that those women who develop recurrent and usually mild elevation of pressure in the later months of pregnancy are those who are particularly liable to turn up again in later life with a raised blood pressure,[52–55] and the sisters of these subjects have a higher blood pressure in pregnancy than the mean for the population.[56] The nature of the stimulus of pregnancy is unknown, and while it is tempting to look at the way in which hypertension may be provoked in patients with obvious underlying renal disease, such as glomerulonephritis, pyelonephritis, and fibromuscular hyperplasia of the renal arteries, and to suggest that there may be an occult renal disorder revealed by pregnancy, there is absolutely no evidence for it. Hypertension in these circumstances certainly seems to be associated with glomerular lesions which are reversible,[57] and the way in which the tendency to hypertension is revealed in these patients must therefore remain a mystery. Another stimulus of considerable interest is that provided by the contraceptive pill, which, in some women, causes a considerable elevation of blood pressure that returns to normal when the drug is stopped.[58] It is uncertain whether this stimulus is the same as that provided by pregnancy and whether there is a similar familial relationship.

My conclusions from this whole survey would be that it is possible to recognize hypertension of renal origin in certain restricted categories, i.e., in those only where it is possible to show a functional or histologic change in the kidneys. Obviously it is impossible ever to say with conviction that the kidney may not play a part in raising the pressure in any given patient, because the tools we use are too crude and at present it is not possible to state in any one case exactly how the blood pressure is raised by renal disease. This is a common situation in medicine, however, and it is still necessary to demand good evidence about participation of the kidneys and not to rely merely on the negative statement that it is impossible to disprove.

References

1. Goldblatt, H., Lynch, J., Hanzal, R. F., and Summerville, W. W.: Studies on experimental hypertension. I. The production of persistent elevation of systolic blood pressure by means of renal ischemia. J. Exp. Med. 59:347, 1934.
2. Peart, W. S.: Hypertension and the kidney. I. Clinical, pathological, and functional disorders, especially in man. Br. Med. J. 2:1353, 1959.
3. Peart, W. S.: Hypertension and the kidney. *In* Black, D. A. K. (Ed.): Renal Disease, 2nd ed. Oxford: Blackwell, 1967, pp. 638–664.
4. Corcoran, A. C., and Page, I. H.: Renal blood flow in experimental renal hypertension. Am. J. Physiol. 135:361, 1942.
5. Berliner, R. W., Bricker, N. S., Brod, J., Gifford, R. W., Hoobler, S. W., Kincaid-Smith, P., Maxwell, M. H., McCormack, L. J., Meaney, T. F., Shapiro, A. P., and Dustan, H. P.: Renal arterial stenosis and parenchymal diseases. *In* Page, I. H., and McCubbin, J. W. (Eds.): Renal Hypertension. Chicago: Year Book, 1968, pp. 306–349.
6. Fahr, T.: Zusammenhangstrennungen und durch Gewalteinwirkungen bedingte Krankhafte veranderungen der Niere, des Nierenbachens unde des Harnleiters. *In* Henke, F., and Lubarsch, O. (Eds.): Handbuch der speziellen pathologischen Anatomie und Histologie, vol. 6, part 2. Berlin: Springer, 1934, pp. 748–774.
7. Kincaid-Smith, P.: Vascular obstruction in chronic pyelonephritic kidneys and its relation to hypertension. Lancet 2:1263, 1955.
8. Poutasse, E. F.: Surgical treatment of renal hypertension. Am. J. Surg. 107:97, 1964.
9. Connor, T. B., Thomas, W. C., Haddock, L., and Howard, J. E.: Unilateral renal disease as a cause of hypertension: Its detection by ureteral catheterization studies. Ann. Intern. Med. 52:544, 1960.
10. Brown, J. J., Peart, W. S., Owen, K., Robertson, J. I. S., and Sutton, D.: The diagnosis and treatment of renal-artery stenosis. Br. Med. J. 1:327, 1960.
11. Dustan, H. P., Poutasse, E. F., Corcoran, A. C., and Page, I. H.: Separated renal

functions in patients with renal arterial disease, pyelonephritis, and essential hypertension. Circulation 23:34, 1961.

12. Richardson, J. R., Jr., Hagedorn, C. W., Hartley, B. J., and Hulet, W. H.: The function of the individual kidneys in hypertension of renal vascular origin. J. Lab. Clin. Med. 65:49, 1965.

13. Benraad, H. B., Benraad, T. J., and Kloppenborg, P. W. C.: Transient hypertension caused by segmental renal artery occlusion. Br. Med. J. 4:408, 1969.

14. Giese, J.: Monograph: The Pathogenesis of Hypertensive Vascular Disease. Copenhagen: Munksgaard, 1966.

14a. Fisher, E. R., Hatt, P.-Y., Pirani, C. L., and Lazzarini-Robertson, A.: Relationship of hypertension to vascular changes. I. Renal and extrarenal vascular changes. *In* Page, I. H., and McCubbin, J. W. (Eds.): Renal Hypertension. Chicago: Year Book, 1968, pp. 372–385.

15. Peart, W. S.: Persistence of hypertension after removal of phaeochromocytoma, where excretion of adrenaline and noradrenaline is normal. *In* Wolstenholme, G. E. W., and Cameron, M. P. (Eds.): Ciba Foundation Symposium on Hypertension, Humoral and Neurogenic Factors. London: Churchill, 1954, pp. 104–116.

16. Baldwin, D. S., Hulet, W. H., Biggs, A. W., Gombos, E. A., and Chasis, H.: Renal function in the separate kidneys of man. II. Hemodynamics and excretion of solute and water in essential hypertension. J. Clin. Invest. 39:395, 1960.

17. Stamey, T. A.: Some observations on the filtration fraction, on the transport of sodium and water in the ischemic kidney, and on the prognostic importance of R.P.F. to the contralateral kidney in renovascular hypertension. *In* Gross, F. (Ed.): Antihypertensive Therapy (Principles and Practice). Berlin: Springer, 1966, pp. 555–579.

18. Maxwell, M. H., Lupu, A. N., and Franklin, S. S.: Clinical and physiological factors determining diagnosis and choice of treatment of renovascular hypertension. Circ. Res. 21 (Suppl. 2):201, 1967.

18a. Berliner, R. W., Bricker, N. S., Brod, J., Gifford, R. W., Hoobler, S. W., Kincaid-Smith, P., Maxwell, M. H., McCormack, L. J., Meaney, T. F., Shapiro, A. P., and Dustan, H. P.: Renal arterial stenosis and parenchymal diseases. I. Renal arterial stenosis. D. Function tests of individual kidneys. *In* Page, I. H., and McCubbin, J. W. (Eds.): Renal Hypertension. Chicago: Year Book, 1968, pp. 317–325.

19. Connor, T. B., Berthrong, M., Thomas, W. C., and Howard, J. E.: Hypertension due to unilateral renal disease with a report of a functional test helpful in diagnosis. Bull. Johns Hopkins Hosp. 100:241, 1957.

20. Blackman, S. S., Jr.: Arteriosclerosis and partial obstruction of the main renal arteries in association with "essential" hypertension in man. Bull. Johns Hopkins Hosp. 65:353, 1939.

21. Pickering, G. W.: High Blood Pressure, 2nd ed. London: Churchill, 1968.

21a. Bohr, D. F., Doyle, A. E., Friedman, S. M., McGiff, J. C., Mendlowitz, M., and Khairallah, P. A.: Vascular reactivity: Experimental and clinical. F. Reactivity of isolated blood vessels from hypertensive animals. *In* Page, I. H., and McCubbin, J. W. (Eds.): Renal Hypertension. Chicago: Year Book, 1968, pp. 179–180.

21b. Brod, J., Hoobler, S. W., Ledingham, J. M., and Frohlich, E. D.: Hemodynamics. *In* Page, I. H., and McCubbin, J. W. (Eds.): Renal Hypertension. Chicago: Year Book, 1968, pp. 350–370.

22. Brod, J., Fencl, V., Hejl, Z., Jirka, J., and Ulrych, M.: General and regional haemodynamic pattern underlying essential hypertension. Clin. Sci. 23:339, 1962.

23. Frohlich, E. D., Ulrych, M., Tarazi, R. C., Dustan, H. P., and Page, I. H.: A hemodynamic comparison of essential and renovascular hypertension. Cardiac output and total peripheral resistance in supine and tilted patients. Circulation 35:289, 1967.

24. Frohlich, E. D., Ulrych, M., Tarazi, R. C., Dustan, H. P., and Page, I. H.: Hemodynamics of renal arterial diseases and hypertension. Am. J. Med. Sci. 255:29, 1968.

25. Bianchi, G., Campolo, L., Vegeto, A., Pietra, V., and Piazza, U.: The value of plasma renin concentration per se, and in relation to plasma and extracellular fluid volume in diagnosis and prognosis of human renovascular hypertension. Clin. Sci. 39:559, 1970.

26. Werkö, L., and Lagerlöf, H.: Studies on the circulation in man. IV. Cardiac output and blood pressure in the right auricle, right ventricle and pulmonary artery in patients with hypertensive cardiovascular disease. Acta Med. Scand. 313:427, 1949.

27. Sannerstedt, R.: Hemodynamic response to

exercise in patients with arterial hypertension. Acta Med. Scand. 180(Suppl. 458):1, 1966.

28. Lund-Johansen, P.: Hemodynamics in early essential hypertension. Acta Med. Scand. (Suppl. 482):1, 1967.

28a. Brod, J., Hoobler, S. W., Ledingham, J. M., and Frohlich, E. D.: Hemodynamics. E. Essential hypertension. *In* Page, I. H., and McCubbin, J. W. (Eds.): Renal Hypertension. Chicago: Year Book, 1968, pp. 364–370.

29. Borst, J. G. G., and Borst-de Geus, A.: Hypertension explained by Starling's theory of circulatory homeostasis. Lancet 1:677, 1963.

30. Ledingham, J. M.: Mechanisms in renal hypertension. Proc. R. Soc. Med. 64:409, 1971.

31. Coleman, T. G., Granger, H. J., and Guyton, A. C.: Whole-body circulatory autoregulation and hypertension. Circ. Res. 28(Suppl. 2):76, 1971.

32. Folkow, B.: The haemodynamic consequences of adaptive structural changes of the resistance vessels in hypertension. Clin. Sci. 41:1, 1971.

33. Bianchi, G., Tilde Tenconi, L., and Lucca, R.: Effect in the conscious dog of constriction of the renal artery of a sole remaining kidney on haemodynamics, sodium balance, body fluid volumes, plasma renin concentration and pressor responsiveness to angiotensin. Clin. Sci. 38:741, 1970.

33a. Del Greco, F., Grollman, A., Ledingham, J. M., Merrill, J. P., Muirhead, E. E., and Masson, G. M. C.: Renoprival hypertension. *In* Page, I. H., and McCubbin, J. W. (Eds.): Renal Hypertension. Chicago: Year Book, 1968, pp. 276–295.

34. Dahl, L. K.: Effects of chronic excess salt feeding. Induction of self-sustaining hypertension in rats. J. Exp. Med. 114:231, 1961.

35. Gross, F.: Adrenocortical function and renal pressor mechanisms in experimental hypertension. *In* Bock, K. D., and Cottier, P. T. (Eds.): Essential Hypertension, An International Symposium. Berlin: Springer, 1960, pp. 92–111.

36. Conn, J. W.: Primary aldosteronism. J. Lab. Clin. Med. 45:661, 1955.

37. Conn, J. W.: Aldosteronism and hypertension. Arch. Intern. Med. 107:79, 1961.

38. Conn, J. W., Rovner, D. R., and Cohen, E. L.: Normokalemic primary aldosteronism. A frequent cause of curable essential hypertension. J. Lab. Clin. Med. 66:863, 1965.

39. Genest, J., Nowaczynski, W., Koiw, E., Sandor, T., and Biron, P.: Adreno-cortical function in essential hypertension. *In* Bock, K. D., and Cottier, P. T. (Eds.): Essential Hypertension, An International Symposium. Berlin: Springer, 1960, pp. 126–146.

40. Laragh, J. H., Ulick, S., Januszewicz, V., Deming, Q. B., Kelly, W. G., and Lieberman, S.: Aldosterone secretion in primary and malignant hypertension. J. Clin. Invest. 39:1091, 1960.

41. Fourth Annual ASCP Research Symposium, Chicago, September 1969. Am. J. Clin. Pathol. 54:287, 1970.

42. Brown, J. J., Davies, D. L., Lever, A. F., and Robertson, J. I. S.: Renin and angiotensin. Postgrad. Med. J. 42:153, 1966.

43. McAllister, R. G., Jr., Van Way, C. W., Dayani, K., Anderson, W. J., Temple, E., Michelakis, A. M., Coppage, W. S., Jr., and Oates, J. A.: Malignant hypertension: Effect of therapy on renin and aldosterone. Circ. Res. 28(Suppl. 2):160, 1971.

44. Laragh, J. H., Angers, M., Kelly, W. G., and Lieberman, S.: Hypotensive agents and pressor substances. The effect of epinephrine, norepinephrine, angiotensin II and others on the secretory rate of aldosterone in man. JAMA 174:234, 1960.

45. Genest, J., Lemieux, G., Davignon, A., Koiw, E., Nowaczynski, W., and Steyermark, P.: Human arterial hypertension, a state of mild chronic hyperaldosteronism. Science 123:503, 1956.

45a. Davis, J. O., Denton, D. A., Laragh, J. H., Mulrow, P. J., and Masson, G. M. C.: The renin-angiotensin-aldosterone system. D. Aldosterone-induced hypertension. E. The renin-angiotensin-aldosterone system in experimental renal hypertension. F. The renin-angiotensin-aldosterone system in clinical hypertensin. *In* Page, I. H., and McCubbin, J. W. (Eds.): Renal Hypertension. Chicago: Year Book, 1968, pp. 229–242.

46. Stockigt, J. R., Collins, R. D., and Biglieri, E. G.: Determination of plasma renin concentration by angiotensin I immunoassay. Diagnostic import of precise measurement of subnormal renin in hyperaldosteronism. Circ. Res. 28(Suppl. 2):175, 1971.

47. Creditor, M. C., and Loschky, U. K.: Incidence of suppressed renin activity and of normokalemic primary aldosteronism in hypertensive Negro patients. Circulation 37:1027, 1968.

48. Peart, W. S.: Renin and angiotensin in relation to aldosterone. Am. J. Clin. Pathol. 54:324, 1970.

49. Melby, J. C., Dale, S. L., and Wilson, T. E.: 18-Hydroxy-deoxycorticosterone in human hypertension. Circ. Res. 28(Suppl. 2):143, 1971.
50. Pickering, G. W.: The Nature of Essential Hypertension. London: Churchill, 1961.
51. Hamilton, M., Pickering, G. W., Roberts, J. A. F., and Sowry, G. S. C.: Arterial pressures of relatives of patients with secondary and malignant hypertension. Clin. Sci. 24:91, 1963.
52. Browne, F. J., and Dodds, G. H.: The remote prognosis of the toxaemias of pregnancy. J. Obstet. Gynaecol. Br. Commonw. 46:443, 1939.
53. Browne, F. J., and Sheumack, D. R.: Chronic hypertension following pre-eclamptic toxaemia. The influence of familial hypertension on its causation. J. Obstet. Gynaecol. Br. Commonw. 63:677, 1956.
54. Dieckmann, W. J.: The Toxemias of Pregnancy, 2nd ed. St. Louis: Mosby, 1952.
55. Gibson, G. B., and Platt, R.: Incidence of hypertension after pregnancy toxaemia. Br. Med. J. 2:159, 1959.
56. MacGillivray, I.: Hypertension in pregnancy and its consequences. J. Obstet. Gynaecol. Br. Commonw. 68:557, 1961.
57. Pollak, V. E., and Nettles, J. B.: The kidney in toxemia of pregnancy: A clinical and pathologic study based on renal biopsies. Medicine 39:469, 1960.
58. Laragh, J. H., Sealey, J. E., Ledingham, J. G. G., and Newton, M. A.: Oral contraceptives. Renin, aldosterone, and high blood pressure. JAMA 201:918, 1967.
59. Benraad, H. B., Benraad, Th. J., and Kloppenborg, P. W. C.: Transient hypertension caused by segmental renal artery occlusion. Br. Med. J. 4:408, 1969.

PART IX. MISCELLANEOUS HYPERTENSION

Hypertensive Diseases in Pregnancy

By Mary Jane Gray, M.D., D.M.S.

HYPERTENSION IS FOUND in the pregnant woman either as a reflection of basic pathology of the cardiovascular or renal system or as a result of the stress of pregnancy itself—the specific "toxemia" of pregnancy, better designated "preeclampsia-eclampsia." At any particular point in the gestation, the differential diagnosis of these may be very difficult. The following discussion will consider some of the physiologic alterations in normal pregnancy and the characteristics of the various hypertensive states found during pregnancy, utilizing the definitions suggested by the Committee on Terminology of the American College of Obstetricians and Gynecologists.

Physiologic Changes of Pregnancy

If one considers the magnitude of the changes affecting the cardiovascular and renal systems of the pregnant woman, it is more remarkable that she has difficulty so rarely than that the precarious balance sometimes topples.

Renal Function

Dilatation of the entire renal collecting system characterizes a change beginning about the third month and returning to normal within 2 to 12 weeks postpartum. A progesterone effect on smooth muscle is primarily responsible but mechanical obstruction may contribute. Thus, all pyelograms in pregnant women show hydronephrosis and hydroureter and are difficult to interpret. Another drawback of the pyelographic examination, in addition to the difficulty of interpretation, is that the fetus is subjected to significant radiation. Except in an emergency, such evaluations should be deferred until 3 months postpartum.

From the Department of Obstetrics and Gynecology, University of Vermont College of Medicine, and Medical Center Hospital of Vermont, Burlington, Vermont.

Sims and Krantz [1] have shown that glomerular filtration is increased by about 50 percent during pregnancy and that renal blood flow and plasma flow are up 25 percent. Possibly as a result of this increased flow, the normal blood urea nitrogen in the pregnant woman is only 8.7 ± 1.5 S.D. mg per 100 ml compared with 13.0 ± 3.0 mg per 100 ml in the nonpregnant. Creatinine is reduced to 0.46 ± 0.06 mg per 100 ml and serum uric acid is also lower.

Posture exerts striking changes in renal function in pregnant women. Assali, Dignam, and Dasgupta [2] have demonstrated a marked fall in glomerular filtration on quiet standing. Chesley and Sloan [3] found a reduction in sodium excretion of 50 percent in supine pregnant women compared to women studied in the lateral position. The changes in the kidney in pregnancy have recently been reviewed by Sims,[4] by Chesley,[5] and by Lindheimer and Katz.[6]

Sodium and Water Balance

Radioisotope techniques have shown that normal, nonedematous pregnant women retain 500 to 700 mEq of sodium during pregnancy, an amount easily accounted for in the products of conception and the markedly expanded material plasma. Hytten, Thomson, and Taggart [7] and Thomson, Hytten, and Billewicz [8] found that their studies showed no excess water retention until the last 10 weeks of pregnancy but found that edema during this period was not necessarily of pathologic origin.

As mechanisms governing sodium balance have become better known, it has become apparent that the physiologic changes of pregnancy involve factors leading to sodium loss as well as sodium retention (Table 1). The previously mentioned 50-percent augmentation in glomerular filtration increases the amount of sodium filtered by the kidney, and, if unbalanced, would lead to sodium depletion.

Progesterone, a powerful antagonist to aldo-

TABLE 1.—*Factors Affecting Sodium Balance in the Pregnant Woman*

Leading to Sodium Loss	*Leading to Sodium Retention*
1. Increased progesterone	1. Increased estrogen
2. Increased glomerular filtration	2. Increased aldosterone
3. Fetal requirements	3. Postural edema

sterone at the renotubular level, is produced in vast quantities by the placenta. Levels of aldosterone secretion are increased about 10-fold during pregnancy to an average of 1,100 μg per day.[9] Despite this, responsiveness to change in dietary sodium is maintained. Rigid sodium restriction increases aldosterone secretion up to an average of 7,800 μg per day, suggesting maximal response to stress of sodium loss. Pike, Miles, and Wardlaw [10] have demonstrated a greater effect of sodium restriction on the juxtaglomerular apparatus of pregnant rats than in nonpregnant controls.

A pregnancy effect on the colonic absorption of sodium, potassium, and water has recently been demonstrated by Parry, Shields, and Turnbull.[11] This may be secondary to an aldosterone effect or to decreased motility.

Some of these relationships are shown in Figure 1. Obviously, the balance is a precarious one and may be easily disturbed.

Cardiovascular Changes

The blood volume gradually expands in pregnancy to about 45 percent above the normal nonpregnant volume, reaching a peak at about 25 weeks and maintaining this increase to term. This includes expansion of both plasma volume and red cells. Several coagulation factors are elevated including fibrogen. Cardiac output and stroke volume are somewhat increased. The large placental circulation is considered by some to act as an arteriovenous shunt. Venous pressure in the pelvis and legs is elevated because of the obstruction of the vena cava by the pregnant uterus.

PREECLAMPSIA–ECLAMPSIA

"Preeclampsia is the development of hypertension with proteinuria or edema, or both, due to pregnancy or the influence of a recent pregnancy. It occurs after the 20th week of gestation but may develop before this time in the presence of trophoblastic disease. Preeclampsia is predominantly a disorder of primigravidas. Eclampsia is the occurrence of one or more convulsions not attributable to other cerebral

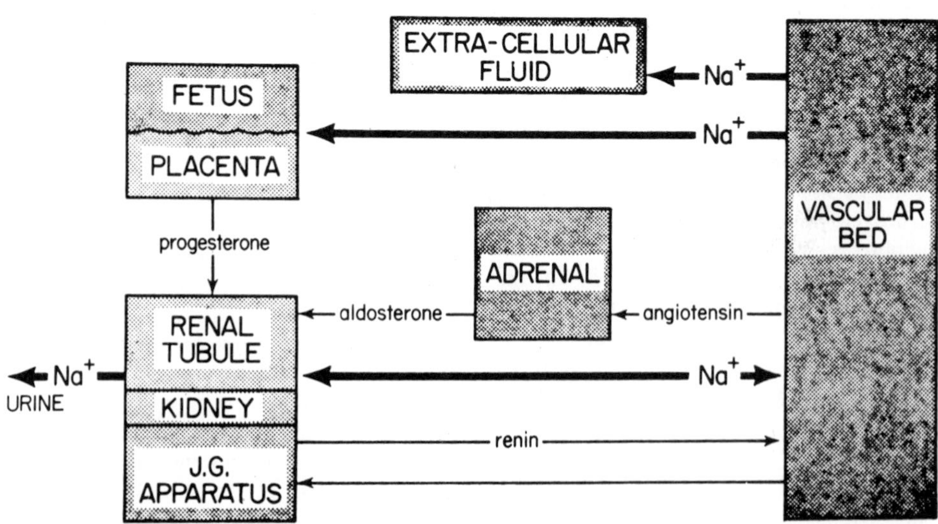

FIG. 1.—Diagrammatic representation of some of the relationships involved in sodium balance in pregnancy.

conditions such as epilepsy or cerebral hemorrhage in a patient with preeclampsia." *

Etiology

Despite claims to the contrary, the cause of preeclampsia–eclampsia remains unclear. Multiple theories have been brought forward, supported by a bewildering body of evidence derived from the study of various organs and enzyme systems, all abnormal in the advanced stages of the disease.

Any theory which attempts to explain the specific toxemia of pregnancy must take into account the circumstances surrounding its occurrence. The disease is found primarily in primigravidas, and among these, the young teenager is the most vulnerable. It is specific for the pregnant human and has not been completely duplicated in any research animal. Convulsions can occur antepartum, intrapartum, or up to 2 days postpartum. In spite of the necessity of pregnancy, the fetus appears to be irrelevant because the condition is even more common in molar pregnancies, where only the trophoblastic tissue develops. Multiple pregnancies greatly increase the likelihood of preeclampsia. Erythroblastosis fetalis, the result of fetal Rh incompatibility, with its hydropic overdeveloped placenta, is commonly associated with acute preeclampsia. And a number of underlying medical conditions such as essential hypertension, renal disease, and diabetes are complicated by superimposed preeclampsia. Although Chesley, Annitto, and Cosgrove [12] have found the rate of development of diabetes to be increased 10-fold in the long-term follow-up of eclamptic multigravids, a recent study [13] involving electron microscopy of renal biopsies in diabetic women with the clinical diagnosis of preeclampsia points up the difficulty in making this diagnosis. The interrelationship between these two entities will require further clarification.

Sims has suggested that the pregnant woman is physiologically so precariously balanced that the syndrome of preeclampsia may be triggered in a number of ways.[14] One of the oldest theories holds that uteroplacental ischemia leads to either the increased production of pressor agents, or the decreased ability to detoxify these substances in the circulation. Increased sensitivity to norepinephrine has been documented in preeclamptic women,[15,16] but does not occur in those with essential hypertension. Hunter and Howard [17] and more recently Zuspan and Abbott [18] have identified pressor agents in amniotic fluid.

Plasma fibrinogen levels are elevated about 50 percent in normal pregnant women to a range of 300 to 600 mg per 100 ml. Several other clotting factors are also increased. McKay [19] has gathered evidence of disseminated intravascular clotting in preeclampsia–eclampsia, initially triggered by degenerating trophoblasts in the placenta and resembling a generalized Shwartzman reaction. Thrombocytopenia and fibrin deposits in the glomeruli have been demonstrated. The mechanism seems important in the rare but grave complication of acute renal corticonecrosis. The Birmingham Eclampsia Study Group [20] has recently demonstrated pulmonary changes suggestive of widespread intravascular clotting. Reid and co-workers [21] have also confirmed the presence of a consumption coagulopathy in preeclamptics.

Brewer [22] has recently redirected attention to the liver, postulating that malnutrition leads to liver damage such that the normal conjugation of hormones is interfered with and suggests that this precipitates the syndrome of preeclampsia. The predominance of male infants in toxemic pregnancies suggests an immune mechanism possibly triggered by histoincompatibility of fetus and mother due to antigens on the Y chromosome.[23,24]

The theory that preeclampsia is caused by sodium retention has lingered long after the evidence to the contrary seems conclusive. While it is true that once the syndrome has developed, the damaged kidney is unable to handle a sodium load and thus the preeclamptic has an increased amount of total-body sodium,[25] several investigators [26–28] have been unable to produce preeclampsia by increasing dietary sodium. Horrobin and Lloyd [29] have shown that salt protects against the hypertensive effect of progesterone in rabbits. Sodium depletion in pregnancy acts as a stimulus to activate the renin-angiotensin system ac-

* All definitions quoted are those suggested by the Committee on Terminology of the American College of Obstetricians and Gynecologists.

TABLE 2.—*The Direction of Changes in Renin and Aldosterone in Pregnancy*

	Normal Pregnancy		*Abnormal Pregnancy*	
	Normal Salt	*Low Salt*	*Preeclampsia*	*Eclampsia*
Renin	+	++	+	–
Aldosterone	+	++	+	–

cording to Gordon, Parsons, and Symonds.[30] Aldosterone, angiotensin, and renin are markedly elevated in the normal pregnant woman compared with the nonpregnant, but are decreased toward normal nonpregnant values in severe preeclampsia with sodium retention (Table 2).[31,32] The decreased reactivity of the normal pregnant woman toward angiotensin is lost in preeclampsia.[33] Ehrlich [34] has confirmed the important role of aldosterone in conserving sodium in normal pregnancy.

Physiologic Alterations

Hypertension in preeclampsia is defined as a rise of at least 30 mm Hg over the usual systolic pressure and a rise of 15 mm Hg in the diastolic pressure or an absolute systolic pressure of 140 mm Hg or more or a diastolic pressure of 90 mm Hg or more. Duncan and Ginsburg [35] have demonstrated an increase in peripheral vascular resistance at both resting and peak levels of blood flow and have postulated a reversible abnormality in the vessel wall. According to Seligman [36] there is an interference of baroreceptor function, possibly on a mechanical basis. The vascular reactivity to pressor substances is increased. The spasm of vessels in the retina may readily be observed. The blood volume is decreased as is the absolute amount of serum protein.[37] In severe disease, the hematocrit may be markedly elevated as fluid is rapidly shifted out of the vascular bed.

Impairment of renal function, manifested initially by generalized edema and later by proteinuria of increasing severity, is usual. The glomerular basement membrane acts as a molecular sieve, allowing immunoglobulins IgG and IgD to escape into the urine.[38] The diagnosis of mild preeclampsia is sometimes made in the absence of proteinuria but must be held suspect. Patients with severe preeclampsia and eclampsia frequently manifest oliguria or even anuria. Tests of renal function reflect this diminished glomerular filtration. In evaluating the BUN and other tests of renal function, care must be taken to compare the results with *pregnant* normals, which are significantly altered from the nonpregnant. In women who had not been given thiazide diuretics, Pollack and Nettles [39] found that the elevation in serum uric acid roughly parallels the severity of the disease, although Pritchard and Stone [40] were unable to demonstrate this.

Sudden excessive weight gain of 2 to 10 pounds within 1 week reflects fluid retention, usually secondary to electrolyte retention due to the diminished glomerular filtration. The excess fluid is usually apparent as generalized edema. Facial swelling is common in severe disease. The effect of the pregnant uterus on the venous return from the legs makes ankle and pretibial edema of little diagnostic aid.

Central nervous system irritability manifested by headache, restlessness, and increased deep-tendon reflexes including clonus usually signifies impending convulsions. Epigastric pain, possibly indicating hepatic involvement and intravascular clotting, frequently precedes convulsions.

Pathologic Changes

The major pathologic changes found in eclampsia are the result of vasospasm, fibrin deposition, or both. The characteristic hepatic lesion, once thought to be pathogenetic of the disease, is periportal necrosis occurring around fibrin thrombi. These lesions are now considered to be a late effect of the systemic disease. Subcapsular hemorrhage with rupture of the liver occurs infrequently, but is often fatal.

More specific in preeclampsia–eclampsia are the renal glomerular changes. Endothelial cells swell so as to block the capillary lumina.

Electron microscopy has shown that the lesion previously described as thickening of the basement membrane does not exist, but confirms glomerular endotheliosis (Fig. 2) with fibrin or fibrinogen deposits. These deposits have been demonstrated by immunofluorimetry.[41] Pollack and Nettles [39] and Altchek, Albright, and Sommers [42] have described increased granularity of the juxtaglomerular apparatus and spasm of the afferent arterioles. Serial renal biopsies suggest that these glomerular lesions appear before the onset of clinical signs and symptoms and regress postpartum. The renal biopsy may be the only sure way to make the differential diagnosis of preeclampsia, but risks of the procedure during pregnancy preclude its routine use. Paul et al.[43] suggest limitations in the diagnostic specificity of the procedure. Rarely in severe preeclampsia or eclampsia, thrombosis of the renal intralobular arteries leads to corticonecrosis with renal failure.

Although placental ischemia has been proposed as an etiologic factor in preeclampsia and placental infarcts and lesions of the spiral arterioles have been described in conjunction with the disease,[44] the correlation of placental lesions with symptoms remains tenuous.

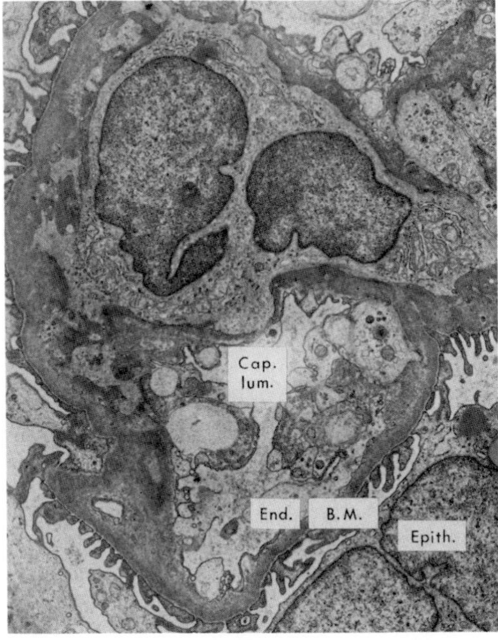

FIG. 2.—Renal lesion found in severe preeclampsia–eclampsia by electron microscopy. **Cap. lum.,** capillary lumen decreased; **End.,** capillary endothelium; **B.M.,** basement membrane; **Epith.,** epithelial cell. (Courtesy Charles P. McCartney, M.D.)

Descriptions of the cerebral lesion come from autopsy material and include edema, thrombi, and hemorrhage, the last being one of the common causes of death. The convulsions of eclampsia are generally thought to be due to cerebral anoxia, secondary to vasospasm or thrombi. Adrenal corticonecrosis and hemorrhage are also common terminally and may be related to the generalized Shwartzman phenomenon with disseminated intravenous clotting described previously.

Prevention

Much mischief has been done by the use of thiazide diuretics as a prophylactic measure against preeclampsia in pregnancy. Early reports were conflicting, but the excellent double-blind study by Kraus, Marchese, and Yen [45] showed conclusively that this measure did not reduce the incidence of preeclampsia although the amount of edema was reduced. The widely quoted series by Finnerty and Bepko,[46] supporting the use of diuretics, was poorly designed, with a large group of patients being transferred to the control group for noncooperation! The results of the major studies relating to this are summarized in Table 3. The hazards associated with the prophylactic use of diuretics are listed in Table 4, and have been discussed elsewhere.[47]

The increased incidence of preeclampsia in the young and the indigent suggests that improved nutrition with special attention to increased protein, both in the underweight and in the malnourished, obese woman, may be of value. New recommendations of the Committee on Maternal Nutrition of the National Academy of Sciences and the National Research Council [48] have just been released suggesting an average weight gain of 24 pounds during pregnancy as desirable.

Any measures that delay pregnancy beyond the midteens will also reduce the incidence of preeclampsia. As in any condition involving hypertension, a relaxed outlook toward life with minimal stress is desirable.

TABLE 3.—*The Use of Prophylactic Thiazides in Pregnancy*

Authors	*No. of Women*	*Double Blind*	*Prevents Edema*	*Decreases Toxemia*
Weseley, A. C., and Douglas, G. W. (1962)	267	Yes	Yes	No
Flowers, C. E., Grizzle, J. E., Easterling, W. E., and Bonner, O. B. (1962)	519	Yes	Yes	No
Cuadros, A., and Tatum, H. J. (1964)	1,771	No	Yes	Yes
Finnerty, F. A., and Bepko, F. J. (1966)	3,083	No *	Yes	Yes
Kraus, G. W., Marchese, J. R., and Yen, S. S. C. (1966)	1,030	Yes	Yes	No

From Gray, M. J.,[47] with permission.
* All patients who did not take pills were moved to the control group.

Differential Diagnosis

The diagnosis of the specific toxemia of pregnancy is easy in the young primigravida who has been seen early in pregnancy, who has been known to be normotensive and in good general health and who then develops the classic triad of hypertension, edema, and proteinuria. Even some of these will have the renal lesion of nephritis if biopsy is done.[39] In the multigravida seen late in pregnancy, without adequate history, the differentiation from chronic hypertensive vascular disease and/or renal disease may be very difficult. Many women show a transient drop in blood pressure during the midtrimester of pregnancy with elevation to previous levels as they approach term. McCartney,[49] using renal biopsy, found that 75 percent of multigravidas who were clinically diagnosed as having "toxemia of pregnancy" had renal lesions of arteriolar sclerosis, or chronic renal disease, or failed to show the glomerular endotheliosis which he considers pathognomonic of preeclampsia.

TABLE 4.—*Hazards of Diuretics During Pregnancy*

Maternal
- Hemorrhagic pancreatitis (four deaths reported)
- Hyponatremia (two deaths reported)
- Hypokalemia
- Metabolic alkalosis
- Hyperuricemia
- Diabetogenic effect

Fetal
- Hyponatremia
- Thrombocytopenia (?)

The diagnosis of preeclampsia in the older patient will always be suspect, and therefore subject to modification after a more complete history and an adequate postpartum evaluation of the renovascular system have been obtained. It is unfortunate that the two most useful tests in the differential diagnosis, the renal biopsy and the Dieckman salt load, in which the patient with essential hypertension is found to handle an intravenous load without difficulty whereas the preeclamptic becomes acutely worse, are each too hazardous to use routinely. Sarles et al.[50] recently confirmed this difference in response to salt-loading between the hypertensive and the preeclamptic.

In the patient who has convulsed, the diagnosis of eclampsia is made if hypertension, proteinuria, and edema are present. Obtaining a history will usually help in diagnosing the epileptic although the young patient who has never previously convulsed may be difficult to evaluate. An occasional severe hypertensive with a cerebral hemorrhage may confuse the clinician, but autopsy usually clarifies these cases.

Therapy

Studies involving serial renal biopsies suggest what clinicians have long suspected, that the symptoms of preeclampsia may abate with treatment, but that the underlying lesion usually regresses only after delivery.[42] All treatment other than the induction of labor remains symptomatic, and the vigor and pattern with which this is carried out will depend upon the severity of the syndrome and the duration of the gestation at the time the diagnosis is made. Mild preeclampsia frequently responds to increased rest. The position in which the rest is obtained is of great importance. Chesley and Sloan [3] have shown that renal clearance in pregnant women is 25 percent greater when they lie on their sides as compared to their backs and has recently reviewed the effect of posture on renal function in preeclampsia.[51] Noble [52] has found that blood pressure in hypertensive pregnant women is lowest in the left lateral position. Mild sedation such as phenobarbital may help the patient relax and increase the amount of bed rest she will tolerate. In picking a time for delivery the hazards of prematurity must be weighed against those of intrauterine fetal death.

If the woman has demonstrated difficulty in handling salt and water by a sudden weight gain and/or generalized edema, dietary salt should be restricted and rest in the lateral position recommended to improve renal function and decrease the loss of fluid and electrolytes into edema fluid on a postural basis. Diuretics may be used cautiously and intermittently with these three warnings:

1. The edema will improve but the underlying disease process will not. This may lull the physician into a false sense of security.
2. Patients frequently complain of weakness after diuresis, suggesting that they have been salt-depleted. Such patients may actually be hypovolemic.
3. Thiazides increase the serum uric acid and interfere with this as a rough indicator of the severity of the disease.

Mathews, Patel, and Sengupta [53] have increased the safety of outpatient management of mild preeclampsia by giving all patients Albustix for the daily testing of urine for proteinuria, and then admitting only those patients who showed more than a trace of albumin. Fetal progress was followed with weekly urinary estriol determinations.

Preeclampsia is considered severe if the blood pressure reaches 160 mm Hg systolic or 110 mm Hg diastolic on at least two occasions, 6 hours apart, or if the woman has proteinuria of 5 gm or more in 24 hours, or is oliguric, has cerebral disturbances, or develops pulmonary edema. Such patients must be hospitalized immediately, sedated, and stabilized and plans made for delivery. Oversedation to the point of near coma should be avoided. Hyperreflexia is best treated with magnesium sulfate. Hypertension which does not respond to rest and sedation but remains a threat to cerebral vessels should be treated with antihypertensive agents such as hydralazine or reserpine. Rapid or combined use of these drugs may lead to vascular collapse and in all cases these agents tend to diminish the blood supply to the uterus, and may impair fetal oxygenation. In severe preeclampsia the kidney is usually unable to respond to diuretic agents because of the renal lesion.

Eclampsia

Although the development of convulsions pushes the patient abruptly from preeclampsia to eclampsia, the underlying disease process is a continuous one and some patients with severe preeclampsia are more gravely ill than some who convulse. Nonetheless, with the onset of convulsions, concern over the associated 5-percent maternal mortality and 25-percent fetal mortality mounts.

Therapy remains symptomatic with attention directed first to maintaining oxygenation during the convulsions, and then to prevention of further seizures. Intravenous administration of 2 to 4 gm of magnesium sulfate given carefully as a bolus will reduce the hyperreflexia immediately. A maintenance dose of magnesium sulfate may be given either intravenously or intramuscularly. Too rapid administration may depress respirations. Magnesium is excreted rapidly by normal kidneys but in cases with renal failure, care must be taken not to raise the serum level too high. Recent evidence shows an effect of magnesium on the generalized Shwartzman reaction.[54] Diazepam has been used by some as an anticonvulsant. Diphenylhydantoin is not always effective and is rarely employed. Morphine has been overused in the past and has a limited place in modern therapy, but small doses of meperidine (Demerol) may be used for sedation.

As soon as the convulsions are under control and the patient is stabilized, delivery should be planned. Induction of labor and vaginal delivery is preferable to cesarean section, if this can be accomplished easily. The renal status must be constantly assessed, grossly by urinary output, and more precisely later by other tests. If oliguria heralds possible renal failure, fluids must be monitored and the patient treated as if she had renal failure from any other cause.

Because of the presence of intravascular clotting in severe preeclampsia and eclampsia, heparin has been suggested [55,56] for the treatment and is occasionally used. It is too hazardous a drug to use in the large numbers of women (up to 10%) who develop mild preeclampsia, and in severe preeclampsia, preparations for delivery preclude its use. A rational place for the heparinization of the toxemia patient may eventually emerge.

After delivery, the natural course of the disease is toward improvement even though, in about 25 percent of patients, the first convulsion occurs postpartum. Careful symptomatic therapy is needed until the renal lesion reverses, the patient diureses, and the blood pressure gradually returns to normal. This may occur within the first 24 hours or require as long as 2 weeks. The renal biopsy usually returns to normal within 6 weeks, but some residual change has been reported over several months.[40]

In women with severe preeclampsia and eclampsia, an adverse effect on the fetus is to be expected. Chakravorty [57] found the infants to be small for dates although this effect did not parallel the albuminuria. The fetoplacental ratio was not abnormal despite changes in placental vessels. Growth retardation of various viscera was pinpointed to a subnormal amount of cytoplasm by Naeye.[58] Many laboratories have attempted to correlate urinary estriol secretion in the mother with fetal well-being, but such correlation is not as good in preeclampsia as in other maternal diseases such as diabetes.[59] When magnesium sulfate is used in treatment, the fetus must be checked for depression secondary to increased serum magnesium levels. This mode of therapy, however, may be less hazardous to the fetus than hypotensive agents involving possible interference with placental blood supply.[60]

Prognosis. Chesley, Annitto, and Cosgrove [12] have followed 268 eclamptic women for an average of 25 years. Women who have had eclampsia have a 25-percent chance of hypertensive complications during future pregnancies but only about 2 percent have full-blown eclampsia again. Of pregnancies carried to 28 weeks or more, 93 percent had a favorable outcome. White women having eclampsia as primigravidas were found to have the same distribution of hypertension and death as the general population. Black women and white women having eclampsia as multigravidas had a mortality about three times the expected rate, the result of an increased incidence of hypertensive disease. Diabetes developed in five times the expected rate in primigravidas and 10 times the expected rate in those having eclampsia as multigravidas. Chesley, Annitto, and Cosgrove concluded that preeclampsia did not cause chronic hypertension. Tillman [61] had previously reached a similar conclusion.

Pregnancy in Hypertensive Women

"Chronic hypertensive disease is the presence of persistent hypertension of whatever cause, before pregnancy, or before the 20th week of gestation or persistent hypertension beyond the 42nd postpartum day." Essential hypertension is the most common medical condition seen in pregnant women, especially in the older multigravida. Many women show a transient fall in blood pressure during the midtrimester of pregnancy, and this may make the diagnosis difficult. Mild labile hypertension confers only a minimally increased risk during pregnancy, reflected chiefly in an increased fetal mortality. The fetal risk can be monitored with estriol determinations and labor induced, usually at about 37 weeks.

In more severe chronic hypertension the risks involve superimposed preeclampsia, premature separation of the placenta, and cerebral hemorrhage. "Superimposed preeclampsia or eclampsia is the development of preeclampsia or eclampsia in a patient with chronic hypertensive vascular or renal disease. When the hypertension antedates the pregnancy as established by previous blood pressure recordings, a rise in the systolic pressure of 30 mm Hg or a rise in the diastolic pressure of 15 mm Hg and the development of proteinuria or edema or both are required during pregnancy to establish the diagnosis."

Although the diagnosis of superimposed preeclampsia is frequently hard to differentiate from an exacerbation of the underlying vascular disease and is always somewhat suspect, there are several bits of evidence for its existence. Altchek, Albright, and Sommers [42] and McCartney [49] have each found biopsy evidence of capillary endotheliosis in addition to arteriolar disease in some of these patients. Similarly, Robertson, Brosens, and Dixon [44] can distinguish coexisting placental lesions of both hypertension and preeclampsia. Plentl and Gray [62] found that women with hypertensive vascular disease with superimposed preeclampsia had an increase in total-body sodium and sodium space similar to preeclamptics but unlike the patients with uncomplicated but severe essential hypertension. With the development of superimposed preeclampsia, the fetal loss increases to about 15 percent. Once a pregnancy with superimposed preeclampsia has occurred, the chance of its recurrence in a future pregnancy is about 80 percent and future pregnancies should be discouraged.[63]

In general, the maternal and fetal prognosis is impaired in patients with cardiac damage, with reduced renal function, advanced retinal changes, a systolic blood pressure of 200 mm Hg or diastolic of 120 mm Hg, or a history of previous superimposed preeclampsia. Such women should be advised against pregnancy and considered as candidates for interruption of pregnancy should it occur. These risks, together with the entire subject of hypertensive complications of pregnancy, are considered elsewhere.[64]

Other rare causes of hypertensive disease in pregnancy include coarctation of the aorta, unilateral renal arterial disease, hyperaldosteronism, and pheochromocytoma. These have been recently reviewed by Sims [14] and by Schewitz.[65] Although the differential diagnoses are established in the usual manner, the presence of the pregnancy increases the difficulties and hazards involved. The subject of renal disease in pregnancy cannot be considered here but the physician must remember the great frequency with which basic renal pathology has been found in kidney biopsies performed on patients clinically diagnosed as having preeclampsia. Chronic pyelonephritis may not only be difficult to differentiate from preeclampsia, but may predispose to its development.

Summary

Hypertension is one of the most common complications of pregnancy. When found occurring de novo together with edema and proteinuria in the young primigravida, the diagnosis is usually preeclampsia, a disease involving many systems and cured only by delivery. In the older multigravida, search must be made for underlying systemic disease such as essential hypertension, diabetes, or renal disease even though the specific lesion of preeclampsia may be superimposed.

Acknowledgment

I would like to thank my colleagues Ethan A. H. Sims, M.D., C. Irving Meeker, M.D., and Lester Silberman, M.D. for their help in preparing this manuscript.

References

1. Sims, E. A. H., and Krantz, K. E.: Serial studies of renal function during pregnancy and the puerperium in normal women. J. Clin. Invest. 37:1764, 1958.
2. Assali, N. S., Dignam, W. J., and Dasgupta, K.: Renal function in normal pregnancy. II. Effects of venous pooling on renal hemodynamics and water, electrolyte, and aldosterone excretion during normal gestation. J. Lab. Clin. Med. 54:394, 1959.
3. Chesley, L. C., and Sloan, D. M.: The effect of posture on renal function in late pregnancy. Am. J. Obstet. Gynec. 89:754, 1964.
4. Sims, E. A. H.: The kidney in pregnancy. *In* Strauss, M. B., and Welt, L. G. (Eds.): Diseases of the Kidney. Boston: Little, Brown, 1971, pp. 1155–1205.
5. Chesley, L. C.: Kidney, fluids and electrolytes. *In* Assali, N. S. (Ed.): Pathophysiology of Gestational Disorders. New York: Academic Press. (In press.)
6. Lindheimer, M., and Katz, A. I.: Kidney function in pregnancy. *In* Wynn, R. M. (Ed.): Obstetric-Gynecologic Annual, vol. 1.

New York: Appleton-Century-Crofts, 1972, pp. 139–166.
7. Hytten, F. E., Thomson, A. M., and Taggart, N.: Total body water in normal pregnancy. J. Obstet. Gynaec. Br. Commonw. 73:553, 1966.
8. Thomson, A. M., Hytten, F. E., and Billewicz, W. Z.: The epidemiology of oedema during pregnancy. J. Obstet. Gynaec. Br. Commonw. 74:1, 1967.
9. Watanabe, M., Meeker, C. I., Gray, M. J., Sims, E. A. H., and Solomon, S.: Secretion rate of aldosterone in normal pregnancy. J. Clin. Invest. 42:1916, 1963.
10. Pike, R. L., Miles, J. E., and Wardlaw, J. M.: Juxtaglomerular degranulation and zona glomerulosa exhaustion in pregnant rats induced by low sodium intakes and reversed by sodium load. Am. J. Obstet. Gynec. 95:604, 1966.
11. Parry, E., Shields, R., and Turnbull, A. C.: The effect of pregnancy on the colonic absorption of sodium, potassium and water. J. Obstet. Gynaec. Br. Commonw. 77:616, 1970.
12. Chesley, L. C., Annitto, J. E., and Cosgrove, R. A.: Long-term follow-up study of eclamptic women. Am. J. Obstet. Gynec. 101:886, 1968.
13. Gonzalez-Gonzalez, L., Lopez-Llera, M., Gonzalez-Angulo, A., Linares, G. R., and Sheider, G. B.: Diabetes mellitus and toxemia of pregnancy: Electron microscopic study of renal biopsies. J. Reprod. Med. 7:123, 1971.
14. Sims, E. A. H.: Preeclampsia and related complications of pregnancy. Am. J. Obstet. Gynec. 107:154, 1970.
15. Raab, W., Schroeder, G., Wagner, R., and Gigee, W.: Vascular reactivity and electrolytes in normal and toxemic pregnancy. J. Clin. Endocrinol. 16:1196, 1956.
16. Zuspan, F. P., Nelson, G. H., and Ahlquist, R. P.: Epinephrine infusions in normal and toxemic pregnancy. Am. J. Obstet. Gynec. 90:88, 1964.
17. Hunter, C. A., Jr., and Howard, W. F.: A pressor substance (hysterotonin) occurring in toxemia. Am. J. Obstet. Gynec. 79:838, 1960.
18. Zuspan, F. P., and Abbott, M.: Identification of a pressor substance in amniotic fluid. Am. J. Obstet. Gynec. 107:664, 1970.
19. McKay, D. G.: Disseminated Intravascular Coagulation: An Intermediate Mechanism of Disease. New York: Harper & Row, 1965.
20. Starkie, C. M., Harding, L. K., Fletcher, D. J., and Stuart, J.: Intravascular coagulation and abnormal lung scans in preeclampsia and eclampsia. Lancet 2:889, 1971.
21. Reid, D. E., Frigoletto, F. D., Tullis, J. L., and Hinman, J.: Hypercoagulable states in pregnancy. Am. J. Obstet. Gynec. 111:494, 1971.
22. Brewer, T. H.: Metabolic Toxemia of Late Pregnancy—A Disease of Malnutrition. Springfield, Ill.: Thomas, 1966.
23. Vara, P., Sakari, T., and Lokki, O.: Toxemia of late pregnancy. Acta Obstet. Gynec. Scand. 44(Suppl. 3):3, 1965.
24. Toivanen, P., and Hirvonen, T.: Sex ratio of newborns: Preponderance of males in toxemia of pregnancy. Science 170:187, 1970.
25. Chesley, L. C.: Sodium retention and preeclampsia. Am. J. Obstet. Gynec. 95:127, 1966.
26. Robinson, J.: Salt in pregnancy. Lancet 1:178, 1958.
27. Bower, D.: The influence of dietary salt intake on preeclampsia. J. Obstet. Gynaec. Br. Commonw. 71:123, 1964.
28. Gray, M. J., Munro, A. B., Sims, E. A. H., Meeker, C. I., Solomon, S., and Watanabe, M.: Regulation of sodium and total body water metabolism in pregnancy. Am. J. Obstet. Gynec. 89:760, 1964.
29. Horrobin, D. F., and Lloyd, I. J.: Preeclamptic toxemia: Possible relevance of progesterone, salt, and furosemide. J. Obstet. Gynaec. Br. Commonw. 77:253, 1970.
30. Gordon, R. D., Parsons, S., and Symonds, E. M.: A prospective study of plasma-renin activity in normal and toxaemic pregnancy. Lancet 1:347, 1969.
31. Watanabe, M., Meeker, C. I., Gray, M. D., Sims, E. A. H., and Solomon, S.: Aldosterone secretion rates in abnormal pregnancy. J. Clin. Endocrinol. Med. 25:1665, 1965.
32. Cresley, L. C.: Vascular reactivity in normal and toxemic pregnancy. Clin. Obstet. Gynec. 9:871, 1966.
33. Talledo, O. E., Rhodes, K., and Livingston, E.: Renin-angiotensin system in normal and toxemic pregnancies. Am. J. Obstet. Gynec. 97:571, 1967.
34. Ehrlich, E. N.: Heparinoid-induced inhibition of aldosterone secretion in pregnant women. Am. J. Obstet. Gynec. 109:963, 1971.
35. Duncan, S. L. B., and Ginsburg, J.: Arteriolar distensibility in hypertensive pregnancy. Am. J. Obstet. Gynec. 100:222, 1968.
36. Seligman, S. A.: Baroreceptor reflex function in preeclampsia. J. Obstet. Gynaec. Br. Commonw. 78:413, 1971.

37. Blekta, M., Hlavaty, V., Trnkova, M., Bendl, J., Bendova, L., and Chytil, M.: Volume of whole blood and absolute amount of serum proteins in the early stage of late toxemia of pregnancy. Am. J. Obstet. Gynec. 106:10, 1970.
38. Studd, J. W. W.: Immunoglobulins in normal pregnancy, preeclampsia and pregnancy complicated by the nephrotic syndrome. J. Obstet. Gynaec. Br. Commonw. 78:786, 1971.
39. Pollack, V. E., and Nettles, J. B.: The kidney in toxemia of pregnancy: A clinical and pathological study based on renal biopsies. Medicine 39:469, 1960.
40. Pritchard, J. A., and Stone, S. R.: Clinical and laboratory observations on eclampsia. Am. J. Obstet. Gynec. 99:754, 1967.
41. Vassalli, P., Morris, R. H., and McCluskey, R. T.: The pathogenic role of fibrin deposition in the glomerular lesions of toxemia of pregnancy. J. Exp. Med. 118:467, 1963.
42. Altchek, A., Albright, W. L., and Sommers, S. C.: The renal pathology of toxemia of pregnancy. Obstet. Gynec. 31:595, 1968.
43. Paul, R. E., Hayashi, T. T., Pardo, V., and Fisher, E. R.: Evaluation of renal biopsy in pregnancy toxemia. Obstet. Gynec. 34:235, 1969.
44. Robertson, W. B., Brosens, I., and Dixon, H. G.: The pathological response of the vessels of the placental bed to hypertensive pregnancy. J. Pathol. 93:581, 1967.
45. Kraus, G. W., Marchese, J. R., and Yen, S. S. C.: Prophylactic use of hydroclorothiazide in pregnancy. JAMA 198:1150, 1966.
46. Finnerty, F. A., and Bepko, F. J.: Lowering the perinatal mortality and prematurity rate. JAMA 195:429, 1966.
47. Gray, M. J.: Use and abuse of thiazides in pregnancy. Clin. Obstet. Gynec. 11:568, 1968.
48. Committee on Maternal Nutrition, National Research Council: Maternal Nutrition and the Course of Pregnancy. Washington, D.C.: National Academy of Sciences, 1970.
49. McCartney, C. P.: The acute hypertensive disorders of pregnancy classified by renal histology. Gynaecologia 167:214, 1969.
50. Sarles, H. E., Hill, S. S., LeBlanc, A. L., Smith, G. H., Canales, C. O., and Remmers, A. R., Jr.: Sodium excretion patterns during and following intravenous sodium chloride loads in normal and hypertensive pregnancies. Am. J. Obst. Gynec. 102:1, 1968.
51. Chesley, L. C., and Duffus, G. M.: Preeclampsia, posture and renal function. Obstet. Gynec. 38:1, 1971.
52. Noble, A. D.: The effect of posture on the blood pressure of pregnant women with hypertension. J. Obstet. Gynaecol. Br. Commonw. 78:110, 1971.
53. Mathews, D. D., Patel, I. R., and Sengupta, S. M.: Out-patient management of toxemia. J. Obstet. Gynaec. Br. Commonw. 78:6110, 1971.
54. Nasu, K., Latour, J. G., and McKay, D. G.: Modification of the generalized Shwartzman reaction by therapeutic agents. Am. J. Obstet. Gynec. 109:991, 1971.
55. Maeck, J. V. S., and Zilliacus, H.: Heparin in the treatment of toxemia of pregnancy. Am. J. Obstet. Gynec. 55:326, 1948.
56. Reid, D. E., Frigoletto, F. D., Tullis, J. L., and Hinman, J.: Hypercoagulable states in pregnancy. Am. J. Obstet. Gynec. 111:493, 1971.
57. Chakravorty, A. P.: Foetal and placental weight changes in normal pregnancy and preeclampsia. J. Obstet. Gynaec. Br. Commonw. 74:247, 1967.
58. Naeye, R. L.: Abnormalities in infants of mothers with toxemia of pregnancy. Am. J. Obstet. Gynec. 95:276, 1966.
59. Muller, K., and Nielsen, J. C.: The prognostic importance of oestrial excretion in preeclampsia. Dan. Med. Bull. 14:165, 1967.
60. Zuspan, F. P.: Toxemia of pregnancy. J. Reprod. Med. 2:116, 1969.
61. Tillman, A. J. B.: The effect of normal and toxemic pregnancy on blood pressure. Am. J. Obstet. Gynec. 70:589, 1955.
62. Plentl, A. A., and Gray, M. J.: Total body water, sodium space and total exchangeable sodium in normal and toxemic pregnant women. Am. J. Obstet. Gynec. 78:472, 1959.
63. Chesley, L. C.: Prognostic significance of recurrent toxemia of pregnancy. Obstet. Gynec. 23:847, 1964.
64. Chesley, L. C.: Hypertensive disorders in pregnancy. *In* Hellman, L. M., and Pritchard, J. A. (Eds.): Williams Obstetrics, 14th ed. New York: Appleton-Century-Crofts, 1971, pp. 685–747.
65. Schewitz, L. J.: Hypertension and renal disease in pregnancy. Med. Clin. North Am. 55:47, 1971.

Management of Hypertension in Toxemia of Pregnancy

By Frank A. Finnerty, Jr., M.D.

Except for the necessity of delivering the fetus, the management of the pregnant patient with acute hypertensive crisis should differ little from the management of the non-pregnant patient. Understanding of the underlying mechanisms involved allows for a rational therapeutic approach.

Hypertensive encephalopathy, whether complicating toxemia pregnancy, acute glomerulonephritis, or essential hypertension, is associated with generalized vasoconstriction and sodium retention. Sodium retention plays a more important role in the pathogenesis of toxemia and glomerulonephritis than in the other types. Vasoconstriction, by decreasing the blood supply to particular areas, accounts for all the important abnormalities (Fig. 1). Thus an increase in cerebral vasoconstriction causes cerebral ischemia, which leads to coma and convulsions. Cerebral ischemia rather than the rise in arterial pressure is, therefore, the important abnormality in inducing coma and convulsions. These same abnormalities are observed in patients with postural hypotension or Stokes-Adams syncope where there is a decrease in cardiac output with a resultant decrease in the amount of blood going to the brain.

From the Department of Medicine, Georgetown University School of Medicine, and the Departments of Medicine and Obstetrics/Gynecology, Georgetown University Medical Division, District of Columbia General Hospital, Washington, D.C.

When the retinal arteries of an eclamptic patient are inspected, they are found to be extremely narrow. Immediately following effective therapy, the arteries are seen to be full again. Indeed, blindness in acute hypertensive states has been shown by ophthalmoscopic examination to be accompanied by complete spastic obliteration of the retinal arteries, which later become patent, with restoration of vision, as the vasoconstriction subsides.

Whatever the underlying disease, the constancy of association of hypertensive encephalopathy with increased blood pressure and the frequency of a sharp rise in arterial pressure preceding the attack suggest that the hypertension or the phenomena that are concerned in its production are causally related to the cerebral syndrome. Increased constriction of the peripheral vessels seems to account for the elevated arterial pressure. The increase in

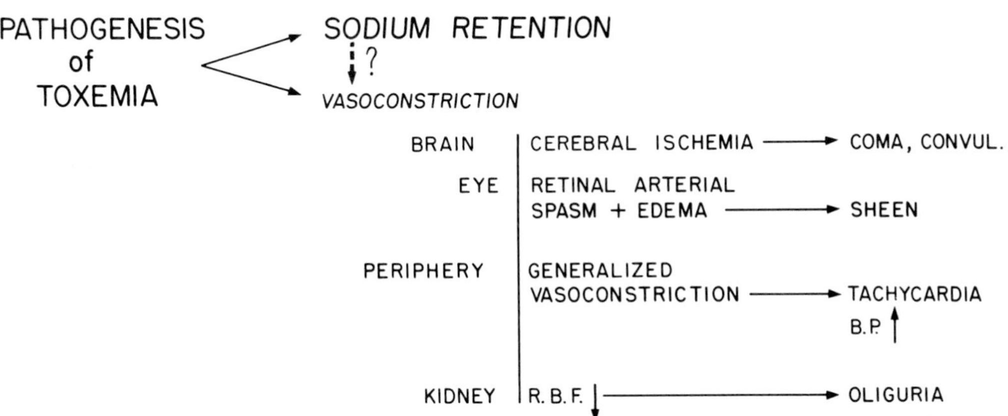

Fig. 1.—Note that the important physiologic abnormalities are a direct result of vasoconstriction.

arterial pressure in toxemia is not associated with a change in cardiac output.

The increased vasoconstriction in the renal circulation, particularly in the afferent vessels, as noted by Assali et al.,[1] accounts in part at least for the decrease in urinary output. The decrease in urinary output is part of the toxemic process and not necessarily a complication.

In the great majority of cases when encephalopathy complicates hypertension, the elevation of arterial pressure is extreme. In encephalopathy complicating acute nephritis, particularly in children, and in eclampsia convulsions may occur with a normal arterial pressure. When the charts of these patients are critically analyzed, however, it is noted that the arterial pressure is about 140/90 mm Hg. Although this figure is the conventional upper limit of normal for subjects over 25 years of age, a diastolic pressure of 90 mm Hg is certainly abnormal for most pregnant women and for all children. The average normal diastolic pressure in these groups is 60 to 70 mm Hg. It is apparent, therefore, that a rise in diastolic pressure from 60 to 80 mm Hg or from 70 to 90 mm Hg is very significant in the particular patient—as significant, indeed, as a rise in diastolic pressure from 90 to 110 mm Hg.

It is plausible to say, therefore, that hypertension per se is not responsible for the encephalopathy, since similar cerebral syndromes can be produced without any elevation of arterial pressure. The common denominator for hypertensive encephalopathy and postural hypotension—the sine qua non of all the above conditions—is a decreased cerebral blood flow due to cerebral vasoconstriction. Whether the multiple small thrombi noted postmortem are a result of or the cause of the cerebral vasoconstriction is unknown. (It is my opinion that the multiple thrombi are caused by the vasoconstriction.)

Since the encephalopathy is always accompanied by an increased vascular resistance—best reflected clinically by a high diastolic pressure—and since clinical experience has shown that clearing of the sensorium, cessation of convulsions, and release of vasoconstriction follow reduction in arterial pressure, the primary aim of therapy should be reduction of arterial pressure.

Since most potent antihypertensive agents produce sodium retention and sodium retention plays an important role in the pathogenesis of encephalopathy of toxemia, insurance and maintenance of an adequate urinary output are also essential in these patients.

From the practical standpoint, the drug chosen to reduce the arterial pressure depends on the clinical condition of the patient, particularly on the degree of cerebral ischemia present. If the condition of the patient is such that a 1½- to 2-hour delay in reducing the arterial pressure would not be harmful, parenteral administration of reserpine, methyldopa, or hydralazine can be used. The lack of a standard dosage of methyldopa and the high incidence of headache, flushing, and tachycardia upon hydralazine administration would seem to make reserpine the drug of choice in this regard. When immediate reduction in arterial pressure is necessary, e.g., when the patient is convulsing or on the verge of a convulsion, intravenously administered trimethaphan camphorsulfonate, sodium nitroprusside, or diazoxide may be useful. The lack of standard dosage necessitates individual titration of dose for both trimethaphan camphorsulfonate and sodium nitroprusside, and the necessity for special preparation of sodium nitroprusside for each administration makes the use of these agents difficult and time-consuming.

Parenteral reserpine has now been available for more than a decade and has become recognized as the most useful agent for the management of acute hypertension. The average effective intramuscular dose is 2.5 mg. There is no advantage in administering the drug intravenously. Although increasing the dosage of reserpine to 5 to 10 mg slightly increases the antihypertensive effect, it also greatly increases its toxicity. Following intramuscular injection, there is a delay in onset of action of at least 1½ hours; the maximal antihypertensive effect is not noted for 3 to 4 hours. The average duration of action is 7½ to 8 hours. At the time of the maximal antihypertensive effect there is a 20- to 25-percent average reduction in mean arterial pressure, and a slight reduction in heart rate usually occurs.

Just as important as the fall in arterial pressure following parenteral reserpine is the calming effect of the drug. This effect becomes apparent 45 minutes following injection, reaches its height at the time of the maximal antihypertensive response, and lasts 11 to 12 hours. Excitable, tense patients commonly are found in a normal sleep; if not spoken to or disturbed, they remain in this state until the effect of the medication has worn off.

The treatment of edema, prevention of sodium retention, and maintenance of a good urinary output are best accomplished by furosemide. In patients who have not received prior diuretics, furosemide is administered intravenously in doses of 40 mg. If the patient has been receiving diuretics, furosemide may be initiated in a dosage of 80 mg. In 2 hours the dose may be repeated if diuresis has not occurred (see below). In addition to a prompt sodium diuresis, this combination of reserpine plus furosemide results in a 25- to 30-percent reduction in mean arterial pressure which frequently lasts for 10 to 12 hours.

Although a very useful agent, reserpine given parenterally has many limitations:

1. Since there is a delay in onset of action of 1½ to 2 hours, reserpine cannot be relied on as the sole therapy in patients who show signs of severe cerebral ischemia.

2. It can be used only for short-term therapy. After 48 hours, nasal congestion, flushing of the face, and lethargy become objectionable to the patient.

3. Nasal congestion and increased tracheobronchial secretions occasionally occur in infants delivered to mothers treated with the drug. To prevent serious fetal complications, the nursery personnel should be alerted to this possibility, so that the infant is kept on its side and nasal congestion is promptly corrected.

4. Occasionally, signs of parkinsonism have been noted when reserpine has been continued for more than 72 hours.

5. Since reserpine frequently potentiates the sedative and occasionally the antihypertensive action of the barbiturates, these two drugs should not be administered concomitantly.

6. Local and, particularly, general anesthesia may occasionally potentiate the antihypertensive effect of reserpine, causing profound falls in arterial pressure. Knowledge of this possible potentiation and the prompt administration of norepinephrine or phenylephrine usually restores the arterial pressure promptly.

Despite these limitations, parenterally administered reserpine and furosemide remain the most useful agents in the treatment of encephalopathy when a delay in action of 2 hours would not be harmful to the patient.

During the past 7 years we have had experience with diazoxide, an agent that chemically resembles chlorothiazide but pharmacologically is quite different (Fig. 2). When administered by mouth, diazoxide reduces arterial pressure only slightly and causes sodium retention and hyperglycemia. When administered by vein, however, it is a very potent antihypertensive agent. The average effective dose is 300 mg undiluted and given rapidly.[2]

Experience has shown that the speed of injection is important in determining both the magnitude of the blood pressure fall and duration of antihypertensive effect. When less than 300 mg of diazoxide is administered in a 10- to 15-second period, only a brief antihypertensive response is noted. In a few hypertensive patients weighing over 150 pounds, 300 mg of diazoxide may produce only a slight reduction in arterial pressure. If a satisfactory fall in arterial pressure does not follow administration of 300 mg of diazoxide, the dosage should be increased to 5 mg per kilogram of body weight.

To date, over 400 patients with various types of hypertensive encephalopathy have been treated with diazoxide. A 35-percent average reduction in mean arterial pressure occurs during the first 2 minutes. During the next 3 to 5 minutes the arterial pressure increases gradually, leveling off at an average 20 percent below control levels (Fig. 3). No signs of postural hypotension, cerebral ischemia, or col-

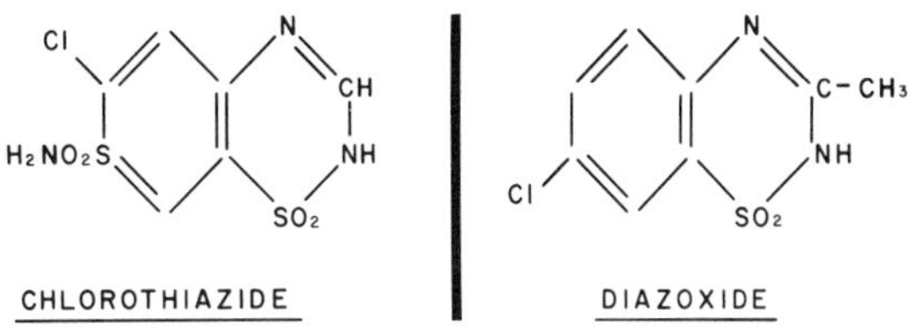

FIG. 2.—Chemical formulas of chlorothiazide and diazoxide.

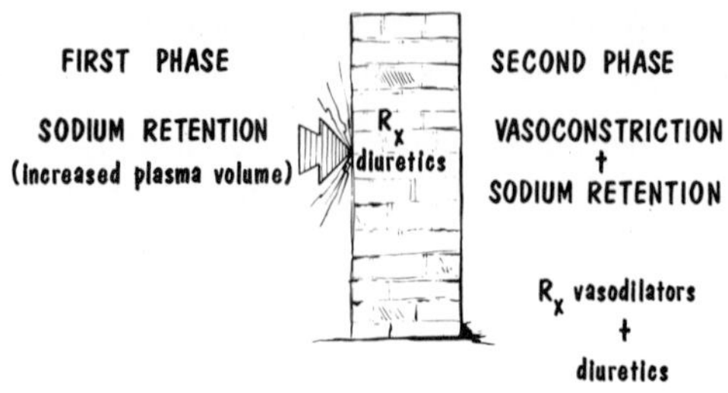

FIG. 3.—Effect of a single dose of 300 mg of diazoxide on arterial pressure and heart rate.

lapse are noted. The average duration of action is 9 to 11 hours.

Although the fall in arterial pressure with diazoxide is associated with an increase in cardiac output and a decrease in total peripheral resistance, there is a decrease in renal blood flow and urinary output and an increase in sodium retention. The decrease in urinary output and sodium retention can be prevented by the concomitant use of thiazide diuretics in most patients with normal renal function. In patients with azotemia and in most patients with toxemia the more potent diuretics such as furosemide are usually needed to guarantee an adequate urinary output.[3]

During the past several years 61 pregnant patients with either severe toxemia or severe toxemia superimposed on chronic hypertension have received diazoxide plus furosemide. Two of these patients had eclampsia. The aim of therapy was to maintain the diastolic pressure continuously below 90 mm Hg (below 80 mm Hg in patients 18 years of age and under) and the urinary output over 1 liter per day. Twelve to 24 hours after these goals were accomplished, labor was induced or a cesarean section was performed. Undiluted diazoxide was rapidly administered intravenously and repeated as often as necessary to maintain the arterial pressure at this level. Thirty-eight patients required one 300-mg dose of diazoxide, 20 patients required two doses and three patients four doses. Furosemide was initiated in a dose of 40 mg, given intravenously to those patients who had not received prior diuretic therapy. If the patient had been receiving diuretic therapy, furosemide was initially given intravenously in a dose of 80 mg. These dosages were increased every 1 or 2 hours until diuresis occurred. Eighty to 100 mg given twice daily was the usual effective dose.

In the two patients with eclampsia the acute reduction of arterial pressure with diazoxide promptly controlled the convulsions. Prior to delivery there was complete clearing of edema in all patients with an average weight loss of 16 pounds. The mean arterial pressure fell from an average of 141 to an average of 92 mm Hg, a 35 percent average reduction (Fig. 4). Albuminuria completely cleared in 14 patients who went into labor spontaneously. In 20 patients the administration of diazoxide temporarily halted labor, which was readily restarted by the use of oxytocics. In the 18 other patients it was necessary to induce labor.

A cesarean section was performed in two patients because the cervix was unfavorable for delivery. All mothers did well postdelivery. Thirty-four mothers delivered entirely normal infants including one set of triplets and four sets of twins. Four infants were born dead; 23 were premature, i.e., weighing less than 5½ pounds.

Forty-four mothers delivered infants under anesthesia. Thirty-four underwent general anesthesia lasting from 5 minutes to 2 hours; in the 14 others anesthesia was induced by pudendal or caudal block or by local infiltration. Thirty of these women delivered normal infants.

Although the immediate onset of action, maintenance of cardiac output and urinary flow, and release of vasoconstriction without causing harm to the mother or fetus make diazoxide and furosemide extremely valuable agents for the treatment of acute hypertension, certain limitations are still present:

1. Transitory hyperglycemia lasting no more than 12 hours occasionally follows intravenous

EFFECT OF RX ON MOTHERS (61 PATIENTS)

35% ↓ in MAP

Urinary output > 1 liter/day in all patients

Complete clearing of edema in all patients

Albuminuria — Complete clearing (14 patients)
Albuminuria — 4+ to 1+ (9 patients)

FIG. 4.—Note the prompt improvement in cardiovascular renal function.

EFFECT OF RX ON INFANTS	
Normal Infants	34
Dead Infants	4 (6%)
Premature Infants	23 (37%)

FIG. 5.—Despite improvement in cardiovascular function, note the high incidence of fetal mortality and prematurity.

administration of diazoxide. Recent reports of Wolff, Grant, and Wales [4] and studies in our laboratory [5] have demonstrated that pretreatment of patients with tolbutamide will effectively prevent the hyperglycemic effect of diazoxide. Although pretreatment with tolbutamide need not be routine, monitoring of blood sugar in these patients is advised.

2. The alkaline nature of the diazoxide solution makes any extravasation outside the vein painful. Although such extravasation is associated with a severe burning sensation which lasts from 1 to 2 hours, no sloughing of tissues has occurred.

3. In 50 percent of the patients who were in labor, the fall in arterial pressure following diazoxide administration was associated with temporary cessation of labor. This probably represents part of a generalized relaxation of smooth muscle and is not a toxic reaction of the drug. This property of diazoxide has recently been evaluated as a possible treatment of premature labor by Landesman and Wilson.[6] Awareness of this development and institution of oxytocics promptly restarted labor.

4. Although the fall in arterial pressure following diazoxide by itself is not associated with postural hypotension, the addition of furosemide to diazoxide by decreasing the plasma volume commonly produces postural hypotension.[3] Awareness of the possibility of this complication and maintenance of the patient in the supine position are all that is necessary.

Although the patients with encephalopathy were rapidly made better candidates for surgery and/or induction of labor (e.g., the arterial pressure was lowered, edema and albuminuria had either disappeared or significantly decreased and the urinary output was maintained above 1 liter per day), the 37-percent incidence of prematurity and the four fetal deaths are still evidence of the inherent dangers of this disease (Fig. 5). These data serve to emphasize that once full-blown toxemia has been allowed to develop, no form of therapy seems capable of reducing the perinatal mortality or prematurity rate. The only effective method for improving the fate of the fetus is the prevention of the vasoconstrictive phase of toxemia, e.g., treating the patient before the rise in arterial pressure and before the development of albuminuria. The value of prophylactic thiazides in this regard has been the subject of several previous reports from our clinic.[7–9]

REFERENCES

1. Assali, N. S., Kaplan, S. A., Fomon, S. J., and Douglass, H. A.: Renal function studies in toxemia of pregnancy. J. Clin. Invest. 32: 44, 1953.
2. Finnerty, F. A., Jr., Kakaviatos, N., Tuckman, J., and Magill, J.: Clinical evaluation of diazoxide, a new treatment for acute hypertension. Circulation 28:203, 1963.
3. Mroczek, W. J., Davidov, M., Gavrilovich, L., and Finnerty, F. A., Jr.: The value of aggressive therapy in the hypertensive patient with azotemia. Circulation 40:893, 1969.
4. Wolff, F. W., Grant, A. M., and Wales, J. K.: Reversal of diazoxide effects by tolbutamide. Lancet 1:1137, 1967.
5. Davidov, M., Kakaviatos, N., and Finnerty, F. A., Jr.: Unpublished data.
6. Landesman, R., and Wilson, K. H.: The relaxant effect of diazoxide on isolated gravid and non-gravid human myometrium. Am. J. Obstet. Gynec. 101:120, 1968.
7. Finnerty, F. A., Jr.: Lowering the perinatal mortality and the prematurity rate. JAMA 195:429, 1966.
8. Finnerty, F. A., Jr.: A decade with Diuril (chlorothiazide). *In* Lyght, C. E. (Ed.): Chlorothiazide in Obstetrics and Gynecology. West Point, Pa.: Merck, 1968.
9. Finnerty, F. A., Jr.: Treatment of mild toxemia. Clin. Obstet. Gynec. 9:944, 1966.

Oral Contraceptive Agents and Hypertension

By Arunabha Ganguly, M.D.

THE ORAL CONTRACEPTIVE agent is presently the most important modality in use for birth control in the advanced countries. It is hard to estimate the number of women using it but it probably is close to twenty million. Despite its wide acceptance it has not been found to be innocuous: A large number of adverse reactions have been reported to date. Hypertension is considered to be an occasional complication.

Although some scattered reports appeared earlier,[1,2] hypertension was established as a complication of oral contraceptive use only recently. This presumably was due to the fact that hypertension is a fairly common condition, and a cause and effect relationship between the use of oral contraceptives and high blood pressure was not appreciated. In 1967 Laragh and his associates,[3] and soon after, Woods [4] raised the possibility that the use of oral contraceptives and the development of hypertension might be related. That the hypertension was not coincidental was borne out by the fact that previously normotensive subjects became hypertensive within weeks or months of taking oral contraceptive drugs and in most of them blood pressure either returned to normal or decreased upon cessation of the drugs. In some women, hypertension reappeared on reinstitution of the oral contraceptive agent, subsiding again on their withdrawal. Somewhat similar observations have also been reported by Weinberger et al.[5] Their observations suggest a causal influence of oral contraceptives in the genesis of hypertension in some subjects. A case of malignant hypertension has been reported by Harris [6] in a young woman taking an oral contraceptive agent for 30 months. Complete reversal of the hypertension followed discontinuance of the drug.

Although hypertension as a complication of the "pill" is being recognized increasingly, the actual incidence of hypertension developing in women taking oral contraceptives is not precisely known. Tyson [7] in a prospective study reported that seven of 45 normotensive women followed over a period of 8 months had significant increases of blood pressure, an incidence of 15.5 percent. Kunin, McCormack, and Abernathy [8] noted a slightly increased mean systolic and diastolic blood pressure by statistical analysis in a group of 496 women already taking oral contraceptives when compared with those not on oral contraceptives and adjusted for various variables in the two groups. But 1 year later, in a second survey in a smaller population drawn from their previous one, they were unable to detect any statistically significant rise in mean blood pressure between oral contraceptive users and nonusers. Saruta, Sorade, and Kaplan [9] noted a 19-percent incidence in 80 women in a somewhat recent prospective study and Spellacy and Birk [10] reported that 15.2 percent of their 57 subjects developed hypertension observed during the sixth cycle. But Weir and associates,[11] in a prospective study from Scotland, noted that although 50 of 66 women had a mean rise of 6.6 mm Hg in systolic blood pressure at the end of 1 year, none had developed actual hypertension. The mean diastolic pressure had not changed significantly.

Most of the studies, however, are retrospective and therefore do not lend themselves to definite conclusions. The issue is further complicated by the variable definition and degree of blood pressure elevation reported by different authors. Also, there have been differences in size between the control group and the group in question and sometimes absence of any control group in some studies. Besides, the

---

From the Department of Medicine, Division of Endocrinology, Stanford University School of Medicine, Stanford, California.

The work reported here was performed during Dr. Ganguly's tenure as a Fellow in Medicine (Training Grant AM–5021, Dr. John A. Luetscher) from the National Institute of Arthritis and Metabolic Diseases, National Institutes of Health, U.S. Public Health Service.

type of drug used for contraception is yet another variable. Therefore, in the absence of a large, well-controlled, prospective study over a reasonably long period of time, the exact incidence of this complication remains elusive.

If the incidence of hypertension caused by oral contraceptives is not clear, the mechanism involved in its development is even more obscure. Various mechanisms, however, have been suggested. Since estrogen has the propensity to cause salt and water retention it conceivably can be involved in the evolution or aggravation of hypertension. Secondly, development of hypertension could be mediated through the renin-angiotensin-aldosterone system. Thirdly, altered, vascular smooth-muscle reactivity induced by the sex hormones may very well be implicated. Lastly, estrogen may have direct effects on the cardiovascular system.

Sodium retention is known to occur in pregnancy and estrogen reportedly [12] reduces renal sodium excretion. The sodium retention can well be due to increased mineralocorticoid activity which estrogen is said to produce. However, Johnson et al.,[13] from their studies on dogs, suggest this might be due to a different mechanism. Michelakis, Stant, and Brill [14] reported no significant change in exchangeable sodium space during various phases of the menstrual cycle. Natural progesterone has a natriuretic and antialdosterone effect [15] although some progestational compounds have been reported to cause salt retention. It is, therefore, unlikely that progesterone could be implicated as causing hypertension in this manner. Horrobin, Lloyd, and Burstyn,[16] however, claim to have induced hypertension in rabbits with progesterone injections. Curiously enough, increased salt intake prevented the development of hypertension. In rabbits pretreated with progesterone, these observers found intravenous infusion of aldosterone caused a rise in blood pressure twice as much as in untreated animals. The relevance of this observation to humans is unclear at present. It is believed that the salt-retaining effect of estrogen probably does not predispose one to hypertension.

Sensitization of vascular smooth muscle brought about by estrogen or progesterone does not seem to be operative, since Chesley and Tepper [17] reported that progesterone did not alter the pressor effect of angiotensin II. Chesley and his associates [18] also noted that pregnant women required two to three times as much angiotensin as did nonpregnant women to induce pressure responses of similar magnitude. Woods [4] was unable to demonstrate any shift in the dose-response curve of rats given estrogen-progesterone combinations. Douglas, Hull, and Langford,[19] in fact, reported a decreased blood pressure response in rats treated with large amounts of an oral contraceptive.

Although increased vascular sensitivity has not been shown to follow the use of either estrogen or progesterone, or both, estrogen has been shown to increase stroke volume and cardiac output. Lim et al.[20] noted no rise in peripheral resistance but an increase in blood pressure in normal subjects who were injected with naturally occurring estrogens, thereby concluding that blood pressure elevation was a result of increased cardiac output. It also has been suggested that estrogen may have a glycosidic effect [21] or might increase the efficiency of myocardial contraction by altering the actomyosin-adenosine triphosphate mechanism.[22] An increase in stroke volume may also be related to increased venous return, resulting from expanded plasma volume which possibly follows secondary hyperaldosteronism. Theoretically, however, all these effects could conceivably be counterbalanced by the effect of estrogen on venous distensibility as the latter is known to reduce venous tone in humans and this recently has been confirmed by the studies of Goodrich and Wood.[23] Walters and Lim,[24] on the other hand, recently reported increased cardiac output during the first 2 to 3 months in six patients taking oral contraceptives. Although systolic blood pressure increased slightly in most of their subjects, the diastolic blood pressure did not show any significant change. This mechanism, therefore, has not been able to shed any light on the etiology of diastolic hypertension.

This now brings us to examine yet another mechanism that conceivably could be implicated in the induction of hypertension associated with the use of oral contraceptives. It was Helmer and Griffith [25] who first noted that estrogen increased the renin substrate level in rats. Subsequently, Layne and his colleagues [26] reported increased aldosterone secretion rates in women taking estrogen or progestational compounds. Further, Crane et al.[27] observed that plasma renin activity was significantly increased in subjects taking ethinyl estradiol or oral contraceptives. It was left to Newton et al.[28] to present a somewhat comprehensive picture of the renin-angiotensin system in a group of 11 subjects with hypertension who were taking oral contraceptives. They noted that the most striking abnormality was marked elevation of renin substrate or angiotensinogen in their subjects. This was a consistent finding. They also observed increased plasma renin activity in these women. Similar observations have been confirmed by others.[5,9,27,30]

Menard, Cain, and Catt [29] reported that in rats the renin substrate level increased within 6 hours of treatment with estrogen, and plasma renin activity was high after 12 hours. In women taking oral contraceptives they noted a marked elevation of the angiotensin II level within 5 days, emphasizing the rapidity of the changes induced by the oral contraceptive agents.

Contrary to previous belief, the renin substrate level seemed to be a rate-limiting factor in the velocity of reaction between renin and angiotensinogen. Interestingly, Newton et al.[28] showed that the observed increase in renin substrate was associated with enhanced rate of angiotensin production in response to a fixed amount of exogenous renin in vitro, thereby implying that the elevated renin substrate level might indeed have some accelerating influence in angiotensin generation. Estrogen per se did not seem to alter the reaction. Skinner, Lumbers, and Symonds [30] were unable to show any qualitative difference in the substrate from normal plasma and plasma from subjects while taking oral contraceptives, velocity of reaction in the two being identical. They noted, though, that maximum velocity of reaction was not reached with the existing substrate level.

The effect of contraceptive agents on aldosterone secretion is not as clear-cut. Newton and associates [28] noted that the influence on aldosterone was transient and less consistent although aldosterone excretion remained elevated in some. Crane and Harris [31] were unable to find good correlation between aldosterone output and renin activity. Weinberger et al.,[5] on the contrary, found a clear correlation between them. The raised aldosterone level returned to normal on terminating the medications in all.

Since the changes in the renin-angiotensin system observed in subjects developing hypertension also occurred in those who remained normotensive on oral contraceptives, it becomes an intriguing problem to explain the causative role, if any, of these changes in the development of hypertension. Skinner, Lumbers, and Symonds [30] noted that during the use of oral contraceptives the rise in renin substrate was associated with a fall in plasma renin concentration as if tending to keep plasma renin activity close to normal. They postulated that this compensatory adjustment perhaps failed to occur in those who became hypertensive. Saruta, Sorade, and Kaplan [9] observed that in their oral contraceptive-induced hypertensives those who developed hypertension had a higher plasma renin concentration than those who did not and, hence, they supported Skinner's thesis of inadequate suppression of renin release in the face of increased substrate as a possible mechanism. On the other hand, Beckerhoff et al.[32] showed that hypertension could be induced with an intact buffer-feedback mechanism but those who remained hypertensive had higher plasma renin activity and less suppression of renin concentration.

Although various biochemical changes described above have now been reported widely and tend to focus our attention on a causal role for the renin-angiotensin system, their precise significance in the genesis or aggravation of hypertension remains enigmatic. Possibly some individuals are unduly susceptible to hypertension in the presence of the altered milieu of renin-angiotensinogen. What exactly is the nature of this susceptibility remains unknown. Hereditary factors may be involved. Some intrarenal vascular alteration may conceivably initiate the process. Laragh [33] has speculated about the possible role of activator or inhibitor of renin-substrate reaction or a qualitative alteration in substrate or an effect of estrogen on the kidney function. These and other questions presently remain unanswered.

In summary then, a small number of women,

perhaps less than 20 percent, show a rise in blood pressure while taking estrogen-containing oral contraceptives. The degree of hypertension is variable and accelerated hypertension can develop. Hypertension can appear after weeks or months of taking the drugs and in most cases is reversible on cessation of use of these drugs, although in some hypertension is reduced but persists. The pathophysiology of this variety of hypertension is not entirely clear but it is believed to be mediated through the renin-angiotensin system in an individual who in some way has inherent or acquired susceptibility.

Acknowledgment

The author wishes to express his gratitude to Dr. John A. Luetscher for his encouragement and advice in the preparation of this chapter, and also to Mrs. Laurie Marson and Miss Sandra Karsen for their superb technical assistance.

References

1. Owen, G.: Hypertension associated with oral contraceptives (Letter to the editor). Can. Med. Assoc. J. 95:167, 1966.
2. Swaab, L. I.: Blood pressure and oral contraception. *In* Proceedings of Second International Congress on Hormonal Steroids, Milan, Italy. Quoted by Laragh et al.[3]
3. Laragh, J. H., Sealey, J. E., Ledingham, J. G. G., and Newton, M. A.: Oral contraceptives. JAMA 201:918, 1967.
4. Woods, J. W.: Oral contraceptives and hypertension. Lancet 2:653, 1967.
5. Weinberger, M. H., Collins, R. D., Dowdy, A. J., Nokes, G. W., and Luetscher, J. A.: Hypertension induced by oral contraceptives containing estrogen and gestagen. Ann. Intern. Med. 71:891, 1969.
6. Harris, P. W. R.: Malignant hypertension associated with oral contraceptives. Lancet 2:466, 1969.
7. Tyson, J. E. A.: Oral contraception and elevated blood pressure. Am. J. Obstet. Gynec. 100:875, 1968.
8. Kunin, C. M., McCormack, R. C., and Abernathy, J. R.: Oral contraceptives and blood pressure. Arch. Intern. Med. 123:362, 1969.
9. Saruta, T., Sorade, G. A., and Kaplan, N. M.: A possible mechanism for hypertension induced by oral contraceptives. Diminished feedback suppression of renin release. Arch. Intern. Med. 126:621, 1970.
10. Spellacy, W. N., and Birk, S. A.: The development of elevated blood pressure while using oral contraceptives: A preliminary report of a prospective study. Fertil. Steril. 21:301, 1970.
11. Weir, R. J., Briggs, E., Mack, A., Taylor, L., Browning, J., Naismith, L., and Wilson, E.: Blood-pressure in women after one year of oral contraception. Lancet 1:467, 1971.
12. Katz, F. H., and Kappas, A.: The effects of estradiol and estriol on plasma levels of cortisol and thyroid-binding globulins and on aldosterone and cortisol secretion rates in man. J. Clin. Invest. 46:1768, 1967.
13. Johnson, J. A., Davis, J. O., Baumer, J. S., and Schneider, E. G.: Effects of estrogens and progesterone on electrolyte balances in normal dogs. Am. J. Physiol. 219:1691, 1970.
14. Michelakis, A. M., Stant, E. G., and Brill, A. B.: Sodium space and electrolyte excretion during the menstrual cycle. Am. J. Obstet. Gynec. 109:150, 1971.
15. Landau, R. L., and Lugibihl, K.: The catabolic and natriuretic effects of progesterone in man. Recent Progr. Hormone Res. 17:249, 1961.
16. Horrobin, D. F., Lloyd, I. J., and Burstyn, P. G.: Oral contraceptives and hypertension (Correspondence). Br. Med. J. 3:285, 1970.
17. Chesley, L. C., and Tepper, I. H.: Effects of progesterone and estrogen on the sensitivity to angiotensin II. J. Clin. Endocrinol. Metab. 27:576, 1967.
18. Chesley, L. C., Talledo, E., Bohler, C. S., and Zuspan, F. P.: Vascular reactivity to angiotensin II and norepinephrine in pregnant and nonpregnant women. Am. J. Obstet. Gynec. 91:837, 1965.
19. Douglas, B. H., Hull, R. P., and Langford, H. G.: Effect of an oral contraceptive agent on blood pressure response to renin. Proc. Soc. Exp. Biol. Med. 133:1142, 1970.
20. Lim, Y. L., Lumberg, E. R., Walters, W. A. W., and Whelan, R. F.: Effects of oestrogens on the human circulation. J. Obstet. Gynaec. Br. Commonw. 77:349, 1970.
21. Ueland, K., and Parer, J. T.: Effects of estrogens on the cardiovascular system of the ewe. Am. J. Obstet. Gynec. 96:400, 1966.
22. Csapo, A.: Actomyosin formation by estrogen action. Am. J. Physiol. 162:406, 1950.
23. Goodrich, S. M., and Wood, J. E.: The effect of estradiol-17β on peripheral venous distensibility and velocity of venous blood flow. Am. J. Obstet. Gynec. 96:407, 1966.

24. Walters, W. A. W., and Lim, Y. L.: Cardiovascular dynamics in women receiving oral contraceptive therapy. Lancet 2:879, 1969.
25. Helmer, O. M., and Griffith, R. S.: The effect of the administration of estrogens on the renin-substrate (hypertensinogen) content of rat plasma. Endocrinology 51:421, 1952.
26. Layne, D. S., Meyer, C. J., Vaishwanar, P. S., and Pincus, G.: The secretion and metabolism of cortisol and aldosterone in normal and in steroid-treated women. J. Clin. Endocrinol. Metab. 22:107, 1962.
27. Crane, M. G., Heitsch, J., Harris, J. J., and Johns, V. J.: Effect of ethinyl estradiol (Estinyl) on plasma renin activity. J. Clin. Endocrinol. Metab. 26:1403, 1966.
28. Newton, M. A., Sealey, J. E., Ledingham, J. G. G., and Laragh, J. H.: High blood pressure and oral contraceptive changes in plasma renin and renin substrate and in aldosterone excretion. Am. J. Obstet. Gynec. 101:1037, 1968.
29. Menard, J., Cain, M. D., and Catt, K. J.: Rapid effects of estrogen on the renin-angiotensin system. Clin. Res. 19:377, 1971.
30. Skinner, S. L., Lumbers, E. R., and Symonds, E. M.: Alteration by oral contraceptives of normal menstrual changes in plasma renin activity, concentration and substrate. Clin. Sci. 36:67, 1969.
31. Crane, M. G., and Harris, J. J.: Plasma renin activity and aldosterone excretion rate in normal subjects. I. Effect of ethinyl estradiol and medoxyprogesterone acetate. J. Clin. Endocrinol. Metab. 29:550, 1969.
32. Beckerhoff, R., Wilkinson, R., Nokes, G. W., and Luetscher, J. A.: (To be published.)
33. Laragh, J. H.: (Editorial) Oral contraceptives and hypertensive disease: A cybernetic overview. Circulation. 42:983, 1970.

PART X. COMPLICATIONS AND SPECIAL CONSIDERATIONS IN THE TREATMENT OF HYPERTENSION

Medical Versus Surgical Treatment of Renovascular Hypertension

By Harriet P. Dustan, M.D.

HYPERTENSION THAT ACCOMPANIES renal arterial stenosis often remits following surgical treatment; also, it can usually be successfully controlled by antihypertensive drug treatment. Given these two types of therapy, there are a number of factors which determine the physician's choice of one as opposed to the other. First there is the lesion itself: its type, whether atherosclerotic or nonatherosclerotic; its natural history, whether progressive or nonprogressive; and its extent, whether sharply localized in a main renal artery or extensive, involving branches as well. Next there is the patient's age, because surgical treatment carries a much higher risk in older patients. In addition to this, when the lesion is atherosclerosis, symptoms of extrarenal occlusive arterial disease are to be considered because presence of symptomatic coronary and/or cerebral atherosclerosis increases the risk of operation. Finally, there is usually some assessment as to whether the lesion is causing the hypertension or is merely coexistent with it.

Aside from these points, there are two others that enter into the decision concerning therapy. One is that when a surgical procedure is successful, hypertension is cured, while antihypertensive drugs merely control it but do not provide a cure.[1] The other concerns the possibility of as yet unknown late side effects of drug treatment during decades of use. Although these drugs have proved surprisingly safe during several years, it must be remembered that they have not been used long enough to assure their safety over decades. Thus, there really isn't a choice to be made since operation is the treatment of choice whenever it is technically feasible and not contraindicated by presence of extrarenal occlusive arterial disease and the hypertension seems likely to be caused by the stenosis.

From the Research Division, The Cleveland Clinic Foundation and The Cleveland Clinic Educational Foundation, Cleveland, Ohio.

This study was supported in part by Grant HE-6835 from the National Heart and Lung Institute, National Institutes of Health.

Type of Lesion

Knowing the type of lesion influences the decision concerning treatment because lesions differ in natural history; most are potentially progressive while one, medial fibroplasia, seems to have reached its maximum stenosis by the time it is discovered.[2] To a certain degree, the timing of a surgical procedure, if it is to be done at all, will depend on what is known concerning the potential for progressive stenosis and this in turn depends on a diagnosis of the type of lesion based on arteriographic and clinical features (see below).

Another point of importance in this consideration concerns the differential diagnosis between atherosclerosis and fibrous dysplasias. This is because, as a group, patients with atherosclerotic stenoses do not benefit as much from surgical treatment in regard to relief of hypertension as do patients with fibrous or fibromuscular dysplasia. The evidence is very clear on this point. Thus, a 1968 review[3] of all studies that separated surgically treated patients into those with atherosclerosis and those with fibrous dysplasias reported that, among 140 patients with atherosclerotic stenosis, hypertension was cured or improved in 74 percent but for the group of 104 with fibrous dysplasias this figure was 92 percent. It is anticipated that results of the Cooperative

Study of Renovascular Hypertension will provide excellent data on this point because of the large number of patients investigated and followed in a similar fashion. Although these results have not yet been published in detail, the report on clinical characteristics [4] compares findings in 339 essential hypertensives with 175 patients with renovascular hypertension cured by surgical treatment. Ninety-one of these patients had atherosclerotic stenoses and 84 fibrous dysplasia. Here again one finds a difference in arterial pressure responses to operation because the former represented 56 percent of the original group with atherosclerosis and the latter 71 percent of those with nonatherosclerotic lesions.

The type of lesion can usually be reliably determined by arteriographic features, as we have repeatedly emphasized.[2,5,6] Most often renal arterial lesions are said to be either atherosclerosis or fibromuscular hyperplasia. However, to lump all nonatherosclerotic stenoses into the category of fibromuscular hyperplasia overlooks the fact that within this category are several distinct lesions having particular age and sex distributions and different natural histories.[2] As indicated elsewhere in this volume,[7] the Mayo Clinic and the Cleveland Clinic pooled their experience with the pathology of renal arterial disease to provide a classification of lesions based on the predominant location in the arterial wall and the predominant tissue type.[8] There are two intimal lesions: atherosclerosis and intimal fibroplasia; and four medial lesions—medial fibroplasia with aneurysms, medial hyperplasia (either fibrous and/or muscular), medial dissection and perimedial fibroplasia. Finally, there is one rare lesion, periarterial fibroplasia.

Atherosclerosis occurs primarily in men after the age of 40. It is usually situated in the proximal centimeter of the renal artery and presents as a circumferential, symmetrical stenosis or as an asymmetrical lesion (Fig. 1). If the stenosis is marked, there is poststenotic dilatation. Complications of this lesion are thrombotic occlusion and dissection. In the former, the column of contrast material ends abruptly after the take-off of the artery and sometimes there is late filling of the distal arterial branches by collateral flow. In the latter circumstance, the artery is irregularly dilated beyond the stenosis, in contrast to the smooth poststenotic dilatation, and rarely the extra lumen is seen.

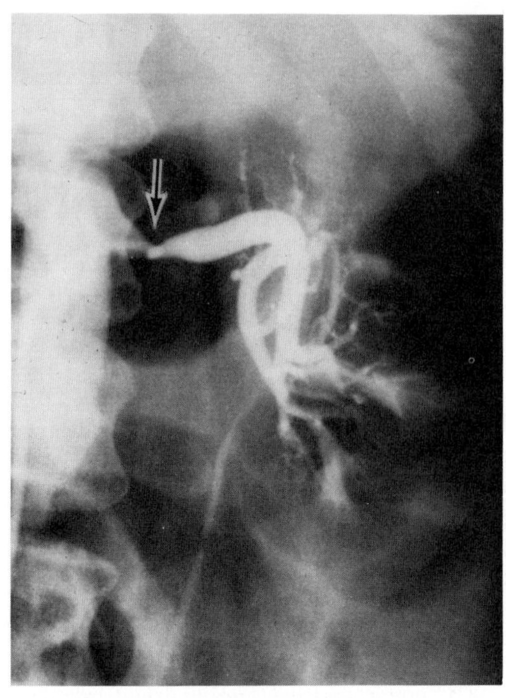

FIG. 1.—Selective renal arteriogram shows asymmetrical narrowing (**arrow**) by an atherosclerotic plaque in the first portion of the artery, with poststenotic dilatation. Presence of this plaque was confirmed at operation when an endarterectomy was performed. (From McCormack, L. J., et al.,[5] with permission.)

Intimal fibroplasia occurs in children and young adults. It presents as a symmetrical stenosis of the main renal artery or its primary branches (Fig. 2). Sometimes the origin of the celiac artery is affected and there may be a long narrowed segment of the abdominal aorta as well. Usually, there is poststenotic dilatation.

Medial fibroplasia is found primarily in the most common nonatherosclerotic type of renal arterial disease. It occurs more often in women than men and usually is found between the ages of 30 and 50 years. This is the lesion which produces the "string-of-beads" arteriogram (Fig. 3). The beads are aneurysms which result from sharply localized deficits of intima and media; these defects alternate with irregular

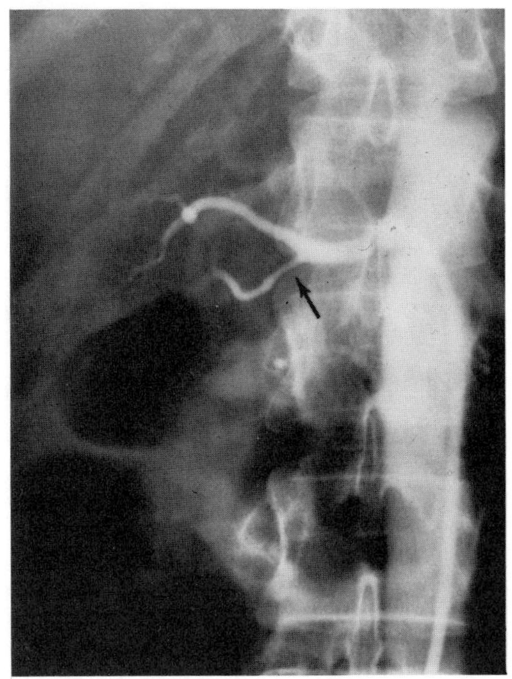

FIG. 2.—Selective renal arteriogram of intimal fibroplasia affecting a primary branch (**arrow**) of the right renal artery. This is an early film taken just after contrast material was injected, which accounts for the poor filling of the distal renal arterial system.

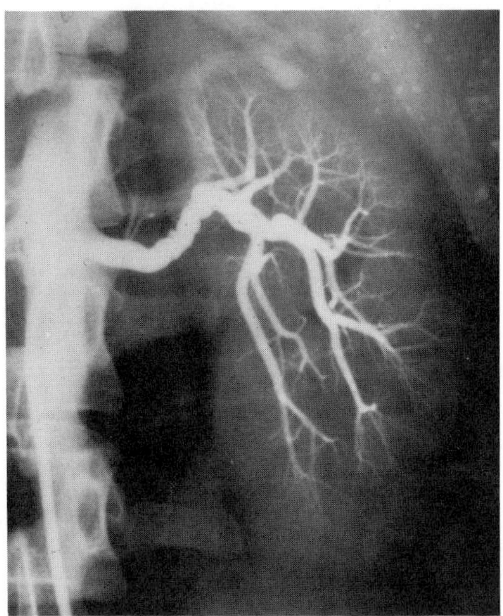

FIG. 3.—Selective renal arteriogram of medial fibroplasia of the left renal artery shows the string-of-beads characteristic of this lesion.

ridges composed primarily of fibrous tissue. The aneurysms are the "beads"; the ridges are the "string." Usually the first portion of the renal artery is spared as the lesion occurs in the distal two-thirds and often involves branches.

Medial hyperplasia represents an increased amount of either fibrous and/or muscular tissue in the media. Arteriographically, it cannot be distinguished from intimal fibroplasia and presents as a symmetrical stenosis of the main renal artery or a primary branch (Fig. 4). Also, it is found in children and young adults, as is intimal fibroplasia.

Medial dissection occurs at any point along the main renal artery and may extend into branches. It is a localized dissecting aneurysm that sometimes is associated with proliferation of intimal tissue, as found in intimal fibroplasia, and sometimes with some degree of muscular hyperplasia. The arteriogram is distinctive

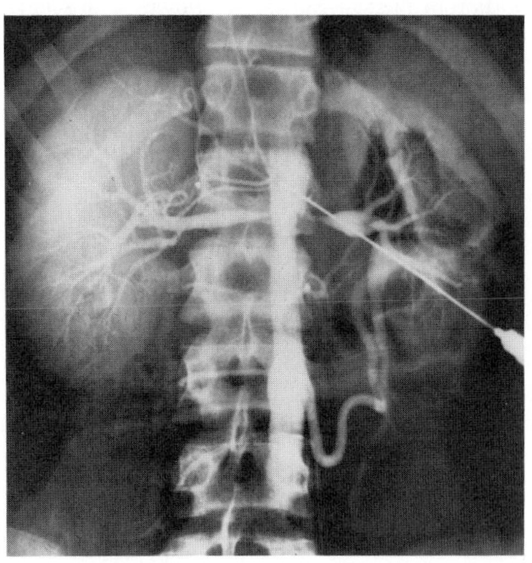

FIG. 4.—A translumbar aortogram of exceptionally good quality shows symmetrical stenoses of the first portion of both renal arteries produced by medial hyperplasia. It also shows other features sometimes seen in association with renal arterial disease in young people: a long, coarcted segment of the abdominal aorta, a network of fine collaterals to the right kidney, and an enlarged inferior mesenteric artery supplying collateral flow to the left kidney. (From McCormack, L. J., et al.,[5] with permission.)

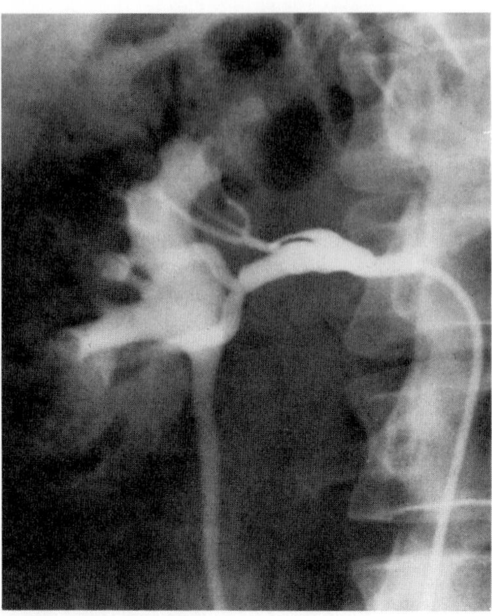

FIG. 5.—Selective arteriogram shows medial dissection of the right renal artery which involves the distal two-thirds of the main trunk and the first portion of the superior polar branch. The segment of that branch distal to the dissection is narrowed by intimal fibroplasia.

(Fig. 5). At first glance, it may be confused with poststenotic dilatation but closer inspection shows an uneven, sometimes jagged, dilatation in contrast to the smooth appearance exhibited in the poststenotic type. It is not to be confused with medial fibroplasia, with its multiple, round aneurysms.

Perimedial fibroplasia is a disease of young women; in our experience [6] it is usually found in patients less than 35 years of age (Fig. 6).

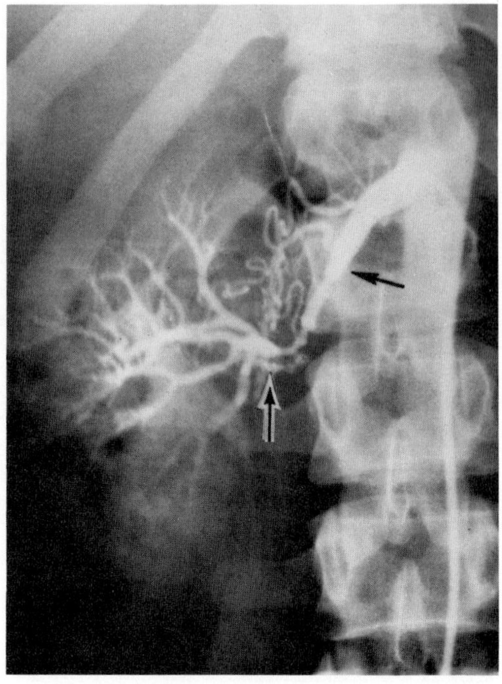

FIG. 7.—Perimedial fibroplasia of the right renal artery (between **arrows**); the stenosis is severe and accompanied by prominent collateral blood supply. Characteristically the stenosis is variable, giving the impression of beading; however the beads are not aneurysmal as in medial fibroplasia (see Fig. 3 for comparison). (From McCormack, L. J., et al.,[5] with permission.)

It is a severely stenosing lesion, seems to have a predilection for the right renal artery and, when it occurs bilaterally, is usually more severe on the right side. The lesion is a dense collar of collagen which develops in the peripheral region of the media and extends into the

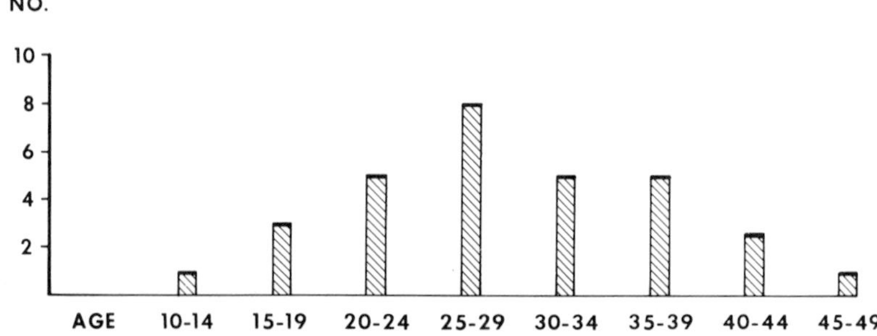

FIG. 6.—Age distribution of 26 women with perimedial fibroplasia shows that most were less than 35 years of age when the lesion was discovered.

more central regions; somewhere in the process of its development the external elastic membrane becomes frayed and may disappear entirely. As the scar tissue increases it entraps muscle bundles and probably because of this it has been classified as fibromuscular hyperplasia.[9] The amounts of collagen vary throughout the affected segment and this variation accounts for the arteriographic features (Fig. 7). Perimedial fibroplasia, like medial fibroplasia, produces a beaded artery. These two lesions are the most common nonatherosclerotic renal arterial diseases and since both produce arterial beading, this probably explains why the term *string-of-beads arteriogram* has been used to describe both.[10] The difference in the natural history of the two lesions [2] makes the distinction between them of paramount importance. Whereas the beads of medial fibroplasia represent aneurysms, the beads of perimedial fibroplasia represent localized areas when the collar of collagen is not so thick as in the adjacent areas—the string. The two can usually be differentiated easily because the aneurysms of medial fibroplasia are larger than the unaffected proximal artery while the segment affected by perimedial hyperplasia is always narrower.

Natural History of Renal Arterial Lesions

During the early experience with renal arterial diseases, there was much concern that either stenoses would progress leading to irreparable renal damage or aneurysms would rupture if operation was not performed promptly. However, not all patients were candidates for surgical treatment because lesions were so extensive that repair was not possible, presence of severe extrarenal atherosclerosis made operation too risky, or stenoses were considered too slight to be a factor in hypertension. Repeated arteriography in such patients has provided information concerning the natural history of these arterial lesions.

Information is reasonably good in regard to atherosclerosis and medial fibroplasia since these are the most common diseases. Thus in our follow-up study [2] we found that in 14 of 39 patients with atherosclerosis, stenosis had become more severe on repeated examination 6 months to 10 years after the first arteriogram, while in only two of 40 patients with medial fibroplasia was there any suggestion of progression. This experience with medial fibroplasia has allayed the concern over potential for rupture of these aneurysms and it seems likely that the reason they do not rupture is that the external elastic membrane remains intact. Since the other lesions occur much less frequently there has not been an opportunity to study so many sequentially as was possible for atherosclerosis and medial fibroplasia. Further, since these lesions predominantly affect young people and are often sharply localized and thus operable, proportionately more patients are treated surgically than those having the more common lesions. However, we have obtained follow-up studies in three patients with perimedial fibroplasia and four with either intimal fibroplasia or medial hyperplasia (it is to be remembered that they cannot be distinguished arteriographically). In two of the former and all of the latter, either the stenosis became more severe or a new lesion developed in a previously unaffected artery. Obviously much more information concerning these two diseases is needed, but this fragmentary evidence suggests that they may be inexorably progressive.

The Extent of the Lesion

The extent of the lesion certainly influences decisions concerning medical versus surgical treatment. Usually atherosclerosis, intimal fibroplasia and medial hyperplasia affect the first portion of the renal artery and are thus amenable to endarterectomy, resection, or bypass grafting. In contrast, both medial and perimedial fibroplasia occur in the distal two-thirds of the main renal artery, usually affect a fairly long segment, and sometimes extend into branches. Further, they are frequently bilateral. Accordingly, it may be difficult or impossible to remove or bypass the obstruction. This adds another factor for consideration because if a unilateral operation fails and nephrectomy is necessary, the remaining kidney is also affected and the possibility of a worsening hypertension cannot be excluded. If medial dissection is localized to the main renal artery it usually does not present any technical difficulty but if it extends into branches it may not be correctable.

Age and Associated Vascular Disease

For a number of reasons a patient's age figures significantly in making a decision about the type of treatment. Most young hypertensive patients with renal arterial disease are basically healthy. They can withstand a major operation and have more potential for benefiting from it than someone older. Not only are patients with nonatherosclerotic stenoses more likely to be cured of hypertension than those with atherosclerosis (see above) but also they can be returned to complete health if the operation is successful.

Patients with atherosclerotic renal arterial disease usually have lesions elsewhere and may have already sustained a stroke or myocardial infarction or have angina. For them the risk of operation is greatly increased. This risk is exemplified by our experience with the surgical treatment of renovascular hypertension in 99 patients; 10 died in the immediate postoperative period and seven of the deaths occurred in patients with atherosclerosis of the renal artery who suffered thrombotic occlusions elsewhere.[11] Also, one of the reports from the Cooperative Study of Renovascular Hypertension indicates that operative mortality of 124 patients with nonatherosclerotic lesions was 5 percent while in 188 with atherosclerosis it was 14 percent.[4]

In weighing risk against potential benefit of a surgical procedure, consideration should be given to duration of possible benefit. For a young person with a nonatherosclerotic lesion, technically successful operative treatment has a 70 to 80 percent chance of curing hypertension for a lifetime.[4,6] For an elderly patient with an atherosclerotic stenosis, a surgical procedure has only about a 50 percent chance of curing hypertension and the duration of benefit is likely to be cut short by extrarenal atherosclerotic complications.[11]

It seems common sense to suggest that patients with the malignant phase of renovascular hypertension not be operated upon until they have been treated with antihypertensive drugs. Even though arterial pressure may not be normalized, some reduction is usually achievable and whatever can be accomplished is as beneficial in this type of malignant hypertension as in any other. Certainly, if cardiac failure is present, it should be controlled preoperatively.

Given lesions for which surgical corrective procedures are feasible, a simple, practical dictum is that those patients chosen for operative treatment should have good enough general health to withstand a major surgical procedure and be young enough to achieve long-range benefit.

Diagnosis of Renovascular Hypertension

It is now widely recognized that finding a renal arterial stenosis in a hypertensive patient does not establish the diagnosis of renovascular hypertension. Until the prognostic value of renal vein renin levels can be determined, or some other method found, this diagnosis will remain a retrospective one based on the cure of hypertension by a surgical procedure.

Since it may be that function tests of the individual kidneys are still being used occasionally for diagnosis of renovascular hypertension, they should be mentioned here. In 1951, Mueller et al.[12] reported that, in dogs, narrowing one renal artery reduced urine flow and sodium excretion on that side and in 1954, Howard et al.[13] reported similar findings in a patient with unilateral main renal arterial stenosis. Two years later Howard, Connor, and Thomas [14] suggested function tests of the individual kidneys for diagnosis of renovascular hypertension and then,[15] having had more experience with the procedure, concluded that if a kidney is the cause of hypertension, urine flow from it, compared with that of the opposite kidney, is reduced by 50 percent and urine sodium concentration by 15 percent. These reports were the beginning of several years of interest in "split-function" tests for diagnosis of renovascular hypertension and they were widely used for this purpose. By 1961, we had shown [16] that bilateral renal arterial lesions are more severe on one side than the other and thus split-function test findings are indistinguishable from those of unilateral stenosis. Further, we found that lesions of an arterial branch affect urine production only quantitatively yet cause hypertension just as surely as main arterial stenoses that affect the quality of urine formed (sodium and creatinine concentrations) as well as its quantity. From that study, as well as all others, there has never been any suggestion that renal excretory function and hypertension are causally associated either in dogs with experimental renal arterial narrowings or patients with stenosing lesions.

After Howard's original descriptions of the separated-function test, several modifications were introduced designed to increase its diagnostic capability.[3] However, these resulted in technical improvements, but did not improve diagnosis and now split-function tests have been largely replaced by measurement of renal vein renin activity.

Helmer and Judson [17,18] first proposed that if comparison of renin activity in blood from the two renal veins showed a larger amount on the affected side this would indicate presence of a renal pressor factor in the associated hypertension which should, then, respond to surgical treatment. Generally speaking, this seems to be the case [19–25] although the published reports present more data on patients whose hypertension was cured by operation than on those in whom it was not, suggesting that patients were chosen for operation on the basis of this test before testing its validity. For a number of reasons it seems doubtful that measurement of renal venous renin activity will clearly distinguish all patients who will respond to surgical treatment. It has been known for a long time that, in dogs with one renal artery constricted, renal venous renin activity, although initially high, falls to normal levels during the chronic phase of hypertension. Further, angiotensin II is not just a direct-pressor hormone but has a number of effects on central and peripheral adrenergic nervous mechanisms.[26] Together, these two observations suggest the possibility that once hypertension has been produced by overproduction of the renal pressor system and the whole series of abnormalities that characterize hypertension has been established, i.e., hemodynamic, volume, adrenal steroid, and neural, it can be maintained by apparently normal amounts. Further, there are likely other factors important in renovascular hypertension that are either not yet recognized or have not yet been widely investigated. One has only to be reminded of the neutral lipid of renal origin that protects against renoprival hypertension,[27] of prostaglandins of renal origin,[28] and of the factor in plasma of hypertensive patients that is thought to influence responsiveness to angiotensin II [29] to realize that the comparison of values for renin in the two renal venous plasmas may not indicate, unequivocally, the presence or absence of renovascular hypertension in a patient who has renal arterial stenosis.

Medical Treatment of Renovascular Hypertension

The effectiveness of antihypertensive drug treatment in controlling hypertension that accompanies renal arterial disease has been clearly shown.[11,30,31] This means that there is an alternative form of therapy available if surgical treatment is not feasible. Several years ago, there was the general opinion that renovascular hypertension is more resistant to the drug therapy than is essential hypertension but subsequent experience has shown this not to be the case since both Sheps et al.[30] and we [11,31] have shown that in most patients arterial pressure can be reduced to normal or near-normal levels and maintained at such levels for years. It is common experience that the malignant phase of renovascular hypertension may be poorly responsive to drug treatment but since malignant hypertension is sometimes very poorly responsive anyway, the presence of a renal artery lesion seems to add nothing distinctive.

Repeatedly, in reports of surgical treatment, comment is made that even if hypertension is not cured by operation it becomes more easily controllable with drugs. On the one hand, this possibility is difficult to assess because if a patient is a suitable candidate for surgical treatment, drug therapy is often not given a thorough trial preoperatively. Then, if hypertension does not remit postoperatively, the physician's commitment to securing a good response to drugs is greater than it was preoperatively and treatment is more likely to be effective. On the other hand, it is possible that in patients who sustain improvement—but not a cure—through operation, a renal pressor factor is eliminated, allowing enhanced responsiveness to drugs. However, until there is a careful study of the effectiveness of drug treatment pre- and postoperatively, the possibility that surgery increases responsiveness to medical therapy will remain speculative.

Summary

There are two types of treatment for the hypertension accompanying renal arterial stenosis. Surgical treatment is designed to remove a renal pressor factor either by nephrectomy or a revascularization procedure. When it is successful, hypertension is cured. Drug therapy controls hypertension but does not cure it.

Surgical treatment is more successful in patients with fibrous dysplasias than in those with atherosclerosis. A number of factors influence choice of treatment. These include the type of lesion, whether atherosclerosis or fibrous dysplasia, whether the lesion is potentially progressive, the extent of the lesion, whether it is sharply localized or involves a long segment of renal artery and extends into primary branches, the age of the patient, presence of extrarenal atherosclerosis and whether there is elevation of renin activity in renal or peripheral venous blood.

References

1. Dustan, H. P., Page, I. H., Tarazi, R. C., and Frohlich, E. D.: Arterial pressure responses to discontinuing antihypertensive drugs. Circulation 37:370, 1967.
2. Meaney, T. F., Dustan, H. P., and McCormack, L. J.: Natural history of renal arterial disease. Radiology 91:881, 1968.
3. Dustan, H. P.: Renal arterial stenosis and parenchymal diseases. *In* Page, I. H., and McCubbin, J. W. (Eds.): Renal Hypertension. Chicago: Year Book, 1968, pp. 306–349.
4. Simon, N. M., Franklin, S., Bleifer, K. H., and Maxwell, M. H.: Clinical characteristics of renovascular hypertension. JAMA 220: 1209, 1972.
5. McCormack, L. J., Poutasse, E. F., Meaney, T. F., Noto, T. J., and Dustan, H. P.: A pathologic-arteriographic correlation of renal arterial disease. Am. Heart J. 72:188, 1966.
6. McCormack, L. J., Noto, T. J., Meaney, T. F., Poutasse, E. F., and Dustan, H. P.: Subadventitial fibroplasia of the renal artery, a disease of young women. Am. Heart J. 73: 602, 1967.
7. McCormack, L. J.: Morphologic abnormalities of the renal artery associated with hypertension. This volume.
8. Harrison, E. G., Jr., and McCormack, L. J.: Pathologic classification of renal arterial disease in renovascular hypertension. Mayo Clinic Proc. 46:161, 1971.
9. Wellington, J. S.: Fibromuscular hyperplasia of renal arteries in hypertension. Am. J. Pathol. 43:955, 1963.
10. Palubinskas, A. J., and Wylie, E. J.: Roentgen diagnosis of fibromuscular hyperplasia of the renal arteries. Radiology 76:634, 1961.
11. Dustan, H. P., Page, I. H., Poutasse, E. F., and Wilson, L. L.: An evaluation of treatment of hypertension associated with occlusive renal arterial disease. Circulation 27:1018, 1963.
12. Mueller, C. B., Surtshin, A., Carlin, M. R., and White, H. L.: Glomerular and tubular influences on sodium and water excretion. Am. J. Physiol. 165:411, 1951.
13. Howard, J. E., Berthrong, M., Gould, B. M., and Yendt, E. R.: Hypertension resulting from unilateral vascular disease and its relief by nephrectomy. Bull. Johns Hopkins Hosp. 94:51, 1954.
14. Howard, J. E., Connor, T. B., and Thomas, W. C., Jr.: A functional test for detection of hypertension produced by one kidney—preliminary studies. Trans. Assoc. Am. Physicians 49:291, 1956.
15. Connor, T. B., Thomas, W. C., Haddock, L., and Howard, J. E.: Unilateral renal disease as a cause of hypertension: Its detection by ureteral catheterization studies. Ann. Intern. Med. 52:544, 1960.
16. Dustan, H. P., Poutasse, E. F., Corcoran, A. C., and Page, I. H.: Separated renal function in patients with renal arterial disease, pyelonephritis and essential hypertension. Circulation 23:34, 1961.
17. Helmer, O. M., and Judson, W. E.: The presence of vasoconstrictor and vasopressor activity in renal vein plasma of patients with arterial hypertension. Hypertension 8:38, 1960.
18. Judson, W. E., and Helmer, O. M.: Diagnostic and prognostic values of renin activity in renal venous plasma in renovascular hypertension. Hypertension 13:79, 1965.
19. Michelakis, A. M., Foster, J. H., Liddle, G. W., Rhamy, R. K., Kuchel, O., and Gordon, R. D.: Measurement of renin in both

renal veins; its use in diagnosis of renovascular hypertension. Arch. Intern. Med. 120: 444, 1967.

20. Winer, B. M., Lubbe, W. F., Simon, M., and Williams, J. A.: Renin in the diagnosis of renovascular hypertension. Activity in renal and peripheral vein plasma. JAMA 202:121, 1967.
21. Fitz, A. E.: Renal venous renin determinations in the diagnosis of surgically correctable hypertension. Circulation 36:942, 1967.
22. Bath, N. M., Gunnells, J. C., Jr., and Robinson, R. R.: Plasma renin activity in renovascular hypertension. Am. J. Med. 45:381, 1968.
23. Woods, J. W., and Michelakis, A. M.: Renal vein renin in renovascular hypertension. Arch. Intern. Med. 122:392, 1968.
24. Simmons, J. L., and Michelakis, A. M.: Renovascular hypertension: The diagnostic value of renal vein renin ratios. J. Urol. 104:497, 1970.
25. Pawsey, C. G. K., Vandongen, R., and Gordon, R. D.: Renal venous renin ratio in the diagnosis of renovascular hypertension: Measurement during active secretion of renin. Med. J. Aust. 1:121, 1971.
26. McCubbin, J. W.: Neurogenic factors. *In* Page, I. H., and McCubbin, J. W. (Eds.): Renal Hypertension. Chicago: Year Book, 1968, pp. 244–263.
27. Muirhead, E. E., Booth, E., Brooks, B., Kosinski, M., Daniels, E. G., and Hinman, J. W.: Renomedullary antihypertensive principle in renal hypertension. J. Lab. Clin. Med. 64:989, 1964.
28. McGiff, J. C., Crowshaw, K., Terragno, N. A., and Lonigro, A. J.: Release of a prostaglandin-like substance into renal venous blood in response to angiotensin II. Hypertension 18:121, 1970.
29. Mizukoshi, H., and Michelakis, A. M.: Evidence for the existence of a sensitizing factor in pressor agents in hypertension. (Abstract) Circulation 43–44(Suppl. II):121, 1971.
30. Sheps, S. G., Osmundson, P. J., Hunt, J. C., Schirger, A., and Fairbairn, J. F.: II. Hypertension and renal artery stenosis: Serial observations on 54 patients treated medically. Clin. Pharmacol. Ther. 6:700, 1965.
31. Dustan, H. P., Meaney, T. F., and Page, I. H.: Conservative treatment of renovascular hypertension. *In* Gross, F. (Ed.): Antihypertensive Therapy: Principles and Practice, An International Symposium. Berlin: Springer, 1966, pp. 544–554.

Long-term Evaluation of Surgery for Renal Arterial Hypertension

By Walter M. Kirkendall, M.D., and Annette Fitz, M.D.

Since 1962, 94 PATIENTS with hypertension and renovascular lesions have been operated on and followed up in a systematic fashion at the University Medical Center, Iowa City, Iowa. Short-term follow-up studies on the 50 initial patients have been reported previously.[1] The total patient group has been recently reviewed in an attempt to determine the efficacy of various operative procedures, and to evaluate the long-term benefits of renovascular repair or nephrectomy on blood pressure and on patient survival. The current report deals with our experiences over a 9-year period and contrasts our experience with our first 40 patients with that of our next 54.

Materials and Methods

Clinical Diagnosis

Our diagnostic evaluations of these patients followed the same outline reported previously in our short-term study.[1]

The work-up included a complete history and physical examination with blood pressures taken in the standing and supine positions. Laboratory work included a urinanalysis, complete blood count, blood urea nitrogen, creatinine, electrolytes, uric acid, blood lipids, fasting or postprandial blood sugar, electrocardiogram, and chest x-ray. Additional special studies, such as intravenous pyelography, aortography or renal angiography, split-renal function tests, and split-renal vein renins, were also performed in the evaluation process.

The intravenous pyelogram is a good screening test, but it cannot diagnose renal artery stenosis. Consequently, the abnormalities found by this procedure were further evaluated by renal arteriography. In taking the history and performing the diagnostic work-up, particular attention was paid to the severity of the hypertension, the resistance of blood pressure to previous drug management, the documentation of the time of onset of hypertension, and the appearance of the optic fundi, especially regarding segmentation of the retinal arterioles. Emphasis was also placed on abdominal bruits, particularly those of long duration and of lateral location.

Special Procedures

In a few patients in whom renal artery stenosis was strongly suspected, such as the patient under 25 with an abdominal bruit, intravenous pyelography was not performed, but aortography with washout films was obtained. Since the presence of the renovascular lesion does not in itself assure significance of that lesion, our patients were also evaluated with split-renal function tests and with split-renal vein renin determinations. Renal vein renin determinations were carried out after the administration of thiazides and methyldopa. This program was believed to be necessary because the majority of our patients were severely hypertensive and it was not reasonable to withhold therapy throughout the diagnostic work-up. On many occasions the split renal vein renins were also performed before and after hydralazine stimulation.[2] Split-renal function tests were also performed in most cases.

Follow-up

Patients have been followed up at the University Hospitals for a minimum of 1 year after operation. Follow-up after this was in some cases performed by the patient's referring physician. Patients are classed as cured if their blood pressure was less than 140/90 mm Hg without drugs, or as improved if mean blood pressure fell 20 mm Hg or more without additional drugs. All other patients were considered unimproved. In some tables, the cured and improved patients are grouped for

From the Renal-Hypertension-Electrolyte Division, Department of Medicine, College of Medicine, University of Iowa, Iowa City, Iowa.

Supported in part by Grant 1 T12 HE-05918-01 from the National Institutes of Health.

TABLE 1.—*Renal Artery Obstruction with Hypertension*

Disease	No. of Patients	Sex		Average Age (in yr)	Operation		Results	
		M	F		N	G	I	UI
Atherosclerosis	63	36	27	52.2	25	38	43	20
F.M.D.	20	8	12	36.3	4	16	16	4
Trauma to renal artery or kidney	6	5	1	32.5	5	1	3	3
Congenital	5	0	5	16.8	4	1	5	0
Total	94	49	45		38 *	56	67	27

Abbreviations used: F.M.D., fibromuscular dysplasia; N, nephrectomy; G, graft; I, patients cured or improved 12 months after surgery; UI, patients unimproved 12 months after surgery.

* In nine of these patients a graft was performed initially, but nephrectomy was later required.

ease of presentation, since it is probable that the ischemia was relieved if blood pressure was decreased substantially at the end of 1 year.

RESULTS

Lesions

Ninety-four patients were found to have stenosis or disruption of a main or branch renal artery (Table 1). Of this group, 22 had bilateral renal artery stenosis due to renal artery atherosclerosis, 41 had unilateral atherosclerotic renal artery stenosis, and 20 had fibromuscular dysplasia. An additional 11 patients had assorted vascular lesions impairing renal blood supply (Table 2). More men than women had atherosclerotic and traumatic lesions, and women predominated in the groups with fibromuscular dysplasia or congenital lesions (Table 1). Patients with atherosclerosis were also older (Table 1).

Fibromuscular dysplasia is used as a group designation to include those patients with subintimal, medial, and subadventitial dysplasia or fibrosis as described by McCormack et al.[3] Twelve of these patients had arteriographic evidence of bilateral involvement.

Operations

Sixty-three operations were done on patients with unilateral or bilateral atherosclerotic renal artery stenosis (Table 3). Forty-one patients underwent a vascular repair with endarterectomy and patch graft, Dacron bypass graft, or saphenous vein graft as the initial operation. Twenty-two patients under-

TABLE 2.—*Miscellaneous Renal Artery Disease with Hypertension*

Sex	Age	Lesion	Operation	Result
Male	19	Traumatic aneurysm	N	I
Male	36	Fractured kidney	N	I
Male	22	Traumatic aneurysm	G	U
Male	29	Fractured kidney	N	U
Female	44	Ligated accessory renal artery	N	I
Male	45	Fractured kidney	N	U
Female	13	Congenital malformation	N	I
Female	21	Aneurysm and stenosis	G	I
Female	31	Aneurysm and stenosis	N	I
Female	2	Thrombus	N	I
Female	17	Neurofibroma	N	I

Abbreviations used: N, nephrectomy; G, graft; I, patients improved after surgery; U, patients unimproved after surgery.

TABLE 3.—*Atherosclerosis*

	M	F	Graft	Results of Graft		Neph-rectomy	Results of Nephrectomy	
				I	U		I	U
Single renal artery	26	15	21	13	8	20	19	1
Bilateral renal artery	10	12	17	8	9	5	3	2

Abbreviations used: M, male; F, female; I, patients cured and improved after surgery; U, patients unimproved after surgery.

went nephrectomy as the initial operative procedure. Three patients with initial grafts later required nephrectomy.

In patients with fibromuscular dysplasia, 18 had a vascular repair or graft as the initial procedure. The remaining patients in this group, and two who originally had a graft, underwent unilateral nephrectomy (Table 4). In one additional patient with fibromuscular dysplasia a secondary nephrectomy was required because of extension of the disease process.

Survival of grafts was generally good. A secondary nephrectomy was required after unsuccessful repair, or graft failure in nine patients of the 66 who had vascular repair. Clotting of the graft or the repaired artery occurred in the immediate postoperative period in two other patients, who died. In one of the nine, an immediate nephrectomy was performed, in another a nephrectomy was performed 2 months later. Seven other patients developed graft failure between 6 months and 4 years after the initial grafting procedure. One of these patients sustained an occlusion of an artery, on which an endarterectomy had been done 6 years before. In all nine patients a nephrectomy was performed when it became evident that the graft was nonfunctional.

Three patients, one with segmental atherosclerotic lesion and two with traumatic fracture of the kidney, had partial nephrectomies; in all cases, this procedure was unsuccessful in relieving the hypertension, and in one instance a secondary nephrectomy was necessitated. Nephrectomies were performed as the initial operative procedure in seven patients with miscellaneous lesions (Table 2).

In 38 patients with atherosclerosis who received grafts, 21 were improved and 17 were unimproved. Twenty-five patients had nephrectomies performed as the initial or secondary procedure. Of these, 22 were improved, and only three were unimproved by the procedure.

Although deterioration in renal function was observed in some of the patients with atherosclerotic renal artery stenosis and nephrosclerosis, progression of fibromuscular dysplasia was rare in patients who had received a graft. In those patients with fibromuscular dysplasia in whom a nephrectomy has been

TABLE 4.—*Fibromuscular Dysplasia*

	M	F	Graft	Results of Graft		Neph-rectomy	Results of Nephrectomy	
				I	U		I	U
Unilateral renal artery lesion	4	4	7	5	2	1	1	0
Bilateral renal artery lesion	4	8	9	7	2	3	3	0

Abbreviations used: M, male; F, female; I, patients cured and improved after surgery; U, patients unimproved by surgery.

performed, progression of the disease in the opposite kidney has not been observed.

Losses

Seven patients have been lost to follow-up between 4 and 12 months postoperatively. The remaining patients were followed for a minimum of 1 year. When all of the patients with vascular lesions are considered as a group, 67 of the 94 patients were considered to be improved by their operative procedure (71.5%) at the end of 1 year, or at their last follow-up visit. Five patients died in the immediate postoperative period; all of these deaths occurred early in the study period, prior to 1965.

Long-term Studies

We studied the 40 patients 3½ years later who were originally evaluated at the end of 18 months (Table 5). At this time, 45 percent of the original 40 patients had died, and the number cured had decreased from 20 to 12 percent. The total of cures and improved results had fallen from 49 to 30 percent. It is of interest that of those patients considered cured 5 years after operation, none had atherosclerosis as a cause of their stenosis.

Recent Studies

In our 54 patients who had operations after 1965 there was no operative mortality, and only two deaths occurred during the follow-up period (Table 5). In this group 39 percent were cured, 40 percent were improved, and only 17 percent were considered unimproved. In contrast, in those patients who were operated on prior to 1965, operative mortality and mortality during the follow-up period were higher. In this group only 49 percent of patients were considered cured or improved after 18 months of follow-up.

Discussion

In Table 5 we have compared our results with those of other representative series. Dustan et al.[4] compared the results in 432 patients operated upon before May of 1964 with 195 gleaned from the literature after that date. Eighty-one percent of the patients were cured or improved before May of 1964, 86 percent after that date. These figures may be somewhat misleading, since they come from many different clinics, from physicians who used different criteria for improvement and cure, and from programs where methods of follow-up were varied and not rigid. These results probably represented a most optimistic evaluation of surgery done at that time for renal artery hypertension.

Shapiro et al.[5] studied a group of 43 patients and noted that 54 percent were cured or improved immediately postoperatively. This improvement was maintained for almost 3 years in 49 percent. It is of interest in this study that 35 percent of the patients were dead at

TABLE 5.—*Results of Surgical Therapy for Hypertension from Renal Artery Disease*

Investigators	*No. of Patients*	*Mortality (%)*	*Follow-Up (in months)*	*Blood Pressure (%)* Normal	*Improved*	*Unimproved*
Before May 1964 [4]	432	7	12–120	41	40	19
After May 1964 [4]	195	4	< 18	57	29	14
Shapiro, A. P., et al., 1969 [5]	43	6	PO	26	28	40
Shapiro, A. P., et al., 1969 [5]	43	35	34	28	21	16
Foster, J. H., et al., 1969 [6]	41	12	12–72	54	17	17
Kaufman, J. J., Lupu, A. N., and Maxwell, M. H., 1968 [7]	137		6	39	38	23
Kirkendall, et al., 1967 [1]	40	30	18	20	29	22
Fitz, A. E., Thompson, E., and Kirkendall, W. M., 1969 [8]	40	45	> 60	12	18	25
Kirkendall, W. M., et al., 1971	54	4	12	39	40	17
Kirkendall, W. M., et al., 1971	94	15	12	31	35	19

34 months, a mortality rate which was duplicated almost exactly by medical management in a more severely ill group of patients. Foster et al.[6] followed up 41 patients from 12 to 72 months, and noted a 73-percent rate of improvement after operation. These patients were, as a group, somewhat younger than those of Shapiro et al.[5] and had fewer problems with atherosclerosis. Kaufman et al.[7] reported a large series of patients, a fairly large percentage of whom had fibromuscular dysplasia and vascular repair, and noted that 77 percent were either cured or improved by the operation.

Approximately 79 percent of our patients in the later study had improvement from surgery for renal artery hypertension; 39 percent were cured. This represents a substantial increase in good results over those obtained when patients were less well selected as in our first study, when only 49 percent had either improvement or cure at the end of 18 months. Although surgical techniques had unquestionably improved during our second study, we believe that better selection of patients was primarily responsible for the good results. We did not suggest operation for those who did not have a clearly significant lesion, those who had severe generalized atherosclerosis, diabetics with microangiopathy, or for those patients with single renal artery lesions who had azotemia. It was our belief that azotemia in a patient with one well-perfused kidney indicated the kidney on the contralateral side was severely nephrosclerotic and there was little chance for long-term benefit. Five of the patients who died in the postoperative period or shortly thereafter in the 1967 study had azotemia and derived no benefit from the operation.

It is of interest that over two-thirds of our patients had atherosclerosis and only 17 percent had fibromuscular dysplasia. This reflects a different distribution of cases as compared with the cases in literature.[3,7] Because patients with atherosclerosis generally do less well after operation than those with fibromuscular dysplasia, our results probably were worsened by this predominance of atherosclerotic patients. Thirty-four of the 94 patients had bilateral lesions and had surgical procedures on both renal arteries, or had a unilateral nephrectomy. Patients with bilateral lesions, as expected, did not do as well with the operation as did those who had a single artery lesion.

Our results with nephrectomy, particularly in the patients with single renal artery lesions, were quite good. Twenty of the 21 with atherosclerotic stenosis were either cured or improved. Nevertheless, it was our decision to preserve renal tissue when at all possible. We believe this particularly important since we do not have a great deal of information on the natural history of either atherosclerosis or fibromuscular dysplasia of the renal arteries. A reflection of our interest in preserving renal tissue is the fact that nine of our patients who had grafts had failure of the grafts and later nephrectomy.

As is pointed out in more detail elsewhere,[5,6,8] the majority of patients who die after the postoperative period succumb from atherosclerotic complications, such as myocardial infarction or strokes. Although progression of atherosclerosis in the contralateral renal artery did not occur frequently, it was identified in three; in one patient a second surgical procedure had to be carried out for a significant lesion which developed in the remaining renal artery. These observations make it obvious that renal artery disease is only one facet of the general vascular disease that occurred in many of our patients with atherosclerosis. The progression of atherosclerotic disease points out clearly the need for therapy to be applied not only for hypertension but for atherosclerosis as well.

The disappointing results of surgical therapy in patients with far-advanced atherosclerotic disease led us to trials of medical therapy early in the study. Thirteen of the patients operated upon had been assigned initially to a medical management group. The surgery was done later because of unresponsiveness to antihypertensive agents in eight, and progression of stenosis with a reduction of renal mass in five. Interestingly, eight of the 13 were improved by the surgical therapy. Five had little or no improvement in blood pressure control.

Several groups [5,9–11] have demonstrated that long-term benefit can be achieved with medical therapy for patients with renal artery stenosis. For instance, Sheps et al.[9] noted that 9 percent of 54 patients treated medically for 8 to 14 years died, while 80 percent of the patients had their blood pressure lowered to diastolic figures below 100 mm Hg. Five of their patients had worsening of the stenosis, increase in blood pressure, or both. Dustan et al.[10] reported that two-thirds of 23 patients followed up from 1 to 6 years had diastolic blood pressures under 100 mm Hg. It is of interest that in 11 of 23 patients, there was evidence of worsening of the lesion, decrease in the renal mass, development of more severe hypertension, or all three. It is evident, therefore, that good blood pressure control by medical management does not preclude continued progression of the stenotic lesion. In five of Dustan's patients, an accompanying fall in renal excretory function was noted, a finding also suggestive of progression of disease. Shapiro et al.[5] reported that 40 percent of 69 patients treated medically were dead at the end of 34 months. This figure is to be compared with the fact that in their surgically treated patients, 35 percent were dead at the end of 34 months. Kaufman and Lupu[11] reported that 22 percent of 36 patients treated medically were dead in from 1 to 8 years. They reported that only 28 percent of this group were able to be maintained with a diastolic blood pressure under 100 mm Hg, while 42 percent could not be controlled medically. They noted that only four of their patients worsened during the period of follow-up, a somewhat surprising figure in view of their relatively poor success rate for lowering blood pressure.

It is clear that if a patient with renal artery stenosis is assigned to a medical program, it is necessary to maintain therapy continuously for long periods, if not for life. During this time, regular observations are necessary to make certain that blood pressure is controlled, and that renal function does not worsen. Should the patient prove to be unresponsive to medical management, or if renal mass or renal function decreases, the decision not to operate must be reevaluated.

Summary and Conclusions

In approximately 80 percent of patients with renal artery stenosis, blood pressure is substantially benefited by surgical therapy using patient-selection criteria developed over the past 10 years. These results in our series have been obtained in a group of whom two-thirds had atherosclerotic causes for their renal artery disèase. Twenty-one of 54 patients had normal blood pressure without drugs at the end of the year and were considered cured. Surgical techniques used to treat these patients varied and were dependent upon the degree of stenosis, the associated disease, and the judgment and ability of the surgeon.

Our results reemphasize that those patients who are young, who have a short history of hypertension, and who have a single lesion of a major renal artery caused by nonatherosclerotic disease almost invariably benefit from operation if there is clear evidence of a significant lesion and good renal function. Our data also indicate that those patients who are unresponsive to medical therapy may benefit from a properly designed operation.

It is important to recognize that those hypertensives who are old, and who have a long history of hypertension, lesions in both renal arteries, evidence of generalized vascular disease, and no clear evidence for the significance of the lesion do poorly when selected for operation. Such patients have not only a high operative morbidity, but also die early in the postoperative period of atherosclerotic events, such as myocardial infarctions and cerebral thrombosis. In this group, medical management may be preferable to surgery, despite the problems of long-continued drug therapy.

References

1. Kirkendall, W. M., Fitz, A. E., and Lawrence, M. S.: Renal hypertension: Diagnosis and surgical treatment. N. Engl. J. Med. 276:479, 1967.
2. Kirkendall, W. M., and Kioschos, J. M.: Studies on patients with renal artery stenosis. Trans. Am. Clin. Climat. Assoc. 82:101, 1970.
3. McCormack, L. J., Poutasse, E. F., Meaney, T. F., Noto, T. J., Jr., and Dustan, H. P.: A pathologic-arteriographic correlation of renal arterial disease. Am. Heart J. 72:188, 1966.
4. Dustan, H. P., Berliner, R. W., Bricker, N. S., Brod, J., Gifford, R. W., Hoobler, S. W., Kincaid-Smith, P., Maxwell, M. H., McCormack, L. J., Meaney, T. F., and Shapiro, A. P.: Renal artery stenosis and parenchymal diseases. *In* Page, I. H., and McCubbin, J.

(Eds.): Renal Hypertension. Chicago: Year Book, 1968, p. 306.

5. Shapiro, A. P., Perez-Stable, E., Scheib, E. T., Bron, K., Moutsos, S. E., Berg, G., and Misage, J. R.: Renal artery stenosis and hypertension. Am. J. Med. 47:175, 1969.
6. Foster, J. H., Rhamy, R. K., Oates, J. A., Klatte, E. C., Burko, H. C., and Michelakis, A. M.: Renovascular hypertension secondary to atherosclerosis. Am. J. Med. 46:741, 1969.
7. Kaufman, J. J., Lupu, A. N., and Maxwell, M. H.: Renovascular hypertension: Clinical characteristics, diagnosis, and treatment. Cardiovasc. Clin. 1 (No. 1):79, 1969.
8. Fitz, A. E., Thompson, E., and Kirkendall, W. M.: Long-term results of operative treatment for renal hypertension. Circulation 40 (Suppl. 3):80, 1969.
9. Sheps, S. G., Osmundson, P. J., Hunt, J. C., Shirger, A., and Fairbairn, J. F.: Hypertension and renal artery stenosis: Serial observations in 54 patients treated medically. Clin. Pharmacol. Ther. 6:700, 1965.
10. Dustan, H. P., Meaney, T. F., and Page, I. H.: Conservative treatment of renovascular hypertension. *In* Gross, F., Naegeli, S. R., and Kirkwood, A. H. (Eds.): Antihypertensive Therapy. New York: Springer, 1966, pp. 544–554.
11. Kaufman, J. J., and Lupu, A. N.: Renovascular surgery. *In* Alken, C. E., Dix, V. W., Goodwin, W. E., and Wildbolz, E. (Eds.): Encyclopedia of Urology. New York: Springer, 1970, pp. 1–33.

Treatment of Malignant Hypertension Associated with Renal Insufficiency

By Allan B. Schwartz, M.D.

THE CLINICAL SYNDROME of the malignant phase of hypertension is a reflection of the diffuse vascular alterations, specifically, fibrinoid necrosis and the resultant compromised perfusion of vital organs, i.e., the kidneys, brain, heart, and eyes. Malignant hypertension associated with renal failure is a devastating combination. That this process is reversible is a thesis gaining support each year. The blood pressure must be reduced to allow vascular changes to heal. The resistance vessels may return to their normal caliber, perfusion will improve, and the syndrome will abate.

The aggressive treatment of the malignant hypertension by lowering the blood pressure to normal levels often results in worsening of the renal failure very early in the treatment program. This further decrease of renal function should be only a transient one. However, the physician faced with such a situation frequently finds himself doubting the reversibility of his patient's condition. The physician is presented with the dilemma of whether to withdraw antihypertensive medication and "stabilize" the blood urea nitrogen (BUN) or to treat aggressively to lower the blood pressure to a normal level. The physician faces the risk of almost certain worsening of renal function and possibly uremia during early treatment in the hope of gradual improvement of renal function over the long course of time. It is the purpose of this chapter to present the clinical and histopathologic correlation of effective treatment of malignant hypertension associated with uremia, demonstrating the reversibility of the uremia and significant improvement of glomerular filtration.

Emphasis is placed on two major points: (1) prompt confirmation of the diagnosis of "primary" nephroangiosclerosis with fibrinoid necrosis by the use of the renal biopsy and, once this has been done, (2) rapid achievement and maintenance of normal blood pressure levels through the use of potent antihypertensive agents in combination to permit the healing of the necrotizing arteriolar lesions. Normal blood pressure levels must be achieved even in the presence of worsening renal insufficiency and uremia requiring dialytic support if improvement of renal function is to occur.

The prognosis of malignant hypertension is definitely better today than 20 years ago, or even 10 years ago. The apparent reasons for this improvement are twofold: (1) the availability of relatively safe, potent antihypertensive agents which have been developed for clinical use during the period; (2) an increasing knowledge and understanding of the use of the antihypertensive agents in the presence of renal insufficiency associated with the malignant phase of hypertension.

Before the advent of such early therapy as sympathectomy, malignant hypertension was consistently a fatal disease within 4 or 5 years, and 80 percent fatal in the first year.[1–3] In 1938, Page reported on beneficial results of anterior nerve root section.[4] He was the first to show some evidence of improvement of cardiac parameters, eye grounds, and renal function in the course of malignant hypertension. The patient still eventually succumbed to the disease, however.

The advent of ganglionic blocking agents and adrenergic blocking agents brought about an improvement in the survival statistics. Encephalopathic and cardiac causes of death associated with malignant hypertension declined. However, the percentage of renal causes of death increased, demonstrating a failure to arrest the arteriolar fibrinoid necrosis within the kidney.

In 1956, McCormack et al.[5] showed definite evidence of healing of acute destructive lesions of malignant nephroangiosclerosis in patients treated with potent antihypertensive agents in-

From the Division of Nephrology and Hypertension, Department of Medicine, Hahnemann Medical College and Hospital, Philadelphia, Pennsylvania.

cluding hexamethonium, pentolinium, chlorisondamine, mecamylamine, reserpine, and hydralazine. Although this was an autopsy study, there had been some transient clinical remissions effected in these patients with malignant nephroangiosclerosis by intensive treatment with the agents noted above. Renal failure was the primary cause of death in 14 out of 19 treated patients. There was a definite "cessation of activity and a regression in both arteriolar necrosis and thrombonecrosis." This was associated with disappearance of most of the foci of fibrin accumulation and of the evidence of acute vascular damage.

McCormack noted in his review that in some patients treatment was not wholly effective and minimal active lesions of malignant nephroangiosclerosis persisted and were apparently progressive, although certainly not nearly as rapidly as in the untreated patient.

McCormack's word was not heeded and for the next few years, physicians feared treatment of malignant hypertension associated with renal insufficiency.

The relationship of renal insufficiency to survival rate of patients with malignant hypertension has been interesting to follow through the evolution of successful antihypertensive therapy.

In 1959, Harrington, Kincaid-Smith, and McMichael [6] reported that malignant hypertension associated with a BUN level of greater than 60 mg per 100 ml before therapy correlated with only a 10-percent survival by two years. Those patients with BUN levels less than 60 mg per 100 ml had a 55-percent survival by 2 years.

In 1961, Dollery [7] expressed the opinion that progressive renal failure could not be halted by antihypertensive therapy. With respect to the blood urea level, Dollery reported only a 15-percent, 1-year survival if malignant hypertension was accompanied by a blood urea level of over 60 mg per 100 ml (a BUN greater than 30 mg per 100 ml). The 1-year survival for patients having malignant hypertension and a blood urea level less than 60 mg per 100 ml was 73 percent.

In a report by Mohler and Freis in 1960,[8] a correlation of the 5-year survival rate was made with normal or nearly normal levels of nonprotein nitrogen prior to treatment.

Sokolow and Perloff [9] reported a 5-year survival of five of 11 patients who had creatinine clearance values greater than 45 ml per minute before therapy with ganglionic blocking agents. Of 15 patients with poor renal function prior to treatment, none survived even 3 years.

In 1961, Kirkendall [10] wrote that successful lowering of blood pressure improved signs of necrotizing arteriolitis that allowed histologic improvement. To produce the same improvement of histology in the kidney, "one must reduce the blood pressure and blood flow to the kidneys so that glomerular filtration rate and renal excretory function are reversibly decreased. Thus, one is on the horns of a dilemma." [10] Kirkendall, as were many others, was faced with the fact that the closer to normotension the patient came, the worse the renal function became during the early treatment phase of the malignant hypertension. The key to the above quotation is that aggressive reduction of blood pressure might initially lower renal function, but this initial decline is a functional one that is "reversible."

Throughout the 1960s, physicians were still unable to cope with malignant hypertension coexisting with significant renal insufficiency. Therapy was often withheld or ineffectively administered at the first hint of BUN rise. As recently as 1966, Langford and Bonar [11] advocated that when a rise in blood urea nitrogen occurs, it is usually best to hold the pressure at the level that has been obtained or even let the blood pressure go slightly higher, rather than immediately pressing on to further blood pressure reduction.[11]

Langford did, however, recognize the need to continue antihypertensive therapy in treating malignant hypertension despite the rise in BUN levels to permit healing of the necrotizing arteriolitis. He also agreed, as we and others have, that it may be necessary to utilize dialysis while hypotensive therapy was being given in the face of worsening renal function.

Schroeder [12] claimed that if improvement in renal function does not occur early, the treatment can be considered only life-extending and he predicted a steadily progressive mortality. He did, however, recognize the value of effective lowering of blood pressure of malignant hypertension with mild to moderate renal insufficiency and noted that in his experience, one-quarter of such treated patients survive 5 years.

Woods and Blythe, in 1967,[13] reported an encouraging recent experience dealing with survival of patients having malignant phase of hypertension complicated by severe renal insufficiency. These advocates of aggressive therapy treated 20 patients with malignant hypertension and a BUN level of 50 mg per 100 ml or higher, and noted a 55-percent, 1-year survival; a 35-percent, 2-year survival; and a 25-percent, longer-term survival.[13]

In 1969, it was again reported that aggressive treatment of accelerated hypertension in patients with azotemia resulted in slight worsening of renal function during the first 2 weeks. However, by 3 months of effective treatment, renal function had improved to levels better than pretreatment values.[14]

One abstract of a case report by Cestero, Pabico, and Freeman in 1969 [15] and a single case report by Eknoyan and Siegel in 1971 [16] have confirmed the improvement of renal function following aggressive lowering of the blood pressure despite the presence of uremia requiring dialytic support.

The case report included in this chapter adds not only convincing clinical evidence of the reversibility of the uremia, but also follow-up renal biopsy evidence of the reversibility of the necrotizing arteriolar lesion of the malignant phase of hypertension in a totally rehabilitated patient.

Conclusions

It is obvious to us that the only way to attack the malignant phase of hypertension associated with primary nephroangiosclerosis is by prompt aggressive lowering of the blood pressure to normotensive levels, despite the presence of renal insufficiency and even uremia.

Reduction of blood pressure to normal levels in patients with malignant phase of hypertension complicated by renal insufficiency does not necessarily result in irreversible deterioration of renal function and may actually improve renal function in a large proportion of patients.

However, primary renal parenchymal disease such as chronic glomerulonephritis and lupus nephritis may be associated with a secondary form of malignant hypertension which presents entirely different considerations. The physician is now faced with the necessity of considering two separate prognostic aspects in one patient, i.e.: What is the prognosis of the primary renal parenchymal disease and what is the prognosis of the secondary and coexisting malignant hypertension? Renal insufficiency might be a definite feature of either.

A clear distinction must be made early between malignant hypertension due to primary nephroangiosclerosis versus malignant hypertension due to primary renal parenchymal disease. Often, the only means by which the distinction can be made is the kidney biopsy.

Once the diagnosis of primary nephroangiosclerosis is established, the treatment program for the malignant phase of hypertension with renal insufficiency is clear-cut: Normal blood pressure levels must be achieved and maintained.

A normal blood pressure provides the only setting in which the necrotizing arteriolar changes within the kidney will heal. Normal blood pressure must be maintained even if renal insufficiency appears to worsen in the early phase of treatment. This further loss in glomerular filtration rate, manifested in a rise in serum creatinine and BUN levels, is a functional, reversible loss.

The sudden decrease in perfusion pressure resulting from the antihypertensive agent will result in a decreased glomerular filtration rate. A transient worsening of azotemia and even uremia may occur during the early vascular healing phase. A need for supportive peritoneal dialysis or hemodialysis therapy may become apparent in some patients. Certainly, if the diagnosis is made early and treatment initiated early, this need will be transient. Once the fibrinoid vascular changes have healed and renal arterioles are again patent, the glomerular perfusion will improve and glomerular filtration rate will gradually increase.

Case Report

The patient is a 32-year-old black woman who presented on June 12, 1970 with a 1-week history of rapidly progressing dizziness, severe suboccipital headache, and nausea. On the day of admission, she had several episodes of vomiting. There was no past history of renal disease, hypertension, cardiovascular disease, or diabetes. The family history was negative for hypertension. No oral contraceptive agent had been taken.

The physical examination demonstrated the blood pressure to be 230/156 mm Hg in the right arm and 228/152 mm Hg in the left arm. Pulse rate was 96 beats per minute and regular. Temperature was 98.6 F, orally. Funduscopic examination revealed severe arteriolar spasm, soft cotton-wool exudates, and flame-shaped hemorrhages and papilledema bilaterally. The heart examination demonstrated the point of maximal impulse in the sixth intercostal space in the anterior axillary line. A prominent left ventricular heave was noted. An atrial gallop was present. A grade III/VI early systolic ejection murmur was noted at the second right intercostal space. The lung fields were clear. On abdominal examination, the liver, spleen and kidneys were not palpable. No costovertebral angle tenderness or abdominal bruit was present. Femoral pulses were strong bilaterally. All peripheral pulses were found to be normal. There was a trace of pretibial and pedal edema bilaterally. The neurologic evaluation showed the patient to be moderately lethargic, but she was well oriented for time, place, and person. There was no nuchal rigidity and no localizing neurologic abnormality.

Laboratory evaluation demonstrated the BUN to be 109 mg per 100 ml, serum creatinine 11.5 mg per 100 ml, serum sodium 137 mEq per liter, serum potassium 3.8 mEq per liter, serum chloride 98 mEq per liter, and serum carbon dioxide combining power 20.9 mEq per liter. Urinalysis demonstrated 8 to 10 red blood cells per high-power field, and a 1+ reaction for protein. Tests for urine sugar and acetone were negative. Urine specific gravity was 1.005. Complete blood count showed a hematocrit of 29 percent, hemoglobin of 9.6 gm per 100 ml, white blood count of 5,150 per cubic millimeter with 65 percent segmented forms, 5 percent bands, and 30 percent lymphocytes. The peripheral plasma renin activity was 5,000 ng per 100 ml (method of Boucher). The initial therapy consisted of 500 mg of alpha-methyldopa and 80 mg of furosemide given intravenously. The alpha-methyldopa was repeated in a 500-mg dose given intravenously every 6 hours for four

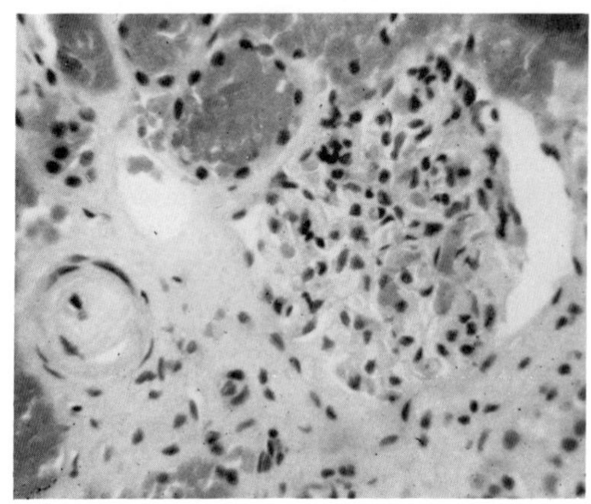

FIG. 1.—Renal biopsy during acute phase shows fibrinoid necrosis of arteriole and nonspecific thickening and proliferation of glomerulus. Hematoxylin and eosin; original magnification, ×360.

doses. At that time, the patient was started on oral therapy consisting of 500 mg of alpha-methyldopa given every 6 hours in combination with 50 mg of hydralazine given every 6 hours and 80 mg of furosemide given every 12 hours. Within 12 hours after the patient's admission, the blood pressure was reduced to 120/80 mm Hg, and within 24 hours the oral medication described above was maintaining a blood pressure of 100/70 mm Hg in the supine posture.

By June 15, 1970 the BUN had increased to 150 mg per 100 ml and the serum creatinine had risen to 16.2 mg per 100 ml. A renal arteriogram demonstrated patent main renal

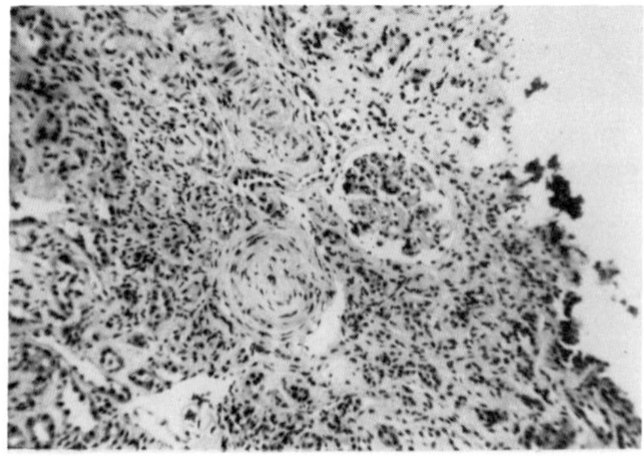

FIG. 2.—Renal biopsy during acute phase. Obliteration of interlobular artery by onion-skin effect. Hematoxylin and eosin; original magnification, ×180.

arteries bilaterally. There was moderate arcuate and interlobular arterial narrowing within the renal cortex. The transit time of the radiopaque material was delayed and there was absence of nephrogram effect. On June 17, the BUN was noted to have increased to 193 mg per 100 ml and the serum creatinine was 15.3 mg per 100 ml. The patient had developed further evidence of uremia, and peritoneal dialysis was instituted for the ensuing 48-hour period. Open renal biopsy was then performed. The renal biopsy demonstrated evidence of fibrinoid necrosis of the afferent arterioles and interlobular arterioles (Fig. 1). There was also a typical onion-skin effect in arterioles diffusely throughout the kidney (Fig. 2). The interstitium was moderately involved with round-cell inflammatory reaction, edema, and a mild degree of fibrosis. The glomeruli were nonspecifically thickened and minimally proliferative (Fig. 3). Only a few of the glomeruli were entirely hyalinized. The 24-hour urine excretion rates for vanillylmandelic acid (VMA) were 6 or 7 mg per 24 hours. Repeated urinary cultures demonstrated no significant growth.

The clinical course was marked by normotensive response to the medications consisting of: furosemide, hydralazine, and alpha-methyldopa in the dosages described above. The patient showed continuous improvement in overall well-being. Over the next 3 weeks, there was a stabilization of the BUN at 142 mg per 100 ml and the serum creatinine at 11.3 mg per 100 ml.

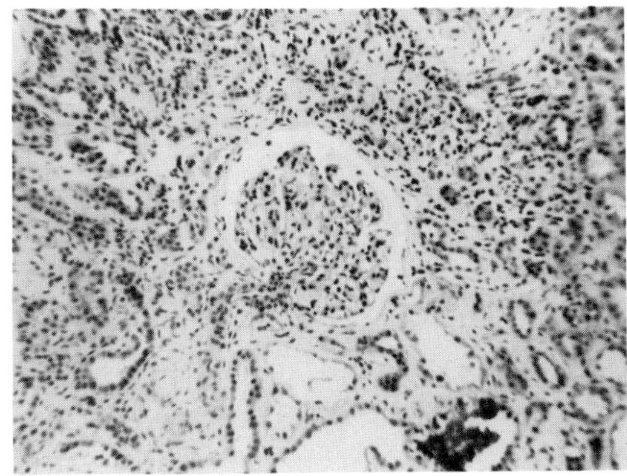

FIG. 3.—Renal biopsy during acute phase with mild nonspecific thickening and proliferation of glomerulus. Hematoxylin and eosin; original magnification, ×180.

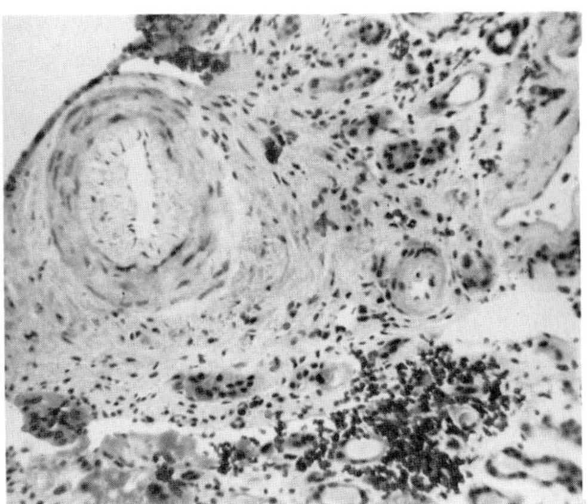

FIG. 4.—Renal biopsy after 7 months of treatment shows afferent arteriolar patency and interlobular arteriolar patency although both arterioles are still thickened. Hematoxylin and eosin; original magnification, ×360.

An orthostatic response to the medications was noted, as the blood pressure was consistently lower in the standing posture than in the supine posture. The average blood pressure in the standing posture was 115/80 mm Hg and the average blood pressure in the supine posture was 170/100 mm Hg during the patient's hospitalization. For this reason, the patient's bed was tilted 30 degrees upright at the head.

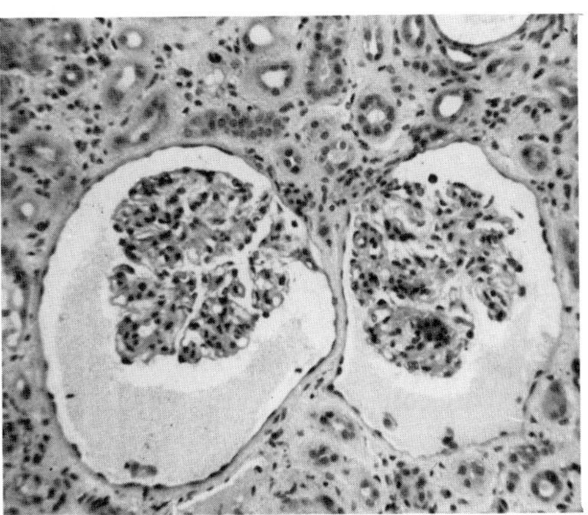

FIG. 5.—Renal biopsy after 7 months of treatment. Glomerular capillary loops are more delicate; however, size of glomeruli is mildly shrunken and increase in Bowman's space is present. Hematoxylin and eosin; original magnification, ×360.

The patient was discharged and followed up at frequent intervals as an outpatient. Medications were continued and occasional adjustments were made to maintain normotensive blood pressure levels. Associated with the marked orthostatic response noted, three episodes of dizziness did occur during the next few months. However, there was no syncope. Again, the supine blood pressure was consistently higher than the normotensive to slightly hypotensive standing blood pressure. The patient's bed at home was placed in the 30-degree, head-up, tilt position to avoid the mild blood pressure elevations while she slept.

During the outpatient follow-up period, the patient was trained to record her own blood pressures at home. She kept an extremely accurate record which corresponded with the in-office readings very well.

The funduscopic picture cleared over the initial 3 months of outpatient follow-up and her residual funduscopic changes consist of mild arteriolar narrowing with no evidence of hemorrhages or exudates.

The patient returned to work in September 1970 and maintained full employment following that date.

The BUN and serum creatinine progressively decreased over the next few months, and the creatinine clearance increased to 30 ml per minute by November 1970.

In January 1971, the patient was readmitted to the hospital for elective evaluation of her renal status after having maintained a steady improvement while normotensive for 7 months. A repeat kidney biopsy showed definite evidence of afferent and interlobular arteriolar patency (Fig. 4). There was no evidence of the typical onion-skin effect and fibrinoid necrosis which had been noted in the initial biopsy. Many glomeruli did show some evidence of shrinking and there was an increase of Bowman's space (Fig. 5). However, the glomerular capillaries were no longer thickened and the degree of proliferation was less than had been noted in the initial biopsy. The creatinine clearance was 30 ml per minute and the serum creatinine was 3.6 mg per 100 ml.

Repeated evaluation of the peripheral plasma renin activity demonstrated values below 1,000 ng per 100 ml in contrast to the initial value of 5,000 ng per 100 ml during the initial hospitalization.

After discharge, the patient was seen at monthly intervals. She maintained a normotensive blood pressure in the upright posture, and a minimum degree of hypertension was recorded only occasionally in the supine posture. The medication was continued rigidly by the patient. By July 1971, the BUN was 42 mg per 100 ml and the serum creatinine was 2.9 mg per 100 ml and the creatinine clearance was 35 ml per minute 13 months following the initial treatment (Fig. 6). The patient has maintained full employment since September 1970, in the capacity of laboratory technician. The antihypertensive prescription at present is: 80 mg of furosemide taken twice daily; 100 mg of hydralazine; and 500 mg of alpha-methyldopa, taken four times each day.

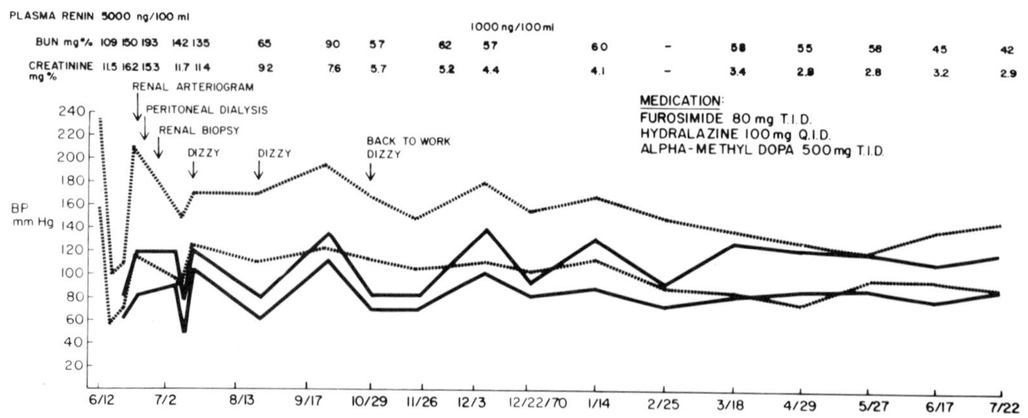

FIG. 6.—Graphic summary of patient's clinical course and treatment.

REFERENCES

1. Bjork, S., Sannerstedt, R., Angervall, G., and Hood, B.: Treatment and progression in malignant hypertension. Clinical follow-up study of 93 patients on modern medical treatment. Acta Med. Scand. 166:175, 1960.
2. Keith, N. M., Wagener, H. P., and Barker, N. W.: Some different types of essential hypertension: Their course and prognosis. Am. J. Med. Sci. 197:332, 1939.
3. Kincaid-Smith, P., McMichael, J., and Murphy, E. A.: The clinical course and pathology of hypertension with papilledema (malignant hypertension). Q. J. Med. 27:117, 1958.
4. Page, I. H.: Medical aspects of surgical treatment of hypertension. JAMA 110:1161, 1938.
5. McCormack, L. J., Beland, J. E., Schneckloth, R. E., and Corcoran, A. C.: Effect of antihypertensive treatment on the evaluation of the renal lesions in malignant nephrosclerosis. Am. J. Pathol. 34:1011, 1958.
6. Harington, M., Kincaid-Smith, P., and McMichael, J.: Results of treatment in malignant hypertension. A seven-year experience in 94 cases. Br. Med. J. 2:969, 1959.
7. Dollery, C. T.: Malignant hypertension in treatment of hypertension. *In* Pickering, G. W., Cranston, W. I., and Pears, M. A. (Eds.): American Lectures in Living Chemistry. Springfield, Ill.: Thomas (Bonnerstone Division), 1961, p. 47.
8. Mohler, E. R., Jr., and Freis, E. D.: Five-year survival of patients with malignant hypertension treated with antihypertensive agents. Am. Heart J. 60:329, 1960.
9. Sokolow, M., and Perloff, D.: Five-year survival of consecutive patients with malignant hypertension treated with antihypertensive agents. Am. J. Cardiol. 6:858, 1960.
10. Kirkendall, W. M.: The management of the hypertensive patient with renal insufficiency. *In* Brest, A. N., and Moyer, J. H. (Eds.): Hypertension: Recent Advances. The 2nd Hahnemann Symposium on Hypertensive Disease. Philadelphia: Lea & Febiger, 1961, pp. 554–564.
11. Langford, H. G., and Bonar, J. R.: Treatment of the uremic hypertensive patient. Mod. Treat. 3:62, 1966.
12. Schroeder, H. A.: Azotemic malignant hypertension. N. Engl. J. Med. 277:491, 1967.
13. Woods, J. W., and Blythe, W. B.: Management of malignant hypertension complicated by renal insufficiency: Further experience. Trans. Am. Clin. Climat. Assoc. 79:108, 1967.
14. Mroczek, W. J., Davidov, M., Gavrilovich, L., and Finnerty, F. A., Jr.: The value of aggressive therapy in the hypertensive patient with azotemia. Circulation 40:893, 1969.
15. Cestero, R. V. M., Pabico, R. C., and Freeman, R. B.: Reversible terminal renal failure in malignant hypertension. Abstracts Am. Soc. Nephrol. 3:10, 1969.
16. Eknoyan, G., and Siegel, M. B.: Recovery from anuria due to malignant hypertension. JAMA 215:1122, 1971.

The Concept of Basal Sodium Excretion in the Management of Hypertension of Primary Renal Disease

By J. C. Rocha, M.D., R. C. Davidson, M.D., J. Milutinovic, M.D., and B. H. Scribner, M.D.

We recently have published data which demonstrate a marked reduction in sodium excretion when dietary sodium restriction is used to treat hypertension in patients with primary renal disease.[1] Contrary to the generally accepted opinion that salt-wasting is the major problem in chronic renal disease and therefore sodium-restricted diets are contraindicated,[2–5] this study demonstrated that most patients with primary renal disease excrete less than the minimum practical dietary intake of sodium (40 mEq per 24 hours) when they are normotensive.[1] If dietary sodium intake exceeds this value, the corresponding increase in sodium excretion required to stabilize sodium balance is accompanied by severe treatment-resistant hypertension despite very little increase in total-body sodium.[1] Finally, this study demonstrated that chronic administration of furosemide can increase the daily level of sodium excretion in the normotensive kidney patient, thereby permitting a more liberal dietary intake of sodium without the development of hypertension.[1]

In the present study we have extended these observations to additional patients, and in so doing have evolved the concept of the basal sodium excretion (BSE), which we define as the highest 24-hour urinary excretion of sodium measured when the patient is normotensive.

From the Department of Medicine, University of Washington School of Medicine, Seattle, Washington.

Supported in part by National Institutes of Health Grant AM-06741 and by a grant from Hoechst Pharmaceutical Co., Somerville, N.J. A portion of this work was performed through Grant RR-37 from the General Clinical Research Centers Program of the Division of Research Resources, National Institutes of Health. Dr. Milutinovic's work was supported by Public Health Service Training Grant T01 AM-06221.

Method

The patients selected for study all had primary renal disease with varying degrees of chronic renal failure. Since each patient was to serve as his own control, and therefore had to be followed for long periods of time partly as an outpatient, these subjects were carefully selected according to the following criteria: (1) demonstrated ability to cooperate and to measure 24-hour urine, blood pressure, and body weight when an outpatient; (2) demonstrated ability to control daily sodium intake accurately at the prescribed level; (3) absence of congestive heart failure or other end-organ damage secondary to hypertension. During the initial phase of therapy, some of the patients were studied in the Clinical Research Center at the University of Washington so that a more accurate measurement of dietary sodium could be obtained.

Daily measurements were made of blood pressure, body weight, 24-hour sodium excretion and creatinine clearance. At appropriate intervals, serum electrolytes were measured by standard methods. Plasma renin activity was measured by the method of Gunnels.[6] The normal value for this method is < 500 ng per 100 ml.

Furosemide in daily doses ranging from 40 to 480 mg was used. Spironolactone, alpha-methyldopa, ethacrynic acid, and reserpine also were used occasionally in standard dosages in some patients.

To conserve space in the tables, averages of daily values for the intervals indicated are shown with single days included when appropriate. The following assumptions were made in analyzing and interpreting the data:

1. That in a stable, cooperative patient whose weight remains constant, measured ex-

TABLE 1.—*Classification of Patients*

Age	*Sex*	*Patient*	*Diagnosis*	*BSE* *	*Sensitivity to Furosemide*	*Class*
42	F	JM	Interstitial nephritis	> 200	Not tested	A
28	F	LR	Renotubular acidosis	> 200	Not tested	A
52	M	DC	Polycystic kidney disease	> 20	Very sensitive	B
24	F	JO	Chronic pyelonephritis	> 20	Very sensitive	B
27	M	RM	Chronic pyelonephritis	> 20	Very sensitive	B
34	M	CN	Chronic glomerulonephritis	> 20	Very sensitive	B
16	F	LJ	Chronic glomerulonephritis	4.5	Moderately sensitive	C
30	M	HL	Polycystic kidney disease	2.5	Moderately sensitive	C
44	M	PA	Chronic glomerulonephritis	6.0	Moderately sensitive	C

* Basal sodium excretion in mEq per 24 hours is the highest measured excretion while the patient is normotensive.

cretion of sodium should reflect approximately the actual intake of sodium.

2. That an aliquot of the daily 24-hour urine output as collected and measured by the patient will measure sodium excretion with sufficient accuracy to demonstrate changes in the renal handling of sodium. Gross collection errors were detected by daily measurement of 24-hour creatinine excretion.

3. That provided serum sodium remains stable, significant changes in extracellular volume and therefore of total-body sodium will be reflected by changes in body weight over periods of less than one week.

RESULTS

In Table 1 we have attempted to illustrate the importance of the concept of BSE by listing the patients in this study according to the level of BSE. Note that the higher the BSE, the more sensitive the patient is to the natruretic action of furosemide and the easier the control of blood pressure, as indicated by the class into which the patient is placed. Class A patients are normotensive on a sodium-free diet and usually require sodium supplements to maintain normal balance. A Class B patient is considered to have a moderately difficult problem with control of hypertension and a Class C patient is the most difficult to manage. Examples of patients in each class are given below.

Actual measurement of BSE is difficult since the precise conditions are hard to arrange. The highest level of sodium excretion per 24 hours achieved while the patient is normotensive is the BSE. The values for BSE shown in Table 1 represent approximations in all but the Class C patients. However, we feel the concept of BSE is more important than the precise measurement, since it facilitates a classification of patients according to the dif-

TABLE 2.—*Sodium Excretion in Class A Patients*

		Sodium-Free Diet				*Sodium Load*			
Patient	*Diagnosis*	*Blood Pressure (mm Hg)*	*Sodium Intake (mEq per 24 hr)*	*Sodium Excretion (mEq per 24 hr)*	*Serum Creatinine (mg per 100 ml)*	*Blood Pressure (mm Hg)*	*Sodium Intake (mEq per 24 hr)*	*Sodium Excretion (mEq per 24 hr)*	*Serum Creatinine (mg per 100 ml)*
JM	Interstitial nephritis	100/60	300	270		148/82	700	669	4.5
LR	Renotubular acidosis	104/65	150	110	8.0	110/76	300	276	6.5

TABLE 3.—*Data on Class B Patient J.O.*

Days	*Weight (in kg)*	*Blood Pressure (mm Hg)*	*Average Urinary Sodium (mEq per 24 hr)**	*Serum Creatinine (mg per 100 ml)*	*Creatinine Clearance (ml per min)*	*Serum Sodium (mEq per liter)*	*PRA (ng per 100 ml)*	*Furosemide (mg per 24 hr)*
1–7	46.8	158/109	73.7	3.2	18.9	139		0
8–13	46.6	150/102	79.2	3.2	17.2	139		0
14–20	45.8	129/96	112.5	3.3	18.7	139	1,482	40
21–27	45.9	118/86	83.5	3.4	18.2	138		40
28–35	45.9	125/86	77.7	3.9	17.0	140		40

* Average of daily excretions for the interval.
Abbreviation used: PRA, plasma renin activity.

ficulty with therapy. Let us now characterize the 3 classes of patients.

Class A

For a patient with chronic renal disease to be placed in Class A, he must be normotensive on a sodium-free diet. As shown in Table 2, our two patients in this class had a very large BSE. In fact, with a sodium load it was not possible to reach basal sodium excretion. In patient J.M., a sodium load that increased sodium excretion to nearly 700 mEq per 24 hours still did not cause hypertension, even though the blood pressure did rise but remained within the range of normal. Hence, the BSE must be somewhat higher than 669 mEq per 24 hours. By the same reasoning, BSE for patient L.R. must be higher than the 276 mEq per 24 hours achieved with a more modest sodium load.

Class A patients are relatively uncommon, numbering in our series around 10 to 20 percent of patients with renal failure due to primary renal disease. Almost invariably they have tubular as opposed to glomerular disease.

Class B

For a patient with primary renal disease to qualify for Class B, his hypertension must be controlled by furosemide alone with or without moderate restriction of sodium intake. In Tables 3 through 5, we present pertinent data on patients that fall into this classification. Note that in each case the hypertension responded well to the institution of furosemide therapy.

TABLE 4.—*Data on Class B Patient D.C.*

Days	*Weight (in kg)*	*Blood Pressure (mm Hg)*	*Average Urinary Sodium (mEq per 24 hr)**	*Serum Creatinine (mg per 100 ml)*	*Creatinine Clearance (ml per min)*	*Serum Sodium (mEq per liter)*	*PRA (ng per 100 ml)*	*Furosemide (mg per 24 hr)*
Renal Clinic		170/130						
1–13	97.3	150/110	130.9	3.0	48.9	143	170	
14–16	96.8	146/114	160.2	2.8	48.7	144		80
17–21	96.8	150/120	140.3	3.0	50.0	142		160
22–49	95.6	150/117	142.3	3.0	48.7	141		240
60–65	93.1	126/92	161.8	3.4	42.6	143	1,608	320
66–72	92.6	123/96	103.3	3.3	40.4	138		320
73–85	93.2	133/92	124.5	3.4	42.4	140		160

* Average of daily excretions for the interval.
Abbreviation used: PRA, plasma renin activity.

In patient J.O. (Table 3), who habitually ate a low-sodium diet, blood pressure control was achieved with only 40 mg of furosemide per day. A transient increase of sodium excretion during days 14 through 20 was enough to produce a slightly negative sodium balance that was associated with control of blood pressure. Note that the weight loss was less than 1 kg, which indicates how *very sensitive* these patients are to slight changes in total-body sodium, a fact noted previously.[1] Blood pressure control was achieved despite elevation of plasma renin activity to 1,482 ng per 100 ml. In patient D.C. (Table 4), who was ingesting a larger amount of sodium, the blood pressure did not drop until the dose of furosemide was increased to 320 mg per day. The initial blood pressure measurements in this patient permit us to make the important point that a Class B patient can be severely hypertensive if he ingests enough sodium. Patient C.N. also responded well to a moderate dose of furosemide, ingesting and excreting about 120 mEq of sodium per 24 hours. In all three patients, after a fall in blood pressure, the chronic administration of furosemide could maintain the same sodium excretion that these patients had when hypertensive. It is noteworthy that there was at most only a slight decrease in renal function as measured by serial creatinine clearance (or serum creatinine) when blood pressure control was accomplished by this manipulation of total-body sodium.

Class C

Patients in Class C are those who are the most difficult to manage. They require severe dietary sodium restriction in addition to large doses of furosemide for control of blood pressure. Often antihypertensive drugs are needed in addition. In our limited experience, these patients usually have had severe blood pressure problems in the past and are referred to us because they have become resistant to all therapy. The early phase of treatment often is complicated by severe adverse reactions to attempts to control blood pressure. These reactions usually are characterized by severe weakness, apathy, lack of energy, and at times dizziness on standing. Conduct of the therapy is very difficult and requires skill, patience, and conviction that the basic therapeutic tools, diet and furosemide, will work if properly used over a sufficient length of time. Because of these considerations, patients in this class usually should be treated in a hospital during the early stages or seen daily until control is achieved.

TABLE 5.—*Data on Class B Patient C.N.*

Days	*Weight (in kg)*	*Blood Pressure (mmHg)*	*Average Urinary Sodium (mEq per 24 hr)**	*Serum Creatinine (mg per 100 ml)*	*Serum Sodium (mEq per liter)*	*Dietary Sodium (mEq per liter)*	*Furosemide (mg per 24 hr)*
1	63.9	174/112	111	4.5	136	120	0
2	63.9	172/110	155			120	0
3	63.9	166/110	116			120	0
4	63.6	170/110	97			120	0
5		160/110	110			120	0
6	62.5	150/100	270	4.4	138	120	160
7	62.3	140/90	112			120	160
8	61.4	148/98	29			120	0
9	61.4	146/92	165			120	160
10	61.8	152/100	93			120	160
11	61.4	130/85	137.5	5.1	138	120	160
12	61.8	138/92	149			120	160
13–30	62.1	134/86	116	4.7		120	160

* Average of daily excretions for the interval.

The core of the problem with Class C patients is the very low BSE. As shown in Table 1, it was below 10 mEq in each of our three examples, which means that an impossible degree of dietary sodium restriction would be required to control blood pressure were it not for furosemide. This point is well illustrated by patient L.J., who was the first patient in our program to receive furosemide.

Patient L.J. (Table 6) was a 15-year-old girl with chronic glomerulonephritis, progressive azotemia, and hypertension which had been nearly impossible to control. This patient's blood pressure was brought under fairly good control by reducing her dietary intake of sodium to the nearly intolerable level of 20 mEq per day and by using alpha-methyldopa (days 1 through 21). An increase of dietary sodium to only 40 mEq per day on day 28 was followed by a marked increase in blood pressure to the level of 165/130 mm Hg in spite of the use of 10 mg of guanethidine, which was started on day 22 in anticipation of this change in diet. This increase in blood pressure was associated with only a 1- to 2-kg increase in body weight, which again demonstrates the extreme sensitivity of these patients to small changes in total-body sodium. Furosemide, started on day 65, produced an increase of sodium excretion on days 66 and 67, and blood pressure control beginning on day 69. Note that eventually, on day 100, the chronic administration of furosemide permitted the intake of sodium to again be increased from 20 mEq per 24 hours to the barely acceptable level of 40 mEq per 24 hours, and after day 110 blood pressure was very well controlled without any other antihypertensive drugs. On day 74, her serum creatinine had risen to 8 mg per 100 ml, suggesting some degree of extracellular volume depletion that was easily corrected, stabilizing her serum creatinine at around 6.7 mg per 100 ml.

In Table 7, data are presented from a patient (H.L.), a 30-year-old man with polycystic kidney disease, who had been an invalid for over 3 years because of severe hypertension. His hypertension had been resistant to a series of treatments that included alpha-methyldopa, guanethidine, hydralazine, and reserpine. However, no treatment involving a sodium-restricted diet had been administered. When he first came to us, his blood pressure was 180/120 mm Hg in spite of therapy with 750 mg of alpha-methyldopa and 75 mg of hydralazine. Severe sodium restriction and furosemide were not able to control this patient's blood pressure at the begin-

TABLE 6.—*Data on Class C Patient L.J.*

Days	*Average Daily BP (mmHg)*	*Sodium Intake (mEq per day)*	*Average Sodium Excretion (mEq per day)*	*Average Weight (kg)*	*Average Serum Creatinine (mg per 100 ml)*	*Serum Sodium (mEq per liter)*	*F (mg per day)*	*A (gm per day)*	*G (mg per day)*
1–21	145/95	20	23	46.2	4.8	139	0	1.0	0
22–27	148/98	20	26	46.5	4.9		0	1.0	10
28	150/90	40	33	46.5	4.9	141	0	1.0	10
29–64	165/130	40	37	47.7	5.6	138	0	1.0	10
65	160/120	20	33	47.6	7.0	140	80	1.25	5
66	165/116	20	61	46.9	7.0		80	1.25	5
67	150/106	20	50	46.6	—		80	1.25	5
68		20	45	—	—		160	1.25	5
69–73	140/90	20	30	46.4	—	138	240	1.25	5
74	132/94	20	20	46.0	8.0		240	0.75	5
75	130/90	ad lib.	4.5	45.5	—	136	0	0.75	5
76–99	130/86	20	24	46.3	6.7		120	0.75	5
100–110	124/86	40	38	45.5	6.8		120	0	5
110–190	130/88	40	41	45.6	6.7		120	0	0

Abbreviations used: BP, blood pressure; F, furosemide; A, Aldomet; G, guanethidine.

TABLE 7.—*Data on Class C Patient H.L.*

Days	Average Blood Pressure (mmHg)		Sodium Intake (mEq per day)	Average Sodium Excretion (mEq per day)	Average Weight (kg)	Creatinine Clearance (ml per min)	Serum Sodium (mEq per liter)	PRA (ng per 100 ml)	F (mg per 24 hr)	R (mg per 24 hr)
	Lying	Sitting								
1	178/120	168/120	Free	79.6	67.7	74.5	138	560		
2–13	152/118	144/120	20	12.8	64.7	65.3	133			
14	160/110	145/115	20	8.2	64.3	76.3	138			
15	154/110	150/114	20	142.6	64.1	73.1	135		60	
16	146/115	142/118	20	120.1	63.1	65.3	139		180	
17–19	148/115	120/85	20	22.7	62.2	54.0	129	1,515	80	
20	150/118	100/80	20	0.8	61.6	56.1	140		60	
21–23	124/101	122/96	20	48.2	60.9	69.3	128		360	
24	118/110	104/?	80	29.6	59.8	52.8	133		480	
25	124/100	114/?	40	13.5	60.4	58.7	129	1,825	480	
26–31	132/104	122/98	40	47.0	60.3	54.5	127	3,000	300	
32	110/80	114/78	40	1.9	60.1	52.8	125		160	
33–57	118/83	121/89	40	10.0	62.1	75.0	126		120	
58–104	140/97	156/107	40	46.5	65.6	70.0	132		320	
105–126	139/104	140/115	40		65.7			670	320	
127–131	150/110	140/116	40	64.2	62.1	56.6	137	1,840	320	
132–140	131/104	129/?	40	21.2	61.7	62.3	137	2,090	320	
141	126/100	128/100	Free	18.0	62.4	64.7	136	1,355	0	
142–145	130/92	130/92	Free	87.5	65.3	73.2	140	475	0	
146	130/80	130/90	Free	623.4	68.7	100.8	144		80	
147–152	137/84	135/94	Free	198.3	65.8	88.9	142		80	
153–164	140/100	140/106	120	148.5	64.9	70.3	138	220	320	
165–170	140/104	140/110	120	114.2	64.4	71.7	136		320	25
171	140/84	120/80	120	102.3	67.1	67.6	136		320	25
172–197	130/85	135/85	120	52.1	66.7	80.9	136		80	25
198–205	120/86	130/90	120						80	

Abbreviations used: PRA, plasma renin activity; F, furosemide; R, reserpine.

ning, and very low sodium excretion despite furosemide therapy can be observed on days 20 and 32, which explains the severity of his disease. The increase of furosemide to 480 mg per day was enough to produce an increase in sodium excretion which was greater than sodium intake on days 21 through 23. The blood pressure control from days 32 through 57 was not followed by an improvement in the patient's well-being, and he remained weak and tired with a recurrence of the hypertension during the weeks that followed.

Undoubtedly we should have used antihypertensive drugs earlier in the management of this patient. On day 165, a modest dose of reserpine was started, and the response was remarkable indeed. Either because of or in spite of the drug, the patient became much easier to manage, and at the time of this writing he has moved up to Class B. He currently is ingesting approximately 120 mEq of sodium per 24 hours and is taking only 80 mg of furosemide. The reserpine has been discontinued.

The third Class C patient (P.A., Table 8) had had severe hypertension for more than 1 year and was referred to us because he had become resistant to treatment. The high level of blood pressure on admission, associated with a grade-IV retinopathy, is consistent with the diagnosis of the accelerated phase of hypertension. At the outset, we felt certain this patient would have a very low BSE, since he was excreting only 75 mEq per 24 hours with a blood pressure in the 220/140 mm Hg range. Attempts to control blood pressure with diet and furosemide alone failed. However, he did lose several kilograms, and this desalting probably was responsible for the fact that his blood pressure responded well to modest doses of alpha-methyldopa and reserpine, which were started on day 7. It is important to note what happened to his 24-hour sodium excretion when his blood pressure fell. Despite continued administration of furosemide, it fell as blood pressure dropped and reached a low of 8.7 mEq per 24 hours on day 12. Evidently he was eating less sodium than the prescribed 40 mEq per 24 hours, since his weight remained relatively constant. However, the important point is that if this patient had not been under close supervision with respect to sodium retention, this fall in sodium excretion would have resulted in sodium retention, which might either have made him resistant to the modest doses of drugs or caused congestive heart failure. These two eventualities have been described many times by others.

Patient P.A. now has been followed for 9 months since the data in Table 8 were compiled. He remains well controlled but on an extremely low salt diet. Hence, he still remains a Class C patient, since whenever he deviates from his 20- to 30-mEq sodium diet he becomes severely hypertensive.

A Paradoxical Response to Changes in Total Body Sodium

In the course of this study we have encountered what is for us a new and very interesting phenomenon, which, for lack of a better term, we are calling a "paradoxical response to changing total-body sodium."

We first encountered this problem in patient H.L. early in the course of treatment. On about day 16 (Table 7) he became weak, very tired, and somewhat dizzy on standing. He did not develop a postural blood pressure drop, but his pulse pressure began to narrow. By day 25 it was nearly impossible to measure his diastolic pressure when standing, and even though the standing systolic pressure was 114 mm Hg, it was barely audible. There was no auscultatory gap. The phenomenon was associated with definite elevation of peripheral renin activity to levels as high as 3,000 ng per 100 ml (normal <500). The phenomenon eventually disappeared, but problems with blood pressure control continued, and on about day 105 more vigorous control of sodium balance was undertaken. During the period from days 132 through 141, he again became very weak, with a narrow pulse pressure and a barely measurable diastolic pressure. Plasma renin activity again was elevated. On day 141 he was placed on a sodium-free diet, and furosemide was stopped. Note that despite a 7-kg weight gain and the appearance of slight edema, his blood pressure fell to nearly normal levels, and he felt markedly improved. Resumption of furosemide and a sodium-restricted diet now resulted in good control of blood pressure. The increase in creatinine clearance suggested a marked fall in renovascular re-

TABLE 8.—*Data on Class C Patient P.A.*

Days	*Average Blood Pressure (mm Hg)*		*Sodium Intake (mEq per day)*	*Average Sodium Excretion (mEq per day)*	*Average Weight (kg)*	*Creatinine Clearance (ml per min)*	*Serum Sodium (mEq per liter)*	*PRA (ng per 100 ml)*	*F (mg per day)*	*A (mg per day)*	*R (mg per day)*
	Lying	*Sitting*									
1	220/130	220/140	Free	75.0	70.3	26.3	136	860			
2–5	200/120	210/140	120	114.4	68.1	23.5	138		160		
6	195/140	200/180	40	32.4	67.5	24.3	136		160		
7–11	148/112	144/129	40	19.6	67.7	23.4	133	1195	160	1000	0.25
12	130/110	120/108	40	8.7	67.8	23.8	132		160	1000	0.25
13–18	136/100	118/103	40	20.5	66.8	22.8	135	1290	320	750	0.25
19–22	142/100	120/103	40	29.3	66.4	22.3	128		400	1000	
23	120/93	99/94	40		65.9		128	3300	400	1000	
24–29	120/90	116/92	40	29.3	66.1	22.4	132		400	1000	
30–38	120/92	110/92	80	64.8	66.2	24.2	138		400	1000	

Abbreviations used: PRA, plasma renin activity; F, furosemide; A, alpha-methyldopa; R, reserpine.

TABLE 9.—*Data on Class B Patient R.M.*

Day	Average Blood Pressure (mm Hg) Lying	Average Blood Pressure (mm Hg) Sitting	Average Sodium Excretion (mEq per day)	Average Weight (kg)	Creatinine Clearance (ml per min)	Serum Sodium (mEq per liter)	PRA (ng per 100 ml)	F (mg per day)
19	130/90	130/90	102.9	62.3	20.2	145	200	160
20	120/82	106/72	88.1	61.6	19.0	139.5	190	160
21	122/94	108/82	67.6	61.3	22.4	137	415	160
22	130/100	126/110	28.5	60.7	22.9	140.5		0
23	132/76	128/86	117.1	62.2	25.4	140.5		80
24	130/84	120/90	166.0	62.6	24.9	141.5	365	80
25	132/84	130/104	182.6	62.2	25.6	146	L 345	80
							S 320	80
26	120/78	104/70	123.3	62.1	25.3	143	710	80

Abbreviations used: PRA, plasma renin activity; F, furosemide; L, lying; S, standing.

sistance. His subsequent course was remarkable in that he moved from Class C to Class B.

Patient P.A. developed the paradoxical response syndrome early in the course of therapy, and on day 6 had a standing blood pressure of 200/180 mm Hg. Again the systolic pressure was barely audible, and the diastolic pressure was nearly impossible to measure. It is of considerable interest that alpha-methyldopa seemed to abort the syndrome and subsequently controlled blood pressure in the face of persistently elevated plasma renin activity.

We have noted this paradoxical response syndrome in one patient who may not have developed elevations in plasma renin activity (Table 9). However, plasma renin activity was not measured on day 20 at the height of the syndrome. Note the fall in blood pressure that accompanied salt-loading and an increase in weight from day 20 to day 23.

DISCUSSION

The present study provides further documentation for the recently formulated thesis that the crucial factor which determines the incidence and severity of hypertension in patients with primary renal disease is the renal handling of sodium: the more sodium excreted by the damaged kidney when the patient is normotensive, the less problem there is with hypertension.[1] To this basic idea now can be added an additional factor, namely, the responsiveness of the damaged kidney to the natruretic effect of furosemide; the more responsive, the greater the sodium excretion and the easier the blood pressure control (Table 1).

We have introduced the concept of BSE in order to focus attention on the crucial role that the renal handling of sodium plays in determining the incidence and severity of hypertension in patients with primary renal disease. This concept also helps clarify the role of furosemide in the management of these patients, which is to increase basal sodium excretion and prevent an increase in blood pressure.

In learning how to use furosemide to increase BSE we have encountered a new problem which as yet we do not understand or know how to avoid, namely, that of a paradoxical hypertensive response to lowering total body sodium. The sequence of events in patient H.L., who developed the syndrome twice, clearly indicates the potential seriousness of the problem (see Table 7, days 16 through 32 and 105 through 142).

The hallmark of this paradoxical response seems to be extreme weakness and chronic fatigue with dizziness on standing. The blood pressure remains elevated without a postural drop, but the pulse pressure is very narrow, and, in the severest cases, the diastolic pressure, particularly when standing, may move up very close to the systolic and become nearly impossible to measure by auscultation. Although the peripheral renin activity often is elevated, this finding may not be a constant feature of the syndrome if the observation in patient R.M. (Table 9) can be confirmed. Temporarily increasing total-body sodium markedly improves well-being and usually is associated with a fall in diastolic pressure and a return to a more normal pulse pressure. At the same time, the glomerular filtration rate increases abruptly, perhaps due to an increase in renal blood flow resulting from a marked decrease in renal peripheral resistance. However, this latter point is based on indirect evidence in only one patient (H.L.) and simply points out the need for further elucidation of the pathophysiology and management of this interesting syndrome.

We have defined BSE as the maximum amount of sodium a patient can excrete per 24 hours while remaining normotensive. Let us now restate this concept in a different way: The presence of hypertension in a patient with primary renal disease indicates that the patient's 24-hour intake of sodium exceeds his BSE. To treat the hypertension, one can either reduce his sodium intake or increase his BSE, or both. This fact emphasizes the importance of constantly relating dietary sodium intake to daily sodium excretion by measuring daily excretion and relating this to any abrupt changes in body weight. Such measurements are particularly important during the initial phase of treatment, when sodium excretion can fall to extremely low levels as blood pressure is brought down. The sequence of events in the early phase of treatment of patient P.A. is a case in point. This patient with chronic glomerulonephritis had been severely hypertensive for several months and was referred because he had become resistant to treatment. When first seen by us, he was in the malignant phase of hypertension. We suspected that his BSE would be very low because he excreted only 75 mEq of sodium per 24 hours with a blood pressure of 220/140 mm Hg. He therefore would be a Class C patient in the classification in Table 1. His initial response to desalting was to lose about 2 kg (Table 8, days 1 through 6). At this point he seemed to develop the paradoxical response syndrome to an extreme degree: his standing blood pressure was 200/180 mm Hg! On day 7, modest doses of alpha-methyldopa and reserpine were begun with a very favorable effect on his blood pressure (days 7 through 23). However, note the fall in urinary sodium excretion that accompanied the fall in blood pressure. It fell as low as 9 mEq per 24 hours on day 12 despite continued administration of furosemide. Had this patient not been on a carefully measured low-sodium diet and under daily observation, he might have increased his total-body sodium and regained his lost weight. If that had happened, he would have apparently continued to be "treatment-resistant" or would have been reported to become "tolerant" to the low dose of alpha-methyldopa. Finally, if his sodium intake had been excessive at that point, his total-body sodium might have increased so much that he might well have developed congestive heart failure. In other words, the drop in sodium excretion that accompanies the drop in blood pressure in these circumstances undoubtedly is responsible for the development of so-called "treatment-resistant hypertension" as well as the edema and congestive heart failure that are said to be "complications" of antihypertensive drug therapy. The only way to avoid these complications is to be sure that the patient's weight remains stable by adjusting the dietary intake of sodium so that it roughly matches the daily excretion as measured. Increasing the dose of furosemide as well as passage of time seems to restore some natruretic response. In this case, the patient eventually stabilized on a 60 to 80-mEq sodium diet, with 400 mg of furosemide daily.

This phenomenon of increasing sensitivity to furosemide is better illustrated by the sequence of events in the case of patient H.L. (Table 7). This patient with polycystic kidney disease, who had suffered from disabling treatment-resistant hypertension for 3 to 4 years, was indeed difficult to control at the outset. Typically, his BSE was very low (below 10 mEq per 24 hours), and even on full doses of furosemide he excreted less than 5 mEq sodium per 24 hours on one occasion. It was all we could do to get his diastolic pressure below 100, even with a 40-mEq sodium intake plus large doses of furosemide. It was on this regimen that he twice developed the paradoxical response syndrome (days 16 through 52; 105 through 142). Then, strangely, after day 142, he rather quickly became tolerant of a 120-mEq sodium diet and eventually required only 80 mg of furosemide. What role the use of

0.25 mg of reserpine from day 165 to 197 had is not clear, but its use was associated with the resolution of the paradoxical syndrome. Had this drug, plus perhaps alpha-methyldopa, been used earlier, he might have been easier to control during the early weeks and perhaps the two episodes of paradoxical response to sodium deprivation might have been aborted or avoided, since alpha-methyldopa seemed to work well in patient P.A. (Table 8) despite elevated plasma renin activity.

How antihypertensive drugs should be used in the management of these patients remains to be determined. Clearly they are not needed in the Class A or B patients. They were valuable in patient P.A. and probably should have been used sooner in patient H.L. If they are to be used, they should be used only in modest dosages. Before starting these drugs, it is important to optimally control body sodium and to maintain control of it after sodium excretion drops with the fall in blood pressure so that the patient remains responsive to low doses of these potentially toxic drugs.

The three patients in Class B illustrate the value of furosemide in increasing BSE to control hypertension in primary renal disease. In the beginning, each of three patients was hypertensive because dietary sodium exceeded BSE. When furosemide was administered, the BSE was increased to the point where the same sodium intake could be excreted without the development of hypertension. None of these patients showed the paradoxical hypertensive response described above, and none required other hypertensive drugs.

It is important to emphasize that patients in Class B, even though they have a higher BSE than patients in Class C, can still develop severe treatment-resistant hypertension if they ingest enough sodium each day. Patient D.C. (Table 4) had severe hypertension at the outset, presumably because he was ingesting about 150 mEq of sodium, which was far in excess of his BSE of 38 mEq. Furosemide increased his BSE to match this intake, and he became normotensive.

The two patients in Class A, with a BSE greater than 200 mEq of sodium, illustrate the fact that patients with chronic renal failure and a significant "sodium leak" rarely have hypertension. Nevertheless, hypertension probably could be produced by greatly increasing the sodium intake to exceed the high BSE.

The patients reported support the hypothesis that the BSE is inversely related to the severity of the hypertension and the difficulty with which it is controlled in chronic renal failure. When dietary sodium exceeds BSE, severe resistant hypertension is the consequence, in spite of the fact that the body sodium is not greatly increased.[1] This observation offers further support to Borst's thesis that hypertension represents a physiologic compensatory mechanism which the body uses to increase sodium excretion.[7] Borst believes that in essential hypertension there may be a basic defect in sodium excretion which is compensated for by an elevated blood pressure. In hypertension associated with chronic renal disease the inability to excrete sodium is imposed by the renal disease itself.

Our patients also provide evidence that furosemide is an effective new modality in the treatment of hypertensives with chronic renal disease. It increases BSE, and thus allows a tolerable sodium intake while maintaining adequate blood pressure control. That furosemide works well even in patients with severe chronic renal failure has been demonstrated by Muth.[8] He demonstrated that it is effective over a wide range of arterial pH and electrolyte abnormalities, but must be used in increasingly larger doses as the glomerular filtration rate declines; that is, generally, the lower the glomerular filtration rate, the greater the dose of furosemide required. Further, furosemide is as effective as the thiazide diuretics in lowering blood pressure in essential hypertension.[9]

What relevance, if any, these concepts with respect to sodium have in the management of essential hypertension is not clear. On the one hand, Tarazi, Frohlich, and Dustan,[10] and Dustan and Page [11] have emphasized the difference in the status of sodium balance in patients with hypertension due to primary renal disease when compared with that of patients with essential hypertension. In the former, changes in blood pressure correlate very well with changes in total body sodium which is consistent with our results using diet and furosemide as the major therapeutic tools. In the latter group, Dustan and Page [11] found an inverse correlation between total-body sodium and blood pressure. Hence, one would not expect much benefit from using diet and furosemide as the primary therapeutic tools in essential hypertension. Yet Kempner's regimen,[12] which, despite the mystery, was probably nothing more than an extremely low sodium diet,[13] proved successful in 60 percent of patients. In fact, it is interesting to speculate whether the rice-fruit regimen would have been nearly 100 percent successful if Kempner [12] or Chapman [13] had been able to use diuretics to increase sodium excretion. Patients on the Kempner regimen sometimes reduced their sodium excretion to as low as 1 to 2 mEq of sodium per day.[12] Hence, no matter how low the intake, it would still require several weeks to lose the 140 mEq of sodium contained in only 1 liter of extracellular fluid. In this connection, it is interesting to note that in a series of patients with essential hypertension treated by Chapman with the rice-fruit diet, the two patients who were resistant to the regimen stabilized their extracellular volume (sodium thiocyanate spaces) at 24 percent and 26 percent of their body weight.[13] In contrast, the two patients who responded had extracellular volumes when stable on the regimen which were 21 percent and 17 percent of body weight. Hence, it is possible that a much higher success rate with the Kempner rice-fruit regimen would have been possible had powerful saluretics been available in that era. This speculation suggests that control of sodium balance probably is important in the management of essential hypertension, and yet those experienced in the field seem to pay little attention to this variable, and the literature on the subject remains confused.

For example, the early publications on alphamethyldopa describe weight gain and edema due to a fall in sodium excretion, yet they fail to recognize the enormous therapeutic importance of this fact. Instead, they list congestive heart failure as a "side effect" or "complication" of alpha-methyldopa treatment and indicate that when it develops, the drug should be stopped. Similarly, they fail to correlate increasing drug "resistance" or therapeutic failure with the degree of sodium retention, while at the same time acknowledging the fact that thiazides increase the sensitivity of the patient to these drugs. Perhaps the most important source of confusion in articles on the use of drugs in treatment of essential hypertension stems from the failure to understand that diuretic therapy is much more effective if some limit is placed on sodium intake. In some texts, dietary sodium restriction is not even mentioned, yet thiazides are advised, which is like trying to bail out a boat without plugging the leak. Careful control of sodium balance with diet and diuretics may yet become the cornerstone in the management of essential hypertension just as it is in patients with hypertension complicating primary renal disease—at least extrapolation into the diuretic era of the experience of Kempner [12] and Chapman [13] points in this direction. And the recent work of Finnerty et al., which demonstrates that an increase in extracellular volume is at least partly responsible for the development of resistance to antihypertensive drugs, may signal another rediscovery of the importance of paying attention to sodium balance in all patients with hypertension.[14] At the very least, limiting sodium intake in patients with essential hypertension should materially reduce the cost of drugs and eliminate many of the side effects of drug therapy, all of which might make the diet attractive enough for patients to follow. They should be given that option.

It is well to emphasize again the fact that the combination of dietary sodium restriction and furosemide is a powerful therapeutic combination that can produce sodium depletion and uremia in patients with chronic renal failure. The potential dangers of this complication quite rightly have been emphasized in the literature on the subject.[1–5] We probably produced this complication in patient L. J. on about day 74 (Table 6). It is equally important to emphasize that the effects of the depletion are readily reversed by increasing total-body sodium slightly, as was done with patient L. J.

Finally, the combination of furosemide and dietary sodium restriction can produce severe potassium depletion in some cases. A high potassium intake and 25-mg doses of spironolactone usually can correct this problem.

Summary

We recently have published data which demonstrate a marked reduction in sodium excretion when dietary sodium restriction is used to treat hypertension in patients with primary renal disease. From these data has emerged the concept of *basal sodium excretion*, which we define as the highest 24-hour sodium excretion measured when the patient is normotensive. In the present report data are presented which support the following impressions relative to basal sodium excretion:

1. The lower the basal sodium excretion, the more severe is the problem of hypertension.
2. The patients with the most difficulty in controlling hypertension have a basal sodium excretion rate which usually is far below the minimum practical dietary intake of sodium, i.e., 50 mEq per 24 hours.
3. When dietary sodium intake exceeds basal sodium excretion, increase in sodium excretion to restore sodium balance usually is accompanied by severe treatment-resistant hypertension despite very little increase in total-body sodium.
4. In many patients, chronic daily administration of furosemide can raise basal sodium excretion sufficiently to permit control of blood pressure by means of only modest dietary sodium restriction.
5. In those patients with the most treatment-resistant hypertension, basal sodium excretion, even with furosemide, can still remain below minimum dietary intake, making blood pressure control extremely difficult.
6. During the initiation of treatment of severe hypertension with dietary sodium restriction and furosemide it is possible to evoke a paradoxical response to decrease in total-body sodium, with an increase in peripheral vein renin activity, high fixed diastolic pressure, and very low pulse pressure. Temporarily increasing total-body sodium reduces renin levels and blood pressure falls.

Based on these preliminary studies, it is believed that a better understanding of the complicated interplay between sodium intake, sodium excretion, and hypertension is necessary before management of hypertension in patients with primary renal disease can be further improved.

Acknowledgment

The authors would like to acknowledge the valuable technical assistance of Miss Patricia Hoover, whose untiring efforts to help our patients follow the protocols made this study possible.

References

1. Ulvila, J. M., Kennedy, J. A., Lamberg, J. D., and Scribner, B. H.: Blood pressure in chronic renal failure. JAMA 220:233, 1972.
2. Relman, A. S.: Chronic renal insufficiency. *In* Beeson, P. B., and McDermott, W. (Eds.): Cecil-Loeb Textbook of Medicine. Philadelphia: Saunders, 1963, pp. 814–820.
3. Epstein, F.: Chronic renal failure. *In* Harrison, T. C. (Ed.): Principles of Internal Medicine, 5th ed. New York: McGraw-Hill, 1966, p. 859.
4. Merrill, J. P.: Management of chronic renal failure. Am. J. Med 36:763, 1964.
5. Reiss, E.: Diet in renal disease. *In* Papper, S. (Ed.): The Kidney, vol. 1. New York: National Kidney Foundation, 1967, pp. 1–6.
6. Gunnels, J. C., Jr., Grim, C. E., Robinson, R. R., and Wildermann, N. M.: Plasma renin activity in healthy subjects and patients with hypertension. Arch. Intern. Med. 119:232, 1967.
7. Borst, J. G. G., and Borst-de Geus, A.: Hypertension explained by Starling's theory of circulatory homeostasis. Lancet 1:677, 1963.
8. Muth, R. G.: Diuretic properties of furosemide in renal disease. Ann. Intern. Med. 69: 249, 1968.
9. Wertheimer, L., Finnerty, F. A., Bercer, B. A., and Hall, R. H.: Furosemide in essential hypertension. Arch. Intern. Med. 127:934, 1971.
10. Tarazi, R. C., Frohlich, E. D., and Dustan, H. P.: Plasma volume in man with essential hypertension. N. Engl. J. Med. 278:762, 1964.
11. Dustan, H. P., and Page, I. H.: Some factors in renal and renoprival hypertension. J. Lab. Clin. Med. 64:948, 1964.
12. Kempner, W.: Treatment of hypertensive vascular disease with rice diet. Am. J. Med. 4:545, 1948.
13. Chapman, C. B.: Some effects of the rice-fruit diet in patients with essential hypertension. *In* Bell, E. T., Clawson, B. J., and Fahr, G. E. (Eds.): Hypertension—A Symposium. Minneapolis: University of Minnesota Press, 1950.
14. Finnerty, F. A., Jr., Davidov, M., Mroczek, W. J., and Gavrilovich, L.: Influence of extracellular fluid volume on response to antihypertensive drugs. Circ. Res. 26–27 (Suppl. I):I-71, 1970.

Hypertension and Cerebrovascular Disease

By Jack P. Whisnant, M.D.

In 1954, Kirby and Hollenhorst[1] noted that ligation of one internal carotid artery resulted in decreased retinal vascular manifestations of hypertension on the side of the ligation and was associated with a decrease in pressure in the corresponding retinal artery. Subsequently, a relative lack of progression of retinal vascular changes also was noted on the side of the ligation. Since then, a number of clinicians have noted that hypertensive changes in the retina were less marked on the side of severe atherosclerotic occlusive disease in one internal carotid artery. These observations give direct evidence of the local effect of decreasing the blood pressure on arterioles comparable to the cerebral arterioles.

In addition, a number of observers have noted improvement in retinal lesions of hypertension in association with reduction of blood pressure by drug treatment. However, the most pertinent evidence that decreasing the blood pressure in hypertensive patients decreases the frequency of occurrence of strokes comes from the randomized drug treatment of hypertension by Freis and his associates.[2,3]

Since the introduction of effective drugs for decreasing the blood pressure, a concern of physicians treating patients who have hypertension has been the threat of localized or generalized ischemia of the brain. However, the autoregulatory mechanism of the brain blood vessels is such that, within a wide range of systemic blood pressures, the cerebral blood flow and therefore the cerebral perfusion is unchanged. Only when there is profound hypotension does cerebral ischemia occur, and it usually is reversible unless it persists over some minutes. Meyer and associates[4] have shown that cerebral blood flow may actually increase slightly when hypotensive drugs are given to hypertensive patients.

In rhesus monkeys, Brierley and associates[5] have noted that, when the cerebral perfusion pressure does not fall below 25 mm Hg in the presence of adequate oxygenation of arterial blood, brain damage does not occur. Below this level, infarcts develop in some animals at the boundary zones of the supply of specific arteries in the brain and more diffuse cerebral damage occurs in others.

In spite of these protective mechanisms of the brain, concern has continued, particularly in regard to the patient with hypertension who also has marked stenosis of part of the vascular tree leading to the cerebral circulation. This concern is related to the presumed more severe ischemia which may occur in the distribution of the stenosed artery when the blood pressure is decreased.

As an example, I cite one patient, a 55-year-old man, who began to have decreased ability to sweat and impotency over the period 1961 to 1966. From 1968 to 1970 he began to note faintness with prolonged standing or sitting, and in 1970 a diagnosis of idiopathic orthostatic hypotension was made and treatment with hydroxyamphetamine (Paredrine hydrobromide), tranylcypromine (Parnate), and fludrocortisone (Florinef) was begun. From February to March of 1971, this patient had four spells of weakness in the right leg and arm associated with an odd feeling on the right side of the face. In one spell there was inability to speak. There was no alteration of consciousness and the symptoms were promptly relieved by lying down. In March, during our observation, the blood pressure was noted to be 180/100 mm Hg while the patient was supine. Within 2½ minutes after he stood up, the blood pressure decreased to 75/50 mm Hg and at this point there was the onset of a similar spell as noted above with weakness of the right extremities and a right-sided Babinski sign. This spell was promptly relieved when the patient

From the Department of Neurology, Mayo Clinic and Mayo Graduate School of Medicine (University of Minnesota), Rochester, Minnesota.

This investigation was supported in part by Research Grant NS-6663 from the National Institutes of Health, Public Health Service.

lay down. After additional treatment with the same drugs, the orthostatic hypotension was satisfactorily controlled, the patient was able to return to work, and no further focal ischemic episodes occurred through the period of observation ending in October 1971.

This is a rather dramatic example of focal cerebral ischemia apparently directly related to a decrease in perfusion pressure from a decrease in blood pressure, comparable to what might occur with hypotensive drugs. Its importance lies in the fact that it is a rare example of this type. It is most unusual for focal ischemia to be manifested even when there is an appreciable drop in the blood pressure in spite of the fact that occlusive cerebrovascular disease and hypertension are commonly associated. Therefore, as a matter of practical consideration, the presence of cerebrovascular disease should not affect the treatment which is recommended for decreasing blood pressure in hypertensive patients.

When hypertensive patients also have transient focal cerebral ischemic attacks, the proper method of approach is antihypertensive medication plus treatment for the transient ischemic attacks; the latter might be anticoagulant therapy or surgical treatment if an appropriate surgical lesion can be detected. If the treatment is to be anticoagulant therapy, my preference is to start anticoagulant treatment and antihypertensive therapy at the same time.

In the last few years we have undertaken a study of stroke in the population of Rochester, Minnesota, and several observations bear on this subject. This population of 50,000 is ideal for this purpose since the primary source of care for the population is the Mayo Clinic and its physicians, and the diagnostic indexing and record retrieval system used at the Mayo Clinic has been implemented in the other medical-care facilities in the city. Therefore, case ascertainment is nearly complete and considerable detail concerning the patient's prior health is available in the records.

When long-term survival of those who were living 1 month after the stroke occurred is plotted according to groupings of systolic blood pressure prior to stroke occurrence in the period 1945 through 1954 (Fig. 1), there is no difference in survival at 1 year but there is a significant difference between the group with the lowest systolic pressure and the two other groups at 10 years. For diastolic blood pressure groupings, there is no difference in survival at 1 year, but there is a significant difference between the highest group and the two others at 10 years. These are compared to the expected survival of the 1950 Minnesota population with the same age distribution and there is a significant difference from expected survival for each blood pressure group.

When the same group of patients who survived a first stroke is examined in regard to the

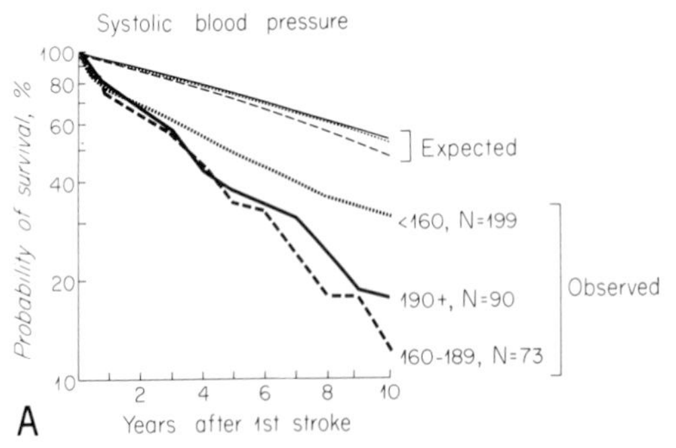

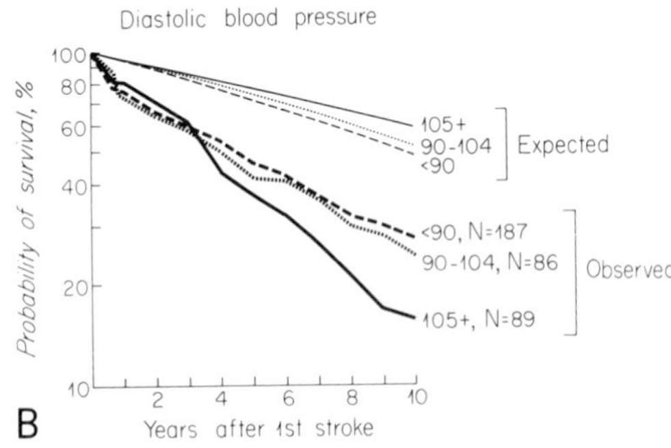

FIG. 1.—Life table analysis of Rochester, Minnesota residents who had their first stroke in the period 1945 through 1954 and survived at least 1 month, according to three groupings of blood pressure prior to the stroke. These are compared to expected survival for the 1950 Minnesota population for the same age distribution. *A*, Systolic blood pressure. *B*, Diastolic blood pressure.

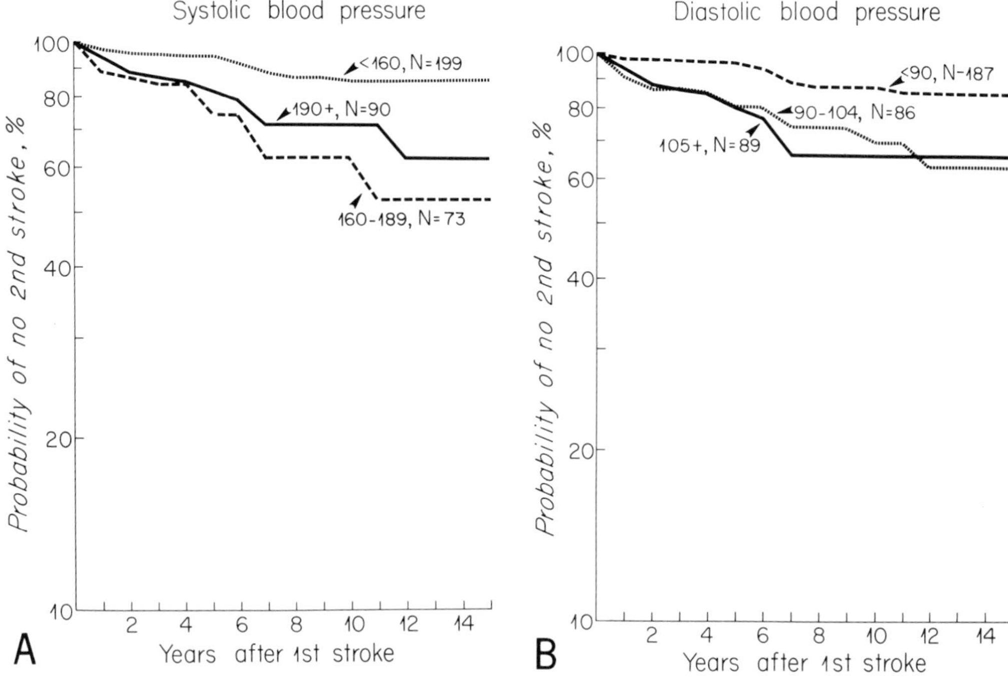

FIG. 2.—Life table analysis, using a second stroke as the end-point, for Rochester, Minnesota residents who had their first stroke in the period 1945 through 1954 and survived at least 1 month, according to three groupings of blood pressure prior to the first stroke. *A*, Systolic blood pressure. *B*, Diastolic blood pressure.

probability of not having a second stroke, there is no gradient among the three levels of blood pressure, as one might expect, but at 5 years after the first stroke there is a significant difference between the lowest systolic pressure group in which about 95 percent had not had a second stroke and the two other groups in which about 80 percent had not had a second stroke (Fig. 2). For diastolic blood pressure, it was about the same.

Therefore, starting with patients who have had a stroke and survived and who also have hypertension, there is not a sharp difference in prognosis determined by the level of blood pressure. The prognosis is already considerably altered by the occurrence of the stroke which may be the overriding consideration even in the presence of hypertension.

Among the patients in the community who had their first transient ischemic attack between 1955 and 1969, we have not been able to demonstrate a significant gradient in terms of survival or in terms of probability of stroke occurrence when the patients are divided into three groups according to the blood pressure at the time of the first transient ischemic attack. The same considerations may apply here as for survivors of the first stroke. (For treatment of hypertensive encephalopathy see the chapter entitled, "Treatment of Hypertensive Emergencies.")

REFERENCES

1. Kirby, T. J., Jr., and Hollenhorst, R. W.: Asymmetric hypertensive retinal changes after ligation of the internal carotid artery. Acta XVII Concilium Ophthalmologicum 1:335, 1955.
2. Veterans Administration Cooperative Study Group on Antihypertensive Agents: Effects of treatment on morbidity in hypertension: Results in patients with diastolic blood pres-

sures averaging 115 through 129 mmHg. JAMA 202:1028, 1967.

3. Veterans Administration Cooperative Study Group on Antihypertensive Agents: Effects of treatment on morbidity in hypertension. II. Results in patients with diastolic blood pressure averaging 90 through 114 mmHg. JAMA 213:1143, 1970.
4. Meyer, J. S., Sawada, T., Kitamura, A., and Toyoda, M.: Cerebral blood flow after control of hypertension in stroke. Neurology 18:772, 1968.
5. Brierley, J. B., Brown, A. W., Excell, B. J., and Meldrum, B. S.: Brain damage in the rhesus monkey resulting from profound arterial hypotension. I. Its nature, distribution, and general physiological correlates. Brain Res. 13:68, 1969.

Treatment of Hypertensive Emergencies

By Ray W. Gifford, Jr., M.D.

THERE ARE TIMES when prompt reduction of blood pressure by parenteral administration of antihypertensive agents can be lifesaving or prevent disabling cardiovascular catastrophes.

Sometimes it is the extremely high level of blood pressure which poses the threat to the cardiovascular system. Such crises include acute hypertensive encephalopathy complicating hypertension from any cause, some cases of malignant hypertension, and severe paroxysmal hypertension associated with pheochromocytoma or the release of tissue catecholamines by certain drugs or foods in patients receiving monamine oxidase (MAO) inhibitors.

In some cases an abrupt rise in blood pressure seems to be more important in the production of symptoms than the level to which it rises. Children with acute glomerulonephritis and women with eclampsia may develop hypertensive encephalopathy and convulsions when the blood pressure is no higher than 160/110 mm Hg. A common denominator in these cases seems to be fluid retention with cerebral edema. Similarly, uremic patients may have convulsions when blood pressure is only moderately elevated.

There are some conditions which qualify as hypertensive emergencies, not so much because of the height of the blood pressure, but because of coexisting complications which make even moderate hypertension dangerous. These include acute left ventricular failure associated with hypertensive heart disease, intracerebral or subarachnoid hemorrhage, and acute dissecting aneurysm of the aorta.

Antihypertensive Drugs for Parenteral Administration

The drugs which can be administered parenterally to reduce blood pressure in managing hypertensive crises are listed in Tables 1 and 2. One of the most important considerations in treating patients with hypertensive emergencies is the rapidity of onset and duration of drug action. Sodium nitroprusside, diazoxide, and phentolamine produce an abrupt depressor response within seconds, while it may take 2 or 3 hours for reserpine (whether administered intravenously or intramuscularly) or methyldopa to have a significant depressor effect. Intermediate between these two extremes are hydralazine and pentolinium, which will usually produce an appreciable reduction in blood pressure within 30 minutes following an intramuscular injection and within 10 minutes when given intravenously.

Route of Parenteral Administration. Sodium nitroprusside, diazoxide, trimethaphan, and methyldopa can only be administered intravenously. The others can be administered intravenously or intramuscularly and the choice of the route affects the rapidity with which blood pressure is reduced by either hydralazine or pentolinium, but not by reserpine. It is preferable to give phentolamine by intravenous injection because it is more rapidly and consistently effective than when given intramuscularly.

Diazoxide must be given very rapidly intravenously in a single bolus, within 15 seconds, otherwise avid binding by serum protein will inactivate the drug.[1] Phentolamine must also be injected rapidly when it is given as a single dose intravenously. Methyldopa should be administered by intravenous infusion over a period of 30 to 60 minutes. Because of their evanescent duration of action, sodium nitroprusside and trimethaphan must be given by continuous intravenous infusion, the rate of the administration being governed by the response of the blood pressure. Hydralazine or pentolinium can be given as a single dose intravenously by slow injection from a 20- or 50-ml syringe or as a continuous intravenous infusion (Tables 1 and 2). Sometimes it is advantageous to give the first dose intravenously from a syringe to obtain a prompt depressor response and then maintain the blood pressure at the desired level by continuous

From the Department of Hypertension and Nephrology, The Cleveland Clinic Foundation, Cleveland, Ohio.

TABLE 1.—*Direct Vasodilating Drugs for Parenteral Administration in the Management of Hypertensive Emergencies*

Drugs	*Intra-muscular* * *(mg)*	*Intravenous*		*Advantages*	*Disadvantages*
		Single Dose (mg)	*Continuous Infusion* † *(mg per liter)*		
Hydralazine (Apresoline)	10–50	10 ‡	100	Rapidly effective; seldom produces hypotension; does not reduce renal blood flow	Increases cardiac output and rate; is not as consistently effective as reserpine or pentolinium in controlling crises associated with essential hypertension
Sodium nitroprusside §			50–100	Rapidly and consistently effective; blood pressure can be titrated to any level by careful adjustment of rate of infusion	Requires constant supervision; best given in intensive care unit with monitoring of blood pressure every 3 to 5 minutes. Not available commercially
Diazoxide § (Hyperstat)		300–600 mg (rapid injection essential)		Rapidly and consistently effective (but not as much so as sodium nitroprusside); does not require as close supervision as does sodium nitroprusside; does not reduce renal blood flow; standardized dose	Blood pressure cannot be controlled at predetermined level by titrating dose; rapid injection of bolus commits one to whatever result is obtained

* Start with the smallest dose shown. Subsequent doses and intervals of administration should be adjusted according to the response of the blood pressure.

† Start the infusion slowly and adjust the rate according to the response of the blood pressure. Constant surveillance is mandatory. The concentration of the solution can be adjusted according to the patient's fluid requirements.

‡ The total dose should be contained in a volume of at least 20 ml and the solution should be administered from a 20- or 50-ml syringe. The blood pressure should be monitored continuously while the injection is being made. The rate of injection should not exceed 0.5 ml per minute, and to avoid hypotension the injection should be stopped frequently when the blood pressure is falling.

§ Not available commercially. Diazoxide has been under investigation for nearly 10 years and its therapeutic potential and toxic effects have been well studied and described. A stock solution of sodium nitroprusside for intravenous administration can be made by dissolving 2 gm of sodium nitroprusside crystals AR (sodium nitroferricyanide-Mallinckrodt) in freshly prepared distilled water sufficient to make 200 ml. The solution is made in a sterile, 200-ml glass-stoppered flask. Since the solution does not tolerate heat, sterilization is accomplished by filtration through a Millipore syringe filter (0.22μ) into previously stoppered, sterilized amber vials (50 ml of solution in 100-ml vials). The stock solution is kept under refrigeration at an average temperature of about 15 C. Usually 5 ml of stock solution (containing 50 mg of sodium nitroprusside) is added to a liter of distilled water containing 5% dextrose and the infusion is started at a rate of 10 drops per minute.

TABLE 2.—*Sympathetic Blocking Drugs for Parenteral Administration in Management of Hypertensive Emergencies*

Drugs	*Intra-muscular* * (*mg*)	*Intravenous*		*Advantages*	*Disadvantages*
		Single Dose (*mg*)	*Continuous Infusion* † (*mg per liter*)		
Pentolinium (Ansolysen)	1–20	10 ‡	40–200	Fairly rapidly and fairly consistently effective; reduces central venous pressure by action to relax large veins	Primary orthostatic effect, requiring large doses to reduce supine blood pressure. Reduces renal blood flow and GFR acutely; bowel and bladder atony in bedfast patients
Trimethaphan camsylate (Arfonad)			1000		
Reserpine (Serpasil, Sandril)	1–5			Rather consistently effective; gradual rather than abrupt decline in blood pressure	Sedation and somnolence interfere with clinical evaluation of sensorium in patients with strokes or hypertensive encephalopathy; delayed onset of action not desirable in acute emergency; cumulative effect can lead to severe hypotension
Methyldopate hydrochloride (Aldomet ester)		250–500 §		Gradual rather than abrupt decline in blood pressure	Similar to reserpine, but less consistently effective and less likely to produce profound somnolence or severe hypotension
Phentolamine (Regitine)	5–15	5–15 (rapid injection essential)	200–400	Specific for hypertension associated with pheochromocytoma, or catecholamine release from tissue stores in patients receiving MAO inhibitors	Not effective except when excessive circulating catecholamine is present; effect is transient

* Start with the smallest dose shown. Subsequent doses and intervals of administration should be adjusted according to the response of the blood pressure.

† Start the infusion slowly and adjust the rate according to the response of the blood pressure. Constant surveillance is mandatory. The concentration of the solution can be adjusted according to the patient's fluid requirements.

‡ The total dose should be contained in a volume of at least 20 ml and the solution should be administered from a 20- or 50-ml syringe. The blood pressure should be monitored continuously while the injection is being made. The rate of injection should not exceed 0.5 ml per minute, and to avoid hypotension the injection should be stopped frequently when the blood pressure is falling.

§ Administered in 100 ml of a 5% solution of dextrose in distilled water over a period of 30 to 60 minutes.

Abbreviation used: GFR, glomerular filtration rate.

intravenous infusion or by intermittent intramuscular injections.

The advantage of intravenous injections of hypotensive drugs is the achievement of rapid blood pressure reduction. The intermittent intravenous method is cumbersome and usually requires the presence of a physician to give the injection. Continuous intravenous infusions of hypotensive drugs result in smoother control of blood pressure than do intermittent injections, but they require constant supervision by trained personnel, preferably in an intensive care unit.

The chief advantage of the intramuscular route is simplicity, for nurses may give these injections whenever the blood pressure rises above a certain level determined by the physician; in many hospitals nurses are not permitted to give intravenous injections. The disadvantages of the intramuscular route are the slower onset of action of the administered drug and the danger of prolonged hypotension from overdosage, for it is difficult, if not impossible, to retard absorption from an intramuscular depot. The effects of overdosage from intravenous injections can usually be reversed by stopping the injection. This is not true, however, for diazoxide, because a single intravenous injection may reduce the blood pressure for periods up to 18 hours.

Role of Diuretic Therapy. The antihypertensive action of all of the drugs used in the management of hypertensive emergencies is enhanced by simultaneous administration of a diuretic, and this is particularly true if the patient is edematous from congestive heart failure or any other cause. Under these circumstances, the diuretic of choice is furosemide (Lasix) because it can be given intravenously, is rapidly effective, and does not cause an acute decrease in glomerular filtration rate which is characteristic of the benzothiadiazine derivatives. The usual dose of furosemide for this purpose is 40 to 80 mg. Ethacrynic acid (Edecrin) can also be given intravenously in doses of 50 to 100 mg and is just as rapidly effective and as potent as furosemide. Nerve deafness has been reported in some azotemic patients who have received intravenous injections of either furosemide or ethacrynic acid too rapidly.

Pharmacology and Side Effects. The drugs which are available for parenteral administration to combat hypertensive crises can be classified according to their mechanisms of action into those which directly dilate the resistance vessels and therefore reduce peripheral resistance (Table 1) and those which act to interfere with sympathetic innervation of the cardiovascular system (Table 2).

Direct Vasodilating Drugs

Hydralazine. For reasons that are not clear, hydralazine is more effective in managing hypertensive encephalopathy complicating acute or chronic glomerulonephritis or eclampsia than it is in managing other types of emergencies. The onset of antihypertensive action is usually apparent within 30 minutes following an effective intramuscular dose and within 10 minutes when it is given intravenously. As the blood pressure declines there is a reflex increase in cardiac rate and output. The net result could be an increase in cardiac work. Consequently, this agent should not be administered to patients with compromised myocardial reserve and/or coronary disease as it has the potential to aggravate or to precipitate congestive heart failure or coronary insufficiency. On the other hand, a reduction in blood pressure induced by hydralazine is not accompanied by a commensurate decrease in renal blood flow; therefore this agent is especially suited for managing hypertensive emergencies associated with renal insufficiency. In addition to tachycardia and palpitations which result from the reflex increase in cardiac output, side effects include flushing, headache, and vomiting.

Sodium Nitroprusside. In my experience the intravenous infusion of sodium nitroprusside has proved to be the most consistently reliable method for reducing blood pressure promptly in hypertensive emergencies, irrespective of etiology.[2] It has been effective when other drugs, including diazoxide, have failed. The hypotensive response occurs within seconds after the infusion is started and is dissipated almost as rapidly when the infusion is stopped. Although it is a direct-dilating agent, unlike hydralazine it does not increase cardiac output and rate.[3] The nitroprusside ion is converted to thiocyanate and serum levels of thiocyanate should be determined every other day if the infusion must be continued for longer than 72 hours. The infusion should be discontinued if the serum concentration of thiocyanate exceeds 12 mg per 100 ml in order to avoid acute toxicity including psychosis and confusion. Because of the precipitous fall in blood pressure that it causes, it should be used cautiously if at all in patients with overt cerebrovascular and/or coronary insufficiency.

In addition to thiocyanate intoxication which occurs only after several days, if at all, acute side effects include nausea, vomiting, muscle twitching, apprehension, and sweating. These symptoms usually accompany rapid reduction of blood pressure by sodium nitroprusside and can be relieved promptly by reducing the rate of infusion or stopping it temporarily. A more gradual reduction of blood pressure can usually be accomplished without producing these symptoms.

Unfortunately, sodium nitroprusside is not available commercially but a solution for intravenous administration can easily be prepared in any pharmacy (Table 1).

Diazoxide. Like hydralazine, diazoxide is a direct vasodilating drug which causes an increase in cardiac output and rate but it does not compromise renal blood flow as much as do the ganglion-blocking agents when given parenterally. Its effect on the blood pressure is so profound that the net result is usually a decrease in cardiac work and consequently it can be administered to patients with decreased myocardial reserve. It may also be given safely to patients with renal insufficiency. In spite of the fact that it is related chemically to chlorothiazide, it causes sodium retention and therefore it is advantageous to administer a diuretic with it, especially when patients are edematous from either cardiac or renal failure. The drug must be administered rapidly (within 15 seconds) intravenously in doses of 300 to 600 mg. The blood pressure usually falls promptly within the first 2 minutes and the maximal hypotensive effect is usually realized within 5 minutes. The duration of effect of a single dose ranges from less than an hour to as long as 18 hours. The abrupt decrease in blood pressure could conceivably be detrimental to patients with cerebrovascular or coronary insufficiency. Side effects include nausea, vomiting, flushing, and hyperglycemia. The last has not been a deterrent to its use for short periods to control hypertensive emergencies, even in diabetic patients.

Because it is consistently effective and has a rather long duration of action, diazoxide will be the agent of choice in the management of hypertensive encephalopathy including that associated with eclampsia, when it becomes commercially available. It probably should not be used in management of dissecting aneurysm of the aorta because it tends to increase cardiac output.

Sympathetic-Blocking Drugs

Ganglion-Blocking Agents. Pentolinium and trimethaphan block both the sympathetic and parasympathetic systems at the autonomic ganglia. Their effect is primarily an orthostatic one, hence large doses must be employed to reduce blood pressure in supine patients. Elevation of the head of the bed augments their antipressor activity. Inhibition of the parasympathetic system leads to atony of the bowel and bladder. Indwelling catheters are necessary for most men and many women receiving large doses of these agents for more than 2 or 3 days. The physician must be constantly vigilant for signs of paralytic ileus and these drugs are not recommended in the immediate postoperative period for they almost always prolong the bowel and bladder paralysis that characterizes this state. Neither of these drugs should be administered to pregnant women near term because of the danger of producing meconium ileus in the newborn. Inactivation of pupillary reflexes by ganglioplegic drugs may cause confusion in the neurologic evaluation of the patient with hypertensive encephalopathy or intracranial hemorrhage, but this is less of a problem than the somnolence induced by reserpine or methyldopa. When blood pressure is reduced by parenteral administration of ganglion-blocking agents, there is an accompanying commensurate, acute decrease in glomerular filtration rate; thus, it is preferable to use other agents when renal insufficiency complicates hypertensive crisis. The ganglion-blocking drugs relax large veins and this makes them uniquely suited for managing hypertensive crises associated with congestive heart failure and elevated central venous pressure.

Following an effective intramuscular dose of

pentolinium the blood pressure begins to fall within 30 minutes and the maximal effect is usually realized within an hour. Trimethaphan cannot be given intramuscularly. A significant hypotensive effect is usually apparent within 5 to 10 minutes after starting an intravenous injection of either of these drugs.

Reserpine. In parenteral doses large enough to reduce blood pressure, reserpine causes profound somnolence in most patients, presumably because it depletes the stores of catecholamine and serotonin in the central nervous system. This is a major deterrent to its use in hypertensive encephalopathy and intracranial hemorrhage because it interferes with the clinical assessment of the sensorium which is so important in evaluating the progress of these patients. The delayed onset of the antihypertensive action of reserpine is not desirable when a true emergency exists. Moreover, repetition of doses at intervals of less than 3 hours can lead to cumulative effect and profound hypotension. Large doses of reserpine cause bradycardia which can be misinterpreted as digitalis intoxication. Reserpine may activate peptic ulcers leading to acute gastrointestinal bleeding, and may cause a Parkinson-like syndrome, especially in older patients. Nasal stuffiness is an annoying side effect for some patients. In spite of these many disadvantages, reserpine is probably the most widely used drug to manage hypertensive crises, simply because it is rather consistently effective, it can be given intramuscularly, and its administration does not require as close supervision and as frequent monitoring of the patient as does the administration of drugs by intravenous infusion. I predict that the present undeserved popularity of reserpine will wane when diazoxide becomes available.

Methyldopa. Methyldopa depletes the stores of norepinephrine in the central nervous system and in the peripheral sympathetic system by displacing some of the norepinephrine with a "false transmitter," alpha-methyl-norepinephrine. Although the depletion is less complete than that induced by reserpine, methyldopa given intravenously may cause enough drowsiness to interfere with the evaluation of the patient's sensorium. Like reserpine, methyldopa has a delayed onset of action (2 to 3 hours). It is not as popular as reserpine, probably because it has to be given intravenously and is less consistently effective than is reserpine.

Phentolamine. The alpha-receptor blocker, phentolamine, is specifically indicated for managing hypertensive crises associated with increased circulating catecholamines, whether from a pheochromocytoma or from sudden release of tissue catecholamine stores by certain drugs or foods containing tyramine in patients receiving MAO inhibitors. Phentolamine is ineffective in managing hypertensive crises from other causes. The effect of phentolamine is short-lived, usually lasting less than 15 minutes; consequently it is desirable to administer either phentolamine or sodium nitroprusside by intravenous infusion after the blood pressure has been controlled initially by rapid intravenous injection of 5 to 15 mg of phentolamine from a syringe. Phentolamine has an almost instantaneous depressor effect when it is given rapidly intravenously in the presence of increased circulating catecholamine. Side effects include tachycardia and flushing.

Clinical Aspects

Some of the hypertensive emergencies which demand prompt reduction of blood pressure are listed in Table 3 along with the drugs of choice for their management.

Acute Hypertensive Encephalopathy. At times the course of hypertension is punctuated by sudden, unexplained rises of blood pressure that are accompanied by neurologic signs and symptoms which constitute the syndrome of hypertensive encephalopathy. The characteristic feature is subacute onset of alteration in consciousness, progressing from drowsiness to stupor and disorientation, and finally to coma; these developments are usually accompanied by severe headache, nausea, vomiting, visual blurring or blindness, and transient neurologic disturbances including focal and generalized seizures. It can be a complication of hypertension from almost any cause, with the possible exceptions of coarctation of the aorta and primary aldosteronism. It is seen in patients with essential hypertension, as well as in those with hypertension secondary to renal parenchymal disease, including acute and chronic glomerulonephritis, renovascular disease, pheo-

TABLE 3.—*Choice of Drugs for Parenteral Administration in the Management of Hypertensive Emergencies*

Hypertensive Emergency	*Preferred Drugs*	*Drugs to Avoid or To Use with Extra Caution*
Acute hypertensive encephalopathy *	Sodium nitroprusside Pentolinium Trimethaphan	Reserpine Methyldopate
Severe hypertension associated with acute or chronic glomerulonephritis *	Hydralazine Methyldopate Sodium nitroprusside	
Eclampsia and preeclampsia *	Hydralazine Reserpine Methyldopate	Pentolinium Trimethaphan
Acute left ventricular failure associated with hypertensive heart disease	Pentolinium Trimethaphan	Hydralazine
Acute coronary insufficiency	Reserpine Methyldopate	Hydralazine Sodium nitroprusside Diazoxide
Intracerebral or subarachnoid hemorrhage	Pentolinium Trimethaphan Hydralazine Sodium nitroprusside	Reserpine Methyldopate
Malignant hypertension *	Pentolinium Trimethaphan Reserpine Sodium nitroprusside	
Pheochromocytoma or MAO inhibition †	Phentolamine Sodium nitroprusside	All others
Acute dissecting aneurysm of aorta	Reserpine Pentolinium Trimethaphan	Hydralazine

* Diazoxide will undoubtedly become the drug of choice when it is commercially available.

† Hypertensive crisis due to sudden release of tissue catecholamine stores when patients receiving MAO inhibitors are given preparations containing ephedrine, amphetamines, tyramine, etc., or consume foods rich in tyramine such as aged cheeses, Chianti wine, some foreign beers, pickled herring, chicken livers, etc.

chromocytoma, or toxemia of pregnancy. In patients with renal failure, the role of uremia in the production of the cerebral signs is difficult to assess; uremia without hypertension and overhydration, however, rarely if ever causes the entire syndrome.

Characteristically, the blood pressure is exceedingly high, usually above 250 mm Hg systolic and 150 mm Hg diastolic. The manifestations of hypertensive encephalopathy appear at lower levels of blood pressure in patients whose hypertension develops rather suddenly (children and adolescents with acute glomerulonephritis and women with toxemia of pregnancy) than in patients with long-standing hypertension.

Hypertensive encephalopathy is a medical emergency requiring prompt reduction of blood pressure to normal or near-normal levels. The agents of choice are diazoxide, sodium nitroprusside, pentolinium, or trimethaphan. When hypertensive encephalopathy complicates acute glomerulonephritis or eclampsia, hydralazine is also effective.

Acute Left Ventricular Failure. When hypertension is suddenly complicated by acute left ventricular failure, it is imperative to reduce the work load of the incompetent left ventricle.

Prompt reduction of blood pressure is probably more important than administration of digitalis although the latter should be given if the patient is not already taking it. Before reducing the blood pressure abruptly, the physician should be certain that the heart failure is due to hypertensive heart disease and not to unrecognized atherosclerotic heart disease with or without acute myocardial infarction. Prompt reduction of blood pressure to normal levels is not advisable for patients with acute coronary insufficiency with or without myocardial infarction. There is a particular indication for the use of either of the ganglion-blocking drugs in managing hypertension associated with acute left ventricular failure from hypertensive heart disease, because these agents reduce systemic blood pressure and right ventricular pressure simultaneously, resulting in increased cardiac output. Furosemide (Lasix) in doses of 40 to 80 mg should be administered either by mouth or intravenously along with pentolinium or trimethaphan. In addition to the administration of a ganglion-blocking agent, digitalis and a diuretic, bed rest, dietary sodium restriction, and the administration of oxygen and morphine are important adjuncts to the therapeutic regimen.

Acute Coronary Insufficiency. Acute coronary insufficiency with or without myocardial infarction can be accompanied by such spectacular increases in blood pressure that the diagnosis of pheochromocytoma may be erroneously suspected. The sequence of events in the few cases that I have observed would indicate that the hypertension followed rather than preceded the onset of coronary insufficiency and was perhaps the result of extreme anxiety. Horwitz and Sjoerdsma [4] have observed the same sequence in one of the patients they reported and postulated that myocardial ischemia initiated a reflex increase in blood pressure. Irrespective of whether the hypertension is the result or the cause of the coronary insufficiency, the extremely elevated blood pressure may embarrass an ischemic left ventricle and should be reduced to more moderate levels. Reserpine is the agent of choice since it brings about a gradual reduction of blood pressure, and the accompanying sedation which it induces is beneficial in this situation.

Intracranial Hemorrhage. When hypertension is complicated by subarachnoid or intracerebral hemorrhage, it is usually advisable to reduce blood pressure by the use of hypotensive drugs given parenterally. Because of the arterial spasm which has been demonstrated angiographically in the area around the bleeding site, there has been some controversy about the advisability of promptly reducing blood pressure and thereby running the risk of decreasing cerebral blood flow in these areas. Certainly, if reduction of blood pressure seems to aggravate or to produce focal neurologic deficits, the physician should be less aggressive in his attempt to lower it. Usually, however, reduction of blood pressure is well tolerated and in some cases it may be desirable to maintain the blood pressure at low normal if not hypotensive levels. Preferred agents include pentolinium, trimethaphan, hydralazine, or sodium nitroprusside since all are promptly effective and do not produce somnolence that might interfere with neurologic evaluation of the patient.

Before reducing the blood pressure abruptly, the physician should be certain that the patient has intracranial bleeding and not an atherothrombotic cerebral infarct. Drastic reduction of blood pressure in patients with acute cerebral infarct might aggravate ischemia with worsening of the neurologic deficit.

Malignant Hypertension. The malignant phase of hypertension is a semi-emergency, for irreversible vascular deterioration occurs at an accelerated rate and will be arrested only when blood pressure is reduced. To gain control of the hypertension rapidly, and especially if oral medication is poorly tolerated due to nausea and vomiting, one may administer diazoxide, sodium nitroprusside, pentolinium or reserpine parenterally for several days until oral medication can be tolerated and is effective.

Pheochromocytoma and Hypertensive Crises Associated with MAO Inhibition. The rapid intravenous injection of 5 or 10 mg of phentolamine will serve both as a diagnostic test and a therapeutic measure for patients with pheochromocytoma. Intravenous infusion of sodium nitroprusside is equally effective in controlling hypertension associated with pheochromocytoma.

Some patients receiving MAO inhibitors will have an acute hypertensive crisis if they should also take ephedrine, amphetamine, tyramine, or any other drug which releases the increased tissue stores of catecholamine. The ingestion of certain beverages or foodstuffs which contain significant amounts of tyramine may also produce hypertensive crises in patients who are taking MAO inhibitors. These include Chianti wine and some foreign beers, unpasteurized cheeses, pickled herring, and chicken livers. The severity of the paroxysm of hypertension so induced and the accompanying symptoms are similar to those of pheochromocytoma since both syndromes are the result of excessive circulating catecholamine. Management of this drug-induced hypertensive crisis is the same as for pheochromocytoma.

Acute Dissecting Aneurysm of the Aorta. Until the recent introduction of hypotensive therapy for the management of acute dissecting aneurysm,[5] the only satisfactory treatment was surgical intervention before exsanguination occurred. Survival rate has been better with medical than with surgical management. The regimen of choice is trimethaphan, administered intravenously, reserpine, administered intramuscularly, and guanethidine (Ismelin) and propranolol (Inderal), administered orally, to maintain the systolic blood pressure between 100 and 120 mm Hg. These drugs are chosen because of their ability to decrease myocardial contractility, thereby lessening the force that the cardiac impulse transmits to the dissecting hematoma. Because hydralazine increases cardiac output and sometimes also increases stroke volume, it should not be used in the management of acute dissecting aneurysm.

Summary

Parenteral administration of hypotensive agents may be life-saving when hypertension acutely threatens the integrity of the cardiovascular system. Unfortunately, at the present time the two most useful agents for managing hypertensive emergencies, diazoxide and sodium nitroprusside, are not commercially available. Reserpine, administered intramuscularly, is enjoying undeserved popularity probably because it is convenient to administer. The slow onset of its antihypertensive action and the profound somnolence that accompanies its administration are major deterrents to its use.

Whatever the indications for using hypotensive drugs parenterally, the physician should strive to substitute the oral for the parenteral route as soon as it is feasible to do so.

References

1. Seller, E. M., and Koch-Weser, J.: Protein binding and vascular activity of diazoxide. N. Engl. J. Med. 281:1141, 1969.
2. Gifford, R. W., Jr.: Hypertensive emergencies and their treatment. Med. Clin. North Am. 45:441, 1961.
3. Schlant, R. C., Tsgaris, T. S., and Robertson, R. L., Jr.: Studies on the acute cardiovascular effects of intravenous sodium nitroprusside. Am. J. Cardiol. 9:51, 1962.
4. Horwitz, D., and Sjoerdsma, A.: Some interrelationships between elevation of blood pressure and angina pectoris. Hypertension: Proceedings of the Council for High Blood Pressure Research of The American Heart Association 13:39, 1964.
5. Wheat, M. W., Jr., Harris, P. D., Malm, J. R., Kiser, G., Bowman, F. O., Jr., and Palmer, R. F.: Acute dissecting aneurysms of the aorta. Treatment and results in 64 patients. J. Thorac. Cardiovasc. Surg. 58:344, 1969.

Selected References

Gifford, R. W., Jr., and Richards, N. G.: Hypertensive encephalopathy. Parts I, II. Curr. Concepts Cerebrovasc. Dis.—Stroke 5:43, 1970.

Finnerty, F. A., Jr.: Hypertension due to toxemia of pregnancy. *In* Brest, A. N., and Moyer, J. H. (Eds.): Cardiovascular Disorders. Philadelphia: Davis, 1968, pp. 1000–1004.

Freis, E. D.: Hypertensive crisis. JAMA 208:338, 1969.

Hamby, W. M., Jankowski, G. J., Pouget, J. M., Dunea, G., and Gantt, C. L.: Intravenous use of diazoxide in the treatment of severe hypertension. Circulation 37:169, 1968.

Miller, W. E., Gifford, R. W., Jr., Humphrey, D. C., and Vidt, D. G.: Management of severe hypertension with intravenous injections of diazoxide. Am. J. Cardiol. 24:870, 1969.

Rationale for Early Treatment of Hypertension

By Sir F. Horace Smirk, K.B.E., M.D.

BEFORE EARLY TREATMENT of hypertension is undertaken we should consider the likelihood of benefit, because, as far as we know, treatment, to remain effective, must be continued for a lifetime.

Most hypertensives go through a symptomless stage with only moderate elevation of the blood pressure. But once exudative retinal changes (grade 3 or grade 4) or one or more of the major complications of hypertension have developed then the outlook has been impaired and, although treatment at this stage will reduce mortality, and reduce it a lot, the eventual results, though less dramatic, will not be as good as those obtainable by treatment if administered before any such complications develop.

Therefore we must ask: Can the incidence of complications be reduced? My answer is unequivocally yes! The evidence is that it is unusual for well-treated patients with retinal grades 1 or 2 to develop advanced retinal changes while on effective treatment, whereas this is not unusual with inadequately treated patients, or in those who stop treatment. Well-treated hypertensive patients seldom develop general or left ventricular failure. The experience of our clinic is that nonfatal and fatal strokes occur less frequently but are not abolished in persons on effective treatment.

There are now many confirmations of early reports that effective treatment by hypotensive agents decreases (1) the occurrence of cerebrovascular accidents,[1–7] and (2) the recurrence of cerebrovascular accidents in those who start treatment after a previous stroke.[2,3,8]

It is therefore surprising that even in recent years many of those who write about the management of strokes concern themselves at length with such subjects as rehabilitation, aspects of personal care, and anticoagulants but make little or no reference to the use of antihypertensive drugs. Most of these papers come from doctors whose professional interests would not normally involve them in the use of antihypertensive drugs.

In two extensive surveys by the Veterans Administration,[9,10] matched hypertensive patients received either active hypotensive drugs or placebos for up to 5 years. In the placebo group the number of adverse events, such as the development of severe retinal changes, heart failure, strokes or coronary disease increased with higher levels of the casual diastolic blood pressure.

Hamilton, Thompson, and Wisniewski[11] compared the number of adverse events experienced by 30 treated and 31 untreated symptomless hypertensives having at least three casual diastolic blood pressures of over 110 mm Hg.

Wolff and Lindeman[12] made a double-blind study comparing the results in 45 patients receiving active drugs with 42 on placebos. These were comparatively mild hypertensive patients lacking threatening complications. Their results are shown in Table 2.

Such valuable observations show that treatment could not be postponed without considerable risk in the patients studied whose disease was not very severe, but certainly not mild.

For many years we have undertaken treatment in patients at an early stage. Treatment is essentially by blood pressure reduction;

Table 1.—*Results from the Veterans Administration Study*

Diastolic Blood Pressures (mm Hg)	*Percentage of Adverse Events*	
	Treated	*Untreated*
115–129	3	38
105–114	8	31.8
90–104	16.3	25.0

From the Department of Medicine, Wellcome Medical Research Institute, Dunedin, New Zealand.

This work was supported by the Medical Research Council of New Zealand.

TABLE 2.—*Results of Hamilton, Thompson, and Wisniewski,*[11] *and of Wolff and Lindeman*[12]

		Percentage of Adverse Events	
		Treated	Untreated
Hamilton, Thompson, and Wisniewski	Men	0	67
	Women	25	42
Wolff and Lindeman	Men and women	13	45

therefore we should consider at what level of blood pressure we begin to reduce the blood pressure by hypotensive drugs.

It seems from Tables 3 and 4 that when in this series casual diastolic pressures are within or above the 90- to 109-mm Hg range or the casual systolic blood pressures are in or above the range 200 to 239 mm Hg, then the 5-year mortality is considerably less in our treated than in our untreated group, in males and in females.

A reduction in the 5-year mortality with treatment also is apparent when the basal systolic pressure is at or above the range of 160 to 179 mm Hg in females or 140 to 159 mm Hg in males. Only 13 men with basal systolic pressures below 140 mmHg were treated; their casual systolic pressures would have been appreciably higher than this. It is difficult to interpret these results, as is also the case when the casual diastolic pressures are above and the basal diastolic pressures below 90 mmHg.

It seems probable, however, that men will derive benefit from treatment at lower levels of the blood pressure than those at which treatment appears to lessen mortality in women.

Furthermore, from results already available, extrapolation warrants the anticipation that, with longer follow-up periods of observation, we may expect to find a reduction in morbidity and mortality in men and women with hypertension of a milder degree than is ordinarily treated at the present time.

Almost from the outset our group has been prepared to treat males earlier and at lower

TABLE 3.—*Effect of Treatment on Mortality in Females*

Casual Systolic Pressure Female (mm Hg)

	240+			200–239			160–199			<160			All		
	D	N	%	D	N	%	D	N	%	D	N	%	D	N	%
T	7	50	14	12	94	13	6	30	20	0	0		25	174	14.4
U	13	29	45	15	60	25	3	28	11	0	4		31	121	25.6

Basal Systolic Pressure Female (mm Hg)

	180+			160–179			140–159			<140			All		
	D	N	%	D	N	%	D	N	%	D	N	%	D	N	%
T	9	48	19	4	57	7	10	45	22	2	24	8	25	174	14.4
U	14	27	52	7	29	24	7	34	21	3	31	10	31	121	25.6

Casual Diastolic Pressure Female (mm Hg)

	130+			110–129			90–109			<90			All		
	D	N	%	D	N	%	D	N	%	D	N	%	D	N	%
T	11	63	18	12	95	13	2	16	13	0	0		25	174	14.4
U	17	45	38	10	56	18	4	18	22	0	2		31	121	25.6

Basal Diastolic Pressure Female (mm Hg)

	110+			90–109			<90			All		
	D	N	%	D	N	%	D	N	%	D	N	%
T	7	53	13	12	83	15	6	38	16	25	174	14.4
U	15	33	46	11	48	23	5	40	13	31	121	25.6

Abbreviations: T, treated; U, untreated; D, dead; N, number at risk.

TABLE 4.—*Effect of Treatment on Mortality in Males*

Casual Systolic Pressure Male (mm Hg)

	240+			*200–239*			*160–199*			*<160*			*All*		
	D	*N*	*%*	*D*	*N*	*%*	*D*	*N*	*%*	*D*	*N*	*%*	*D*	*N*	*%*
T	5	20	25	9	50	18	8	22	36	0	0		22	92	23.9
U	8	12	67	15	25	60	9	35	26	2	5	40	34	77	44.2

Basal Systolic Pressure Male (mm Hg)

	180+			*160–179*			*140–159*			*<140*			*All*		
	D	*N*	*%*	*D*	*N*	*%*	*D*	*N*	*%*	*D*	*N*	*%*	*D*	*N*	*%*
T	8	22	36	7	32	22	5	25	20	2	13	15	22	92	23.9
U	6	7	86	8	13	62	10	20	50	10	37	27	34	77	44.2

Casual Diastolic Pressure Male (mm Hg)

	130+			*110–129*			*90–109*			*<90*			*All*		
	D	*N*	*%*	*D*	*N*	*%*	*D*	*N*	*%*	*D*	*N*	*%*	*D*	*N*	*%*
T	9	38	24	11	45	24	2	9	22	0	0		22	92	23.9
U	13	23	57	13	28	46	7	23	30	1	3	33	34	77	44.2

Basal Diastolic Pressure Male (mm Hg)

	110+			*90–109*			*<90*			*All*		
	D	*N*	*%*	*D*	*N*	*%*	*D*	*N*	*%*	*D*	*N*	*%*
T	7	34	21	14	42	33	1	16	6	22	92	23.9
U	10	15	67	11	25	44	13	37	35	34	77	44.2

Abbreviations: T, treated; U, untreated; D, dead; N, number at risk.

levels of the blood pressure than females, and we feel this has been worthwhile.

The results of the build and blood pressure study of the American Society of Actuaries [13] indicate that slightly elevated levels of the blood pressure, even below those just discussed, have an adverse effect on mortality, in the long term. Indeed blood pressures below the mean population levels for the various age groups are associated with a better than average life expectancy, due mainly to a reduction in the cardiovascular mortality.

It has been mentioned in another chapter in this symposium that the 5-year mortality increases as the number of complications present at the outset of the follow-up period increases from 0 to 1 to 2, is usually higher in older than in younger decades and is greater in males than in females.

A possible explanation is that the occurrence of complications may not only be the direct effect of elevation of the blood pressure but may be due in part to increased vulnerability of the heart and blood vessels to a high blood pressure. No doubt the structural damage associated with certain complications also contributes to the increase in mortality.

Were we able to discover, in terms of family history or other factors, that certain classes of patient were more vulnerable to the adverse effects of blood pressure increase than others, this might indicate that the treatment of such persons should start earlier and at lower blood pressures than is customary. An obvious example is that males are more vulnerable to the adverse effects of a raised blood pressure than are females. Another example is evidence of predisposition to coronary artery disease. A very high incidence of stroke in close relatives might also suggest a decrease in the capacity to withstand a high blood pressure.

Perera [14] has shown that the course of untreated hypertension is long, often covering a period of 20 years, so that a 5-year follow-up is inadequate. Although there was a long survival in many of Perera's relatively mildly affected, untreated hypertensive patients, the brutal fact remains that the mean age at death was 44 years in the nonlabile and 56 in his labile group; and this included females as well as males.

Sooner or later we will need to develop screening programs to discover untreated persons with levels of the blood pressure which would benefit by treatment, or alternatively who would merit the institution of periodic checks on the blood pressure. Such a program would also uncover frank hypertensives as well as borderline cases.

I believe a pilot scheme in a small community with a limited objective and all doctors cooperating would stand a good chance of obtaining and demonstrating worthwhile results.

One might begin by screening the first-degree relatives of substantial hypertensives. In our study,[15] to which I have already referred, we had 519 first-degree relatives of substantial hypertensives and 290 controls, thought to be representative of the general population. There were 88 relatives and 35 controls in the 40 to 59 age group.

In this age group 14.3 percent of the controls had casual systolic blood pressures exceeding 160 mm Hg, the corresponding figure for the relatives being 34.1 percent.

The separation between the incidence of high-ranking blood pressures in first-degree relatives and controls was better using basal systolic blood pressures. As shown in Table 5, there were only 2.9 percent of male controls with a basal systolic blood pressure of 140 mm Hg or more and 19.3 percent of the first-degree relatives. I have presented previously the evidence that the 5-year mortality in males has already started to increase at basal systolic blood pressure levels of 140 to 159 mm Hg.[16]

My guess is that in a pilot scheme, 1000 first-degree male relatives of substantial hypertensives aged 40 to 69 would yield about 200 persons with a basal systolic pressure of 140 mm Hg or more. Were these maintained on treatment and followed for 5 years, I should be disappointed if the saving in mortality were fewer than 15 and gratified if it were as many as 60.

TABLE 5.—*Percentage of Males Aged 40–59 with Basal Systolic Pressures Above Certain Stated Levels*

	Controls	*First-degree Relatives*
160+ mm Hg	0.0	5.7
140+ mm Hg	2.9	19.3
120+ mm Hg	11.4	46.6

A consideration of importance is that in effectively treated hypertensive males and females the character of the mortality picture, with treatment, has changed out of recognition. From 1950 to 1958 coronary artery disease was comparatively low on the list of hypertensive disorders causing deaths, accounting for 19 percent of deaths. Since 1959, coronary disease and sudden death probably due to coronary disease in our series accounted for 42 percent of all the causes of death; [17] and other clinics [18] are reporting similar experience. One may enquire whether, since heart failure and stroke have been diminished by relatively early treatment, we could diminish the incidence of coronary deaths were we to treat hypertension at a still earlier stage, particularly in men but also in women.

One must also ask the question whether the routine measures ordinarily recommended for decreasing coronary artery mortality should be adopted, namely, strong advice on the avoidance of smoking, encouragement of exercise, a comparatively low-calorie diet, and especially a diet low in saturated fats.

To sum up, I think the stage has come when we should try to devise methods of ensuring, as far as is practicable, that persons, at least those over 40, are screened for hypertension and recommended for treatment when there is a likelihood of benefit. Screening should start earlier in the first-degree relatives of substantial hypertensives.

I think it right that attempts to prevent hypertensive disease should not exclude either young or old persons. It should aim, not only at the relief of any symptoms, but at decreasing the incidence of important complications and, in the long run, improving life expectancy.

Many factors such as the patient's ability to cooperate, family history, etc. need consideration before deciding whether treatment should be undertaken or if further periodic checks should be arranged.

Some patients with a moderate casual blood

pressure increase have near to normal basal pressures. There is little justification for subjecting such persons to a lifetime of hypotensive drug treatment unless thereby symptoms such as substantial headache or giddiness are found to be relieved by blood pressure reduction. Otherwise the appropriate measure would appear to be a periodic check on the blood pressure level at intervals of, say, 6 months to 1 year, electrocardiograms at 2- to 3-year intervals, and perhaps chest x-rays for heart size.

REFERENCES

1. Hodge, J. V., McQueen, E. G., and Smirk, F. H.: Results of hypotensive therapy in arterial hypertension. Br. Med. J. 1:1, 1961.
2. Lee, R. E., Seligmann, A. W., Clark, M. A., and Rousseau, P. A.: Freedom from cerebral vascular accidents during drug-induced blood pressure reduction in "benign" hypertensive disease. Am. J. Cardiol. 11:738, 1963.
3. Douglas, R. M.: Hypertensive cerebrovascular disease considered in relation to treatment with hypotensive drugs. Med. J. Aust. 2:525, 1964.
4. Hood, B., Aurell, N., Falkheden, T., and Bjork, S.: Analysis of mortality in hypertensive disease. *In* Gross, F. (Ed.): Antihypertensive Therapy. Berlin: Springer, 1966, p. 370.
5. Smirk, F. H.: High Arterial Pressure. Oxford: Blackwell, 1957, pp. 104, 378, 401, 430.
6. Hodge, J. V., and Smirk, F. H.: The effect of drug treatment of hypertension on the distribution of deaths from various causes. A study of 173 deaths among hypertensive patients in the years 1959 to 1964 inclusive. Am. Heart J. 73:441, 1967.
7. Smirk, F. H.: The prognosis of untreated and of treated hypertension and advantages of early treatment. Am. Heart J. 83:825, 1972.
8. Marshall, J.: A trial of long-term hypotensive therapy in cerebrovascular disease. Lancet 1:10, 1964.
9. Veterans Administration Cooperative Study Group on Antihypertensive Agents: Effects of treatment on morbidity in hypertension: Results in patients with diastolic blood pressures averaging 115 through 129 mmHg. JAMA 202:1028, 1967.
10. Veterans Administration Cooperative Study Group on Antihypertensive Agents: Effects of treatment on morbidity in hypertension: Results in patients with diastolic blood pressure averaging 90 through 114 mmHg. JAMA 213:1143, 1970.
11. Hamilton, M., Thompson, E. N., and Wisniewski, T. K. M.: The role of blood pressure control in preventing complications of hypertension. Lancet 1:235, 1964.
12. Wolff, F. W., and Lindeman, R. D.: Effects of treatment in hypertension. Results of a controlled study. J. Chronic Dis. 19:227, 1966.
13. Society of Actuaries: Build and blood pressure study. Chicago, 1959.
14. Perera, G. A.: Relation of blood pressure lability to prognosis in hypertensive vascular disease. J. Chronic Dis. 121, 1955.
15. Smirk, F. H.: Blood pressure in families: Preliminary communication. N. Z. Med. J. 71:355, 1970.
16. Smirk, F. H.: Observations on the mortality of 270 untreated and 199 untreated retinal grade 1 and 2 hypertensive patients followed in all instances for five years. N. Z. Med. J. 63:413, 1964.
17. Smirk, F. H., and Hodge, J. V.: Causes of death in treated hypertensive patients. Br. Med. J. 2:1221, 1963.
18. Breckenridge, A., Dollery, C. T., and Parry, E. H. O.: Prognosis of treated hypertension. Q. J. Med. 39:411, 1970.

Effects of Therapy of the Prognosis of Hypertensive Patients

By Edward D. Freis, M.D.

IT HAS BEEN KNOWN for some time that antihypertensive drug treatment will reverse many of the manifestations of malignant hypertension. Isolated reports appeared even before 1950 [1,2] using the drugs then available. However, it was not until a few years later, when hexamethonium became available, that antihypertensive agents were generally accepted as an effective treatment for malignant hypertension.[3–7]

Until recently it had not been conclusively demonstrated that treatment with antihypertensive drugs would favorably influence the prognosis in benign essential hypertension. Although clinical reports indicating that drug treatment reduced mortality in patients with essential hypertension had appeared in the sixties the interpretation of these results was open to some question. The control groups for these studies were made up from either patients observed prior to the drug treatment era [8] or else from those who had refused treatment.[9] Because of questions relating to the controls the results were not universally accepted and the question of therapeutic effectiveness in reducing morbidity and mortality remained a matter of medical controversy.[10,11]

From the Veterans Administration Hospital and the Department of Medicine, Georgetown University School of Medicine, Washington, D. C.

In 1964 Hamilton, Thompson, and Wisniewski [12] reported on the first prospective controlled trial of treatment in patients with moderately severe essential hypertension. Selecting only those with diastolic blood pressures averaging 110 mm Hg or higher they assigned 61 patients alternately to either active drugs or placebos. Over an 8-year period of follow-up, 16 of the untreated patients had complications, primarily strokes, compared with five of the treated group. However, four of the five latter patients exhibited a poor blood pressure response to treatment. Of the group whose blood pressure had been effectively controlled only one sustained a major complication.

A prospective randomized trial also was carried out by Wolff and Lindeman [13] in 87 patients with moderately severe hypertension attending the outpatient clinic at Johns Hopkins Hospital. Twelve percent defaulted. Over the 2-year period of follow-up the incidence of morbid events in the treated group was one-third that observed in the patients who were given placebos.

The Veterans Administration Cooperative Study comprised 523 male patients with initial diastolic blood pressures averaging between 90 and 129 mm Hg over several outpatient visits. Because the patients were chosen from those presenting at Veterans Administration

Table 1.—*Summary of Controlled Therapeutic Trials in Essential Hypertension*

Source	No. of Patients	Diastolic Range (mm Hg)	Morbid Events: Control Group	Morbid Events: Treated Group
Hamilton, Thompson, and Wisniewski [12]	61	110+	16	5
Wolff and Lindeman [13]	87	110+	31	12
Veterans Study I [14]	143	115+	27	1
Veterans Study II [15]	380	90–114	56 *	22

* Value does not include 20 patients who were dropped because of diastolic elevations to 125+ mm Hg.

Superscript numbers refer to reference list at end of this chapter.

Hospitals they exhibited a greater prevalence of cardiovascular disease than would be expected in a random sampling of the general population of hypertensive patients. Although the median age was 49 years approximately 20 percent were between the ages of 60 and 75 years. Patients were excluded if they had curable forms of hypertension or presented with a history of a severe hypertensive complication such as malignant hypertension, cerebral or subarachnoid hemorrhage, or severe congestive heart failure requiring continuous use of diuretics for its control. However, patients with a past history of cerebral thrombosis, congestive heart failure controlled with digitalis alone, or healed myocardial infarction were permitted in the trial.

The antihypertensive regimen consisted of a combination of 100 mg of hydrochlorothiazide plus 0.2 mg of reserpine daily to which 75 or 150 mg of hydralazine was added. The control group received placebos of these agents.

The results are presented with respect to two main subgroups of patients as follows: (1) those with initial diastolic blood pressures averaging between 115 and 129 mm Hg,[14] and (2) the less severe group with prerandomization diastolic levels averaging between 90 and 114 mm Hg.[15] The trial was terminated in the first group of 143 patients with the higher levels of diastolic blood pressure after an average follow-up of only 20 months. During this relatively brief period, four patients in the control group died of cardiovascular complications versus none in the treated group. Nonfatal but major cardiovascular complications occurred in 23 additional patients in the control group as compared to only one in the treated patients. Thus, the ratio of morbid events was 27 in the 73 control patients to one in the 70 treated patients. Since the patients were randomly assigned to either regimen and their prognostic characteristics prior to randomization were not significantly different, the beneficial result can be ascribed to the effects of treatment.

The second group of 380 patients, whose initial levels of diastolic blood pressure prior to randomization averaged between 90 and 114 mm Hg, remained in the trial for an average period of 3.3 years, the longest period of observation being 5.5 years. Nineteen deaths related to cardiovascular disease occurred among the 194 control patients as compared with eight cardiovascular deaths in the treated group. Seven of the patients in the control group died of strokes compared with only one in the treated series. The most frequent cause of death was coronary artery disease, of which 11 fatal events occurred in the control series and six in the treated patients.

The percentage of patients developing major complications, either fatal or nonfatal, was 28.9 in the control patients and 11.8 in the treated series. Life table analysis indicated that morbid events were occurring at a more or less constant rate throughout the period of postrandomization follow-up, and that over a 5-year period the risk of developing a major cardiovascular complication was reduced from 55 to 18 percent by treatment. In addition to those developing morbid events, 20 patients, all in the control group, were removed from the trial because of persistent elevations of diastolic blood pressure to levels of 125 mm Hg or higher.

The most frequent complication was stroke, which occurred in 20 patients in the control group and five in the treated. Congestive heart failure, renal failure, dissecting aneurysm, and accelerated hypertension occurred only in the control group. The complications of coronary artery disease, that is, myocardial infarction or sudden death, occurred with nearly equal frequency in the control and treated groups of patients.

As would be expected, the greater the age of the patients at entry the higher was the incidence of morbid events. However, treatment was effective in all age groups. The results were analyzed separately for the three subgroups of patients below age 50, between 50 and 59 years, and age 60 or above. The incidence of major complications was more than twice as high in the control as compared to the treated patients in each of these subgroups of patients.

The incidence of morbid events following randomization was considerably higher in the patients who exhibited clinical electrocardiographic, x-ray, or laboratory evidence of cardiovascular damage at the time of entry. Over the relatively brief period of follow-up, the effectiveness of treatment was most evident in the patients entering with signs of organic disease. However, the trend in the patients without evidence of cardiovascular damage also indicated benefit, the incidence of major complications in the latter being twice as high in the control compared to the treated group.

The difference in the incidence of morbid events between control and treated groups was greatest in the patients with the higher levels of systolic blood pressure. With respect to diastolic blood pressure the difference between control and treated groups was highly significant in the subgroups with diastolic levels averaging 105 through 114 mm Hg and was favorable toward treatment, although not statistically significant, in those entering with diastolic levels of 90 through 104 mm Hg. A longer period of follow-up in this milder group might have revealed a more significant difference between control and treated patients.

These results obviously are of great importance in the practical treatment of hypertensive patients. They demonstrate conclusively that treatment is effective in patients exhibiting any evidence of cardiovascular disease as well as in those with diastolic blood pressures averaging 105 mm Hg or higher on repeated office or clinic visits. Surveys carried out by Wilber and Barrow [16] and Stamler et al.[17] indicate that many such patients are not presently receiving adequate treatment. Intensive educational efforts are needed to alert both the profession and the public to the importance of long-term, unremitting, effective antihypertensive therapy in such patients.

Other groups of hypertensive patients, such as those with borderline hypertension and female patients with mild hypertension, are not at such a high risk of developing major complications. As yet, no controlled therapeutic trials have been carried out in the latter groups to determine whether the benefits of treatment outweigh the disadvantages of side effects and other difficulties associated with life-long drug treatment. However, extrapolating the results of epidemiologic studies (which indicate that even mild hypertension is associated with a significant shortening of life expectancy [18]), it would appear reasonable to treat all patients whose diastolic blood pressures are consistently above 95 mm Hg with antihypertensive agents. If antihypertensive drugs are not used in the more borderline patients regular follow-up still is indicated to detect evidence of progression. Also, treatment of blood lipid disorders when present, institution of appropriate schedules of regular exercise, and other general health measures are advisable since patients with even borderline hypertension tend to develop atherosclerosis at an accelerated rate.[19]

References

1. Freis, E. D., and Wilkins, R. W.: Effect of pentaquine in patients with hypertension. Proc. Soc. Exp. Biol. Med. 64:455, 1947.
2. Freis, E. D., and Stanton, J. R.: A clinical evaluation of Veratrum Viride in the treatment of essential hypertension. Am. Heart J. 36:723, 1948.
3. Restall, P. A., and Smirk, F. H.: Treatment of high blood pressure with hexamethonium iodide. N. Z. Med. J. 49:206, 1950.
4. Campbell, A., and Robertson, E.: Treatment of severe hypertension with hexamethonium bromide. Br. Med. J. 2:804, 1950.
5. Johnson, R. L., Freis, E. D., and Schnaper, H. W.: Clinical evaluation of 1-hydrazinophthalazine (C-5968) in hypertension: With special reference to alternating treatment with hexamethonium. Circulation 5:833, 1952.
6. Perry, H. M., Jr., and Schroeder, H. A.: The effect of treatment on mortality rates in severe hypertension. A comparison of medical and surgical regimens. Arch. Intern. Med. 102: 418, 1958.
7. Dustan, H. P., Schneckloth, R. E., and Corcoran, A. C.: The effectiveness of long-term treatment of malignant hypertension. Circulation 18:644, 1958.
8. Leishman, A. W. D.: Hypertension, treated and untreated: A study of 400 cases. Br. Med. J. 1:1361, 1959.
9. Hodge, J. W., McQueen, E. G., and Smirk, F. H.: Results of hypotensive therapy in arterial hypertension. Br. Med. J. 1:1, 1961.
10. Goldring, W., and Chasis, H.: Antihypertensive therapy: An appraisal. Arch. Intern. Med. 115:523, 1965.
11. Relman, A. S.: Editorial comment. *In* Ingelfinger, F. J., Relman, A. S., and Finland, M. (Eds.): Controversy in Internal Medicine. Philadelphia: Saunders, 1966, pp. 101–102.
12. Hamilton, M., Thompson, E. N., and Wisniewski, T. K. M.: The role of blood pressure control in preventing complications of hypertension. Lancet 1:235, 1964.
13. Wolff, F. W., and Lindeman, R. D.: Effects

of treatment on hypertension. Results of a controlled study. J. Chronic Dis. 19:227, 1966.

14. Veterans Administration Cooperative Study Group on Antihypertensive Agents: Effect of treatment on morbidity and mortality. Results in patients with diastolic blood pressures averaging 115 through 129 mmHg. JAMA 202:1028, 1967.
15. Veterans Administration Cooperative Study Group on Antihypertensive Agents: II. Results in patients with diastolic blood pressure averaging 90 through 114 mmHg. JAMA 213:1143, 1970.
16. Wilber, J. A., and Barrow, J. G.: Reducing elevated blood pressure. Experience found in a community. Minn. Med. 52:1303, 1969.
17. Stamler, J., Schoenberger, J. A., Lindberg, H. A., Shekelle, R., Stoker, J. M., Epstein, B., De Boer, L., Stamler, R., Restivo, R., Gray, D., and Cain, W.: Detection of susceptibility to coronary disease. Bull. N.Y. Acad. Med. 45:1306, 1969.
18. Society of Actuaries: Build and Blood Pressure Study, vol. I. Chicago, 1959.
19. Freis, E. D.: Hypertension and atherosclerosis. Am. J. Med. 46:735, 1969.

Effects of Antihypertensive Therapy on Target Organs

By Kwan Eun Kim, M.D.

EXTENSIVE EVALUATION of life insurance statistics indicates not only that life expectancy decreases with any elevation of blood pressure above the lowest normal levels, but also that the complications of hypertension are directly related to the level of the blood pressure.[1] However, the fact that increased arterial blood pressure is associated with increased morbidity and mortality does not permit the conclusion that blood pressure reduction by drug therapy will necessarily improve the life expectancy and decrease the morbidity.

The value of antihypertensive therapy has been clearly demonstrated for both men and women with malignant hypertension[2–7] and moderately severe essential hypertension.[8–11] The Veterans Administration Cooperative Study[12] showed that antihypertensive therapy reduced morbidity and mortality even in mildly hypertensive male patients. However, the value of therapy for mild hypertension in females has not yet been clearly demonstrated.

Hypertension is a generalized vascular disease. However, the vascular deterioration especially involves the heart, the brain, the retinae, and the kidneys.

The purpose of this chapter is to review the effect of antihypertensive therapy on target organs and ultimate prognosis.

From the Division of Nephrology and Hypertension, Department of Medicine, Hahnemann Medical College and Hospital, Philadelphia, Pennsylvania.

Overall Mortality and Morbidity

Malignant Hypertension

Table 1 shows the mortality in three series of untreated patients with malignant hypertension. In these different series of patients, 79, 80, and 90 percent died in the first year, and 99 percent of the patients in all series died within 5 years after diagnosis.[5,13,14] In contrast, the mortality in five series of treated patients with malignant hypertension was markedly reduced (Table 1).[3–7] The mortality at 1 year and at 5 years in treated patients with malignant hypertension ranged between

Table 1.—*Mortality in Untreated and Treated Patients with Malignant Hypertension*

Authors	*Year of Report*	*Percentage of Mortality*	
		One Year	*Five Years*
Untreated Patients			
Keith, Wagener, and Barker[13]	1939	79	99
Kincaid-Smith, McMichael, and Murphy[14]	1958	90	99
Björk et al.[5]	1960	80	99
Treated Patients			
Dustan et al.[3]	1958	30	67
Harrington, Kincaid-Smith, and McMichael[4]	1958	50	78
Björk et al.[5]	1960	24	50
Mohler and Freis[6]	1960	—	78
Farmer, Gifford, and Hines[7]	1963	35	71

From Moyer, J. H., and Kim, K. E.: The effect of antihypertensive therapy on ultimate prognosis. *In* Russek, H. I., and Zohman, B. L. (Eds.): Cardiovascular Therapy. Baltimore: Williams & Wilkins, 1971, pp. 181–192, with permission.

24 and 50 percent, and between 50 and 78 percent, respectively.

Even among treated patients, however, those whose blood pressure is well controlled and who do not have advanced vascular damage—especially renal damage—at the beginning of treatment have a much better prognosis than those whose blood pressure is not well controlled and who have advanced renal damage. Björk and associates [5] divided their treated patients into two groups, denoted as inadequately and adequately treated. They found that the results were better in the latter group. Mohler and Freis [6] also found that the group surviving for 5 years or longer was characterized by: (1) normal or nearly normal levels of nonprotein nitrogen prior to treatment, indicating good renal function; and (2) by significantly greater reductions of both systolic and diastolic blood pressure as a result of treatment, when compared with the nonsurviving group of treated patients.

Similarly, in the series of Sokolow and Perloff,[15] out of 11 patients presenting with satisfactory renal function (creatinine clearance greater than 45 ml per minute), four survived for 5 years or longer when treated with ganglionic-blocking agents. With the same treatment, none of 15 patients presenting with poor renal function survived for 3 years. The correlation between survival and degree of control of the diastolic blood pressure was also reported by Farmer, Gifford, and Hines.[7]

All these studies indicate that survival is related directly to the extent of blood pressure reduction during antihypertensive therapy and to kidney function at the beginning of therapy.

With the advent of the artificial kidney and renal homotransplantation, even patients who have malignant hypertension with uremia can be sustained for prolonged periods of useful life. Bilateral nephrectomy in the malignant phase of hypertension with uremia invariably results in a marked reduction of blood pressure and clinical improvement.[16] We have several patients with malignant hypertension and uremia who have had bilateral nephrectomy and have been on maintenance hemodialysis. During this time they have had only mild hypertension, even without medication.

Benign Hypertension

Hodge, McQueen, and Smirk,[8] over a period of 1 to 8 years of observation, found a 50-percent reduction in mortality in their treated group of patients with grade II hypertensive retinopathy as compared with those who received no treatment. The untreated control group was composed of patients who refused to undertake treatment. Therefore, the validity of the comparison was questionable, since the untreated subjects were probably more neglectful of their health.

A controlled therapeutic trial was carried out by Hamilton, Thompson, and Wisniewski,[9] who alternately assigned 61 patients with diastolic blood pressures of 110 mm Hg or higher to treated and control (placebo) groups. Thirty patients were treated with antihypertensive drugs, and 31 were not treated. Over an 8-year period of follow-up, 16 (52%) of the untreated patients had complications (primarily cerebrovascular accidents) as compared to 5 (17%) of the treated group. Of those five, four had poor blood pressure control despite antihypertensive therapy; therefore, only one of the patients who responded well to treatment had a severe complication.

Wolff and Lindeman [10] carried out a double-blind study over a 2-year period in 87 patients with mild to moderately severe hypertension. The incidence of morbidity in the treated patients was one-third of that observed in the placebo group (six of 45 patients, or 13%, in the treatment group and 19 of 42 patients, or 45%, in the placebo group).

A carefully designed, prospective, controlled study was reported by the Veterans Administration Cooperative Study Group,[11] who studied 143 male hypertensive patients with diastolic blood pressures averaging between 115 and 129 mm Hg. Severe complications developed in 27 of 70 (39%) of the patients given placebo, but in only one of the 73 patients actively treated, or 1 percent. Four deaths (6%) occurred in the placebo group and none in the treated group.

More recently Veterans Administration Cooperative Study [12] has demonstrated that active antihypertensive treatment significantly reduced morbidity and mortality in male hypertensive patients with diastolic pressure averaging 90 to 114 mm Hg. In this study, the difference in the incidence of morbid events between control and treated group was highly significant in the subgroups with diastolic levels, averaging 105 to 114 mm Hg, and was favorable toward treatment, although not statistically significant, in those entering with diastolic levels of 90 through 104 mm Hg.

At the present time there are no prospective control studies on the value of antihypertensive drug therapy for mildly hypertensive female patients (diastolic pressure below 110 mm Hg).

Effect on the Kidneys

The renal function of patients with mild essential hypertension may be normal during the early stages. As the disease progresses, the renal function gradually becomes impaired. Moyer and associates [17] demonstrated a direct correlation between renal damage and the severity of blood pressure elevation above diastolic pressures of 110 mm Hg. The more severe the arterial pressure elevation, the lower the glomerular filtration rate, indicating that high arterial pressure causes renal damage. They [2] also demonstrated that effective reduction of the blood pressure with antihypertensive drugs arrested the deterioration of renal function in patients with severe, moderately severe, and malignant hypertension.

Woods and Blythe [18] demonstrated that the glomerular filtration rate could be increased or at least maintained by aggressive therapy with antihypertensive drugs in patients with malignant hypertension complicated by renal insufficiency. Recently Mroczek and associates [19] showed that aggressive antihypertensive therapy resulted in a slight worsening of renal function during the first 2 weeks of treatment in patients with the accelerated phase of hypertension with azotemia. Three months later, however, maintenance of reduced arterial pressure was associated with improvement of renal function above control (pretreatment) values. Twenty-six months later, renal function was markedly improved in the surviving patients.

Harrington, Kincaid-Smith, and McMichael [4] reported that after treatment with antihypertensive drugs, the main changes in the kidneys were a conversion of cellular intimal hyperplasia in the interlobular arteries to fibrous intimal thickening and the healing of fibrinoid degeneration to hyaline and fibrous tissue. McCormack and associates [20] concluded that treated patients with malignant nephrosclerosis, especially after long periods of treatment, almost always exhibited remission and healing of the acute arteriolar lesions.

More recently Eknoyan and Siegel [21] reported that with effective antihypertensive therapy, a single patient with malignant hypertension and anuria underwent diuresis and had enough improvement in renal function to maintain life without dialysis over 2 years. We also have a patient with the malignant phase of essential hypertension and uremia whose creatinine clearance rose to 30 ml per minute with effective antihypertensive therapy. She has been alive more than 18 months without dialysis. The experience with these patients demonstrates that the malignant phase of essential hypertension with uremia is not always irreversible. Therefore, vigorous therapy with dialysis and antihypertensive drugs is indicated in management of even uremic patients with the malignant phase of essential hypertension.

In patients with mild to moderate hypertension, the rate of renal deterioration per year is very small and does not differ significantly in treated and untreated patients.[2] In summary, the deterioration of renal function in patients with malignant or severe hypertension can be arrested or prevented with effective antihypertensive therapy. There is some evidence that impaired renal function may be improved with aggressive antihypertensive therapy. Some question exists as to the efficacy of treatment in arresting the slow deterioration of renal function seen with mild and moderate hypertension. Observations of this type must perhaps be extended over a longer follow-up period before the value of such therapy can be demonstrated. It seems reasonable to suppose, however, that early treatment of mild or moderately severe hypertension would be of even greater value in delaying or preventing the vascular deterioration in the kidney.

Effect on the Cardiovascular System

The increased work load on the heart due to increased peripheral resistance leads to cardiac enlargement, hypertrophy and eventually cardiac failure in hypertensive patients. With effective antihypertensive therapy, heart size has been reduced in about 25 percent of patients with malignant hypertension,[4,7] and the electrocardiogram has shown improvement in 20 to 50 percent of the patients in different studies.[4,7,15] Effective therapy also prevents or relieves congestive heart failure, so that this has become an uncommon cause of death in hypertensive patients treated with antihypertensive agents.

A relationship between elevated blood pressure levels and an increased rate of atherogenesis has been definitely established.[22] Kannel and his associates [23] (in the Framingham study) noted that hypertension increased the risk of coronary artery disease 2.6 times in men 40 to 59 years of age and was associated with a sixfold increase of risk in women the same age.

In the series of Wolff and Lindeman,[10] eight of 19 complications in the placebo control group were episodes of congestive heart failure, which cleared or improved with therapy. In none of the treated patients did congestive heart failure occur. There were two cases of sudden death, presumably due to coronary artery disease, in the treated group; and angina pectoris developed in two patients of the placebo control group.

Cerebrovascular Effects

The overall incidence of cerebrovascular accident has been reduced by effective antihypertensive therapy. Hodge and Smirk [24] concluded that effective treatment decreases the incidence of death caused by cerebrovascular accidents. Dustan and associates [3] found that in patients with malignant hypertension, cerebral hemorrhage was associated with poor control of the blood pressure, whereas myocardial infarction was not.

Leishman [25] also concluded that in patients with benign hypertension (diastolic blood pressure 130 mm Hg or higher), treatment reduced the mortality mainly by preventing cerebral hemorrhage and renal failure. Nevertheless, fatal cerebrovascular accidents occurred despite control of hypertension. Leishman postulated that there were two causes of cerebrovascular accident, one preventable by lowering blood pressure (cerebral hemorrhage) and the other not preventable (cerebral thrombosis). The patients who died were victims primarily of cerebral thrombosis, and reduction of blood pressure did not protect them from this.

Perry and associates [26,27] assigned all deaths to one of the following three categories: (1) "hypertensive," by which they meant renal failure or hemorrhagic stroke; (2) "atherosclerotic," by which they meant myocardial infarction or thrombotic stroke; and (3) "other," which included all causes of death outside of the first two categories. They concluded that hypertensive causes of death were clearly related to the level of blood pressure, whereas atherosclerotic causes of death were not obviously influenced by the efficacy of antihypertensive therapy.

Hypertensive encephalopathy, a cerebrovascular complication primarily of malignant hypertension, can be prevented and also be successfully treated with effective antihypertensive therapy.

Effects on the Retina

As the vessels and other structures of the optic fundi are easily seen, the observation of retinal changes has yielded considerable information concerning the degree and nature of the vascular damage in essential hypertension, its progression during the natural course of the disease, and its regression during antihypertensive therapy.

With effective antihypertensive therapy, papilledema, as well as retinal hemorrhages and exudates, can be prevented or reversed if already present when treatment is started. Smirk [28] found that papilledema disappeared only after 3 to 4 months of intensive treatment in patients with malignant hypertension. He stated that a clear reduction in the amount of papilledema should be evident in 3 to 4 weeks, with reappearance of a physiologic cup or of a part of the disc edge; the last residues of edema take longest to disperse. He also stated that within the first month of effective treatment, soft exudates should resolve and there should be no fresh hemorrhage. However, substantial dispersal of hard exudate is unlikely in less than 6 months, and some might remain after 12 months, but it would be absorbed in most patients who had been under effective treatment for 12 to 18 months.

Dollery, Ramalho, and Paterson[29] concluded that lowering the blood pressure to normal did not usually bring about any dramatic change in the focal or general narrowing of the larger arterioles. Their careful measurement of these retinal vessels revealed that there was often a substantial increase in caliber of the smallest vessels, accompanied by a small decrease in size of the largest arterioles near the optic disc. More recently Ramalho and Dollery[30] found that small arterioles dilated when pressure was reduced, whereas the larger retinal arterioles dilated in only three young hypertensive patients but were unchanged or narrowed in the remainder of the group studied.

Changes in the Cause of Death

Effective antihypertensive therapy not only reduces mortality, but also changes the relative incidence of various causes of death. As Table 2 shows, uremia is the most common cause in untreated patients with malignant hypertension. Congestive heart failure and cerebrovascular accident are the next most common causes of death.[2,14,31,32] Effective treatment greatly reduces the incidence of death from congestive heart failure and somewhat reduces mortality due to uremia (depending on the status of renal function at the beginning of treatment), whereas coronary artery disease appears to increase in incidence.[3,7]

Table 3 shows the percentage distribution of deaths among untreated and treated patients with all grades of hypertensive disease from the Dunedin Hospital hypertension clinic.[24] The treated patients are divided into two

Table 2.—*Causes of Death in Untreated and Treated Patients with Malignant Hypertension*

	Causes of Death				
Authors	*Uremia* (%)	*Cardiac Failure* (%)	*Cerebro-vascular Accident* (%)	*Coronary Artery Disease* (%)	*Other* (%)
Untreated Patients					
Smith, Odel, and Kernohan[31]	59	21	16	1	3
Kincaid-Smith, McMichael, and Murphy[14]	65 *	13	20	1	1
Milliez et al.[32]	67 †	—	26	—	7
Moyer et al.[2]	65	12	23	—	—
Treated Patients					
Dustan et al.[3]	42	—	25	14	19
Harrington, Kincaid-Smith, and McMichael[4]	54 ‡	6	24	2	14
Mohler and Freis[6]	29	—	33	27 §	11
Farmer, Gifford, and Hines[7]	28	4	40	9	19 ¶
Björk et al.[5]	43	5	36	11	5

From Moyer, J. H., and Kim, K. E.: The effect of antihypertensive therapy on ultimate prognosis. *In* Russell, H. I., and Zohman, B. L. (Eds.): Cardiovascular Therapy. Baltimore: Williams & Wilkins, 1971, pp. 181–192, with permission.

* Forty-eight percent due to uremia and heart failure.
† Twenty-six percent due to uremia and heart failure.
‡ Nineteen percent due to uremia and heart failure.
§ "Cardiac death" (authors' designation).
¶ Cause of death unknown in 13 percent.

TABLE 3.—*Causes of Death Among Untreated and Treated Hypertensive Patients*

Cause of Death	*Untreated 1950–1958*	*Treated 1950–1958*	*Treated 1959–1964*
Coronary artery disease and sudden cardiac death	17.1	19.2	42.0
Cerebrovascular accident	39.6	33.1	22.5
Congestive heart failure	23.2	12.7	6.1
Uremia	12.2	20.5	9.5
Other	7.9	14.6	19.9

From Moyer, J. H., and Kim, K. E.: The effect of antihypertensive therapy on ultimate prognosis. *In* Russell, H. I., and Zohman, B. L. (Eds.): Cardiovascular Therapy. Baltimore: Williams & Wilkins, 1971, pp. 181–192, by permission; the data are from Hodge and Smirk.[24]

groups on the basis of when they were treated, because the advent of new drugs improved the treatment of hypertension and gave better results. Comparing the untreated group to the treated group during the period of 1950 to 1958, it can be seen that the incidence of death from congestive heart failure was greatly reduced and that from cerebrovascular accident was somewhat reduced in the treated group. Marked reduction in congestive heart failure and cerebrovascular accident and marked increase in coronary artery disease are striking changes in the causes of death in the group treated between 1959 and 1964, as compared to both the untreated patients and those who were treated between 1950 and 1958. In the group treated from 1959 to 1964 coronary artery disease, together with sudden cardiac death probably due to coronary artery disease, was the most common cause of death. It accounted for 42 percent of all deaths, or 50.9 percent of deaths when causes not related to hypertension were excluded. These studies show that effective treatment of hypertension decreases the incidence of deaths due to cerebrovascular accidents and congestive heart failure. The authors [24] also indicate that the percentage of deaths from unrelated causes such as malignancy for 1962 to 1964 was more than twice that for the previous 3 years, reflecting presumably an overall reduction in deaths due to the vascular complications of hypertension. Nevertheless, it appears that with the effective treatment of hypertension, atherosclerotic complications have emerged as the most important problem.

RESULTS OF DISCONTINUING ANTIHYPERTENSIVE THERAPY

With the potent antihypertensive drugs an increasing number of hypertensive patients can be maintained at normal or nearly normal levels of blood pressure. This ability to reduce arterial pressure for prolonged periods has suggested the possibility that in some patients the pressure might "reset" at a lower level, so that therapy would no longer be necessary.[33]

Thurm and Smith [34] found that 16 of 69 hypertensive patients with an average mean blood pressure of 122 mm Hg before treatment remained normotensive (average diastolic pressure below 90 mm Hg) for 10 to 42 months after antihypertensive drugs were discontinued. However, Dustan and associates [35] recently reported that after antihypertensive drugs were discontinued in a group of 60 hypertensive patients, the blood pressure returned to pretreatment levels in 21 and rose toward pretreatment levels in 37. In only two patients did the diastolic hypertension not reappear in more than 8 years. These two patients, apparently cured, were among the nine (out of 27) patients that Page and Dustan [33] reported in 1962 whose hypertension seemed to have been cured after therapy was discontinued following long-term treatment. In six of the nine patients treatment was subsequently restarted because the blood pressure again rose to hypertensive levels, and in one the pressure was found to vary spontaneously enough so that the effects of discontinuing drugs could not be assessed.

Dustan's group [35] found that the rate at

which the blood pressure rose after treatment was stopped seemed related to the type of hypertension, height of diastolic pressure, and severity of vascular disease before treatment. In six of nine patients who had had malignant hypertension and six of another nine with renal artery disease, the blood pressure rose promptly and treatment was restarted within a month. Among patients with essential hypertension, those who were able to remain off treatment for 2 to 6 months had significantly lower pretreatment pressure than those whose hypertension returned in less than 2 months. In reporting this study, the authors also pointed out that the differences between the small percentage of cured patients in their series [35] and the large percentage of cured patients in the series reported by Thurm and Smith [34] are probably due to differences in severity of the hypertension and resulting vascular damage among the patients studied. Many of those included in their series had high diastolic pressure and severe vascular disease, whereas those in the Thurm and Smith series were mildly hypertensive, as shown by a group average mean arterial pressure of 122 mm Hg. They concluded that most hypertensive patients require continuous treatment for good pressure control, and that permanent downward resetting of pressure by treatment is rare.

Summary

Effective antihypertensive therapy greatly reduces morbidity and mortality for both men and women with malignant and moderately severe hypertension. Therapy also reduces morbidity and mortality in mildly hypertensive male patients. Even among treated patients, however, those whose blood pressures are well controlled and in whom vascular damage—especially renal damage—is not severe when treatment is started have a much better prognosis than those whose blood pressures are not well controlled and have advanced renal damage.

Not only can effective treatment of hypertension arrest further renal damage, but also there is some evidence that it may even improve renal function. The advent of the artificial kidney and renal homotransplantation has made it possible to treat malignant hypertension with uremia by means of bilateral nephrectomy, which results in a marked reduction of blood pressure and consequent clinical improvement, so that even patients in the malignant phase of hypertension with uremia can have prolonged periods of useful life.

Effective treatment reduces heart size, improves the electrocardiographic findings and prevents or relieves congestive heart failure.

The overall incidence of cerebrovascular accident has been reduced by effective therapy. Effective therapy can also prevent and reverse papilledema, as well as retinal hemorrhages and exudates.

Although at present there is no convincing evidence available from prospective, well-controlled studies that would specifically indicate the value of antihypertensive therapy of female patients with mild hypertension (diastolic blood pressure less than 110 mm Hg), it seems entirely reasonable to treat mildly hypertensive patients on the assumption that reduction of the blood pressure in an early stage of the disease may prevent the complications of hypertension from developing, including many of the atherosclerotic complications.

Effective antihypertensive therapy not only reduces mortality but also changes the incidence of the causes of death. In the patient with malignant hypertension, effective treatment markedly reduces the incidence of death from congestive heart failure and uremia, whereas the incidence of coronary artery disease increases.

In patients with all grades of hypertension, effective treatment greatly reduces the incidence of death from congestive heart failure and cerebrovascular accident and increases the incidence of death from coronary artery disease. It appears that the atherosclerotic complications have emerged as the most important problem in the treatment of hypertensive patients. The percentage of deaths unrelated to causes associated with hypertension also increases in patients effectively treated.

Most hypertensive patients require continuous antihypertensive treatment for good pressure control, since permanent downward resetting of pressure by treatment is rare.

References

1. Society of Actuaries: Build and Blood Pressure Study, vol. 1. Chicago, 1959.
2. Moyer, J. H., Heider, C., Pevey, K., and Ford, R. V.: The effect of treatment on the vascular deterioration associated with hypertension, with particular emphasis on renal function. Am. J. Med. 24:177, 1958.
3. Dustan, H. P., Schneckloth, R. E., Corcoran, A. C., and Page, I. H.: The effectiveness of long-term treatment of malignant hypertension. Circulation 18:644, 1958.
4. Harrington, M., Kincaid-Smith, P., and McMichael, J.: Results of treatment in malignant hypertension. A seven-year experience in 94 cases. Br. Med. J. 2:969, 1959.
5. Björk, S., Sannerstedt, R., Angervall, G., and Hood, B.: Treatment and prognosis in malignant hypertension. Clinical follow-up study of 93 patients on modern medical treatment. Acta Med. Scand. 166:175, 1960.
6. Mohler, E. R., Jr., and Freis, E. D.: Five-year survival of patients with malignant hypertension treated with antihypertensive agents. Am. Heart J. 60:329, 1960.
7. Farmer, R. G., Gifford, R. W., Jr., and Hines, E. A.: Effect of medical treatment of severe hypertension. A follow-up study of 61 patients with group 3 and group 4 hypertension. Arch. Intern. Med. 112:118, 1963.
8. Hodge, J. V., McQueen, E. G., and Smirk, H.: Results of hypotensive treatment in arterial hypertension. Based on experience with 497 patients treated and 156 controls, observed for periods of one to eight years. Br. Med. J. 1:1, 1961.
9. Hamilton, M., Thompson, E. N., and Wisniewski, T. K. M.: The role of blood pressure control in preventing complications of hypertension. Lancet 1:235, 1964.
10. Wolff, F. W., and Lindeman, R. D.: Effects of treatment in hypertension. Result of a controlled study. J. Chronic Dis. 19:227, 1966.
11. Veterans Administration Cooperative Study Group on Antihypertensive Agents: Effects of treatment on morbidity in hypertension. Results in patients with diastolic blood pressures averaging 115 through 129 mmHg. JAMA 202:1028, 1967.
12. Veterans Administration Cooperative Study Group on Antihypertensive Agents. Effect of treatment on morbidity and mortality. II. Results in patients with diastolic blood pressures averaging 90 through 114 mmHg. JAMA 213:1143, 1970.
13. Keith, N. M., Wagener, H. P., and Barker, N. W.: Some different types of essential hypertension. Their course and prognosis. Am. J. Med. Sci. 197:332, 1939.
14. Kincaid-Smith, P., McMichael, J., and Murphy, E. A.: The clinical course and pathology of hypertension with papilloedema (malignant hypertension). Q. J. Med. 27: 117, 1958.
15. Sokolow, M., and Perloff, D.: Five-year survival of consecutive patients with malignant hypertension treated with antihypertensive agents. Am. J. Cardiol. 6:858, 1960.
16. Onesti, G., Kim, K. E., Brest, A. N., and Swartz, C.: Evidence for the renal origin of the malignant phase of essential hypertension. Circulation 40(Suppl. III):157, 1969.
17. Moyer, J. H., Heider, C., Pevey, K., and Ford, R. V.: The vascular status of a heterogeneous group of patients with hypertension, with particular emphasis on renal function. Am. J. Med. 24:164, 1958.
18. Woods, J. W., and Blythe, W. B.: Management of malignant hypertension complicated by renal insufficiency. N. Engl. J. Med. 277: 57, 1967.
19. Mroczek, W. J., Davidov, M., Gavrilovich, L., and Finnerty, F. A., Jr.: The value of aggressive therapy in the hypertensive patient with azotemia. Circulation 40:893, 1969.
20. McCormack, L. J., Béland, J. E., Schneckloth, R. E., and Corcoran, A. C.: Effects of antihypertensive treatment on the evolution of the renal lesions in malignant nephrosclerosis. Am. J. Pathol. 34:1011, 1958.
21. Eknoyan, G., and Siegel, M. B.: Recovery from anuria due to malignant hypertension. JAMA 215:1122, 1971.
22. Freis, E. D.: Hypertension and atherosclerosis. Am. J. Med. 46:735, 1969.
23. Kannel, W. B., Dawber, T. R., Kagan, A., Revotskie, N., and Stokes, J.: Factors of risk in the development of coronary heart disease. Six-year follow-up experience. The Framingham Study. Ann. Intern. Med. 53:33, 1961.
24. Hodge, J. V., and Smirk, F. H.: The effect of drug treatment of hypertension on the distribution of deaths from various causes. A study of 173 deaths among hypertensive patients in the years 1959 to 1964 inclusive. Am. Heart J. 73:441, 1967.
25. Leishman, A. W. D.: Merit of reducing high blood pressure. Lancet 1:1284, 1963.
26. Perry, H. M., Schroeder, H. A., Catanzaro, F. J., Moore-Jones, D., and Camel, G. H.: Studies on the control of hypertension. VIII. Mortality, morbidity, and remissions dur-

ing twelve years of intensive therapy. Circulation 33:958, 1966.

27. Perry, M., Wessler, S., and Avioli, L. V.: Survival of treated hypertensive patients. JAMA 210:890, 1969.

28. Smirk, F. H.: Results of methonium treatment of hypertensive patients. Based on 250 cases treated for periods up to 3½ years, including 28 with malignant hypertension. Br. Med. J. 1:717, 1954.

29. Dollery, C. T., Ramalho, P. S., and Paterson, J. W.: Retinal vascular alterations in hypertension. *In* Gross, F. (Ed.): Antihypertensive Therapy. Berlin: Springer, 1966, pp. 152–163.

30. Ramalho, P. S., and Dollery, C. T.: Hypertensive retinopathy. Caliber changes in retinal blood vessels following blood pressure reduction and inhalation of oxygen. Circulation 37:580, 1968.

31. Smith, D. E., Odel, H. M., and Kernohan, J. W.: Causes of death in hypertension. Am. J. Med. 9:516, 1950.

32. Milliez, P., Tcherdakoff, P., Samarcq, P., and Rey, L. P.: The natural course of malignant hypertension. *In* Bock, K. D., and Cottier, P. T. (Eds.): Essential Hypertension. An International Symposium. Berlin: Springer, 1960, pp. 214–230.

33. Page, I. H., and Dustan, H. P.: Persistence of normal blood pressure after discontinuing treatment in hypertensive patients. Circulation 25:433, 1962.

34. Thurm, R. H., and Smith, W. M.: On resetting of "barostats" in hypertensive patients. JAMA 201:301, 1967.

35. Dustan, H. P., Page, I. H., Tarazi, R. C., and Frohlich, E. D.: Arterial pressure responses to discontinuing antihypertensive drugs. Circulation 37:370, 1968.

Carotid Sinus Nerve Stimulation in the Treatment of Hypertension

By Albert N. Brest, M.D., Leslie Wiener, M.D., and Benjamin Bacharach, M.D.

Bilateral carotid sinus nerve stimulation has proved to be an effective means for controlling diastolic hypertension in certain instances. Although the exact clinical indications for this therapeutic modality have yet to be established, its potential is considerable. This chapter will review the historical background for its application, and its clinical use in the treatment of severe diastolic hypertension which was poorly responsive to antihypertensive drug therapy.

Historical Background

In the early 1920s the classic experiments of Hering established a firm basis for the role of the carotid sinuses in the maintenance of blood pressure. These baroreceptors have become recognized as major sentinels in the homeostatic system of blood pressure control. Specifically, the carotid sinuses monitor intra-arterial blood pressure and then alter accordingly the traffic of sympathetic nerve impulses to vasomotor centers in the medulla. Thus, when the blood pressure rises, afferent impulse traffic is increased and, correspondingly, the vasomotor centers reduce the flow of sympathetic impulses to peripheral vasomotor sites in the arterioles, venules, and heart. The physiologic end-result includes blood pressure lowering and bradycardia. The reverse effect follows blood pressure reduction. Harnessing of this homeostatic mechanism would seem to be a physiologic approach to the treatment of hypertension.

In 1956, McCubbin, Green, and Page [1] suggested the implication of the carotid sinus reflex as a factor in the persistence of elevated blood pressure. Carotid sinus baroreceptors demonstrated a marked reduction in threshold response in hypertensive dogs as compared with normotensive animals when they were subjected to different levels of steady pressure or to standard pulsatile pressure of different mean levels. In 1965, Tuckman, Slater, and Mendlowitz [2] reported that the carotid sinus reflexes in hypertensive man do not function at their full capacity. Subsequently, Bristow and co-workers [3] provided evidence to indicate that carotid sinus activity is depressed in systemic hypertension. Theoretically, if these baroreflexes could be "reset," hypertension would either remit or, at the least, be controlled more easily.

In 1958, Warner [4] proposed electrical stimulation of the carotid sinus nerve as a method of producing hypotension and effected a decrease in systemic arterial pressure in normotensive dogs for periods up to 90 minutes. In 1964, Griffith and Schwartz [5] demonstrated a sustained 40-mm reduction in systolic pressure and a 35-mm decrease in diastolic pressure in hypertensive animals subjected to unilateral stimulation of the carotid sinus nerve with the opposite nerve intact. When the opposite nerve was transected, the animals responded maximally to exogenous electrical stimulation with a sustained reduction in systolic pressure of 90 mm Hg and in diastolic pressure of 60 mm Hg. In 1965, Schwartz and Griffith [6] and Bilgutay and Lillehei [7] reported the effectiveness of chronic electrical stimulation of the carotid sinus nerve in the treatment of hypertensive man. These early studies employed implanted electrical carotid sinus discs and sinus nerve stimulators. It soon became apparent, however, that the use of completely implantable stimulators which apply an identical and fixed level of stimulation to all patients and in all positions was impracticable. Contrariwise, it seemed evident that if this technique were to be clinically useful the levels of stimulation would have to be easily controllable and capable of titration. Accordingly, radio frequency-coupled stimulators were applied to these investigations, and Neufeld et al.[8] first reported

From the Jefferson Medical College and Hospital, Philadelphia, Pennsylvania.

on their use in 1965. Subsequently, more detailed studies were reported by Neistadt and Schwartz,[9] Parsonnet and associates,[10] and Tuckman and co-workers.[11]

Thus far, the most extensive trials of carotid sinus nerve stimulation in hypertensive man have been reported by Tuckman and co-workers [11] and by Schwartz.[12]

Tuckman and associates [11] reported clinical studies in 12 severely hypertensive patients. Group A consisted of nine patients who responded inadequately to trials of antihypertensive agents, in that drug treatment failed to keep the supine diastolic pressures below 140 mm Hg. Group B consisted of three accelerated essential hypertensive patients with severe and rapidly progressing uremia. In six of the nine patients in the first group, stimulation chronically reduced the arterial pressure in both the supine and the erect positions without the use of adjuvant antihypertensive drugs or salt-restricting diets. In another patient, the blood pressure was controlled with a combination of carotid sinus nerve stimulation and adjuvant therapy with hydrochlorothiazide and methyldopa. Blood pressure was not adequately controlled in any of the three patients with accelerated hypertension.

Schwartz [12] described his clinical results in 11 hypertensive subjects. In each instance, the lesions amenable to other surgical procedures were excluded and the patients were either not responsive to medication or could not tolerate the side effects of drugs. The minimal resting blood pressures were 190/110 mm Hg. One patient with advanced renal failure at the time of surgery died 2 months postoperatively; however, a 20-mm Hg reduction in systolic and diastolic pressures had been achieved. One patient required removal of the stimulator 2 months after implantation, because of an unrelated chest burn; but, during the 2-month period of stimulation, the blood pressure was reduced from the preoperative level of 250/140 mm Hg to a mean level of 150/100 mm Hg. Another patient was lost to follow-up. The other eight patients were followed for periods ranging from 20 months to 4½ years. Six of these eight patients achieved reductions in blood pressure ranging between 30 and 100 mm Hg systolic and 24 and 80 mm Hg diastolic with a mean of 48 and 42 mm Hg, respectively; none received any antihypertensive medication. The two remaining patients, who had previously been refractory to all medication, had minimal response to carotid sinus nerve stimulation alone but reinstitution of medication resulted in a marked reduction in blood pressure.

Clinical Experiences

We studied the clinical effectiveness of bilateral carotid sinus nerve stimulation in eight patients with severe essential hypertension. In each instance, the diastolic hypertension was uncontrolled despite a triple-drug regimen of furosemide (80 mg daily), guanethidine (50 mg daily, minimum), and methyldopa (2 gm daily, minimum). Two of the eight patients had malignant hypertension (with grade IV hypertensive retinopathy and serum creatinine greater than 5 mg per 100 ml in each instance).

Stimulation was induced with a Barostat Carotid Sinus Nerve Stimulator (CSNS) (Medtronic, Inc.). The Barostat CSNS consists of an implanted receiver/electrode assembly and an externally worn transmitter/antenna assembly. The transmitter assembly includes a battery-powered pulse generator and an attached antenna coil. The subcutaneously implanted receiver contains two electrically isolated receiving coils and circuits, each supplying impulses to an electrode which is attached to a carotid sinus nerve bundle. The transmitter antenna coil is placed on the skin directly over the receiving coils contained within the implanted receiver. The transmitter supplies stimulus power to the receiver by radio frequency-inductive coupling through the skin. The rate and amplitude of the generated pulses can be physician-adjusted by controls located inside the transmitter case.

The clinical data are summarized in Table 1. Follow-up ranged from 1 to 24 months. It should be noted that the reported blood pressures before stimulation represent, in each instance, the average of three weekly blood pressures obtained while the patient was receiving antihypertensive drug therapy. The blood pressures reported after stimulation represent the average of three weekly blood pressures obtained during the last month of stimulation.

Diastolic normotension was achieved with

TABLE 1.—*Clinical Data: Eight Patients Treated with Bilateral Carotid Sinus Nerve Stimulation (BCSNS)*

				Before BCSNS		*After BCSNS*			
Patient	*Age*	*Sex*	*Race*	*Therapy*	*Blood Pressure* * *(mmHg)*	*Therapy*	*Blood Pressure* † *(mmHg)*	*Follow-up (months)*	*Comments*
M. B.	61	M	C	FSM, MD, GUAN	190/140	FSM	145/90	24	
D. S.	49	M	C	FSM, MD, GUAN	200/130	None	130/90	22	
A.D.	43	M	C	FSM, MD, GUAN	200/120	FSM	140/90	21	
J. S.	30	M	C	FSM, MD, GUAN	190/120	FSM	145/85	19	
E. W.	52	M	N	FSM, MD, GUAN	190/130	FSM, MD	140/85	18	Pre-BCSNS creatinine, 2.3 mg per 100 ml; post-BCSNS creatinine, 2.3 mg per 100 ml.
V. J.	44	F	N	FSM, MD, GUAN	190/145	FSM, MD, GUAN	160/120	7	Patient discontinued BCSNS, suffered stroke, expired 4 days later
D. J.	37	F	N	FSM, MD, GUAN	220/180	FSM, MD, GUAN	180/130	3	Malignant hypertension. Pre-BCSNS creatinine 5.6 mg per 100 ml. Expired, renal failure.
H. S.	29	F	N	FSM, MD, GUAN	280/160	FSM, MD, GUAN	175/125	1	Malignant hypertension. Pre-BCSNS creatinine 6.4 mg per 100 ml. Expired, renal failure.

Abbreviations used: FSM, furosemide; MD, methyldopa; GUAN, guanethidine; C, Caucasian; N, Negro.
* Average of three weekly blood pressures before BCSNS.
† Average of three weekly blood pressures during the last follow-up month after BCSNS.

bilateral carotid sinus nerve stimulation alone in one patient with nonmalignant hypertension. Diastolic normotension was achieved (and maintained) with a combination of stimulation and antihypertensive drug therapy in four others; and, in each instance, the amount of drug therapy was substantially less than that employed prior to stimulation. The sixth patient with nonmalignant hypertension obtained significant blood pressure reduction (mean arterial pressure reduced more than 20 mm Hg), but diastolic normotension was not achieved despite the additional use of antihypertensive drug treatment. There was little disparity between the supine and erect blood pressure reductions obtained in each of the six subjects. In contrast, both patients with malignant hypertension obtained significant blood pressure reduction, but arterial pressures remained substantially elevated; and both had a rapidly progressive downhill clinical course, terminating in death secondary to renal failure.

Hemodynamic Studies

Acute cardiac hemodynamic studies were performed during the postabsorptive basal state in five of the eight patients. A No. 7 bipolar pacing catheter with lumen was introduced into the coronary sinus. Cardiac output was measured by the indicator-dilution method. Intra-arterial pressure was measured directly from the brachial artery via an indwelling 17-gauge Teflon catheter needle, using a P 23db Statham strain-gauge transducer. Mean isovolumic pressure rate (an indirect index of myocardial contractility) was determined from the formula

$$\text{MIPR} = \frac{\text{diastolic pressure}}{\text{pre-ejection period}}$$

The pre-ejection period was calculated from simultaneous recordings of the electrocardiogram, phonocardiogram, and carotid artery pulse. Total peripheral resistance was calculated, in arbitrary units, from the arterial pressure and the cardiac output, as

$$\frac{\text{mean arterial pressure} - \text{mean coronary sinus pressure}}{\text{cardiac output}}$$

To eliminate the chronotropic influence of bilateral carotid sinus nerve stimulation, the aforementioned hemodynamic studies were subsequently repeated while the control heart rate was maintained at a constant rate (98 per minute, average) by coronary sinus pacing.

The acute hemodynamic response (Table 2) consisted of a sharp reduction in arterial pressure (81/35 mm Hg) with accompanying decreases in heart rate (19.8 beats per minute), cardiac index (1.67 liters per minute), and mean isovolumic pressure rate (230.3 mm Hg per second) while the systemic resistance increased (11.6 units).

The hemodynamic response obtained while the heart rate was maintained at a constant rate, by coronary sinus pacing, is reported in Table 3. Under this condition, the reduction in arterial pressure (60/31 mm Hg) was accompanied by decrease in cardiac index (0.85 liters per minute) and mean isovolumic pressure rate (303.4 mm Hg per second) but without any significant change in systemic resistance.

Discussion

In our study, significant blood pressure reduction (mean blood pressure reduced >20 mm Hg) was achieved in each of the eight patients. Normotension was obtained in five of the six patients with nonmalignant hypertension, while the sixth patient in this category had significant blood pressure reduction, albeit without achievement of normotension. The latter patient succumbed to a cerebrovascular accident, several days after she discontinued bilateral carotid sinus nerve stimulation (presumably because of neck discomfort secondary to stimulation). The two patients with malignant hypertension also obtained a significant antihypertensive response (mean arterial blood pressure reached >20 mm Hg); however, despite the blood pressure reduction, both patients experienced a rapidly progressive downhill clinical course, ultimately succumbing to renal failure. It is noteworthy that each of the five patients who achieved normotension has continued to sustain this effect for prolonged periods, ranging from 18 to 24 months, thus denying the theoretic consideration that chronic carotid sinus nerve stimulation might lose its effectiveness.

The acute hemodynamic response to such stimulation has been studied by Tuckman and

TABLE 2.—*Acute Hemodynamic Response to Bilateral Carotid Sinus Nerve Stimulation (BCSNS)*

Patient	Blood Pressure (mm Hg)		Heart Rate (beats per minute)		Cardiac Index (liters per minute)		Systemic Resistance (units)		Mean Isovolumic Pressure Rate (mm Hg per second)	
	C	*B*	*C*	*B*	*C*	*B*	*C*	*B*	*C*	*B*
A. D.	270/144	150/95	79	68	—	2.22	—	49.5	1107	593
J. S.	210/120	160/110	80	76	4.9	1.8	29.6	72.2	706	733
D. S.	215/120	120/60	80	48	3.12	2.04	48.1	44.1	667	300
E. W.	230/132	—	89	—	2.86	—	57.8	—	733	—
V. J.	240/135	180/115	96	68	4.0	2.2	45.0	61.1	675	563
Average	233/130	152/95	84.8	65.0	3.72	2.05	45.1	56.7	777.6	547.3

Abbreviations used: C, control; B, with BCSNS.

TABLE 3.—*Acute Hemodynamic Response to Bilateral Carotid Sinus Nerve Stimulation (BCSNS) (Heart Rate Maintained by Coronary Sinus Pacing)*

Patient	Blood Pressure (mm Hg)		Heart Rate (beats per minute)		Cardiac Index (liters per minute)		Systemic Resistance (units)		Mean Isovolumic Pressure Rate (mm Hg per second)	
	P	*PB*	*P*	*PB*	*P*	*PB*	*P*	*PB*	*P*	*PB*
A. D.	280/160	150/95	95	95	3.46	2.32	59.3	47.4	1230	528
J. S.	210/122	170/98	90	90	4.3	3.0	36.0	40.0	718	490
D. S.	230/120	160/85	85	85	3.12	2.54	51.3	43.3	705	472
E. W.	220/130	215/122	110	110	3.57	3.06	44.8	49.0	722	610
V. J.	220/140	165/118	108	108	3.3	2.6	52.7	51.3	778	536
Average	232/134	172/103	97.6	97.6	3.55	2.7	48.8	46.2	830.6	527.2
P		>0.05		N.S.		> 0.05		N.S.		> 0.05

Abbreviations used: P, atrial pacing, without BCSNS; PB, atrial pacing, with BCSNS; N.S., not significant.

associates [11] and by Epstein and co-workers.[13] Tuckman et al.[11] reported that stimulation in the supine position reduced the average mean arterial pressure from 165 to 132 mm Hg (−21%) and heart rate from 89 to 75 beats per minute; these changes were associated with average reductions of minus 11 percent in cardiac output and minus 10 percent in peripheral vascular resistance. Epstein and associates [13] studied the effects of carotid sinus nerve stimulation at rest and found that mean arterial pressure fell 23 percent and cardiac output decreased 8 percent while total peripheral resistance decreased by 14 percent and heart rate fell an average of 7 beats per minute; during exercise, mean arterial pressure fell 16 percent but no significant change occurred in cardiac output. Epstein et al.[13] concluded that the fall in blood pressure could be attributed to a reflexly induced decrease in peripheral vascular resistance and cardiac output.

In contrast with the previously cited studies, conventional hemodynamic studies obtained in the present investigation revealed an increase in peripheral resistance while reductions in cardiac output, heart rate, and calculated myocardial contractility accompanied the sharp decrease in arterial pressure. The modest increase in peripheral resistance in the present study, as contrasted with the findings of Tuckman and Epstein, probably reflects the more profound reduction in blood pressure, cardiac output, and heart rate induced in our investigation. When heart rate was controlled by coronary sinus pacing, the marked blood pressure fall was not accompanied by any significant change in peripheral resistance; considering the sharp reduction in blood pressure induced, as well as the decline in cardiac output, the absence of the anticipated rise in peripheral vascular resistance indicates that there was a profound reflexly induced block in vasomotor response. Taking all data into consideration, it appears that the antihypertensive response to bilateral carotid sinus nerve stimulation represents a combination effect of suppression in peripheral vasomotor tone plus reduction in myocardial contractility.

From a physiologic standpoint, carotid sinus nerve stimulation results both in a decrease in beta stimulation of the heart and a reduction in alpha stimulation to the arterioles. The combined effect results in blood pressure reduction. Recent reports [14] indicate the beneficial effects of beta-adrenergic blockade in the treatment of diastolic hypertension, and the effectiveness of alpha-adrenergic blockade is well substantiated. Hence, the dual antihypertensive mechanism exhibited by bilateral carotid sinus nerve stimulation can be regarded as highly advantageous.

There is now convincing evidence, from several clinical studies, to indicate that such stimulation is an effective means of reducing diastolic hypertension. This therapeutic modality should have particular usefulness in hypertensive patients who are poorly responsive to combination antihypertensive drug therapy or others in whom blood pressure reduction is achieved with drug treatment but at the expense of serious untoward effects.

Conclusions

1. Bilateral carotid sinus nerve stimulation can induce long-term reduction of both supine and erect arterial pressures, without incapacitating postural hypotension.
2. Such stimulation can lower blood pressure significantly in many patients poorly responsive to antihypertensive drug regimens.
3. Responsiveness to stimulation is generally accompanied by enhanced effectiveness of antihypertensive drug therapy.
4. Bilateral carotid sinus nerve stimulation induces its antihypertensive effect via decrease in beta stimulation to the heart and reduction in alpha stimulation to the arterioles.
5. Bilateral stimulation of the carotid sinus nerves should be particularly useful in hypertensive patients who are poorly responsive to combination antihypertensive drug therapy, or those in whom blood pressure reduction is achieved with drug treatment but with a high incidence of serious untoward effects.

References

1. McCubbin, J. W., Green, J. H., and Page, I. H.: Baroreceptor function in chronic renal hypertension. Circ. Res. 4:205, 1956.
2. Tuckman, J., Slater, S. R., and Mendlowitz, M.: Carotid sinus reflexes. Am. Heart J. 70:119, 1965.
3. Bristow, J. D., Honour, A. J., Pickering, G.

W., Sleight, P., and Smyth, H. S.: Diminished baroreflex sensitivity in high blood pressure. Circulation 39:48, 1969.

4. Warner, H. R.: The frequency-dependent nature of blood pressure regulation by the carotid sinus studied by an electric analog. Circ. Res. 6:35, 1958.
5. Griffith, L. S. C., and Schwartz, S. I.: Reversal of renal hypertension by electrical stimulation of the carotid sinus nerve. Surgery 56:232, 1964.
6. Schwartz, S. I., and Griffith, L. S. C.: Reduction of hypertension by electrical stimulation of the carotid sinus nerve. Proceedings of an International Symposium held at Dayton, Ohio, November, 1965. *In* Kezdi, P. (Ed.): Baroreceptors and Hypertension. New York: Pergamon Press, 1967.
7. Bilgutay, A. M., and Lillehei, C. W.: Treatment of hypertension with an implantable electronic device. JAMA 191:649, 1965.
8. Neufeld, H. N., Goor, D., Nathan, D., Fischler, H., and Yerusalmi, S.: Stimulation of the carotid baroreceptors using a radio-frequency method. Israel J. Med. Sci. 1:630, 1965.
9. Neistadt, A., and Schwartz, S. I.: Effects of electrical stimulation of the carotid sinus nerve in reversal of experimentally induced hypertension. Surgery 61:923, 1967.
10. Parsonnet, V., Myers, G. H., Holcomb, W. G., and Zucker, I. R.: Radio-frequency stimulation of the carotid baroreceptors in the treatment of hypertension. Surg. Forum 17:125, 1966.
11. Tuckman, J., Reich, T., Lyon, A. F., Goodman, B., Mendlowitz, M., and Jacobson, J. H., II: Electrical stimulation of the carotid sinus nerves in hypertensive patients. *In* Hypertension, vol. 16. New York: The American Heart Association, Inc., 1968.
12. Schwartz, S. I.: Clinical applications of carotid sinus nerve stimulation. Cardiovasc. Clin. 1(3):208, 1969.
13. Epstein, S. E., Beiser, J. D., Goldstein, R. E., Stampfer, M., Wechsler, A. S., Glick, G., and Braunwald, E.: Circulatory effects of electrical stimulation of the carotid sinus nerves in man. Circulation 40:269, 1969.
14. Prichard, B. N. C., and Gillam, P. M. S.: Treatment of hypertension with propranolol. Br. Med. J. 1:7, 1969.

Survival Rates Following Splanchnicectomy for Essential and Malignant Hypertension

By Reginald H. Smithwick, M.D., and
Charles W. Robertson, M.D.

BECAUSE OF THE very high mortality among patients having essential or malignant hypertension and because there was no effective medical treatment, a number of operations upon the sympathetic nervous system were developed in an attempt to lower blood pressure. The unusual variability of blood pressure in hypertensive patients, especially in response to stimuli such as pain, cold, emotion, and change of posture appeared to implicate the sympathetic nervous system in the development and perpetuation of hypertension and suggested that resection of vasoconstrictor nerves might result in a lowering of blood pressure levels and a reduction in reflex responses to stimulation.

Among the first procedures to be utilized was the subdiaphragmatic splanchnicectomy of Craig,[1] and the supradiaphragmatic splanchnicectomy of Peet.[2] After a number of years' experience with these operations, a technique for splanchnicectomy was developed by one of us (R.H.S.) which appeared to combine the advantages of the Craig and Peet operations. It was called lumbodorsal splanchnicectomy.[3] The early results were encouraging, so beginning in 1938 the operation was offered to patients with the more severe forms of continued hypertension on the basis that it offered a reasonable chance for relief of symptoms, a slowing of the progress of vascular disease, and increased life expectancy. Other operations upon the sympathetic nervous system have also been employed, but they were either performed in relatively small numbers of patients or the follow-up studies were of relatively short duration.[4–7]

Since the onset of this study, one of us (R.H.S.), together with various associates, has published numerous reports dealing with methods of study, surgical technique, selection of patients for operation, and describing the effect of splanchnicectomy on blood pressure levels and responses, cardiovascular disease, and life expectancy. A representative number of these articles is referred to.[8–31] The purpose of this chapter is to summarize the results of lumbodorsal splanchnicectomy in terms of its effect upon the survival rates of hypertensive patients. Included are all patients operated upon during the years 1938 through 1966 and followed through 1967. In addition to the surgical cases are many patients who were studied, who were found suitable for surgery, to whom operation was offered but who decided not to be operated upon. These patients will be referred to as controls and the outcome, in terms of survival, will be compared with that of the patients who elected to be operated upon. This is a prospective follow-up study since it was planned to keep in touch with all of these patients for as many years as possible. Since they were referred to us by physicians from all parts of the world, it was impossible for us to follow them personally. All patients and/or their physicians were written to on the anniversary of the date of operation or study, and have been followed with great care until the time of death or loss to follow-up. We will also compare the survival of our patients with suitable control data from the literature and, where possible, with the survival of patients treated with antihypertensive drugs. The survival of treated and untreated patients will also be compared with that of the population as a whole of comparable age and sex.

We would like to call attention to the year 1950, which is the time when antihypertensive drugs became generally available as a method of treating hypertension. We have arranged our material in such fashion as to show the

From the Department of Surgery, Boston University School of Medicine, Boston, Massachusetts.

TABLE 1.—*Survivals—Essential and Malignant Hypertension*

a. Keith, Wagener and Barker Series Versus Smithwick Controls

Classification of Eye-ground	A. K.W.B. Series (1927–1932)					B. Smithwick Controls (1941–1945)					Statistical Significance of Group B Versus Group A at 5 to 9 yr
	No. of Patients	Alive at 5 yr		Alive at 5 to 9 yr		No. of Patients	Alive at 5 yr		Alive at 5 to 9 yr		
		No.	%	No.	%		No.	%	No.	%	
Group I	10	7	70	6	60	111	79	71	65	59	0
Group II	26	14	54	9	35	69	40	58	32	46	0
Group III	37	7	20	3	8	73	22	30	9	12	0
Group IV	146	1	1	1	1	38	0	0	0	0	0

b. Keith-Wagener-Barker Plus Smithwick Controls Versus Smithwick Surgical Patients

Classification of Eye-ground	C. K.W.B. Series (A) + Smithwick Controls (B)					D. Smithwick Surgical Cases (1938–1944)					Statistical Significance of Group D versus Group C at 5 to 9 yr	
	No. of Patients	Alive at 5 yr		Alive at 5 to 9 yr		No. of Patients	Alive at 5 yr		Alive at 5 to 9 yr			
		No.	%	No.	%		No.	%	No.	%	X^2	P
Group I	121	86	71	71	59	251	228	91	210	84	26.2	$< .001$
Group II	95	54	57	41	43	147	124	84	108	74	21.1	$< .001$
Group III	110	29	26	12	11	161	110	68	84	52	46.9	$< .001$
Group IV	184	1	1	1	1	78	37	47	29	37	68.9	$< .001$

A. These are the original Keith, Wagener, and Barker patients.

B. Contains Smithwick control patients with comparable mortality rates.

C. The patients in A and B are combined in order to have adequate numbers in each group for comparison with survival rates of cases in D.

D. Smithwick surgical patients. The increased survival of the surgical patients is highly significant statistically for all four groups. None of the patients received antihypertensive drugs. The patients in C and D are compared in Figure 1 by means of survival curves. The survival rates were calculated by the ad hoc or direct method.[32] The X^2 test with Yates correction was used to determine the significance of differences between survival rates throughout this chapter.

possible influence of drugs upon the survival of surgically treated patients, upon the survival of controls, and upon the survival of patients treated adequately with drugs alone. It is of interest that the hypotensive effect of the great majority of the drugs which have been developed during the past 20 years is due, directly or indirectly, to a depressant effect upon the sympathetic nervous system. One of the first articles on the use of antihypertensive drugs was entitled " 'Medical sympathectomy' in hypertension." [32]

Mortality Among Hypertensives Prior to Splanchnicectomy or the Use of Antihypertensive Drugs

In 1930, Blackford, Bowers, and Baker [33] found that the mortality among 202 cases followed up for 5 to 11 years was 50 percent for that group as a whole, and 70 percent for males and 39 percent for females. In 1939, Keith, Wagener, and Barker [34] reported that the mortality for 219 patients followed up for 5 to 9 years averaged 91 percent, being 93 percent for males and 88 percent for females. They also divided their cases into four groups on the basis of their eyeground classification. Survival curves were constructed which clearly demonstrated different survival rates for each group. These two reports point out the importance of sex and eyeground changes as guides to prognosis. In Table 1 (part A), we have listed the Keith-Wagener-Barker patients according to the four eyeground groups, giving survival rates at 5 years and 5 to 9 years. Because their series is heavily weighted in groups III and IV we have included a substantial number of our early control cases (Table 1, part B). These cases were studied in the years 1941–1945 and followed up for 5 to 9 years. The outcome could not have been influenced by antihypertensive drugs. Our series contains relatively large numbers of Group I and II patients. The survival rates for the four groups in both series are essentially the same. We have therefore combined the two series (Table 1, part C). This accomplishes two purposes. It gives adequate numbers of patients in each group to establish survival rates uninfluenced by splanchnicectomy or antihypertensive drugs and to serve as a basis for judging the effectiveness of a particular form of treatment. With this in mind we have compared the survival rates at 5 to 9 years of a series of our earliest patients treated

SURVIVALS – ESSENTIAL & MALIGNANT HYPERTENSION

K.W.B. + SMITHWICK CONTROLS vs. SMITHWICK SURGICAL CASES

Keith, Wagener & Barker Eyeground Groups

MALES & FEMALES COMBINED

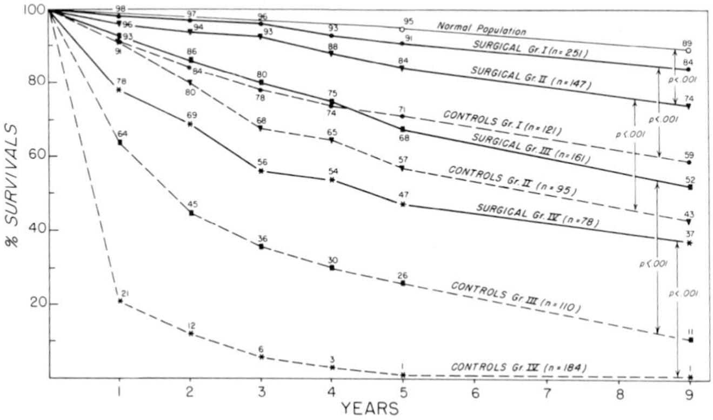

Fig. 1.—The controls establish the survival rates for hypertensive patients prior to the advent of splanchnicectomy or antihypertensive drugs for up to 9 years of observation. The curves for the surgical patients indicate that there has been a highly significant increase in survival rates for all four groups following splanchnicectomy. The 9-year survival rate of the Group 1 surgical patients approximates that of the population as a whole of comparable age, while that of the Group 1 controls is significantly lower.

by splanchnicectomy (Table 1, part D) with the combined Keith-Wagener-Barker and Smithwick controls (Table 1, part C). The differences are highly significant statistically for all four groups. This clearly establishes the effectiveness of splanchnicectomy in prolonging life. Since the patients were operated upon in the years 1938–1944, and followed up for 5 to 9 years, the outcome could not have been influenced by the use of antihypertensive drugs. The data contained in Table 1 (parts C and D) are presented in Figure 1 in the form of survival curves. The curves for the controls (Table 1, part C) are almost identical with the original Keith-Wagener-Barker curves for their patients alone.[34] In Figure 1, the percentages of survival are given at 1-year intervals and at the end of 9 years for the surgical patients as well as the controls. The data contained in Table 1 and Figure 1 clearly establish the importance of dividing patients into four categories on the basis of the Keith-Wagener-Barker eyeground groups. Other systems for dividing hypertensive patients into categories have also been devised [35–37] including that of one of us.[38] The purpose is to take changes in the cerebral, cardiac, and renal areas into consideration as well as resting blood pressure levels and the response to sedation in an attempt to arrange patients into more comparable groups. We have arranged large numbers of our patients according to these various systems and find the prognosis is surprisingly similar for all systems. Björk et al.[39] have also compared the various systems. It would therefore seem best to adopt the Keith-Wagener-Barker plan for grouping since it is simple and meaningful. The eyegrounds should, however, be examined and the findings described by an experienced ophthalmologist. The findings serve as an excellent guide to prognosis. Our version of the Keith-Wagener-Barker eyeground groups is as follows:

Group I. Any findings other than arteriovenous compression, hemorrhages, exudate, or papilledema.

Group II. The emphasis is on sclerosis. All patients have arteriovenous compression, but do not have hemorrhages, exudates, or papilledema.

Group III. Hemorrhages or exudates and any type of vascular change are present. Papilledema is absent.

Group IV. Papilledema is present and usually most of the other abnormalities as well.

Keith, Wagener, and Barker also divided their patients according to sex. Table 2 (part A) contains their male patients and part B contains a group of Smithwick's controls. There is no significant difference in the mortality rate of the two series. They are combined in part C and the survival rates compared with Smithwick's surgical series in part D. There is a highly significant increase in the survival of the surgical patients. The survival rates of the surgical patients are compared with those of the male population as a whole of comparable age, showing that for all four groups the survival of the surgical patients is significantly decreased. The findings for female patients divided into the four groups are shown in Table 3, with the patients arranged in parts A,B,C, and D as in Table 2. Again, the surgical survival rates are significantly different from those of the controls. By contrast with males, there is no significant difference in the survivals of Group I and II surgical patients and those of the female population as a whole of comparable age. This again emphasizes the advisability of dividing patients by sex as well as by group classifications when discussing prognosis or effect of treatment. Reference to Figure 1, in which the patients are divided by groups but not by sex, indicates that the survival of Group I surgical patients does not differ significantly from that of the population of comparable age. Reference to Tables 2 and 3 indicates that this does not hold for Group I males but does hold for Group I females.

Twenty-year Survival Rates As Influenced by Partial Exposure to Antihypertensive Drugs

The discussion thus far has been concerned with untreated and splanchnicectomized hypertensive patients uninfluenced by exposure to and therefore the possible (or probable) use of antihypertensive drugs. Because of the small number of cases in Keith-Wagener-Barker groups I and II and the comparatively short period of follow-up, Breslin, Gifford, and Fairbain [40] carried out another study of Mayo

TABLE 2.—*Five- to 9-Year Survivals in Male Hypertensive Patients Classified According to Keith, Wagener, and Barker Eyeground Groups*

Classification of Eye-ground	*A. K.W.B. Series (1927–1932)*			*B. Smithwick Controls (1941–1945)*			*Statistical Significance*
		Alive at 5 to 9 yr			*Alive at 5 to 9 yr*		
	No. of Patients	*No.*	*%*	*No. of Patients*	*No.*	*%*	*Group B Versus Group A*
Group I	7	4	57	64	32	50	0
Group II	14	4	29	36	11	31	0
Group III	22	2	9	48	4	8	0
Group IV	99	0	0	26	0	0	0
Total	142			174			

Classification of Eye-ground	*C. K.W.B. Series + Smithwick Controls (1927–1945)*			*D. Smithwick Surgical Patients (1938–1944)*			*Statistical Significance*			
		Alive at 5 to 9 yr			*Alive at 5 to 9 yr*		*Group D Versus Group C*		*Group D Versus Normals*	
	No. of Patients	*No.*	*%*	*No. of Patients*	*No.*	*%*	X^2	*P*	X^2	*P*
Group I	71	36	51	101	77	76	11.0	$< .001$	6.0	$< .05$
Group II	50	15	30	60	37	62	9.7	$< .01$	11.6	$< .001$
Group III	70	6	9	96	41	43	21.6	$< .001$	45.0	$< .001$
Group IV	125	0	0	43	13	30	36.8	$< .001$	30.4	$< .001$
Total	316			300						

The increased survival rate for the surgical patients (D versus C) is highly significant for all four groups. On the other hand, the survival rates of all four groups of surgical patients are significantly lower than those of the male population of comparable age (88%). Thus the survival rate for Group I patients with sexes combined, when compared with normals as indicated in Figure 1, does not apply to males, but does apply to females (Table 3), again emphasizing the advisability of evaluating the sexes separately.

TABLE 3.—*Five- to 9-Year Survivals in Female Hypertensives Classified According to Keith, Wagener, and Barker Eyeground Groups*

Classification of Eye-ground	A. K.W.B. Series (1927–1932)			B. Smithwick Controls (1941–1945)			Statistical Significance
	No. of Patients	Alive at 5 to 9 yr		No. of Patients	Alive at 5 to 9 yr		Group B Versus Group A
		No.	%		No.	%	
Group I	3	2	67	47	33	70	0
Group II	12	5	42	33	21	64	0
Group III	15	1	7	25	5	20	0
Group IV	47	1	2	12	0	0	0
Total	77			117			

Classification of Eye-ground	C. K.W.B. Series + Smithwick Controls (1927–1945)			D. Smithwick Surgical Patients (1938–1944)			Statistical Significance			
	No. of Patients	Alive at 5 to 9 yr		No. of Patients	Alive at 5 to 9 yr		Group D Versus Group C		Group D Versus Normals	
		No.	%		No.	%	X^2	P	X^2	P
Group I	50	35	70	150	133	89	8.4	$< .01$	.03	$< .90$
Group II	45	26	58	87	71	82	7.5	$< .01$	1.7	$< .20$
Group III	40	6	15	65	43	66	24.0	$< .001$	8.7	$< .01$
Group IV	59	1	2	35	16	46	25.8	$< .001$	14.9	$< .001$
Total	194			337						

The survival rates of all groups treated surgically are significantly higher than those of the controls (D versus C). The survival rates of Groups I and II, surgical series, do not differ significantly from those of the female population of comparable age (90%). Those of Groups III and IV, however, are significantly lower.

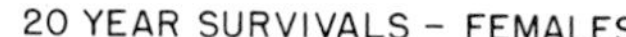

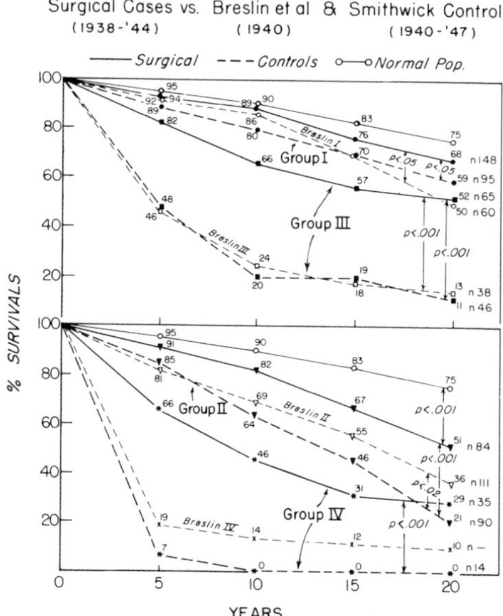

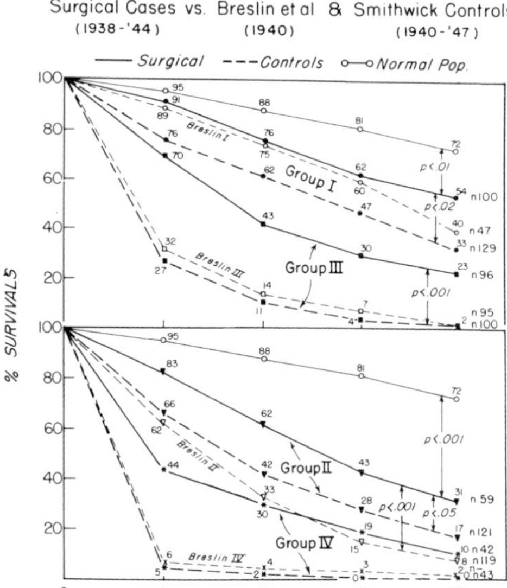

FIG. 2.—There are no important differences between the survival rates of the two control series of patients. The surgical survival rates are higher than those of one or both of the control series. The differences are statistically significant for Group I, II and III cases. The survival rate of Group I males is significantly lower than that of the male population of comparable age. For the first 10 years, the survival rate of the Breslin, Gifford, and Fairbain series [40] is uninfluenced by antihypertensive drugs. Thereafter (from 1950) the survivors in all three series were exposed to drugs and we presume many received them. The direct or ad hoc method was used to calculate the survival rates.

FIG. 3.—The 20-year survival rates of the two control series are similar for Group I, III, and IV while that of the Breslin, Gifford, and Fairbain [40] Group II is higher. The survival rates of all four surgical groups are higher than those of one or both control groups. The differences are statistically significant for Group I, II, and III patients. The survival rate for Group I surgical females is not significantly different from that of the female population of comparable age, but that of the Group I controls is significantly lower. All survivors could have received antihypertensive drugs from 1950 onward. The direct or ad hoc method was used to calculate survival rates.

Clinic patients in which the 20-year survival rates were determined for 540 traced patients in whom the diagnosis of hypertension was made in the year 1940. The cases were divided by sex and the four eyeground classifications. This material is presented in Figure 2 for males and in Figure 3 for females. We have added comparable numbers of Smithwick's control surgical patients for comparison. Survival rates are given at 5-year intervals for 20 years. Since antihypertensive drugs came into general usage in 1950, it is probable that the series of Breslin, Gifford, and Fairbain [40] was influenced by their use in the last 10 years of the follow-up period. For our patients, the period of exposure was even greater since we had to include patients studied during the years 1940–1947 and operated upon during the years 1938–1944 in order to obtain adequate numbers for comparison with the Breslin series. Thus the curves do not truly represent the natural history of the disease. They are useful, however, for judging survival partially influenced by drugs and for judging the effectiveness of splanchnicectomy as a method of treatment.

Twenty-five-Year Survival Rates As Influenced By Exposure to Antihypertensive Drugs

The survival rates for Smithwick's control patients studied during the years 1938–1945

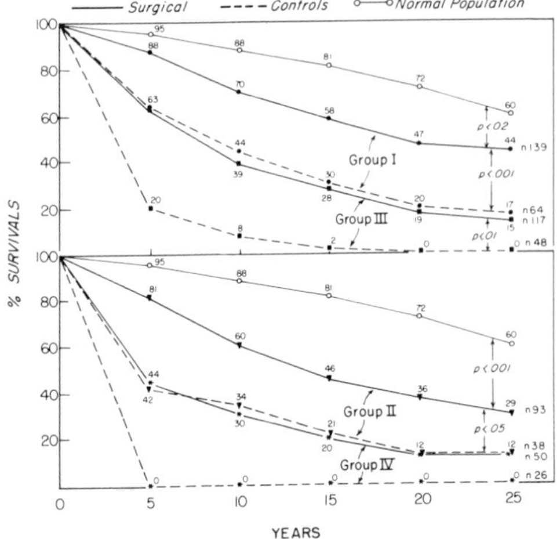

FIG. 4.—The 25-year survival rates of the surgically treated patients are higher than those of the controls in all four groups significantly so for Group I, II, and III patients. The survival rate of the surgical Group I patients is significantly lower than that of the male population of comparable age. The actuarial method was used to calculate the survival rates.

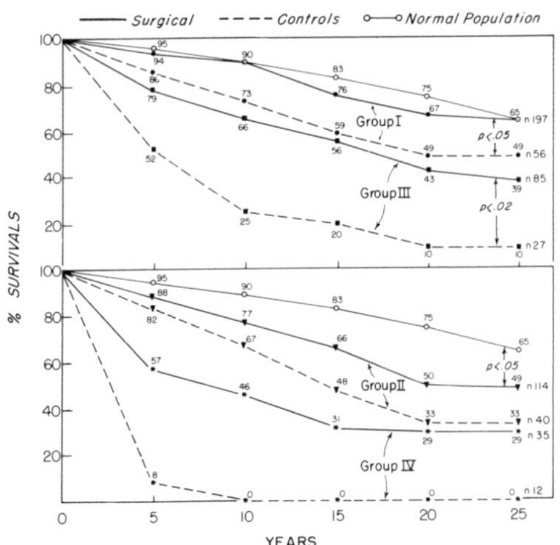

FIG. 5.—The survival rates of the surgical patients are significantly higher than those of the controls in all four groups. The differences are statistically significant for Groups I, III, and IV. The 25-year survival rate of Group I surgical females is almost identical with that of the female population of comparable age, but that of the Group I female controls is significantly lower. The actuarial method was used to calculate survival rates.

are compared with those of his surgical cases operated on during the years 1938–1945 in Figures 4 (males) and 5 (females). These were the earliest reported patients in both series and consequently had minimal (but equal) exposure to the possible use of antihypertensive drugs from 1950 onward. As indicated by Figure 4 the survival rates of all male surgical groups are higher than those of the corresponding control groups. The differences are statistically significant for patients in Groups I, II, and III. The survival rates for all male surgical patients and controls are significantly different from those of the male population as a whole of comparable age. This is in contrast to the findings in Figure 5, which show that there is no difference between the survival rates of the female surgical Group I cases and those of the female population as a whole of comparable age. The survival rate of the Group I female controls is, however, significantly lower. This is of course also true for the Group II, III, and IV controls. The survival rates of all groups of female surgical patients are higher than those of the corresponding controls. The differences are statistically significant for Groups I and III.

ONE- TO 25-YEAR SURVIVAL RATES AS INFLUENCED BY MAXIMAL EXPOSURE TO ANTIHYPERTENSIVE DRUGS

The patients who had maximal exposure to antihypertensive drugs are those studied or operated upon during the years 1938–1966 and followed up through 1967. This is especially true of the controls since 1,135 (57%) were first seen between 1950 and 1966 when antihypertensive drugs became available, while 878 (31%) of the surgical patients were operated upon during that period. The findings are shown in Figures 6 (males) and 7 (females). The outstanding finding in Figure 6 is that for the first time in any of our surveys, the survival rates of the Group I controls did not differ

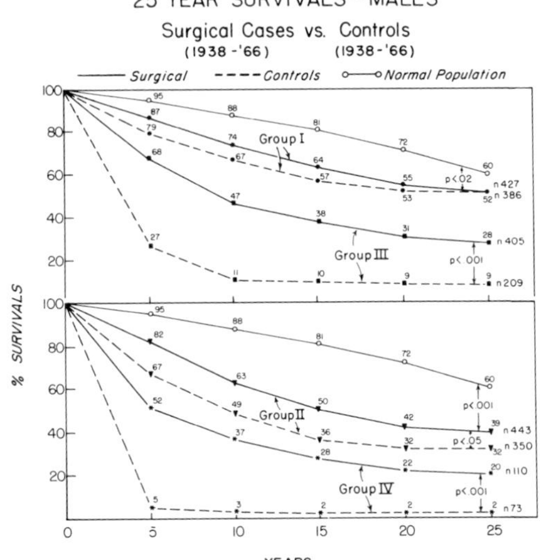

FIG. 6.—This figure contains survival curves covering our entire experience with male hypertensive patients. Every patient who was operated on or studied during the years 1938–1966 and followed through 1967 is included. There were 1,385 male surgical patients and 1,018 male controls. The 25-year survival rates were calculated by the actuarial method and are given at 5-year intervals.

The outstanding finding has to do with the Group I patients in whom for the first time the survival rate of the controls at the end of the period of observation did not differ significantly from that of the surgical patients. The survival rates of both Group I surgical patients and controls were significantly lower than those of the male population as a whole of comparable age. The survival rates of the Group II, III, and IV surgical patients were significantly higher than those of the corresponding control patients. The difference between the survival rates of the Group II, III, and IV surgical patients, and the control patients as well, is significantly lower than that of the male population of comparable age. Deaths from all causes are included in calculating survival rates. The operative mortality rates were: Group I, 1.9 percent; Group II, 3.2 percent; Group III, 4.7 percent; and Group IV, 5.5 percent.

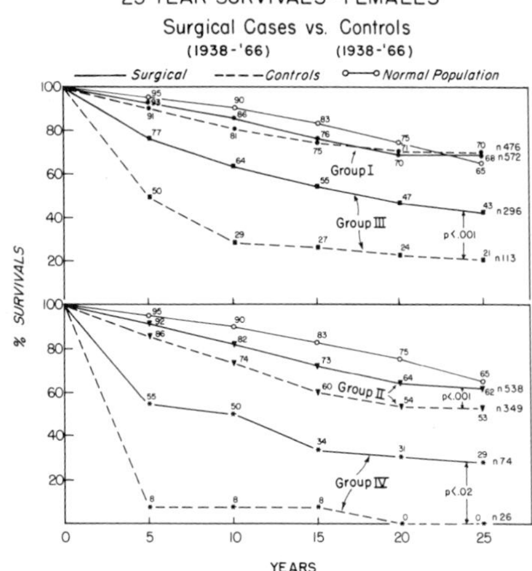

FIG. 7.—This figure contains survival curves covering the entire experience with female hypertensive patients. Every patient who was operated on or studied during the years 1938–1966 and followed through 1967 is included. There were 1,480 surgical and 964 control patients. The actuarial method was used for calculating 25-year survival rates. These are given at 5-year intervals. The outstanding finding was that, as with the males, the survival rate of the Group I female controls was not significantly different from that of the Group I female surgical patients.

The survival rate of the Group I surgical females was not different significantly from that of the female population as a whole of comparable age. However, that was noted before in previous comparisons (Table 3, Figs. 3 and 5). The survival rate of Group II surgical females did not differ significantly from that of the female population as a whole. This also had been noted previously (Table 3). The difference between the survival rates of the Group II, III, and IV surgical patients and those of the corresponding controls is significant. On the other hand, the difference between the survival rates of the Group III and IV surgical patients and Group II, III, and IV controls is significantly below that of the female population of comparable age.

Deaths from all causes are included in calculating survival rates. The operative mortality was: Group I, 0.9 percent; Group II, 1.3 percent; Group III, 5.7 percent; and Group IV, 6.7 percent.

materially from those of the Group I surgical patients; in fact, at 25 years the rates were the same, i.e., 52 percent. By contrast, in Figure 4, the survival rates for Group I control and surgical patients were 17 and 44 percent ($P < 0.001$) respectively. These patients did not have as much exposure to antihypertensive drugs. Figure 7 reveals the same findings for females. The 25-year survival rates for Group I controls and surgical patients were 70 and

68 percent respectively. In Figure 5, which contains females who had much less exposure to the use of drugs, the corresponding rates were 49 and 65 percent ($P < 0.05$). In the other comparisons we have made (Tables 2 and 3, and Figs. 2 and 3) a significant difference between control Group I and the surgical Group I survival rates was apparent. The patients either had no exposure to effective drugs or were exposed to them for a much shorter period of time. The fact that the prognosis for our patients followed up for 5 years improved significantly for those studied after 1950, by comparison with those studied before, has previously been noted.[41] Figure 6 also shows that survival rates of the males in Group I are significantly lower for controls and surgical patients alike than are rates for the normal population of comparable age. Of course, those of Groups II, III, and IV are very markedly lower. The survival rates of the Group II, III, and IV surgical patients are significantly higher than those of the corresponding controls. Figure 7 shows that the survival rate of the Group I surgical patients is not significantly different from that of the female population at 25 years. The same is true of the controls. The survival rate of the Group II female surgical patients also is virtually the same as that of the female population as a whole at 25 years. That of the Group II controls and, of course, those of Group II and IV patients are significantly lower. The survival rates of the Group II, III, and IV surgical patients were significantly higher than those of the corresponding controls.

We feel that the material in Figures 6 and 7 is most representative of the results of splanchnicectomy and of the outcome of the controls so far as survival rates are concerned. The results are influenced without doubt by the patients' exposure to antihypertensive drugs from 1950–1967. The extent to which drugs were used is unknown but we believe most patients received them during this portion of the follow-up. The data contained in Figures 6 and 7 will be used to compare the survival rates following splanchnicectomy and of the controls with those of series of patients selected from the literature who had adequate antihypertensive drug treatment.

Splanchnicectomy

Extent of Operation

Before comparing the results of surgery with those of antihypertensive drug treatment, a few comments about splanchnicectomy would seem appropriate. When the operation of lumbodorsal splanchnicectomy was developed,[3] its extent was based upon physiologic evidence of postoperative postural hypotension, in order to be sure that the splanchnic bed was thoroughly denervated. Our previous studies had revealed that partial denervation was not as effective. There were no effective antihypertensive drugs at that time to supplement the effect of splanchnicectomy. The operation was performed in two stages, 10 days to 2 weeks apart. Shortly after it became apparent that effective antihypertensive drugs were available (soon after 1950), we decided to decrease the magnitude of the operation somewhat and to supplement it with antihypertensive drugs as needed. We then modified the operation [28,31] by removing the sympathetic trunks from D9 through D12 bilaterally, which included the lesser and least splanchnic nerves as well, and the great splanchnic nerves from the celiac ganglion to the midthoracic regions. We were able to perform this operation bilaterally in one stage. Postural hypotension was mild, the hospital stay averaged about 2 weeks, the convalescent period thereafter was comparatively short, i.e., a month or so for most patients, and persistent untoward secondary side effects were negligible. This combination of a less extensive splanchnicectomy with supplementary drugs as needed has worked out well. Of 585 of the surgical patients we followed up in 1970 on whom we have data regarding drugs, 354 (61%) were receiving medication and 39 percent were not. Most commonly, a modest amount of a diuretic was used. This was sometimes supplemented by one of the *Rauwolfia* compounds. The combination of a conservative splanchnicectomy, with supplementary use of drugs as needed, makes a satisfactory substitute for treatment with antihypertensive drugs alone in cases that are difficult to control or when patients will not follow the regimen conscientiously or when the combined regimen is preferred by the patient.

TABLE 4.—*Percentage of Survivals in Group I Hypertensives*

		Males						*Females*					
			Alive at						*Alive at*				
Author	*Treatment*	*No. of Patients*	*5 yr*	*10 yr*	*15 yr*	*20 yr*	*25 yr*	*No. of Patients*	*5 yr*	*10 yr*	*15 yr*	*20 yr*	*25 yr*
a.													
Breslin controls (Figs. 2 and 3)	Unknown	47	89	75	60	40		60	96	86	70	50	
Smithwick controls (Figs. 6 and 7)	Unknown	385	79	67	57	53	52	476	91	81	75	71	70
			++				O						O
Smithwick surgical patients	Splanchnicectomy	427	87	74	64	55	52	572	93	86	76	70	68
		+++				+++	+++	++	+				+++
							+++						+
					Group II								
b.													
Breslin controls (Figs. 2 and 3)	Unknown	119	62	33	15	8		111	81	69	55	36	
Smithwick controls (Figs. 6 and 7)	Unknown	350	67	49	36	32	32	349	86	74	60	54	53
							+						+++
Smithwick surgical patients (Figs. 6 and 7)	Splanchnicectomy	443	82	63	50	42	39	538	92	82	72	64	62
					Groups I and II								
c.													
Breslin controls (Figs. 2 and 3)	Unknown	166	70	45	29	17		171	86	75	60	41	
			O						O				
Smithwick controls (Figs. 6 and 7)	Unknown	735	73	58	47	43	42	825	89	78	67	64	63
			++						+++				
Smirk controls [42]	None	77	56					122	75				
			++						O				
Smirk controls [42]	Antihypertensive drugs	92	76					178	85				
			O						+++				
			+										
Breckinridge, Dollery and Parry [43]		362	83					422	94++				
			O						O				
Smithwick surgical patients (Figs. 6 and 7)	Splanchnicectomy	870	85	68	57	48	45	1110	92	84	74	67	65

The symbols O, +, ++, and +++ relate to statistical significance of comparisons: O, not significant; +, P < .05; ++, P < .01; +++, P < .001. See text for further comments.

Five- to 10-year Survival Rates in Controls and Patients Treated By Drug Therapy or Surgery

We have been unable to find a follow-up study giving survival rates for Group I or II patients, divided according to the two sexes, and adequately treated with antihypertensive drugs. We have therefore selected two series of patients treated with drugs, divided by sex and eyeground classifications, with Groups I and II combined to compare with controls and surgically treated patients (Table 4, part c). In Table 4 (part a) we have repeated the data for the controls of Breslin et al. (Figs. 2 and 3) and for Smithwick's controls and surgical patients (Figs. 6 and 7) in Group I. In Table 4 (part b) similar data are tabulated for Group II patients. We have done this in order to emphasize the marked difference between Group I and II patients' survival rates. Some of the differences which have statistical significance are indicated. As previously stated, the difference between the two groups is that all Group II patients have arteriovenous compression and this finding occurs in all Group I patients. In other words, Group II patients have clear-cut evidence of sclerosis. Breslin, Gifford, and Fairbain [40] have also emphasized that the differentiating feature between Group I and II patients is evidence of sclerosis.

With regard to the comparisons made in Table 4 (part c) where Groups I and II are combined, the marked differences in survival rates according to sex are obvious. At 5 years, the survival rate of Smirk's controls is significantly lower than that of the Breslin or Smithwick controls. This applies equally to males and females. The survival of Smirk's treated males is significantly higher than that of his controls. For males, the survival rate of Smirk's treated series is not significantly different from that of the Breckinridge series, but is significantly lower than that of Smithwick's surgical series. There is no significant difference between the survivals of Breckinridge's patients and Smithwick's surgical male patients. For females, the survival of Smirk's controls is significantly lower than that of the Breslin or Smithwick controls. Also, the survival rate of Smirk's treated patients is significantly lower than that of the Breckinridge series or the Smithwick surgical patients, while there is no significant difference in the survival rates of the latter two series. How they will compare after 25 years of observation time alone will tell.

In Table 5 (part a) the survival rates of the controls of Breslin and Smithwick are compared with those of the treated Group III patients of Farmer, Gifford, and Hines,[44] and Breckinridge, Dollery, and Parry,[43] and Smithwick. At 5 years, the survival rates of treated male patients were significantly higher than those of the controls. The survival rate of the series of Beckinridge et al. was significantly higher than that of the Smithwick surgical series at 5 years. This is the only comparison in which the survival rate of patients treated with antihypertensive drugs exceeded by a significant percentage that of patients treated by splanchnicectomy. What the comparisons would show at 25 years cannot be predicted. At 6 years, the surgical survivals significantly exceeded those of the antihypertensive-drug-treated patients of Farmer, Gifford, and Hines.[44] At 5 years, the treated female patients fared significantly better than the controls and there was no significant difference in the survival rates of the drug and surgical series. At 6 years the survival rate of the surgical cases was significantly higher than that of the drug series of Farmer, Gifford, and Hines.[44] At 25 years the survival rates of Smithwick's surgical patients were significantly higher than those of the controls.

In Table 5 (part b) we have summarized the data for Group IV patients, those with so-called "malignant" hypertension. Here the difference between the sexes is not so apparent because the results are so much poorer than those of the Group I, II, and III patients. The difference in the 5-year survival rates of patients in Simpson's and Smirk's series is significant and would be so even at 10 years if the number of patients were larger. Generally, treated patients did much better than the controls and at 5 years there was little difference in efficacy between drug and surgical treatment. At 6 years the survival rate of the male and female surgical patients was significantly higher than that of the drug series of Farmer, Gifford, and Hines.[44] At 10 years the survival rate of the Smithwick surgical patients was significantly higher than that of the drug-treated

TABLE 5.—*Percentage of Survivals in Group III and IV Hypertensives*

		Group III Males							Group III Females						
			Alive at							*Alive at*					
Author	*Treatment*	*No. of Patients*	*5 yr*	*6 yr*	*10 yr*	*15 yr*	*20 yr*	*25 yr*	*No. of Patients*	*5 yr*	*6 yr*	*10 yr*	*15 yr*	*20 yr*	*25 yr*
a.															
Breslin controls (Figs. 2 and 3)	Unknown	95	32		14	7	2		38	46		24	18	13	
Smithwick controls (Figs. 6 and 7)	Unknown	209	27	20	11	10	9	9	113	50	42	29	27	24	21
				O							O				
Farmer, Gifford, and Hines [44]	Antihypertensive drugs	67		27				+++	27		48				
			+++							+++					
Breckinridge, Dollery, and Parry [43]	Unknown	83	81	+++					64	86	+				+++
			+							O					
Smithwick surgical patients (Figs. 6 and 7)	Splanchnicectomy	405	68	63	47	38	31	28	296	77	73	64	55	47	43

		Group IV Males							Group IV Females						
			Alive at							*Alive at*					
Author	*Treatment*	*No. of Patients*	*5 yr*	*6 yr*	*10 yr*	*15 yr*	*20 yr*	*25 yr*	*No. of Patients*	*5 yr*	*6 yr*	*10 yr*	*15 yr*	*20 yr*	*25 yr*
b.															
Breslin controls (Figs. 2 and 3)	Unknown	53	6		4		2		22	19		14	12	10	
Smithwick controls (Figs. 6 and 7)	Unknown	73	5	3	3	2	2	2	26	8	8	8	8	0	O
Farmer, Gifford, and Hines [44]	Antihypertensive drugs	41	+++	24					20	+++	20				+++
Simpson and Smirk [45]	Antihypertensive drugs	43	36		19			+++	27	62		31			
			O	++						O	+				
Breckinridge, Dollery, and Parry [43]	Antihypertensive drugs	49	47 O		+				50	48		O			
			O							O					
Smithwick surgical patients (Figs. 6 and 7)	Splanchnicectomy	110	52	47	37	28	22	20	74	55	53	50	34	31	29

The symbols O, +, ++, and +++ relate to statistical significance of comparisons; O, not significant; +, $P < 0.05$; ++, $P < 0.01$; +++, $P < 0.001$. See text for further comments.

series of Simpson and Smirk. The drop of about 50 percent in the 10-year survival rate of both males and females in the Simpson and Smirk series by comparison with that at 5 years is of interest since all patients who did not remain on antihypertensive drugs were eliminated from consideration. In Tables 4 (part c) and 5 (parts a and b), 16 comparisons have been made between the 5- and 10-year results of antihypertensive drug treatment and splanchnicectomy. Antihypertensive drug treatment was significantly better in one patient, the two methods were equally effective in eight, and the results of splanchnicectomy were significantly better in seven.

In Table 6, we have summarized data from the literature pertaining to survival rates for Group IV patients with the sexes combined. While the outlook for females is better than for males, the difference is not so significant statistically as it is for patients in Groups I, II, and III. The marked improvement in the survival of patients treated medically or surgically by comparison with that of the controls is very obvious.

Comment

Before any effective treatment for essential or malignant hypertension became available, the mortality rate for these patients was significantly higher than that of the population as a whole of comparable age. It was also higher for males than for females.

Splanchnicectomy was the first form of treatment which significantly increased the survival rates of patients with essential and malignant hypertension.

The statistical significance of its effect is indicated by comparisons of survival rates of control and surgical patients divided according to the four eyeground groups of Keith, Wagener, and Barker and followed up 5 to 9 years (Table 1 and Fig. 1) and for these same patients divided by sex as well (Tables 2 and 3). These comparisons establish the survival rates for untreated patients (controls) and also establish the value of splanchnicectomy since they were made prior to the availability of antihypertensive drugs (1950). There is a highly significant improvement in the survival rates of the surgical cases in all four groups for both sexes. The survival rates for Group I and II female surgical patients were improved so that they did not differ significantly from those of the female population of comparable age.

In Figures 2 (males) and 3 (females), comparisons are made between control patients of Breslin et al., controls of Smithwick, and Smithwick's surgical patients, all followed up for 20 years. The survival rates of the surgical patients are higher than those of the controls in all four groups, significantly so for the surgical patients of both sexes in Groups I, II, and III. Breslin's patients were followed up through 1960, the Smithwick surgical patients through 1964, and the Smithwick control patients through 1967, so that the results would have been influenced by antihypertensive drug usage from 1950 onward.

In Figures 4 (males) and 5 (females) survival rates are given at 5-year intervals for 25 years. Smithwick's controls and surgical patients operated on during the years 1938–1945 and followed up through 1965 are compared. All these patients were studied or operated upon prior to the advent of antihypertensive drugs but the results could have been influenced by them from 1950 through 1965. The exposure to the possible effect of drugs is, however, considerably less than that of the patients included in Figures 6 and 7. This represents a 20- to 27-year follow-up of the 575 males (Fig. 4) and the 566 females (Fig. 5). The results have been described.

In Figures 6 (males) and 7 (females), survival rates are also given at 5-year intervals for 25 years. Smithwick's controls and surgical patients operated on during the years 1938–1966 and followed up through 1967 are compared. This is a summary of our entire experience. Figure 6 shows the treatment results in 2,403 males and includes all of those shown in Figure 4 plus an additional 1,828 (76%) studied or operated on after 1945. The treatment results of 2,444 patients are shown in Figure 7, including all of those seen in Figure 5 plus 1,878 patients (77%) studied or operated on after 1945.

The overall exposure of the patients shown in Figures 6 and 7 to the possible effects of antihypertensive drugs was much greater than that of the patients in Figures 4 and 5. The 4,847 patients described in Figures 6 and 7 were followed up from 1 to 29 years. The

TABLE 6.—*Percentage of Survivals in Group IV Hypertensives (Sexes Combined)*

Author	*Treatment*	*No. of Patients*	*Alive at* 5 yr	6 yr	8 yr	10 yr	12 yr	15 yr	20 yr	25 yr	
Keith, Wagener, and Barker (Table 1)	None	146	1								
Smithwick (Table 5b)	Unknown	99	5			4	4	3	1	1	Controls
Breslin (Table 5b)	Unknown	75	10			7			4		
Harrington [46]	Antihypertensive drugs	82	23								
Farmer (Table 5b)	Antihypertensive drugs	61		23							
Simpson and Smirk (Table 5b)	Antihypertensive drugs	70	45			23					Drugs
Perry et al.[47]	Antihypertensive drugs	97	48				41				
Breckinridge (Table 5b)	Antihypertensive drugs	99	48								
Björk et al.[48]	Antihypertensive drugs	93	50								
Peet and Isberg [49]	Splanchnicectomy	143	22			10					
Sellers et al.[7] *	Splanchnicectomy and adrenalectomy	68 22				53	 45				Surgery
Smithwick (Table 5b)	Splanchnicectomy	184	53	49		42	40	30	24	22	

* Smithwick Group IV (similar prognosis). The prognosis for treated cases is greatly improved over that of the controls. No statistical comparisons were attempted since the proportion of males and females is unknown for the most part, and there are other important differences in the patient material contained in the different series.

duration of follow-up was from 10 to 29 years in 92 percent of the patients and less than 10 years in 8 percent. A follow-up of 4,470 of 4,847 patients for 10 to 29 years is adequate to bring out any significant differences between the survival rates of control and surgical patients. We believe that the survival rates, based on the use of all of our patient material as shown in Figures 6 and 7, are the most accurate and representative of any of the data we have presented. These are the rates which will be used in the various comparisons to be made.

A comparison of the survival curves in Figures 6 and 7 reveals clear-cut differences from those seen in Figures 4 and 5, especially as regards the Group I controls. The fact that at 25 years, for the first time in any of the comparisons we have made, there is no difference between the survival rates of Group I controls and the corresponding surgical patients indicates that a very significant improvement in the prognosis of Group I patients has taken place. We believe that this is due to greater exposure to (and use of) antihypertensive drugs. It is not thought to be related to the statistical calculations.

The data in Figure 7 suggest that Group I female patients, if adequately treated with antihypertensive drugs, could very well have a normal life expectancy for 25 years or more. This has been the case for the Group I and II surgical patients. Figure 6 reveals that the Group I surgical and control males, with identical survival rates (52%), did not have a normal (60%) survival rate. The rate for the controls was markedly improved over that shown in Figure 4 (17%). This is further evidence of the fact that the male does not tolerate hypertension as well as the female. To achieve a normal survival rate for males it may be necessary to institute treatment earlier, in the stage of intermittent hypertension (resting or home diastolic blood pressure readings below 90 mm Hg, ambulatory readings elevated). The patients described in Figures 6 and 7 and, in fact, in all of Smithwick's control and surgical series, were regarded as having continued hypertension, that is, a diastolic blood pressure of 90 mm Hg or more in the resting horizontal position throughout a period of several days' hospitalization and study, except for levels during the sedative test. In a recent Veterans Administration Cooperative Study,[50] it was found that among males, whose ambulatory diastolic pressures averaged 90 to 114 mm Hg during their last two clinic visits, there was a statistically significant ($P < 0.001$) progression of cardiovascular disease (incidence of morbid events) among controls followed up an average of 3.9 years compared with that noted among patients treated with antihypertensive drugs for an average of 3.7 years. When the diastolic levels averaged 115 to 129 mm Hg, an equally significant progression of vascular disease developed in about half the time.[51] The extent to which antihypertensive drugs have altered survival rates is indicated by the data contained in Tables 4 through 6. Unfortunately the follow-up studies are of comparatively short duration.

Summary and Conclusions

Splanchnicectomy is the first form of treatment which significantly increased the survival rate of patients with essential and malignant hypertension. The differences between the survival rates of surgical and control patients are statistically significant for all four Keith, Wagener, and Barker eyeground groups (Table 1 and Fig. 1) and for all comparisons when divided by sex as well (Tables 2 and 3). These observations were made prior to the advent of effective antihypertensive drugs (1950). They involve comparatively small numbers of cases followed for relatively short periods of time.

The advent of antihypertensive drugs has modified the natural history of the disease. It has influenced the survival rate of controls and surgical patients as well. It, therefore, is not possible to describe our entire experience with the problem of hypertension from 1938 through 1967 except as influenced by exposure to (and the use of) drugs.

We have attempted to describe the results by comparing relatively small numbers of control and surgical patients studied and operated upon prior to the appearance of the drugs, but whose course was influenced by exposure to them for a portion of the follow-up period of 20 to 27 years (Figs. 2 through 5).

We have also described the outcome when all our patient material, concerning patients studied or operated upon during the years 1938–1966 and followed up through 1967, is used. This involves much larger groups of patients having a far greater exposure to antihypertensive drugs. In 92 percent of the patients, the follow-up period ranged from 10 to 29 years. We feel that calculations involving our entire experience with hypertensive patients are the ones upon which conclusions regarding survival rates of our control and surgical patients should be based (Figs. 6 and 7).

On this basis, there has been a striking and highly significant improvement in the prognosis of the Group I controls. The 25-year survival rates of the control and surgical Group I patients are virtually identical (Figs. 6 and 7) and significantly higher than those of the Group I controls shown in Figures 4 and 5. The 25-year survival rates of the female Group I control and Group I and II surgical patients are not significantly different from those of the female population as a whole of comparable age. The 25-year survival rates of the Group II, III, and IV surgical patients were significantly higher than those of the controls.

Survival rates for series of patients treated with antihypertensive drugs are compared with those of Smithwick's surgical patients in Tables 4 through 6. The comparisons are for short periods of time, 5 to 10 years. Longer follow-up studies of patients treated with antihypertensive drugs are needed, especially for Groups I and II. The findings indicate that antihypertensive drugs as well as splanchnicectomy have significantly increased the survival rates of hypertensive patients. Both have their limitations, and when treatment is instituted in the more advanced stages, nothing approximating a normal life expectancy should be expected.

A conservative splanchnicectomy, supplemented by antihypertensive drugs as needed, has been helpful in the management of hypertension which is difficult to control with drugs or when patients will not follow a medical regimen.

The extraordinary improvement in the prognosis which we have observed over the years among our Group I controls leads us to suspect that antihypertensive drug treatment, if instituted early enough, may result in a normal or near-normal life expectancy for cooperative patients for a period of 25 years or more. It may, however, be necessary to institute treatment earlier in males than in females to obtain such results.

Acknowledgments

Acknowledgment of great indebtedness to hundreds of persons who have helped with this project over a period of some 35 years is very much in order. Among these are large numbers of interns, residents, nurses, technicians, and secretaries, as well as close medical and surgical associates who have helped with the study and care of these patients. The late G. P. Whitlaw, M.D., who supervised the surgical management of these patients, was of inestimable assistance, as was Dera Kinsey, M.D., who supervised the medical management of these patients. Grants-in-aid have been received and acknowledged over the years from various private, state, and federal sources. Many patients have made generous donations as well. Without this support this study could not have been continued. Sincere thanks are due Miss Rita Waldron for many years of faithful and skillful assistance with technical and statistical matters and to Miss Katherine Kirrane, who has been present from start to finish and who has supervised the follow-up studies, the management of personnel, and various other very important aspects of the project. Sincere thanks are also due Mr. John Alman, Director, Computer Center, Boston University, and Professor Herbert Kayne of the Boston University School of Medicine for their invaluable advice regarding the interpretation and use of and assistance with the handling of the statistical material. Most sincere thanks are due the Trustees of the University Hospital (formerly the Massachusetts Memorial Hospital), who approved the establishment of the Smithwick Foundation in 1946 and through it have given continued support to this project. Without their help and understanding, this study could not have been carried on to its conclusion.

References

1. Craig, W. M.: Surgical approach to and resection of the splanchnic nerves for relief of hypertension and abdominal pain. West. J. Surg. 42:146, 1934.
2. Peet, M. M.: Splanchnic resection for hypertension. A preliminary report. Univ. Mich. Med. Bull. 1:17, 1935.
3. Smithwick, R. H.: A technique for splanchnic resection for hypertension. Preliminary report. Surgery 1:1, 1940.

4. Crile, G.: The Surgical Treatment of Hypertension. Philadelphia: Saunders, 1936.
5. Grimson, K. S.: Total thoracic and partial to total lumbar sympathectomy and celiac ganglionectomy in treatment of hypertension. Ann. Surg. 114:753, 1941.
6. Grimson, K. S.: Sympathetic ganglionectomy. Results of treatment. *In* Moyer, J. H. (Ed.): Hypertension. The First Hahnemann Symposium on Hypertension. Philadelphia: Saunders, 1959, pp. 690–694.
7. Sellers, A. M., Barrett, J. S., Wolferth, C. C., Sr., Lopez, R., Itskovitz, H. D., Blakemore, W. S., and Zintel, H. A.: Adrenalectomy and sympathectomy for hypertension. Ten-year survival. Arch. Surg. 89:880, 1964.
8. Castleman, B., and Smithwick, R. H.: The relation of vascular disease to the hypertensive state. Based on a study of renal biopsies from 100 hypertensive patients. JAMA 121: 1256, 1943.
9. Talbott, J. H., Castleman, B., Smithwick, R. H., Melville, R. S., and Pecora, L. J.: Renal biopsy studies correlated with renal clearance observations in hypertensive patients treated by radical sympathectomy. J. Clin. Invest. 22:387, 1943.
10. Rojas, F., Smithwick, R. H., and White, P. D.: Nonspecific major operations and lumbodorsal sympathectomy. A comparison between their effects on the blood pressure. JAMA 126:15, 1944.
11. White, P. D., Smithwick, R. H., Mathews, M. W., and Evans, E.: The electrocardiogram in hypertension. Am. Heart J. 30:165, 1945.
12. Bridges, W. C., Johnson, A. L., Smithwick, R. H., and White, P. D.: Electrocardiography in hypertension. Study of patients subjected to lumbodorsal splanchnicectomy. JAMA 131:1476, 1946.
13. Newell, J. H., and Smithwick, R. H.: Pregnancy following lumbodorsal splanchnicectomy for essential and malignant hypertension and hypertension associated with chronic pyelonephritis. N. Engl. J. Med. 236:851, 1947.
14. Smithwick, R. H.: The surgical treatment of continued hypertension. Some suggestions about the selection of cases for this form of therapy. J. Med. Soc. N. J. 44:304, 1947.
15. Freis, E. D., and Smithwick, R. H.: The effect of lumbodorsal splanchnicectomy for the blood volume and "thiocyanate space" of patients with essential hypertension. Am. J. Med. Sci. 214:363, 1947.
16. Smithwick, R. H.: Surgical treatment of hypertension. Am. J. Med. 14:744, 1948.
17. Smithwick, R. H.: Continued hypertension: Prognosis for surgically treated patients. Br. Med. J. 2:237, 1948.
18. Wilkins, R. W., Culbertson, J. W., and Smithwick, R. H.: The effects of various types of sympathectomy upon vasopressor responses in hypertensive patients. Surg. Gynec. Obstet. 87:661, 1948.
19. Smithwick, R. H.: Surgical treatment of hypertension. *In* Andrus, W. DeW. (Ed.): Advances in Surgery, vol. 11. New York: Interscience, 1949, pp. 81–153.
20. Smithwick, R. H., and Robertson, C. W.: The phenomenon of hyperreactivity. Definition and illustrations. Angiology 2:143, 1951.
21. Whitelaw, G. P., and Smithwick, R. H.: Effect of extensive sympathectomy upon blood pressure response and levels. Angiology 2: 157, 1951.
22. Smithwick, R. H.: Hypertensive cardiovascular disease. The effect of thoracolumbar splanchnicectomy upon mortality and survival rates. JAMA 147:1611, 1951.
23. White, J. C., Smithwick, R. H., and Simeone, F. A.: The Autonomic Nervous System. Anatomy, Physiology and Surgical Application, 3rd ed. New York: Macmillan, 1952, pp. 296–350; 420–430.
24. Smithwick, R. H., and Thompson, J. E.: Splanchnicectomy for essential hypertension. Results in 1266 cases. JAMA 152:1501, 1953.
25. Smithwick, R. H., Bush, R. D., Kinsey, D., and Whitelaw, G. P.: Hypertension and associated cardiovascular disease. Comparison of male and female mortality rates and their influence on selection of therapy. JAMA 160: 1023, 1955.
26. Smithwick, R. H.: Splanchnicectomy in the treatment of essential hypertension. *In* Moyer, J. H. (Ed.): Hypertension. The First Hahnemann Symposium on Hypertension. Philadelphia: Saunders, 1959, pp. 681–690.
27. Smithwick, R. H., Whitelaw, G. P., and Kinsey, D.: Surgical measures in the present day management of hypertension. *In* Brest, A. N., and Moyer, J. H. (Eds.): Hypertension. Recent advances, The Second Hahnemann Symposium on Hypertensive Disease. Philadelphia: Lea & Febiger, 1961, pp. 603–618.
28. Smithwick, R. H.: Thoracic and thoracolumbar sympathectomy and vagotomy. *In* Gibbon, J. H., Jr. (Ed.): Surgery of the Chest. Philadelphia: Saunders, 1962, pp. 300–325.

29. Kinsey, D., Whitelaw, G. P., Walther, R. W., Theophilis, C. A., and Smithwick, R. H.: The long-term follow up of malignant hypertension. JAMA 181:571, 1962.
30. Whitelaw, G. P., Kinsey, D., and Smithwick, R. H.: Factors influencing the choice of treatment in essential hypertension. Surgical, medical, or a combination of both. Am. J. Surg. 107:219, 1964.
31. Smithwick, R. H.: Splanchnicectomy. *In* Cooper, P. (Ed.): The Craft of Surgery. Boston: Little, Brown, 1971, pp. 1723–1726.
32. Turner, R.: "Medical sympathectomy" in hypertension. A clinical study of methonium compounds. Lancet 2:353, 1950.
33. Blackford, J. M., Bowers, J. M., and Baker, J. W.: A follow-up study of hypertension. JAMA 94:328, 1930.
34. Keith, N. M., Wagener, H. P., and Barker, N. W.: Some different types of essential hypertension: Their course and prognosis. Am. J. Med. Sci. 197:332, 1939.
35. Berkson, J., and Gage, R. P.: Calculation of survival rates for cancer. Mayo Clin. Proc. 25:270, 1950.
36. Palmer, R. S., Loofbourow, D., and Doering, C. R.: Prognosis in essential hypertension: Eight-year follow-up study of 430 patients on conventional medical treatment. N. Engl. J. Med. 239:990, 1948.
37. Hammarstrom, S., and Bechgaard, P.: Prognosis in arterial hypertension: A comparison between 251 patients after sympathectomy and a selected series of 435 non-operated patients. Am. J. Med. 8:53, 1950.
38. Smithwick, R. H.: Hypertensive cardiovascular disease. Effect of thoracolumbar splanchnicectomy on mortality and survival rates. JAMA 147:1611, 1951.
39. Björk, S., Sannerstedt, R., Falkheden, T., and Hood, B.: An analysis of survival rates in 381 cases on combined treatment with various hypotensive agents. Acta Med. Scand. 169:673, 1961.
40. Breslin, D. J., Gifford, R. W., Jr., and Fairbain, J. F.: Essential hypertension. A twenty year follow-up study. Circulation 33:87, 1966.
41. Kinsey, D., Sise, H. S., and Whitelaw, G. P.: Changes in mortality rates of treated hypertensive patients in a decade. Geriatrics 16: 397, 1961.
42. Smirk, F. H.: Observations on the mortality of 270 treated and 199 untreated retinal Grade I and II hypertensive patients followed in all instances for 5 years. N. Z. Med. J. 63: 413, 1964.
43. Breckinridge, A., Dollery, C. T., and Parry, E. H.: Prognosis of treated hypertension. Changes in life expectancy and causes of death between 1952 and 1967. Q. J. Med. 39: 411, 1970.
44. Farmer, R. G., Gifford, R. W., Jr., and Hines, E. A., Jr.: The effect of medical treatment of severe hypertension. A follow-up study of 161 patients with Group 3 and Group 4 hypertension. Arch. Intern. Med. 112:118, 1963.
45. Simpson, F. O., and Smirk, F. H.: The treatment of malignant hypertension. Am. J. Cardiol. 9:868, 1962.
46. Harrington, M.: Ganglion-blocking agents in hypertension. Med. Clin. North Am. 45:395, 1961.
47. Perry, H. M., Jr., Schroeder, H. A., Catanzaro, F. J., Moore-Jones, D., and Camel, G. H.: Studies on the control of hypertension. VIII. Mortality, morbidity and remissions during twelve years of intensive therapy. Circulation 33:958, 1966.
48. Björk, S., Sannerstedt, R., Angerwall, G., and Hood, B.: Treatment and prognosis in malignant hypertension. A clinical follow-up study of 93 patients on modern medical treatment. Acta Med. Scand. 166:175, 1960.
49. Peet, M. M., and Isberg, E. M.: The problem of malignant hypertension and its treatment by splanchnic resection. Ann. Intern. Med. 28:755, 1948.
50. Freis, E. D.: Effects of treatment on morbidity in hypertension. II. Results in patients with diastolic blood pressure averaging 90 through 114 mmHg. Veterans Administration Cooperative Study Group on antihypertensive agents. JAMA 213:1143, 1970.
51. Freis, E. D.: Effects of treatment on morbidity in hypertension. Results in patients with diastolic pressures averaging 115 through 129 mmHg. Veterans Administration Cooperative Study Group on antihypertensive drugs. JAMA 202:116, 1967.

The Role of Combined Adrenalectomy-Sympathectomy in the Treatment of Severe Arterial Hypertension

By Alfred M. Sellers, M.D.

BETWEEN THE YEARS of 1950 and 1959, at a time when available antihypertensive therapy was often ineffective, combined adrenalectomy and sympathectomy were performed in 171 patients with severe intractable hypertension.[1] With the advent of newer, more effective antihypertensive agents, primarily the thiazide diuretics and guanethidine, we have not found it necessary to employ this surgical treatment of hypertension since 1959. However, the excellent long-term survival of these patients with advanced vascular disease has prompted publication of these results as well as reëvaluation of the possible usefulness of this procedure in certain patients.

Historical Background

The first attempt to utilize subtotal adrenalectomy in the treatment of hypertension was by Crile in 1914.[2] In 1930 Pieri performed resection of the abdominal sympathetics as treatment of hypertension.[3] In 1934, DeCourcy evaluated bilateral subtotal adrenalectomy in eight patients based on his theory that their hypertension was due to excess secretion of epinephrine.[4] In 1935, Adson and Peet described the sympathectomies, subdiaphragmatic and thoracic respectively, which now bear their names.[5,6] Smithwick began thoracolumbar sympathectomy in 1938, and over the ensuing years the Smithwick-type sympathectomy became the most widely used form of surgical treatment for hypertension.[7] An evaluation of thoracolumbar sympathectomy at this hospital disclosed major problems with postoperative morbidity which included severe postural hypotension and incisional back pain.[8] In addition, although there was some evidence for relief of headaches associated with hypertension and a tendency to halt the progression of hypertensive retinopathy, there was a frequent late recurrence of hypertension. In 1949 Green, Nelson, and Dodds [9] observed marked amelioration of severe hypertension and diabetes mellitus following subtotal adrenalectomy. In March 1950 a group at our hospital, headed by Charles C. Wolferth, Sr., embarked upon this study of the effects of combined adrenalectomy and sympathectomy as treatment for severe hypertension.[10] All of the initial operations from 1950 to 1954 were performed by Dr. Harold A. Zintel and subsequent operations by Drs. William T. Fitts, Jr., and William S. Blakemore. Drs. William A. Jeffers, Francis Lukens, Joseph H. Hafkenschiel, A. Gorman Hills, Harold D. Itskovitz, and William C. Frayer were major contributors to this project. Many others in the Departments of Surgery, Medicine, Anesthesiology, and Ophthalmology in the Hospital of the University of Pennsylvania have participated in this work.

Rationale for Adrenalectomy

Dysfunctional diseases of the adrenal gland are usually associated with abnormal blood pressure levels: hypertension with adrenal hyperfunction and hypotension with hypofunction.[11] Hypotension is one of the cardinal features of Addison's disease. When adrenal insufficiency develops, the blood pressure of patients with essential hypertension may revert toward normal.[12] Hypertension then may be induced in such patients by administration of desoxycorticosterone (DOC) and salt.[13] There is evidence that the adrenal cortex may influence the formation of pressor substances, and in the presence of adrenocortical failure, a deficiency in formation of renin substrate has been observed.[14] In Cushing's syndrome, hypertension may be present in up to 85 percent of patients; except in patients with advanced

From the Section on Clinical Pharmacology and Hypertension, The Edward B. Robinette Foundation, and the Cardiopulmonary Division, Department of Medicine, Hospital of the University of Pennsylvania, Philadelphia, Pennsylvania.

renovascular impairment, the hypertension usually disappears following adrenalectomy.[15]

When the adrenal dysfunction relates principally to androgens or estrogens, significant influence upon blood pressure is less common. Congenital adrenal hyperplasia and hypertension have been associated with the adrenogenital syndrome [16] as well as the syndrome of primary amenorrhea and hypokalemia described by Biglieri, Henon, and Brust.[17] Primary hyperaldosteronism is attributed to increased adrenal secretion of aldosterone due either to a functioning adrenocortical adenoma or to adrenal hyperplasia. With adrenalectomy, the hypertension and other manifestations of this disorder usually disappear. The syndrome of primary hyperaldosteronism had not yet been described by Conn when this adrenalectomy series began in 1950. However, in a retrospective review of the histologic examination of adrenal glands removed at operation, adrenocortical adenomas were found in only two of 184 patients, and no patients were cured of their hypertension as a result of unilateral adrenalectomy and removal of an adrenocortical tumor.

Much of the evidence linking the adrenals to hypertension has been uncovered since we began adrenalectomy for hypertension. However, even then, there was sufficient clinical evidence to suggest that a critical reduction of functioning adrenal tissue might lead to amelioration of hypertension. Incubation studies performed by Cooper et al.[19] on adrenal tissue removed at these operations disclosed an inverse relationship between the secretion of cortisol per gram of adrenal tissue and the height of the diastolic blood pressure. The recent isolation of 18-hydroxydeoxycorticosterone (18-OH-DOC) from the adrenal venous effluent of hypertensive patients has led to increased speculation of an active rather than a permissive role for the adrenals in hypertension.[20]

TABLE 1.—*Type of Operation and Survival 12 to 21 Years*

Type of Operation	*No. of Patients Operated on*		*No. of Patients Surviving*	
SA alone	12		3	
SA and Peet	1		0	
SA and Adson	68		16	
TA and Adson	88	171	32	51(29%)
SA or TA and SMWK	15		3	
Total	184		54	(29%)

Abbreviations used: SA, subtotal adrenalectomy; TA, total adrenalectomy; SMWK, Smithwick sympathectomy.

INDICATIONS AND CONTRAINDICATIONS FOR SURGERY

Indications for surgical treatment of hypertension have included (1) failure to respond to medical therapy, with persistence of diastolic pressures over 120 mm Hg, and (2) evidence of progressive vascular damage to the target organs of hypertension. The Smithwick classification was used as a basis for grading the severity of the hypertensive vascular disease in these patients.[21] No patients in Smithwick Group I, i.e., those with the mildest degree of hypertension, were considered candidates for this operation. Sixty-eight patients (40%) were in Smithwick Group IV, representing the most advanced vascular disease and the poorest prognosis. The remaining patients were divided evenly between Groups II and III.

Surgery has not usually been attempted for

TABLE 2.—*Twelve- to 21-Year Survival Related to Smithwick's Classification*

Smithwick's Classification	*No. of Patients Operated on*	*No. of Patients Living*	*No. of Patients Dead*	*Percentage of Patients Surviving*
II	57	27	30	47
III	46	8	35	17
IV	68	16	50	24
Total	171	51	115	29

patients over 55 years of age or on those who have suffered a myocardial infarction or cerebrovascular accident with less than 6 months' convalescence. A further contraindication for surgery was a blood urea nitrogen (BUN) greater than 20 mg per 100 ml or phenolsulphonphthalein (PSP) excretion of less than 15 percent in 15 minutes. A degree of emotional maturity and reliability was considered a requirement for those who were subsequently to depend upon adrenal replacement therapy for the remainder of their lives.

Types of Operations Performed

In Table 1, data are presented to include the types of operations performed and the survival rates from each. The operations were done in two stages, usually about 10 days to 1 month apart. The 12 patients subjected to adrenalectomy alone represented the first patients operated on, many of whom had advanced renal disease with little hope for survival by any form of treatment then available. Among the 15 patients subjected to adrenalectomy and thoracolumbar sympathectomy were six who had adrenalectomy only after thoracolumbar sympathectomy had failed to relieve their hypertension. One hundred seventy-one patients with severe arterial hypertension were subjected to total or subtotal adrenalectomy combined with Adson- or Smithwick-type of sympathectomy. Throughout this chapter, attention will be directed to these 171 patients who form a more homogeneous group for evaluation.

Survival

Table 2 presents the 12- to 21-year survival as related to the preoperative Smithwick classification. Fifty-one of the original 171 patients operated on are living today and have survived from 12 to 21 years following operation. A total of 113 patients (67%) survived 5 or more years (Table 3). In Smithwick Class III and IV, the 5-year survival rate was 61 and 56 percent respectively; in Smithwick Group II the 5-year survival was 81 percent. Eighty-nine patients (52%) survived 10 or more years; the 10-year survival rate in Smithwick Group II was 65 percent; Group III, 47 percent; and Group IV, 44 percent.

TABLE 3.—*Five- to 20-Year Survival Rates*

5-Year Survival

Smithwick's Classification	*No. of Patients Operated on*	*5-Year Survivors*	*Percentage of Patients Surviving 5 Years*
II	57	47(27)	81
III	46	28(8)	61
IV	68	38(16)	56
Total	171	113	67

10-Year Survival

Smithwick's Classification	*No. of Patients Operated on*	*10-Year Survivors*	*Percentage of Patients Surviving 10 Years*
II	57	37(27)	65
III	46	21(4)	47
IV	68	31(16)	44
Total	171	89	52

15-Year Survival

Smithwick's Classification	*No. of Patients Operated on*	*15-Year Survivors*	*Percentage of Patients Surviving 15 Years*
II	48	28(23)	58
III	38	10(6)	26
IV	64	19(16)	30
Total	150	57	38

20-Year Survival

Smithwick's Classification	*No. of Patients Operated on*	*20-Year Survivors*	*Percentage of Patients Surviving 20 Years*
II	4	0(0)	0
III	4	1(1)	25
IV	14	3(3)	21
Total	22	4	18

The numbers in parentheses represent those alive now.

Fifty-seven patients (38%) survived for 15 years or more. The 15-year survival rate in Smithwick Group II was 58 percent, falling to 26 percent in Group III, and to 30 percent in Group IV. Four patients (18%), one in Smithwick Group III and three in Group IV, out of a total of 22 operated on prior to 1951, have now survived for 20 years. It must be noted that survival data in Tables 2 and 3 include patients who survived for the specified length of time and subsequently may have died. The numbers in parentheses in survival Table 3 indicate those actually alive at the time this chapter was written.

Mortality

Of 171 patients subjected to combined adrenalectomy and sympathectomy, 115, or 67 percent, have now died (Table 4). Nine patients survived less than 30 days postoperatively and are considered as operative deaths; the operative mortality was 5 percent. As might be anticipated the largest number of patients who died were those whose preoperative classification was Smithwick Group IV. Thirty-six patients died of cerebrovascular accidents, 33 of myocardial infarction, and five of uremia. The deaths from uremia occurred mainly in patients whose preoperative renal function was below the levels eventually established as adequate to permit surgery. There have been only two deaths from adrenal insufficiency. It is noteworthy that not a single death in this entire series resulted from congestive heart failure. Attention is called to the noncardiac deaths which may occur in any group of patients in this age group. The average age of all patients at the time of operation was 38 years; the present survivors are in the age range of 55 to 70.

TABLE 4.—*Cause of Death Following Adrenalectomy*

Cause	*No. of Patients*	*Percentage of Patients*
Stroke	36	31
Myocardial infarction	33	29
Uremia	5	4
Bleeding ulcer	3	3
Cancer	6	5
Adrenal insufficiency	2	2
Aortic dissection	2	2
Pulmonary embolism	2	2
Miscellaneous and unknown	26	22
Total	115	100%

Clinical Results of Surgery

Blood pressures after operation were classified by an arbitrary system into A, B, C, and D groups, A indicating an excellent result and D a poor one (Table 5). It was thought preferable to classify the results in relation to a normal pressure rather than with respect to the fall from preoperative levels. Of those patients now alive, 94 percent have had an excellent or good blood pressure response (Table 6). Only 6 percent failed to respond and maintain blood pressures greater than 220/120 mm Hg. A number of these patients had further improvement in their blood pressures by the addition of newly developed antihypertensive agents. Responsiveness to these agents has appeared to be enhanced by adrenalectomy and sympathectomy. We have found that hypotensive responses to chlorothiazide after sympathectomy and adrenalectomy may be dramatic; patients who were operative failures occasionally may be converted into normotensive patients.[22] The falls in blood pressure noted in patients subjected to adrenalectomy have tended to be permanent in contrast with the gradual rise toward the preoperative level often observed after sympathectomy alone.

Improvement in blood pressure change seemed to bear surprisingly little relationship to the patient's preoperative Smithwick classification. Seventy percent of those in Smithwick Group II had an excellent or A response, 88 percent in Smithwick Group III and, surprisingly, 69 percent of the Smithwick Group IV survivors achieved an excellent blood pressure result. With an ascending Smithwick rating, the mortality has increased, while, as might

TABLE 5.—*Classification of Results According to Blood Pressure Response*

(A)	Excellent	150/100 mm Hg supine; equal or less standing
(B)	Good	150 to 180/100 to 110 mm Hg supine; equal or less standing
(C)	Poor	180 to 200/110 to 120 mm Hg supine; equal or less standing
(D)	Failure	200/120 mm Hg or more; equal or less standing

TABLE 6.—*Blood Pressure Response in 51 Survivors*

Smithwick Classification	*A*	*B*	*C*	*D*
II	21	5	0	1
III	7	1	0	0
IV	11	3	0	2
Total	39	9	0	3
(%)	76	18	0	6

be anticipated, the mortality rate correlated inversely with the degree of blood pressure improvement. Among those achieving an excellent or good result, the mortality was 41 and 48 percent respectively. Where the result was classed as poor or a failure, the mortality was 95 percent. The occurrence of some deaths among patients who had been doing well since operation remains a matter for concern. It has become clear that control of blood pressure in hypertensives affords far from complete protection from lethal arterial episodes, especially in those with advanced vascular deterioration prior to operation.

Responses Measured by Electrocardiogram, Heart Size, and Optic Fundi

Recognizing that a reduced blood pressure alone was not the full measure of a patient's response to adrenalectomy and sympathectomy, further evaluation of improvement in vascular disease in the target organs was done. Examinations were performed at 6-month intervals and the degree of vascular disease was studied in the heart, brain, eyes, and kidneys. The ECG improved in 40 percent of patients in whom signs of left ventricular hypertrophy had been present preoperatively. Heart size, measured by orthodiagram, was reduced in 47 percent. The most dramatic improvement occurred in hypertensive retinopathy which improved in 62 percent and remained unchanged in 38 percent.[23] Hemorrhages, exudates, or papilledema, present preoperatively in many patients, completely disappeared, and progression of hypertensive retinopathy was not observed.

Cardiac Failure, Myocardial Infarction, Angina, and Stroke

In approximately 25 percent of the patients symptoms or signs of cardiac failure were noted prior to operation. Following adrenalectomy and sympathectomy, dramatic improvement occurred; currently, no patients receive digitalis for cardiac failure; two patients require digitalis for control of atrial fibrillation. Disappearance of cardiac failure occurred independently of the degree of postoperative reduction in blood pressure. Probably the enhanced ability of the adrenalectomized patient to excrete salt and water accounted in large measure for this improvement.

Eighteen patients were subject to the anginal syndrome before operation and 12 of these have improved. However, angina has appeared as a new symptom in 12 other patients since operation. Similarly, 38 patients sustained myocardial infarction postoperatively, 32 males and six females; 33 episodes proved to be fatal. Only four of 25 patients dying in the postoperative year died of myocardial infarction, whereas death due to stroke accounted for 48 percent of deaths during the same period. Forty-three strokes occurred after operation and 36 (84%) were fatal. Twenty-nine, or 77 percent, of the myocardial infarctions occurred postoperatively in patients with excellent or good blood pressure responses. These data would favor the current trend toward early, energetic therapy of hypertension before evidence of vascular disease is noted in the target organs.

Renal Function

Preoperative evaluation of renal function was limited mainly to measurement of BUN and PSP excretion. Following adrenalectomy the BUN became a less reliable index of renal function because of the effects of adrenal insufficiency on prerenal azotemia. As a rule those with advanced renal disease were excluded from this operative series, but occasionally, patients with BUN between 20 to 30 mg per 100 ml were accepted and in several instances the long-term survival appeared to justify this decision. Survival for more than 10 years occurred in a patient whose BUN was 28 mg per 100 ml and whose urea clearance was less than 50 percent of normal prior to operation. As further indication of the remarkable long-term preservation of renal function, only two patients have died of uremia beyond the first year after operation. In a small, selected group of patients studied before operation by creatinine, para-aminohippuric acid, and inulin clearance, similar levels of renal function were measured 7 to 8 years after operation.[24]

Renovascular Hypertension

Most of these operations were performed before modern techniques were available for the diagnosis of renal artery stenosis as a cause of hypertension. Subsequently, no patients were subjected to adrenalectomy in whom renal artery stenosis was not first ruled out by arteriography. A review of five patients whose blood pressure response to adrenalectomy was unsatisfactory led to the discovery of renal artery stenosis in four. In two of these, normal blood pressure levels were obtained following unilateral nephrectomy.

Adrenal Replacement Therapy

No adrenal steroid replacement has been required during or after the first-stage operation. Patients subjected to total adrenalectomy have been maintained on an average of 37.5 mg of cortisone and 0.05 mg of 9-α-fluorohydrocortisone (Florinef) daily. Following subtotal adrenalectomy it has been possible to maintain patients on as little as 12.5 to 25.0 mg of cortisone daily. Several patients who underwent only subtotal adrenalectomy have felt well without steroid replacement, showing no evidence of adrenal insufficiency unless subjected to severe stress or infection. Because of the potent salt-retaining effects of Florinef, supplementary sodium chloride tablets have not been necessary, although liberal use of the saltshaker has been suggested. During the hot summer months when sodium loss through perspiration may be enough to precipitate mild adrenal insufficiency, we have asked our patients to increase their Florinef dosage to 0.1 mg daily. The desired level of adrenal replacement therapy for each patient was based on the minimal amount of steroid required to maintain a state of well-being without overt symptoms of adrenal insufficiency. In patients with renal insufficiency, it has been our experience that the diastolic blood pressure may not fall even when severe adrenal insufficiency occurs although the pulse pressure may diminish.

Complications of Adrenalectomy

Among the late complications of this operation, we have encountered peptic ulcer with roentgenographic confirmation in 16 patients and bleeding in 11. In three patients, gastrointestinal hemorrhage was a cause of death. In some of these patients a history of peptic ulcer preceded adrenalectomy. The incidence of peptic ulcer among the adrenalectomy-sympathectomy patients does not exceed the natural occurrence of this disease in the United States.[25]

Raynaud's phenomenon, with varying degrees of pain, numbness, and pallor of the fingertips, occurred in approximately 10 percent upon exposure to cold. In only one instance, a patient who earned his living as a telephone lineman, did these complaints cause the patient to change his occupation. No treatment beyond the use of warm gloves has proved necessary. A possible explanation for this phenomenon involves hyperactivity of the upper thoracic sympathetic fibers following extirpation of the lower thoracic and lumbar ganglia. However, a normal capacity for blood flow to the fingers was demonstrated by vasodilatation tests. It was not clear why this complaint did not occur in all patients subjected to the same degree of sympathectomy.

Gouty arthritis occurred in 11 patients and hyperuricemia in approximately two-thirds of those studied.[26] The etiology appeared unrelated to adrenalectomy or sympathectomy operations or to the dosage of steroid-replacement therapy administered. Decreased renal clearance of uric acid was measured and was thought to be secondary to the renotubular effect of increased lactic acid production from the ischemia of severe vascular disease as present in patients with severe hypertension, as well as myocardial infarction, and arteriosclerosis obliterans. The incidence of gout and hyperuricemia was independent of therapy with thiazide diuretics and occurred in patients whose uric acid clearance was diminished out of proportion to creatinine clearance.

Increased skin pigmentation, an expected sequel to adrenalectomy, occurred in approximately one-third of these patients and appeared unrelated to any other clinical or laboratory evidence of adrenal insufficiency or to the dose of adrenal replacement therapy.[27] Fortunately, it has not presented a cosmetic problem.

The incidence of diabetes was studied in 40 patients utilizing a 4-hour glucose tolerance test.[27,28] Although three patients with diabetes demonstrated a decreased insulin requirement following adrenalectomy, 13 patients with normal preoperative blood sugars developed hyperglycemia postoperatively. The incidence of a positive family history for diabetes was no greater among those patients who were free from diabetes postoperatively. Fourteen patients demonstrated hypoglycemia at 4 hours with unresponsiveness to hypoglycemia thought to be characteristic of adrenocortical inadequacy. In three patients hyperglycemia at the 1- or 2-hour interval was followed by hypoglycemia at the 4-hour point. Apparently cortisone, administered for a prolonged period, even in the small doses commonly used for adrenal replacement therapy, may have diabetogenic properties in susceptible patients.[27]

Four patients also developed hypothyroidism postoperatively, but most patients were euthyroid. One of the more troublesome problems encountered following adrenalectomy related to the appetite-stimulating effect of cortisone. The resultant weight gain which in many patients amounted to 10 to 20 percent of their preoperative weight occurred in spite of their receiving minimal adrenal replacement dosage plus our advice to follow low-calorie and, particularly, low-fat diets.

No pituitary tumors have been discovered at autopsy as might have been anticipated in association with increased melanophore-stimulating hormone (MSH) production and marked skin pigmentation. All patients were screened for pheochromocytoma with phentolamine tests prior to operation and none were found subsequently at the time of adrenalectomy. More than 50 episodes of adrenal insufficiency have occurred, most of them mild and not requiring hospitalization. Two deaths occurred due to adrenal insufficiency in patients with severe pneumonia. Many patients have safely undergone both elective and emergency surgery and by increasing their adrenal replacement therapy at the time of this stress, no complications have occurred which could be attributed to their prior adrenalectomy.

Discussion

As a result of the development of more effective antihypertensive agents, it has not been necessary to perform bilateral adrenalectomy for hypertension since 1959. However, we continue to be impressed that many patients with severe, advanced vascular disease who were operated upon when antihypertensive therapy was much less effective have responded favorably to combined adrenalectomy and sympathectomy. The Smithwick classification has been useful in evaluating the survival results of this operative procedure, as well as comparison with survival following thoracolumbar sympathectomy.[21] The use of a nationally accepted classification of hypertension would further facilitate comparison with survival results obtained with current medical regimens. After thoracolumbar sympathectomy, the Smithwick survival rate was 50 percent in 5 years and 36 percent in 10 years. This compares with 67 percent in 5 years and 52 percent in 10 years following adrenalectomy and sympathectomy for patients with similar degrees of vascular disease. The survival of 38 percent of our patients for 15 years has been most encouraging. Some of the success of the adrenalectomy procedure may be attributed to the presence of a well-integrated medical and surgical team prepared to deal not only with surgical complications, but with manifestations of severe hypertensive cardiovascular disease or adrenal insufficiency. Long-term follow-up examinations continue to be done twice annually. Unlike those with Addison's disease of medical etiology, our patients do not appear to lack energy and vigor for their full work loads unless they have cardiovascular complications.

It has been difficult to obtain data of equivalent long-term survival following medical therapy of hypertension. In many reports, the classification of hypertensive severity was related to the author's choice of criteria, making it almost impossible to compare results with those of any other investigator. In 1939 Keith,

Wagener, and Barker[29] published data to show a 5-year survival rate of only 2 percent in hypertensive patients with papilledema. In 1963, Farmer, Gifford, and Hines reported a 6-year survival rate of 23 percent for patients with malignant hypertension who had received modern antihypertensive therapy.[30] Simpson and Smirk have reported the 5-year survival of 34 percent of patients with malignant hypertension treated medically.[31] In 1966, Perry reported a 7- to 13-year survival rate of 41 percent utilizing modern antihypertensive therapy in patients with malignant hypertension, but no azotemia.[32] Generally, 5-year survival rates after medical therapy of severe hypertension have ranged from 22 to 50 percent. Admittedly, the long-term results of treatment of severe hypertension with those antihypertensive agents used most commonly today has still not been evaluated. It is certainly possible that the use of newly developed and more energetically applied medical therapy may yield results equal to those obtained with combined adrenalectomy and sympathectomy. At this time our 10-year survival rate of 52 percent compares quite favorably with the results of medical therapy reported to date.[33] The fact that surgery represents a form of built-in treatment has made unnecessary the type of strict medical supervision required of patients receiving complex and costly regimens of three or four different antihypertensive agents. In the light of these excellent survival rates during 20 years of treatment with combined adrenalectomy and sympathectomy, it may be worth reassessing the role of this type of surgical treatment for the patient with severe hypertension, unresponsive to medical therapy, whose renal function is still well preserved. No successful procedure has thus far been devised for selecting patients capable of a highly favorable response to adrenalectomy and sympathectomy and such operations should be limited to those with an urgent need for control of their hypertensive disease, but who have responded poorly to antihypertensive drugs or have been unable to tolerate them.

Summary

Between 1950 and 1959, adrenalectomy and sympathectomy were performed in 171 patients who had failed to respond to medical treatment and who demonstrated evidence of progressive vascular damage to the heart, brain, eyes, and kidneys. A total of 64 percent have survived 5 years and 52 percent for 10 years, 38 percent for 15 years, and four patients (18%) have survived for 20 years. Seventy-six percent have had an excellent and 18 percent a good blood pressure response. Improvement has also occurred in heart size, electrocardiographic signs of left ventricular hypertrophy, and particularly in the degree of hypertensive retinopathy. Cardiac failure, often present before operation, was never observed subsequently in these patients. Late deaths from coronary occlusion have occurred despite good blood pressure response and may reflect the advancing age of these patients as well as the need for early treatment of hypertension before evidence of vascular damage has appeared in the target organs. The total effects of combined adrenalectomy and sympathectomy upon the blood pressure, symptoms, and physical findings, and degree of rehabilitation of severe hypertensives refractory to other methods of treatment have been beneficial to some extent in nearly all survivors. These favorable results have not yet been equalled over extended periods of time by medical antihypertensive therapy.

References

1. Sellers, A. M., Barrett, J. S., Wolferth, C. C., Lopez, R., Itskovitz, H. D., Blakemore, W. S., and Zintel, H. A.: Adrenalectomy and sympathectomy for hypertension: Ten-year survival. Arch. Surg. 89:880, 1964.
2. Crile, G.: Surgical Treatment of Hypertension. Philadelphia, Saunders, 1938.
3. Pieri, G.: La resezione dei nervi splanchni. Ann. Ital. Chir. 6:678, 1927.
4. DeCourcy, J. L.: Subtotal bilateral adrenalectomy for hyperadrenalism (essential hypertension). Ann. Surg. 100:310, 1934.
5. Adson, A. W., Craig, W. McK., and Brown, G. E.: Surgery in its relation to hypertension. Surg. Gynec. Obstet. 62:314, 1936.
6. Peet, M. M.: Splanchnic section for hypertension: A preliminary report. Univ. Mich. Med. Bull. 1:17, 1935.
7. Smithwick, R. H.: A technique for splanchnic resection for hypertension. Surgery 7:1. 1940.
8. Zintel, H. A., Sellers, A. M., Wolferth, C. C.,

Jeffers, W. A., Hafkenschiel, J. H., Hills, A. G., Mackie, J. A., and Langfeld, S. B.: Experiences with thoracolumbar sympathectomy and with combined adrenalectomy-sympathectomy in the treatment of patients with essential hypertension. Surgery 37:928, 1955.
9. Green, D. M., Nelson, J. N., and Dodds, G. A.: Effects of adrenal resection on hypertension and diabetes. Fed. Proc. 8:60, 1949.
10. Wolferth, C. C., Fitts, W. I., Jeffers, W. A., and Sellers, A. M.: The place of adrenalectomy in the treatment of severe arterial hypertension. Bull. N. Y. Acad. Med. 33:151, 1957.
11. Sellers, A. M., Jeffers, W. A., Wolferth, C. C., Blakemore, W. S., and Itskovitz, H. D.: The adrenal cortex in hypertension: Cause and effect. Am. J. Cardiol. 9:704, 1962.
12. Perera, G. A.: The relation of the adrenal cortex to hypertension; observations on the effect of hypoadrenalism on a patient with hypertensive vascular disease. JAMA 129: 537, 1945.
13. DeGermes, L., Deschamps, H., Bricaire, H., and Fossey, B. M.: Arterial hypertension during desoxycorticosterone acetate therapy. Ann. Endocrinol. 13:314, 1952.
14. Lewis, H. A., and Goldblatt, H.: Studies on experimental hypertension. XVII. Experimental observations on the humoral mechanism of hypertension. Bull. N. Y. Acad. Med. 18:459, 1942.
15. Raker, J. W., Cope, O., and Ackerman, I. P.: Surgical experience with the treatment of hypertension of Cushing's syndrome. Am. J. Surg. 107:153, 1964.
16. Eberlein, W. R., and Bongiovanni, A. M.: Congenital adrenal hyperplasia with hypertension. Unusual steroid pattern in blood and urine. J. Clin. Endocrinol. 15:1531, 1955.
17. Biglieri, E. G., Henon, M. A., and Brust, W.: 17-Hydroxylation deficiency in man. J. Clin. Invest. 45:1946, 1966.
18. Conn, J. W.: Primary aldosteronism. J. Lab. Clin. Med. 45:661, 1955.
19. Cooper, D. Y., Touchstone, J. C., Roberts, J. M., Blakemore, W. S., and Rosenthal, O.: Steroid formation by adrenal tissue from hypertensives. J. Clin. Invest. 37:11524, 1958.
20. Melby, J. C., Dale, S. L., and Wilson, T. E.: 18-Hydroxy-deoxycorticosterone in human hypertension. Circ. Res. 29(Suppl. II):II–143, 1971.
21. Smithwick, R. H., Whitelaw, G. P., and Kinsey, D.: Surgical approach to treatment of essential hypertension. Am. J. Cardiol. 9:893, 1962.
22. Sellers, A. M., Barends, F. J., Goldman, M. E., Lindauer, M. A., and Jeffers, W. A.: Effect of chlorothiazide on severe arterial hypertension including patients previously subjected to sympathectomy and adrenalectomy. Circulation 18:779, 1958.
23. Frayer, W. C.: Improvement in hypertensive retinopathy following adrenal resection and sympathectomy. Arch. Ophthalmol. 58:331, 1957.
24. Crosley, A. P., Jr., Barker, E. S., and Clark, J. K.: Long-term follow-up of renal function of hypertensive patients treated by adrenalectomy. J. Lab. Clin. Med. 54:801, 1959.
25. Kirsner, J. B.: Drug-induced peptic ulcer. Ann. Intern. Med. 47:666, 1957.
26. Itskovitz, H. D., and Sellers, A. M.: Gout and hyperuricemia after adrenalectomy for hypertension. N. Engl. J. Med. 268:1105, 1963.
27. Hills, A. G., Zintel, H. A., and Parsons, D. W.: Observations of human adrenal cortical deficiency. Am. J. Med. 21:358, 1956.
28. Bryfogle, J. W., Sellers, A. M., and Itskovitz, H. D.: Diabetes mellitus following adrenalectomy for hypertension. Presented at a regional meeting of the American College of Physicians, Philadelphia, Penna., Nov. 4, 1965.
29. Keith, N. M., Wagener, H. P., and Barker, N. W.: Some different types of essential hypertension: Their course and prognosis. Am. J. Med. Sci. 197:332, 1939.
30. Farmer, R. G., Gifford, R. W., Jr., and Hines, E. A.: Effect of medical treatment of severe hypertension. Arch. Intern. Med. 112:118, 1963.
31. Simpson, F. O., and Smirk, F. H.: Treatment of malignant hypertension. Am. J. Cardiol. 9: 868, 1962.
32. Perry, H. M., Schroeder, H. A., Catanzaro, F. J., Moore-Jones, D., and Camel, G. H.: Studies on the control of hypertension. VIII. Mortality, morbidity, and remissions during twelve years of intensive therapy. Circulation 33:958, 1966.
33. Freis, E. D.: The value of antihypertensive therapy. Bull. N. Y. Acad. Med. 45:951, 1969.

Guidelines to Medical and Surgical Therapy of Patients with Pheochromocytoma

By Karl Engelman, M.D.

SELF-EVIDENT AS IT may appear, the cornerstone of successful management of the patient suspected of harboring a pheochromocytoma is the establishment of a valid diagnosis. While the details of diagnosing this condition are given in this book (see the chapter entitled "Pheochromocytoma: Incidence, Pathophysiology, and Diagnosis"), a few points deserve reemphasis because of the frequency with which mistakes in diagnosis produce either false-positive or false-negative results. Most mistakes occur either because the diagnosis of pheochromocytoma was not considered or because the results of laboratory tests were aberrant and misled the physician. In this regard, it should be emphasized that most laboratory errors (particularly for catecholamine and vanillylmandelic acid assays) result in higher than normal values. This often leads to needless surgery for a tumor. The only protection which the physician has from these latter problems is to be sure that the laboratory which he uses for these tests is competent to perform these procedures accurately. Another potential source of error with diagnosing this disease is reliance on the now outdated pharmacologic tests (histamine, phentolamine, tyramine, or glucagon) which may lead to either false-positive or false-negative results in a significant number of instances. Despite the shortcomings of some clinical pathology laboratories, there are available today to physicians in all areas of the country accurate biochemical assays. As a general principle it should be emphasized that no patient should undergo therapy (especially surgery) for pheochromocytoma unless chemical evidence of excessive urinary excretion of catecholamines and metabolites has been documented.

Once assured of the diagnosis, the physician is faced with defining the proper course of therapy to insure a successful result in this usually curable but often dangerous disease. Therapy is designed to reverse the cardiodynamic and metabolic complications of excessive catecholamine secretion.

Primary among the treatable hemodynamic consequences are hypertension, orthostatic hypotension, tachycardia and arrhythmias, and congestive heart failure either due to prolonged hypertension or to catecholamine cardiomyopathy.[1,2] Although the cardiomyopathy is of as yet undefined pathogenesis, it seems probable that it is due to the metabolic effects of catecholamines on the myocardium rather than due to the hypertensive state. Other metabolic derangements prevalent in patients with pheochromocytoma are hyperglycemia or glucose intolerance, increased perspiration, hypermetabolism (elevated basal metabolism rate) and an elevation of plasma free-fatty acid concentrations. The last three may be related[3] but rarely are these problems of pressing clinical consequence as compared to the hemodynamic changes.

While surgical removal of the tumor is the preferred course of action in most instances, some patients will have to undergo long-term medical therapy because of circumstances which contraindicate surgery (metastatic spread, recent myocardial infarction, severe cardiomyopathy, etc.). However, regardless of whether surgery is to be the mode of therapy, all patients should be subjected to pharmacologic control of their disease on an acute or chronic basis. This may be achieved either through the use of the more conventional and generally available peripherally acting adrenergic-blocking drugs or through the use of still experimental inhibitors of catecholamine synthesis. Either mode of therapy has proved successful for preoperative and intraoperative management of patients or for chronic definitive therapy.

From the Section on Hypertension and Clinical Pharmacology, University of Pennsylvania School of Medicine, Philadelphia, Pennsylvania.

Two classes of peripheral adrenergic-blocking drugs are now available—the α- and β-adrenergic blockers. Phentolamine (Regitine) and phenoxybenzamine (dibenzyline) are the two α-adrenergic blockers which have clinical usefulness. Both drugs are used primarily to counteract the hypertensive effects of the catecholamines, with phentolamine being reserved for acute intravenous use. Despite the fact that phentolamine is also available in tablet form (50 mg) for oral administration, its relatively short duration of action (2 to 4 hours) and frequent side effects of gastrointestinal upset and tachycardia are contraindications for subacute or chronic therapy in patients with pheochromocytoma. Dibenzyline, on the other hand, is not commercially available for intravenous use, but the oral form (10-mg capsule) is the preferred agent in preoperative preparation and chronic therapy. Dibenzyline has a reasonably rapid onset of action (1 to 2 hours) with a duration of action for at least several days so the drug may be given in a single, oral daily dose and the effect is smooth and sustained. Nasal congestion, orthostatic tachycardia, sedation, and retrograde ejaculation are common minor complaints of patients receiving dibenzyline, but other serious side effects are uncommon.

The primary therapeutic effects of the α-blockers are to reduce the blood pressure and to prevent sudden hypertensive crises which may occur spontaneously or during surgery. The goal of preoperative preparation is to achieve relative normalization of blood pressure and marked blunting of attacks during a period of about a week before surgery. This assures a safer operative course since the stimuli of induction of anesthesia and intubation usually precipitate extremely severe elevations of blood pressure in unprepared patients. The usual daily dose of dibenzyline required to achieve this degree of control ranges from 30 to 80 mg although doses as high as 200 mg per day or more may be required in rare patients. At the onset of therapy the effective dose may be approximated by giving incremental doses several times daily over the first several days until the desired effect of controlling blood pressure and sweating is achieved. In the patient strongly suspected of having a pheochromocytoma, but for whom biochemical corroboration is still lacking, such a therapeutic trial of dibenzyline may be very helpful in gaining insight into the diagnosis and possibly treating the patient.

The therapeutic program in the preoperative patient should be continued to the day of surgery without fear of adverse consequences during surgery. Despite apparently adequate α-adrenergic blockade with dibenzyline, some patients may still manifest considerable increases in blood pressure at the time of induction or during manipulation of the tumor. Rapidly administered, intravenous doses of phentolamine (1 to 10 mg, given as necessary) are used for additive therapy at this time. It is important to be aware of the possibility of severe hypotensive responses with the use of either α-blocker in certain patients whose tumors secrete significant amounts of epinephrine as well as norepinephrine. This results from blockade of the α-adrenergic vasoconstrictor effects leaving unopposed and exaggerating the significant β-adrenergic vasodilating effects of the epinephrine.

Chronic use of dibenzyline has also proved very successful as definitive therapy for both the hypertension and the cardiomyopathy. We now have experience with patients receiving the drug for 10 years with excellent results. The acute and subacute effects of phentolamine and dibenzyline in an 11-year-old girl with metastatic pheochromocytoma are shown in Figure 1. The more even control with dibenzyline is evident. Annual progress reports from the mother over the next 10 years document the sustained therapeutic effect in this patient. Of additional interest is the fact that there was little discernible growth of the metastases during the period of observation. It is difficult to attribute this lack of tumor progression to the α-blocker therapy, and it seems more likely that this represents the natural history and innate biology of this often very slow-growing cancer, which usually kills by virtue of the cardiovascular effects of its hormone secretion, rather than by the progressive growth of the metastases.

More recent introduction of effective β-adrenergic blocking agents permits pharmacologic control of the other major hazards of this disease—tachyarrhythmias. While propranolol, the only commercially available β-

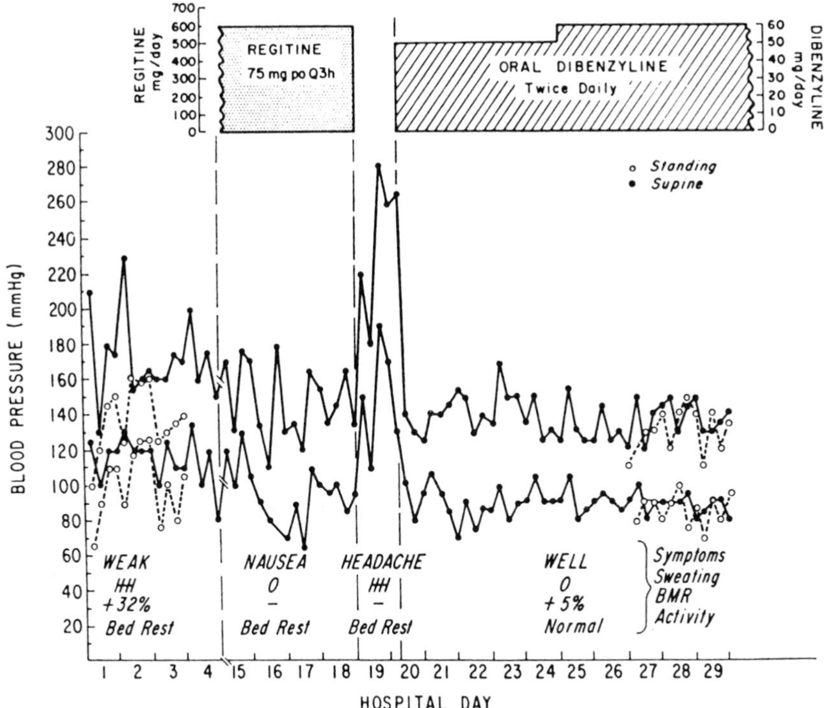

FIG. 1.—Results of therapy on the blood pressure and clinical condition of an 11-year-old girl with malignant pheochromocytoma.

blocker in this country, has not generally been necessary on a long-term basis, its use during surgery as an acutely administered specific antiarrhythmic agent has been especially worthwhile. Because the β-blockers are specific antagonists for these catecholamine-induced arrhythmias, patients with pheochromocytoma are unusually sensitive to their therapeutic effects. Oral doses of propranolol as small as 5 to 10 mg given every 4 to 6 hours often suffice to completely suppress ventricular ectopic activity or other arrhythmias. Similarly, great care must be taken during surgery when intravenous doses of 1 to 2 mg often reverse bizarre tachyarrhythmias within less than a minute. If excessive doses are used, congestive failure may quickly result because these patients (especially those with cardiomyopathy) are also very sensitive to the negative inotropic effects of the drug. Since the onset of activity is so rapid after intravenous use, if is frequently wiser to use a smaller dose initially, followed by a second dose if the desired effects are not achieved. As newer β-adrenergic blocking agents with more selective antiarrhythmic effects and less negative inotropic activity become available, this may be less of a problem.

Another approach to the pharmacologic therapy of the patient with excessive catecholamine secretion has been the use of drugs which block the synthesis (Fig. 2) rather than the peripheral effects of these hormones. Compounds such as alpha-methyldopa and others were initially developed in the hope that by virtue of their ability to inhibit the aromatic-L-amino acid decarboxylase or dopamine-β-hydroxylase enzymes, they might reduce catecholamine synthesis and be useful drugs, not only in pheochromocytoma, but also in other conditions. Experience in animals and man revealed that these agents were generally ineffective in terms of their primary goal. These results were explained by the studies of Udenfriend, Zaltzman-Nirenberg, and Nagatsu [4] which showed the rate-limiting step in catecholamine synthesis to be the hydroxylation of tyrosine. Their demonstration that a number

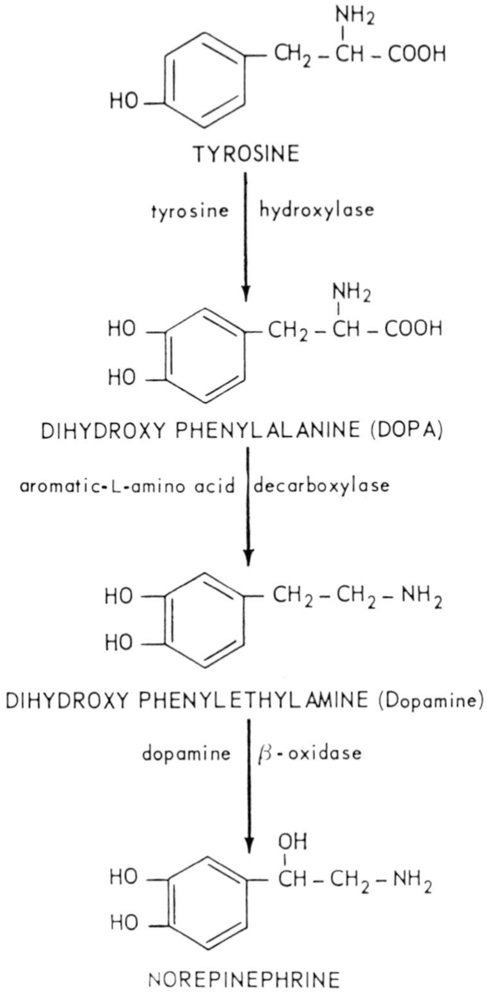

TYROSINE

tyrosine hydroxylase

DIHYDROXY PHENYLALANINE (DOPA)

aromatic-L-amino acid decarboxylase

DIHYDROXY PHENYLETHYLAMINE (Dopamine)

dopamine β-oxidase

NOREPINEPHRINE

FIG. 2.—Biosynthetic pathway for norepinephrine.

of analogs of tyrosine and phenylalanine were potent competitive inhibitors of tyrosine hydroxylase both in vitro and in vivo led to clinical trials with several of these compounds.

Two of these compounds, α-methyltyrosine [5] and α-methylphenylalanine,[6] have proved to be effective in treating patients with pheochromocytoma. The more potent of the two, α-methyltyrosine, has been used more extensively and has proved sufficiently potent to reduce catecholamine secretion by the tumors by as much as 80 to 90 percent. The resulting clinical response has been gratifying in that not only has the hypertension been controlled, but the associated findings including cardiomyopathy and intraoperative complications have been remarkably improved.[7] This drug has been useful both for chronic and subacute (preoperative) therapy, and were it not for the fact that α-methyltyrosine is still an investigational drug, it would be the treatment of choice for the preparation of the patient for surgery. Complications of therapy have been minor, consisting mainly of sedation and the danger of crystalluria due to the insolubility of the drug in urine. While the use of inhibitors of catecholamine synthesis is more intellectually satisfying and in some regards is more clinically effective than the use of peripheral competitive antagonists, it seems unlikely at the present time that such agents will become generally available in a commercially marketed rather than research category.

Surgery for pheochromocytoma presents special problems which can be handled quite successfully if they are anticipated and the surgical team is prepared beforehand with the necessary drugs and devices to ensure proper monitoring and control. First among the uncertainties of surgery for this condition is the exact location of the tumor. This rarely presents serious difficulty since more than 95 percent of tumors arise from sites situated between the diaphragm and the floor of the pelvis. Exact localization of these intra-abdominal tumors (mostly adrenal in origin) is not necessary as long as the proper surgical approach is carried out. Therefore, it is the exclusion of extra-abdominal tumors which bears paramount importance in the presurgical evaluation. Intrathoracic tumors can almost always be identified if the conventional and oblique views of the thorax are obtained to carefully look for the characteristic posterior mediastinal paravertebral mass arising from the thoracic sympathetic chain. Other rare tumors such as those arising from the carotid body or from the glomus jugulare tissue of the base of the skull can usually be detected by careful physical examination and appropriate radiologic investigation if it appears indicated.

Rarely are special radiographic or other studies indicated in this disease since they are often misleading and may be quite hazardous in these fragile patients. Arteriographic studies in an attempt to define a site of tumor origin are perhaps most useful in demonstrating adrenal tumors, but since all tumors must be expected to arise from the adrenal glands until proved otherwise, this hardly seems a maneuver worth the risk to the patient. Furthermore, arteriograms are not very useful for identifying small, yet functional, tumors which may arise from the adrenal medulla bilaterally or from the periaortic sympathetic chain and other less common sites of neural crest-tissue deposition. Similarly, retroperitoneal gas studies used in an attempt to define adrenal or other tumors are not indicated since they are difficult to perform and are likely to identify only the larger tumors that are easily found at surgery. Vena cava catheterization to obtain venous plasma samples for catecholamine assay as a means of localizing the site of a tumor may be exceptionally helpful in those rare cases where the tumors are not found at the time of surgery, but the procedure must still be considered a research technique available at only a few institutions.

The best means of localizing the tumor or tumors (they are multicentric in origin in 10 to 20% of patients) still remains careful surgical exploration with adequate patient monitoring to document changes in pulse rate or rhythm and blood pressure which occur when these tissues are carefully palpated. These changes in vital signs are so useful because they often occur even when the surgeon is unaware that he is touching tumor tissue.[7]

Successful surgery for pheochromocytoma depends more on the activities cephalad to the anesthetist's drapes than those in the operative field. The main difference between surgery for this tumor and a similar exploration for adrenalectomy or abdominal exploration rests on the manifold physiologic derangements induced by the increased circulating catecholamines. Adequate control of these problems can only be achieved if the problems which may occur are all understood and anticipated with methods available to counteract any crisis encountered in the operating room. The immediate recognition of evolving problems is provided by electronic monitoring techniques (see below). The ability to reverse problems during surgery is provided by the availability in the same room for immediate use of large quantities of phentolamine (at least 100 mg), propranolol, adequate supplies of volume-expanding fluids (see below), and cardiac pacing and defibrillating devices.

The adequacy of the constant monitoring not only permits the sensitive localization of the tumor, but enables the physicians manipulating the anesthetic and other pharmacologic agents to treat the patient's hemodynamic status with a greater degree of accuracy and control. Three parameters should be constantly recorded for immediate observation: intra-arterial blood pressure, central venous pressure, and an EKG lead to record a readily identifiable P wave. Since induction of anesthesia is often accompanied by arrhythmias and hypertensive episodes even in apparently adequately prepared patients, it is necessary to institute the monitoring procedures before general anesthesia is begun. The intraarterial line is especially important, and it should be placed by percutaneous techniques or by a direct surgical procedure under local anesthesia.

Premedication of patients undergoing surgery for pheochromocytoma is important. While sedatives and tranquilizers have been used, atropinization prior to entrance into the operating room may be hazardous since these patients often have a baseline tachycardia. Induction may be performed with thiopental, and intubation facilitated with succinylcholine. The latter drug must be given with careful attention, however, since in several patients it has precipitated cardiac arrest or serious arrhythmias, especially when a second dose was required. Though theoretic considerations have indicated the possibility of problems related to histamine release with the use of *d*-tubocurarine, we have not encountered problems when this drug has been used routinely as a muscle relaxant.

The selection of general anesthetic agents most suitable for patients with pheochromocytoma has been the subject of much discussion and controversy. However, the use of β-adrenergic blocking drugs and adequate presurgical preparation of the patient has simplified the problem to a considerable degree. There is general agreement that cyclopropane is contraindicated for surgery in this condition due to its remarkable sensitization to catecholamine-induced arrhythmias. Combinations of nitrous oxide, ether, and oxygen, while having been favored in the past, are not currently used so widely because of the explosion hazard of the ether and the relatively slow rate of withdrawal of this agent after prolonged procedures. Some of the newer halogenated anesthetic agents have been found to be advantageous because of their antiadrenergic effects. Halothane has proved to be an excellent agent for use in this disease since it can be increased or decreased in effect rapidly and it is a very useful adjunct in the control of the blood pressure. Its use, however, is also accompanied by an increased sensitivity to arrhythmias which can be well controlled with either lidocaine or, preferably, propranolol.[8] Methoxyflurane, another halogenated anesthetic gas related to halothane, has been advocated for use in patients with pheochromocytoma since it is reported to produce less potentiation to catecholamine-induced arrhythmias. Like halothane it may produce a profound reduction of blood pressure at full anesthetic levels, a useful property in these hypertensive patients. However, its increased blood:gas partition ratio results in a slower onset of activity, and a much more prolonged withdrawal period is required for reversal of effect. This latter property has proved troublesome in some patients with pheochromocytoma who characteristically show a hypotensive response to removal of the tumor, and the limited ability to rapidly reverse the hypotensive effects of methoxyflurane at this stage of the operation has proved to be disadvantageous as opposed to the use of halothane.[8,9]

The choice of surgical approach to exploration is of great importance. Urologists and other surgeons initially favored retroperitoneal flank incision since this provides an easier approach to the adrenal gland and results in less postoperative morbidity. Unfortunately, this approach does not permit adequate exploration of alternative potential tumor-bearing areas aside from the single adrenal gland on that side, a point of great importance in a condition where multiple primary tumors occur commonly and must always be excluded by complete exploration. For this reason surgeons now generally prefer an anterior transabdominal approach which permits exploration and tumor removal from any site between the diaphragm and the pelvis.[7] For the rare extra-abdominal tumor, conventional surgical incisions are made depending on the site. An interesting palliative procedure has recently been described for those extremely rare cases where a functioning glomus jugulare tumor enters the jugular vein.[10]

In addition to intraoperative problems of arrhythmia and hypertension, another serious hazard involves the hypotension which usually occurs within 2 to 3 minutes of complete tumor removal. For some time this phenomenon was treated with large doses of pressor drugs (usually norepinephrine), but frequently patients succumbed with "refractory shock" despite increasing dosages. To explain this phenomenon, it was suggested that patients with pheochromocytoma might be hypovolemic, and preoperative infusion of blood was advocated for this problem.[11] More recent studies in a much larger group of patients indicate that most patients with pheochromocytoma have normal plasma volumes and red cell mass.[7] An alternative and more tenable explanation for the hypotension evolved from studies of the physiologic basis of orthostatic hypotension in patients with pheochromocytoma. It was found that these patients suffer from markedly abnormal and attenuated sympathetic reflexes, probably as a result of chronic catecholamine secretion by the tumor.[12] As a result, normal sympathetic vasoconstriction does not occur in response to tilting, Valsalva's maneuver, deep breathing, and other stimuli known to activate this reflex. The hypotension after tumor removal could then be explained by an inadequate reflex vasoconstrictor response in the face of a rapidly falling plasma catecholamine concentration in addition to the suppression of reflexes produced by most general anesthetics. Under these circumstances, infusion of large doses of exogenous norepinepherine would merely perpetuate the condition existent when the tumor was in situ, and weaning of the patient from the pressor support usually took many hours, and sometimes days.

Despite the fact that these patients are not hypovolemic, immediately following tumor resection they represent a situation of relative hypovolemia; i.e., an imbalance between a normal blood volume and an expanded intravascular space. Therefore, rapid overexpansion of the blood volume at the time of tumor removal should result in better maintenance of the blood pressure and no need for pressor agents. Blood loss should be replaced as it occurs during the operation, and approximately 10 minutes before total removal of the tumor an infusion is begun with 5% human albumin in normal saline. The objective is to rapidly expand the intravascular volume to the point that systolic blood pressure remains in the 90 to 100 mm Hg range. An excess of 1,000 to 2,000 ml over estimated fluid losses is usually necessary to achieve this effect. Among more than 30 patients treated by this technique none have required any pressor agents during the period after tumor removal. The use of simulated plasma (5% albumin) also permits easy diuresis of the excess fluid during the immediate postoperative period so as to reduce the postoperative hypertension which transiently occurs in these patients even when they have been cured of the tumor.

Following surgery it is always necessary to collect urine specimens for documentation of cure or recurrence of the disease. Specimens should not generally be collected earlier than 4 to 5 days after surgery since increased values can be observed earlier either due to the postoperative stress or to delayed excretion of residual tumor products. Periodic yearly collections should be made thereafter to check for tumor recurrence (metastases) or the growth of previously unrecognized primary tumors.

As satisfying as it is to effect a cure of this rare and dramatic condition, the physician should never be complacent until he has also fully excluded the possibility of certain associated conditions in the patient and his family. Careful examination of the patient should be made to determine whether the tumor developed in association with one of the associated familial syndromes. Evidence for von Recklinghausen's neurofibromatosis, Lindau-von Hippel disease, and other neuroectodermal disorders should be sought with special attention paid to the presence of multiple neuromas or thyroid nodules which could indicate the presence of the dominantly inherited triad of Sipple's syndrome—multiple, bilateral adrenal pheochromocytomas, medullary carcinoma of the thyroid, and hyperparathyroidism.[13,14] Finding of any of these familial conditions should precipitate a careful evaluation of all family members to enable adequate treatment of all afflicted individuals. Genetic counseling to such a group is obviously of extreme importance.

With careful attention to the many complicated problems which may arise in the treatment of patients with pheochromocytoma and by following the guidelines enumerated above, the physician faced with this task should be able to provide his patient with an excellent prospect of success. The course of treatment should be interesting and, at times, exciting, and the results should be gratifying to all concerned.

References

1. Szakas, J. E., and Cannon, A.: L-Norepinephrine myocarditis. Am. J. Clin. Pathol. 30:425, 1958.
2. Engelman, K., and Sjoerdsma, A.: Chronic medical therapy for pheochromocytoma. Ann. Intern. Med. 61:1302, 1966.
3. Engelman, K., Mueller, P. S., and Sjoerdsma, A.: Elevated plasma free fatty acid concentrations in patients with pheochromocytoma. N. Engl. J. Med. 270:865, 1964.
4. Udenfriend, S., Zaltzman-Nirenberg, P., and Nagatsu, T.: Inhibition of purified beef adrenal tyrosine hydroxylase. Biochem. Pharmacol. 14:837, 1965.
5. Engelman, K., Horwitz, D., Jequier, E., and Sjoerdsma, A.: Biochemical and pharmacologic effects of α-methyltyrosine in man. J. Clin. Invest. 47:577, 1968.
6. Engelman, K., and Sjoerdsma, A.: Unpublished data.
7. Sjoerdsma, A., Engelman, K., Waldman, T. A., Cooperman, L. H., and Hammond, W. G.: Pheochromocytoma: Current concepts of diagnosis and treatment. Ann. Intern. Med. 65:1302, 1966.
8. Cooperman, L. H., Engelman, K., and Mann, P. E. G.: Anesthetic management of pheochromocytoma employing halothane and beta-adrenergic blockade. Anesthesiology 28:575, 1967.
9. Engelman, K.: Unpublished data.
10. Chretien, P. B., Engelman, K., Hoye, R. G., and Geelhoed, G. W.: Surgical management of intravascular glomus jugulare tumor. Am. J. Surg. 122:740, 1971.
11. Brunjes, S., Johns, V. J., Jr., and Crane,

M. G.: Pheochromocytoma post-operative shock and blood volume. N. Engl. J. Med. 262:393, 1960.

12. Engelman, K., Zelis, R., Waldmann, T., Mason, D. T., and Sjoerdsma, A.: Mechanism of orthostatic hypotension in pheochromocytoma. Circulation 38(Suppl. VI):VI-72, 1968.

13. Sipple, J. H.: Association of pheochromocytoma with carcinoma of thyroid gland. Am. J. Med. 31:163, 1961.

14. Catalona, W. J., Engelman, K., Ketcham, A. S., and Hammond, W. G.: Familial medullary thyroid carcinoma, pheochromocytoma and parathyroid adenoma (Sipple's syndrome). Cancer 28:1245, 1971.

Index